MW01236124

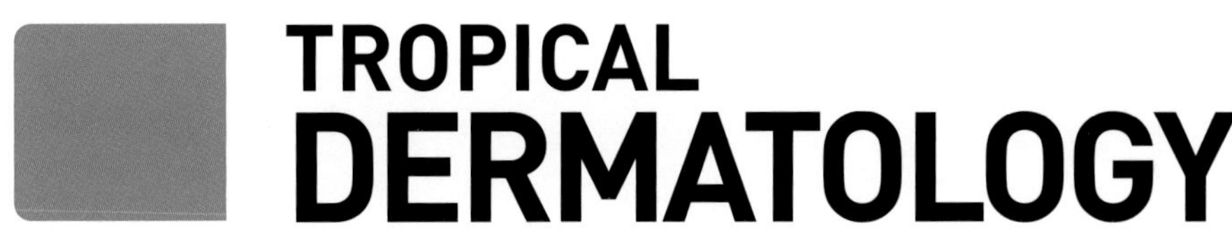
TROPICAL
DERMATOLOGY

Commissioning Editor: *Sue Hodgson*
Project Development Manager: *Belinda Kuhn*
Editorial Assistant: *Amy Lewis*
Project Manager: *Jess Thompson*
Design Manager: *Andy Chapman*
Illustration Manager: *Mick Ruddy*
Illustrator: *Paul Banville*
Marketing Manager(s) (UK/USA): *Jorinde Dirkmaat and Megan Carr*

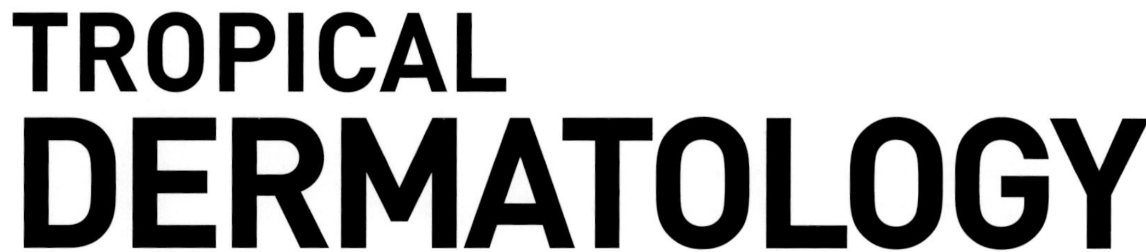

TROPICAL DERMATOLOGY

Stephen K. Tyring MD PhD MBA
Professor of Dermatology, Microbiology/Molecular Genetics
and Internal Medicine
University of Texas Health Science Center
Houston, Texas
USA

Omar Lupi MD MSc PhD
Associate Professor of Dermatology
Federal University of the State of Rio de Janeiro (UNIRIO)
Adjunct Professor of Medical Clinics
Rio de Janeiro State University (UERJ)
Professor of Dermatology
Post-Graduate Course of Dermatology (UFRJ, IDRDA and PGRJ)
Rio de Janeiro
Brazil

Ulrich R. Hengge MD MBA
Professor of Dermatology
Department of Dermatology
Heinrich-Heine University
Düsseldorf
Germany

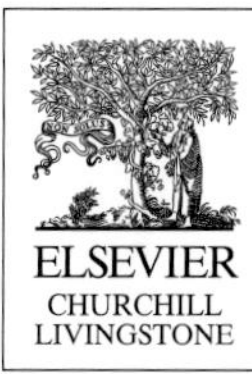

ELSEVIER
CHURCHILL
LIVINGSTONE
An affiliate of Elsevier Inc.

First published 2006

ISBN 0-443-06790-2

British Library Cataloguing in Publication Data
A catalogue record for this book is available from the British Library

Library of Congress Cataloging in Publication Data
A catalog record for this book is available from the Library of Congress

Notice
Medical knowledge is constantly changing. Standard safety precautions must be followed, but as new research and clinical experience broaden our knowledge, changes in treatment and drug therapy may become necessary or appropriate. Readers are advised to check the most current product information provided by the manufacturer of each drug to be administered to verify the recommended dose, the method and duration of administration, and contraindications. It is the responsibility of the practitioner, relying on experience and knowledge of the patient, to determine dosages and the best treatment for each individual patient. Neither the Publisher nor the authors assume any liability for any injury and/or damage to persons or property arising from this publication.
The Publisher

Printed in China
Last digit is the print number: 9 8 7 6 5 4 3 2 1

Contents

List of Contributors

Valeria Aoki MD PhD
Adjunct Professor of Dermatology
Department of Dermatology
Faculty of Medicine
The University of São Paulo (FMUSP)
University of São Paulo
São Paulo
Brazil

Jennifer Aranda MD
Resident Physician
Department of Dermatology
University of Texas Southwestern
Medical Center
Dallas, Texas
USA

Francis T. Assimwe MD
Department of Dermatology
Mbara University Hopsital
Mbara
Uganda

Rubem David Azulay MD PhD
Professor Emeritus of Dermatology
Federal University of Rio de Janeiro
(UFRJ)
Fluminense Federal University (UFF)
Rio de Janeiro
Brazil

Arival Cardoso de Brito MD PhD
Titular Professor
Federal University of the State of Pará
(UFPA)
Belém do Pará
Brazil

Fatima Bacellar PhD
Centre for Vectors and Infectious
Disease Research
National Institute of Health Dr Ricardo
Jorge
Águas de Moura
Portugal

Col Paul M. Benson MD
Department of Dermatology
Walter Reed Army Medical Center
Washington DC
USA

Ross Barnetson MD
Professor of Dermatology
Department of Medicine (Dermatology)
University of Sydney
Sydney, New South Wales
Australia

G. Todd Bessinger MD PhD MPH
Chief, Dermatology Service
Tripler Army Medical Center
Honolulu, Hawaii
USA

Michelle Gralle Botelho MD PhD
Dermatologist
Federal University of Rio de Janeiro
(UFRJ)
Rio de Janeiro
Brazil

Francisco G. Bravo MD
Assistant Professor of Dermatology and
Pathology
Alberto Hurtado Faculty of Medicine
Alexander von Humboldt Institute of
Tropical Medicine
Peruvian University Cayetano Heredia
Lima, Peru

Mathijs Brentjens MD
Chief Resident
Department of Dermatology
University of Texas Medical Branch
Galveston, Texas
USA

Anne E. Burdick MD MPH
Professor of Dermatology and Director
Telemedicine Program
Department of Dermatology and
Cutaneous Surgery
University of Miami School of Medicine
Miami, Florida
USA

Mark Burnett MD
Department of Pediatrics
Walter Reed Army Medical Center
Washington DC
USA

Juan Cabrera MD
Assistant Professor of Neurology
Department of Neurology
Alberto Hurtado Faculty of Medicine
Peruvian University Cayetano Heredia
Lima
Peru

Virginia A. Capó MD PhD
Professor of Pathology
Department of Pathological Anatomy
"Pedro Kourí" Tropical Medicine
Institute
Habana
Cuba

Iphis Campbell MD PhD
Staff of Dermatology Department
University of Brasília (UnB)
Brasília
Brazil

Ana Maria Mosca de Cerquiera MD
Head of Pediatric Dermatology Sector
Hospital Jesus
Professor of Dermatology
Policlínica Geral do Rio de Janeiro
Rio de Janeiro
Brazil

Bart Currie MD FRACP DTM+H
Professor of Medicine and Head
Tropical and Emerging Infectious
Diseases Division
Menzies School of Health Research
Charles Darwin University and Northern
Territory Clinical School
Flinders University
Royal Darwin Hospital
Casuarina, Northern Territory
Australia

Denise M. Demers MD
Chief, Division of Pediatric Infectious
Diseases
Department of Pediatrics
Tripler Army Medical Center
Honolulu, Hawaii
USA

Luis A. Diaz MD
Professor and Chair
Department of Dermatology
The University of Carolina at Chapel Hill
Chapel Hill, North Carolina
USA

Dirk M. Elston MD
Associate in Dermatology and Pathology
Department of Dermatology
Geisinger Medical Center
Danville, Pennsylvannia
USA

Charles D. Ericsson MD
Professor and Clinical Director
Division of Infectious Diseases
University of Texas Houston Medical School
Houston, Texas
USA

Wânia Mara del Favero MD PhD
Professor of Pediatric Dermatology
Federal University of Rio de Janeiro (IPPMG/UFRJ)
Rio de Janeiro
Brazil

Gunter Hans Filho MD PhD
Titular Professor of Dermatology
University of Mato Grosso
Campo Grande
Brazil

Ryssia Alvarez Florião MD PhD
Dermatologist
IASERJ Hospital
Rio de Janeiro
Brazil

Fábio Francescone MD
Dermatologist
Amazônia
Brazil

Stacy Frankel MD
Dermatology Resident
Department of Dermatology and Cutaneous Surgery
University of Miami School of Medicine
Miami, Florida
USA

Eduardo Gotuzzo MD
Professor of Medicine
Alberto Hurtado Faculty of Medicine
Director
Alexander von Humboldt Institute of Tropical Medicine
Peruvian University Cayetano Heredia
Lima
Peru

Maria G. Guzman MD PhD
Professor
Head Virology Department
"Pedro Kourí" Tropical Medicine Institute (IPK)
Department of Virology
Habana
Cuba

Vidal Haddad Junior MD PhD
Adjunct Professor of Dermatology
The University of the Whole State of São Paulo (UNESP)
Botucatu, São Paulo
Brazil

Julio Hilario-Vargas MD
Post-Doctoral Research Associate
Department of Dermatology
School of Medicine
University of North Carolina
Chapel Hill, North Carolina
USA

David B. Huang MD PhD MPH
Assistant Professor
Baylor College of Medicine
Department of Internal Medicine
Division of Infectious Diseases
Houston, Texas
USA

Dieter Häussinger MD
Professor and Director
Department of Gastroenterology, Hepatology and Infectious Diseases
Heinrich-Heine University
Düsseldorf
Germany

Ulrich R. Hengge MD MBA
Professor of Dermatology
Department of Dermatology
Heinrich-Heine University
Düsseldorf
Germany

Márcio Lobo Jardim MD PhD
Titular Professor of Dermatology
Federal University of Pernambuco (UFPE)
Recife
Brazil

Renata A. Joffe MD
Dermatologist
Department of Dermatology
Federal University of Rio de Janeiro (UFRJ)
Rio de Janeiro
Brazil

Sam Kalungi MBChB MMed
Honorary Lecturer
Department of Pathology
Makerere University Medical School
Kampala
Uganda

Ratnakar Kamath MD
Department of Dermatology, Venereology and AIDS Medicine
G. T. Hospital, Grant Medical College
Mumbai
India

Christine Ko MD
Clinical Instructor
Department of Medicine (Dermatology)
University of California
Los Angeles, California
USA

Gustavo Kouri MD PhD DRSc
Head Professor and Head Researcher
Department of Virology
"Pedro Kourí" Tropical Medicine Institute (IPK)
Habana
Cuba

Patricia Lee MD
Center for Clinical Studies
Houston, Texas
USA

Peter Leutscher MD
Danish Bilharziasis Laboratory
Jaegersborg
Charlottenlund
Denmark

Omar Lupi MD MSc PhD
Associate Professor of Dermatology
Federal University of the State of Rio de Janeiro (UNIRIO)
Adjunct Professor of Medical Clinics
Rio de Janeiro State University (UERJ)
Professor of Dermatology
Post-Graduate Course of Dermatology (UFRJ, IDRDA and PGRJ)
Rio de Janeiro
Brazil

Jackson Machado-Pinto MD PhD MSc
Titular Professor and Head of Dermatology
Department of Dermatology
Belo Horizonte Mercy Hospital
Belo Horizonte
Brazil

Pascal Magnussen MD DTM+H
Senior Researcher
Danish Bilharziasis Laboratory
Jaegersborg
Charlottenlund
Denmark

Claudia Pires do Amaral Maia MD MSc
Assistant Professor of Dermatology
Policlínica Geral do Rio de Janeiro
Rio de Janeiro
Brazil

Janak Maniar MD
Professor
Department of Dermatology, Venereology and AIDS Medicine
G. T. Hospital, Grant Medical College
Mumbai
India

Antoine Mahé MD PhD
Head of the Department of Dermatology and Sexually Transmitted Infections
Institute of Social Hygiene
Dakar-Fann
Senegal

Michael R. McGinnis PhD
Director, Medical Mycology Research Center
Professor of Pathology, Dermatology, Microbiology and Immunology
Department of Pathology
University of Texas Medical Branch
Galveston, Texas
USA

Jeffrey Meffert MD
Department of Dermatology
59th Medical Wing/MMID
Lackland AFB, Texas
USA

Jeffery A. Meixner PhD
Post Doctoral Fellow Medical Mycology
Department of Pathology
University of Texas Medical Branch
Galveston
Galveston, Texas
USA

Beatriz Meza-Valencia MD
Staff Pediatrician
Department of Pediatrics
Tripler Army Medical Center
Honolulu, Hawaii
USA

Charles Moon MD
Staff Dermatologist
Department of Dermatology
Ireland Army Community Hospital
Ft. Knox, Kentucky
USA

Rogerio Neves Motta MD MSc
Assistant Professor of Internal Medicine and Infectious Diseases
Federal University of State of Rio de Janeiro (UNIRIO)
Rio de Janeiro
Brazil

Frank Mwesigye MD
Senior Consultant Ophthalmologist
Department of Ophthalmology
Mulago National Referral Hospital
Kampala
Uganda

Leninha Valério do Nascimento MD PhD
Titular Professor of Dermatology
Rio de Janeiro State University (UERJ)
Rio de Janeiro
Brazil

Joao Paulo Niemeyer-Corbellini MD
Dermatologist
Federal University of Rio de Janeiro (UFRJ)
Rio de Janeiro
Brazil

René Garrido Neves MD PhD
Titular Professor of Dermatology
Department of Dermatology
Federal University of Rio de Janeiro (UFRJ)
Rio de Janiero
Brazil

Josephine Nguyen MD
Department of Dermatology
Stanford University
Stanford, California
USA

Juan P. Olano MD
Assistant Professor
Department of Pathology
Director, Residency Training Program
Member, Center for Biodefense and Emerging Infectious Diseases
University of Texas Medical Branch
Galveston, Texas
USA

Martin Ottolini MD
Director of the Pediatric Infectious Disease Fellowship
F. Edward Hébert School of Medicine
Uniformed Services University of the Health Sciences
Bethesda, Maryland
USA

Katie R. Pang MD
Resident Physician
Department of Dermatology
Wayne State University School of Medicine
Detroit, Michigan
USA

Mauro Romero Leal Passos MD PhD
Professor and Head of the Sexually Transmitted Diseases Sector
Fluminenese Federal University (UFF)
Rio de Janeiro
Brazil

Seema Patel MD
Visiting Scientist
Department of Pathology
University of Texas Medical Branch
Galveston,Texas
USA

Dominique Fausto Perez MD
Resident
Federal University of Rio de Janeiro (UFRJ)
Rio de Janeiro
Brazil

Andréa Neiva dos Reis MD
Resident
Federal University of the State of Rio de Janeiro (UNIRIO)
Rio de Janeiro
Brazil

Wingfield Rehmus MD MPH
Clinical Instructor, Co-Director of Clinical Trials Unit
Department of Dermatology
Stanford University
Stanford, California
USA

Karl Heinz Richter MD (Deceased)
Professor Emeritus
Düsseldorf
Germany

Joachim Richter MD
Assistant Professor
Specialist, Tropical and Internal Medicine
Tropical Medicine Unit
Department of Gastroenterology, Hepatology and Infectious Diseases
Heinrich-Heine University
Düsseldorf
Germany

Evandro Rivitti MD PhD
Titular Professor of Dermatology
Department of Dermatology
University of São Paulo (FMUSP)
São Paulo
Brazil

Sebastião A. P. Sampaio MD PhD
Professor Emeritus of Dermatology
Department of Dermatology
University of São Paulo (FMUSP)
São Paulo
Brazil

Omar da Rosa Santos MD PhD
Titular Professor of Nephrology
Federal University of Rio de Janeiro (UNIRIO)
Rio de Janeiro
Brazil

Ivan Semenovitch MD MSc
Assistant Professor of Dermatology
Policlínica Geral do Rio de Janeiro
Rio de Janeiro
Brazil

Michael B. Smith MD
Director
Division of Clinical Microbiology
Department of Pathology
University of Texas Medical Branch
Galveston, Texas
USA

Leticia Spinelli MD
Dermatologist
Rio de Janeiro Mercy Hospital
Rio de Janeiro
Brazil

Rita de Sousa MSc
Center for Vectors and Infectious Disease Research
National Institute of Health Dr Ricardo Jorge
Águas de Moura
Portugal

Karan K. Sra MD
Center for Clinical Studies
Houston, Texas
USA

Carolina Talhari MD
Dermatologist
Federal University of the Amazon
Amazônia
Brazil

Sinésio Talhari MD PhD
Titular Professor and Head of Dermatology
Federal University of the Amazon
Amazônia
Brazil

Lynnette K. Tumwine MBChB MMED
Honorary Lecturer
Department of Pathology
Faculty of Medicine
Makerere University
Kampala
Uganda

Maria L. Turner MD
Chief, Consultation Service
Dermatology Branch, NIH
Bethesda, Maryland
USA

Stephen K. Tyring MD PhD MBA
Professor of Dermatology, Microbiology/Molecular Genetics and Internal Medicine
University of Texas Health Science Center
Houston, Texas
USA

Renata de Queiroz Varella MD
Sexually Transmitted Diseases Section
Fluminese Federal University (UFF)
Niterói, Rio de Janeiro
Brazil

Antônio Carlos Francescone do Valle MD PhD
Senior Researcher
Evandro Chagas Hospital
Oswaldo Cruz Foundation (FIOCRUZ)
Rio de Janeiro
Brazil

Luciano Vera-Cabrera MD
Professor
Department of Dermatology
University Hospital
University Autónoma de Nuevo León
Madero Y Gonzalitos Col. Mitras Centro
Monterrey
México

Govinda S. Vivesvara PhD
Research Microbiologist
Division of Parasitic Diseases
National Center for Infectious Diseases
Centers for Disease Control and Prevention
Atlanta, Georgia
USA

Olivera Welsh MD DrSc
Professor
Coordinator of Basic Research
Dermatology Department
University Hospital
University Autonoma de Nuevo León
Monterrey
México

Anthony White MBBS FACD
Clinical Senior Lecturer
University of Sydney
Bondi Junction
Sydney, New South Wales
Australia

Jashin J. Wu MD
Dermatology Resident
Department of Dermatology
University of California, Irvine
Irvine, California
USA

Mauricio Younes-Ibrahim MD PhD
Associate Professor of Nephrology
Federal University of the State of Rio de Janeiro (UNIRIO)
Professor of Nephrology Rio de Janeiro State University (UERJ)
Rio de Janeiro
Brazil

Clarisse Zaitz MD PhD
Professor of Dermatology
São Paulo Mercy Hospital
São Paulo
Brazil

Preface

Patients with tropical diseases present to physicians in temperate parts of the world with increasing frequency. Many of these patients are native to the temperate country but have traveled to tropical destinations for work and/or tourism. Examples in the United States during the past year include lassa fever in New Jersey, tanapox in New Hampshire, *Penicillium marneffei* in Texas as well as hundreds of cases of leishmaniasis in American and allied troops returning from Iraq and Afghanistan. On the other hand, the patient may not have a history of recent travel, but may have been infected by a pet from a tropical country (e.g., monkeypox in Wisconsin), food from tropical waters (e.g., *Vibrio vulnificus* septicemia in persons eating raw oysters shipped from the Gulf of Mexico) or imported animal hides (i.e., anthrax). In other cases, the patient may be an immigrant or an adoptee.

Some tropical diseases were common in temperate lands until recently. For example, measles was commonly diagnosed in North America and Europe until late in the 20th century, but now is rarely seen in these regions. Measles, however, is a major cause of morbidity and mortality in the tropics. Therefore, most measles reported in North America and Europe is imported, such as in unvaccinated citizens of these areas returning from tropical destinations.

Conversely, other tropical diseases rarely seen in the United States in the 20th century have become widespread in the 21st century. The most notable example of this situation is the spread of the West Nile virus to almost all states since 1999.

While infectious diseases are frequently the source of cutaneous problems in the returned traveler, non-infectious skin diseases usually predominate. Such non-infectious sources of cutaneous problems include excessive sun exposure and mucocutaneous reactions to medications taken for prophylaxis or therapy (including phototoxic reactions). Exposure to tropical plants and animals (especially invertebrates), marine and freshwater organisms and other irritants are also frequent causes of cutaneous complaints.

It is important to remember, however, that most physician visits for cutaneous problems are unrelated to the patient's travel or national origin but are the same conditions seen daily in patients who have never left their local communities.

Therefore, the goal of *Tropical Dermatology* is to provide a guide to the mucocutaneous manifestations of tropical diseases. In order to formulate a differential diagnosis, the morphology of the skin lesions must be considered in view of the patient's symptoms, physical examination, general medical and exposure history as well as their vaccination and medicine record. Laboratory and/or biopsy results can often be used to reach a diagnosis and to help determine the appropriate management.

Stephen K. Tyring
Houston
Omar Lupi
Rio de Janeiro
Ulrich R. Hengge
Düsseldorf

Acknowledgments

We wish to thank Nancy Bell, PhD for proofreading the text. We deeply appreciate the contribution of clinical photographs from physicians throughout the world. We would also like to thank Prof. René Garrido Neves for his magnificent work on tropical dermatology in Brazil, for the last 25 years. Most of all, we wish to thank the patients who allowed their photographs to be used. Without their contribution, the publication of *Tropical Dermatology* would not be possible.

Part I

Introduction

Chapter 1

Syndromal tropical dermatology

Stephen K. Tyring

- Sexually transmitted diseases
- Fever and rash
- Rash and eosinophilia
- Ulcers and other specific skin lesions

Introduction

With increasing numbers of persons from industrialized, temperate countries traveling and/or working in tropical lands, there is a marked need for physicians to be able to diagnose accurately and treat tropical diseases with mucocutaneous manifestations. While some studies demonstrate that approximately one-third to two-thirds of travelers returning from tropical countries experience some health problem, diarrhea is the most prevalent complaint. Mucocutaneous problems, however, are among the top five health complaints of the returned traveler, and comprise 10–15% of health concerns of persons returning from the tropics.[1]

During international conflicts, soldiers from North America, Europe, and Australia are often required to serve in tropical lands and sometimes develop diseases not familiar to physicians of their home countries. This was the case for French soldiers serving in Vietnam in the 1950s and American soldiers serving there in the 1960s and 1970s. Recently hundreds of American and allied troops serving in Iraq and Afghanistan have developed "Baghdad boils," i.e., leishmaniasis, transmitted by sand fly bites (Fig. 1.1).

Likewise, millions of persons from tropical countries now live and work in temperate lands and may present with medical problems with which the physician is not familiar. Whereas the cutaneous problems in the returned traveler are frequently the result of infectious diseases, skin diseases of non-infectious etiologies usually predominate. Such non-infectious sources of skin problems include excessive sun exposure, cutaneous reactions to medications taken for prophylaxis (including phototoxic reactions) or exposures to marine, freshwater or other irritants. Furthermore, whether it is the traveler or the immigrant presenting to the physician, many cutaneous complaints are unrelated to the person's travel or national origin, but are the same conditions seen daily in every physician's office. Therefore, the physician should not ignore the common sources of dermatological problems while searching for an exotic etiology.

Another, somewhat recent source of patients with tropical skin diseases are adoptees who frequently originate in Central America or Southeast Asia. These children could be infected with organisms having a long incubation period that may not have been detected by physical examinations and not preventable by available vaccines.

Tropical infections in temperate lands, however, are not totally unique to travelers. For example, the outbreak of monkeypox in Wisconsin, USA, in 2003 was a result of prairie dogs acquiring the virus from Gambian rats housed in adjacent cages in pet stores. The prairie dogs then transmitted the infection to humans who had never been near the usual range of monkeypox, i.e., central Africa.

Occasionally, the patient with a tropical disease is neither the traveler nor exposed to an animal carrying an infectious agent. The carrier may be a friend or relative who is a returned traveler who has acquired a tropical infection and who has not yet developed signs or symptoms. This possibility has recently been given much attention due to the potential spread of severe acute respiratory syndrome (SARS) or avian influenza virus. On the other hand, the contaminated food may have originated in a tropical or subtropic area, such as when oysters from the Gulf of Mexico are shipped to

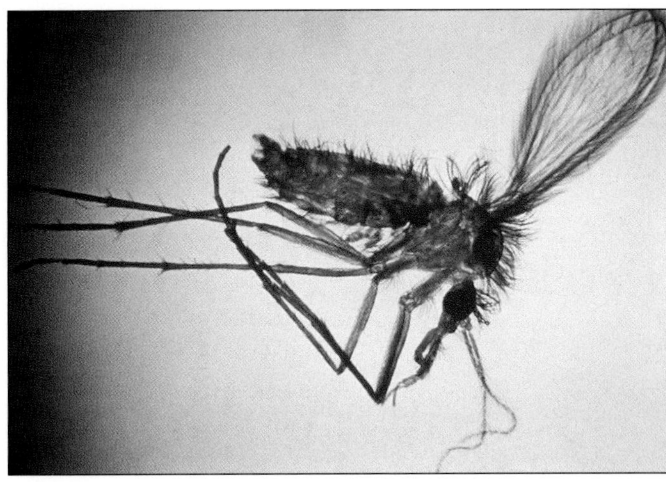

Figure 1.1 Female *Phlebotomus* spp. sand fly, a vector of leishmaniasis. (Courtesy of World Health Organisation.)

the Midwest USA and are consumed raw. The resulting *Vibrio vulnificus* or hepatitis A infection thus produces gastrointestinal and cutaneous manifestations in persons who may not have visited the source of the shellfish. Therefore, it is always important to ask about new pets, changes in diet, or any other change in persons with a suspected tropical disease. On the other hand, the traveler may have purchased non-consumable items which are the source of their dermatoses. For example, animal skins used for rugs or blankets may be the source of anthrax. A non-infectious cause may include nickel-containing jewelry, to which the patient has developed contact dermatitis.

Whereas travelers naturally fear large carnivores while on camera safari or sharks and a variety of other aquatic animals while swimming or diving, it must be remembered that the animal (indirectly) responsible for most morbidity and mortality is the mosquito (i.e., malaria, dengue, etc.) (Fig. 1.2). An example of a mosquito-borne disease that was considered primarily "tropical" in the recent past but is now relatively common in much of North America is infection with the West Nile virus (Fig. 1.3).

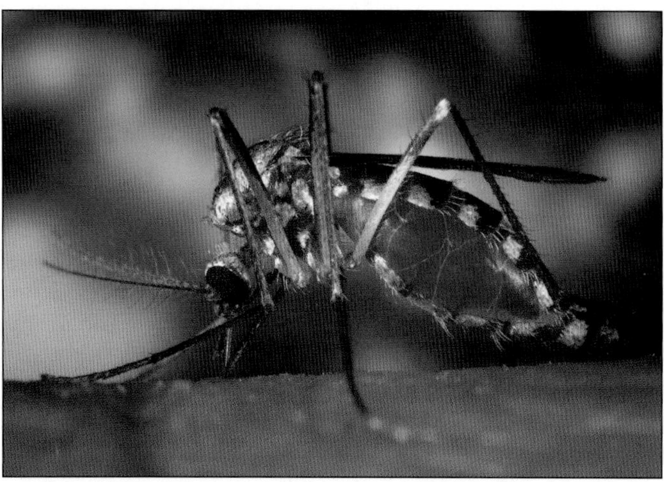

Figure 1.2 Ochlerotatus (*Aedes*) triseriatus mosquito feeding on a human hand. (Courtesy of Centers for Disease Control and Prevention.)

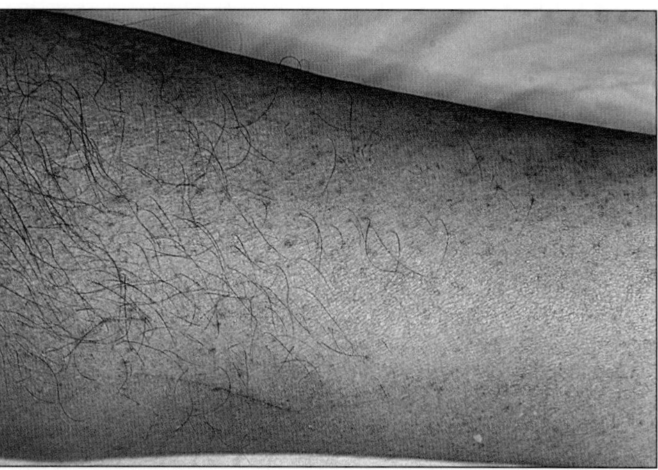

Figure 1.3 Erythematous macules associated with West Nile virus infection. (Courtesy of Dr. David Huang.)

Sometimes the skin findings on physical examination are not the reason for the physician visit or even the patient's complaint. Such skin findings may be cultural, such as tattoos, scarification, or the result of the use of kava or of chewing betel nuts. Some cultural practices, however, would be considered abuse in industrialized countries, but are widely accepted religious/cultural practices in certain lands. An example of such practice is female circumcision, which is practiced in many countries in sub-Saharan Africa. On the other hand, the skin changes may be much more benign, transient, and may even be the result of previous therapies, such as cupping and coining, widely practiced by immigrants from Southeast Asia.

Considerations for deciding the differential diagnosis of cutaneous manifestations of tropical diseases and/or of diseases acquired while traveling must be based not only on the type of lesions and systemic symptoms but also on the patient's history of travel. Because the incubation period of various infectious diseases differs widely, it is important to know when the patient traveled. For frequent travelers, the history may become complex if they report having visited many destinations within the past few months. Because vectors differ with the climate, the season of travel is also noteworthy. Even in a tropical country where the temperature is always hot or warm, there may be a dry season and a rainy season. Because seasons are reversed north and south of the Equator, it is important to know the season at the destination. The duration of the stay is significant, not only because it increases the chance of acquiring an infectious disease but also because it tells the physician if the person was in the tropics during the incubation period of the suspected disease. Whether the visitor was only in an urban environment or also in a rural area is relevant. Whereas a sexually transmitted disease could be acquired in either location, an arbovirus or a zoonosis might be more likely in a rural situation. The altitude of the destination could provide a clue to the etiology of the skin condition, as could the type of sleeping condition. For example, a sexually transmitted disease could easily be acquired in a five-star hotel, but an infection transmitted by a flea, louse, or mite would be more likely in someone who slept on the ground and/or in a tent.

The type and preparation of food and drink consumed by the traveler would not only help explain gastrointestinal symptoms; it could also be a clue to cutaneous signs, i.e., unsafe drinking water or milk or raw or undercooked meat, fish, or shellfish.

A list of the patient's current and recent medications can be very useful and should include prescription drugs, illicit drugs, and herbal remedies, because the source of the cutaneous problem may not be directly related to the travel destination, but rather may be due to medications taken to prevent travel-related illnesses. For example, many antimalarials, such as chloroquine, mefloquine, proguanil, quinine, and halofantrine, can cause cutaneous reactions, and chloroquine, doxycycline, and quinine can cause photosensitivity. Interestingly, chloroquine can worsen psoriasis. A number of agents taken to treat or prevent diarrhea can also cause cutaneous reactions, such as quinolones (ciprofloxacin, ofloxacin, sparfloxacin, levofloxacin), furazolidone, metronidazole, trimethoprim-sulfamethoxazole and bismuth sulfate; quinolones are particularly likely to produce photosensitivity. Antihelmintic medications, such as ivermectin, albendazole, and diethylcarbamazine, can also produce pruritus and rash. Even diethyltoluamide (DEET), used to prevent arthropod bites, can cause an irritant dermatitis when used in high concentrations.

Because many medications in tropical countries are sold over the counter and/or have different trade names than in industrialized lands, patients are not always certain what they received if treated during their travel. Likewise, an injection or transfusion given in a tropical country might also carry an increased risk of contamination. A similar risk might be taken by having acupuncture, tattoos, or body piercing in tropical lands, but these procedures can be hazardous even in industrialized countries, because the first intervention is occasionally done by non-medical personnel and the other two are almost never done by medically trained persons.

A history of pre-travel vaccinations and/or immunoglobulins would be useful for possible exclusion of certain suspected etiologies. For example, if the yellow fever vaccine and the hepatitis A and/or B vaccine series were administered in sufficient time before the travel, it is less likely that these viruses were the source of the medical complaint.

The traveler's occupational or recreational exposure to dirt, water, or animals can be an important component of the history. An animal bite or scratch should be easy to remember, but the bite of many arthropods may not even be noticed until after a cutaneous reaction has appeared and the responsible fly, mite, or flea has moved on to the next victim. Exposure to some animals may be more indirect. For example, the spelunker (cave-explorer) may inhale aerosolized bat guano and develop rabies without ever touching a bat. A history of swimming, boating, or surfing can be a clue to an aquatic/marine etiology. Such fresh- or brackish-water activities may increase the risk of infection with schistosomiasis or with free-living ameba, while marine activities may be associated with jellyfish stings, contact with the venomous spines of certain fish, or irritant dermatitis from fire coral. A preexisting skin abrasion or laceration or a puncture wound from a sea urchin or sting ray may result in a secondary bacterial infection.

Thus, a complete medical and travel history and physical examination is imperative in helping to narrow the differential diagnoses in the returned traveler, the immigrant, or the adoptee with a tropical origin. The qualitative and quantitative nature of the skin lesions are very important and are discussed in detail later in this chapter. Specific attention must be given to the age of the patient as well as to the person who is immunocompromised due to human immunodeficiency virus (HIV), internal malignancy, organ transplantation, or other iatrogenic source of immunocompromise. Blood tests, e.g., liver/kidney function tests, complete blood counts with differentials, urinalysis, skin scraping, biopsy, and/or culture are often necessary to confirm the diagnosis. A recent example of the importance of knowing both the patient's national origin and their immune status was seen when an HIV-seropositive man from Myanmar presented with the first case of *Penicillium marneffei* reported from Houston, TX (Fig. 1.4).

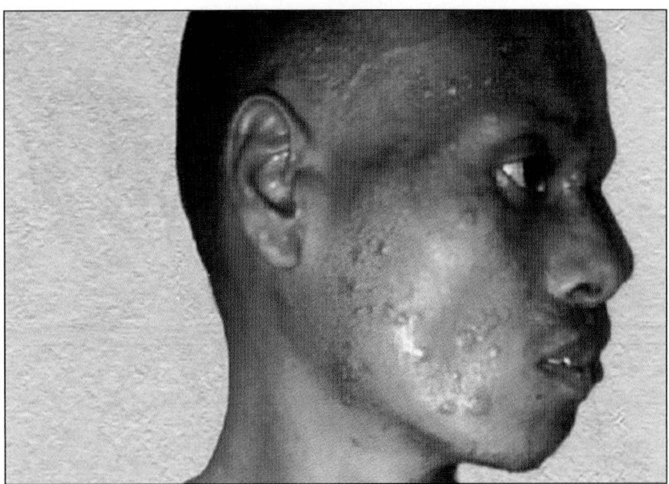

Figure 1.4 Umbilicated papules of the face secondary to *Penicillium marneffei* in a human immunodeficiency virus (HIV)-seropositive patient from Myanmar who presented to a clinic in Houston, TX. (Courtesy of Dr. Khanh Nguyen.)

Many viral diseases that were not considered "tropical" 50 years ago are now much more frequently seen in immigrants from tropical countries or in travelers who did not receive their recommended childhood vaccines. Three common examples are measles, rubella, and hepatitis B. Until the 1960s measles and rubella were very common sources of infection in temperate countries, but in the twenty-first century they have become rare in industrialized countries, except for imported cases. Worldwide, however, almost one million children die of measles annually (Fig. 1.5) and rubella still causes many congenital abnormalities. Measles is still the number one vaccine-preventable killer of children in the world. Morbidity and mortality are often the result of secondary bacterial infections developing in malnourished infants with measles (Fig. 1.6). In east Asia, sub-Saharan Africa, and many other parts of the tropical world, hepatitis B is very common and a major source of morbidity and mortality. Although measles, rubella, and hepatitis B should not be a problem in the immunized traveler, many travelers have not received the proper immunizations because they or their parents had unfounded concerns about the safety of the vaccines. This problem continues to grow as more people reach child-bearing age without ever knowing anyone who has suffered from the childhood diseases common in the first half of the 20th century. Therefore, they do not understand that the approved vaccines are a million-fold safer than the diseases they are designed to prevent.

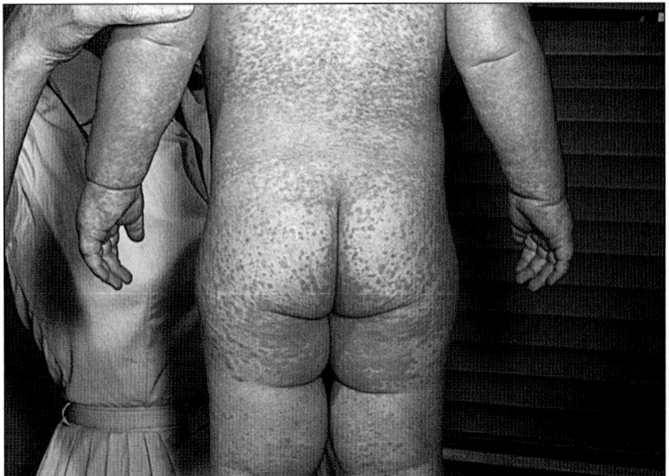

Figure 1.5 Erythematous macules of measles on day 3 of the rash. (Courtesy of Centers for Disease Control and Prevention.)

Sexually transmitted diseases

Sexually transmitted diseases (STDs) should be considered at the top of the differential diagnoses when a patient presents with

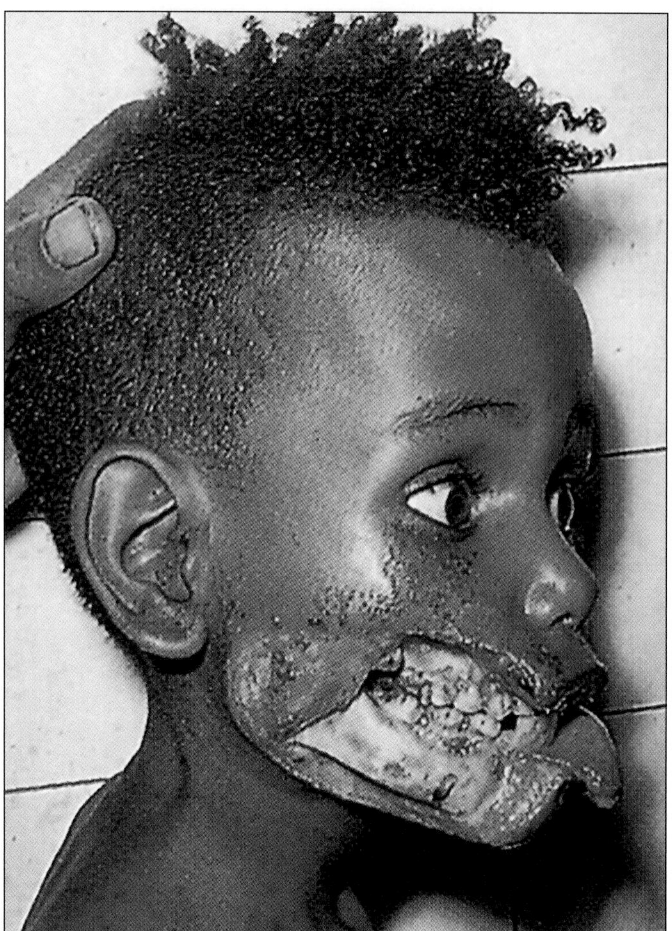

Figure 1.6 Cancrum oris (Noma) of the facial region is associated with malnutrition and poor oral hygiene in the presence of *Treponema vincentii* plus Gram-negative bacteria following a systemic disease such as measles. (Reproduced from Peters W and Pasvol G (eds). Tropical Medicine and Parasitology, 5th edition, Mosby, London 2002, image 870.)

genital lesions and/or urogenital discharge.[2–4] Although many of the same considerations would be true whether the patient was a recent traveler or not, certain factors should be given attention in travelers:

- Was the person traveling without his/her spouse/family and therefore outside his/her usual social structure?
- Did the person travel to countries where sex workers are readily available? While sex workers are available in most parts of the world, legally or illegally, the traveler might be less likely to acquire an STD in Mecca during a haj than in Amsterdam, Bangkok, or Nairobi, where sex workers are very prevalent.
- Did the person attend parties where large amounts or alcohol and/or drugs were consumed (e.g., "spring break" in the USA)?
- If the traveler is strongly suspected of having an STD, did he/she visit a destination where chancroid, granuloma inguinale (GI), or lymphogranuloma venereum (LGV) (L serovars of *Chlamydia trachomatis*) is prevalent? If so, the diagnostic tests and therapy might need to be expanded beyond those under consideration for STDs acquired in temperate lands.

When one STD is confirmed, there is an increased possibility of acquisition of additional STDs. Not only is this the case because the source partner(s) may have had multiple STDs, but also because having certain STDs makes a person more susceptible to other STDs. The best example of this phenomenon is the two- to fivefold greater risk of acquiring HIV if the person with a genital ulcer disease (GUD) has sex with an HIV-positive individual. The reasons for this increased risk include the reduced epithelial barrier in all GUDs as well as the infiltrate of CD4+ cells in certain GUDs such as genital herpes. These CD4+ cells are the targets for HIV infection. Genital herpes is the most prevalent GUD in industrialized countries. In fact, the Centers for Disease Control and Prevention estimate that there are 45 million herpes simplex virus type 2 (HSV-2)-seropositive persons in the USA. In the tropics, chancroid has been the most frequently diagnosed GUD, followed by syphilis and genital herpes, but the last two diseases are becoming more prevalent in certain tropical countries. Depending on the travel destination, LGV and GI must also be considered. The dates and duration of travel are important components of the history because the primary clinical presentation of all these GUDs ranges between 2–3 days (genital herpes and chancroid) and 4 weeks (syphilis and GI).

Currently, the World Health Organization (WHO) estimates that there are 46 million HIV-seropositive persons in the world. Many of these people have GUD, which may be changed both qualitatively and quantitatively by HIV. Therefore the traveler may have a "non-classical" presentation of GUD. In addition, it should be remembered that the signs and symptoms of GUD can also appear on the perianal area/buttock or in or around the mouth. Other locations are possible, but less likely.

In general, however, multiple, painful, usually bilateral vesicles which progress to ulcers on skin or start as ulcers on mucous membranes, then heal over after 3–4 without therapy or within 2–3 weeks with antiviral therapy, are consistent with genital herpes. Because most true primary cases of genital herpes recur, a history of multiple recurrences of the vesicles or ulcers is highly consistent with genital herpes. This diagnosis can be confirmed by viral culture or serology. In the absence of these tools, a useful test is the Tzanck smear, which usually demonstrates multinucleated giant cells in herpetic lesions, but is of low sensitivity and specificity. Genital herpes, however, can present many diagnostic dilemmas because the first recognized clinical occurrence is often not the result of a recent infection but rather represents a first-episode, non-primary outbreak. Whereas a true primary outbreak of genital herpes is usually consistent with acquisition of the virus 2 days to 2 weeks previously, a first-episode, non-primary outbreak may be consistent with an infection any time in the past. In this case, the patient's recent travel history may be of less importance than his/her sexual encounters of the most distant past.

Although syphilis is much more common in many developing countries than in the USA, western Europe or Australia, the lack of travel certainly does not exclude syphilis. This diagnosis should be suspected when the patient presents with a single, non-tender, genital, perianal, or lip ulcer associated with non-tender lymphadenopathy. While chancroid is uncommonly reported in industrialized countries, it is very common in the tropics. It is usually characterized by one or more painful genital ulcers and painful lymphadenopathy. In LGV the primary lesion is usually very transient and is often not seen. The clinical presentation is usually that of tender inguinal lymphadenopathy, sometimes with a suppurating bubo. The diagnosis of GI is very rarely made outside the tropics. The presentation is usually that of one or more non-tender genital ulcers with inguinal swelling. If any of these bacterial GUDs is suspected, the appropriate diagnostic tests must be initiated, i.e., serology for syphilis and LGV, culture for chancroid and LGV, tissue examination for GI, and the appropriate antibiotic started.

Whereas a history of multiple recurrences of genital vesicles or ulcers would be consistent with genital herpes, a more difficult scenario is represented by the patient who reports a single outbreak of non-specific genital signs and symptoms that are resolved by the clinic visit. A western blot or type-specific serological test for HSV-2 would determine whether the person was infected with this virus, but it would not be definitive proof that that HSV-2 was responsible for the resolved outbreak. For example, a HSV-2 serologically positive person may acquire syphilis, but the genital ulcer may resolve without therapy, or with inadequate treatment, before the clinic visit at home. Thus, a careful history may reveal the need for serology for HSV-2 as well as for syphilis. Because HIV can be acquired concomitantly with or subsequently to these GUDs, but not produce genital manifestations, HIV testing should be conducted as well. Although many patients may be hesitant to admit sexual activity that puts them at risk for STDs, others will worry about these activities following travel (or any time) and ask to be tested for "everything." If the sexual encounter with a new partner has been very recent, the serological test may be false-negative because serology for syphilis, HIV, or HSV-2 may require weeks to become positive in the majority of persons after initial infection.

Patients who ignore their primary genital lesions because of denial or difficulty finding medical care during their travels may believe that the problem is gone because the lesion has resolved. If syphilis is the cause of the GUD, it may reappear weeks or months later as non-genital cutaneous manifestations in the form of secondary (or tertiary) syphilis (Fig. 1.7). A careful history regarding the primary lesion may lead to the appropriate diagnostic tests and therapy. Some STDs may not produce any genital signs or symptoms and the disease may be diagnosed long after the travel (or the non-travel acquisition), making it more difficult to find the source of the infection. Although over 90% of HIV-seropositive persons eventually develop indirect mucocutaneous manifestations of infection, the primary rash of seroconversion (if present) is not noticed by most patients. Therefore, the diagnosis is usually made when the patient develops systemic signs and symptoms (fever, chills, diarrhea, weight loss, lymphadenopathy) and/or develops one or more of the opportunistic infections, neoplasms, or inflammatory skin problems frequently seen in HIV patients. Similar to HIV, primary infection with hepatitis B rarely produces genital lesions. Diagnosis is usually made long after infection due to systemic symptoms or non-specific skin changes such as jaundice. It is noteworthy that hepatitis B is the only STD for which a prophylactic vaccine is available. Therefore, a history of successful hepatitis B vaccination makes this diagnosis less likely.

Although the pustules of disseminated gonococcemia are distinctive, the consequences of untreated *Neisseria gonorrhoeae* (gonococcus) are usually pelvic inflammatory disease, epididymitis,

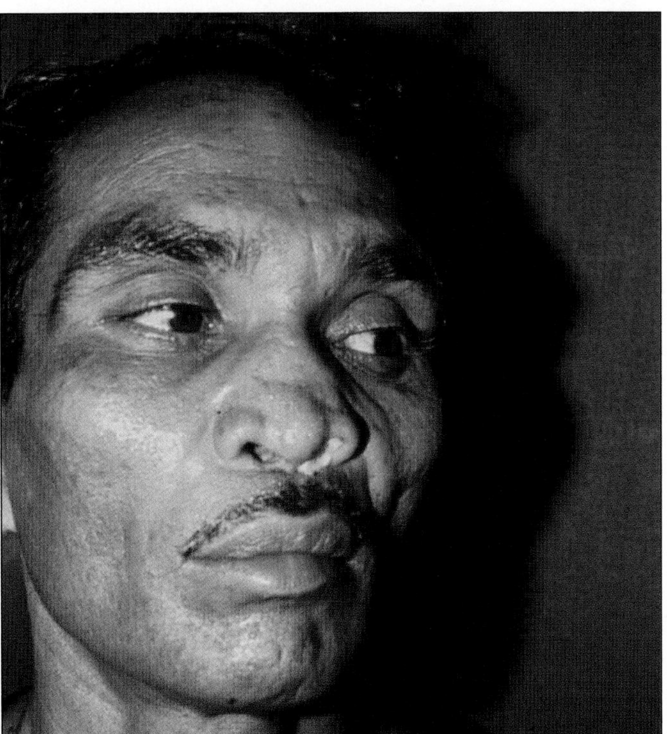

Figure 1.7 Saddle-nose deformity due to tertiary syphilis in a human immunodeficiency virus (HIV)-seropositive man in India. (Courtesy of Dr. J. K. Maniar.)

proctitis, pharyngitis, or conjunctivitis. Pelvic inflammatory disease can also be caused by *Chlamydia trachomatis* (non-L serovars), *Mycoplasma hominis*, or various anaerobic bacteria. The non-L serovars of *C. trachomatis* can also cause epididymitis, proctitis, and conjunctivitis. Pharyngitis can also be due to HSV-2 or *Entamoeba histolytica*. The initial presentation of GC, *C. trachomatis* (non-L serovars), *Ureaplasma urealyticum*, *Mycoplasma genitalium*, *Trichomonas vaginalis*, or even HSV-2 may be urethritis. Vaginal discharge can be caused by any of these organisms as well as *Candida albicans*, *Gardnerella vaginalis*, peptostreptococci, *Bacteroides* spp. or *Mobiluncus* spp. These organisms can usually be diagnosed by smear, wet-mount, DNA detection, serology, or culture. Antimicrobial therapy is usually initiated based on the physical examination and smear or wet-mount and modified, as needed, when other laboratory studies are completed.

Infection with human papillomaviruses (HPV) is one of the most common STDs in the world, but the clinical implications of the infection vary widely. There are over 20 HPV types that can cause genital lesions, but most infections do not result in any visible lesions. Because the incubation period of HPVs can be months, or even years, if and when genital lesions do develop, it is often very difficult for the patient to determine the source partner. Therefore, it is usually a challenge for the physician to relate HPV lesions to travel, especially recent travel. Non-oncogenic genital HPV, such as types 6 and 11, result in condyloma acuminatum, which can be treated with cytodestructive therapy, surgery, or with the immune response modifier, imiquimod. Oncogenic genital HPV, such as types 16 and 18, can result in anogenital cancer, the most prevalent of which is cervical cancer. Cervical cancer is the second most prevalent cancer killer of women in the world and over 99% of all cervical cancer is caused by HPV. Most cervical cancer deaths are in tropical countries, making HPV one of the world's deadliest tropical diseases (although rarely listed with the other major tropical diseases). There are many reasons why more cervical cancer deaths occur in tropical countries. First, in industrialized countries most women receive regular Pap smears, which result in early detection and subsequent therapy of cervical abnormalities, thus reducing progression to cervical cancer. If cancer is detected, surgery, radiation therapy, or chemotherapy is available. In most tropical countries, regular Pap smears are not the standard of care. Therefore, cervical cancer is often detected too late for successful intervention, even if it is available. Second, there appears to be a genetic susceptibility that allows oncogenic HPV to progress to malignancy. This genetic susceptibility appears to be more prevalent in certain tropical countries. The rarity of male circumcision in many tropical countries appears to be a risk factor for the development of cervical cancer in these males' partners. Third, most of the world's estimated 46 million HIV-seropositive individuals live in tropical countries where no antiretroviral therapy is available. Not only is cervical cancer an acquired immunodeficiency syndrome (AIDS)-defining illness in HIV seropositive women, the same HPV can cause anal cancer, which is a major problem in homosexual men with HIV.

Molluscum contagiosum (MC) is a poxvirus that can be sexually transmitted, resulting in wart-like lesions on the genitalia. In contrast to HPV, however, MC does not progress to malignancy. Like condyloma acuminatum, however, MC can be treated with cytodestructive therapy, surgery, or imiquimod.

Ectoparasites such as scabies, *Sarcoptes scabiei*, and pubic lice, *Phthirus pubis*, can be sexually transmitted. In contrast to many STDs, however, these ectoparasites can be easily treated with topical medications such as lindane or permethrin. Like all STDs, if the sexual partner is not treated concomitantly, reinfection is common.

Fever and rash

The most common cause of fever after tropical travel is malaria, which usually does not have specific cutaneous manifestations. Dengue fever is the second most common cause of fever in the traveler and does have somewhat specific cutaneous manifestations, making dengue fever the leading cause of fever with rash in the traveler returning from a tropical destination (Fig. 1.8). Other common causes of fever and rash include hepatitis viruses, rickettsia, and some enteric fevers. It should always be kept in mind, however, that fever in the returned traveler may not be due to exposure during travel. For example, the fatigue of travel, i.e., jet lag, may make one more susceptible to influenza or other common infections in temperate lands.

When both fever and rash are seen, the time between travel and onset of signs and symptoms becomes increasingly important. If travel preceded fever and rash by less than 1–2 weeks, considerations should include anthrax, dengue fever, diphtheria, ehrlichiosis, hemorrhagic fever viruses, leptospirosis, Lyme disease, measles, meningococcal infections, plague, rickettsia, toxoplasmosis, trichinosis, tularemia, typhoid fever, and yellow fever. If the period between travel and fever/rash is up to a month, the list should be expanded to include hepatitis viruses (A, C, and E), HIV, rubella,

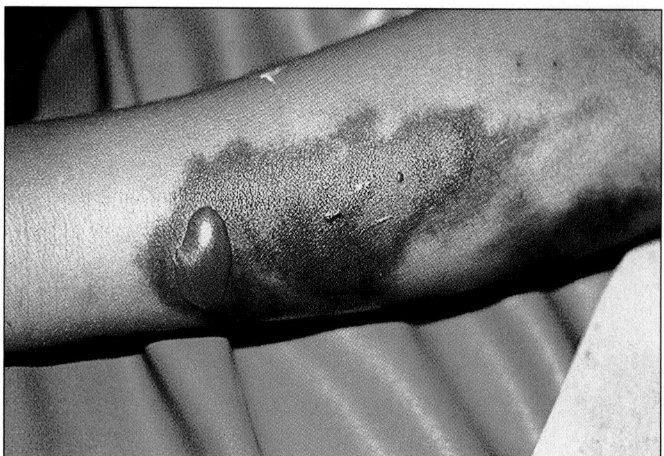

Figure 1.8 Hemorrhagic bullae in dengue virus infection. (Reproduced with permission from WHO.)

schistosomiasis and trypanosomiasis. If at least 3 months separate travel from fever/rash, the following infections should be considered: bartonellosis, filariasis, gnathostomiasis, hepatitis viruses (B and C), histoplasmosis, HIV, leishmaniasis, Lyme disease, melioidosis, penicilliosis, syphilis, trypanosomiasis, and tuberculosis. In each case, however, the nature of the fever, the type of rash, the destination of the travel, and any other symptoms must be considered.

Because many infections producing fever with rash can be rapidly fatal and/or easily spread, it is imperative immediately to initiate diagnostic tests and antimicrobial therapy for the presumed cause of the infection. Such infections include anthrax, bartonellosis, *Candida* (macronodules), diphtheria, disseminated gonorrhoeae (papules and pustules over joints), hepatitis viruses, leptospirosis, meningitis (asymmetrical, scattered, petechiae, and purpura), plague, *Pseudomonas* (ecthyma gangrenosum), relapsing fevers, rickettsia (scattered petechiae and purpura), *Staphylococcus* (Osler's nodes, diffuse toxic erythema), *Streptococcus* (Janeway lesions, diffuse toxic erythema), *Strongyloides* (migratory petechiae and purpura), syphilis, tuberculosis, typhoid fever (rose spots) (Fig. 1.9), various Gram-negative bacteria (i.e., peripheral gangrene), *Vibrio* (especially *V. vulnificus*), and viral hemorrhagic fevers (petechiae, purpura, hemorrhage).

Rash and eosinophilia

Eosinophilia may be due to diverse processes, such as allergic, neoplastic, and infectious diseases.[5] Although an allergic reaction could easily result from an exposure during travel, eosinophilia in the returned traveler may have nothing directly to do with the travel. On the other hand, it may be due to an infectious process or to a drug taken for prophylaxis or therapy during travel. If an infection is the cause of the eosinophilia, it is usually a parasitic disease, especially due to a helminth. Only a few viral, bacterial, or fungal diseases are associated with both rash and eosinophilia, e.g., streptococcal (i.e., scarlet fever), tuberculosis, HIV, and coccidioidomycosis. Protozoa only rarely provoke eosinophilia.

The principal helminth that causes eosinophilia is *Strongyloides*. When *Strongyloides* is disseminated such as in the hyperinfection

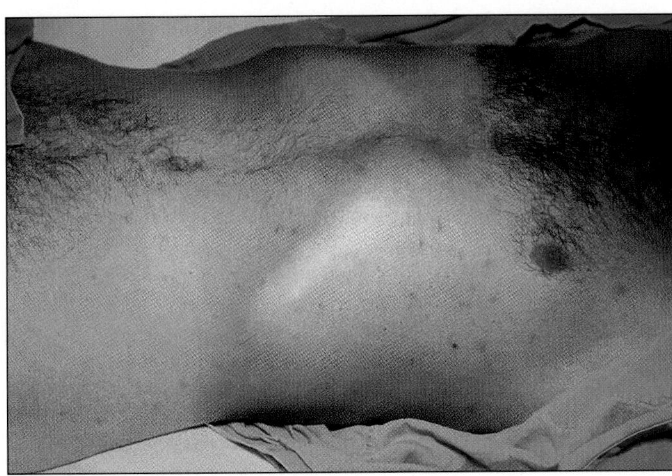

Figure 1.9 Rose spots in a patient with typhoid fever due to *Salmonella typhi*. (Courtesy of Centers for Disease Control and Prevention/Armed Forces Institute of Pathology, Charles N. Farmer.)

syndrome, skin lesions such as urticaria, papules, vesicles, petechiae, and migratory serpiginous lesions become common, especially if the patient is given systemic corticosteroids (because *Strongyloides* was not considered).

Pruritic, erythematous papules can be seen as a result of schistosomal cercariae, as in swimmer's itch. Eosinophils may be seen in the skin biopsy as well as in the blood.

Pruritic lesions of the skin and subcutaneous tissues are commonly associated with eosinophilia in onchocerciasis. Lymphangitis, orchitis, and epididymitis are also commonly observed.

In loiasis, fever and eosinophilia are typically seen. Migratory lesions, especially angioedema, are usually erythematous and pruritic.

Likewise, gnathostomiasis produces recurrent edema after ingestion of raw fish. The skin lesions are usually erythematous, pruritic, and/or painful.

Drug hypersensitivity is a relatively common cause of eosinophilia and may be associated with non-specific skin changes such as urticaria and/or phototoxic reactions. Although most drugs that cause eosinophilia may not be taken for purposes related to traveling, increased sun exposure during travel may make the problem clinically apparent. Because antibiotics may be taken for prophylaxis or therapy more frequently during traveling, they should be given careful consideration when eosinophilia is detected. Such antibiotics include penicillins, cephalosporins, quinolones, isoniazid, rifampin, and trimethoprim-sulfamethoxazole.

Ulcers and other specific skin lesions

Pruritus and urticaria

Non-specific cutaneous manifestations of tropical diseases may include pruritus and urticaria. Frequently, more specific signs may accompany pruritus and urticaria, which are useful in narrowing the differential diagnoses. If eosinophilia is found with the pruritus and urticaria, helminthic infections should be considered. Therefore, consideration should be given to trichinellosis, strongyloidiasis, schistosomiasis, onchocerciasis, loiasis, hookworms, gnathostomiasis, dracunculiasis, and cutaneous larva migrans. Pinworms, as well as protozoa such as amebiasis, giardiasis, and trypanosomiasis, are less likely to produce eosinophilia. Pruritus and urticaria are possible with spirochetes such as *Borrelia* (e.g., relapsing fevers), *Spirillum* (e.g., rat-bite fever) and *Treponema* (i.e., syphilis and pinta). *Yersinia* (e.g., plague) is another bacteria that produces pruritus and urticaria, which can be present before buboes form. The hepatitis viruses (e.g., A, B, and C) can produce pruritus and urticaria, as can a number of ectoparasites and biting arthropods, e.g., ticks, scabies, bedbugs, lice, fleas, mites, and flies.[6–10]

Jaundice

Although hepatitis viruses can produce pruritus and urticaria, jaundice is a more specific indication that the problem has a hepatitic etiology. Not only can all the hepatitis viruses (A–E) produce jaundice, other tropical viruses also do so commonly, e.g., yellow fever and Rift Valley fever. Less frequently, dengue and Epstein–Barr viruses can cause jaundice, as can such bacteria as *Leptospira* (i.e., leptospirosis), *Coxiella* (i.e., Q fever) and *Treponema* (i.e., syphilis). Protozoa, such as malaria, and drug reactions can also be responsible.

Vesicles and bullae

Although vesicles and bullae can appear as a result of contact dermatitis or drug eruption, including photodermatitis and photo-exacerbated drug eruptions as well as toxic epidermal necrolysis, many cases represent the early stages of a viral or bacterial infection. The most common viral etiology in the traveler or non-traveler includes the herpesviruses, especially herpes simplex virus 1 and 2, as well as varicella-zoster virus, both primary varicella and herpes zoster. Measles and many enteroviruses (e.g., hand, foot, and mouth disease) can present with vesicles, as can certain alphaviruses. A number of poxviruses, such as vaccinia, variola, orf, tanapox, and monkeypox, can produce vesicles. Less commonly, vesicles comprise an early stage of certain bacterial diseases such as *Vibrio vulnificus*, *Bacillus anthracis*, *Brucella* spp., *Mycobacteria tuberculosis*, *Mycoplasma* spp., *Rickettsia akaru* and *Staphylococcus* (bullous impetigo). Other organisms such as fungi that cause tinea pedis, protozoa (e.g., *Leishmania brasiliensis*), and helminths (e.g., *Necator americanus*) can occasionally cause vesicles.

Macules and papules

A wide variety of infectious and non-infectious etiologies are related to both macules and to papules. Almost any of the vesicular diseases listed above may initiate first as a macule, then a papule, before becoming a vesicle. A number of drugs, arthropod bites (e.g., mosquito or flea) and infestations (e.g., scabies and other mites) commonly cause macules and/or papules. The range of terrestrial, freshwater, and marine contactants can elicit these cutaneous reactions, as can a spectrum of drugs. Viral etiologies include HIV, as in the HIV seroconversion syndrome, Epstein–Barr virus (infectious mononucleosis), human herpesvirus 6 (roseola), parvovirus B-19 (fifth disease), measles, rubella, and various hemorrhagic fever viruses. Many bacteria can be responsible, such as *Rickettsia*, *Bacillus anthracis*, spirochetes (*Spirillum*, *Leptospira*, *Borrelia*, *Treponema*), *Coxiella burnetii*, *Yersinia pestis*, *Salmonella typhi*, *Bartonella bacilliformis*, and *Brucella*. Histoplasmosis and coccidioidomycosis are fungal diseases commonly associated with macules and/or papules. Certain protozoa such as *Toxoplasma gondii* and *Leishmania* can also induce these types of lesions. Among helminths, hookworm disease, strongyloidiasis, and onchocerciasis can be associated with macules and/or papules.

Nodules

Although otherwise similar, papules are usually less than 0.5–1.0 cm, while nodules are larger than 0.5–1.0 cm in diameter. Except for certain poxviruses which cause orf and milker's nodules, as well as warts and malignancies induced by HPV, viruses rarely form nodules. On the other hand, all subcutaneous and systemic mycoses can induce nodules. Bacterial causes of nodules include *Bartonella* (verruga peruana and cat-scratch disease), *Buckholderia mallei* (glanders), *Calymmatobacterium granulomatis* (GI), *Chlamydia trachomatis* (LGV), *Klebsiella rhinoscleromatis* (rhinoscleroma), *Leptospira autumnalis* (leptospirosis), *Mycobacteria* spp. (atypical mycobacteria, cutaneous tuberculosis, leprosy, etc.), *Nocardia brasiliensis* (and other bacterial causes of mycetoma) and *Treponema pallidum* (bejel, yaws). Protozoan causes of nodules include amebiasis, leishmaniasis, and trypanosomiasis. Almost all helminthic infections that have mucocutaneous manifestations can induce nodules, e.g., coenurosis, cysticercosis, dirofilariasis, dracunculiasis, echinococcosis, filariasis, gnathostomiasis, loiasis, onchocerciasis, paragonimiasis, schistosomiasis, sparganosis, and visceral larval migrans. If the helminthic nodule contains sufficient fluid, it will produce a cyst. Cysts can be seen in helminthic infections such as coenurosis, echinococcosis, filariasis, gnathostomiasis, loiasis, and onchocerciasis. There are also arthropod causes of nodules such as myiasis, scabies, tick granulomas, and tungiasis.

Ulcers

Whereas ulcers can form as a result of breakdown of previously normal skin, they frequently develop from nodules after inflammation destroys the epidermis and papillary layer of the dermis. Herpes simplex virus is a very common cause of ulcers in both tropical and temperate regions of the world. Other causes of GUD are bacterial, e.g., chancroid, GI, LGV, and primary syphilis. Other bacterial diseases that commonly cause ulcers include anthrax, bacterial mycetomas, diphtheria, glanders, melioidosis, mycobacterial diseases (e.g., Buruli ulcer, leprosy, tuberculosis), plague, rickettsia, tropical ulcers, tularemia, and yaws. A number of fungi can form nodules that break down into ulcers, or they can induce ulcers from systemic spread: blastomycosis, chromomycosis, coccidioidomycosis, cryptococcosis, histoplasmosis, lobomycosis, mycetomas, paracoccidioidomycosis, penicilliosis, and sporotrichosis. The most common helminthic cause of cutaneous ulcers is dracunculiasis, when the worm erupts from the skin. Two protozoan diseases cause ulcers – amebiasis and leishmaniasis. Arthropod causes of ulcers include myiasis and tungiasis. Many bites (e.g., brown recluse spiders and various snakes), stings (e.g., insect, jellyfish, and scorpion) or venomous spines of various fish can also induce ulcers.

Eschars

An eschar can be seen in both temperate and tropical lands due to *Pseudomonas aeruginosa* (i.e., ecthyma gangrenosum), but the most common causes of eschars are *Rickettsia*. Eschars due to anthrax can be seen in persons who work with animal skins, but anthrax has received much attention recently due to its potential use in bioterrorism. The best-recognized etiology of a non-infectious eschar is a bite from a brown recluse spider.

Petechiae and purpura

Petechiae and purpura can result from adverse reactions to a number of drugs. The most important infectious cause of petechiae and/or ecchymoses with fever is meningococcemia, which has a high rate of morbidity and mortality and is widespread throughout the tropical world and found sporadically in industrialized countries. Other bacterial causes include *Borrelia, Burkholderia, Enterococcus, Haemophilus, Leptospira, Pseudomonas, Rickettsia, Streptobacillis, Treponema, Vibrio,* and *Yersinia.* A number of hemorrhagic fever viruses can cause petechial or purpuric lesions, but the most prevalent viral causes are enteroviruses, cytomegalovirus, dengue, and yellow fever. Protozoal diseases (e.g., malaria and toxoplasmosis) and helminths (e.g., trichinellosis) can also induce this clinical presentation.

Hypopigmentation and hyperpigmentation

Changes in pigmentation can be seen after a variety of medications, many of which are taken for prophylaxis or therapy related to travel. These agents include a spectrum of drugs such as antibiotics, antidiarrheals, anthelmintics, and antimalarials, many of which can also elicit photosensitization. A number of infectious agents can also alter pigmentation. Leishmaniasis, pinta, and tinea versicolor may be associated with hypopigmentation or hyperpigmentation. Leprosy, onchocerciasis, syphilis, and yaws are more often associated with hypopigmentation. Erythrasma, HIV, and loiasis are more frequently causes of hyperpigmentation.

Migratory skin lesions

With the exception of the movements of larvae of myiasis, mucocutaneous migratory lesions are usually due to infections with helminths. The best-recognized example is cutaneous larval migrans, but migratory lesions can also be due to dracunculiasis, fascioliasis, gnathostomiasis (Fig. 1.10), hookworms, loiasis, paragonamiasis, sparganosis, or strongyloidiasis.

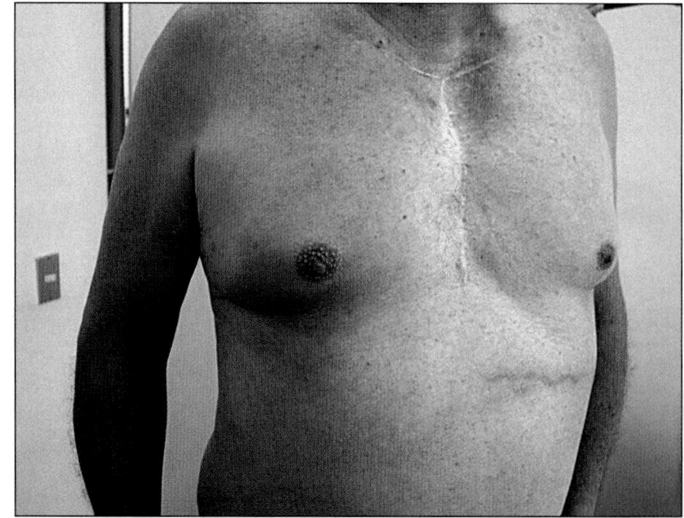

Figure 1.10 Migratory erythema secondary to gnathostomiasis in a patient in Peru. (Courtesy of Dr. Francisco Bravo.)

In conclusion, the differential diagnoses of mucocutaneous lesions in the returned traveler, immigrant, or adoptee should be based on the morphology of the lesions, but the patient's symptoms, general medical, and exposure history must all be considered.[11–17] The physical examination and laboratory results must be integrated with the patient's vaccination and medication record. The travel destination(s), travel duration, living, work/recreation conditions, food and drink ingestion, and activities while traveling must all be taken into consideration. It must not be forgotten, however, that many mucocutaneous problems in the returned traveler or the immigrant/adoptee are not related to the travel or the country of origin but can be the same disorders seen daily in patients who have never left their local communities.

References

1. Steffen R, Rickenbach M, Wilhelm U. Health problems after travel to developing countries. J Infect Dis 1987; 156:84.
2. Brown TJ, Yen-Moore A, Tyring SK. An overview of sexually transmitted diseases. Part I (bacterial STDs). J Am Acad Dermatol 1999; 41:511–529.
3. Brown TJ, Yen-Moore A, Tyring SK. An overview of sexually transmitted diseases. Part II (viral STDs). J Am Acad Dermatol 1999; 41:661–677.
4. Czelusta A, Yen-Moore A, Vander Straten M et al. An overview of sexually transmitted diseases. Part III. Sexually transmitted diseases in HIV infected patients. J Am Acad Dermatol 2000; 43:409–432.
5. Weller PF. Eosinophilia in travelers. Med Clin North Am 1992; 76:1413.
6. Caumes E, Carriere J, Guermonprez G. Dermatoses associated with travel to tropical countries: a prospective study of the diagnosis and management of 269 patients presenting to a tropical disease unit. Clin Infect Dis 1995; 20:542–548.
7. Chaudhry AZ, Longworth DL. Cutaneous manifestations of intestinal helminthic infections. Dermatol Clin 1989; 7:275–290.
8. Colven RM, Prose NS. Parasitic infections of the skin. Pediatr Ann 1994; 23:436–442.
9. Lockwood DN, Keystone JS. Skin problems in returning travelers. Med Clin North Am 1992; 76:1393–1411.
10. Mackey SL, Wagner KF. Dermatologic manifestations of parasitic disease. Infect Dis Clin North Am 1994; 8:713–743.
11. Jong EC, McMullen R, eds. The travel and tropical medicine manual. Philadelphia, PA: Saunders; 1995:1–644.
12. Geraminejad P, Memar O, Aronson I et al. Kaposi's sarcoma and other manifestations of human herpesvirus 8. J Am Acad Dermatol 2002; 47:641–655.
13. Sterling J, Tyring SK, eds. Human papillomaviruses. London: Oxford Press University; 2001:1–153.
14. Tyring SK, ed. Mucocutaneous manifestations of viral diseases. New York: Marcel Dekker; 2002:1–574.
15. Lupi O, Tyring SK. Tropical dermatology: viral tropical diseases. J Am Acad Dermatol 2003; 49:979–1002.
16. Hengge UR, Tannapfel A, Tyring SK et al. Lyme borreliosis. Lancet Infect Dis 2003; 3:489–500.
17. Wilson ME, Chen LH. Dermatologic infectious diseases in international travelers. Curr Infect Dis Rep 2004; 6:54–62.

Chapter 2

Issues for travelers

David B. Huang, Jashin J. Wu and Charles D. Ericsson

- Introduction
- Pretravel advice
- Advice while traveling
- Post-travel advice

Introduction

Both tropical and non-tropical diseases are commonly reported problems among travelers to a developing country.[1,2] Among tropical diseases, malaria and traveler's diarrhea are the two most common health issues encountered during travel to a developing country. Malaria is an important risk in some frequently visited areas such as tropical Africa (up to 95% of infections are due to *Plasmodium falciparum*),[3] Asia, and Latin America, whereas traveler's diarrhea can practically occur in any country associated with poor hygiene (the incidence rate is 20–90% depending on country visited).[4] As for non-tropical diseases, dermatosis (12%) has been reported to be one of the three most common reasons a traveler sought consultation from a physician.[2] Bacteria and fungal skin infections (often from contact with coral and shells) and scabies accounted for 4.4%, 1.9%, and 2%, respectively, among 860 travelers who sought medical care.[2] Among travelers to the Maldives and Fiji, dermatoses (including sunburns and superficial injuries) were the most frequent reasons for seeking physician care.[5] Sunburns and insect bites were the most common dermatological problems occurring in 10% and 3% of Finnish travelers (n = 2665), respectively.[6] Table 2.1 lists the most common dermatoses in one prospective study of 269 consecutive patients (out of 7886) with short-term travel who presented to a French tropical disease unit during a 2-year period.[2] In 61% of these cases, the dermatoses presented during travel and in 39% of the cases after return from travel.

Physicians with patients who travel should be familiar with potential travel-related dermatoses, infectious diseases, and environmental hazards (Table 2.2) specific to the area of patient travel. The physician should also discuss general preventive measures of dermatoses, infectious diseases, and environmental hazards, including vaccinations that are recommended to the traveler (Tables 2.3 and 2.4).

Pretravel advice

Pretravel preparation

One month prior to travel, individuals with a preexisting medical condition, especially immunosuppressed travelers, should be examined by their primary care physician. Immunosuppressed travelers may be at increased risk of acquiring intestinal protozoa, including *Giardia lamblia*, *Isospora belli*, *Entamoeba histolytica*, and *Cryptosporidium parvum*.[7,8] In addition, special precautions should be discussed with those patients with allergies, diabetes, cardiac, pulmonary, or gastrointestinal disorders.[9] These patients should wear engraved bracelets listing their existing medical conditions, and take with them past electrocardiograms or chest radiographs when appropriate. Patients with chronic illnesses should bring adequate supplies of necessary drugs. Also, travelers should make sure that their health insurance will be able to cover medical care, hospitalization, or medical evaluation in the area of travel destination. In addition, the traveler should prepare a list of physicians and specialists who speak English and have respectable qualifications in case of emergencies.

Travel instructions should be prepared and include specific details concerning the prevention and care of common dermatoses (e.g., sunburns), infectious diseases (e.g., malaria and traveler's diarrhea), and injuries related to environmental hazards. The physician should also discuss vaccinations appropriate to the area of travel (Table 2.3).

Travel medical kit

Travelers should bring a medical kit that includes a thermometer, bandages and gauze, adhesive tape, antiseptic or bactericidal soap solution, aspirin, antacids, antimotion sickness drug, antihistamines for allergies, decongestant for those prone to nasal congestion, sunscreen, water purification material, insect repellents, and a mild oral laxative or suppository for constipation. In general,

Table 2.1 Travel-associated dermatoses diagnosed in 269 French travelers presenting to a tropical disease unit in Paris in 1991–1993[2]

Diagnosis	Number of cases (%)
Cutaneous larva migrans	67 (24.9)
Pyodermas	48 (17.8)
Arthropod-related pruritic dermatitis	26 (9.7)
Myiasis	25 (9.3)
Tungiasis	17 (6.3)
Urticaria	16 (5.9)
Rash with fever	11 (4.1)
Cutaneous leishmaniasis	8 (3.0)
Scabies	6 (2.2)
Injuries	5 (1.9)
Cutaneous fungal infections	5 (1.9)
Exacerbation of preexisting illness	5 (1.9)
Sexually transmitted diseases	4 (1.5)
Cutaneous herpes simplex	3 (1.1)
Septicemia	3 (1.1)
Acute venous thrombosis	2 (0.7)
Pityriasis rosea	2 (0.7)
Mycobacterium marinum infection	2 (0.7)
Acute lymphatic filiariasis	1 (0.4)
Traumatic abrasion	1 (0.4)
Lichen planus	1 (0.4)
Erythema nodosum	1 (0.4)
Reiter's syndrome	1 (0.4)
Undetermined	9 (3.3)
Total	269 (100)

Table 2.2 Potential environmental hazards associated with travel

Environment	Factors and potential hazards to consider
Terrain concerns	Traversing safely and maintaining orientation Ability to find camping/safe shelter Exposure to air, wind,and solar radiation Exposure to animals or insects that may cause bites, injury, or infection
Extreme temperatures/ weather	Appropriate clothing for extreme temperatures (i.e., risk for hypothermia and heatstroke) and prevention of solar radiation exposure Carry plenty of water to prevent dehydration
Air	Existing pulmonary disease and airway hyperreactivity Outdoor pollutants Indoor pollutants from fossil fuels/inadequate ventilation High altitudes and mountain sickness
Water	Exposure, including ingestion of and direct contact with contaminated water with waterborne infectious diseases (e.g., schistosomiasis, leptospirosis), industrial waste dumping, chemical toxins Exposure to aquatic life that may cause bites, injury or infection

broad-spectrum antibiotics should not be given to travelers. The exception is in the traveler to remote areas where access to these medications is limited or prophylaxis is recommended. Antimalarial or antidiarrheal antimicrobials may be necessary and may be given with clear instructions of administration and warning labels of potential side-effects. Otherwise, broad-spectrum antibiotics should not be given to travelers.

Vaccine-preventable diseases

Routine and recommended commercially available vaccines for international travel are listed in Table 2.3. Routine vaccines for preventable diseases in childhood should be administered to children who are traveling according to recommended schedules. Certain vaccines are recommended for the prevention of diseases that are common to the area of travel. For some countries, the only required vaccine for international travel is the yellow fever vaccine. For those who do not receive vaccination with yellow fever, individuals may be subject to vaccination, medical follow-up, and/or isolation or even denied entry into the country of destination. An updated list of vaccines required by each country is provided by a Centers for Disease Control and Prevention (CDC) publication.[10] This list of recommended vaccines by country is also listed at the website http://www.cdc.gov/travel/travel.htm.

Live virus vaccines are contraindicated in travelers who are pregnant or immunocompromised. An exception lies with pregnant women who are at substantial risk of exposure to natural infection with yellow fever. Pregnancy and breast-feeding are not contraindications for receiving vaccines that are toxoid, killed, or inactivated.[10] Other contraindications to vaccines include individuals who have had anaphylactic reactions to avian products including eggs. Immunosuppressed persons, including human immunodeficiency virus (HIV)-infected individuals, should not receive live vaccines, including varicella, oral typhoid, and yellow fever.[11]

Advice while traveling

Preventive health advice

Table 2.4 lists general preventive measures for the traveler. Briefly, travelers should be educated and prepared for travel health-related

Table 2.3 Routine and recommended commercially available vaccines for international travel

Vaccine	Antigenic form	Schedule/indications	Adverse effects
Required by law			
Yellow fever	Live-attenuated	One dose, 10 days before travel, with a booster every 10 years for those travelling to endemic areas	Fever (2–5%), headache, myalgia
Routine			
Diptheria–tetanus–pertussis	Inactivated	Three doses at 2, 4, and 6 months of age for all travelers, with a booster every 10 years, as given with tetanus vaccine	Local reactions,[a] occasional risk of systemic reactions[b]
Haemophilus influenzae b	Capsular polysaccharide	Four doses at 2, 4, 6, and 12–15 months of age	Local reactions, occasional risk of systemic reactions
Influenza	Inactivated reactions	One dose annually to travelers at increased risk of complications from influenza	Local reactions, occasional risk of systemic reaction
Measles–mumps–rubella	Live-attenuated	Two doses given to all persons born after 1956	Fever (5–15%), rash (5%), joint pains (up to 40% in postpubertal females), local reactions (4–55%)
Poliomyelitis	Inactivated	Three doses: the first two are given at 4–8-week intervals; the third is given 6–12 months after the second, for non-vaccinated persons > 18 years and immunocompromised hosts at increased risk of exposure to poliovirus	Local reactions
Tetanus–diphtheria	Adsorbed toxoids	Three doses: the first two are given 4–8 weeks apart; the third is given 6–12 months later, with a booster every 10 years for all adults	Local reactions, occasional systemic symptoms
Varicella	Live-attenuated	Two doses 4–8 weeks apart for persons without a history of varicella	Local reactions (25–30%), fever (10%), rash (8%)
Meningococcal (A, C, Y, W-135)	Polysaccharide	One dose, with a booster every 5 years for those traveling to Saudi Arabia or sub-Saharan meningococcal belt, Haj pilgrims, and those who have had a splenectomy	Local reactions, fever (2%)
Recommended			
Encephalitis, Japanese	Inactivated	Three doses, each 1 week apart for all (20%), traveling to endemic areas (Asia and Southeast Asia)	Local reactions 20%, systemic reactions (10%), angioedema, urticaria (0.1%)
Hepatitis A	Inactivated	Two doses, 6–12 months apart for those traveling to developing countries (i.e., Africa, Asia except Japan and Singapore, Latin America, the Caribbean, and remote parts of Eastern Europe)	Local reactions (50%), systemic reactions (10%)
Hepatitis B	Recombinant-derived hepatitis B surface antigen	Three doses: two doses 1 month apart; third dose 5 months after dose 2 for health care workers and persons in contact with blood, body fluids, or potentially contaminated medical instruments, and persons (i.e., expatriates) residing in areas of high endemicity for hepatitis B surface antigen	Local reactions (10–20%), systemic reactions (rare)
Combined hepatitis A/B	Inactivated hepatitis A/ recombinant B surface antigen	Three doses: two doses 1 month apart; third dose 5 months after dose 2 as listed above	Local reactions, systemic reactions (rare)
Pneumococcal	Capsular polysaccharide	One dose for immunocompromised hosts, splenectomy, and the elderly	Local reactions, fever, rash, arthritis, serum sickness
Rabies	Inactivated	Three doses at days 0, 7, and 21 or 28 for travelers to areas for > 1 month where rabies risk is considerable: a booster may be given 1 year later	Local reactions (30%), systemic reactions, immune complex reactions (6%)
Typhoid	Live attenuated	Four doses at days 0, 2, 4, 6 for travelers to endemic areas boost every 5 years	Gastrointestinal symptoms,[c] systemic reactions
	Vi capsular polysaccharide	One dose and a booster every 2–3 years for travelers to endemic areas	Local reactions, systemic symptoms (rare)

[a]Local reactions include pain, swelling, and induration at site of injection.
[b]Systemic symptoms include fever, headaches, and malaise.
[c]Gastrointestinal symptoms include nausea, vomiting, and diarrhea.

Table 2.4 General preventive measures for the traveler

Altitude	All travelers should be encouraged to drink plenty of water, and avoid caffeine and alcoholic beverages and tobacco, especially those who are climbing mountains and traveling to high-altitude destinations. Care should be taken not to participate in excessive exercise. Acetazolamide (Diamox) may be taken 24 hours before ascent and for an additional 2 days after arrival at highest altitude to prevent altitude-related problems
Dehydration	Similar to those traveling to high-altitude destinations, all travelers should be encouraged to drink plenty of water, and avoid caffeine and alcoholic beverages, especially in hot climates. The elderly should not depend on thirst as an indicator of sufficient fluid intake
Envenomation	As a general rule, travelers should not touch or walk on what cannot be seen, especially in areas that contain venomous animals (scorpions, snakes, spiders, or other biting animals). Travelers should wear long-sleeved shirts and pants (trousers) and avoid walking bare-footed. Boots are recommended with pants tucked into them. Snakebite kits containing antivenom against venomous animals should be readily available at local heath clinics and hospitals
Food	Food should be boiled, well-cooked (i.e., served hot), or peeled as appropriate before eating. Uncooked or unfresh food or unpeeled fruits and vegetables should be completely avoided. Careful attention should be taken to ensure that prepared foods are not contaminated by dirty surfaces, water, or insects. Dairy products should be avoided unless it is known that they have been properly refrigerated, and hygienically prepared
Injuries	Travelers should purchase health insurance before traveling. Injuries commonly occur during travel and many accidents can be prevented with common sense. The most common injuries include motor vehicle accidents, violence and aggression, drowning, sports-related injuries, animals, and other accidents
Mosquitoes/other insects	Insect repellents containing diethyltoluamide (DEET) in a 20–35% concentration; long-sleeved shirts and pants should be worn; shirts should be tucked in. Beds covered with mosquito nets and preferably impregnated with permethrin repellent should be encouraged in areas of infected mosquitoes, especially in malarial areas. Home windows and doors should also be well screened. Travelers should be advised to inspect themselves and their clothing for ticks, both during outdoor activity and at the end of the day. Ticks are detected more easily on light-colored or white clothing. Prompt removal of attached ticks can prevent some infections
Sexual activities	The avoidance of casual sexual encounters or, at the least, safe sex with barrier protection (i.e., condoms) should be emphasized, especially in areas with a high risk of contracting human immunodeficiency virus (HIV) and other sexually transmitted diseases and to provide birth control
Sun	Sufficient sun protection should be encouraged in the traveler who spends time outdoors (e.g., hat, cap, sunglasses, and sunblock). Overly strenuous exercise should also be avoided. Sunscreen that blocks both ultraviolet A and B should be applied to the skin 30 min before sun exposure. Sun protection factor 15 is generally safe and should be reapplied every 1–3 h if swimming
Walking	Covered footwear should be encouraged, especially in areas where contaminated soil may contain infected insects (e.g., sand flies), excrement, worm larvae (e.g., hookworm and strongyloides). These areas should be avoided, especially by children
Water/beverages	In areas without clean drinking water, bottled water, bottled beverages, and drinks prepared with boiling water (boiled for at least 3 min) should be encouraged. In these areas, ice cubes may represent a risk of infection due to the unknown purity of the water. Chlorination, iodination, water filters, and disinfectants may also be used in water of unknown purity. Milk should be boiled before drinking. Generally, hot (> 50°C) tap water is relatively safer than cold tap water; although hot tap water can also be contaminated. Beverages mixed with water and non-carbonated drinks should be avoided. Coffee and tea made with boiled water and hot milk, beer, and wine are generally safe

issues, including: the effects of high-altitude destinations, jet lag, acclimatization; potential contaminated water, food and beverages; prolonged exposure to the sun, insect or animal bites; transmission of sexually transmitted diseases; malaria prophylaxis; and traveler's diarrhea.

Jet lag may occur as a result of disturbances to the traveler's circadian rhythm. For every 1–2 h of time change, an average of 1 day is required to adjust. For people who travel to areas with high altitudes, adequate hydration and avoidance of alcoholic beverages and tobacco for the first few days are recommended. Acetazolamide (Diamox) may be taken to prevent altitude-related sickness. Contaminated water and ice can be avoided by boiling for 3 min or treatment with chemicals such as iodine, Lugo's solution, or liquid chlorine bleach. Beverages that contain ice or are mixed with water should be avoided. Coffee, tea, and milk made with boiling water are generally safe, as are carbonated drinks and wine. Dairy products should be avoided unless pasteurization, proper refrigeration, and hygiene preparation are known. Bottled commercial water should be encouraged in areas of questionable water purity. Foods considered for ingestion should be hot, well-cooked, and prepared by a reliable source. Cold foods, raw or improperly cooked meat, salads, custards, and cream pastries should be avoided. Raw fruits can be eaten after peeling, if the skin is unbroken. Green leafy vegetables should be scrubbed with detergent solution and soaked in strong iodine or chlorine solutions. Heat stroke and exhaustion can be avoided with adequate hydration and avoidance of overly strenuous exercise. In addition, protection from the sun can be achieved with the use of sunscreen 30 min before sun exposure with a sunscreen protection factor (SPF) of 15, reapplied every 1–3 h with water exposure. In areas with a high prevalence of insects, long-sleeved shirts and trousers/pants impregnated with permethrin and insect repellent with a 20–35% diethyltoluamide (DEET) should be used.[12] Places of residence should have screened doors and windows and beds covered with mosquito nets. Although often impractical, in areas with venomous animals (e.g., scorpions, snakes), an antivenom kit should be readily available. Long trousers tucked into boots should be worn. In addition, the traveler should avoid areas where one cannot see or walk, especially at nighttime, as mosquitoes and snakes are usually nocturnal in their habits.

Malaria

One of the most important risks of travel to developing countries is malaria. The CDC has country-specific guides to areas where malaria prophylaxis is needed and where areas of chloroquine-resistant falciparum malaria is prevalent.[10] Chloroquine-resistant *Plasmodium falciparum* malaria occurs mostly in the para-Amazon region of South America, South and Southeast Asia, tropical areas of Africa, and Oceania. However, areas of chloroquine-resistant *P. falciparum* must be reviewed regularly as the area of spread of resistance is increasing. Prophylaxis and treatment of malaria are listed in Table 2.5. For areas with chloroquine-sensitive malaria species (Haiti, Dominican Republic, Central America, and parts of the Middle East), the drug of choice in adults is chloroquine (Aralen). The recommended dose is 300 mg base orally once-weekly, beginning 1–2 weeks before departure and weekly while in the endemic area and continued 4 weeks after the last possible exposure to malaria. For children, chloroquine with a dose of 5 mg/kg of base weekly should be used. Chloroquine is safe for infants and pregnant women. For areas with chloroquine-resistant malaria, adult dosages of mefloquine (Lariam) 228 mg base orally once weekly beginning 1–2 weeks before travel is recommended. Mefloquine has an extensive side-effect profile, including insomnia, bad dreams, dizziness, headache, irritability, gastrointestinal symptoms, neuropsychiatric reactions, and seizures. Mefloquine is contraindicated in those with a psychiatric or epileptic history or those with a cardiac conduction disorder. For areas with chloroquine-resistant malaria, adult dosages of atovaquone/proguanil, doxycycline or mefloquine are recommended.[13] In areas with *P. vivax* or *P. ovale*, primaquine can be considered to prevent potentially relapsing malaria from persisting liver forms. The dose of primaquine is 15 mg base orally each day for 14 days.

Traveler's diarrhea

In many areas, traveler's diarrhea is the leading cause of medical illness. The most common bacterial causes of traveler's diarrhea are enterotoxigenic *Escherichia coli*, enteroaggregative *E. coli* and *Campylobacter* spp., depending on the region studied. Other common causes include viruses (rotavirus and Norwalk), bacteria (*Shigella*, and *Salmonella*) and parasitic organisms (amebiasis and giardiasis). Diarrhea should be treated by replacing lost fluids with adequate fluids such as water, tea, broth, and carbonated beverages with electrolyte replacement. Loperamide (Imodium) and diphenoxylate (Lomotil) may be used for non-dysenteric diarrhea. If diarrhea is distressing or mild diarrhea persists for greater than 3 days, with three or more stools with symptoms, consideration can be given to a short course of antibiotics such as a fluorquinolone (norfloxacin 400 mg, ciprofloxacin 500 mg, or levofloxacin 500 mg orally daily for 3 days) or a macrolide (azithromycin 500 mg orally daily for 3 days).[14]

Post-travel advice

Post-travel issues

Diagnoses of dermatoses and travel-related illnesses, both during and after return from travel, often represent a diagnostic dilemma.[15–17] Evaluation of travelers with skin lesions or fevers

Table 2.5 Prophylaxis and treatment of malaria[22]

Type of malaria	Treatment	Prophylaxis
Uncomplicated malaria, *P. vivax* or *P. ovale*	Chloroquine phosphate 600 mg base orally immediately, followed by 300 mg base orally at 6, 24 and 48 hours **plus** primaquine phosphate 30 mg base orally daily for 14 days	Chloroquine phosphate 300 mg base orally once per week
P. falciparum, chloroquine-sensitive	Chloroquine phosphate (as above)	Chloroquine phosphate (as above)
P. falciparum chloroquine-resistant, mild to moderately ill	Quinine sulfate base 542 mg orally three times a day for 7 days **plus** doxycycline 100 mg orally twice a day for 7 dyas, **or** clindamycin 20 mg base/kg/day orally divided three times a day for 7 days	Atovaquone/proguanil 1 tablet orally daily, **or** doxycycline 100 mg orally daily, **or** mefloquine 228 mg base orally once per week
P. falciparum chloroquine-resistant, mild to moderately ill	Mefloquine 684 mg base orally as initial dose, followed by 456 mg base orally given 6–12 hours after initial dose	
P. falciparum chloroquine-resistant, mild to moderately ill	Atovaquone-proguanil 4 tablets orally daily for 3 days	
P. falciparum chloroquine-resistant, severely ill	IV quinidine gluconate **plus** IV doxycycline **or** IV clindamycin. When the patient improves, he/she can change to oral quinine, doxycycline and clindamycin	

(> 38°C) must include an extensive travel history with discussion of epidemiological exposures along with a complete physical examination. Differential diagnosis will depend on travel location, length of stay, exposures, physical exam and clinical presentation, microbiological, serological, and laboratory studies. Skin lesions based on morphology (e.g., macule, papule, vesicle, nodule, etc.) may be the initial clue to the diagnosis of a dermatosis or other travel-related illness. Skin biopsy, cultures, and radiographic imaging may help confirm diagnosis.

In most travelers to developing countries for short periods of time (less than a month), medical examination and laboratory studies are not needed. However, routine medical examination and screening should be considered for expatriate travelers, even in individuals who appear healthy upon return. Screening tests should include urinalysis, liver function tests, tuberculosis skin test, or chest radiographic examination, and a complete blood cell count for evidence of anemia, leukocytosis, leucopenia, or eosinophilia. Eosinophilia and a stool test may provide a good screening test for possible intestinal or systemic helminthic and protozoan infections. One stool examination is not adequate in ruling out parasitic infections. Three stool examinations should be performed and may approximate the absence of infection with 70% certainty. Table 2.6 lists incubation periods for selected febrile illnesses that may affect travelers. In a returning febrile traveler, malaria, enteric fever, dengue fever, hepatitis, and amebic liver abscess should be considered.[18–20] In those with eosinophilia and a possible exposure to helminths, filariasis, schistosomiasis, strongyloides, and other intestinal helminths should be considered. Serological test for these helminths are not routinely available but may be obtained through some state health laboratories or at the CDC. In certain infectious diseases, malaria, hepatitis, schistosomiasis, and intestinal parasites may not present until months and possibly years after a traveler's return.[21]

With increasing international travel over the past few decades, physicians will need to educate travelers better on general preventive measures, including dermatoses, infectious diseases, and potential environmental hazards endemic to specific geographic areas of travel. Increased physician knowledge in travel medicine-related issues will also aid in more prompt diagnoses and treatment of dermatoses and travel-related illnesses.

Table 2.6 Incubation periods for selected febrile illnesses that may affect travelers[23]

Short: <10 days	Intermediate: 7–28 days	Long: >4 weeks	Variable: weeks to years
Anthrax	Bartonellosis	Brucellosis	AIDS
Boutonneuse fever	Brucellosis	Hepatitis A, B, C, E	Melioidosis
Crimean–Congo HF	Chagas diseases	Leishmaniasis	Rabies
Chikungunya fever	Ehrlichiosis	Loiasis	Schistosomiasis
Colorado tick fever	Hepatitis A, C, E	Lymphatic filariasis	Tuberculosis
Dengue	HF with renal syndrome	Malaria	Amebiasis
Histoplasmosis	Lassa fever	Trypanosomiasis gambiense	
Legionellosis	Leptospirosis		
Marburg/Ebola fever	Lyme disease		
Plague	Malaria		
Psittacosis	Q fever		
Rat-bite fever	Rocky Mountain spotted fever		
Relapsing fever	Smallpox		
Rocky Mountain spotted fever	South American HF		
Tularemia	Toxoplasmosis		
Yellow fever	Trichinellosis		
Yersiniosis	Trypanosomiasis		
	Typhoid fever		
	Typhus fevers		

AIDS, acquired immunodeficiency syndrome; HF, hemorrhagic fever.

References

1. Steffen R, Rickenbach M, Wilhelm U et al. Health problems after travel to developing countries. J Infect Dis 1987; 156:84–91.
2. Caumes E, Carriere J, Guermonprez G et al. Dermatoses associated with travel to tropical countries: a prospective study of the diagnosis and management of 269 patients presenting to a tropical disease unit. Clin Infect Dis 1995; 20:542–548.
3. Steffen R, Fuchs E, Schildknecht J et al. Mefloquine compared with other malaria chemoprophylactic regimens in tourists visiting east Africa. Lancet 1993; 22:1299–1303.
4. Manatsathit S, Dupont HL, Farthing M et al. Working party of the Program Committee of the Bangkok World Congress of Gastroenterology 2002. Guideline for the management of acute diarrhea in adults. J Gastroenterol Hepatol 2002; 17 (suppl.):S54–S71.
5. Raju R, Smal N, Sorokin M. Incidence of minor and major disorders among visitor to Fiji. In Lobel HO, Steffen R, Kozarsky PE, eds. Travel medicine 2: proceedings of the second conference on international travel medicine. Atlanta, GA: International Society of Travel Medicine; 1992:62.
6. Peltola H, Kyronseppa H, Holsa P. Trips to the south – a health hazard. Morbidity of Finnish travellers. Scand J Infect Dis 1983; 15:375–381.
7. Ament ME, Rubin CE. Relation of giardiasis to abnormal intestinal structure and function in gastrointestinal immuno-deficiency syndromes. Gastroenterology 1972; 62:216–226.
8. Heyworth MF. Immunology of *Giardia* and *Cryptosporidium* infections. J Infect Dis 1992; 166:465–472.
9. Walker E, Williams G. Travellers requiring special advice. Br Med J 1983; 16:1265–1266.
10. Centers for Disease Control and Prevention. Health information for international travel, 1999–2000. Atlanta, GA: Department of Health and Human Services; 1999.
11. Wilson ME, von Reyn CF, Fineberg HV. Infections in HIV-infected travelers: risks and prevention. Ann Intern Med 1991; 114:582–592.
12. Fradin MS. Mosquitoes and mosquito repellents: a clinician's guide. Ann Intern Med 1998; 128:931–940.
13. Lobel HO, Kozarsky PE. Update on prevention of malaria for travelers. JAMA 1997; 278:1767–1771.
14. Ericsson CD, DuPont HL. Traveler's diarrhea: approaches to prevention and treatment. Clin Infect Dis 1993; 16:616–624.
15. Lucchina LC, Wilson ME, Drake LA. Dermatology and the recently returned traveler: infectious diseases with dermatologic manifestations. Int J Dermatol 1997; 36:167–181.
16. Lockwood DN, Keystone JS. Skin problems in returning travelers. Med Clin North Am 1992; 76:1393–1411.
17. McKendrick M. Infectious diseases and the returning traveler – experience from a regional infectious diseases unit over 20 years. J Appl Microbiol 2003; 94 (suppl.):25S–30S.
18. Klion AD, Nutman TB. Infectious diseases of international travel. Adv Intern Med 2001; 47:265–292.
19. Walker E, Williams G. Infections on return from abroad – II. Br Med J 1983; 286:1197–1199.
20. Schwartz MD. Fever in the returning traveler, part II: a methodological approach to initial management. Wilderness Environ Med 2003; 14:120–130.
21. Wolfe MS. Medication evaluation of the returning traveler. In: Jong EC, Keystone JS, eds. Travel medicine advisor. Atlanta, GA: American Health Consultants; 1991:26.1–26.15.
22. Maitland K, Bejon P, Newton CR. Malaria. Curr Opin Infect Dis 2003; 16:389–395.
23. DuPont HL, Steffen R. Travel medicine and health, 2nd ed. Hamilton, Ontario: BC Decker; 2001.

Chapter 3

Working in the tropics

Ross Barnetson and Anthony White

- Cultural context
- Clinical context
- Traditional therapies
- Equipment
- Pharmaceutical supplies
- Personal preparation
- Geographical considerations

Cultural context

All illness exists in a cultural context. It is essential to understand the cultural background of the society in which one will be working if one is to be effective. Beliefs about the cause and treatment of disease can differ profoundly from scientific orthodoxy. Ignoring or dismissing these beliefs can result in poor compliance, at the very least. At the other extreme, strong offence may be taken at the cultural insensitivities of a well-meaning but ignorant visitor to a community.

Anyone planning medical mission work should begin by reading in depth about the country, its history, religions, culture, and customs. How do people feel about being examined physically? Is an examination by a physician of the opposite sex out of the question? How much eye contact is uncomfortable? Are certain treatments, for example injections, viewed locally as the only worthwhile treatment? An attempt should be made to acquire a basic vocabulary in the local language to cover greetings and simple civilities. The words for a few key clinical terms ("itch," "pain," "getting better/worse," etc.) can, used with a questioning inflexion, greatly speed up the consultation. Of course, the services of an interpreter are essential for explaining the disease and its treatment to the patient or when a detailed history is sought.

An understanding of what is financially affordable for the patient is a concern of all physicians everywhere. Enquiries should be made to ascertain what is a realistic imposition before prescribing treatment in an unfamiliar setting. Due deference and respect should be shown to local power structures of the health providers and civil authorities. Visiting consultants, by the manner in which they deal with local colleagues, can be extremely influential in either strengthening or undermining the way local doctors and nurses are perceived by the population they serve.

As a rule, the straightforward, blunt, time-obsessed approach of westerners needs to be softened considerably when operating in many other cultures. What is required is a calm, courteous, and patient demeanour, unruffled by delays or setbacks.

Clinical context

Every effort should be made to become familiar with the local pattern of skin disease. As a rule, in tropical dermatology, infections of all types and infestations are much more common than in the temperate zones. On the other hand, skin cancer and degenerative disease, common in temperate, western zones, are almost unknown.

One should refresh one's knowledge of the clinical features and management of the prevalent diseases, understanding that they are often much more extensive and severe than what one might be accustomed to, as a result of remaining untreated over a long time.

The intensity of pigmentation can affect the appearance of common skin conditions such as psoriasis and eczema. Clinicians who have little experience in managing patients with deeply pigmented skins should familiarize themselves with the spectrum of disease in non-Caucasian skin.

In most countries, good statistics exist on the prevalence of leprosy and human immunodeficiency virus (HIV). These figures should be sought as a guide as to what to expect in clinics. The particular geographic zone may have a high prevalence of a particular disease such as leishmaniasis.

Some diligent reading on such unfamiliar entities is essential preparation.

Traditional therapies

The term "traditional medicine" encompasses all those modalities of health care that date from the dawn of time to the advent of scientific medicine.

From time immemorial all societies have sought remedies from their immediate surroundings for the illnesses that have afflicted them. Parts of local animals, plants, or various minerals have provided the basis of treatment. Many of the treatments have become well-known household remedies in those societies.

Others are administered by healers who are often highly respected members of their communities. Some treatments involve manipulation or invasive procedures such as acupuncture. Childbirth and mental illnesses have their own traditional specialist healers.

It is still true that most of the populations of developing countries continue to depend on their traditional medicine for primary health care. Practitioners of scientific medicine should therefore accord due respect to traditional healers and those who have faith in them. "Scientific" doctors should seek to understand and work alongside healers rather than denigrating or patronizing them.

Undoubtedly many traditional treatments, hallowed by centuries of use, will, when subjected to scientific evaluation, prove to be effective. Aspirin, quinine, and digoxin, all "traditional" remedies, have become incorporated in mainstream medicine.

At the same time as developing countries are being exposed to scientific medicine, there is an increasing interest in traditional herbal remedies (alternative or complementary medicine) in the populations of developed countries.[1]

The World Health Organization, through its Traditional Medicine Program, is encouraging the compiling of national formularies and the study of efficacy. Plants with medicinal potential are being subject to systematic pharmacological research.

Equipment

Inevitably, this is a trade-off between what is desirable and what is practicable. In general, supplies of all types will be less accessible in most tropical settings. This includes banal items such as pen, paper, and batteries. One should aim to be self-sufficient and impose as little logistical strain on local facilities as possible.

Good management depends on accurate diagnosis. This in turn is the product of a satisfactory clinical examination. The situations in which clinical examinations are performed are often not ideal, with poor lighting. This is a particular problem with the darker skins usually encountered in the tropics. The most important item for the dermatologist is therefore a headlamp with binocular loupe and rechargeable, belt-mounted battery pack. One should ascertain on what voltage the local power system operates and obtain the appropriate adaptors.

Photographic documentation is essential for teaching purposes. One should be familiar with one's camera equipment and carry adequate supplies of batteries and film.

The following list of dermatological equipment may be trimmed or expanded to fit the circumstances, such as available transport and the nature of the host facility:

- Notebook, stationery, and pens
- Local anesthetic: with and without epinephrine (adrenaline); syringes, needles
- Biopsy kit: punch biopsies, 2–8 mm scissors, skin hooks, needle-holders
- Excision kit: scalpels, blades, forceps, needle-holders, suture material
- Corticosteroid for intralesional injection
- Gloves, dressings, antiseptic sachets, alcohol gel hand cleanser
- Cautery/diathermy
- Wood's light
- Pathology:
  - bottles with formalin
  - envelopes for skin scrapings
  - microscope, slides, cover slips, potassium hydroxide
  - culture media (bacterial and fungal).

Pharmaceutical supplies

Topical and systemic drugs are limited in range and availability in most developing countries. It is helpful for any visiting dermatologist to take as much in the way of pharmaceutical supplies as cost and transport facilities permit. The choice of drugs should reflect the local pattern of skin disease. Antifungals (topical and oral) and topical corticosteroids are the most needed. There is still considerable merit in some older preparations which may be regarded as obsolete in western countries. An example is topical gentian violet which is cheap, stable, and effective for candidiasis and the commonly encountered secondarily infected eczema patient.

Pharmaceutical companies are often willing to donate supplies. Several western countries have organizations that collect drugs for distribution to individuals or bodies to take on missions. There is, however, no place for the use of products which have passed their expiration date.

Arrangements will need to be made with the host country, pointing out that the supplies are for dispensing gratis and thus facilitating passage through Customs.

Personal preparation

Visitors on medical missions should be physically, including dentally, healthy. Adequate supplies of personal routine medications should be taken as well as a first-aid kit, insect repellent, and sunscreen. Again, the principle of self-sufficiency applies.

An early visit to a travel medical centre is essential to ensure that the appropriate vaccination program is completed on time. If visiting a malarial area, advice will be given as to the appropriate chemoprophylaxis.

Geographical considerations

Many skin diseases are universal. An obvious example is psoriasis, though it may have a lower incidence in tropical countries, possibly due to the immunosuppressive effect of sunlight. Another disease which comes into this category is atopic dermatitis, which has increasing prevalence in industrialized countries, but is very uncommon in some tropical countries, for instance in Africa. The exact reason for this is unclear, but it is probable that it is related to recurrent infections and worm infestations.[2] Many infections and infestations are also universal. Examples are herpes simplex, varicella and herpes zoster, papillomavirus infections, staphylococcal and streptococcal skin infections, dermatophyte infections, and scabies. Others are mainly confined to the tropics, such as leprosy, deep fungal and protozoal infections. These are usually influenced by the tropical climate, and the presence of certain insects in the area. Clearly it is important when one is in a certain country to find out what diseases are most prevalent there.

Mass air travel has had a major impact on skin diseases, and it is important to take a history of recent travel to hotter climes. Cutaneous leishmaniasis is not uncommonly seen in Australia in children of Middle Eastern families who have paid a visit to their relatives in their country of origin. The children, lacking immunity, acquired the disease through sand fly bites and the cutaneous lesions become apparent after they return. Leprosy, with its long incubation period, is often diagnosed years after the patient has migrated to Australia.

HIV-AIDS (acquired immunodeficiency syndrome) has also had a major impact on skin diseases in the tropics. In a recent study of 1000 such patients in Tanzania, viral infections were the commonest first manifestation of HIV infection, particularly herpes zoster. A total of 97% of patients with herpes zoster between the ages of 20 and 50 were HIV-positive (Fig. 3.1).[3] Atopic eczema, previously rare in Africa, was seen commonly. Other skin diseases prevalent in HIV patients were fungal infections (tinea and candidiasis), bacterial infections and Kaposi's sarcoma. Blue nails are also a distinctive marker for HIV infection.

Australia and Oceania

Australia is unusual. A vast majority of the population have fair skin, having migrated to the continent in the last 200 years.

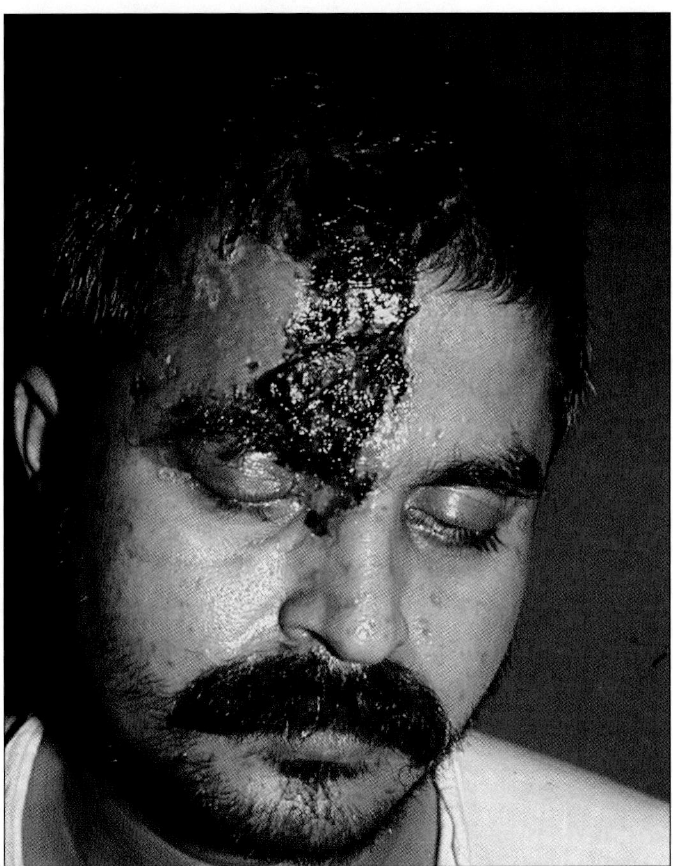

Figure 3.1 Herpes zoster in a human immunodeficiency virus (HIV)-seropositive patient. (Courtesy of Dr. J. K. Maniar.)

However, it must be remembered that the indigenous inhabitants, of whom there are now about 400 000, have darkly pigmented skins. This is not surprising given the climate of Australia, which is in large part tropical or subtropical. The original immigrants were from Europe, but more recently there has been significant migration to Australia from Southeast Asia and Oceania. Skin cancers in the indigenous people are very uncommon but squamous cell carcinomas may occur in areas of inflammation, such as leprosy ulcers or tropical ulcers. Basal cell carcinomas do occur, but uncommonly, in people with black skin.

As a result of the European migration to Australia, the incidence of sun-induced skin cancer is enormous, the highest in the world. It is estimated that there are 384 000 new cases of skin cancer per year, out of a population of 19 million.[4] In all, 256 000 of these are basal cell carcinomas, 118 000 are squamous cell carcinomas, and 10 000 are melanomas. The overall cost of skin cancer in Australia is huge.

As might be expected, skin infections are a major problem: skin diseases are the second commonest group of diseases, after respiratory diseases, seen by health professionals. Of special note are deep fungal infections such as sporotrichosis and chromomycosis, seen particularly in the north of the continent. Leprosy is still endemic in the aboriginal communities, though the number of new patients presenting per year is small. Generally, tuberculosis is not a common condition in Australia, so cutaneous tuberculosis is extremely rare.

Oceania is a composite of many small islands in the Pacific, where care of skin diseases in general is rather basic. For the whole of the South Pacific (except French and American protectorates) there is only one dermatologist, in Fiji. Skin diseases are extremely common, particularly superficial dermatophyte infections.[4] These are commonly in the pant area, probably because in many villages, there are communal washing facilities so the inhabitants have to shower wearing shorts.

Chromomycosis is seen but not commonly. Leprosy is still a problem, but a minor one, and the disease is close to elimination. Scabies is a major problem, though it was reduced by the treatment of some populations with ivermectin in a drive to eradicate filariasis. One other problem is the incidence of hereditary skin diseases, due to the fact that many of the islands (and countries) in Oceania are very small and intermarriages are common. As a result hereditary conditions such as albinism and ichthyosiform erythroderma are not uncommon.

Asia

Asia is the largest continent on the planet, and the spectrum of skin diseases is enormous. As far as tropical skin diseases are concerned, the continent can be usefully divided into: (1) the Middle East; (2) the Indian subcontinent; and (3) the Far East.

The Middle East

The Middle East is less populated than the other areas, and much of the terrain is arid. By far the most important skin disease in this area is cutaneous leishmaniasis, due to *Leishmania tropica* and *L. major*, transmitted by the sand fly. This is the cause of "oriental sore," which is common in children in the Middle East, who usually only get a single lesion, producing a lifelong immunity so that they generally do not get more. It is interesting to note that the Iraqis were aware of this 2000 years ago, and used to inoculate their children with the debris from a sore on the lower leg to prevent the children from getting mutilating sores on their face.

More recently, the irrigation workers from non-leishmanial endemic countries (non-immunes) have posed a major problem because, if they have multiple bites from sand flies at the same time they develop multiple sores – sometimes 50–100 – which certainly require systemic therapy. Oriental sore is generally self-limiting, clearing within a year, but a variant lupoid leishmaniasis (which mimics lupus vulgaris) may go on for many years, because patients have limited immunity to the infection.

Melasma and facial hypermelanosis are common in the Middle East, and throughout Asia in general. This results from sun exposure. This is yet another reason for covering the face and neck, as is the custom in these countries. It is less marked in Africans who have darker skin.

Indian subcontinent

One of the most important diseases in India is leprosy, with 600 000 new cases per year. This is at a time when most countries have been able to minimize the disease or eradicate it. There are still numerous leprosaria in the country. As it is a disease of both skin and nerves, it is a major cause of deformity. It has a very long incubation period (up to 20 years), and is a very chronic disease: however, it rarely kills the patient.

Another common disease in India is the deep fungal infection, mycetoma, sometimes known as Madura foot (Madura is in India) (Fig. 3.2). This may be due to true fungi (eumycetes), or to actinomycetes. It is important to culture the organism if possible, because the treatment varies with the cause. This usually causes swelling of the foot, with discharging sinuses. There is also marked osteomyelitis in those with fungal mycetoma, where itraconazole may be unobtainable due to cost, and amputation of the foot may be necessary. As might be expected, other skin infections and infestations are common, particularly those due to helminths such as dracunculiasis (Fig. 3.3) and filariasis (Fig. 3.4).

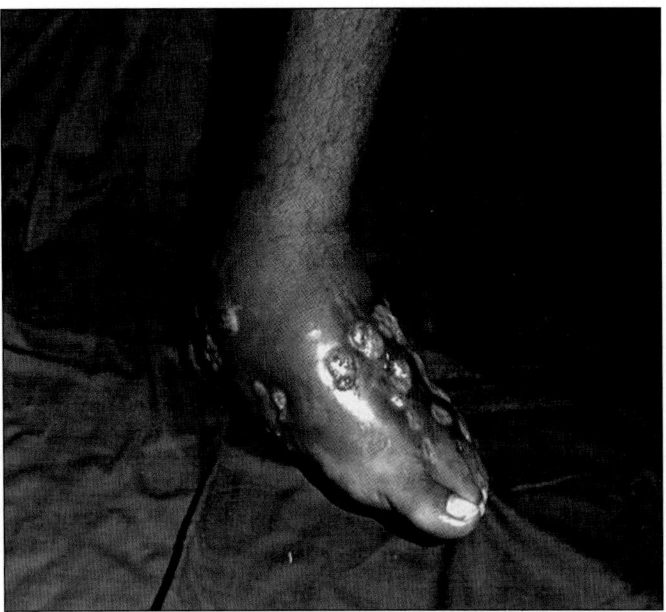

Figure 3.2 Mycetoma. (Courtesy of Dr. J. K. Maniar.)

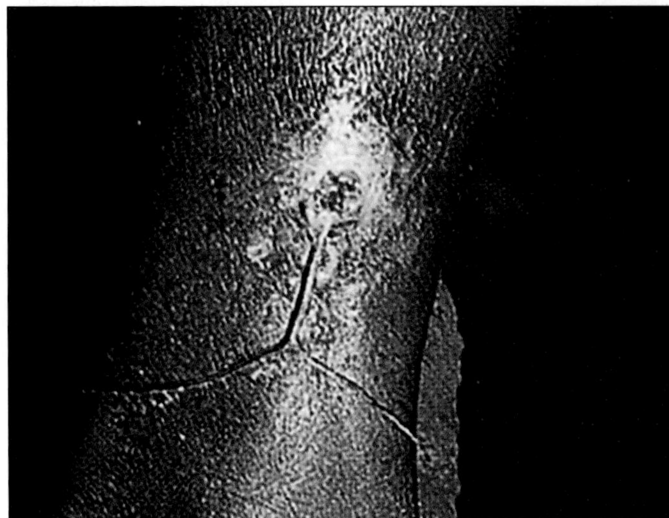

Figure 3.3 Dracunculiasis (Guinea worm infection) extraction method. (Reproduced from Peters W and Pasvol G (eds). Tropical Medicine and Parasitology, 5th edition, Mosby, London 2002.)

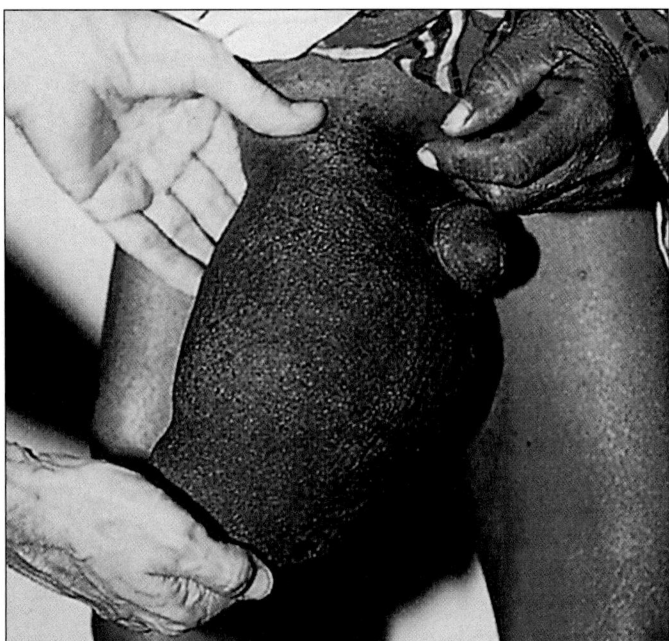

Figure 3.4 Filariasis with hydrocele. (Reproduced from Peters W and Pasvol G (eds). Tropical Medicine and Parasitology, 5th edition, Mosby, London 2002.)

Vitiligo is also common in India, presumably due to some hereditary factor, and it may be very extensive. Many Indians were taken to Fiji in the nineteenth century to cut the sugar cane, and settled there. Vitiligo is also common in these Indians, but not in indigenous Fijians.

There are also, surprisingly, reports of skin cancers in Bangladeshi patients. These are almost certainly due to arsenic in the well water.

Far East

Most of the Far Eastern countries are close to the Equator, and are hot and humid. In some, also, there is abundant tropical rain forest. Worm infestations are common, including strongyloidiasis, a chronic condition which results in urticaria and larva currens. Filiariasis is also a problem due to mosquito-borne *Wuchereria bancrofti* and *Brugia malayi*. This leads to elephantiasis, particularly of the lower leg (elephantiasis of the scrotum is usually due to *Mycobacterium tuberculosis*). Cutaneous larva migrans due to dog hookworm is also common, leading to a self-limiting dermatosis, usually on the buttocks or lower legs.

Leprosy is no longer common in the Far East. Cutaneous tuberculosis is relatively common, because tuberculosis is still a major problem there.

One other disease deserves mention – lichen amyloidosis. This is extremely common in the Far East, and causes an intensely pruritic eruption, usually on the legs. There is clearly a genetic element, but its cause is unknown.

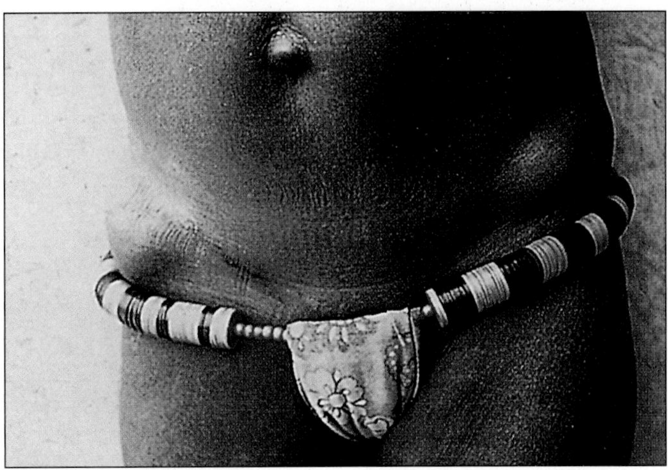

Figure 3.5 Onchocerciasis nodules. (Reproduced from Peters W and Pasvol G (eds). Tropical Medicine and Parasitology, 5th edition, Mosby, London 2002.)

Europe

Most of Europe is temperate. However, the south of Europe and the Mediterranean islands are subtropical and certain skin diseases are common there. Leishmaniasis and leprosy are still a problem in countries bordering the Mediterranean, though a minor one. Endemic Kaposi's sarcoma, which is unrelated to HIV infection, is seen in the southern European countries, particularly in the legs of elderly men.

Africa

Africa is a huge continent with many skin problems. It may be divided into four regions for convenience: North Africa, East Africa and horn of Africa, West Africa and Southern Africa.

North Africa

There are large areas of desert, and the density of populations is generally quite small, apart from in the urban districts. As might be expected in a desert region, leishmaniasis occurs in parts of North Africa, generally of the "oriental sore" presentation. Other skin infections are also common.

East Africa and Horn of Africa

Ethiopia is unusual in that much of the country is at high altitudes. For instance, Addis Ababa is at an altitude of 2800 m. As a result, certain diseases such as malaria are not a major problem. Leprosy is still a problem, though leprosy-control programs have been successful in some areas in reducing the prevalence.

Leishmaniasis is a major problem, and is generally unlike that seen in the Middle East. The skin lesions are much more chronic than the classical "oriental sore," being more like those seen in Central and South America. Mucocutaneous leishmaniasis is common, probably due to direct spread, rather than metastatic spread, as occurs in espundia. Diffuse cutaneous leishmaniasis also occurs, again being similar to leishmaniasis in the Americas. The clinical presentation is very similar to lepromatous leprosy, and many were admitted to leprosaria having been wrongfully diagnosed. The distinction can easily be made by performing a smear or a skin biopsy.

Deep fungal infections are common, including mycetoma, sporotrichosis (easily diagnosed clinically by the sporotrichoid spread), and chromomycosis. Onchocerciasis is a major problem in parts of Ethiopia (Fig. 3.5). This presents with an itchy rash on one limb ("unilateral scabies"), before developing into a generalized pruritic rash, with enlargement of the lymph glands and depigmentation on the shins. Fortunately blindness is uncommon in this form of onchocerciasis (unlike that in West Africa). The reason for this is unknown.

Autoimmune skin diseases are also relatively common, particularly at a young age. Pemphigus is seen in children, as are other bullous diseases such as linear immunoglobulin A (IgA) disease.

Podoconiosis is a unique form of elephantiasis seen in Ethiopia (non-filarial elephantiasis) in non-mosquito (due to the altitude) areas of the country. This is thought to be due to a constituent of the soil causing a reaction in the inguinal lymph nodes, resulting in lymphoedema (Fig. 3.6).

West Africa

Skin diseases are particularly prevalent in West Africa, which is notorious for its helminthic skin diseases. Onchocerciasis is a huge problem because it causes "river blindness" due to invasion of the orbit by microfilariae. It presents as a pruritic skin disease, as in the Ethiopian variety, becoming generalized, and causes much suffering.

Another helminthic disease which affects the skin is loiasis, which causes Calabar swellings. Bancroftian and Malayan filariasis are also seen in West Africa, as is dracunculiasis. Cutaneous larva migrans, due to dog hookworm, and larva currens, due to *Strongyloides*, are also prevalent. Many other tropical skin diseases are also seen commonly in the countries of West Africa, including leprosy, yaws, and tropical ulcers.

Southern Africa

Tropical skin diseases are also common in Southern Africa. HIV-AIDS is a major problem leading to viral, bacterial, and fungal skin infections.

The American continent

As might be expected, there is a tremendous spectrum of skin diseases in the American continent. The skin diseases seen in Canada and the USA are those seen in most developed countries, and are similar to those in Europe.

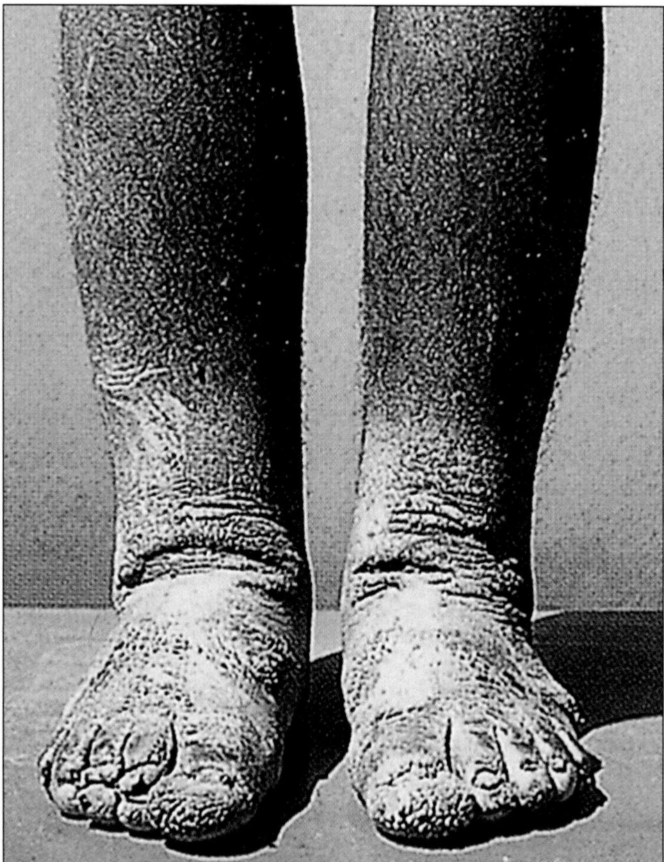

Figure 3.6 Podoconiosis (non-filarial elephantiasis) in an Ethiopian. Podoconiosis is a debilitating condition caused by the passage of microparticles of silica and alumino-silicates through the skin of people who walk bare-footed in terrain with a high content of red laterite of volcanic origin. (Reproduced from Peters W and Pasvol G (eds). Tropical Medicine and Parasitology, 5th edition, Mosby, London 2002, image 1101.)

Central and South America

Tropical skin diseases are mainly seen in Central America, including Mexico and Guatemala, and in northern South America, generally excluding Argentina and Chile.

This part of the world is notorious for its fungal infections. These include infections which are seen elsewhere, such as mycetoma, chromomycosis, sporotrichosis, histoplasmosis and phycomycosis, and some diseases which are only seen in the American continent such as lobomycosis and coccidioidomycosis. Worm infestations affecting the skin are also common in Central and South America, and include onchocerciasis, strongyloidiasis, and cutaneous larva migrans.

Leprosy is still common in Brazil (which has the second highest incidence in the world). A particular complication of leprosy in Mexico is the Lucio reaction, a form of vasculitis caused by *M. leprae*, and which for some reason is almost unknown outside that region.

Leishmaniasis, particularly due to *Leishmania mexicana* and *L. braziliensis*, is also a major problem in Central America. It tends to be a much more chronic disease than Old World leishmaniasis, and may present in many exotic forms such as espundia, chiclero ulcers on the ears, and diffuse cutaneous leishmaniasis, which is also seen in Ethiopia.

Another disease seen in South America is fogo selvagem (Brazilian pemphigus). This form of pemphigus is seen in certain families and certain localities in Brazil, and seems to be connected to the waterways there. The exact pathogenesis is unknown. It is clearly an autoimmune disease frequently associated with endocrine disturbance, but the precipitating agents (with a possible insect vector) are unclear.

Thus, working in the tropics requires preparation of one's equipment and pharmaceutical supplies. Personal preparation, however, is paramount in that everything possible should be done to avoid becoming ill, i.e., proper vaccinations and other prophylaxis (e.g., against malaria), insect repellent, sunscreen, and first-aid kit. Geographical considerations are very important because of the marked differences between the various parts of the tropical world. One must be aware of the diseases that are encountered at the destination and how they have been managed for generations. The local people, however, are a more important consideration than the diseases or the tropical destination, because one must always be aware of their customs, taboos, and traditional healers. Otherwise, the western ideas of therapy and prevention will not be accepted.

References

1. Buchness MR. Alternative medicine and dermatology. Semin Cutan Med Surg 1998; 17:284–290.
2. Flohr C. Dirt, worms and atopic dermatitis. Br J Dermatol 2003; 148:871–877.
3. Naburi AE, Leppard BJ. Herpes zoster and HIV infection. Int J STD AIDS 2000; 11:254–256.
4. White AD, Barnetson RStC. Practising dermatology in the South Pacific. Med J Aust 1998; 169:659–662.

Part 2

Protozoa

Chapter 4 *Trypanosomiasis*

Chapter 5 *Leishmaniasis*

Chapter 6 *Cutaneous manifestations of infection by free-living amebas*

Helminths

Chapter 7 *Nematodal Helminths*

Chapter 8 *Other helminths*

Chapter 9 *Cestodes*

Chapter 10 *Trematodes*

Viral Infections

Chapter 11 *HIV and HIV-associated disorders*

Chapter 12 *Hemorrhagic fevers*

Chapter 13 *Poxviruses*

Chapter 14 *Measles*

Chapter 15 *HTLV-1*

Chapter 16 *Tropical manifestations of common viral infections*

Fungal Infections

Bacterial Infections

Ectoparisitic Diseases

Chapter 4

Trypanosomiasis

Ivan Semenovitch and Omar Lupi

African trypanosomiasis
- Introduction
- History
- Epidemiology
- Pathogenesis and etiology
- Clinical features
- Patient evaluation, diagnosis, and differential diagnosis
- Pathology
- Treatment

American trypanosomiasis
- Introduction
- History
- Epidemiology
- Pathogenesis and etiology
- Clinical features
- Patient evaluation, diagnosis, and differential diagnosis
- Pathology
- Treatment

Protozoa of the genus *Trypanosoma* are responsible for the widespread tropical disease trypanosomiasis. There are African and American forms and they are considered endemic in some regions of these continents.

African trypanosomiasis

Synonyms: African trypanosomiasis, sleeping sickness

Key features:

- Exposure to tsetse flies
- Fever, headache, joint pain, skin rash, lymph node enlargement, skin rash, anemia, and weight loss in the hemolymphatic stage
- Motor and sensory disorders, sleep cycle alteration, white cells, and protein increase in the meningoencephalitic stage

Introduction

Also known as sleeping sickness, African trypanosomiasis is an acute and chronic disease caused by a parasite called *Trypanosoma brucei.* The parasites are transmitted to humans through the bite of tsetse flies (*Glossina* spp.) in some regions of Africa.

Although confined to the African continent, in this time when air travel is continuously increasing, all dermatologists should know the cutaneous manifestations and be aware of the diagnostic tests for African trypanosomiasis, so that prompt diagnosis and proper treatment may follow.

History

The first references to sleeping sickness in Western Africa are from 1734, due to Atkins, and tell of somnolence, dementia, and death. Nepveu (in 1890) found, for the first time, trypanosomes in the blood of a patient in Argel, but did not relate this fact to the disease. Forde and Dutton (1901, 1902) observed, for the first time, trypanosomes in the blood of a patient with irregular fever in Gambia (*T. gambiense*). Castellani, the next year, identified the same parasite in the cerebrospinal fluid (CSF) of a sleeping-sickness patient in Uganda (*T. ugandense*). In 1903, Bruce and Nabarro demonstrated the disease transmission by flies of the genus *Glossina.* In 1910, Stephens and Fantham found another species of trypanosome, in Rhodesia, and named it *T. rhodesiense.* Finally, Kinghorn and Yorke showed, in 1912, that the *T. rhodesiense* transmission was due to bites of tsetse flies of the genus *Glossina.*[1]

Epidemiology

African trypanosomiasis is estimated to infect more than 20 000 and kill more than 5000 Africans annually, representing a risk to more than 50 million people who live near the vector. Approximately 6.5 million square kilometers in Africa remain unpopulated because of the presence of the infection, resulting in a heavy economic burden. The disease is confined to the African continent and its main geographical distribution comprises Senegal, south of Mali, Burkina Faso, Niger, Chad, southeast of Sudan, Ethiopia, Angola, Botswana, Zimbabwe, and Mozambique (Fig. 4.1).

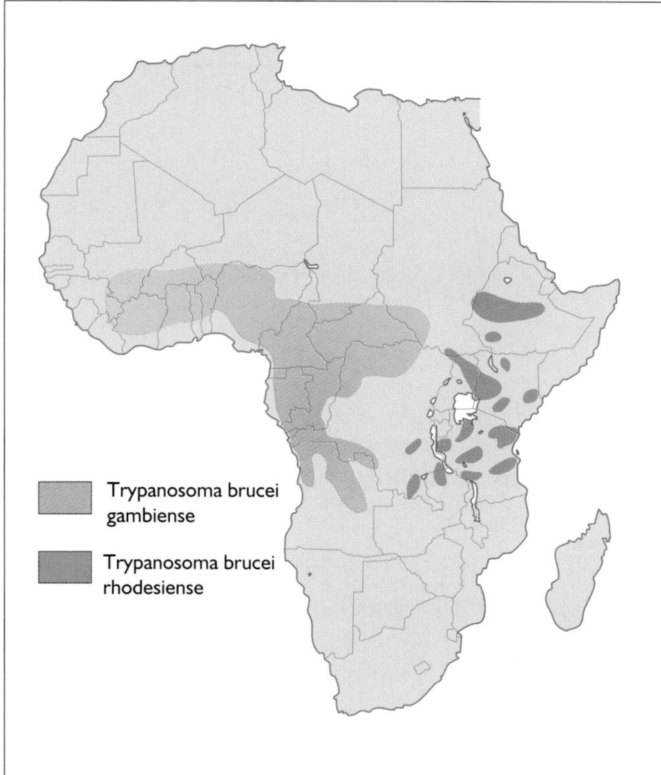

Figure 4.1 Distribution of the two forms of African trypanosomiasis in Africa.

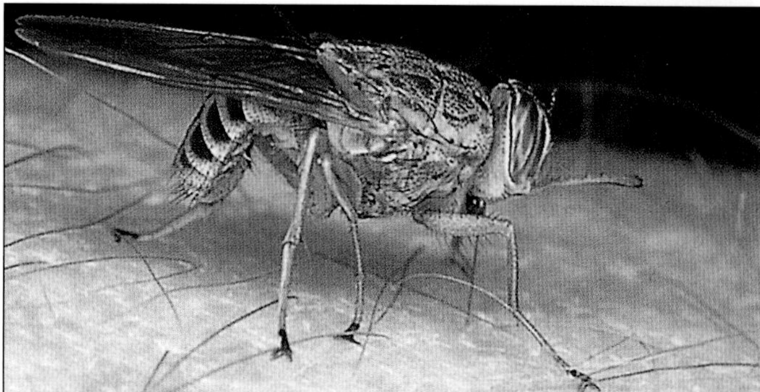

Figure 4.2 Tsetse fly feeding. (Reproduced from Peters W and Pasviol G (eds). Tropical Medicine and Parasitology, 5th edition, Mosby, London 2002, image 163.)

Occasional cases are imported into countries where the parasite is not endemic. Age, sex, and race appear to have no influence on susceptibility to African trypanosomiasis.[2,3]

T. brucei gambiense is found primarily in the west and central regions of sub-Saharan Africa. It primarily infects humans but there may be animal reservoirs, such as pigs, dogs, or sheep. *Glossina palpalis, G. tachinoides,* and *G. fuscipes* are the three main species of tsetse flies involved in the transmission of Gambian sleeping sickness.[4–6]

The more virulent *T. brucei rhodesiense* is a parasite of wild game, therefore humans are only its occasional hosts. It is found primarily in East Africa (from Ethiopia and eastern Uganda south to Zambia and Botswana). Flies of the *G. morsitans* group are responsible for Rhodesian sleeping sickness (including *G. pallidipes* and *G. swynnertoni*). These flies strike individuals visiting an endemic area, such as herdsmen, hunters, photographers, and tourists in general.[3,4]

Intrauterine transmission has been recorded infrequently. Preventive measures have involved the removal of entire villages to testse-free land and mass treatment.[4,5]

Pathogenesis and etiology

Trypanosomes are hemoflagellates that belong to the Salivaria family, *Trypanosoma* genus and *T. brucei* species. There are three subspecies: *T. brucei gambiense, T. brucei rhodesiense,* and *T. brucei brucei*. The first two are responsible for African trypanosomiasis in humans while the third one is an agent of animal trypanosomiasis (nagana). In the peripheral blood of humans, trypanosomes vary in length from 10 to 40 μm. The different subspecies of *T. brucei* can be distinguished by differences in pathogenicity for certain animals, electrophoresis, and DNA hybridization.[4,7]

T. brucei is transmitted by the tsetse fly *Glossina* (Fig. 4.2), within which it undergoes several developmental changes. During the bite of an infected animal or human host, trypomastigotes are ingested and rapidly differentiate into procyclic forms, in the insect midgut, by losing their antigenic surface coats. After 15–20 days of multiplication, these non-infectious epimastigotes migrate to the tsetse fly salivary glands and change morphologically into infectious metacyclic forms. When injected into humans, these metacyclic forms multiply and mature, in about 10 days, in the connective tissue and blood. From the skin, where they produce a local chancre, trypanosomes travel to lymph nodes, where they stimulate antibody production (and enlargement of these nodes). They alter the composition of their surface glycoproteins continuously in order to escape the host immune response. Transmission can also occur via blood transfusion.[3,4]

Tissue damage is induced by either toxin production or immune complex reaction with release of proteolytic enzymes. Immune complexes have been demonstrated in both the circulation and the target organs of infected patients. Autoantibodies are frequently directed against antigen components of red cells, brain, and heart. Anemia due to hemolysis can result in further tissue destruction. Thus the initial response to the infection can result in febrile episodes, lymph node enlargement, myocardial and pericardial inflammation, anemia, thrombocytopenia, disseminated intravascular coagulation, and renal insufficiency in the acute stage of the infection.[3,6,7]

Central nervous system (CNS) changes are most prominent in cases of *T. brucei gambiense* disease. They occur 3–18 months after the infection and consist of infiltrations in the meninges with lymphocytes, plasma cells, and morular cells. Morular cells are modified plasma cells with granular inclusions (immunoglobulins). Neurons undergo variable degeneration with myelin destruction and diffuse glial reaction. Meningeal lesions are usually represented by a diffuse leptomeningitis with congestion, edema, and microhemorrhages.[6–8]

Clinical features

Following the bite of the tsetse fly, blood invasion by trypanosomes is immediate. After an incubation period of a few weeks, first there is the invasion stage (septicemic) with parasites in the circulation, also called the hemolymphatic stage; then there is the meningo-encephalitic stage in which we can find neurological, neuroendocrine, and psychic symptoms. However, electroencephalographic tests have demonstrated invasion of the CNS coinciding with the hemolymphatic stage, but not with CSF alterations, which occur later.[3,9]

Rhodesian sleeping sickness is usually much more virulent and often results in cardiac failure and acute neurological manifestations. On the other hand, Gambian sleeping sickness is typically a chronic disease with primarily neurological features and no initial chancre. When symptoms do appear, usually after months or years, they are so mild that they tend to be ignored by the patient. These differences are not absolute and the opposite can also occur.[4,8]

The initial phase is characterized by the trypanosomal chancre (Fig. 4.3), the earliest sign of disease, which is a local, pruritic, and painful inflammatory reaction at the site of inoculation. The chancre is an indurated red or violaceous nodule, 2–5 cm in diameter, that is accompanied by regional lymphadenopathy and usually appears 48 h after the tsetse bite. A central necrotic eschar may form before the chancre desquamates within 2–3 weeks, leaving no trace. Many patients think of it as an isolated "boil" or simply never notice it. Chancres are rare in patients with Gambian sleeping sickness but are present in 70–80% of people infected with *T. rhodesiense*. Erythematous, urticarial, or macular rashes on the trunk, targetoid in shape, and occurring 6–8 weeks after the onset of illness, represent the most important clinical sign of early disease in light-skinned patients and are called trypanids (Fig. 4.4). Approximately 50% of light-skinned patients show trypanids after fever begins. These lesions may show a hemorrhagic component and are probably caused by type III hypersensitivity. Local lymph node enlargement may occur in the region draining the chancre and usually progresses to generalized lymphadenopathy.[1,3,8]

The hemolymphatic stage normally begins 3–10 days after the chancre with invasion of the blood stream and reticuloendothelial system. High fever, headache, joint pains, and malaise recur at irregular intervals, corresponding to waves of parasitemia. Transient pruritic and papular rashes may be encountered during this stage. The clinical exam reveals enlargement of the liver and spleen, and edema of several causes (peripheral, pleural, ascites). Enlarged, rubbery, and painless lymph nodes occur in 75% of patients. In the Gambian form, the posterior cervical (Winterbottom's sign) (Fig. 4.5) and supraclavicular nodes are most commonly involved. Rhodesian infection usually does not show cervical adenopathy but often reveals axillary and epitrochlear node enlargement. During this secondary stage, edematous facies due to a painless swelling may possibly involve the hands and feet. As the disease progresses, there is increasing weight loss and debilitation. Petechiae are a rare complication that is sometimes accompanied by a generalized cutaneous flush seen more commonly in Rhodesian African trypanosomiasis. Mild presternal and intense generalized pruritus with excoriations, acroparesthesias, erythema nodosum, ichthyosis, icterus, and purpura have been reported in both forms of the disease. Signs of myocardial involvement may appear early in

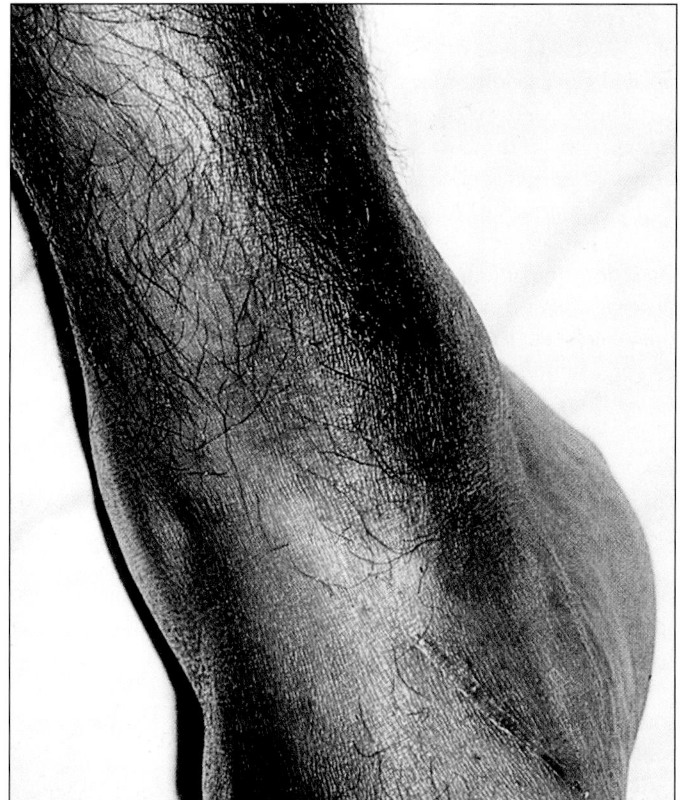

Figure 4.3 Trypanosomal chancre. (Reproduced from Peters W and Pasvol G (eds). Tropical Medicine and Parasitology, 5th edition, Mosby, London 2002, image 169.)

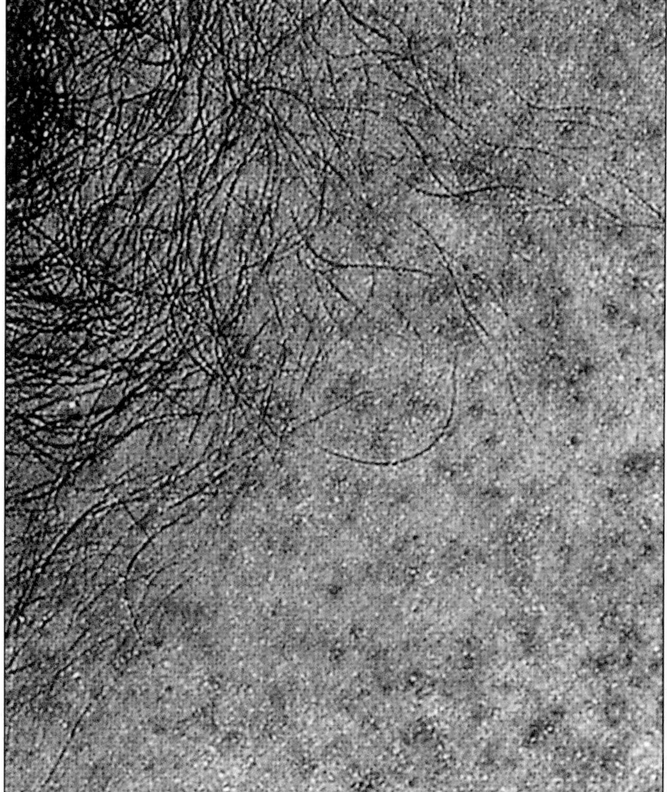

Figure 4.4 Trypanosomal rash due to *T. brucei rhodesiense*. (Reproduced from Peters W and Pasvol G (eds). Tropical Medicine and Parasitology, 5th edition, Mosby, London 2002, image 171.)

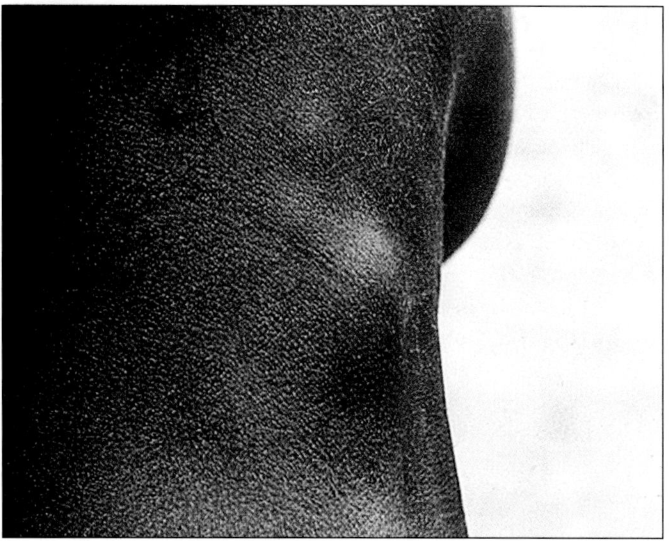

Figure 4.5 Winterbottom's sign: cervical lymphadenopathy due to infection with *T. brucei gambiense*. (Reproduced from Peters W and Pasvol G (eds). Tropical Medicine and Parasitology, 5th edition, Mosby, London 2002, image 172.)

Rhodesian infection and myocarditis may be the cause of death before evidence of CNS invasion appears.[1,8]

The meningoencephalitic stage appears within a few weeks or months of onset of Rhodesian infection, different from Gambian sleeping sickness, which may start 6 months to several years after that. Insomnia, anorexia, behavioral changes, alterations in sleep patterns, apathy, and headaches are among the early findings. A variety of motor or tonus disorders may follow, including tremors and disturbances of speech, gait, and reflexes. Focal lesions may cause paralysis, limited to a few muscular groups, that are transitory or permanent. Epileptic convulsions and hemiplegia are not common. Delayed, bilateral pain out of proportion to a sharp blow or squeeze applied to soft tissues occurs during CNS involvement: this is known as Kerandel's deep delayed hyperesthesia. Somnolence is the classic symptom of the disease. Insomnia precedes it in a transitional period during which patients are sleepy all day but have difficulty in sleeping at night. Deep somnolence appears late and is progressive. At this stage, pruritus andexcoriations from scratching are common. Soon the patient becomes severely emaciated and then comatose, not responding to external stimuli. Death commonly results from intercurrent infection due to immune suppression.[1,3,8]

Patient evaluation, diagnosis, and differential diagnosis

Recent travel to endemic areas of Africa should lead physicians to consider African trypanosomiasis in individuals presenting with acute febrile illnesses. The three most specific signs include the chancre (first stage), the targetoid macular trypanid (second stage), and Kerandel's deep delayed hyperesthesia (third stage).[8]

Definitive diagnosis requires identification of the parasite in the bite lesion (difficult), blood, lymph node, or CSF. Giemsa's or Wright's stain of the buffy coat of centrifuged heparinized blood makes identification easier, since the trypanosomes are often concentrated in the buffy coat. In patients with Gambian sleeping sickness, in which trypanosomes are found less frequently in the blood, concentration methods such as ion exchange chromatography, diethylaminoethyl (DEAE) filtration, culture, or animal inoculation should be used.[1,3,4]

All patients should have a lumbar puncture before and after treatment, to determine whether CNS involvement is present. The CSF shows increased number of lymphocytes and an elevation in protein concentration.[1,9]

Several immunodiagnostic tests have been developed for African trypanosomiasis, including an indirect hemagglutination test, indirect fluorescent antibody test, and an enzyme-linked immunosorbent assay (ELISA). Serologic tests become positive about 12 days after onset of infection. Titers of circulating antibody fluctuate and after high parasitemia, brief periods of excess antigen may depress antibody titers below detectable levels. Because parasites change their antigenic coats so frequently, no serologic test can be relied on for definitive diagnosis.[3,4]

Two new tests for stage determination in the CSF were evaluated on 73 patients diagnosed with hemagglutination tests in Côte d'Ivoire. The polymerase chain reaction (PCR) detecting trypanosome DNA (PCR/CSF) is an indirect test for trypanosome detection whereas the latex agglutination test detecting immunoglobulin M (Latex/IgM) is an indicator for neuroinflammation. Both tests were compared with classically used tests, double centrifugation, and white blood cell count of the CSF. PCR/CSF appeared to be the most sensitive test (96%), and may be of use to improve stage determination.[9]

Trypanosome-specific antibody detection in saliva is also possible. This could lead to the development of a simple, non-invasive, reliable saliva field test for diagnosis of sleeping sickness.[10]

Other laboratory findings include anemia, increased sedimentation rate, thrombocytopenia, reduced total serum protein, increased serum globulin and elevated IgM level which, in the CSF, is pathognomonic for the meningoencephalitic stage of trypanosomiasis.[1,3,11]

African trypanosomiasis should be differentiated from a variety of other diseases, including malaria, influenza, pneumonia, infectious mononucleosis, leukemia, lymphoma, the arbovirus encephalitides, cerebral tumors, and various psychoses. The chancre, exposure to tsetse flies, and the classic somnolence are the cardinal points for distinguishing those diseases from sleeping sickness.[1,3,4]

Pathology

After inoculation, trypanosomes produce a local chancre and then spread through the lymphatics, resulting in enlargement of lymph nodes secondary to reactive plasma cell and macrophage infiltration. The organisms eventually disseminate to the circulatory system, where the parasitemia usually remains low, and they multiply by binary fission.[1,3]

The early pathology is, thereafter, mainly in the lymph nodes, firstly those draining the sore and then generally, but with trypanosomes not easily seen histologically. Hematopoietic organs present hyperplastic reactions in acute cases, and degenerative reactions in chronic ones. The latter cases show infiltration of plasma cells, lymphocytes, histiocytes, and arteritis.[3,4,8]

Hematoxylin and eosin staining of biopsy specimens from trypanids demonstrates superficial perivascular lymphocytic infiltrate with mild lymphocytic spongiosis. Neutrophils and leukocytoclasia can also be found in those targetoid lesions. Degenerative lesions and cell infiltrates are also seen in organs such as the heart, liver, and kidneys, mainly in *T. rhodesiense* infections.[1,3]

CNS lesions are represented by perivascular infiltrations of histiocytes, plasma cells, and Mott cells (abnormal plasma cells). These lesions are most frequently found after 3–18 months from the onset of the infection and are more common in the *T. gambiense* disease. Nerve cells degenerate to complete atrophy with demyelinization, affecting the brain, cerebellum, brain stem, and meningeal membranes.[1,3,4]

Treatment

Suramin is the drug of choice for the early hemolymphatic stage of both *T. b. gambiense* and *T. b. rhodesiense* infections before CNS invasion occurs. The dose is 15–20 mg/kg of body weight per week, given intravenously, up to a maximum single dose of 1 g. Suramin, which is excreted by the kidneys, binds to plasma proteins and may persist in the circulation, at low concentrations, for as long as 3 months. A single course for an adult is usually 5 g, never exceeding 7 g. Its main side-effects are fever, cutaneous rash, conjunctivitis, renal insufficiency, abdominal pain, paresthesia, and muscle pain.[1,12]

Pentamidine is an alternative drug for the treatment of early hemolymphatic disease. The dose is 4 mg/kg given every other day by intramuscular injection for a total of 10 doses. Like suramin, pentamidine does not cross the blood–brain barrier. Its main side-effects are tachycardia, hypotension, and hypoglycemia. Other rare ones are diarrhea, vomiting, sweating, pruritic rash, and seizures.[12,13]

Melarsoprol, an arsenical, is the drug of choice for both Gambian and Rhodesian sleeping sickness once involvement of the CNS has occurred, since it penetrates the blood–brain barrier. The drug is administered in three courses of 3 days each, intravenously, with a recommended dosage of 3.6 mg/kg per day. If signs of arsenical toxicity occur (exfoliative dermatitis, optical nerve inflammation, and arsenical encephalopathy), the drug should be discontinued. The Jarisch–Herxheimer reaction, due to trypanosome lysis, causes a febrile reaction which usually appears early after the therapy is initiated. It has been suggested that corticoids protect patients from melarsoprol encephalopathy but this hypothesis still lacks proper evidence.[12–14]

Nitrofurazone should be used when melarsoprol fails. It is recommended in a dosage of 30 mg/kg, orally, 3–4 times a day, for 5–7 days. Its main secondary effects are joint pains and hemolytic or neurotoxic reactions.[3,4,12,13]

Difluoromethylornithine (eflornithine, DFMO), which is an irreversible inhibitor of polyamine biosynthesis, is also used in patients with CNS involvement. The recommended dosage is 400 mg/kg per day, intravenously, in four divided doses for 2 weeks, followed by 300 mg/kg per day, orally, in four doses for 30 days. The main side-effects are diarrhea and anemia.[12,13,15]

Antimicrobial peptides, which are components of the innate immune system of a variety of eukaryotic organisms, are also being tested, with good initial results, for the treatment of African trypanosomiasis.[16]

Most patients recover after treatment with eflornithine, suramin, or pentamidine for hemolymphatic disease. Lumbar punctures should be performed at 6-month intervals for 2 years. Melarsoprol should be initiated as soon as signs of CNS invasion are found. If therapy is started late or not started at all, irreversible brain damage or death will occur.[1,12,13]

Measures to prevent and control African trypanosomiasis include surveillance and treatment, chemoprophylaxis with pentamidine, and vector control with destruction of tsetse fly habitat, insecticides, repellents, and protective clothing.[1]

References

1. Rocha LAC, Ferreira FSC. Tripanossomíase humana africana. In: Veronesi R, Focaccia R, eds. Tratado de infectologia, vol. 2. São Paulo: Atheneu; 1996:1306–1315.
2. Goldsmith RS. Infectious diseases: Protozoal. In: Tierney LM Jr, Mcphee SJ, Papadakis MA, eds. Current medical diagnosis and treatment. Connecticut: Appleton & Lange; 2002:1463–1465.
3. Quinn TC. African trypanosomiasis. In: Cecil RL, Goldman L, Bennett JC, eds. Cecil textbook of medicine, vol. 2. Philadelphia: WB Saunders; 1996:1896–1899.
4. Bryceson AM, Hay RJ. Parasitic worms and protozoa. In: Champion RH, Burton JL, Ebling FJG, eds. Textbook of dermatology, vol. 2. Oxford: Blackwell Science; 1998: 1407–1408.
5. Stich A, Barrett MP, Krishna S. Waking up to sleeping sickness. Trends Parasitol 2003; 19:195–197.
6. Waiswa C, Olaho-Mukani W, Katunguka-Rwakishaya E. Domestic animals as reservoirs for sleeping sickness in three endemic foci in south-eastern Uganda. Ann Trop Med Parasitol 2003; 97:149–155.
7. Welburn SC, Odiit M. Recent developments in human African trypanosomiasis. Curr Opin Infect Dis 2002; 15:477–484.
8. McGovern TW, Williams W, Fitzpatrick JE et al. Cutaneous manifestations of African trypanosomiasis. Arch Dermatol 1995; 131:1178–1182.
9. Jamonneau V, Solano P, Garcia A et al. Stage determination and therapeutic decision in human African trypanosomiasis: value of polymerase chain reaction and immunoglobulin M quantification on the cerebrospinal fluid of sleeping sickness patients in Côte d'Ivoire. Trop Med Int Health 2003; 8:589–594.
10. Lejon V, Kwete J, Büscher P. Towards saliva-based screening for sleeping sickness? Trop Med Int Health 2003; 8:585–588.
11. Lejon V, Reiber H, Legros D et al. Intrathecal immune response pattern for improved diagnosis of central nervous system involvement in trypanosomiasis. J Infect Dis 2003; 187:1475–1483.

12. Bouteille B, Oukem O, Bisser S. Treatment perspectives for human African trypanosomiasis. Fundam Clin Pharmacol 2003; 17:171–181.
13. Docampo R, Moreno SN. Current chemotherapy of human African trypanosomiasis. Parasitol Res 2003; 90 (suppl. 1): S10–S13.
14. Nok AJ. Arsenicals (melarsoprol), pentamidine and suramin in the treatment of human African trypanosomiasis. Parasitol Res 2003; 90:71–79.
15. Burri C, Brun R. Eflornithine for the treatment of human African trypanosomiasis. Parasitol Res 2003; 90 (suppl. 1):S49–S52.
16. McGwire BS, Olson CL,Tack BF et al. Killing of African trypanosomes by antimicrobial peptides. J Infect Dis 2003; 188:146–152.

American trypanosomiasis

Synonyms: American trypanosomiasis, Chagas disease, South American trypanosomiasis, Cruz trypanosomiasis, Chagas–Mazza disease, schizotrypanosomiasis

Key features:

General features
- Chagas disease is caused by the protozoan parasite *Trypanosoma cruzi*, transmitted by many species of triatomine bugs

Acute stage
- Children with inflammatory lesions at the site of inoculation, fever, tachycardia, hepatosplenomegaly, lymphadenopathy, and signs of myocarditis
- Parasites in peripheral blood, positive serologic tests

Chronic stage
- Heart failure with cardiac arrhythmias; thromboembolism
- Dysphagia, constipation, megaesophagus, megacolon
- Positive xenodiagnosis or hemoculture; positive serologic tests; abnormal electrocardiogram

Introduction

Chagas disease is caused by the flagellate *Trypanosoma cruzi*, a protozoan parasite of humans, as well as wild and domestic animals. *T. cruzi* infection only occurs in rural areas of tropical zones of the Americas and is transmitted by many species of triatomine bugs that become infected by ingesting blood from infected animals or humans. In many countries of Latin America, especially South America, Chagas disease is the most important etiology of heart disease.

Dermatologists should be aware of the earliest signs of the disease, which are the lesions that can be found at the site of inoculation, and therefore initiate proper treatment as soon as possible, in order to avoid serious cardiac and bowel disease.

History

In 1909, Carlos Chagas, a Brazilian physician, described the parasite, *T. cruzi*, in the hindgut of triatomine bugs. After observing trypanosomes in the blood of monkeys that had been bitten by those bugs, he found the same *T. cruzi* in the peripheral blood of a child who was feverish, and who had anemia, lymphadenopathy, and hepatosplenomegaly. In 1909, Chagas published his first notes about this new infection in humans: it was then an endemic illness in the central region of Brazil. It is considered the first and only time in the history of medicine when the agent, the vectors, and the clinical presentation of a new disease were all described by the same investigator.[1,2]

Epidemiology

Chagas disease infects approximately 12 million people and kills about 60 000 each year, mostly in rural areas. *T. cruzi* and its arthropod vectors are widely distributed from the south of the USA to Patagonia, in the south of South America (Fig. 4.6). Human trypanosomiasis in Latin America is primarily an infection of poor people living in mud huts or shacks with crude wooden walls and palm leaf roofs, that provide ideal hiding and breeding places for the bugs (Fig. 4.7). Age, sex, and race do not influence the incidence of the disease, although the acute forms are more frequently observed in children.[3–5]

There are basically two forms in which *T. cruzi* can circulate in nature, known as the sylvatic and the domestic cycles. The sylvatic cycle results from interaction between wild animals and the vector triatomine bugs that associate with them. The main sylvatic reservoirs are marsupials, rodents, small carnivores, armadillos, rabbits, monkeys, and bats. These animals are used to living in the same areas where the sylvatic triatomines are found. Congenital transmission of the parasite is rare in this cycle.[1,4,6]

The domestic cycle is the result of human invasion in wild areas. It occurs under conditions in which infected animals, such as rats and armadillos, living close to human habitations, are bitten by vector bugs that invade houses to search for a blood meal. This situation enables *T. cruzi* to be transmitted from person to person – a domiciliary cycle – turning Chagas disease into a public health problem. Besides humans, small mammals (cats and dogs) and domestic rodents may become infected and thus important reservoirs.[3,4]

American trypanosomiasis vectors are arthropods of the family Reduviidae and subfamily Triatominae. They only feed on blood but sometimes engage in cannibalism or coprophagia, resulting in a possible vector-to-vector transmission of *T. cruzi*. They are known as kissing bugs because of their habit of biting human faces (Figs 4.8 and 4.9). The main species are *Triatoma infestans* (Argentina, Bolivia, Brazil, Chile, Paraguay, Peru, and Uruguay) *Rhodnius prolixus* (Colombia, Guianas, Venezuela, and Central America) and *Panstrongylus megistus* (Brazil).[4,7–9]

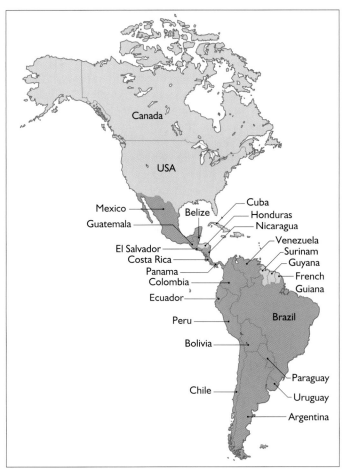

Figure 4.6 Worldwide distribution of Chagas disease.

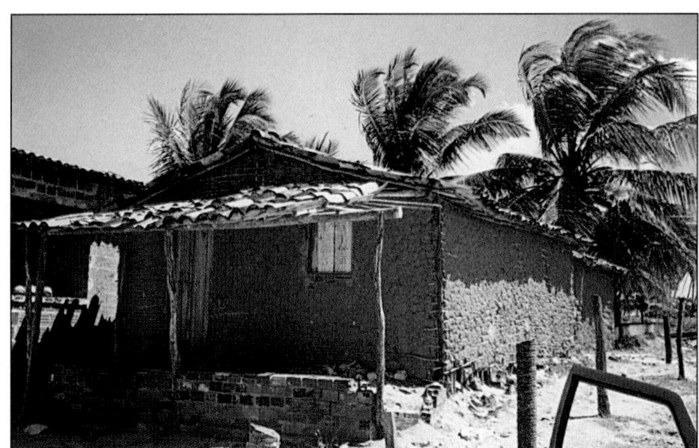

Figure 4.7 Mud hut with crude wooden walls and palm leaf roofs in the Northeast province of Brazil.

Countries with the highest incidence of infection due to *T. cruzi* include Argentina, Brazil, Bolivia, Chile, and Venezuela (Fig. 4.6). In some Latin American countries, positive serologic findings for *T. cruzi* constitute a social stigma; employers may be reluctant to hire someone who may later develop chronic Chagas disease.[8,10,11]

Pathogenesis and etiology

T. cruzi is a flagellate protozoan that belongs to the Mastigophora class, Kinetoplatida order, and Trypanosomatidae family. The parasite is 15–20 μm in length and has a typical undulant membrane and flagellum in an anterior position (Fig. 4.10). It bears some resemblance to the trypanosomes that cause sleeping sickness in Africa. Trypomastigotes in the peripheral blood of vertebrate hosts are ingested after a blood meal by blood-sucking reduviids. Once the insect has been infected, it remains infected for the rest of its life. The parasites transform into epimastigotes and multiply in the midgut of the insect vector, later becoming metacyclic trypomastigotes in the hindgut of the bug. When the infected bug takes a subsequent blood meal, it usually defecates during or after feeding, so that the infective metacyclic forms are deposited on the

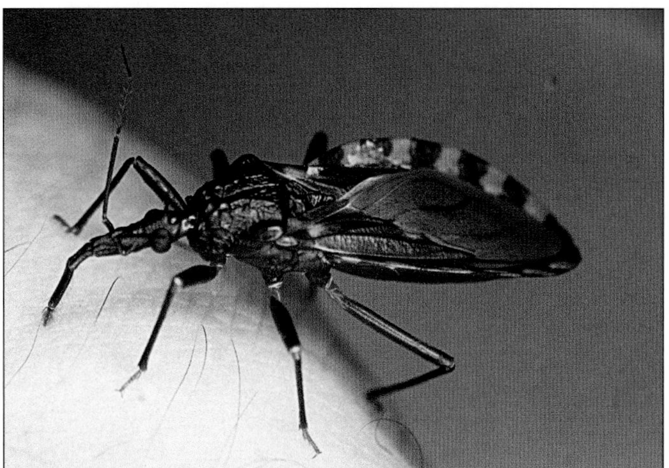

Figure 4.8 *Triatoma infestans*. (Courtesy of G. Vieira/Fiocruz.)

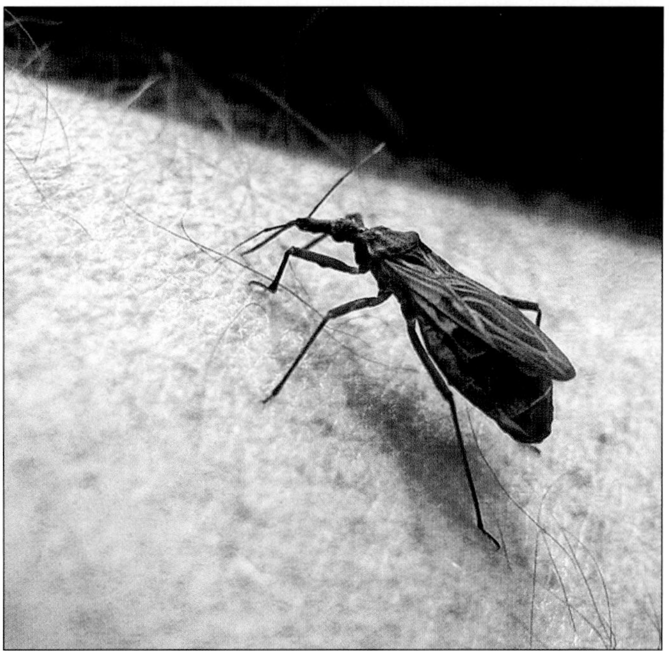

Figure 4.9 *Rhodnius prolixus*. (Courtesy of Centers for Disease Control and Prevention.)

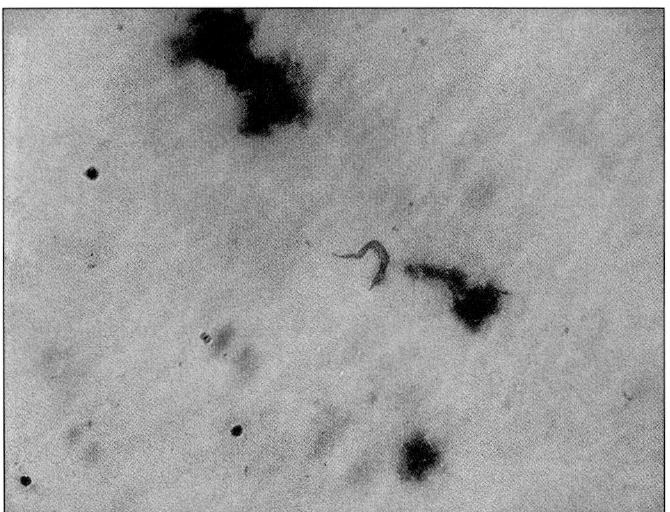

Figure 4.10 *Trypanosoma cruzi* collected from the urine of a *Triatoma infestans*. (Courtesy of MMO Cabral, IOC/FIOCRUZ, Rio de Janeiro, Brazil.)

skin. The parasite penetrates the skin (generally through the bite wound) or the conjunctiva, leaving a local inflammatory lesion. These protozoans can penetrate a large amount of host cell types, where they become intracellular amastigotes. These amastigotes multiply in the cytoplasm and become once again trypomastigotes. Then they rupture out of the cells, infecting new ones, or simply enter the blood stream to initiate new cycles of multiplication or be ingested by new vectors. Transmission can also occur by blood transfusion or congenital infection.[1,4,12]

In the acute phase of Chagas disease, the high level of parasitemia seems to have an important role in the pathogenesis of the inflammatory response. A local inflammatory lesion develops at the site of entry and this is called a chagoma. Enlarged lymph nodes show hyperplasia and amastigotes may be found in reticular cells. Skeletal muscle tissue shows parasites and focal inflammation. In severe cases, myocarditis with enlargement of the heart develops. The CNS can also be invaded by *T. cruzi*.[4,5]

The main affected organs in chronic Chagas disease are the heart, the esophagus, and the intestine. Surprisingly, the parasites might be difficult to find in these affected organs at this stage. The hearts of these patients may even be normal in size but they are usually hypertrophied and dilated. The microscopic findings in the heart are not specific and consist of mononuclear cell infiltrates, hypertrophy of fibers, areas of necrosis, fibrosis, and edema. Fibrosis is considered most responsible for the loss of the contractile activity of the myocardium in chronic patients. The conduction system of the heart usually shows signs of inflammation that correlate well with electrocardiographic changes observed.[3,4,9]

Recently, cell-mediated cytotoxicity has been related to the pathogenesis of inflammation and cell alterations in the chronic phase of the infection. The presence of granulomas, sometimes still in the acute phase, provides evidence to corroborate that hypothesis, which still lacks confirmation.[1,5]

In the chronic phase, the esophagus and the colon show dilatation and hypertrophy that are microscopically similar to the alterations observed in the heart. There is also marked parasympathetic denervation in these and other hollow viscera.

Placental inflammatory lesions and focal necrosis in the chorionic villi, with the presence of amastigotes, are found in congenital *T. cruzi* infection. These findings may result in abortion, stillbirth, acute disease in the fetus, or even no infection at all.

The indeterminate form is represented by patients with antibodies to *T. cruzi* but with no signs or symptoms of infection. These individuals will probably develop the disease later in life, since endocardial biopsies from these cases have recognizable pathologic changes. However, up to half of these patients will die of causes other than Chagas disease according to research done in areas where chronic infection is common.[1,8,9]

Some answers are still needed in order to clarify fully the pathogenesis of Chagas disease. Researchers are not yet able to explain the latency period of up to 30 years before heart or bowel disease initiates or the fact that few intracellular parasites are found in the affected organs in chronic disease. Finally, few reports relate HIV infection to Chagas disease, but some authors believe that some protozoans may persist and reactivate in humans even years after proper treatment and that HIV could be responsible for this reactivation of a dormant *T. cruzi* infection.[13]

Clinical features

The majority of the infected individuals remain asymptomatic. When these patients develop signs of the disease it usually happens after an incubation period of approximately 1 week. Acute Chagas disease is most commonly seen in children and starts with a local inflammatory lesion at the site of inoculation. When *T. cruzi* penetrates through the conjunctiva, the local periorbital swelling is referred to as Romaña's sign (Fig. 4.11). When entry occurs through skin, the local area of erythema and induration is called chagoma.

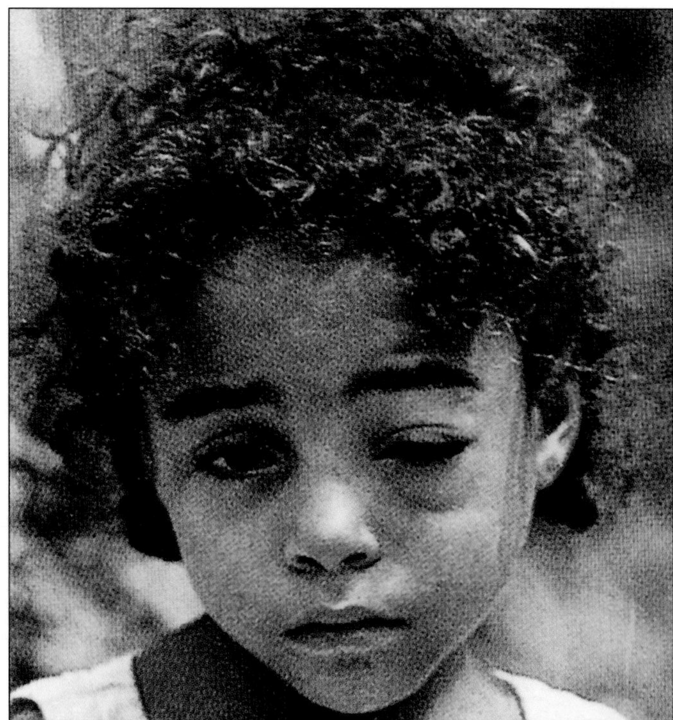

Figure 4.11 Romaña's sign. (Reproduced from Peters W and Pasvol G (eds). Tropical Medicine and Parasitology, 5th edition, Mosby, London 2002, image 195.)

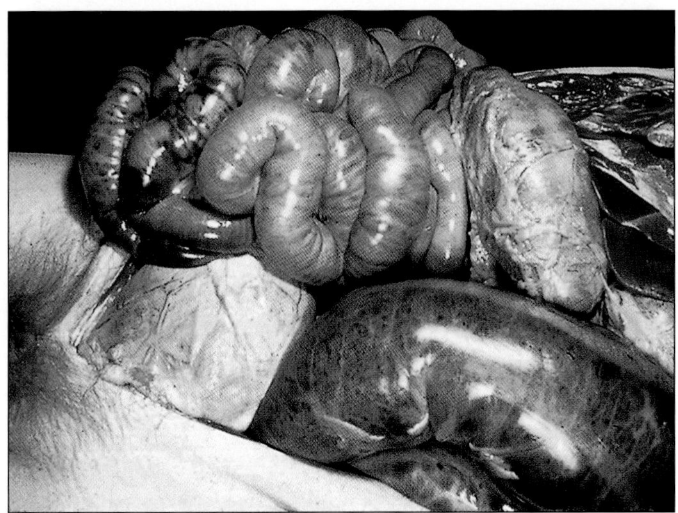

Figure 4.12 Megacolon in a woman who died of chronic Chagas's disease. (Reproduced from Peters W and Pasvol G (eds). Tropical Medicine and Parasitology, 5th edition, Mosby, London 2002, image 203.)

Romaña's sign, also called ophthalmoganglionar complex, develops rapidly and is characterized by unilateral painless bipalpebral edema, conjunctivitis, inflammation of the lacrimal gland, and local lymphadenopathy. Periorbital cellulitis and metastatic chagomas, sometimes with the presence of fatty tissue necrosis, can also be seen.[1,5]

Chagomas (cutaneous adenopathy complex) are furuncle-like violaceous lesions that are accompanied by regional adenopathy, induration, and discrete central edema. These lesions correspond to the site of parasite entry and may last for several weeks. Other signs of acute Chagas disease include fever, malaise, headache, myalgia, hepatosplenomegaly, and transient skin rashes (schizotripanides).[1,5,9]

Acute myocarditis may lead to cardiac insufficiency, but arrhythmias are rare. Meningoencephalitis is a severe complication, usually limited to children with a poor prognosis. Acute pancreatitis due to elevated parasitism has been observed. Death in the acute phase is not a common event.[14]

Within a few weeks or months, signs and symptoms gradually disappear and the patient enters the indeterminate phase. This phase is characterized by apparent recovery with presence of antibodies to *T. cruzi* and low levels of parasitemia in the blood. Years or decades later, a variable amount of these cases develop signs and symptoms of chronic Chagas disease. These patients should never donate blood because their parasitemia is similar to a chronic patient and there is an elevated risk of transfusional transmission.[9,13,14]

The chronic stage is characterized by manifestations of cardiac and esophageal or colon disease. Palpitations, precordial discomfort, arrhythmias, and tachycardia may reflect some degree of heart block and may lead to sudden death. Cardiomegaly and severe cardiac failure sometimes become evident only years after the first episodes of tachycardia. Other signs and symptoms include hepatomegaly, peripheral edema, and systemic or pulmonary embolization originating from mural thrombi. Sudden death due to thromboembolic accidents, blockage of the conduction system of the heart, or chronic heart failure may occur.[1,9,14]

Megacolon (Fig. 4.12) and megaesophagus, caused by damage to nerve plexuses in the bowel or esophageal wall, show dysphagia, a feeling of fullness after eating small amounts, chest pain, and regurgitation. Salivary gland hypertrophy and esophageal cancer are sometimes reported in patients with chagasic megaesophagus. Chagasic megacolon causes chronic constipation and abdominal pain and may be complicated by volvulus, obstruction, and perforation of the intestine. There are few descriptions of an association between chagasic megacolon and colon cancer. Sometimes the chagasic patient stays for 2–3 weeks without bowel movements due to severe megacolon. Megasyndromes are common in Brazil but rare in Venezuela.[5,15]

Patient evaluation, diagnosis, and differential diagnosis

For proper diagnosis, a history of exposure to *T. cruzi,* due to travel to an endemic area or blood transfusion, should be sought. Appropriate selection of tests permits a definitive parasitologic diagnosis in most cases.

In the acute stage, direct microscopic examination of anticoagulated fresh blood or a buffy coat preparation for motile trypanosomes is the main procedure. Parasites should be confirmed in a stained preparation such as thick blood films, buffy coat, and the sediment after centrifuging the supernatant of clotted blood. Blood can also be cultured on Nicolle–Novy–McNeal (NNM) medium and inoculated into laboratory mice or rats. Biopsies of lymph nodes or skeletal muscle are also considered for culture or histologic examination. In the chronic stage the parasite can only be detected by culture or xenodiagnosis.[1,4]

Xenodiagnosis is a procedure that uses the vector, acting as a biological culture medium, for the detection of *T. cruzi* infection in humans. Non-infected laboratory-reared nymphs of triatomines are placed in a cylindric pot, covered with a piece of gauze, and applied to the skin surface (upper limb), supported by a bracelet. These triatomines, which were unfed for the previous 3–4 weeks, stay on the skin surface for about 30 min, become engorged and then are kept in entomological laboratory conditions. After about 30 days, excreta of the insects are microscopically examined for moving *T. cruzi* trypomastigotes. Xenodiagnosis has been shown useful for evaluation of parasitemia and its relationship with clinical conditions of Chagas disease. It is also considered an efficient diagnostic method for *T. cruzi* in the blood stream, and is particularly useful in chronic chagasic infection.[16]

Serologic testing is generally not needed for the diagnosis of acute disease. Antibodies of the IgM class are usually elevated early in the acute stage but are replaced by IgG antibodies as the disease progresses. False-positive reactions can occur in the presence of leishmaniasis or *T. rangeli* (a non-pathogenic parasite found in humans in Central America). Other laboratory tests may show lymphocytic leukocytosis, elevated sedimentation rate, or transient electrocardiographic abnormalities. In certain regions of South America, radiologic examination may show cardiac enlargement with characteristic apical aneurysms, megaesophagus, or megacolon.

The diagnosis of chronic Chagas disease is difficult as it relies upon clinical judgment in excluding other causes of heart or gastrointestinal disease, as well as demonstrating antibodies to *T. cruzi.* Xenodiagnosis is very helpful but comparison between different serologic tests is needed to confirm the infection, as the parasitemia in this stage is characteristically low. The main serologic tests for *T. cruzi* infection are indirect hemagglutination, indirect immunofluorescence, immunoenzymatic (ELISA), direct agglutination with 2-mercaptoethanol (DA-2ME), and complement fixation (Guerreiro–Machado reaction). A positive reaction in at least two of the mentioned tests allows the physician to confirm the chagasic etiology.[17]

Recently, in the chronic stage, PCR has been used to detect the parasite in blood samples. Western blot is another promising technique for future diagnosis of Chagas disease.[4,17]

Acute Chagas disease should be differentiated from other systemic infections such as typhoid fever, visceral leishmaniasis, schistosomiasis, mononucleosis, toxoplasmosis, and dengue fever. Romaña's sign must be distinguished from other causes of unilateral orbital edema such as the reaction to an insect bite, trauma, or orbital cellulitis. Congenital *T. cruzi* infections are very similar to congenital toxoplasmosis, cytomegalic inclusion disease, and syphilis. Chagasic myocardiopathy resembles postpartum, alcoholic, and fibrotic myocardiopathy. Chagasic meningoencephalitis can be differentiated from toxoplasmosis due to the great amount of parasites in the CSF. The value of positive serologic findings for *T. cruzi* in the differential diagnosis of both heart and megadisease will depend upon the prevalence of antibodies in the general population.

Pathology

Histologically, the site of parasite entry (chagoma) shows mononuclear cell infiltration, interstitial edema, and intracellular aggregates of amastigotes in cells of the subcutaneous tissue and muscle. Enlarged lymph nodes show hyperplasia and amastigotes in reticular cells.

Regarding other tissues, invasion by *T. cruzi* is rife. Skeletal and cardiac muscle show organisms and focal inflammation. The CNS may also be parasitized in acute American trypanosomiasis.

In the chronic stage, trypanosomes are hard to find in the affected organs. Microscopic findings in the heart consist of focal mononuclear cell infiltrates, hypertrophy of cardiac fibers with areas of necrosis, fibrosis, and edema. The microscopic changes in the esophagus or colon are very similar to those observed in the heart, with the addition of a great reduction in the number of myenteric ganglion cells, reflecting the characteristic parasympathetic denervation.[1,4,5]

Treatment

Therapy is unsatisfactory. Even proper treatment, in the chronic phase, does not alter the serologic reaction or the cardiac function, although it usually cures the patient in the acute stage.

Currently two drugs are being used for Chagas disease: nifurtimox and benznidazole. Both are active against blood and tissue trypanosomes, and should be administered for a period of at least 30 and up to 90 days of treatment. This long period is necessary due to the difficult task of attempting to eradicate all parasitism from the blood. These drugs are given orally, metabolized in the liver, and excreted through the kidneys. The exact mechanism of action for both of these drugs is unknown.[4,18]

Nifurtimox is available in 120-mg tablets and should be used in a dose of 8–12 mg/kg per day (divided in two doses). Dosage for children is slightly higher and up to 15 mg/kg per day. The main side-effects are anorexia, weight loss, nausea, vomiting, abdominal pain, insomnia, and behavioral changes. With the ingestion of alcohol there is marked antabuse effect.[1,4]

Benznidazole is the alternative drug of choice at a dosage of 5–10 mg/kg per day, in two daily doses. Between 1991 and 1995, in Brazil, a trial showed that a 60-day course of benznidazole treatment of early chronic *T. cruzi* infection in 130 patients was safe and 55.8% effective in producing negative seroconversion of specific antibodies. Its main side-effects are skin urticariform rashes, bone marrow suppression, and peripheral polyneuropathy.[4,18]

The side-effects for both drugs subside when the dosage is reduced or treatment is stopped. Nifurtimox appears to be less effective in parasite strains from certain geographic areas of Brazil than other strains from Argentina or Chile.

Allopurinol is continuously being evaluated at a dosage of 600 mg/day for the treatment of chronic infection. Itraconazole appeared better than allopurinol at preventing the development of cardiopathy in cases that were electrocardiographically normal at baseline, in a recent study done in Chile. However, there is no evidence that the established pathologic changes of chronic Chagas disease can be reversed by any therapy. Whether or not proper treatment would prevent the development of later chronic disease in indeterminate-stage patients is still controversial.[18,19]

The treatment of patients with established chronic heart disease is supportive. Antiarrhythmic drugs, such as amiodarone, or pacemakers may prolong the survival of these patients. Management of megadisease includes special diets, use of laxatives, and surgical procedures.

Prevention of the infection involves sanitary education of the population and the use of residual insecticides directed at domiciliary vectors. Interrupting the transmission of Chagas disease using insecticide-treated materials could be a cost-effective option, particularly for sylvatic vectors, which enter houses at night. Vaccines are still being researched and are not yet available.[20]

References

1. Ferreira MS, Lopes RF, Chapadeiro E et al. Doença de Chagas. In: Veronesi R, ed. Focaccia – Tratado de infectologia, vol. 2. São Paulo: Atheneu; 1996:1175–1213.
2. Morel CM. Chagas disease, from discovery to control – and beyond: history, myths and lessons to take home. Mem Inst Oswaldo Cruz 1999; 94 (suppl. 1):3–16.
3. Goldsmith RS. Infectious diseases: protozoal. In: Tierney LM Jr, Mcphee SJ, Papadakis MA, eds. Current medical diagnosis and treatment. Connecticut: Appleton & Lange; 2003: 1413–1415.
4. Neva FA. American trypanosomiasis (Chagas' disease). In: Cecil RL, Goldman L, Bennett JC, eds. Cecil textbook of medicine, vol. 2. Philadelphia, PA: WB Saunders; 1996: 1899–1903.
5. Bryceson AM, Hay RJ. Parasitic worms and protozoa. In: Champion RH, Burton JL, Ebling FJG, eds. Textbook of dermatology, vol. 2. Oxford: Blackwell Science; 1998: 1408–1410.

6. Gürtler RE, Segura EL, Cohen JE. Congenital transmission of *Trypanosoma cruzi* infection in Argentina. Emerg Infect Dis 2003; 9:29–32.
7. Carvalho ME, Silva RA, Barata JMS et al. Soroepidemiologia da tripanosomíase americana na região do litoral sul, São Paulo/ Chagas' disease in the southern coastal region of Brazil. Rev Saúde Pública 2003; 37:49–58.
8. Dias JCP, Silveira AC, Schofield CJ. The impact of Chagas disease control in Latin America: a review. Mem Inst Oswaldo Cruz 2002; 97:603–612.
9. Siqueira-Batista R, Gomes AP. Infecção por *Trypanosoma cruzi*: revisitando o mal de Chagas/infections by *Trypanosoma cruzi*: revisiting Chagas disease. J Bras Med 2002; 82:28–41.
10. Bar ME, Damborsky MP, Oscherov EB et al. Triatomines involved in domestic and wild *Trypanosoma cruzi* transmission in Concepción, Corrientes, Argentina. Mem Inst Oswaldo Cruz 2002; 97:43–46.
11. Espinoza-Gómez F, Maldonado-Rodríguez A, Coll-Cárdenas R et al. Presence of Triatominae (Hemiptera, Reduviidae) and risk of transmission of Chagas disease in Colima, México. Mem Inst Oswaldo Cruz 2002; 97:25–30.
12. Souza W. A short review on the morphology of *Trypanosoma cruzi*: from 1909 to 1999. Mem Inst Oswaldo Cruz 1999; 94:17–36.
13. Pacheco RS, Ferreira MS, Machado MI et al. Chagas' disease and HIV co-infection: genotypic characterization of the *Trypanosoma cruzi* strain. Mem Inst Oswaldo Cruz 1998; 93: 165–169.
14. Corbett CEP, Scremin LHG, Lombardi RA et al. Pancreatic lesions in acute experimental Chagas' disease. Rev Hosp Clin Fac Med Univ São Paulo 2002; 57:63–66.
15. Adad SJ, Etchebehere RM, Araujo JR et al. Association of chagasic megacolon and cancer of the colon: case report and review of the literature. Rev Soc Bras Med Trop 2002; 35:63–68.
16. Schenone H. Xenodiagnosis. Mem Inst Oswaldo Cruz 1999; 94:289–294.
17. Langhi Júnior DM, Bordin JO, Castelo A et al. The application of latent class analysis for diagnostic test validation of chronic *Trypanosoma cruzi* infection in blood donors. Braz J Infect Dis 2002; 6:181–187.
18. de Andrade AL, Zicker F, de Oliveira RM et al. Randomised trial of efficacy of benznidazole in treatment of early *Trypanosoma cruzi* infection. Lancet 1996; 348:1407–1413.
19. Apt W, Arribada A, Zulantay I et al. Itraconazole or allopurinol in the treatment of chronic American trypanosomiasis: the regression and prevention of electrocardiographic abnormalities during 9 years of follow-up. Ann Trop Med Parasitol 2003; 97:23–29.
20. Kroeger A, Villegas E, Ordoñez-González J et al. Prevention of the transmission of Chagas' disease with pyrethroid impregnated materials. Am J Trop Med Hyg 2003; 68:307–311.

Chapter 5

Leishmaniasis

Jackson Machado-Pinto and Rubem David Azulay

- Introduction
- Etiology
- Epidemiology
- Immunology
- Clinical picture
- Laboratory diagnosis
- Treatment
- Prophylaxis

Synonyms: Leishmaniasis: ulcera de Bauru and botão da Bahia (Brazil), uta (Peru), ulcera de los chicleros (Mexico), pian-bois (French Guyana), bush yaws (Surinam), and forest yaws (Guyana), oriental sore, and bouton d'Orient
Visceral leishmaniasis: kala-azar, dum-dum fever

Introduction

The word "leishmaniasis" refers to a wide variety of pathological manifestations that impact differently on health and that differ in their severity. They are a group of zoonotic infections of men and certain animals caused by several species of a flagellated parasite belonging to the order Kinetoplastidae, genus *Leishmania*, and transmitted by the bite of a fly of the genera *Phlebotomus* and *Lutzomyia*.[1] Once inoculation into the skin takes place, the parasites rapidly locate to the phagolysosomes of the mononuclear phagocyte system.

Etiology

Human infection can be caused by several species of *Leishmania* which are included in four complexes: (1) *tropica* (*L. tropica*, *L. major*, *L. minor*, and *L. aethiopica*); (2) *mexicana* (*L. mexicana*, *L. amazonensis*, *L. pifanoi*, and *L. venezuelensis*); (3) *braziliensis* or *viannia* (*L. brasiliensis*, *L. guyanensis*, *L. panamensis*, and *L. peruviana*); and (4) *donovani* (*L. donovani*, *L. infantum*, *L. chagasi*, *L. sinesis*, and *L. nilotica*).[2] The first three complexes include the species responsible for cutaneous and mucocutaneous lesions while the *donovani* complex includes the species responsible for visceral involvement. Each species shows a marked tendency to occupy a particular zoogeographical zone. There are no morphological differences between any two species: they can only be distinguished through the use of electron microscopy, biochemical analysis, and molecular biology methods.[3,4] All the infecting species live alternately in the blood or other tissues of the vertebrate and the intestine of the insect. In the amastigote stage of its life cycle, which occurs only intracellularly in mammals, the parasite is a non-flagellated round or ovoid organism containing a spherical vesicular nucleus and a smaller kinetoplast complex. The organism in its promastigote stage, seen in insect hosts and cultures but never in humans, is slender and elongated, and has a centrally placed vesicular nucleus and a single anterior flagellum arising from a well-developed kinetoplast.

The biting flies of the genera *Phlebotomus* and *Lutzomyia* are responsible for the transmission of the parasites. They are small and hairy and remain near the breeding areas because their ability to fly is limited.

The fly acquires the parasites by ingesting the infected blood from a reservoir host. In the insect's intestine the microorganisms of *Leishmania* become promastigotes, and when the insect feeds on humans, the promastigotes gain access to tissues of the human body, where they change to amastigotes.[5]

Epidemiology

Leishmaniasis is endemic in 88 countries, 67 in the Old World and 21 in the New World. The worldwide annual incidence is 400 000 cases and the prevalence is 12 million cases. It is estimated that 350 million people all over the world are at risk of acquiring the disease each year. Over 90% of the cases of cutaneous leishmaniasis happen in Afghanistan, Iran, Saudi Arabia, Syria, Brazil, and Peru.[6]

Old-World-type leishmaniasis is endemic in countries bordering the Mediterranean and in Asia Minor.

Visceral leishmaniasis is widely distributed in Asia, along the Mediterranean coast, and in Africa and South America.

Humans, dogs, and rodents are the main reservoirs for the *Leishmania* microorganisms, but natural infection has been observed in cats, dogs, and horses in both Brazil and Argentina.[7]

There is no predilection for race, nationality, sex, or age. However, the great majority of cases are seen in adult males between 20 and 40 years of age. Visceral leishmaniasis, however, is seen most commonly in children in China and in the Mediterranean area while mostly young adults are affected in India. Old-World cutaneous leishmaniasis is seen more often in children.

Immunology

There is considerable evidence that a T-cell-mediated immune response plays a very important role in the cure of leishmaniasis.[8,9] Cure would be related to a Th1 profile with the production of interleukin-2 (IL-2) and gamma-interferon (IFN-γ). Susceptibility to or worsening of the disease would be associated with the lack of such a response, or to the development of a Th2-type response, with the production of IL-4 and IL-10.[10–13]

IFN-γ is the most potent cytokine in the induction of leishmanicide activity of macrophages, increasing the production of oxygen and nitrogen metabolites, activating natural killer (NK) cells and allowing the expression of major histocompatibility complex (MHC) of both classes. CD4+ and NK cells are stimulated by IL-12 to produce IFN-γ, whose presence, together with IL-12, is important for the differentiation of Th1 cells.[14]

Tumor necrosis factor-α (TNF-α) is also important in the control of *Leishmania* infections. It is involved in the resistance to several pathogens. It is produced by activated macrophages and NK cells and amplifies the macrophagic activation triggered by IFN-γ. On the other hand, excessive TNF-α production is associated with worse prognosis in several infectious processes, since it also provokes greater activation and production of nitric oxide that are hazardous to the patient.[15]

IL-12 is a cytokine produced by antigen-presenting cells (monocytes, macrophages, dentritic cells, and B cells). Its main biological activity is on T and NK cells, which are stimulated to produce IFN-γ. It is also involved in the induction of cell proliferation and cytotoxicity, playing a very important role in the differentiation and expansion of CD4+ cells of the Th1 type.[16]

IL-10 is related to the inhibition of Th1 response, thus leading to increased survival of the *Leishmania* inside the macrophages.[17]

Susceptibility to infection has been related to inadequate Th1 response: patients with mucosal lesions have been shown to have increased production of IFN-γ and TNF-α and decreased production of IL-10. They have also been shown to have IL-10 and TNF-β which are unable to downregulate these immune responses efficiently, thus leading to increased tissue damage.[18]

Peripheral blood mononuclear cells of patients with diffuse or anergic leishmaniasis display increased expression of mRNA for IL-2, IL-4, and IL-10 and decreased expression of IFN-γ in the active phase of the disease. After treatment, there is a shift towards Th1, with an increase in IFN-γ and a decrease in IL-10 production. This change is not associated with long-term protection, which suggests that, similarly to what happens in visceral leishmaniasis, in diffuse or anergic leishmaniasis a Th1 response is also protective.[19] Patients who heal spontaneously show a very strong T response and increased production of IFN-γ. Individuals with asymptomatic visceral leishmaniasis show increased production of IFN-γ and decreased production of IL-10.[20]

Although CD4 cells are known to have the importance discussed above, the role of CD8 cells remains controversial.

The delayed skin reaction test (Montenegro or Leishman reaction) is positive in the majority of cases of cutaneous leishmaniasis. Positivity appears while the skin eruption is still active and remains positive long after spontaneous cure. It is usually negative during the febrile phase of visceral leishmaniasis and often becomes positive after cure. In American leishmaniasis, the skin test is an important tool for diagnosis, since the scarcity of parasites in longer-standing lesions is the rule. It is positive in over 90% of cases and invariably negative in patients with diffuse leishmaniasis.[21] The skin test is also important in the recruitment of non-sensitized individuals for tests of vaccines against leishmaniasis.[22] The skin test has been used to predict relapse in American leishmaniasis. It has been observed that patients with a negative skin test and diagnosed and treated for American leishmaniasis have a 3.4 times higher risk of relapse as compared to patients with a positive test before treatment.[23] It seems that a negative skin test is related to perhaps specific immunological deficiencies of the host that impair the mechanisms involved in the cure process of the disease. The skin test consists of the intradermal injection of a phenolated suspension of promastigotes, usually on the volar aspect of the forearm. After 48–72 h, it is considered positive if a papule over 5 mm in diameter is formed at the site of inoculation.

As far as antibodies are concerned, different clinical forms of leishmaniasis will show important peculiarities in the levels of immunoglobulin G (IgG) isotypes. In mucocutaneous, localized cutaneous and visceral leishmaniasis there is a predominance of IgG1 and, less importantly, of IgG2 and IgG3. Patients with diffuse leishmaniasis invariably show high levels of IgG4.[24]

Animals which have recovered from *L. tropica* infection acquire immunity against reinfection, but not against *L. donovani*; however, *L. donovani* infections give an animal immunity against *L. donovani*, but not against *L. tropica*. It has been reported that surviving visceral leishmaniasis confers lifelong immunity against all types of leishmaniasis and patients with the American form of cutaneous leishmaniasis have succesfully been inoculated with *L. tropica* and vice versa. For ethical and practical reasons, no one has challenged patients with *L. donovani*, since its course is so variable and treatment is often ineffective.

Clinical picture

Even though certain disease characteristics may be commonly associated with a particular species, one should not rely on clinical patterns to indicate which species is involved in any one single case. The leishmaniases consist of cutaneous, mucosal, and visceral syndromes.

Old-World leishmaniasis

Cutaneous leishmaniasis of the Old World is caused by *L. major*, *L. tropica*, *L. aethiopica*, and *L. infantum*. Contact infection is reported; the infection is inoculable and autoinoculable. All previously uninfected individuals are susceptible. The lesions are usually found on unclothed regions of the body and the face, neck, and arms are the favored sites of involvement. Six clinical patterns have been recognized thus far: (1) wet (rural, major, zoonotic) type; (2) dry (urban, minor, tropical, anthroponotic) type; (3) cutaneous leishmaniasis due to *L. aethiopica*; (4) cutaneous leishmaniasis due to *L. infantum*; (5) *Leishmaniasis recidivans* (chronic lupoid leishmaniasis); and (6) diffuse cutaneous leishmaniasis (lepromatoid or pseudolepromatous leishmaniasis). The first four tend to evolve with self-healing whereas the last two tend to chronicity and may not heal spontaneously.

Cutaneous leishmaniasis due to *L. major* (wet, rural, or zoonotic type)

After a short incubation period of 1–4 weeks, rarely longer than 2 months, a red furunculoid nodule appears at the site of inoculation. More than 30 lesions may be present. The lesions evolve with ulceration covered by a crust. There may be satellite lymphatic nodules and lymphangitis. Healing takes place in 2–6 months and leaves a scar. Rodents are the usual reservoir of the infection.

Cutaneous leishmaniasis due to *L. tropica* (dry, urban, tropical as above or anthroponotic type)

The incubation period is greater than 2 months and usually over 1 year. A few nodules appear, usually on the face and slowly become plaques and ulcerate. Secondary satellite nodules occur only rarely and healing takes place very slowly, over a period of 8–12 months. Humans and dogs are the most important reservoirs. Infection protects against reinfection.

Cutaneous leishmaniasis due to *L. aethiopica*

A (usually single) lesion on the central face can rarely be followed by satellite papules which may coalesce to form a single nodule that may not ulcerate or become crusted. Lesions evolve to heal slowly over a 5-year period. If the site of inoculation was close to the mucosal border of the mouth or nose, primary mucocutaneous leishmaniasis may ensue with diffuse infiltration, similarly to what may happen in *L. braziliensis* leishmaniasis, but without its potential for gross destruction.

Cutaneous leishmaniasis due to *L. infantum*

Although in children infection with *L. infantum* usually causes visceral disease, adults tend to develop self-healing cutaneous lesions without visceral involvement. There may be solitary mucosal lesions.

Leishmaniasis recidivans (chronic lupoid leishmaniasis)

Brownish-red or yellow papules appear near or in a scar of oriental sore, usually on the face. They slowly coalesce to form a plaque or nodules that strongly resemble lupus vulgaris and may enlarge considerably and ulcerate. The Montenegro skin test is strongly positive.

Diffuse cutaneous leishmaniasis (pseudolepromatous or lepromatoid leishmaniasis)

Symmetrically distributed papules, nodules, and plaques on the face strongly resemble lepromatous leprosy, without involvement of the mucous membranes, viscera, or lymphatic tissue. Parasites (*L. aethiopica*) can easily be found in the lesions inside macrophages. The Montenegro skin test is negative. Treatment leads to some improvement but relapse happens very often.

American leishmaniasis

Clinically the disease presents itself under four main forms: (1) cutaneous; (2) mucocutaneous; (3) diffuse; and (4) visceral.

The cutaneous lesions follow inoculation after an incubation period of 10–90 days and are generally found in exposed areas of the body. This primary erythematous and papular lesion may become ulcerated or boil-like and be followed by regional lymphadenopathy with or without lymphangitis in 12–30% of the cases. According to the parasite involved, the lesion may heal spontaneously or progress to involve other areas of the skin or mucous membranes. While *L. major* and *L. tropica* infections (Old World cutaneous leishmaniasis) tend to be self-healing, *L. braziliensis* infections tend to disseminate hematogenously to cause mucosal lesions of variable impact on health after a period of clinical latency that can last up to several months. In those cases, mucosal involvement happens before the first year of infection in 38.5% of patients and after the first year in 80.9%.[25] Mucosal involvement also occurs with *L. vianna panamensis*. However, most cases of American leishmaniasis due to *L. mexicana mexicana* resolve within 6 months.

Cutaneous lesions

Several types of skin lesions and also varied combinations of the following can be found:

- Ulcerated: the lesion may be frankly ulcerated with raised borders; they may be nodular and ulcerated (gummatous), with a granulomatous bottom sometimes covered by a thick crust (Fig. 5.1).
- Impetigo-like: they start as vesicles or pustules that rupture very fast and are covered by a crust. Parasites are usually extremely abundant in these lesions.
- Lichenoid: isolated or grouped follicular papules are sometimes seen, occasionally around a central atrophic area (Fig. 5.2).
- Sarcoid-like: nodules with a tumid aspect, sometimes resembling sarcoid or tumid lupus erythematosus (Fig. 5.3).
- Nodules: these are only rarely seen, can be subcutaneous or dermal–hypodermal, and bear no relation to regional lymphatic vessels.

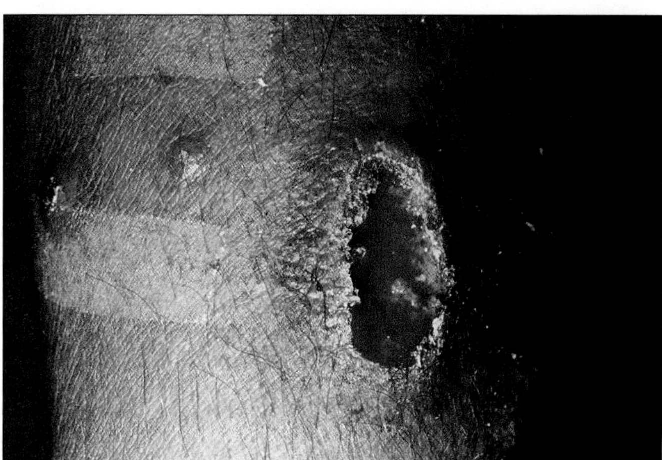

Figure 5.1 Cutaneous leishmaniasis due to *Leishmania braziliensis*. Ulcer with raised borders and small boil-like lesions around the ulcer.

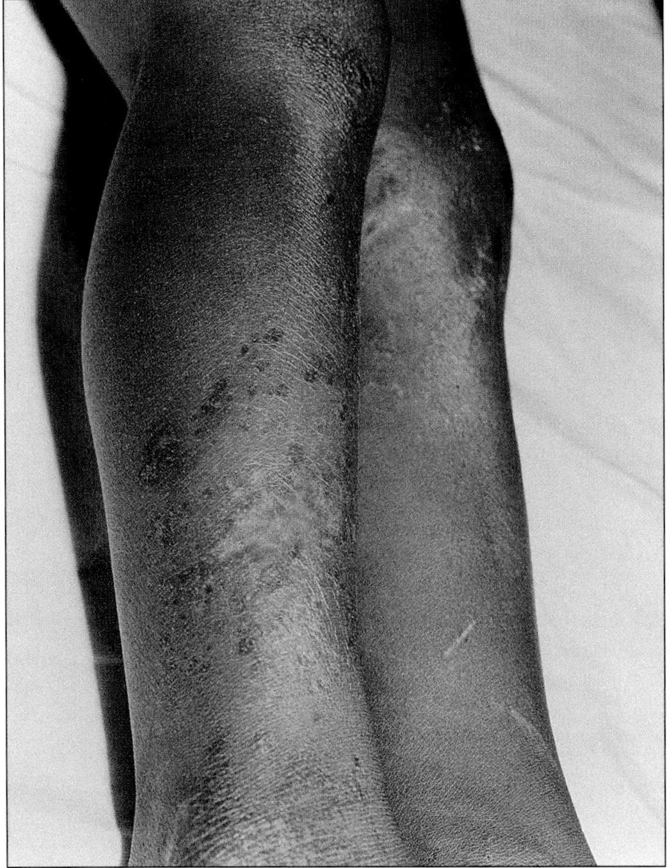

Figure 5.2 Disseminated papules on the legs of a 12-year-old girl.

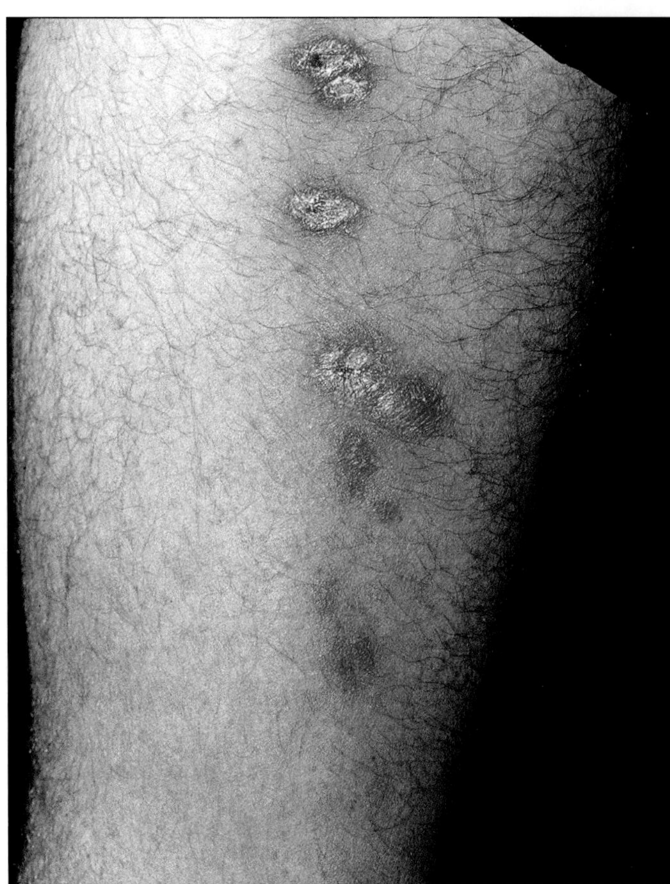

Figure 5.4 Lymphangitic leishmaniasis.

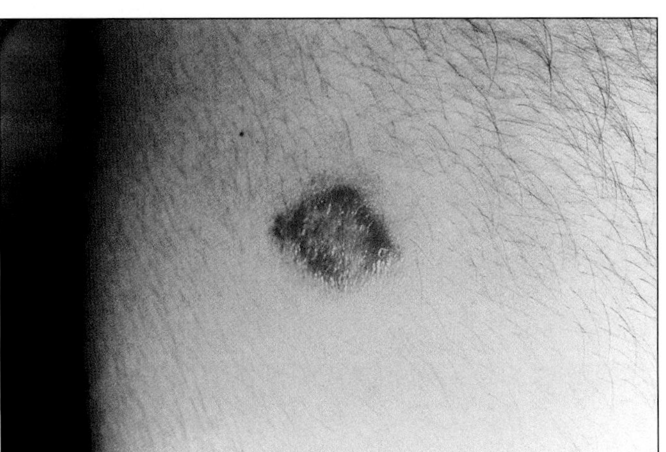

Figure 5.3 Sarcoid-like lesion on the trunk.

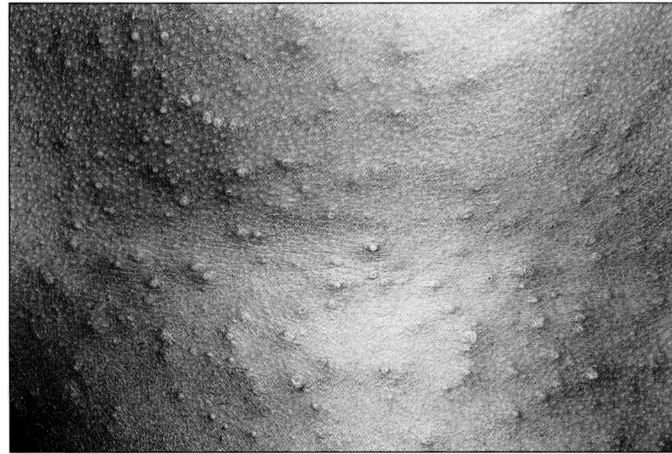

Figure 5.5 Thousands of pustules were seen on the trunk of a 29-year-old rural worker.

- Vegetating: these can look wart-like and are usually seen in the extremities.
- Lymphangitic: sometimes leishmaniasis can be manifested by nodules that disseminate via lymphatic spread, mimicking classic sporotrichosis (Fig. 5.4).
- Furunculoid: boil-like lesions occasionally seen isolated or near ulcerated lesions.
- Miliary: sometimes small pustular lesions in the thousands are seen, even in immunocompetent hosts infected by *L. braziliensis* (Fig. 5.5).

Mucosal lesions

The nose, mouth, and pharynx are often involved by ulcerated or infiltrated or both types of lesion. The nose is usually edematous and has a violaceous hue. Superficial telangiectasias can sometimes be seen. When in the mouth, a grossly granular aspect can sometimes be appreciated, mainly when the palate is involved (Fig. 5.6). Lip lesions are usually ulcerated or assume the aspect of hypertrophic cheilitis (Fig. 5.7). Only rarely are the genital or the eye mucosae affected.

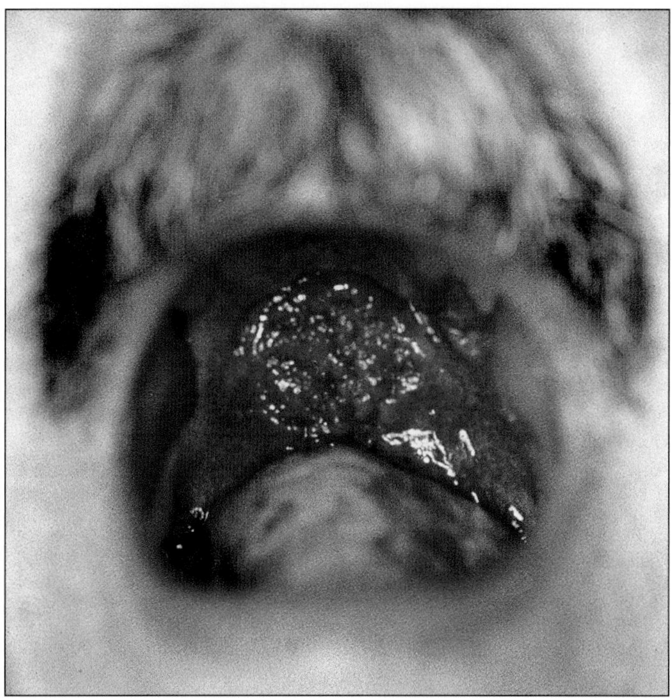

Figure 5.6 Grossly granular vegetation on the palate.

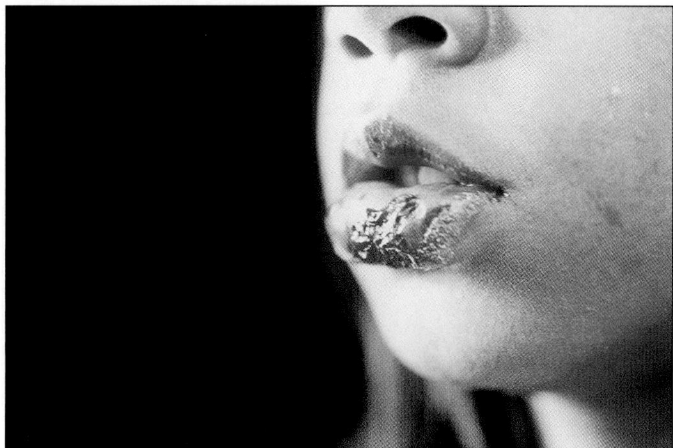

Figure 5.7 Hypertrophic cheilitis.

Diffuse cutaneous leishmaniasis

Also called anergic and lepromatous or pseudolepromatous leishmaniasis, the clinical picture of diffuse leishmaniasis can be caused by both the *aethiopica* complex (*L. aethiopica*) in Africa and the *mexicana* complex (*L. amazonensis*) in the Americas.

Multiple keloid-like lesions associated with nasal infiltration and ulceration without destruction of the nasal septum are usually found. There may be laryngeal and pharyngeal involvement.

The Montenegro skin test is negative and both the histopathological examination and the direct smear show numerous amastigote forms of *Leishmania*.

Visceral leishmaniasis

The incubation period is from 1 to 36 months. Fever, anorexia, weight loss, diarrhea, pallor, abdominal tenderness, cough, and lymphadenopathy develop either suddenly or slowly to progress with hepatomegaly and splenomegaly, oral, nasal, and intestinal hemorrhage, leading to cachexia. Fever and visceral enlargement are the two commonest and most consistent findings. Fever may be continuous or intermittent. In the acute cases, fever starts suddenly, is elevated, and frequently is accompanied by shivers and sweating. Liver enlargement causes abdominal protrusion which is usually proportional to the duration of disease. The spleen is also enlarged and tender to palpation. As the disease process progresses there may be complications such as enteritis, pneumonia, bronchopneumonia, nephritis, and tuberculosis that, together with the severe hemorrhagic phenomena, may lead to death.

Papules or nodules may appear at the inoculation site. Other cutaneous findings may be either non-specific or specific. Non-specific findings include hair abnormalities which are similar to those found in kwashiorkor: yellowish discoloration of fine and brittle hair. Purpura, hyperpigmentation, and xeroderma are found in 7.6% of patients. Specific findings related to skin parasitism include ulcers, papules, and nodules.[26]

Post-kala-azar dermal leishmaniasis (Fig. 5.8) is a sequela of treated, untreated, or symptomless kala-azar in endemic areas. This condition presents with a characteristic cutaneous eruption resulting from infection of the skin by previous visceral infecting organisms. It may be related to an improvement in cellular immunity after cure of visceral disease. All ages, sexes, and races are susceptible. The lesions are depigmented macules, malar erythema similar to the butterfly rash of lupus erythematosus, nodules and, less frequently, the verrucous, papillomatous, hypertrophic, and xanthomatous types.

Established visceral leishmaniasis does not resolve by itself and progresses in a few days or months to death.

Patients concomitantly infected by leishmaniasis and HIV characteristically relapse after treatment.

Laboratory diagnosis

The diagnosis of leishmaniasis is based on the demonstration of the parasite in the stained smears of material aspirated from cutaneous lesions, lymph nodes, bone marrow, or spleen, and from spinal fluid or in stained tissue or in culture. The Giemsa, Wright, or Feulgen stains are used to demonstrate the organisms in smear and tissues. With the use of these stains, the cytoplasm appears blue, the nucleus pink, and the kinetoplast a deep red (Fig. 5.9).

Histopathological examination shows a granuloma with lymphocytes, histiocytes, and many plasma cells around areas with epithelioid cells. In recent cases, multiple *Leishmania* organisms may be found inside histiocytes (Fig. 5.10).

The Nicolle–Novy–MacNeal (NNM) medium, consisting of bactoagar, sodium chloride, sodium hydroxide, distilled water, and rabbit or guinea pig defibrinated blood with added antibiotics, or chick embryo medium, is used for culture. Culture is positive in about 40% of cases and, like hamster inoculation that reproduces the disease in 2–3 months, is not routinely used in clinical practice.

The Montenegro skin test is perhaps the most common tool to complement diagnosis. Its value has already been discussed and the reader is referred to the section on immunology of leishmaniasis.

Infection can also be demonstrated by serological means. Indirect immunofluorescence for *Leishmania* and enzyme-linked

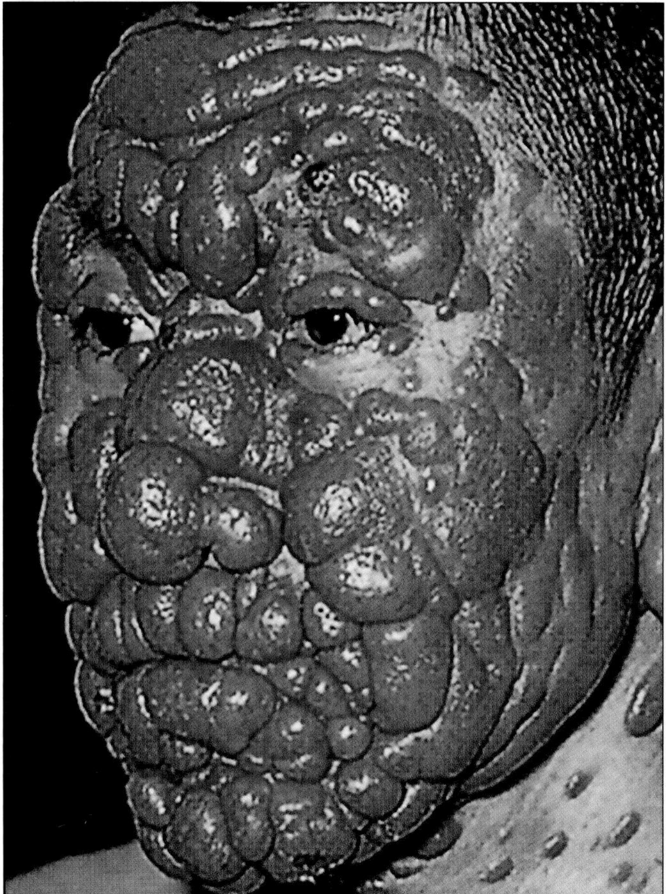

Figure 5.8 Post kala-azar dermal leishmaniasis in a Chinese patient. (Reproduced from Peters W and Pasvol G (eds). Tropical Medicine and Parasitology, 5th edition, Mosby, London 2002, image 228)

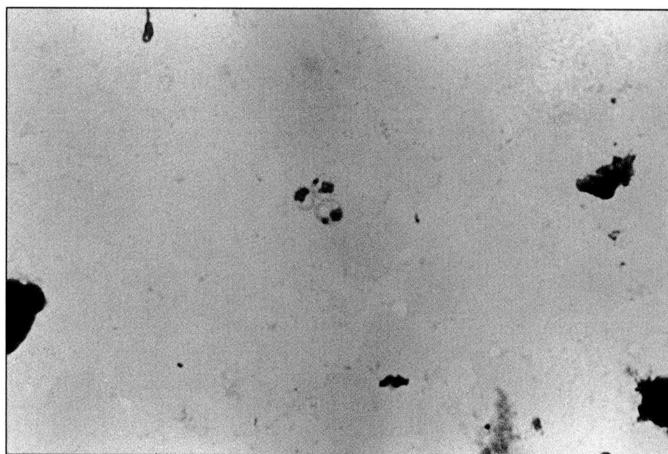

Figure 5.9 Giemsa stain of smear showing typical *Leishmania* bodies.

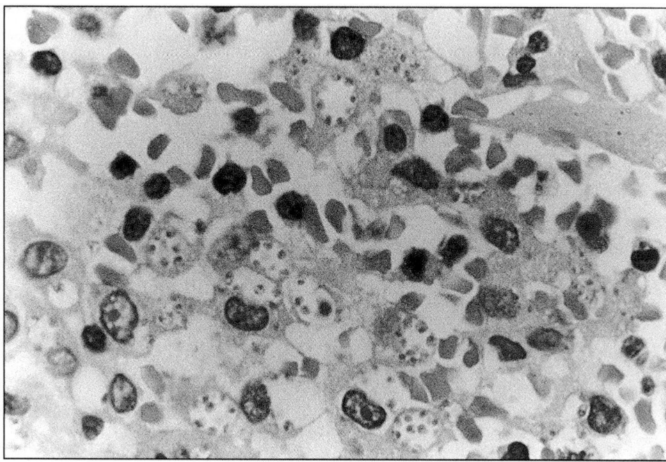

Figure 5.10 Hematoxylin and eosin section of skin with several *Leishmania* organisms inside histiocytes.

immunosorbent assay (ELISA) are sensitive techniques. Indirect immunofluorescence is not specific and yields positivity in 75–100% of patients. It may present cross-reactivity with *Trypanosoma cruzi* infections. Titers over 1:80 favor the diagnosis of leishmaniasis. When available, polymerase chain reaction is 100% sensitive and specific.[27]

Treatment

Old-World leishmaniasis

The treatment for cutaneous disease is non-parenteral therapy or a short course of antimony. The combination of antimony, 8 mg/kg per day for 14 days, plus allopurinol, 20 mg/kg per day, cured 81% of patients studied as compared to a 74% cure rate in the antimony-alone group. Intralesional antimony may also be used. On alternate days 0.5–2.0 ml sodium stibogluconate (100 mg antimony/ml) is injected into all sides of the lesion until it blanches in a total of 10 injections. Cure can be observed in 85% of patients at the 3-month follow-up. If liquid nitrogen is sprayed on the lesions once-monthly for 2 months, the cure rate is 73%.

When oral therapy is preferred, fluconazole, 200 mg daily for 6 weeks, cures 90% of patients.[28]

Paromomycin is a parenteral aminoglycoside antibacterial agent that also has considerable activity against protozoa. It can be used as an ointment and there are those who suggest that 4 weeks of paromomycin ointment could become the first line of treatment for uncomplicated cutaneous leishmaniasis due to *L. major*.[29]

American cutaneous leishmaniasis

Pentavalent antimony remains the standard treatment of American cutaneous leishmaniasis, despite the frequency of adverse reactions related to its use, its requirement for intramuscular or intravenous injection each day, and the development of occasional resistance. *N*-methyl-glucamine and sodium stibogluconate are available in 5-ml vials that contain 1.5 g of antimonial, corresponding to 425 mg of pentavalent antimony. It is recommended that doses between 10 and 20 mg/kg body weight be given each day. As there seems to be wide variation in strain susceptibility to antimony, there is no consensus regarding the duration of each series. There are several papers that demonstrate that a treatment regimen that consists of 10-day series followed by 10-day free-of-treatment intervals is effective and provides the least risk of development of side-effects, which, in most instances, seem to be cumulative and dose-related.[30,31]

Others recommend continuous treatment for 20 days for cutaneous leishmaniasis and 28 days for mucocutaneous leishmaniasis. Among the adverse reactions listed, cardiotoxicity and nephrotoxicity are the most serious. Prolongation of QT interval may be observed on the electrocardiogram and acute renal failure followed by sudden death may occasionally occur, even after only a few injections.[32] Most patients on antimony will develop pancreatitis that in most instances is only subclinical or will present with abdominal pain. Pain at the site of injections and myalgia are commonly seen. The combination of a killed *L. amazonensis* promastigote vaccine with low-dose *N*-methyl-glucamine has been shown to be quite effective and safe in the treatment of cutaneous leishmaniasis.[27]

As TNF-α has been shown to have an important role in the pathogenetic mechanism of leishmaniasis, it seems obvious that the addition of a potent TNF-α antagonist such as pentoxiphylline would improve the response to treatment.[18,33] Controlled trials are needed to confirm the use of pentoxiphylline in association with *N*-methyl-glucamine.

Pentamidine isothianate is a treatment option in many areas. It is available in 300-mg vials. It has been successfully used in the treatment of leishmaniasis caused by *L. guyanensis* or *L. braziliensis*. Renal, cardiologic, and hepatic evaluation should be performed before the administration of 4 mg/kg in three intramuscular injections, one every other day, with a cure rate around 90%.[34] Long-term administration has been shown to provoke permanent hyperglycemia.

Amphotericin B is indicated in cases that do not respond to antimony. Slow intravenous administration is mandatory. It is available in 50-mg vials. The recommended dosage is 0.5–1.0 mg/kg body weight, not exceeding a total daily dose of 50 mg. Renal function needs careful monitoring during the administration of amphotericin B, which also causes loss of potassium, that, if undetected, may lead to cardiac arrhythmias. Its use is not indicated in elderly patients or pregnant women. Liposomal amphotericin B is injected infrequently because of its relatively higher cost but is virtually 100% effective, even when leishmaniasis is associated with human immunodeficiency virus (HIV).[35]

Visceral leishmaniasis

The standard treatment is antimony, 20 mg/kg per day for 28 days. However, resistance is high in some endemic areas. Pentamidine and amphotericin B are options but have the disadvantage of parenteral use and toxicity. Miltefosine is an oral agent that, at 2.5 mg/kg daily for 28 days, cures virtually 100% of the patients studied in India. Diarrhea and vomiting occur rather frequently and the drug has reproductive toxicity in animals. Therefore, women to be treated with miltefosine should be cautioned to practice contraception. Miltefosine probably should not be used alone in the treatment of patients concomitantly infected with visceral leishmaniasis and HIV.[28]

Prophylaxis

Since immunity appears to be lifelong against infections with some strains of parasites of cutaneous and mucocutaneous leishmaniasis, vaccination seems to be effective prophylactically. Indeed, it has been shown in mice, rhesus monkeys, and also in humans that vaccination with a killed *L. amazonensis* promastigote vaccine induces a Th1 response related to significant resistance against *Leishmania*.[36,37] Other vaccines have also shown promising results.[38,39]

References

1. Desjeux P. Information on the epidemiology and control of leishmaniasis by country and territory. WHO/Leish 1991; 91:47.
2. Centers for Disease Control and Prevention. Identification and diagnosis of parasites of public health concern. Home page www.cdc.gov (updated February, 2001; accessed November 11, 2003).
3. Alexander J. Unusual axonemal doublet arrangements in the flagellum of *Leishmania* amastigotes. Trans R Soc Trop Méd Hyg 1978; 72:345–347.
4. Furtado TA. Leishmaniose tegumentar americana. In: Machado-Pinto J, ed. Doenças infecciosas com manifestações dermatológicas. Rio de Janeiro: Editora Medsi; 1994:319–328.
5. Wirth DF, Rogers WO, Barker Jr R et al. Leishmaniasis and malaria: new tools for epidemiologic analysis. Science 1986; 234:975–979.
6. World Health Organization. Division of Control of Tropical Diseases. Leishmaniasis control: home page www.who.int/health-topics/leishmaniasis.htm (updated December, 2000), accessed November 11, 2003.
7. Lainson R. Ecological interactions in the transmission of the leishmaniases. Phil Trans R Soc 1988; 321:389–404.
8. Coutinho SG, Louis JA, Mavel J et al. Induction of specific T lymphocytes of intracellular destruction of *Leishmania major* in infected murine macrophages. Parasit Immunol 1984; 6:157–169.
9. Pirmez C, Cooper C, Paes-Oliveira M et al. Immunologic responsiveness in American cutaneous leishmaniasis lesions. J Immunol 1990; 145:3100–3104.
10. Mossmann TR, Coffman RL. Two types of mouse helper T-cell clones: implications for immune regulation. Immunol Today 1987; 8:223–227.
11. Fiorentino DF, Bond DW, Mossmann TR. Two types of mouse T-helper cell IV Th2 clones secrete a factor that inhibits cytokine production by Th1 clones. J Exp Med 1989; 170:2081–2095.
12. Scott P. Host and parasite factors regulating the development of CD4+ subjects in experimental cutaneous leishmaniasis. Res Immunol 1991; 142:32–35.
13. Pirmez C, Yamamura M, Uyemura K et al. Cytokine patterns in the pathogenesis of human leishmaniasis. J Clin Invest 1993; 91:1390–1395.
14. Reiner SL, Zheng S, Corry DB et al. Constructing polycompetitor cDNAs for quantitative PCR. J Immunol Meth 1994; 175:275.
15. DaCruz AM, de Oliveira MP, de Luca PM et al. Tumor necrosis factor-alpha in human American tegumentary leishmaniasis. Mem Inst O Cruz 1996; 91:225–229.
16. Trinchieri G. Role of interleukin-12 in human Th1 response. Chem Immunol 1996; 63:14–29.

17. Carvalho EM, Correia-Filho D, Bacellar O et al. Characterization of the immune response in subjects with self-healing cutaneous leishmaniasis. Am J Trop Med Hyg 1995; 53:273–277.
18. Bacellar O, Lessa H, Schriefer A et al. Up-regulation of Th1-type responses in mucosal leishmaniasis patients. Infect Immun 2002; 70:6734–6740.
19. Bonfim G, Nascimento C, Costa J et al. Variation of cytokine patterns related to therapeutic response in diffuse cutaneous leishmaniasis. Exp Parasitol 1996; 84:188–194.
20. d'Oliveira Jr A, Costa SR, Barbosa AB et al. Asymptomatic *Leishmania chagasi* infection in relatives and neighbors of patients with visceral leishmaniasis. Mem Inst O Cruz 1997; 95:15–20.
21. Marzochi MCA. Leishmanioses no Brasil. As leishmanioses tegumentares. J Brás Méd 1992; 63:82–95.
22. Mayrink W, Costa CA, Magalhães PA. A field trial of a vaccine against American leishmaniasis. Trans R Soc Trop Med Hyg 1979; 73:385–387.
23. Passos VMA, Barreto SM, Romanha AJ et al. American cutaneous leishmaniasis: use of a skin test as a predictor of relapse after treatment. Bull WHO 2000; 78:968–974.
24. Rodriguez V, Centeno M, Ulrich M. The IgG isotypes of specific antibodies in patients with American cutaneous leishmaniasis: relationship to the T-cell mediated immune response. Parasit Immunol 1996; 18:341–345.
25. Pessoa SB. Profilaxia da leishmaniose tegumentar no estado de São Paulo. Folha Méd 1941; 22:157–161.
26. Diógenes MJN, Alencar JE, Menezes RHO et al. Leishmaniose visceral americana. In: Machado-Pinto J, ed. Doenças infecciosas com manifestações dermatológicas. Rio de Janeiro: Editora Medsi; 1994:328–338.
27. Machado-Pinto J, Pinto J, Costa CA et al. Immunochemotherapy for cutaneous leishmaniasis: a controlled trial using killed *Leishmania (Leishmania) amazonensis* vaccine plus antimonial. Int J Dermatol 2002; 41:73–78.
28. Berman J. Current treatment approaches in leishmaniasis. Curr Opin Infect Dis 2003; 16:397–401.
29. Asilian A, Jalayer T, Nilforooshzadeh M et al. Treatment of cutaneous leishmaniasis with aminosidine (paromomycin) ointment: double-blind, randomized trial in the Islamic Republic of Iran. Bull WHO 2003; 81:353–359.
30. Magalhaes PA, Mayrink W, Costa CA et al. Calazar na zona do Rio Doce – minas gerais. Resultados de medidas profiláticas. Rev Inst Med Trop São Paulo 1980; 22:197–202.
31. Arana BA, Navin TR, Arana FE et al. Efficaccy of a short course (10 days) of high dose meglumine antimoniate with or without interferon-γ in treating cutaneous leishmaniasis in Guatemala. Clin Infect Dis 1994; 18:381–384.
32. Kopke LFF, Café MEM, Neves LB et al. Morte após uso de antimonial pentavalente em leishmaniose tegumentar americana. An Bras Dermatol 1993; 68:259–262.
33. Lessa HA, Machado P, Lima F et al. Successful treatment of refractory mucosal leishmaniasis with pentoxifylline plus antimony. Am J Trop Med Hyg 2001; 65:87–89.
34. De Paula CD, Sampaio JH, Cardoso DR et al. A comparative study between the efficaccy of pentamidine isothianate given in three doses for one week and N-methyl-glucamine in a dose of 20 mgsbv/day for 20 days to treat cutaneous leishmaniasis. Rev Soc Bras Med Trop 2003; 36:365–371.
35. Murdaca G, Setti M, Campelli A et al. Liposomal amphotericin B for the treatment of acute phase and secondary prophylaxis of visceral leishmaniasis in a HIV positive patient. Infez Med 2000; 8:241–244.
36. Mayrink W, Pinto JA, Costa CA et al. Evaluation of the potency and stability of a candidate vaccine against American cutaneous leishmaniasis. Am J Trop Med Hyg 1999; 61:294–295.
37. Kenney RT, Sacks DL, Sypek JP et al. Protective immunity using recombinant human IL-12 and alum as adjuvants in a primate model of cutaneous leishmaniasis. J Immunol 1999; 163:4481–4488.
38. Armijos RX, Weigel MM, Aviles H et al. Field trial of a vaccine against New World cutaneous leishmaniasis in an at-risk child population: safety immunogenicity and eficaccy during the first 12 months of follow-up. J Infect Dis 1998; 177:1352–1357.
39. Sharifi I, Fekri AR, Aflatonian MR et al. Randomized vaccine trial of single dose of killed *Leishmania major* plus BCG against anthroponotic cutaneous leishmaniasis in Bam, Iran. Lancet 1998; 351:1540–1543.

Chapter 6

Cutaneous manifestations of infection by free-living amebas

Francisco G. Bravo, Juan Cabrera, Eduardo Gotuzzo and Govinda S. Vivesvara

- Epidemiology
- Microbiological characteristics and pathogenesis
- Clinical manifestations
- Pathology
- Therapy

Free-living amebas belonging to the genera *Acanthamoeba*, *Balamuthia*, and *Naegleria* are mitochondria-bearing eukaryotic protozoa that cause fatal central nervous system (CNS) disease in humans and other animals. These amebas are also called amphizoic amebas, because of their ability to lead a free-living existence in nature as well as lead an endozoic existence within humans and other animals. Both *Acanthamoeba* and *Naegleria* are ubiquitous and have been isolated from all continents. They are usually found in soil or in fresh water such as ponds, creeks, and pools. The environmental niche of *Balamuthia*, however was not known until recently. It has now been isolated from a soil sample obtained from a potted plant recovered from the house of a fatal case of *Balamuthia* encephalitis.[1] Although these free-living amebas are a well-known cause of neurological disease, little is known about the skin infections they cause.

The taxonomic classification of free-living amebas is in a state of flux. However, *Naegleria fowleri*, the only species of *Naegleria* that is known to cause CNS disease, is included in the class Heterolobosia and family Vahlkampfiidae. Several species of *Acanthamoeba* (*A. castellani*, *A. culbertsoni*, *A. healyi*, *A. polyphaga*, *A. rhysodes*) that are known to cause CNS disease are classified under class Lobosea, family Acanthamoebidae. *Balamuthia mandrillaris*, the only known species, is also included in the family Acanthamoebidae because of its affinities to *Acanthamoeba* based on recent molecular data.[2]

N. fowleri causes a fulminating and acute necrotizing meningo-encephalitis called primary amebic meningoencephalitis (PAM), primarily in healthy children and young adults, leading to death within 5–10 days. Populations at risk are those with a history of swimming in warm freshwater bodies such as lakes, ponds, hot springs, and effluents from factories and power plants.

Acanthamoeba, on the other hand, causes an insidious subacute encephalitis, referred to by some as granulomatous amebic encephalitis (GAE). The affected individuals may or may not have a history of exposure to natural bodies of water, but in many cases they have a history of immunodeficiency whether because of human immunodeficiency virus (HIV) or acquired immuno-deficiency syndrome (AIDS) or debilitation, immunosuppressive drugs, or pregnancy. Occasionally, patients with *Acanthamoeba* infections have skin lesions, commonly described as chronic ulcers. GAE also leads to death after a prolonged course of several weeks to years.

Up until 1990 all GAE infections were considered as due to *Acanthamoeba* because of the presence of cysts in the brain tissue, since *N. fowleri* does not encyst in the brain. However, many of these cases were considered atypical because they were serologically negative in the immunofluorescence (IIF) test for *N. fowleri* and *Acanthamoeba* spp. In 1990, Visvesvara and Stehr-Green reported the isolation of a new species of ameba, provisionally identified as leptomyxid ameba, from the brain of a pregnant baboon at the San Diego Zoo that died after developing lethargy and focal neurological deficits.[3] Visvesvara et al. made antiserum to this ameba and demonstrated, using the IIF test on a series of 16 atypical cases of GAE from different parts of the world (including two from Peru), that most of these cases were caused by the leptomyxid ameba.[4] Five of these 16 cases also manifested cutaneous ulcers. By 1993, Vivesvara et al. had established the characteristic features of this new ameba species and named it *Balamuthia mandrillaris*.[5]

In most cases of *B. mandrillaris* infection, the disease follows a prolonged course with a fatal outcome; commonly the diagnosis is either missed or only made postmortem. Skin lesions, whenever present, precede the development of the CNS symptoms by weeks or months. Therefore the importance of early recognition of the cutaneous involvement cannot be underestimated as it could allow prompt diagnosis and treatment.

Epidemiology

Around 100 cases of *B. mandrillaris* infection have been reported world wide, with approximately half of those cases occurring in the USA.[6] Some have taken place in the context of immunosuppression.[7,8] On the other hand, cases seen in Latin America, Asia, and Australia are mostly seen among immune-competent patients. It is interesting to remark that up to 44% of the US cases reported to the Centers for Disease Control for *Balamuthia* testing had Hispanic ethnicity.[9,10]

Naegleria and *Acanthamoeba* have been repeatedly isolated from nature. However, little is known about the ecology of *B. mandrillaris*. Most isolates have been made from clinical specimens, requiring tissue cultures. Only recently, *Balamuthia* was isolated from flower-pot soil obtained from the home of a child who died of *Balamuthia* encephalitis.[1]

The sporadic appearance of *Balamuthia* as a cause of human disease seems to indicate that this ameba is present in the human environment: this is also corroborated by the presence of antibodies against *Balamuthia* in the normal population.[11]

Besides the USA, the disease has also been reported in Canada,[4] Australia,[12] Eastern Europe,[13] Thailand,[14] and recently in Japan.[15] In Latin America cases have been described in Peru,[16–19] Argentina,[20,21] Venezuela,[22,23] Mexico,[24] Brazil,[25] and Chile.[4] Up to 45 cases of free-living ameba infection have been identified at the Instituto de Medicina Tropical Alexander von Humboldt, at Cayetano Heredia General Hospital, in Lima, Peru; 20 cases have been confirmed by immunofluorescence test as being caused by *Balamuthia*.

Peruvian cases originated from three coastal, semidesert regions such as Piura, Ica, and Lima. Many of these patients were children, mostly male, either farmers or urban dwellers. Frequently there was a history of swimming in small ponds and creeks, although in some patients swimming activities were limited to public pools.

Microbiological characteristics and pathogenesis

Balamuthia mandrillaris, at the light microscope level, is morphologically similar to *Acanthamoeba*, especially in tissue sections. A dense nucleolus, usually single, but sometimes appearing to be fragmented into two or three pieces, appears to be the salient characteristic feature that can be used to differentiate *Balamuthia* from *Acanthamoeba*. *Balamuthia* has two stages in its life cycle: an uninucleated trophozoite, measuring 15–60 μm in diameter, and a cyst which appears to be double-walled at light microscopy but is actually trilaminar when examined by transmission electron microscopy. The cyst measures 15–25 μm in diameter. No flagellated state has been described. Its movements are crab-like, with multiple pseudopodia at a speed of ~0.15 μm/s, which is rather slow when compared to other amebas.[1]

Until recently *Balamuthia* amebas have only been isolated from clinical specimens, either brain or skin, using monolayers of mammalian cell cultures such as monkey kidney or human lung fibroblast.[26] Only recently has it been possible to isolate and culture *Balamuthia* from soil on agar plates coated with bacteria. *Balamuthia* amebas are slow-growers and emerge only after other amebas such as *Acanthamoeba* and *Naegleria* colonize the agar plate. *Balamuthia* do not feed on bacteria; however it feeds on other amebas and multiplies. It can also be grown on non-cellular axenic media, such as BM-3.[27]

Extensive molecular analysis has revealed that there is very little genetic variation among the different clinical and soil isolates of *Balamuthia* and all are included in the only known species, *B. mandrillaris*. By polymerase chain reaction (PCR) assay, primers based on mitochondrial small-subunit-rRNA genes have been shown to amplify a product successfully from whole-cell DNA of *Balamuthia*, allowing differentiation from *Acanthamoeba* and human cells.[28]

Balamuthia may enter the human body either by clinically evident wounds or through microabrasions. Thereafter it may be contained at the skin level, producing a florid granulomatous reaction, or it may pass directly to the blood stream and reach the CNS. It has been postulated that the spread from the cutaneous site to the CNS may also follow a different pathway, traveling throughout the adventitial layer of the vessels that link the nasal region with the brain circulatory system.[17] This is more relevant when one considers the frequent mid facial location of the skin lesions.

Once the ameba reaches the brain tissue, it will cause marked necrosis and a characteristically severe angiitis, involving arteries and veins, with active invasion of the vessel walls by the microorganism. Thrombotic amebic angiitis produces infarcts of the CNS substance, which then becomes infiltrated by amebas.[17]

Clinical manifestations

In Peruvian patients, the populations affected varied in age, ranging from 5 to 63 years old, with 50% being age 15 or younger. The majority of patients came from rural, coastal areas of Peru, which are arid regions with a hot climate; only a few cases were urban dwellers. Many patients did have a history of bathing in local creeks and ponds, as a way to refresh themselves after physical labor or sport activities.

The existence of a skin lesion preceding CNS involvement has been previously reported, but not as commonly as in the Peruvian cases.[4,7,12,14,21,30–34] Some authors have previously described central face lesions,[12] with findings of granulomatous inflammation, but few have reported the observation of the ameba.[7,35] The classical cutaneous lesion is a painless plaque, a few millimeters thick, and 1 to several cm in diameter. The color may be the same as skin tone or dark red, sometimes with an added violet hue. Occasionally, the edges are ill-defined, representing more of an infiltrated area. Most patients will present with a single lesion, although some may have two or three affected areas. Lesions are either asymptomatic or tender to touch, with preservation of local sensation. On palpation, the skin may feel very indurated or rubbery, with an occasional palpable raised border.

Lesions are commonly located on the center of the face and occasionally on the extremities or the trunk. If in the face, the lesion is usually located over the nose and cheek, extending upward or downward to involve either the eyelid or the upper lip (Figs 6.1 and 6.2). As the disease progresses, it may result in a symmetrically diffuse, enlarged nose, eventually leading to massive infiltration and deformity (Fig. 6.3); occasionally there may be central ulcerations.

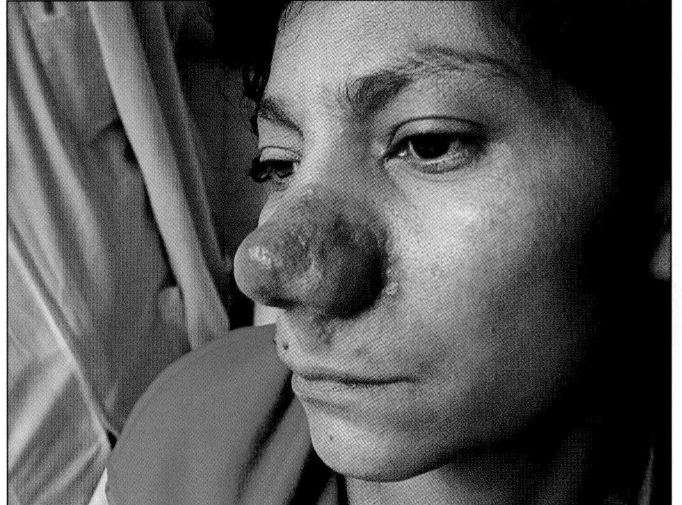

Figure 6.1 Classical plaque on the dorsum of the nose, a location commonly seen in patients infected with *Balamuthia mandrillaris*.

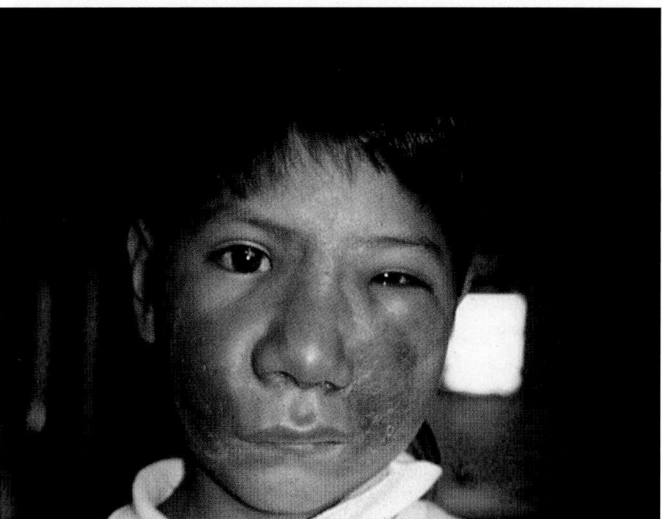

Figure 6.3 Typical progression of the lesion, infiltrating all facial tissue.

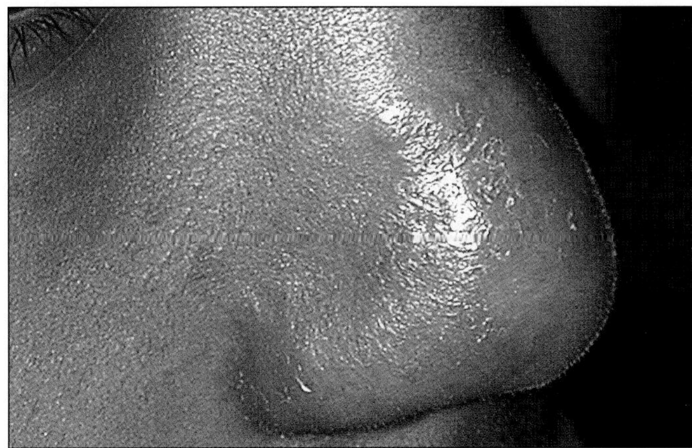

Figure 6.2 Similar lesion in a younger patient.

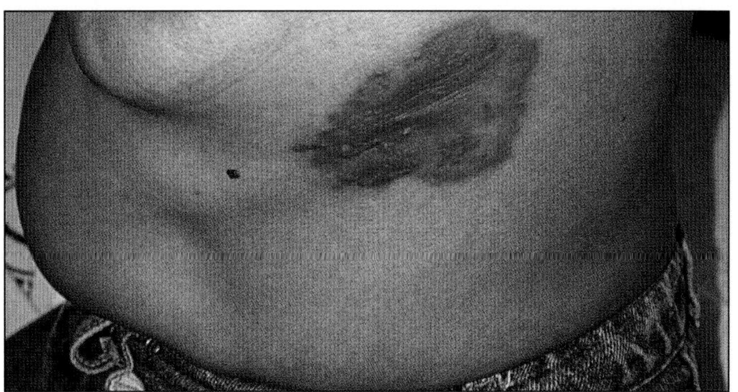

Figure 6.4 Lesion on the chest, excised after a partial response to medical therapy.

In some cases the lesion is a subcutaneous nodule or plaque with no epidermal changes. The history of previous trauma at the lesion site is rather exceptional.

Peripheral lesions manifest as plaques (Fig. 6.4) or nodules, located on the extremities, chest, abdomen, or buttock areas. The same characteristics of color and consistency on palpation also apply to peripherally located lesions. Occasionally, the skin surrounding the lesion feels woody on palpation. Some plaques may ulcerate, although the characteristics described for the primary lesion are always evident around the ulcer.

The general aspect of the facial lesion is rather characteristic, whereas peripheral lesions on extremities can easily be confused with other entities. In our experience, diagnosis is commonly missed or delayed at extrafacial locations. Mucosal involvement, either oral or periorbital, may develop by continuity in a few patients.

For facial lesions the differential diagnosis may include tuberculosis (lupus vulgaris), mucocutaneous leishmaniasis, leprosy, sporotrichosis, paracoccidiomycosis, rhinoscleroma (nose of Hebra) and rhinoentomophtoromycosis. Sarcoidosis (lupus pernio), discoid lupus, and Wegener's granulomatosis may also present with central face lesions. Neoplastic processes such as basal cell carcinomas and lymphomas may be confused with *Balamuthia* infection, although they tend to be destructive rather than infiltrating.

When the cutaneous lesion is located in extrafacial areas, the differential diagnosis should additionally include other proliferating processes, such as peripheral lymphomas and sarcomas.

Some patients may develop regional lymphadenopathy. Five of 15 patients with ganglionar involvement did have amebas in the lymph nodes, as demonstrated by conventional histology, although there is no certainty they were *Balamuthia*.

At a later stage, the patient develops neurological disease.[16] As a rule the cutaneous involvement precedes the CNS involvement. The time frame between the onset of the skin lesion and the neurological symptoms may range from 30 days to 2 years, with an average of 5–8 months. A unique case in our series, with the classical central face lesion, never developed neurological symptoms. His skin lesion eventually disappeared, despite no therapeutic intervention, with complete recovery; in a follow-up visit 8 years later, he continues to do well. Incidentally, his case was the only one showing cysts but no trophozoites on the skin biopsy.

The CNS involvement manifests itself initially with headache and photophobia. Later, other signs of endocranial hypertension, such as seizures, lethargy, and anisocoria, become evident, followed by signs of motor or sensorial deficit. Fever may accompany the CNS disease. Eventually, patients succumb to a profound coma and die.

Neuroradiologic findings include multiple hypodense lesions, some of them with mild peripheral edema. Computed tomography and magnetic resonance imaging studies are very helpful to locate and to follow up the brain involvement.

Pathology

The histopathological findings seen in skin biopsies show a consistent, repetitive pattern, suggestive of this infection.

At first glance a diffuse mixed infiltrate is seen in the reticular dermis (Fig. 6.5), including lymphocytes, plasma cells, and histiocytes. The histiocytes may be distributed either diffusely or forming ill-defined granulomas. Characteristically, a large number of multinucleated giant cells will be seen, located either at the center of the granulomatous aggregates or interstitially, between collagen bundles. Some lesions may have aggregations of eosinophils, neutrophils, or nuclear dust. Foci of vasculitis, defined as fibrin around blood vessels, may be present as well. The giant cells may show phagocytosis of elastic fibers.

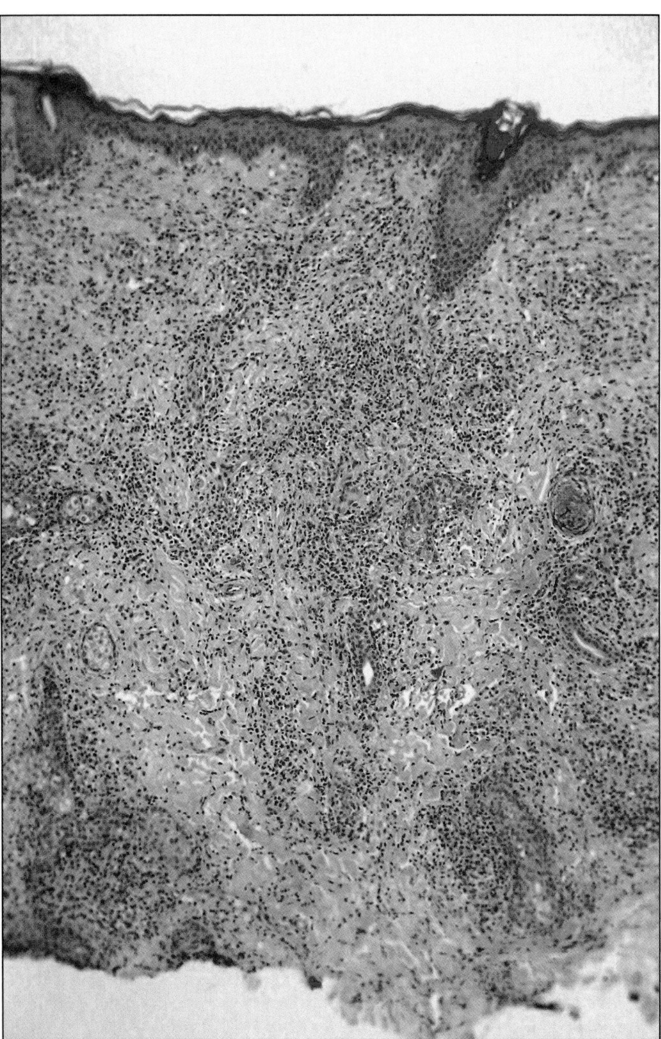

Figure 6.5 Superficial and deep, dense and diffuse, ill-defined granulomas. Hematoxylin and eosin: 40×.

In one particular case, the inflammatory infiltrate was mainly located in the subcutaneous fat, with a pattern of septal lobular panniculitis, and with the cellular components usually seen in the dermal type. An additional finding was the presence of thick bundles of collagen at the periphery of the infiltrate, as seen in dermatofibromas. This patient had a history of a penetrating injury at the inoculation site.

Over two-thirds of the lesions may have scarce amebas, which are nevertheless detectable. They are seen either as trophozoites (the majority of cases) or as cysts (usually intracellular). Multiple cuts are required to find the microorganisms. Identification of the microbe is difficult: if only the cytoplasm is seen, they can easily be confused with histiocytes. However, if the nucleus and nucleolus are seen, the ameba can be identified as such (Figs 6.6 and 6.7). In some occasions, the cytoplasm of the parasite takes a bubbly appearance. We find that hematoxylin and eosin (H&E) staining is adequate to visualize the amebas; however, other authors recommend the use of Mallory, Trichrome and Grocott–Gomori argentic stains.[17] It should be noted, however that routine histology does not allow fully identification of the species.

Differential diagnosis is not difficult if the organisms causing disease are readily seen on H&E or periodic acid–Schiff stains; however, tuberculosis may represent a diagnostic challenge, as its bacilli are difficult to see.

A variety of mycosis fungoides, called granulomatous slack skin, an entity characterized by being very rich in giant cells, should be included in the differential diagnosis.

The diagnosis should be suspected in the context of a classical centrofacial lesion and the finding of a diffuse lymphoplasmocytic infiltrate, with a histiocytic component and numerous giant cells, forming ill-defined granulomas. If the clinical picture is suggestive of free-living ameba infection, multiple cuts are mandatory to increase the likelihood of finding the parasite.

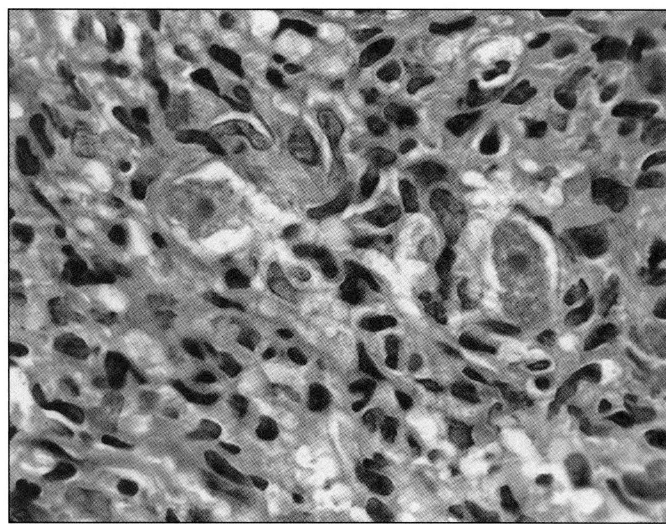

Figure 6.6 Two amebas seen in skin tissue. Hematoxylin and eosin: 1000×.

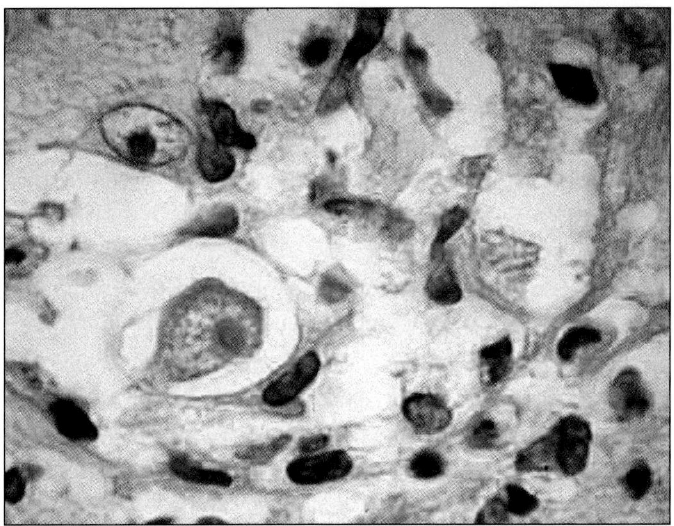

Figure 6.7 A trophozoite seen next to the epidermis. Hematoxylin and eosin: 1000×.

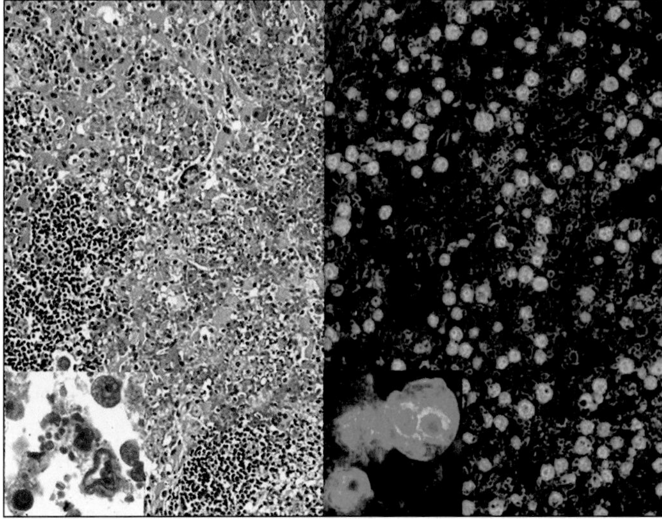

Figure 6.9 Left: a brain section stained with hematoxylin and eosin shows massive numbers of amebas. Inset at lower left: a higher-power view of ameba showing a flattened nucleolus about to fragment. Right: a low-power (×200) view of a brain section reacted first with rabbit anti-*Balamuthia mandrillaris* serum followed by goat antirabbit immunoglobulins in the indirect immunofluorescence assay. Inset at right bottom: a high-power (×1000) view.

With regard to the findings in the brain tissue, striking features in autopsies include hemorrhagic necrotic areas visible both on the surface (Fig. 6.8) and on sagittal cuts.[17] This will be seen in the brain lobules, the brainstem, and cerebellum. Cerebral edema will be consistently present, and a few cases will also have evidence of tonsil herniation. A suppurative process affecting the meninges may be evident on occasions.

Microscopic examination of brain tissue shows large areas of necrosis and hemorrhage. In contrast to the skin, where the amebas are scarce, trophozoites and cysts are readily seen in the brain sections (Fig. 6.9). Great numbers of amebas infiltrate the vascular subadventitial space of arteries, veins, and even capillaries, leading to a real amebic perivasculitis, resulting in thrombosis of capillaries and microinfarcts of the brain tissues.

Besides routine histology, other methods for ameba detection include inmunofluorescent staining of the microorganism in skin or brain tissue, as well as IF testing of the patient's serum.[2,23,36] Culturing of the organism from the affected tissue should be attempted, even though the methodology is fastidious.

Unfortunately, since all of the special techniques are not widely available, a presumptive diagnosis should therefore be made in the context of the clinical and histological findings, as described above. A remarkable difference between published cases and those seen at our institution was the time of diagnosis. In almost all of our cases the diagnosis was made before any evidence of CNS involvement. This was due to early detection based on the identification of the characteristic skin lesion. In theory, such a prompt diagnosis could allow an early and successful therapeutic intervention, even before CNS invasion took place.

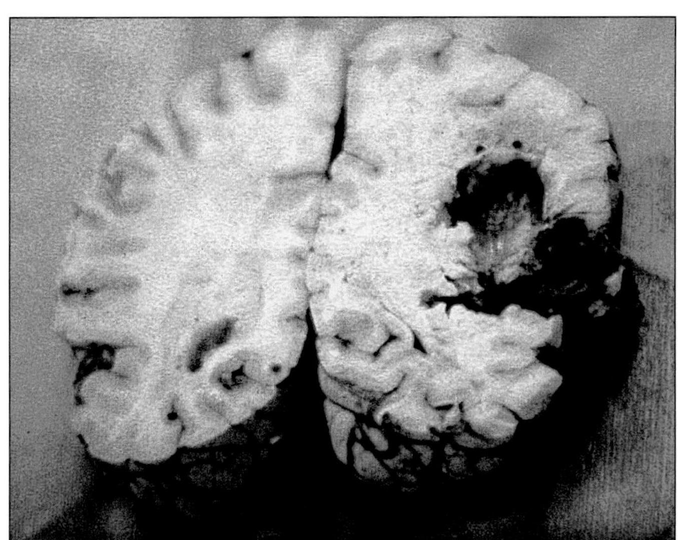

Figure 6.8 A sagittal section of brain, showing necrosis.

Therapy

Once the difficulties involved in diagnosis are overcome, prompt aggressive drug therapy should be considered. Unfortunately, no therapy has been shown to be consistently effective in treating *Balamuthia* infections. A recent report described the successful treatment of two cases. In both patients (one with a cutaneous lesion), the diagnosis was made when the CNS was already involved. Antimicrobial therapy used included fluocytosine, pentamidine, fluconazole, sulfadiazine and a macrolide. Interestingly, phenothiazines were also added in one case to the treatment regimen.[37] Both patients received prolonged oral therapy (up to 5 years). In another recent report, a 72-year-old woman recovered from *Balamuthia* encephalitis after treatment with the regimen described above.[38] Additionally, two of the Peruvian cases with a confirmatory test for *Balamuthia* spp., one with CNS involvement, have also survived after prolonged therapy with albendazole and itraconazole. One of these patients had a very large lesion on the chest wall that was surgically excised as part of her treatment. Thus, surgical excision of the cutaneous lesion, whenever possible, should be considered as a way to reduce the inoculum size.

As more and more cases are reported, this entity should be called to the attention of dermatologists, infectious disease specialists, neurologists, pediatricians, and internists. Cases do occur all over the world, and many diagnoses will be missed unless we have a high index of suspicion. It is very likely that this condition may explain some of the cases previously described as lethal midline granuloma.

References

1. Schuster FL, Dunnebacke TH, Booton GC et al. Environmental isolation of *Balamuthia mandrillaris* associated with a case of amebic encephalitis. J Clin Microbiol 2003; 41:3175–3180.
2. Booton GC, Carmichael JR, Visvesvara GS et al. Genotyping of *Balamuthia mandrillaris* based on nuclear 18S and mitochondrial 16S rRNA genes. Am J Trop Med Hyg 2003; 68:65–69.
3. Visvesvara GS, Stehr-Green JK. Epidemiology of free-living ameba infections. J Protozool 1990; 37:25S–33S.
4. Visvesvara GS, Martinez AJ, Schuster FL et al. Leptomyxid ameba, a new agent of amebic meningoencephalitis in humans and animals. J Clin Microbiol 1990; 28:2750–2756.
5. Visvesvara GS, Schuster FL, Martinez AJ. *Balamuthia mandrillaris*, N. G., N. sp., agent of amebic meningoencephalitis in humans and other animals. J Eukaryot Microbiol 1993; 40:504–514.
6. Schuster FL, Visvesvara GS. Amebic encephalitides and amebic keratitis caused by pathogenic and opportunistic free-living amebas. Curr Treat Options Infect Dis 2003; 5:273–282.
7. Gordon S, Steinberg J, DuPuis MH et al. Culture isolation of *Acanthamoeba* species and Leptomyxid amebas from patients with amebic meningoencephalitis, including two patients with AIDS. Clin Infect Dis 1992; 15:1024–1030.
8. Anzil AP, Rao C, Wrzolek MA et al. Amebic meningoencephalitis in a patient with AIDS caused by a newly recognized opportunistic pathogen. Leptomyxid ameba. Arch Pathol Lab Med 1991; 115:21–25.
9. Bakardjiev A, Azimi PH, Ashouri N et al. Amebic encephalitis caused by *Balamuthia mandrillaris*: report of four cases. Pediatr Infect Dis J 2003; 22:447–453.
10. Schuster FL, Glaser C, Honarmand S et al. *Balamuthia* amebic encephalitis risk, Hispanic Americans (letter). Emerg Infect Dis 2004; August. Available online at http://www.cdc.gov/ncidod/EID/vol10no8/04-0139.htm.
11. Huang ZH, Ferrante A, Carter RF. Serum antibodies to *Balamuthia mandrillaris*, a free living ameba recently demonstrated to cause granulomatous amoebic encephalitis. J Infect Dis 1999; 179:1305–1308.
12. Reed RP, Cooke-Yarborough CM, Jaquiery AL et al. Fatal granulomatous amoebic encephalitis caused by *Balamuthia mandrillaris*. Med J Aust 1997; 167:82–84.
13. Kodet R, Nohynkova E, Tichy M et al. Amebic encephalitis caused by *Balamuthia mandrillaris* in a Czech child: description of the first case from Europe. Pathol Res Pract 1998; 194:423–430.
14. Sangruchi T, Martinez AJ, Vivesvara GS. Spontaneous granulomatous amebic encephalitis : report of four cases from Thailand. Southeast Asian J Trop Med Public Health 1994; 25:309–313.
15. Shirabe T, Monobe Y, Visvesvara GS. An autopsy case of amebic meningoencephalitis. The first Japanese case caused by *Balamuthia mandrillaris*. Neuropathology 2002; 22:213–217.
16. Campos P, Cabrera J, Gotuzzo E et al. [Neurological involvement in free living amebiasis.] Rev Neurol 1999; 29:316–318.
17. Recavarren-Arce S, Verlarde C, Gotuzzo E et al. Amoeba angeitic lesions of the central nervous system in *Balamuthia mandrillaris* amoebiasis. Hum Pathol 1999; 30:269–273.
18. Galarza C, Larrea P, Kumakawa H. Amebiasis cutánea de vida libre. Primer caso reportado en el Hospital Dos de Mayo, Lima, Perú. Dermatol Peruana 1997; 7:65–69.
19. Ballona R, Aquije M. Compromiso cutáneo en encefalitis granulomatosa amebiana fatal causada por *Balamuthia mandrillaris*. Folia Dermatol Peruana 2003; 14:28–30.
20. Taratuto AL, Monges J, Acefe JC et al. Leptomyxid amoeba encephalitis: report of the first case in Argentina. Trans R Soc Trop Med Hyg 1991; 85:77.
21. Galarza M, Cuccia V, Sosa FP et al. Pediatric granulomatous cerebral amebiasis: a delayed diagnosis. Pediatr Neurol 2002; 26:153–156.
22. Martinez AJ, Guerra AE, Garcia-Tamayo J et al. Granulomatous amebic encephalitis: a review and report of a spontaneous case from Venezuela. Acta Neuropathol 1994; 87:430–434.
23. Gonzalez-Alfonzo JE, Martinez AJ, Garcia V et al. Granulomatous encephalitis due to a leptomyxid amoeba. Trans R Soc Trop Med Hyg 1991; 85:480.
24. Riestra-Castaneda JM, Riestra-Castaneda R, Gonzalez-Garrido AA et al. Granulomatous amebic encephalitis due to *Balamuthia mandrillaris* (Leptomyxiidae): report of four cases from Mexico. Am J Trop Med Hyg 1997; 56:603–607.
25. Chimelli L, Hahn MD, Scaravilli F et al. Granulomatous amoebic encephalitis due to leptomyxid amoebae: report of the first Brazilian case. Trans R Soc Trop Med Hyg 1992; 86:635.
26. Schuster FL. Cultivation of pathogenic and opportunistic free-living amebas. Clin Microbiol Rev 2002; 15:342–354.
27. Schuster FL, Visvesvara GS. Axenic growth and drug sensitivity studies of *Balamuthia mandrillaris*, an agent of amebic meningoencephalitis in humans and other animals. J Clin Microbiol 1996; 34:385–388.
28. Booton GC, Schuster FL, Carmichael JR et al. *Balamuthia mandrillaris*: identification of clinical and environmental isolates using genus-specific PCR. J Eukaryot Microbiol 2003; 50 (suppl.):508–509.
29. Deol I, Robledo L, Meza A et al. Encephalitis caused by free-living amoeba *Balamuthia mandrillaris*: case report with literature review. Surg Neurol 2000; 53:611–616.
30. Rowen JL, Doerr CA, Vogel H et al. *Balamuthia mandrillaris*: a newly recognized agent for amebic meningoencephalitis. Pediatr Infect Dis J 1995; 14:705–710.
31. Gotuzzo E, Bravo F, Cabrera J. Amebas de vida livre – enfase na infeccao por *Balamuthia mandrillaris*. In: Cimerman S, Cimerman B, eds. Medicina tropical. São Paulo, Brazil: Atheneu; 2003:59–64.
32. Griesemer DA, Barton LL, Reese CM et al. Amebic meningoencephalitis caused by *Balamuthia mandrillaris*. Pediatr Neurol 1994; 10:249–254.

33. Denney CF, Iragui VJ, Uber-Zak LD et al. Amebic meningoencephalitis caused by *Balamuthia mandrillaris*: case report and review. Clin Infect Dis 1997; 25:1354–1358.
34. Pritzker AS, Kim BK, Agrawal D et al. Fatal granulomatous amebic encephalitis caused by *Balamuthia mandrillaris* presenting as a skin lesion. J Am Acad Dermatol 2004; 50 (suppl.): 38–41.
35. Martinez AJ, Visvesvara GS. *Balamuthia mandrillaris* infection. J Med Microbiol 2001; 50:205–207.
36. Schuster FL, Glaser C, Honarmand S et al. Testing for *Balamuthia* amebic encephalitis by indirect immunofluorescence. In: Lares-Villa F, Booton GC, Marciano-Cabral F, eds. Proceedings of Xth international meeting on the biology and pathogenicity of free-living amebas. Ciudad Obregon, Mexico: ITSON DIEP; 2003: 173–178.
37. Deetz TR, Sawyer MH, Billman G et al. Successful treatment of *Balamuthia* amoebic encephalitis: presentation of 2 cases. Clin Infect Dis 2003; 37:1304–1312.
38. Jung S, Schelper RL, Visvesvara GS et al. *Balamuthia mandrillaris* meningoencephalitis in an immunocompetent patient: an unusual clinical course and a favorable outcome. Arch Pathol Lab Med 2004; 128:466–468.

Chapter 7

Nematodal helminths

- Filariasis ▪ *Sam Kalungi and Lynnette K. Tumwine*
- Onchocerciasis ▪ *Wingfield Rehmus and Josephine Nguyen*
- Loiasis ▪ *Francis T. Assimwe and Ulrich R. Hengge*

Filariasis

Sam Kalungi and Lynnette K. Tumwine

Synonyms:

- *Wuchereria bancrofti:* wuchereriasis, and Bancroft's filariasis
- *Loa loa: loiasis*
- *Onchocerca volvulus:* blinding filarial disease, Roble's disease, craw-craw, river blindness, and gale filarienne
- *Brugia timori*
- *Mansonella ozzardi:* Ozzard's filariasis, mansoneliasis ozzardi
- *Mansonella steptocerca*
- *Brugia malayi: Wuchereria malayi, Microfilaria malayi, Filaria malayi*
- Dirofilariasis

Key features:

- The filariases result from infection with insect-vector-borne tissue-dwelling nematodes. This group of nematodes is characterized by having a microfilaria stage of development between the egg and the fully developed larva
- Depending on the species, adult filariae may live in the lymphatics, blood vessels, skin, connective tissues, or serous membranes
- The females produce larvae (microfilariae) which live in the blood stream or skin
- All true filariae infecting humans are transmitted by dipteran vectors
- A few species of animal filariae may accidentally infect humans
- The transmission of human filariae is confined to warm climates: a high temperature is necessary for the parasites to develop in the vectors

Introduction

The filariases are an important aspect of dermatologic medicine because the skin is one of the commonly affected organs. Filariases which affect the skin include *Wuchereria bancrofti*, *Brugia malayi*, *Loa loa*, and *Onchocerca volvulus*.

The subcutaneous filariases lead to severe skin itch, papules, and scratch marks. Later the whole skin becomes dry and thickened. Skin hypo-, hyper-, and depigmentation may occur. Nodules may be formed.

The lymphatic filariases lead to lymphedema of the extremities, the vulva, scrotum, arms, and breasts. The legs often have a warty appearance with folds and cracks. Lymphatic filariasis is a disfiguring, disabling disease which makes life difficult. The physical consequences are pain, ugly swollen limbs, and bad-smelling skin. Life becomes difficult and simple actions like walking and working become impossible. The more the disease progresses, the more sufferers are shunned by society[1–3] (Fig. 7.1).

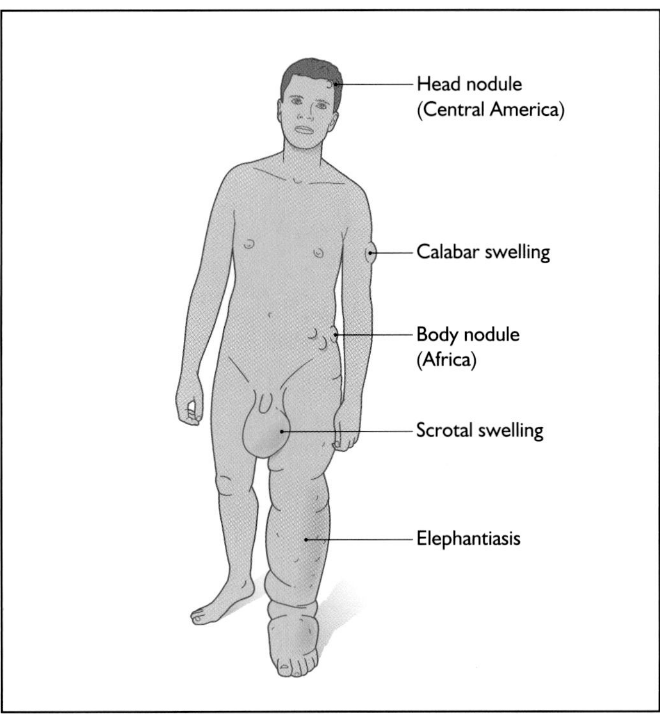

Figure 7.1 Cutaneous manifestations of nematodal infections. (Courtesy of Dr. Daniel Conner.)

History

Filariasis has been a worldwide scourge of civilization for thousands of years. It was depicted on the pharaonic murals of Egypt and in the ancient medical texts of China, India, Japan, and Persia. Elephantiasis and hydrocele were first associated with parasitic filarial worms and their mosquito vectors in the late nineteenth century by French, English, and Australian physicians working with patients from Cuba, Brazil, China, and India. Lichenstein and Brug were the first to observe and describe the microfilaria of *B. malayi*. Macfie and Corson first identified microfilaria of *Dirofilaria streptocerca* in the skin of Ghanaians in 1922. *Mansonella ozzardi* was first described in 1897 by Manson.[4,5]

Epidemiology

Filariasis is only common in some tropical, coastal, and island areas of Africa, Asia, the Pacific, and the Americas. The prevalence of filariasis varies in the endemic communities. The disease has been observed in individuals aged 10 years and above. Men are equally affected as women.[6]

Lymphatic filariasis, also known as elephantiasis and caused by *W. bancrofti* and *B. malayi*, now puts at risk more than a billion people in at least 80 countries. More than 120 million people are affected by lymphatic filariasis. One-third of those infected live in India, another third in Africa, and most of the remainder in South Asia, the Pacific, and the Americas. *B. malayi* is confined to Asia.

Infection by *Loa loa* is limited to West and Central Africa. *Onchocerca volvulus* is endemic in sub-Saharan Africa, Central and northern South America, and in Yemen. In endemic areas the infection occurs throughout life.[7,8]

Globally, the infection has been recognized as the second leading cause of permanent and long-term disability. The deforming, mutilating disease of the limbs and genitals results not only in physical crippling but also in serious psychosocial consequences.

Transmission of *W. bancrofti* is by mosquitoes of the genera *Culex*, *Aedes*, and *Anopheles*, while the vectors for *B. malayi* are mosquitoes of the genera *Aedes*, *Anopheles*, and *Mansonia*. *Loa loa* is transmitted by species of flies of the genus *Chrysops* and *O. volvulus* by species of black flies of the genus *Simulium*.[9]

Pathogenesis and etiology

Attacks of acute lymphangitis caused by filariae cause acute inflammation of part of a limb, joint, or a testicle.

Filarial worms cause a wide variety of clinical pathologies depending on the degree of host immune reaction to adults and microfilariae. In endemic zones for filariasis, studies of cellular and humoral immunity show near-universal seropositivity, indicating prior infection.

In lymphatic filariasis specific immunoglobulin E (IgE) titers are highest in people with tropical eosinophilia, lower in those with chronic lymphedema, and lowest in normal persons in endemic areas and those with asymptomatic microfilaremia. Conversely, asymptomatics have higher IgG titers to filarial antigens than symptomatic patients.

Most people in endemic areas are asymptomatic, probably because of the tolerance induced in utero.

Children of seropositive mothers have cord blood with IgE antifilarial antibodies. This reflects prenatal sensitization since IgE does not cross the placenta.[10,11]

The major filariases – lymphatic filariasis caused by *W. bancrofti* and *B. malayi*, loiasis due to *L. loa*, and onchocerciasis due to *O. volvulus* – are solely human infections but dirofilariasis is zoonotic.

Life cycle and morphology[1]

The filarial worms are transmitted by a variety of blood-sucking insects to humans (see Table 7.1). The life cycle of the parasites is depicted in Figure 7.2.

Pathology

The pathology of filariases results from the presence of adult worms in the tissues. In lymphatic filariasis the adult worms live in lymphatic vessels, mostly of the lymph nodes, pelvis, epididymis, and spermatic cord, and these adult worms cause the most significant lesions.[10,12]

They release microfilariae into the lymph and they circulate in the blood stream with periodicity; the highest densities occur around midnight, coinciding with the time the vector will bite the host. Periodicity may also coincide with the sleeping and waking of the definitive host. It has been shown that the flow of chyle is greatest during sleep, possibly accounting for the surge of microfilariae into the blood at this time.

The periodicity may also depend on the cyclic parturition of the female worm.

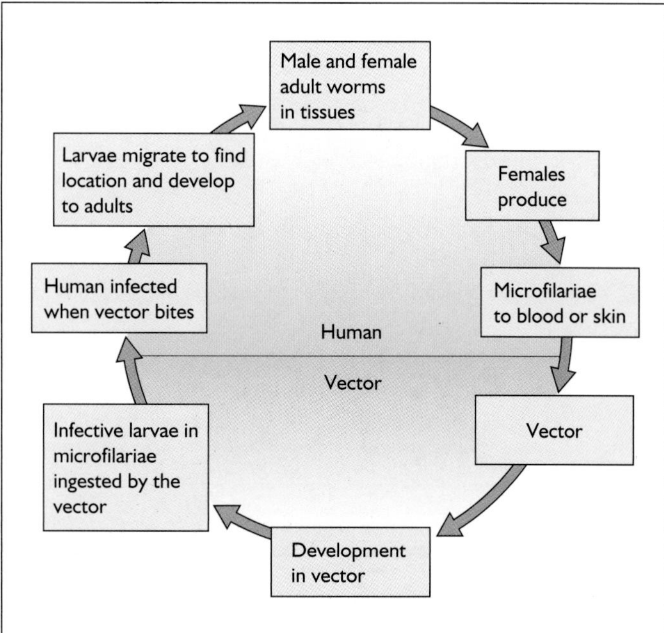

Figure 7.2 The life cycle of *nematodal helminths*. (Adapted from *Encyclopedia Brittanica* by Joanna Chan.)

Table 7.1 Characteristics of microfilaria and the geographical distribution[13]

Species	*Wuchereria bancrofti*	*Brugia malayi*	*Brugia timori*	*Loa loa*	*Mansonella ozzardi*	*Mansonella perstans*	*Mansonella streptocerca*	*Onchocerca volvulus*
Geographical distribution	Tropics and subtropics, worldwide	S.E. Asia, Indian subcontinent	Indian Archipelago, Timor	West and Central Africa	Caribbean, Central and South America	Africa and South America	West and Central Africa	Africa, Yemen and Central and South America
Vectors	Mosquitoes: *Culex, Aedes, Anopheles, Mansonia*	Mosquitoes: *Mansonia, Anopheles, Aedes*	Mosquitoes: *Anopheles*	Tabanid flies: *Chrysops*	Biting midges: *Culicoides* Black flies: *Simulium*	Biting midges: *Culicoides*	Biting midges: *Culicoides*	Black flies
Adult habitat	Lymphatic system	Lymphatic system	Lymphatic system	Subcutaneous tissues, conjunctiva	Subcutaneous tissues	Mesenteric connective tissues of the abdominal organs	Dermis	Subcutaneous
Habit of microfilaria	Blood	Blood	Blood	Blood	Blood	Blood	Skin	Skin
Periodicity	Nocturnal	Nocturnal	Nocturnal	Diurnal	Aperiodic	Aperiodic	–	–
Sheath	Present	Present	Present	Present	Absent	Absent	Absent	Absent
Key features of microfilariae	Short head space; dispersed nuclei; sheath unstained in Giemsa; body in smooth curves	Long head space; sheath stained pink in Giemsa; terminal and subterminal nuclei	Long head space; sheath unstained in Giemsa; terminal and subterminal nuclei	Single row of nuclei to hooked tail filled end of tail; sheath unstained in Giemsa	Small size; long slender tail; aperiodic	Small size; blunt tail filled with nuclei; aperiodic	Slender shape; hooked tail filled with nuclei; occurs in skin	

Initially the worms cause only dilatation of the lymphatic vessels, leading to a thickened vessel endothelial lining, a chronic inflammatory infiltrate consisting of lymphocytes, plasma cells, and eosinophils adjacent to the worm or in the surrounding tissues. A granulomatous reaction occurs, leading to necrosis, degeneration of the worms, fibrosis, and obliteration of the lymphatics, and ultimately causing gross lymphedema (Fig. 7.3).[14,15]

In loiasis, the migration of the adult worm through the dermis or subcutis elicits an eosinophil reaction and edema. There is also dermal fibrosis.

In onchocerciasis, the pathology is due to the host's reaction to microfilariae in the dermis. There is increased dermal edema, perivascular inflammation, and small eosinophil abscesses around the degenerating microfilaria.[5,10]

Clinical features

- In endemic zones the exposure is universal, yet most people are asymptomatic.
- Another common pattern is when individuals are asymptomatic, antibody-positive, and have microfilaremia.
- Patients with acute lymphatic filariasis present with recurring malaise, fever, lymphadenitis, and perilymphadenitis.
- Patients with lymphatic chronic obstructive pathology present with either hydrocele or elephantiasis. The arm, breast, scrotum, or vulva may be involved, and there may be chyluria.
- A small proportion of patients have tropical eosinophilia.
- Patients with *L. loa* may present with swellings known as Calabar or fugitive swellings on any part of the body.
- Dead worms (within nerves) may cause neurological deficits, including parasthesiae or paralysis.
- Itching and scratching are often the first manifestations of onchocerciasis, followed by altered pigmentation. Patients may also present with wrinkling, papules, edema, and a skin that appears like a leopard's or lizard's skin.
- Tumors may also be formed over bony prominences.[1,3,10,11]

Patient evaluation, diagnosis, and differential diagnosis

Patient evaluation

Take a thorough history and examination of the patient.

Most patients present late with features of chronic infection, having acquired the infection a year or so earlier. Clinical manifestations include woody edema, which involves the lower extremities or the genitalia. The upper limbs and mammary glands of women are the next common site. Some patients with elephantiasis develop a crusty, warty skin over the lower extremities and this is called mossy foot.

In the skin, onchocerciasis leads to severe itch as a major presenting complaint. Later the whole skin becomes thickened, dry, and lichenified. There is loss of elasticity (hanging groins, see Fig.7.4).

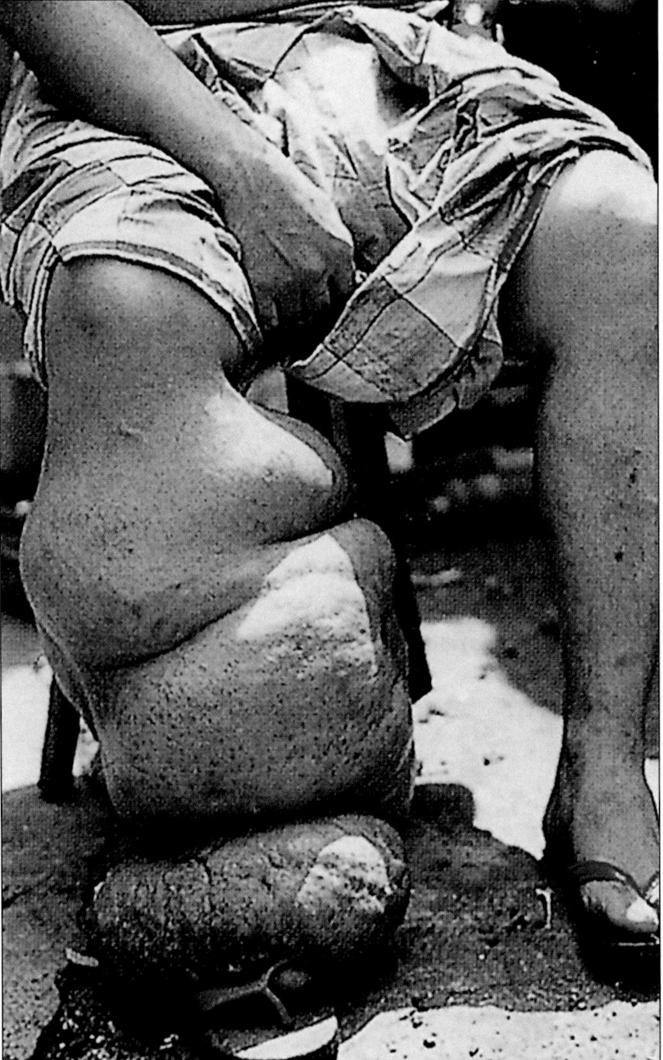

Figure 7.3 Massive elephantiasis due to *Brugia malayi*. (Reproduced from Peters W and Pasvol G (eds). Tropical Medicine annd Parasitology, 5th edition, Mosby, London 2002.)

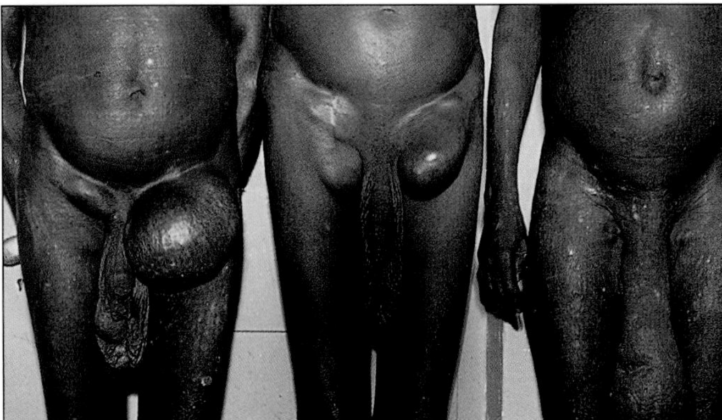

Figure 7.4 Hanging groin and scrotal elephantiasis due to onchocerciasis. (Reproduced from Peters W and Pasvol G (eds). Tropical Medicine annd Parasitology, 5th edition, Mosby, London 2002.)

Onchonodules and tumors can be seen and palpated, in particular above the hip bones, but also elsewhere.

In loiasis an adult worm migrating beneath the conjunctiva or below the skin may be the first indication of infection. Calabar swellings may develop in any portion of the skin but are more frequently seen around the wrists and ankles. Onset is sudden but the swellings regress gradually.

Diagnosis[13]

Microfilariae are found in the blood and skin but they can also be found in bone marrow preparations, cervical smears, urine, fine-needle aspirates, and hydrocele fluid.

Blood examination

The tests here include:

- Stained thick blood films for identification of microfilariae: stains used include Giemsa and hematoxylin.
- Capillary blood examination for the presence of microfilariae.

Skin snips

Skin snips are taken to detect microfilariae of *Onchocerca volvulus* and *Mansonella streptocerca* that reside in the skin (see Onchocerciasis, Patient evaluation, diagnosis, and differential diagnosis, below, for further details).

Urine and hydrocele fluid

The centrifuged sediment is examined for microfilariae. Slides can be stained or fixed.

Other diagnostic methods

- The microhematocrit method is useful for the diagnosis of filarial infections when the numbers of microfilariae are too small.
- Quantitative buffy coat is used as a rapid diagnostic test to detect microfilariae.
- Microfilaria counts.

Differential diagnosis[11, 16, 17]

- Acute bacterial lymphangitis: it spreads centripetally from the periphery towards the lymph glands.
- Chronic infective lymphadenitis (bacterial): patients present with fever and other constitutional symptoms of the associated disease.
- Primary and secondary tumors of the lymph glands: patients present with marked weight loss, recurrent fever, and other constitutional signs related to the tumor, e.g., lymphedema carcinomatosa following breast cancer.
- Other obstructive disorders of the veins and lymphatics: initially the edema is pitting with distinct venodilatation, and ulceration may occur.
- Chronic chemical lymphadenitis: this may occur in elevated areas where there is no filariasis and it is confined to the lower limbs. Lymphangiography shows distorted lymphatic channels.
- Tuberculous lymphadenitis: this is differentiated by constitutional symptoms related to tuberculosis.
- Endemic Kaposi's sarcoma: there are distinct skin nodules on the affected lower limb. It usually occurs in middle-aged or elderly men.

- Maduramycosis: only the foot is usually affected with multiple discharging sinuses.
- Congenital hydrocele: the patient has a thickened tunica vaginalis; the scrotal swelling begins shortly after birth. These hydroceles transilluminate light.
- Hernias: they have a cough impulse.
- Milroy's disease: this is a congenital absence or insufficiency of the lymphatic channels found mostly in young women in temperate countries.
- Differential diagnosis of onchocerciasis includes scabies in which lesions are typically found in the interdigital spaces and the buttocks. It may also resemble superficial fungal infections, leprosy, and skin changes due to long-standing eczema.
- Differential diagnosis of loiasis includes swellings produced by other migrating parasites and guinea worm. *L. loa* may also present with ocular manifestations.

Treatment

Treatment depends on the stage and severity of the disease.

Acute lymphangitis or lymphadenitis

- Rest the patient and elevate the affected part.
- Add dressings if needed.
- Give aspirin 500 mg 4–6-hourly.
- Prescribe antihistamines, e.g., promethazine 25 mg 1–3 times daily.
- Consider antibiotics such as penicillin since the cause also may be bacterial.
- Note: Do not give diethylcarbamazine until the acute stage is over.

Chronic stages

Lymphatic filariasis

- Keep clean and manage intercurrent infections.
- Do excisions to improve lymphatic flow.
- Lymph massage, intermittent compression, elastic compression bandages and stockings or laced boots may be helpful.
- Give diethylcarbamazine 50 mg/kg three times a day for 3 weeks. If there are still microfilariae on the slide after this period, repeat the cycle.
- Administer ivermectin 12 mg plus albendazole 400 mg in a single dose for adults (see onchocerciasis, below). This will kill microfilariae but not the adult worms that have died of old age (3–4 years).
- Give yearly albendazole for 3–4 years.

Onchocerciasis

- Treat secondary infection with antiseptics or antibiotics as impetigo and secondary lichenified eczema as lichen simplex.
- Give diethylcarbamazine orally.
- Give suramin intravenously weekly.
- Administer ivermectin.
- Give mebendazole or levamisole.

Loiasis

- Give diethylcarbamazine.
- Give mebendazole.

References

1. Brown HW, Neva FA. Blood and tissue nematodes of human beings. In: Brown HW, Neva FA, eds. Basic clinical parasitology. CT: Appleton-Century-Crofts; 1983:143–167.
2. Ufomadu GO, Akpa AU, Ekejindu IM. Human onchocerciasis in the lower Jos plateau, central Nigeria: the prevalence, geographical distribution and epidemiology in Akwanga and Lafia local government areas. Ann Trop Med Parasitol 1993; 87:107.
3. World Health Organization. Stop filariasis now. Lymphatic filariasis elimination programme. WHO/CDS/CPE/CEE/ 2001.2b. Geneva: WHO; 2001.
4. Meyers WM, Neafie CR, Connor HD. Bancroftian and Malayan filariasis. In: Chapman HB, Daniel HC, eds. Pathology of tropical and extraordinary diseases. Washington, DC: Armed Forces Institute of Pathology; 1976:340–352.
5. Grove DI. A history of human helminthology. London: CAB International; 1990:597–640.
6. Onapa AW, Simonsen PE, Erling PM et al. Lymphatic filariasis in Uganda: baseline investigations in Lira, Soroti and Katakwi districts. Trans R Soc Trop Med Hyg; 2001:95:161–167.
7. World Health Organization. Lymphatic filariasis. International task force on disease eradication. WHO/CDS/CPE/CEE/ 2000.2. Geneva: WHO; 2000.
8. Yumbe MJ, Sole N, Capote R et al. Prevalence, geographical distribution and clinical manifestations of onchocerciasis on the island of Bioko (Equatorial Guinea). Trop Med Parasitol 1995; 46:13–18.
9. Manson-Barr PEC, Bell DR. Filariais. In: Manson-Barr PEC, Bell DR, eds. Manson's tropical diseases, 19th edn. London: Churchill Livingstone; 1991:353–403.
10. Lucas S. Pathology of tropical infections. In: Mcgee JO'D, Isaacson P, Wright AN, eds. Oxford textbook of pathology. New York: Oxford University Press; 1992:2239–2247.
11. Schull RC. Disorders of the lymphatic system and spleen. In: Common medical problems in the tropics. London: Macmillan Education; 1987:196.
12. Ash JE, Spitz S. Pathology of tropical diseases, an atlas. Philadelphia, PA: WB Saunders; 1945.
13. World Health Organization. Bench aids for the diagnosis of filarial infections. Geneva: WHO; 1997.
14. Ufomadu GO, Akpa AU, Ekejindu IM. Human onchocerciasis in the lower Jos plateau, central Nigeria: the prevalence, geographical distribution and epidemiology in Akwanga and Lafia local government areas. Ann Trop Med Parasitol 1992; 86:637–647.
15. Lucas SB. Diseases caused by parasitic protozoa and metazoa. In: MacSween RNM, Whaley K, eds. Muir's textbook of pathology. New York: Oxford University Press; 1995.
16. Gottlieb JG, Ackerman BA. Atlas of the gross and microscopic features of simulators. In: Kaposi's sarcoma: a text and atlas. Philadelphia, PA: Lea & Febiger; 1998:73–110.
17. Onapa WA, Simonsen PE, Pedersen ME. Non-filarial elephantiasis in the Mount Elgon area (Kapchorwa district) of Uganda. Acta Trop 2001; 78:171–176.

Onchocerciasis

Wingfield Rehmus and Josephine Nguyen

Synonyms: Onchocerciasis, African river blindness, blinding filariasis, craw-craw, sowda

Key features:

- Onchocerciasis affects 18 million individuals worldwide, primarily in Africa
- It is the second leading infectious cause of blindness
- Major dermatologic manifestations include subcutaneous nodules, onchocercal dermatitis, depigmentation, and lymphadenitis
- It has a large socioeconomic impact both by lost productivity due to associated blindness and pruritus and by human migration to avoid infection
- Onchocerciasis control campaigns have limited the public health impact of the disease through coordinated efforts of the World Health Organization, World Bank, non-governmental organizations, governments, and pharmaceutical companies

Introduction

Onchocerciasis is a filarial disease caused by the parasite *Onchocerca volvulus*, which affects 18 million people worldwide. It is the second leading infectious cause of blindness and causes significant morbidity and loss of productivity also due to severe itching. The skin lesions are wide-ranging, varying from a pruritic morbilliform eruption to extensive, degenerative skin changes. Recent research demonstrates that the people of highly endemic communities consider onchocerciasis, especially the unrelenting pruritus, to be among their main health problems. For many years, the skin lesions of onchocerciasis were thought to be of minor consequence compared to its associated eye disease, but the dermatologic aspects of the disease have been found to have major adverse psychosocial and socioeconomic effects as well.

Since 1975, efforts have been aimed at controlling the disease and blocking its transmission though vector-control strategies and, later, through widespread distribution of the antimicrofilarial drug ivermectin. Although these efforts have been able to eliminate onchocerciasis as a major public health problem, eradication has remained an elusive goal. New data, suggesting the coexistence of endosymbiotic bacteria and their role in the etiology of symptoms, offer hope that new treatment strategies may be able to move control efforts one step closer to elimination of the disease.[1]

History

In 1875, John O'Neill in Ghana first reported the presence of *O. volvulus* microfilariae in a case of "craw-craw," a common West African name for onchocerciasis. Fifty years later in Sierra Leone, D.B. Blacklock officially declared the vector to be the black fly, *Simulium*, although the residents of endemic communities had long associated the skin lesions and subsequent blindness with the bite of the fly.[2]

Epidemiology

Onchocerciasis is endemic in 36 countries. Twenty-nine of these are in sub-Saharan Africa, which is a broad band across central Africa. The remaining seven countries have small endemic foci and are located on the Arabian peninsula (Yemen) and in Latin America (Brazil, Colombia, Ecuador, Guatemala, Mexico, and Venezuela).

Eighteen million people, 99% of whom live in Africa, are infected with *O. volvulus* and have dermal microfilariae. Of those infected with the disease, over 6.5 million suffer from severe itching or dermatitis, 270 000 are blind, and another 500 000 suffer from visual impairment. Although blindness is often the primary concern, onchocercal skin disease can also have devastating consequences. Research has found that the socioeconomic impact of skin disease, when measured in terms of disability-adjusted life years, is as great as the burden of blindness. Severe itching has been found to cause both a significant decrease in productivity in those affected and an elevated school drop-out rate in their children.[3]

Onchocerciasis can affect all individuals irrespective of age or gender; however, it is more common in males than in females. It is transmitted by the black fly, *Simulium*, which breeds in rapidly flowing waters, and transmission is most intense in river valleys due to the higher concentration of vectors. These river valleys are often in rural areas that tend to be remote with few resources and little access to health care. In some fertile river valleys, community blindness rates have reached 30%. Fear of blindness has led to such depopulation that socioeconomic development in these regions has been impaired as residents move to regions that are far less fertile.[4] Additionally, deforestation has increased the vector population in many areas, adding to the burden of disease.[2] Despite the localization in remote, poor regions with limited health care, control programs have been able to diminish the public health impact of the disease significantly.

Pathogenesis and etiology

Onchocerciasis is a parasitic infection caused by the filarial nematode, *O. volvulus*, for which humans are the only known reservoir. Black flies of the genus *Simulium* (Fig. 7.5) are the only vectors of *O. volvulus*; however, there are many different species of black flies that can transmit onchocerciasis, and these vary by terrain and geographical distribution (*S. damnosum* in Africa and *S. ochraceum*, among others, in the Americas).

Black fly eggs are laid in the water of fast-flowing rivers, with adult flies emerging after 8–12 days. The flies live for up to 4 weeks and can travel hundreds of kilometers during their life span in wind currents. After mating, the female black fly seeks a blood meal. Ingestion of blood from an infected person allows the microfilariae to enter the gut. The ingested microfilariae differentiate and then molt during the next 6–12 days before moving to the insect's mouth, where they remain until a second blood meal allows them to enter a new human host. The injected larvae migrate to the human's subcutaneous tissue and congregate into nodules, called onchocercomas, where they slowly mature into adult worms (macrofilariae).[2]

The adult female macrofilaria grows to be 30–80 cm in length and remains in these nodules for the remainder of its life. Smaller

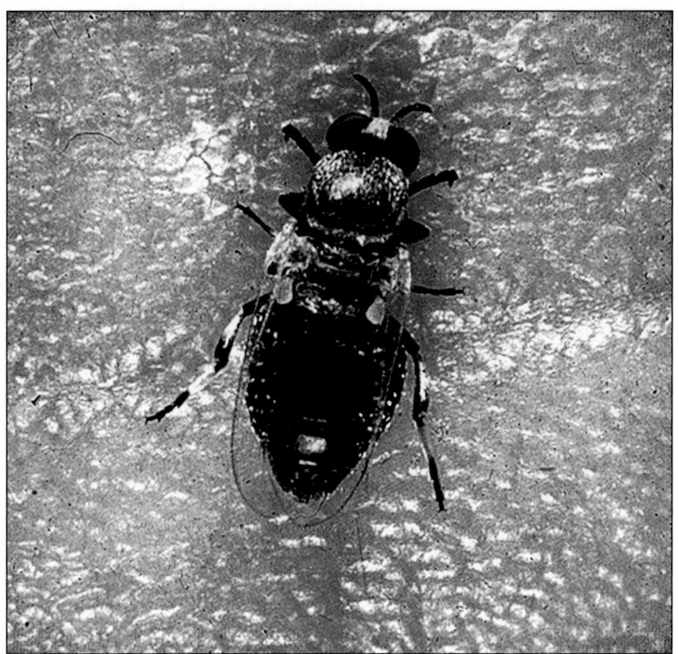

Figure 7.5 A female simulium black fly and an erythematous bite reaction. (Courtesy of Dr. Daniel Conner.)

male worms migrate between nodules to mate. After mating, the eggs develop into microfilariae within the female worm and leave the worm at the rate of approximately 1300–1900 microfilariae per day. Each microfilaria lives for approximately 2 years and never reaches a size greater than several tenths of a micrometer. Microfilariae migrate through the body, awaiting ingestion by a black fly for further development. The majority die without completing their life cycle (Fig. 7.6).

Clinical symptoms can be attributed to the presence of the adult worms in skin nodules, to the migration of microfilariae throughout the body, and to an intense inflammatory response to dead microfilariae. Recent evidence has also shown that endosymbiotic bacteria, *Wolbachia*, may be responsible for much of this inflammation. *Wolbachia* is an essential symbiont of O. *volvulus*. Extracts from worms that have been treated so that they do not harbor *Wolbachia* have been found to evoke minimal immune stimulation. The inflammatory response has been found to be mediated by induction of chemotactic cytokines by functional Toll-like receptor 4 on host cells and may be initiated by release of *Wolbachia* endotoxin-like substances upon the death of the microfilariae.[5]

Clinical features

Multiple chronic, systemic, and localized manifestations may occur in patients suffering from onchocerciasis, including weight loss and growth arrest in addition to the more classic dermatologic and ophthalmologic symptoms. Manifestations typically appear approximately 1–3 years after the bite of the black fly and have been shown to vary by geographic location. For example, blindness is not a common complication in all areas.[6]

The cutaneous changes caused by infection with O. *volvulus* are well-documented and account for significant morbidity caused by

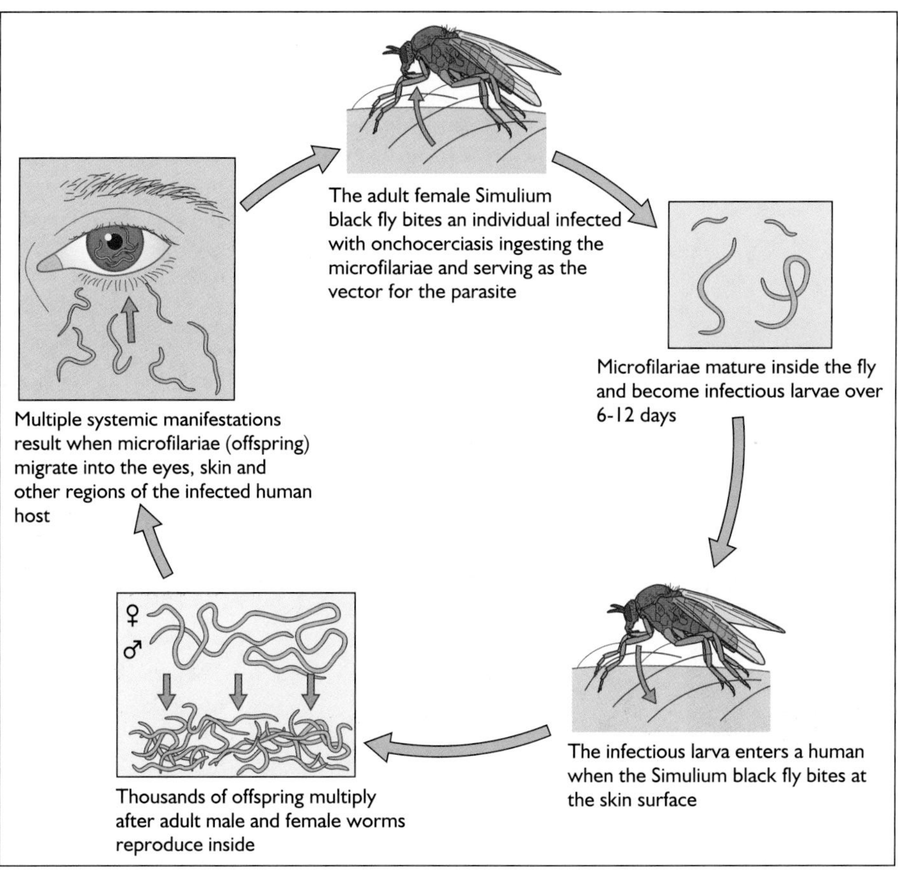

The adult female Simulium black fly bites an individual infected with onchocerciasis ingesting the microfilariae and serving as the vector for the parasite
Microfilariae mature inside the fly and become infectious larvae over 6-12 days
The infectious larva enters a human when the Simulium black fly bites at the skin surface
Thousands of offspring multiply after adult male and female worms reproduce inside
Multiple systemic manifestations result when microfilariae (offspring) migrate into the eyes, skin and other regions of the infected human host
♀
♂

Figure 7.6 Life cycle of *Onchocerca volvulus*. Adapted from Encyclopedia Brittanica by Joanna Chan.

the infection. In addition to causing intense pruritus, onchocercal dermatitis is also causally associated with insomnia, fatigue, and low self-esteem.[7]

A classification scheme for documenting skin disease was developed by Murdoch et al. in 1993[8] to aid in the definition of skin findings and the quantification of the burden of skin disease. Five main categories of skin disease exist:

1. Acute papular onchodermatitis (APOD) consists of pruritic papules that may progress to vesicles or pustules and that is widely distributed. APOD may be associated with erythema or edema. The lesions are most commonly located on the upper extremities or trunk and may be transient.
2. Chronic papular onchodermatitis (CPOD) is characterized by 3–9-mm flat-topped papules, which may have associated pruritus and are often hyperpigmented. These lesions are typically scattered over the buttocks, waist area, and shoulders, and may be accompanied by acute lesions elsewhere (Fig. 7.7).
3. Lichenified onchodermatitis (LOD) is seen most commonly in young patients and tends to be found more often in Yemen than in other geographic areas. In LOD, pruritus is severe and often asymmetrical. Hyperpigmented, lichenified plaques develop, and lymph nodes in the affected region are often enlarged. When a single limb is involved, the condition may be referred to as "sowda".
4. Atrophy (ATR) caused by onchocerciasis often mimics the normal effects of aging, such as loss of elasticity, leaving the skin wrinkled in appearance. It is most frequently noted on the buttocks and may be associated with decreased sweating or hair growth.
5. Depigmentation (DPM) can be seen in infected individuals on the anterior tibialis in large patches, often referred to as "leopard skin". Pigment loss is complete within the patch, except for perifollicular islands of retained normal pigmentation. Depigmented lesions are occasionally pruritic. They can be found on the abdomen or lateral groin in addition to their classic location on the shins[8] (Fig. 7.8).

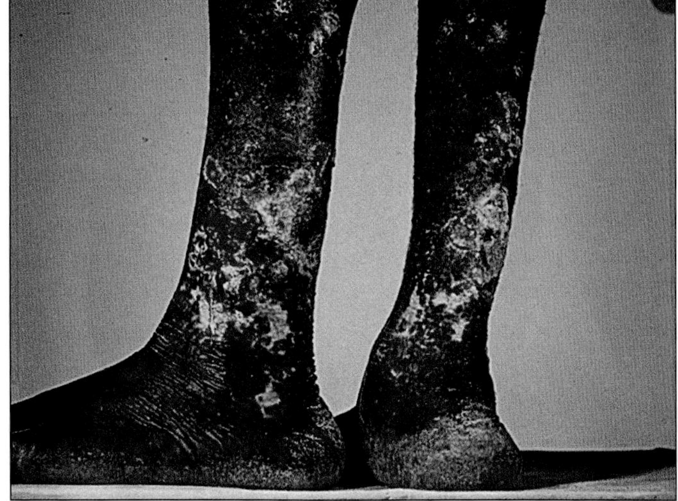

Figure 7.8 Depigmentation caused by onchodermatitis is frequently located on the lower legs. (Courtesy of Dr. Daniel Conner.)

Other dermatologic manifestations may exist in conjunction with these five main categories of skin disease. The onchocercoma is a firm, painless, freely mobile subcutaneous nodule, often located over a bony prominence. It is comprised of 2–3 adult worms surrounded by a thick fibrous coat and ranges in size from 2 to 10 cm (Fig. 7.9)[9]. The distribution of the onchocercoma varies with geographic distribution: in Africa, lesions are found throughout the body, while in the Americas they are more typically isolated to the scalp.[10] Onchocercomas may be particularly palpable when the burden of disease is high and when lesions are located over bony prominences; however, they may also be clinically indistinct.

"Hanging groin" refers to increased inelasticity in the region of the inguinal fold. Lymphadenitis occurs when lymph nodes that drain the areas of involvement become enlarged. After years of infection, degenerative skin changes occur and the skin begins to sag, giving a hanging appearance to the skin (Fig. 7.10). Hanging

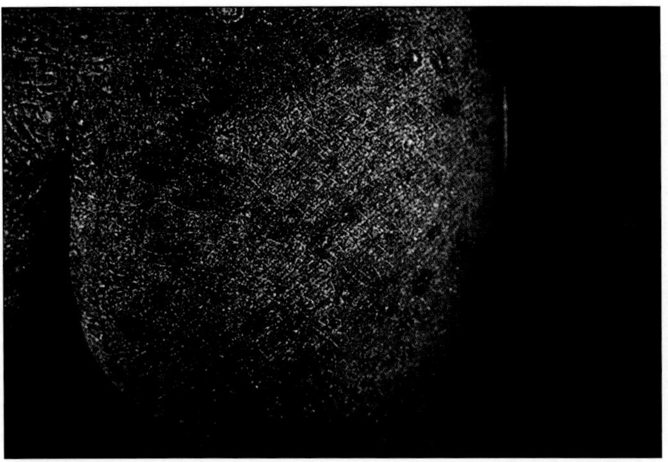

Figure 7.7 Chronic papular onchodermatitis with flat-topped papules, leading to spotty hyperpigmentation on the buttocks.

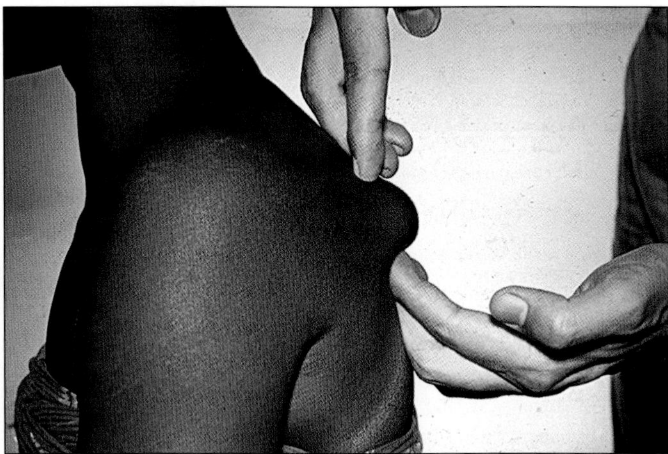

Figure 7.9 An onchocercoma is comprised of several adult worms surrounded by a thick fibrous coat. (Courtesy of Dr. Daniel Conner.)

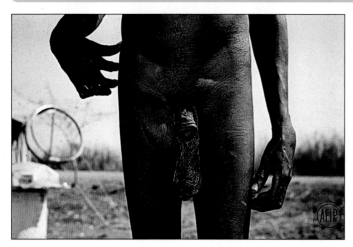

Figure 7.10 Hanging groin is caused by degenerative changes leading to loss of elasticity in the skin of the inguinal fold. (Courtesy of Dr. Daniel Conner.)

groin is seen more commonly in males than in females. Involvement of deeper nodes can lead to lymphedema and elephantiasis.[8]

As connoted by the popular epithet "river blindness," drastic ocular changes may also result from *O. volvulus* infection. Anterior uveitis, conjunctivitis, and punctate keratitis are among early ocular findings, whereas more chronic presentations of onchocerciasis may include optic atrophy and glaucoma. Chronic anterior segment involvement can cause iris atrophy, cataracts, and glaucoma. Posterior uveitis has also been linked to onchocerciasis and, when present chronically, results in retinal and optic disk atrophy. Choroidal involvement may lead to loss of capillaries and pigment. Eye involvement may progress despite the lack of ongoing inflammation. Many patients lose their sight completely, and many others have significant visual loss as a result of the infection.[11]

Patient evaluation, diagnosis, and differential diagnosis

A presumptive diagnosis of onchocerciasis can be made on clinical grounds in a patient with a classic onchocercoma and characteristic skin changes. Evaluation of a patient with suspected onchocerciasis involves a complete skin exam with notation of all skin findings. Ophthalmologic evaluation is crucial, even in patients without ocular symptoms. The presence of microfilariae in the anterior chamber or cornea, which may be clearly visible, is an important component of the initial diagnosis.

Given a classic constellation of signs and symptoms, the diagnosis of onchocerciasis is not difficult to make; however, in many cases, fewer symptoms may be present. The differential diagnosis for onchocercal skin disease depends on the clinical manifestations of the disease in the particular case in question. For patients with acute papular onchodermatitis, miliaria and diffuse insect bites are the main differential diagnoses and can be distinguished from onchocerciasis by the size and location of the lesions. APOD lesions are larger and more widely distributed, than those seen in miliaria but are smaller than arthropod bites, which also may cluster.

Chronic papular onchodermatitis and lichenified onchodermatitis more closely resemble scabies or diffuse atopic dermatitis. Chronic papular onchodermatitis can be distinguished by its characteristic flat-topped papules and lack of burrows, while lichenified onchodermatitis is differentiated by its unilateral and confluent character.

Atrophy is commonly seen in old age, and the characteristics of onchocercal atrophy do not distinguish it from older age, except for its localization to one site (most commonly the buttocks) and its occurrence in young patients.

The differential diagnosis for depigmentation is postinflammatory hypopigmentation, traumatic hypopigmentation, and vitiligo. The depigmentation caused by onchocerciasis is characterized by perifollicular islands of normal pigmentation and occurs most commonly on the shins.[8]

If definitive diagnosis is necessary, as in less characteristic cases, then several laboratory tests exist to confirm the diagnosis. The classic method of determining the prevalence and intensity of onchocercal infection is by a skin snip, whereby small (3–5-mg) pieces of skin are snipped with a scalpel. The sample of skin is placed in a physiologic solution such as saline and the intensity of the infection is determined based on the number of microfilariae seen to emerge from the skin. The snip is most productive when taken from the iliac crest area. Although this test is very specific, it is not sensitive for the detection of early or light infections.

The Mazzotti test involves the administration of 6 mg diethylcarbamizine, which inhibits neuromuscular transmission in nematodes and results in pruritus and inflammation in the area of microfilariae within 2 h. This test is rarely used today due to the side-effects of diethylcarbamizine administration; however, local application of diethylcarbamizine (the Mazzotti patch test) results in pruritus and inflammation at the site of application in the presence of microfilariae and is far less invasive.

Enzyme-linked immunosorbent assay (ELISA) to identify microfilarial antigens and polymerase chain reaction (PCR) to amplify repetitive DNA sequences unique to *O. volvulus* have greater sensitivity than skin snips but are limited by cost. Additionally, ELISA cannot distinguish between current and past infections.

A rapid-format antibody card has recently been developed to detect antibodies to a specific *O. volvulus* antigen and may prove useful for non-invasive diagnosis in the future.[10] This test detects IgG4 antibodies to *O. volvulus* Ov16 antigen in serum and has a high sensitivity and specificity. Like the ELISA, it is limited by its inability to distinguish between active and past infection.[12]

Pathology

The subcutaneous nodule of the onchocercoma has central worms surrounded by a dense wall of fibrous tissue that may extend around and between the worms. In early lesions, a granulomatous or mixed inflammatory infiltrate may exist, but in long-standing lesions, only the dense fibrous tissue remains along with calcification. Microfilariae may be seen in the surrounding tissue.

A punch biopsy from a patient with onchocercal dermatitis usually reveals microfilariae 5 μm in diameter between the collagen of the upper dermis together between the associated tissue eosinophils

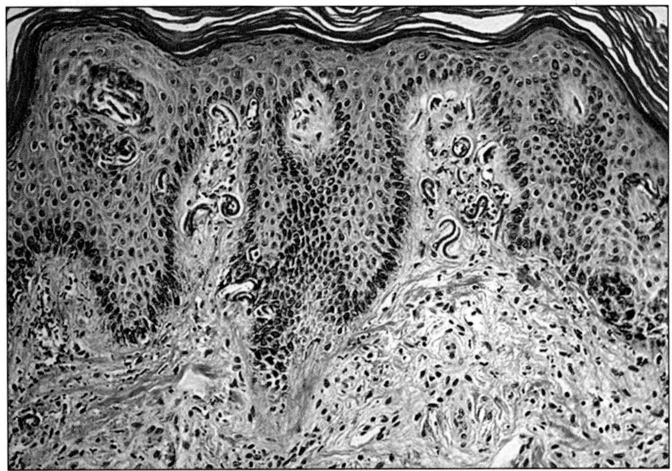

Figure 7.11 Histopathological evaluation of onchodermatitis reveals the presence of microfilariae between the collagen, dermal fibrosis, reactive hyperkeratosis, and a dermal inflammatory infiltrate. (Courtesy of Dr. Daniel Conner.)

and lymphocytes seen in both the superficial and deep dermis (Fig. 7.11). The dermis shows progressive fibrosis and the overlying epidermis is characterized by acanthosis and hyperkeratosis.[9]

Treatment

Ivermectin is the mainstay of therapy for onchocerciasis. Although not capable of killing the adult worm, ivermectin is effective at killing microfilariae without causing the Mazzotti reaction seen after treatment with diethylcarbamazine. A single dose of 150 μg/kg given PO is sufficient to kill microfilariae and temporarily control patients' symptomatology. Ivermectin selectively binds to glutamate-gated chloride channels and causes cell death in invertebrate nerve and muscle cells. Because it does not kill adult worms, which can live for up to 14 years, ivermectin must be given at regular intervals to maintain low microfilarial levels and to prevent progression of the disease. Annual treatment has been demonstrated to prevent progression of eye disease and to improve severe skin involvement.

Adverse reactions to ivermectin include symptoms caused by accelerated microfilarial death at the time of initial dosing, but with diminished adverse effects on subsequent dosings due to a decreased microfilarial load. Its safety in pregnancy has not been established and it is excreted in breast milk. Caution must also be taken when using ivermectin in regions endemic for *Loa loa*, as severe central nervous system dysfunction may arise in patients with *L. loa* following treatment.[13]

Recent evidence has demonstrated that *Wolbachia* endobacteria are both necessary for fertility of their nematode hosts and central to the development of the host's immune reaction after microfilarial death. This discovery has led to the use of commonly used antibiotics for onchocerciasis control. Treatment with doxycycline, 100 mg/day for 6 weeks, is sufficient to disrupt embryogenesis of the female worm by depleting *Wolbachia*. When combined with ivermectin, doxycycline therapy can lead to absence of microfilaridermia that lasts for 18 months. Patients treated with ivermectin alone have a reappearence of dermal microfilariae only 4 months after therapy. Preliminary data suggest that ivermectin combined with 200 mg of doxycycline/day for 4 weeks may have an equivalent efficacy. Although not yet the standard of care, coadministration of doxycycline holds promise in the treatment of onchocerciasis.[1]

As an adjunct to oral therapy, nodulectomy, or surgical removal of the adult worm, may lower the numbers of microfilariae entering the eye. Nodulectomy is more commonly practiced in Latin America than in Africa.

Ivermectin is not only the mainstay of treatment for an individual afflicted with onchocerciasis, but also a key component of control programs aimed at lowering or eliminating the public health burden caused by this disease. The first widespread public health initiative to control the disease was the Onchocerciasis Control Programme (OCP) led by the World Health Organization and established in 1975 to break the cycle of transmission through vector control. It focused initially vector control on the seven countries with the highest historic prevalence rates of onchocerciasis, eventually expanding to a total of 11 countries. Its goal was to interrupt the transmission cycle of the disease for several years longer than the life span of the typical adult worm, which is 14 years. It concluded its efforts in 2002. As a result of these vector-control efforts, the burden of disease in the affected countries has fallen substantially and over 100 000 cases of blindness have been prevented.[14] Once available, mass distribution of ivermectin was added to the program as an additional tool to decrease the overall burden of circulating microfilariae and to control the symptoms of those afflicted with onchocerciasis. While parasite populations in OCP program areas are currently insufficient to maintain transmission, it is anticipated that a recrudescence of onchocerciasis transmission will result from migration of either infected black flies or infected persons into the former OCP area.

The African Programme for Onchocerciasis Control (APOC) began in 1996, covering another 19 countries in Africa where vector control is not practical. Its main focus is the delivery of ivermectin, backed by the commitment of the drug's manufacturer Merck to provide ivermectin free of charge. Self-sustainable community-based treatment programs are the central mechanisms of distribution. With annual dosing of ivermectin in all affected regions, the APOC has been successful in eliminating onchocerciasis as a public health problem. Eradication of *O. volvulus* has remained elusive and is not felt to be possible with current technology given the long life of the adult worm, political unrest in the affected region, and the long flight path of the vector. Still, remarkable progress has been made by both OCP and APOC.

The Onchocerciasis Elimination Program in the Americas was launched in 1992 and covers all six countries with endemic onchocerciasis in the Americas. Like the APOC, it is based primarily on treatment with ivermectin. While elimination of onchocerciasis in Africa remains a distant goal, favorable circumstances in the Americas may allow for complete elimination of the disease. The American vector is inefficient and the disease is localized in small foci with high vector densities, and little migration of vector or infected humans, allowing for possible interruption of the life and transmission cycle.[15]

Research on new treatment methods is continuing with a particular focus on treatments that will kill the adult worm. The risk of resistance to ivermectin developing within *O. volvulus* is real and, once present, could spread quickly given the long distances traveled by the black fly. The recent discovery of the endosymbiotic *Wolbachia* may provide a new opportunity to further decrease the burden of disease and prevent its resurgence as a public health problem.

References

1. Hoerauf A, Butter D, Adjei O et al. Onchocerciasis. Br Med J 2003; 326:207–210.
2. Burnham G. Onchocerciasis. Lancet 1998; 351:1341–1346.
3. The UNDP/World Bank/WHO special programme for research and training in tropical diseases. Onchocerciasis. Available online at: http://who.int/tdr/diseases/oncho.htm. Accessed August 31, 2004.
4. Benton B, Bump J, Seketeli A et al. Partnership and promise: evolution of the African river-blindness campaigns. Ann Trop Med Parasitol 2002; 96:S5–S14.
5. Andre A, Blackwell N, Hall L et al. The role of endosymbiotic *Wolbachia* bacteria in the pathogenesis of river blindness. Science 2002; 295:1892–1895.
6. Kale OO. Onchocerciasis: the burden of disease. Ann Trop Med Parisitol 1997; 92:S101–S115.
7. Hagan M. Onchocercal dermatitis: clinical impact. Ann Trop Med Parisitol 1997; 92:S85–S96.
8. Murdoch ME, Hay RJ, Mackenzie CD et al. A clinical classification and grading system of the cutaneous changes in onchocerciasis. Br J Dermatol 1993; 129:260–269.
9. Weedon D. Helminth infestations in: skin pathology, 2nd edn. London: Churchill Livingstone; 2002:733–734.
10. Okulicz JF, Elston DM. Onchocerciasis (river blindness). In: James W, ed. Emedicine. May 9 2002. Available online at: http://www.emedicine.com/derm/topic637.htm (accessed August 31, 2004).
11. Rathinam SR, Cunningham ET. Infectious causes of uveitis in the developing world. Int Ophthalmol Clin 2000; 40:137–152.
12. Weil GJ, Steel C, Liftis F et al. A rapid-format antibody card test for diagnosis of onchocerciasis. J Infect Dis 2000; 182:1796–1799.
13. The Mectizan Expert Committee. Recommendations for the treatment of onchocerciasis with Mectizan in area co-endemic for onchocerciasis and loiasis. Available online at: http://www.mectizan.org/loarecs.asp (accessed August 31, 2004).
14. Tropical disease research: progress 1995–96. Thirteenth programme report of the UNDP/World Bank/WHO special programme for research and training in tropical diseases. Chapter 7, pages 86-99. Geneva: World Health Organization, 1997. Available oneline at: www.who.int/tdr/diseases/oncho (accessed August 31, 2004).
15. The Carter Center. Final report of the conference on eradicability of onchocerciasis. Jan 2002. Available online at: http://www.cartercenter.org/documents/1047.pdf (accessed August 31, 2004).

Loiasis

Francis T. Assimwe and Ulrich R. Hengge

Synonyms: Calabar (Nigeria) swellings, Cameroon swellings, fugitive swellings, migratory filaria, eye worm

Key features:

- This is a very common disease in sub-Saharan Africa due to the *Loa loa* nematode: it affects approximately 13 million people as of the year 2002[1]
- It causes physical and psychological disability
- The disease is preventable and curable

Introduction

Loa loa is a parasitic filarial nematode that infects human skin and eyes with probable allergic offset, resulting in kidney, lung, and heart disease.[1] It has affected human beings for ages: the earliest reliable documentation was in 1770 in the Carribean.[2] Today it is a disease of Equatorial, West, and East Africa.[3]

Definition

Loiasis is a chronic nematode infection of humans due to adult filariae and microfilariae of *Loa loa*. The disease does not show any sexual preference.

Etiopathophysiology

Humans are the definitive host and the disease is spread by a vector fly (intermediate host): *Chrysops* spp. These deer/antelope flies reside under the canopy of tropical wood/forest adjacent to ponds or slow-moving rivers. They are daytime-biting flies feeding off blood.

When feeding, they ingest microfilariae along with blood from an infected human. Microfilariae develop into infective larvae within the fly and are transmitted to subcutaneous tissue of an uninfected human by another bite.

In subcutaneous tissue, larvae mature into adult worms with males on average half the size of a female, which is 5–7 cm long. These migrate through connective tissue to the rest of the body, and yield microfilariae during the day which may be taken up by a biting *Chrysops* fly to another human before the cycle continues.

Adult worms can persist for more than a decade in subcutaneous tissue. Symptoms often begin about 1 year after infection. Thousands of bites are needed to induce infection, implying that persons from outside an endemic area have to be exposed to bites for at least 3 months to become infected.

Clinical features

Clinical findings are due to filariae and released microfilariae movement in tissues and vessels.

The typical dermatological lesion presents as a recurrent migratory focal angioedema due to adult filariae, often found on the limbs, commonly near large joints, with pain or pruritus. They are also frequently found periorbitally. The lesions last hours or days to weeks (less than 20). The nomenclature has been derived from the lesions: Calabar (Nigeria), Cameroon, and fugitive swellings.

At times a characteristic raised outline of skin due to the underlying mature filariae is visible (migratory filariasis) and the worm may be seen crossing subconjunctivally (Fig. 7.12), causing severe conjunctivitis (eye worm disease). Urticaria due to released microfilariae is also common. There may also be associated arthritis, myalgia, and regional lymphadenopathy of affected body parts.

Systemic symptoms include mainly fever and fatigue, though disease may affect other organ systems as well. An allergic or toxic reaction to microfilariae may cause regional lymphedema (lower limb, hydrocele), peripheral nerve dysfunction, encephalopathy, kidney glomerular disease, pulmonary complications, and cardiomyopathy.

Patients may suffer from multiple infections but generally have fewer than 10 worms at a time. Dead worms may calcify in tissue.

However, oftentimes infection is asymptomatic and only detected by routine physical examination or laboratory investigations.

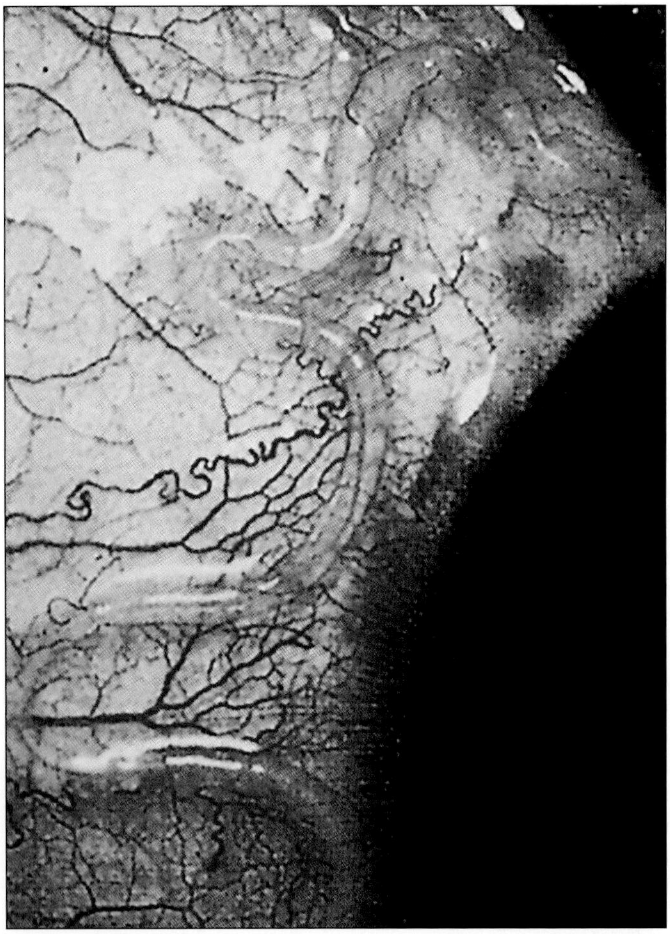

Figure 7.12 Adult *Loa loa* in the conjunctiva. (Reproduced from Peters W and Pasvol G (eds). Tropical Medicine and Parasitology, 5th edition, Mosby, London 2002, image 320).

Diagnosis

Definitive

1. Typically, a worm is extracted from an excised subcutaneous nodule or during subconjuctival migration (Fig. 7.13).
2. Microfilariae can be detected in skin snips by microscopy.
3. Microfilariae can be detected in blood drawn during the day or in other body fluids (urine, cerebrospinal fluid, sputum), as demonstrated by microscopic analysis. This is most relevant to permanent residents of endemic areas who are microfilaremic as compared to infected temporary residents who are mostly amicrofilaremic.
4. X-rays of calcified worms in tissue provide a definitive diagnosis.
5. Serological analysis of blood samples (*Loa*-specific IgG4) will provide a definitive diagnosis.

Empirical

1. Typical clinical findings are diagnostic.
2. Eosinophilia, leukocytosis, and increased serum IgE are also diagnostic.
3. A positive Mazzotti test is diagnostic. A small dose of diethylcarbamazine is given as a challenge, under observation. When positive, the test induces intense itching, presumably due to a microfilaricidal effect in vessels.

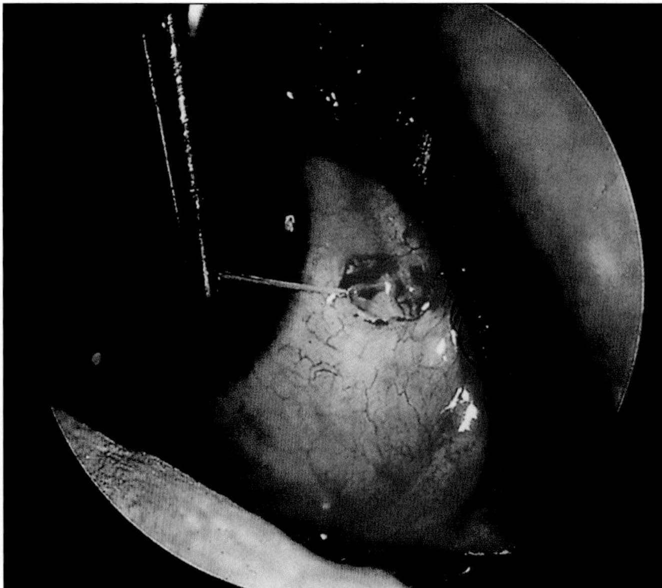

Figure 7.13 Extraction of *Loa loa* from the conjunctiva. (Reproduced from Peters W and Pasvol G (eds). Tropical Medicine and Parasitology, 5th edition, Mosby, London 2002, image 321).

Differential diagnosis

The differential diagnosis includes other filarial infections, gnathistomiasis, toxocariasis, and focal idiopathic angioedema.

Treatment

1. Diethylcarbamazine (Hetrazan) is given for a 3-week oral course with the dose adjusted according to the blood microfilarial load: high microfilarial loads require careful treatment as they may induce idiopathic encephalomeningitis, even when very low doses of diethylcarbamazine are given. In these instances antihistamines/corticosteroids are a necessary adjuvant treatment. Thus, diethylcarbamazine is more often used in patients who are amicrofilaremic.[4]
2. Ivermectin (Mectizan, Stromectol) and albendazole are treatment options. However, ivermectin is also associated with anaphylaxis and encephalopathy if given to patients with high microfilarial blood levels and thus is to be handled with extra caution.[5,6] Note: the above pharmacological treatment may not protect from the appearance of subcutaneous nodules with worms and hematuria.
3. Worms may be surgically removed from the conjuctivae and nodules excised where clinically feasible.

Prognosis

The prognosis is generally good; the morbidity is temporary, though recurrent. Permanent damage such as kidney disease and blindness may occur. Fatalities are due to anaphylactic reactions, secondary to worm rupture in internal tissue, and empirical antifilarial treatment of high microfiliaremic patients.[6] Greater emphasis on health education, focusing on prevention and prophylaxis (vector, habitat, and risk behavior), are vital to controlling this helminthic dermatosis.

References

1. Cox FEG. A history of human parasitology. Clin Microbiol Rev 2002; 15:595–612.
2. Akue JP, Devany E. Transmission intensity affects both antigen-specific and nonspecific T-cell proliferative responses in *Loa loa* infection. Infect Immun 2002; 70:1475–1480.
3. WHO research and training in tropical diseases (TDR), Special programme with UNDP/World Bank. 2001. Available online at: www.who.int/tdr/diseases/oncho. Accessed August 31, 2004.
4. Nutman TB, Miller KD, Mulligan M et al. Diethylcarbamazine prophylaxis for human loiasis. Results of a double-blind study. N Engl J Med 1988; 319:752–756.
5. Chippaux JP, Nkinin SW, Gardon-Wendel N et al. Release of *Loa loa* antigens after treatment with ivermectin. Bull Soc Pathol Exot 1998; 91:297–299.
6. Gardon J, Gardon-Wendel N, Demanga-Ngangwe K et al. Serious reactions after mass treatment of onchocerciasis with ivermectin in an area endemic for *Loa loa* infection. Lancet 1997; 350:18–22.

Chapter 8

Other helminths

- Dracunculiosis ▪ *Francis T. Assimwe and Ulrich R. Hengge*
- Cutaneous larva migrans ▪ *Ulrich R. Hengge*
- Trichinellosis ▪ *G. Todd Bessinger*

Introduction

Nematodal helminths

Nematodal helminths represent infectious agents that are not very infectious, but have developed a delicate strategy to infect human hosts. As such, they manage to overcome the epidermal barrier, enter the human body, and travel by several methods to different places in the body, where they cause disease. These diseases are endemic in Asia, Africa, and Latin America.

Despite the existence of effective and rather cheap therapies, many endemic countries cannot provide these therapies for the vast majority of infected patients. Until this changes, strong emphasis needs to be placed on prevention and patient education.

Dracunculiosis

Francis T. Assimwe and Ulrich R. Hengge

Synonyms: Guinea worm disease, dracunculiasis, dracontiasis, medina worm

Key factors

- Dracunculosis is a very common skin disease in the tropics worldwide due to *Dracunculus medinensis*
- It causes physical and psychological incapacitation
- It is preventable, curable, and can be eradicated

Introduction

Dracunculosis is a parasitic dermatosis that has plagued humans for centuries. Earliest texts date from Ebers papyrus about 1500 BC and particular descriptions of disease have been found in the work of Greek, Roman, and Arab physicians in the tenth and eleventh centuries AD.[1] In the New World it persists in the tropics and is endemic in parts of sub-Saharan Africa (Figs 8.1 and 8.2).

The disease does not have any sexual predisposition. However, it is less commonly encountered in children.[2]

Definition

Dracunculosis is a chronic nematode infection of humans by the female worm *Dracunculus medinensis*.

Etiology and pathophysiology

Thousands of larvae are released into water from females extruding from an ulcerated nodule of an infected human (definitive host). These larvae are then ingested by cyclopoid copepods (tiny aquatic crustaceans, approximately 2–3 mm long) that serve as intermediate hosts, where they mature into infective larvae (Fig. 8.3). Humans unintentionally swallow the crustacea in unsafe (unfiltered, unboiled) drinking water, especially from surface waters – ponds, lagoons, valley dams, reservoirs, streams, or rivers.[3]

The crustaceas are dissolved in the acidic gastric environment, releasing infective larvae which penetrate transluminally into loose connective tissue, often the peritoneal cavity. Larvae then migrate through the interstitium and lymphatics, homing to subcutaneous tissues where they grow, mature, and fertilize in about 1 year (10–18 months). The adult female is 70–120 cm long.

Fertilized females migrate epicutaneously (over approximately 4 weeks) where on contact with water they release larvae to complete the life cycle, before they die (Fig. 8.3).

Clinical features

This condition is asymptomatic during incubation until maturity and fertilization. Symptoms and signs occur due to epicutaneous migration of fertilized females. Systemic features may precede cutaneous manifestations and include nausea, vomiting, diarrhea, syncope, and dyspnea.

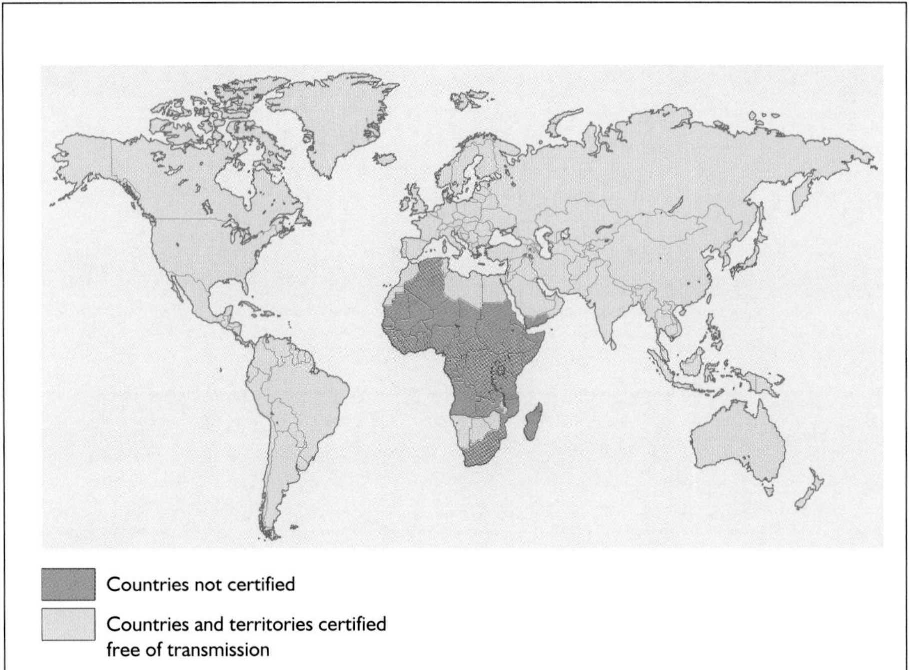

Figure 8.1 Countries and territories certified free of dracunculiasis.

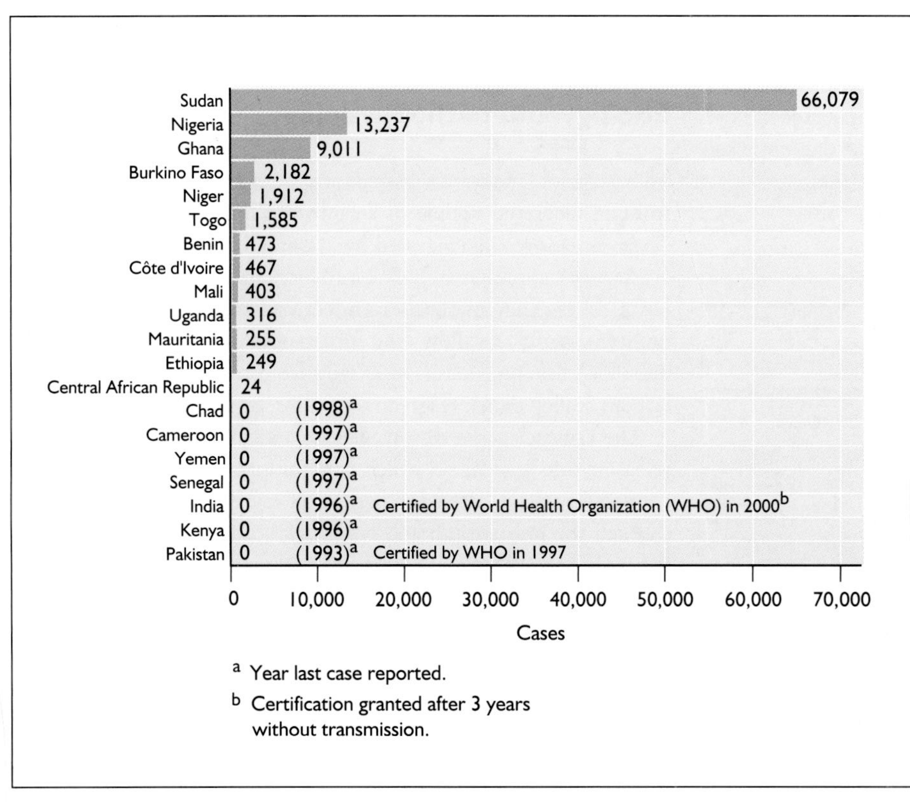

Figure 8.2 Numbers of cases of dracunculiasis per country in 1999.

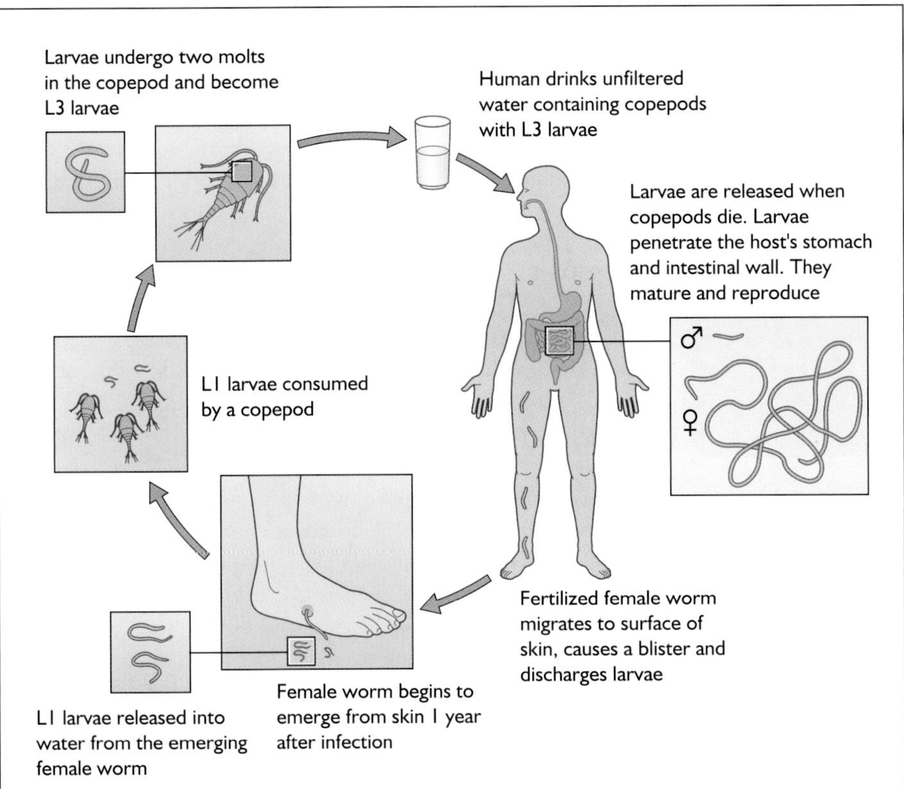

Figure 8.3 Life cycle of the female *Dracunculus medinensis*. Humans become infected by drinking unfiltered water containing copepods (small crustaceas) which are infected with the larvae of *D. medinensis*. Following ingestion, the copepods die and release the larvae, which penetrate the hosts stomach and intestinal wall and enter the abdominal cavity and retroperitoneal space. After maturation into adults and copulation, the male worms die and the females (70–120 cm long) migrate in the subcutaneous tissues towards the skin surface. Approximately 1 year after infection, the female worm induces a blister on the skin, generally on the distal lower extremity, that ruptures. When this lesion comes into contact with water, a contact that the patient seeks in order to relieve the local discomfort, the female worm emerges and releases larvae. The larvae are ingested by a copepod and after 2 weeks (and two molts) develop into infective larvae . Ingestion of the copepods finishes the cycle. i, infective stage; d, diagnostic stage. (Adapted from Centers for Disease Control and Prevention.)

The earliest dermatological manifestations are urticaria and erythematous papulonodular lesions, which are painful but may be preceded by pruritus.

Papules and nodules may develop into vesiculobullous lesions with surrounding induration (Fig. 8.4A), which cause an intense burning sensation that is relieved by submerging the affected body parts in water.

Subsequent skin ulcerations may be colonized by bacterial infections, often leading to pyodermas (Fig. 8.4B).

If the worm ruptures in the tissue, it causes cellulitis or abscess formation or heals with calcification.

The lower legs and feet are the most commonly affected sites but the parasites may extrude from thighs, trunk, upper limbs, or head. They have also been found in soft tissues like pericardium, testicles, and ligaments.

A patient may have more than 20 worms extruding at a time, but usually there are fewer than five. No protective immunity develops and reinfection is therefore common.

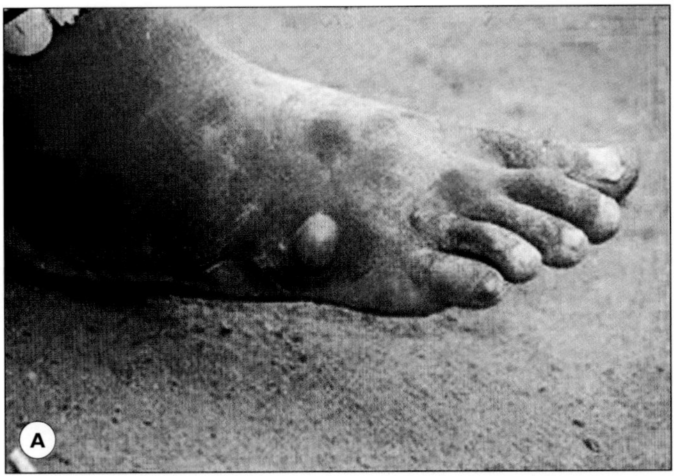

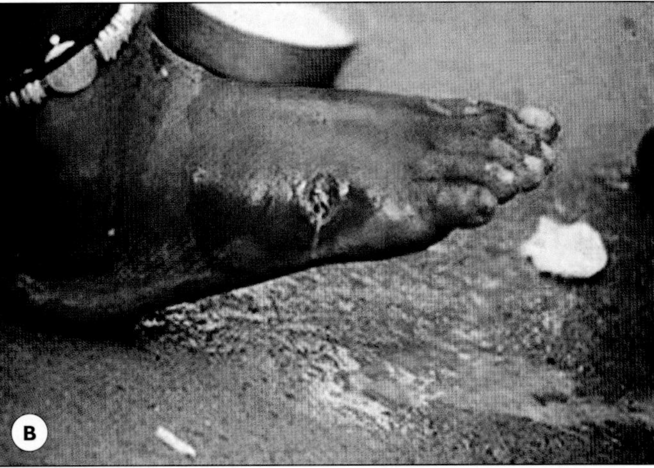

Figure 8.4 Clinical presentation. The female guinea worm induces a painful blister (A); after rupture of the blister, the worm emerges as a whitish filament (B) in the center of a painful ulcer which is often secondarily infected. (Reproduced from Center of Disease Control and Prevention, courtesy of Global 2000/The Carter Center, Atlanta, Georgia.)

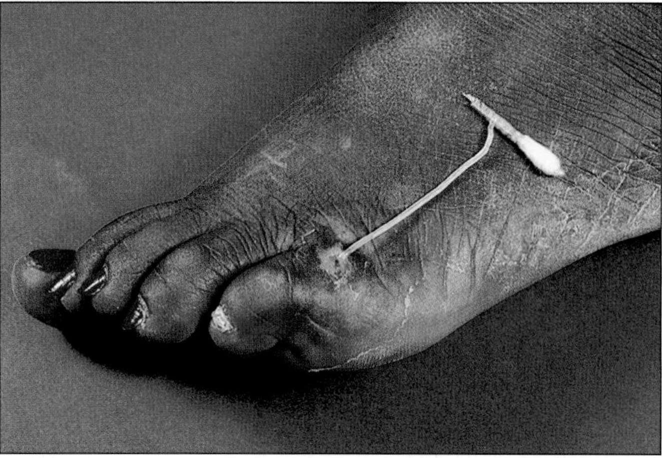

Figure 8.5 An emerged guinea worm is being pulled out from an ulcerated lesion. (Courtesy of World Health Organisation.)

Diagnosis

Definitive

1. Typically, a worm extrudes from a skin lesion (Fig. 8.5).
2. Suspect ulcer: wet smears showing motile larvae on microscopy.

Presumptive

1. Typical clinical findings.
2. Increased erythrocyte sedimentation rate, immunoglobulin E (IgE), and eosinophil count.

Histology reveals mixed inflammatory infiltrate and granulation tissue at the anterior end of the worm with or without fibrosis.

Differential diagnosis

The differential diagnosis includes other filarial diseases before the typical worm emerges.

Treatment

1. Slowly coil out the parasite around a small rod approximately 2–5 mm/day until the worm has come out completely.
2. The lesion should be widely excised to avoid complications, though care must be taken to check that all of the worm has been excised, as remnants may induce a severe inflammatory response.
3. Tiabendazole (Ebendazole) 50 mg/kg per day divided into two doses, for 3 days, and metronidazole 250 mg t.i.d. for 10 days are not parasiticidal but are antiinflammatory and aid healing.

Prognosis

Dracunculosis often causes physical and psychological incapacitation which, though rarely permanent, causes significant loss of work output. Studies in Nigeria[3] and Thailand[4] revealed 21–84% and 28–34% of physical task incapacitation in affected patients, respectively.

Prevention includes avoiding the ingestion of contaminated water through prior sieving and boiling.

Eradication is possible and has been proven in Asia and previously endemic African countries: Senegal, Cameroon, Chad, and Kenya (Fig. 8.2). Only 13 are still affected and statistics are encouraging, as in Uganda, which reduced its incidence to 6 in 2002 from 130 000 in 1990.[5] This requires increased prioritization of public and medical knowledge of the management and preventability of dracunculosis and intermediary host/vector control, especially as this is a disease where a small number of water contacts or low proportion of risk behavior is sufficient to maintain transmission.[6]

References

1. Henderson PL, Fontaine RE, Kyeyune G. Guinea worm disease in Northern Uganda: a major public health problem controllable through an effective water programme. Int J Epidemiol 1988; 17:434–440.
2. Cox FEG. A history of human parasitology. Clin Microbiol Rev 2002; 15:595–612.
3. Okoye SN, Onwuliri CO, Anosike JC. A survey of predilection sites and degree of disability associated with guinea worm (*Dracunculus medinensis*). Int J Parasitol 1995; 25:1127–1129.
4. Hours M, Cairncross S. Long term disability due to guinea worm disease. Trans R Soc Trop Med Hyg 1994; 88:559–560.
5. Wendo C. Uganda leads Africa's charge against guinea worm disease. Lancet 2003; 361:1446.
6. Etard JF, Kodio B, Traora S et al. Water contacts in dracunculiasis-infected patients in Mali: transmission risk activities. Bull Soc Pathol Exot 2002; 95:295–298.

Cutaneous larva migrans

Ulrich R. Hengge

Synonyms: creeping eruption, plumber's itch, sandworm disease, *Ancylostoma brasiliense*

Cutaneous larva migrans is the most common tropical parasite dermatosis. It generally presents as an erythematous serpiginous cutaneous eruption caused by percutaneous penetration and subsequent migration of larvae of various nematodes. It causes a substantial amount of itching and burning. Geographically, it is most commonly found in subtropical areas and southwestern USA. However, increased foreign travel means that cutaneous larva migrans is no longer confined to these areas.

Pathophysiology

The larva cycle begins when eggs are transmitted from animal feces into warm, moist soil, where the larvae hatch. Initially, they feed on soil bacteria. Using their proteases, larvae penetrate through follicles, fissures, or intact skin, generally on the soles of humans. After penetrating the stratum corneum of the host, the larvae shed their natural cuticle before beginning migration.

In their natural animal hosts, the larvae are able to penetrate into the dermis and gain access to the lymphatic and venous system. Upon transport to the lungs, they invade the alveoli and migrate to the trachea, where they are swallowed. In the intestine sexual maturation occurs and the cycle begins again as the eggs are excreted.

Humans are accidental hosts, and the larvae are believed to lack the collagenase enzymes required to penetrate the basement membrane to invade the dermis. As a consequence, the disease remains limited to human skin.

Frequency

Cutaneous larva migrans is very common.

Mortality and morbidity

Cutaneous larva migrans causes a benign disease, but may cause significant pruritus. No predilection of race and gender occurs.

Clinical presentation

The clinical presentation is of erythematous, classically serpiginous linear lesions with advancing edges (Fig. 8.6). There is intense pruritus and tingling, and pruritic, erythematous papules, smaller than 3–4 mm may occur. Slightly elevated, erythematous tunnels track several centimeters from the penetration site. Surrounding non-specific dermatitis and secondary pyoderma may occur. Generally, the tracks advance several millimeters per day. Lesions are located on the dorsa of the feet, interdigital spaces of the toes, the anogenital region, the buttocks, hands, and knees.

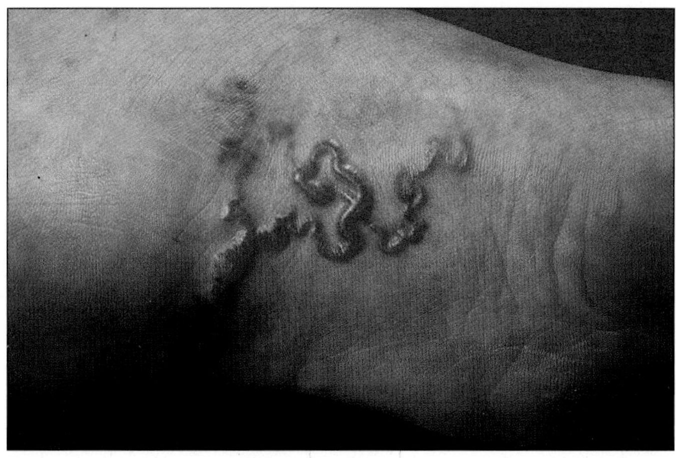

Figure 8.6 Sharply demarcated linear zigzag lesion on the medial aspect of the foot, representing the creeping of the larva.

Patient history

Patients usually report a history of sunbathing, walking barefoot on the beach, or a similar activity in a tropical location. Hobbies and occupations that involve contact with warm, moist, sandy soil, including children in sandboxes, are typical.

Laboratory findings

Diagnosis is mostly based on the classic clinical appearance of the eruption. Laboratory studies have not proven helpful except for occasional peripheral eosinophilia and increased IgE levels.

Etiology

Ancylostoma brasiliense (hookworm in wild and domestic dogs and cats) is the most common cause. It can be found in central and southern USA, Central America, South America, and the Caribbean.

A. caninum (dog hookworm) is found in Australia.

Uncinaria stenocephala (dog hookworm) is found in Europe.

Several others, such as cattle and cat hookworms, or certain parasites (*Strongyloides papillosus*) represent additional causative organisms.

Differential diagnosis

The differential diagnosis includes jellyfish stings, scabies, phyto-photodermatitis, epidermal dermatophytosis, erythema migrans (Lyme borreliosis), migratory myiasis, and photoallergic dermatitis.

Procedures

A skin biopsy taken just ahead of the leading edge of the track may identify the larva (periodic acid–Schiff stain: positive) in a suprabasal burrow associated with spongiosis, intraepidermal vesicles, necrotic keratinocytes, and an epidermal and upper dermal chronic inflammatory infiltrate with eosinophils.

Treatment

Tiabendazole (Mintezol) is currently considered the agent of choice. Topical application is used for early, localized lesions. For widespread lesions or unsuccessful topical treatment, oral administration is advised. Other treatments include albendazole, mebendazole, and ivermectin. The treatment course generally leads to decreased pruritus within 24 h, while lesions/tracts resolve within 1–2 weeks. Antibiotics are indicated when secondary infection occurs. As an alternative topical therapy, liquid nitrogen applied to the progressive end of the larval burrow and 1 cm around it has been successfully used.

Tiabendazole (Mintezol) inhibits the helminth-specific fumarate reductase, which inhibits microtubule formation and leads to impaired glucose uptake. It is one of the third-generation heterocyclic anthelminths. A 10–15% suspension is generally used under an occlusive dressing q.i.d. for 1 week. Sometimes, tiabendazole is administered in a compound with a corticosteroid cream. Alternatively, it is given as 25–50 mg/kg per day PO divided every 12 h for 2–5 days.

Anorexia, nausea, vomiting, diarrhea, hematuria, headache, and dizziness may occur on oral administration. Closely monitor hepatic or renal function.

Ivermectin (Stromectol) is a semisynthetic macrocyclic lactone antiparasitic agent with broad-spectrum action against nematodes, producing flaccid paralysis through binding of glutamate-gated chloride ion channels. It has a good safety profile with low toxicity, and single dosing enhances patient compliance. Adults are treated with 12 mg PO once or 200 μg/kg. Although rare, the drug may cause fever, glandular tenderness, pruritus, muscle aches, and headaches. In immunocompromised patients, repeat courses of therapy may be required.

Albendazole (Albenza) is a broad-spectrum benzimidazole carbamate anthelmintic drug that acts by interfering with glucose uptake and disruption of microtubule aggregation. It is used as an alternative to tiabendazole (400 mg PO q.i.d. for 3 days or 200 mg PO b.i.d. for 5 days).

Mebendazole (Vermox) is a broad-spectrum anthelmintic drug that also inhibits microtubule assembly and irreversibly blocks glucose uptake. The adult dose is 200 mg PO b.i.d. for 4 weeks.

Complications

Secondary bacterial infection, usually with *Streptococcus pyogenes*, may cause cellulitis.

Prognosis

The prognosis is excellent, since the disease is self-limiting. Humans are the accidental dead-end hosts, with the larva dying, sometimes, however, as late as 1 year in rare cases.

Patient education

Persons who travel to tropical regions and pet owners should be aware of this condition.

References

1. Edelglass JW, Douglass MC, Stiefler R et al. Cutaneous larva migrans in northern climates. A souvenir of your dream vacation. J Am Acad Dermatol 1982; 7:353–358.
2. Herbener D, Borak J. Cutaneous larva migrans in northern climates. Am J Emerg Med 1988; 6:462–464.
3. Jelinek T, Maiwald H, Nothdurft HD et al. Cutaneous larva migrans in travelers: synopsis of histories, symptoms, and treatment of 98 patients. Clin Infect Dis 1994; 19:1062–1066.
4. Richey TK, Gentry RH, Fitzpatrick JE et al. Persistent cutaneous larva migrans due to *Ancylostoma* species. South Med J 1996; 89:609–611.
5. Rodilla F, Colomina J, Magraner J. Current treatment recommendations for cutaneous larva migrans. Ann Pharmacother 1994; 28:672–673.
6. Van den Enden E, Stevens A, Van Gompel A. Treatment of cutaneous larva migrans. N Engl J Med 1998; 339:1246–1247.

Trichinellosis

G. Todd Bessinger

Synonyms: Trichinosis, trichinelliasis, trichiniasis

Key features:

- Humans are infected by eating undercooked meat.
- In the enteral stage, the parasite infects the intestine of the host and the main clinical feature is transient diarrhea.
- During the parenteral stage, the parasite migrates through tissue, resulting in pulmonary, cardiac, neurologic, and dermatologic manifestations.
- The primary dermatologic manifestation is periorbital edema.
- The main pathologic finding is encysted larvae in striated muscle.

Introduction

Trichinella species are widely distributed parasites of carnivorous animals. Human trichinellosis is primarily due to infection with the nematode *Trichinella spiralis*, although there are at least six other species and three additional genotypes that may cause human infection.[1] For most of its history, trichinellosis was attributed to eating undercooked pork. Over the last 50 years, there have also been outbreaks associated with eating horsemeat and wild game. The organism has intestinal and tissue phases (Fig. 8.7): most associated morbidity occurs in the tissue phase.

History

James Paget discovered the helminth encysted in a cadaveric muscle specimen in 1835, when he was a first-year medical student.[2] However, it was not until 1860 that the parasite was linked to the consumption of pork and clinical disease.[3] At the time, trichinellosis was a greatly feared disease. Improvements in sanitation and veterinary medicine have decreased transmission from infected swine to humans in some areas but the disease continues to be a major health problem in many parts of the world.

Epidemiology

Trichinella species are distributed worldwide except in desert regions.[4] Domestic and sylvatic infection cycles exist.

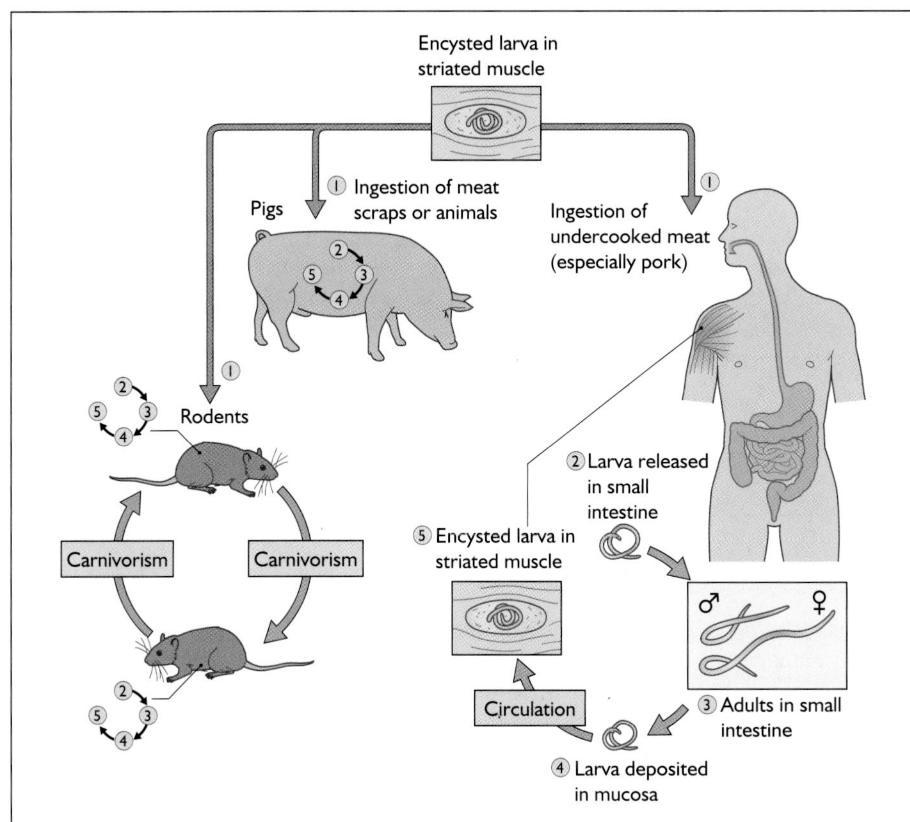

Figure 8.7 Life cycle of trichinellosis. Trichinellosis is acquired by ingesting meat containing cysts (encysted larvae) of *Trichinella*. After exposure to gastric acid and pepsin, the larvae are released from the cysts and invade the small-bowel mucosa where they develop into adult worms (females 2.2 mm, males 1.2 mm in length; life span in the small bowel is 4 weeks). After 1 week, the females release larvae that migrate to the striated muscles where they encyst. *Trichinella pseudospiralis*, however, does not encyst. Encystment is completed in 4–5 weeks and the encysted larvae may remain viable for several years. Ingestion of the encysted larvae perpetuates the cycle. Rats and rodents are primarily responsible for maintaining the endemicity of this infection. Carnivorous/omnivorous animals, such as pigs or bears, feed on infected rodents or meat from other animals. Different animal hosts are implicated in the life cycle of the different species of *Trichinella*. Humans are accidentally infected by eating improperly processed meat of these carnivorous animals (or eating food contaminated with such meat). Geographic distribution is worldwide. i, infective stage; d, diagnostic stage. (Adapted from Centers for Disease Control and Prevention.)

In the domestic cycle, humans are exposed to the parasite by eating undercooked, infected swine. Transmission in the swine herd occurs by feeding the pigs garbage, from pig-to-pig transmission due to tail or ear bites or by failing to remove carcasses promptly, which are then eaten by other herd members, or via synanthropic animals living near the herd.[1] Although rats have been shown to be competent hosts for *T. spiralis*, their role in transmission of the disease to humans and swine is controversial. Horses have also been the source of outbreaks of domestic-cycle trichinellosis in Italy and France.[1] The prevalence of equine infection worldwide is very low.

The sylvatic cycle occurs among scavenger and cannibalistic carnivores throughout the world. It occurs primarily in temperate and tropical regions because the larvae do not survive in frozen carcasses. Examples of animal hosts include wolves, bears, foxes, tigers, mountain lions, wolverines, boars, walruses, birds, raccoon dogs, and domestic dogs and cats. As in the domestic cycle, humans acquire *Trichinella* larvae by ingesting undercooked meat from a host animal.

Infections are most commonly reported in rural areas of Asia and Latin America. Human and animal infections were reported in Mexico, Argentina, and Chile throughout the last century.[5] Recently, Bolivia has also reported outbreaks. The disease is still a public health problem in both Argentina and Chile. In Asia, major outbreaks have occurred in China and Thailand.[6] Prevalence data are not available for northern South America and many parts of Africa.[7]

Increases in trichinellosis also occurred in areas of central and eastern Europe in the 1990s and have led some to designate it a reemerging disease.[7,8] However, its increased prevalence may be due more to improvements in diagnosis and better public health reporting.

Pathogenesis and etiology

Trichinella spp. are obligate intracellular parasites with all stages of the life cycle occurring within the infected host. The disease is clinically and parasitologically separated into enteral and parenteral phases (Table 8.1).

During the enteral phase, the parasite is acquired by ingesting the encysted larvae in the muscles of infected animals. The larvae are released from the tissue and excyst when host gastric juices break down the cyst wall. The first-stage (L1) larvae are passed to the small intestine where they infect a row of columnar epithelium.[9] The larvae molt four times, reach adulthood, and mate. About 5 days later, newborn larvae are produced and penetrate into lymphatic or blood vessels where they are carried throughout the host, thus beginning the parenteral phase of the infection.

Once they reach striated muscle, the larvae leave the capillaries and penetrate the muscle fiber sheaths.[10] In this environment they grow to their full size in about 30 days, surrounding themselves with a sheath derived from the muscle fiber. The encysted larvae remain viable for many years, even after the capsule has calcified.

Each adult female worm can produce 500–1500 larvae over its life span.[10] Eventually, through a combination of cell- and antibody-mediated immunity, the female is expelled from the host intestinal mucosa.[9] In rodent studies, the presence of the adult parasite in

Table 8.1 Progressive symptoms of trichinellosis

Time postinfection	Stage of infection	Progressive disease symptoms
12 h–2 days	Initial penetration and development of larval stages	First symptoms: mild and non-descript
30–32 h 5–7 days	Copulation and female penetration of mucosa	Intestinal inflammation and pain, nausea, vomiting, diarrhea Terminates with facial edema and fever
5 days–6 weeks	Newborn larvae are released into tissues and start migration	Focal or localized edema: face and hands. Pneumonia, pleurisy, encephalitis, meningitis, nephritis, deafness, peritonitis. Death from myocarditis
10 days–6 weeks	Larvae start to penetrate muscle cells	Muscular pain, breathing difficulties, swelling of masseter muscles, weak pulse and low blood pressure, damage to heart. Death as a result of heart failure, respiratory failure, toxemia, or kidney damage

Reproduced from: http://martin.parasitology.mcgill.ca/jimspage/biol/trich.htm.

the intestine induces a type-I hypersensitivity reaction resulting in the production of parasite-specific IgE and increased numbers of mast cells and eosinophils.[8] Murine mast cell-produced protease-1 is vital for expulsion of the worm and the specific IgE produced is protective for rodents. No similar studies have been done in humans.

Diarrhea associated with the enteral phase is directly induced by the parasite and is mediated by the induction of active secretion of water and ions into the intestinal lumen.[8] The persistent diarrhea seen in the enteral phase during some outbreaks may be due to adult worms persisting in the intestines of frequently exposed people.[8]

As the larvae invade the muscles, they directly damage muscle fibers. The inflammation and, in particular, the tissue eosinophilia induced by the parasite further damage the muscle tissue, resulting in myalgia or, when the parasite invades heart muscle, myocarditis.[8] In addition, the wandering larvae may exit the vascular system and either become trapped in non-muscle tissue or attempt to reenter the blood stream, causing a granulomatous tissue reaction or vasculitis.

Clinical features

The severity of the clinical manifestations correlates with parasite burden (the number of larvae ingested). The clinical course is also influenced by the gender, age, ethnic group, infecting *Trichinella* species (*T. pseudospiralis* infection can result in prolonged disease), and immune status of the host.[8] The incubation period is usually 2–7 days after ingestion although duration, like severity, correlates with the number of parasites ingested.[9]

In the enteral phase, lasting about one week, the parasites are released from the ingested meat and penetrate the intestinal mucosa. Most infected individuals are asymptomatic or experience mild transient diarrhea and nausea.[10] However, patients with moderate to severe infections may experience malaise, diarrhea or constipation, nausea, upper abdominal pain, vomiting, and/or low-grade fever lasting several days.[9] These symptoms disappear over the next 2–6 weeks as the parasite enters the parenteral phase.

Most patients experience myalgia.[8–10] The primary dermatologic manifestions are periorbital edema (Fig. 8.8), which can progress to full facial edema, subungual petechiae (Fig. 8.9), and a non-specific macular, papular, or urticarial eruption[9,10] which can mimic measles.[8] The periorbital, facial, and/or extremity edema is thought to be a manifestation of the type-I allergic reaction to the parasite while the petechiae are due to the vasculitis induced by the larval migration into and out of small vessels. Skin desquamation and hair and nail loss have been reported during convalescence.[9]

There is also a reported association between polyarteritis nodosa and trichinellosis.[10] This may be due to cross-reactivity between parasite antigens and host endothelium, deposition of immune complexes in vessel walls, hypereosinophilia-induced tissue damage, or high levels of circulating IgE which initiate or sustain inflammatory vascular disease.

Other clinical manifestations of the parenteral phase include conjunctivitis, fever, headache, dysphagia, a paralysis-like state,

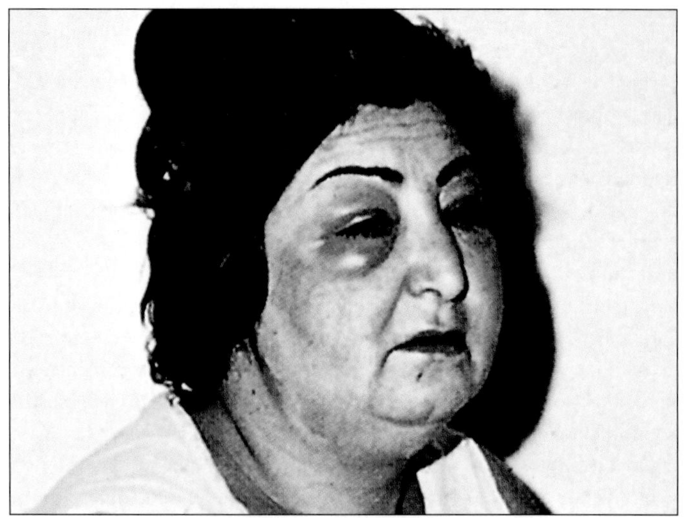

Figure 8.8 Periorbital edema from acute trichinosis. (Reproduced from Peters W and Pasvol G (eds). Tropical Medicine and Parasitology, 5th edition, Mosby, London 2002, image 667.)

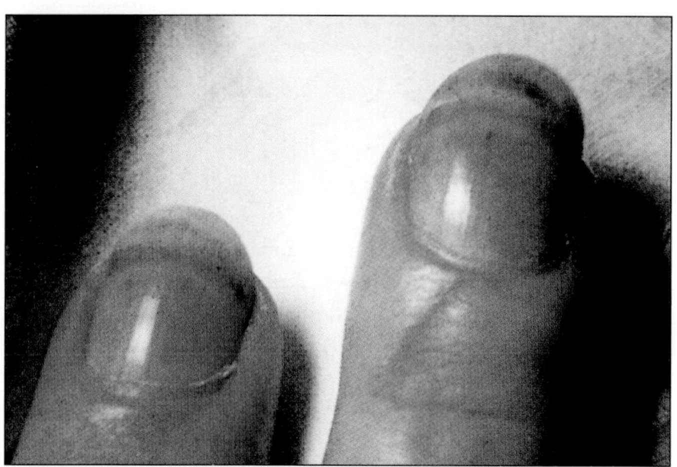

Figure 8.9 Splinter hemorrhages from acute trichinosis. (Reproduced from Peters W and Pasvol G (eds). Tropical Medicine and Parasitology, 5th edition, Mosby, London 2002, image 668.)

insomnia, weight loss, peripheral nerve sensations, hot flashes, coryza, bronchitis, hoarseness, retinal hemorrhages, visual disturbances, and paralysis of ocular muscles.[9] Patients with more severe disease have the same but more prominent symptoms. In particular, these patients have high fever and eosinophilia, severe muscle pain and headaches, more prominent cutaneous eruptions, and marked edema that may involve the eyelids, face, and extremities. They can also develop hypercoagulability leading to arteriolar thrombosis.

Neurologic manifestations occur in 10–24% of cases and usually begin during the second week of the infection. Symptoms include headache, vertigo, tinnitus, deafness, aphasia, and/or seizures.[9,10] These symptoms are thought to be secondary to bystander nerve cell damage by migrating eosinophils and parasite migration-induced vasculitis.[8]

Myocarditis, sometimes resulting in sudden death, occurs between the fourth and eighth week of infection.[8] Myocarditis can lead to arrhythmias, hypotension, and heart failure.

Case fatality is low and usually due to myocarditis and heart failure, pneumonitis, or neurologic complications. Other causes of fatal trichinellosis include hypokalemia, adrenal insufficiency, and occlusive vascular disease.

The convalescent phase begins 6–8 weeks postinfection when the females cease production of larvae and the circulating larvae have encysted in muscle tissue. This phase is marked by progressive disappearance of clinical symptoms, although myalgias may persist for up to 6 months.[11]

Patient evaluation, diagnosis, and differential diagnosis

Patients with mild to moderate disease may have so few or mild symptoms that they often do not seek medical care. In an outbreak, the index cases are usually those with severe infections.

Trichinellosis should be considered in patients presenting with myalgias, periorbital edema, fever, and a peripheral eosinophilia with or without subungual or conjunctival hemorrhages, and/or a history of transient diarrhea. A careful history of the eating habits of the patient and family should be elicited during the interview.

Eosinophilia and leukocytosis are common in trichinellosis. Eosinophilia (up to 19 000/μl) begins early and increases from the second to fifth week. The degree of eosinophilia correlates with the severity of myalgias and is more pronounced in patients with neurological symptoms.[11] The eosinophilia regresses slowly over several weeks to months. A massive drop in eosinophils in patients with severe trichinellosis is a harbinger of a poor outcome or death.[10,11] Leukocytosis occurs early in the course of the disease and subsides in parallel with clinical symptoms.[11]

During the course of trichinellosis, non-specific increases in creatine phosphokinase (CPK), lactate dehydrogenase (LDH), and aldolase occur in 70–90% of infected patients.[11] Although there is a correlation between CPK levels and the intensity of myalgia, there is no corresponding relationship between CPK and the severity of infection.

Electromyographic (EMG) changes may occur during the acute period and gradually disappear over 2–3 months.[8] Although they are not pathognomonic, EMG disturbances may correlate with the degree and severity of infection.[11]

Increased serum IgE frequently occurs but its absence does not exclude the diagnosis of trichinellosis. Elevations occur during the acute parenteral phase but there is a poor correlation between specific IgE levels and degree of infection with *T. spiralis*.[8] Parasite-specific IgE is difficult to detect due to its short half-life in serum.[11]

IgG begins to rise 2–3 weeks after infection and may persist for many years after the resolution of the disease. There are several commercially available kits for detecting IgG antibodies to *Trichinella* spp. An enzyme-linked immunosorbent assay (ELISA) is currently recommended for screening, in combination with Western blotting for confirming the diagnosis in positive ELISAs.[11] A major limitation in tropical areas is that several of the commercially available tests cross-react with other parasite antigens such as *Loa loa* and visceral larva migrans.[8,11]

Muscle biopsy demonstrating the encysted parasite is the definitive diagnostic procedure.[8] It not only confirms the presence but can also quantify the degree of infection. However, muscle biopsy is only recommended when the serology is unclear. Approximately 0.2–0.5 g of muscle (less than pea-sized) should be collected from the deltoid region and should be free of skin and fat.[11] Direct observation of the parasite is done in one of three ways: trichinelloscopy or histologic examination before or after digestion of muscle fibers.

In trichinelloscopy, a small portion of muscle tissue is compressed between two glass slides and examined on a dissecting microscope. The second method, histologic examination after fixation and staining, is more sensitive than trichinelloscopy in the early stages of infection when the larvae are small. It can also demonstrate pathologic changes in the muscle tissue. Digestion of muscle fibers after biopsy with 1% pepsin and 1% hydrochloric acid is much more sensitive than direct observation. However, this method cannot be used until 17–20 days after infection because the cysts are not resistant to digestion until that time.[8]

Direct observation of formalin-fixed and stained specimens shows basophilic transformation of muscle cells and coiled *Trichinella* larvae within the host muscle fiber (the so-called "nurse cell").

The differential diagnosis of the enteral phase of trichinellosis includes food poisoning and viral or bacterial diarrhea. The most common misdiagnosis of the parenteral phase of trichinellosis is influenza. Other differential diagnoses include angioedema, serum sickness, septicemia, allergic reactions to food or drugs, typhoid fever, chronic fatigue syndrome, polio, encephalitis, pneumonia, bronchitis, vasculitides, toxocariasis, schistosomiasis, leptospirosis, and visceral larva migrans.

Treatment and prevention

Antihelmintic treatment is recommended for all infected people during the 4–6 weeks after infection. Current recommendations consist of either mebendazole 5 mg/kg divided b.i.d. for 10–15 days or albendazole 400 mg b.i.d. for 10–15 days. Both are contraindicated in pregnant women and children under 2 years of age, although mebendazole has reportedly been used in younger children when it was deemed necessary.[11]

Glucocorticoids have been used to treat the hypersensitivity reactions in trichinellosis. They should only be used in severe and moderately severe cases and always in conjunction with antihelmintics.[11] In experimental infections, immunosuppressive drugs prolonged the survival of adult worms.[8] They may also prolong the eosinophilia by delaying encapsulation of larvae in the muscle.[11] The recommended glucocorticoid is prednisolone for 10–14 days at 30–60 mg/day divided into multiple doses. Non-steroidal anti-inflammatory drugs can be used in conjunction with antihelmintics in less severe cases.

Because acquisition of the parasite in humans occurs exclusively through the consumption of meat, adequate veterinary screening, freezing, and cooking of meat should prevent transmission.

References

1. Pozio E. New patterns of *Trichinella* infection. Vet Parasitol 2001; 98:133–148.
2. Campbell WC. History of trichinosis: Paget, Owen, and the discovery of *Trichinella spiralis*. Bull Hist Med 1979; 53:520–522.
3. Campbell WC. Historical introduction. In: Campbell WC, ed. *Trichinella* and trichinosis. New York: Plenum Press; 1983:1–30.
4. Dupouy-Camet, J. Trichinellosis: a worldwide zoonosis. Vet Parasitol 2000; 93:191–200.
5. Ortega-Pierres MG, Arriaga C, Yepez-Mulia L. Epidemiology of trichinellosis in Mexico, Central and South America. Vet Parasitol 2000; 93:201–225.
6. Takahashi Y, Mingyuan L, Waikagul J. Epidemiology of trichinellosis in Asia and the Pacific rim. Vet Parasitol 2000; 93:227–239.
7. Geerts S, de Borchgrave J, Dorny P et al. Trichinellosis: old facts and new developments. Verh K Acad Geneeskd Belg 2002; 64:233–248.
8. Bruschi F, Murrell KD. New aspects of human trichinellosis: the impact of new *Trichinella* species. Postgrad Med J 2002; 78:15–22.
9. Capo V, Despommier D. Clinical aspects of infection with *Trichinella* spp. Clin Microbiol Rev 1996; 9:47–54.
10. Markell EK, Voge M, John D, eds. The blood and tissue-dwelling nematodes. In: Medical parasitology. Philadephia, PA: WB Saunders; 1992:327–332.
11. Dupouy-Camet J, Kociecka W, Bruschi F et al. Opinion of the diagnosis and treatment of trichinellosis. Expert Opin Pharmacother 2002; 3:1117–1130.

Chapter 9

Cestodes

Jackson Machado-Pinto

- Introduction
- Biology and life cycle
- Pathogenesis and immunity
- Human cysticercosis
- Hydatid disease
- Sparganosis

Introduction

Tapeworms cause disease in humans in either of the two stages of their life cycle: the adult stage, which takes place in the intestines, where it causes mild or non-existent clinical manifestations, and the larval stage, which causes signs and symptoms secondary to enlarging larval cysts in various tissues of a mammalian host. The four more common human tapeworms are *Taenia solium* (pork tapeworm), *T. saginata* (beef tapeworm), *Diphyllobotrium latum*, and *Hymenolepis nana*. They cause primarily gastrointestinal symptoms in the definitive host. The intermediate host allows penetration of the intestinal mucosa by the larval stage. Humans can only bear the larval stage of *Echinococcus granulosus*, which causes cysts observed in visceral organs.[1] However, besides *T. solium* and *E. granulosus*, cutaneous disease by cestodes can only be caused by larvae belonging to the genus *Spirometra*.

Biology and life cycle

The adult tapeworm can reach considerable length (up to 9 m). Its body has two main parts: the head, or scolex, fit for attachment, and the proglottids, which are hermaphroditic egg machines. Within each proglottid are male and female reproductive organs. The fertilized eggs accumulate in large numbers inside the uterine horns and can be released into the host's intestine, or the entire gravid terminal proglottid can be eliminated. Both the eggs and the proglottids may be found in the stool. Ingestion of the eggs by a susceptible intermediate host will allow the eggs to develop into larvae, which are called oncospheres. The oncospheres of *T. saginata* and *T. solium* further develop into encysted forms called cysticerci, or bladder worms. Cysticercosis thus refers to the disease caused in cattle by cysticerci of *T. saginata* and to the disease caused by the larval stage of *T. solium* in pigs and humans. An oncosphere able to develop germinal membranes, which can generate germinal tissue within a cyst is termed hydatid: it is the typical cyst of echinococcosis. Ingestion of tissues containing cysts by a susceptible definitive host allows the development of the larval stage into an adult and completion of the life cycle.[1]

Pathogenesis and immunity

Adult cestodes within the intestine usually cause no morphological and identifiable changes in the mucosa or submucosa. Some patients may present moderate eosinophilia. Immunity plays only a limited role during adult tapeworm infection. It has little effect on the duration of infection or on the susceptibility to reinfection. However, immunity plays an important role during the intermediate stage of larval development. The inflammatory infiltrate surrounding the cysts starts at the time of larval migration and is markedly intensified as the cyst degenerates. All cellular elements can be seen, including giant cells, fibroblasts, and neutrophils.[2]

The signs and symptoms triggered by this reaction will obviously depend on the site where the reaction takes place. If at the base of the brain, a cysticercic meningitis may ensue. In brain tissue, the cysts may calcify and cause seizures. Involvement of skin, muscle, eyes, and heart has also been described.

Humoral antibody response and complement-mediated organism lysis, delayed hypersensitivity, and protection of immunized animals have been shown experimentally.[3]

Humans are the only definitive host for *T. saginata* (beef tapeworm) and infection takes place when poorly cooked muscle of diseased cattle is ingested. Humans are also the only definitive host for *T. solium* (pork tapeworm) and infection occurs only after the ingestion of contaminated meat.

Larvae of *E. granulosus* enter the portal circulation and the majority are trapped by the liver sinusoids. Some bypass the liver and pass the lungs and heart carried by the blood stream to any other organ or tissue in the body.[4] Within hours an inflammatory response may be seen. If any larvae survive, within 5 days they can develop into hydatids. Cell-mediated immunity controls metastatic dissemination during the early phase of infection. Also, humoral responses and complement activation occur.

E. granulosus persists in nature by infecting dogs, which house the adult worm in their intestinal tract, or sheep or cattle, which become the intermediate hosts by ingesting the contaminated dog feces. The dog ingests the beef or lamb containing larvae and completes the cycle. Humans become involved accidentally by contact with contaminated dog feces, as do sheep, and thereby become the hosts for the gradually enlarging cyst, the hydatid.

Human cysticercosis

Cysticercosis is due to infection with eggs of *T. solium* acquired by contact with contaminated human feces. Contact with food or water contaminated with human feces and autoinfection from anus to mouth by a person with the adult tapeworm are the two most likely routes by which a human may become the intermediate host. Reverse peristaltic and internal infection are less likely to occur. After penetrating the host's intestinal wall, the oncosphere develops rapidly and within 10 weeks matures to a fully developed larva. The cyst is usually 0.5–1.0 cm in diameter and contains a yellow, viscous fluid and the invaginated head, referred to as *Cysticercus cellulosae*.[5] The cyst remains viable for 3–5 years and eventually degenerates. At this time, an inflammatory response is evoked and calcification often takes place.

Cysticercosis is relatively common in Mexico, South America, and certain parts of Africa.

Lesions can develop in almost any organ tissue of the body. In the skin, small-mass lesions can be palpated, more than seen. They are usually multiple and asymptomatic. The brain, eye, heart, other muscles, and peritoneal cavity may also be affected. In a Brazilian study, 64 911 protocols of anatomopathological examinations were reviewed. Thirty (0.05%) had the diagnosis of cysticercosis. Ninety percent had cysticerci in the subcutaneous tissue, skeletal muscle, or mucous membrane, while the CNS was affected in 6.7%.[6]

Diagnosis is often made by an X-ray examination of the head or extremities, which shows small calcifications. Computed tomography of the head or the suspected area will clearly show the space-occupying lesions. Magnetic resonance imaging findings in parenchymal neurocysticercosis depend on the stage of involution of the cysticerci. Enzyme-linked immunosorbent assay and the hemagglutination test using cyst vesicular fluid as antigen are 80–95% sensitive and specific. Immunoblot has been determined to be the serologic test of choice, because its specificity and sensitivity approach 100% and 94%, respectively.[7]

Treatment of old cutaneous lesions is surgical. Patients with active infection with living organisms may be treated with praziquantel, 50 mg/kg per day in three divided doses, for 2 weeks or with albendazole, 15 mg/kg per day, with a maximum of 800 mg, for 8 or more days. Albendazole is cheaper and has 20% more cysticidal activity than does praziquantel.[7]

Prevention of infection by control of deposition of human feces is most important. Continued control of meat inspection of human infection with the adult stage of *T. solium* will also decrease the prevalence of cysticercosis.

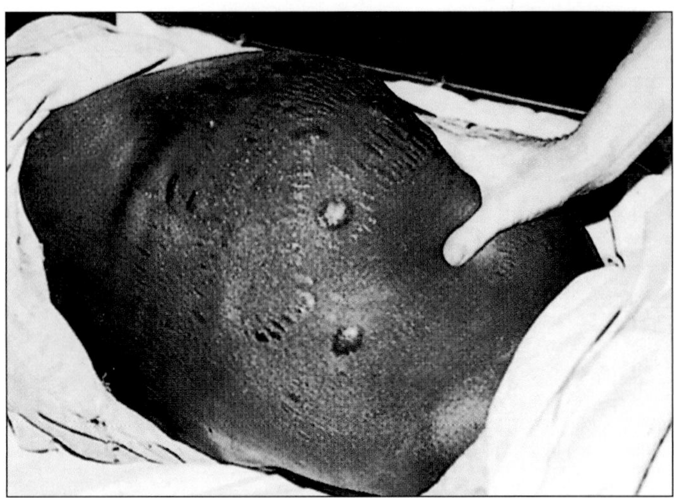

Figure 9.1 Massive hydatid cyst in a Kenyan boy. (Reproduced from Peters W and Pasvol G (eds). Tropical Medicine and Parasitology, 5th edition, London 2002, image 748).

Hydatid disease

Echinococcosis is seen in most sheep- and cattle-raising areas in the world, including Australia, New Zealand, Argentina, Uruguay, Chile, parts of Africa, Eastern Europe and the Middle-East. It is particularly common in Lebanon and Greece.

When humans ingest the eggs of *E. granulosus*, oncospheres penetrate the mesenteric vessels from which they reach the various organs of the body. The liver and lungs are commonly infected and are the sites of development of hydatid cysts. The cyst increases in size at the rate of about 1 cm/year. It is this gradually enlarging mass that compresses adjacent host structures and whose protuberance on the outside can sometimes be appreciated (Fig. 9.1), leading to the signs and symptoms of echinococcosis. Allergic symptoms, such as urticaria, asthma, and anaphylaxis, are rare.[8]

Computed tomography best shows the wall calcification. Magnetic resonance imaging depicts the exact anatomic location of the cyst.[4]

Surgical removal of the intact cyst is the preferred form of therapy. Albendazole has been used in doses of 10 mg/kg per day for 8 weeks in the treatment of inoperable cases or as preoperative therapy for 4 days.[8]

The cycle of infection can be broken by keeping dogs free of infection by proper disposal of carcasses and entrails of dead sheep, cattle, and hogs.

Sparganosis

Sparganosis is an infection caused by the migrating larvae of the cestode genus *Spirometra*. A subcutaneous mass is the most common dermatologic manifestation. Histologically, there is a granulomatous panniculitis and dermatitis, containing a section of a sparganum.[9]

References

1. Smyth JD, Heath DD. Pathogenesis of larval cestodes in mammals. Helm Abstr 1970; 39:1–23.
2. Isaak DD, Jacobson RH, Reed ND. Thymus dependence of tapeworm (*Hymenolepis diminuta*) elimination from mice. Inf Immob 1975; 12:1478–1479.
3. Rickard MD, Arundel JH, Adolph AJ. A preliminary field trial to evaluate the use of immunization for the control of acquired *Taenia saginata* infection in cattle. Res Vet Sci 1981; 30:104–108.
4. Kurugoglu S, Kizilkilic O, Ogut G et al. Cross-sectional imaging features. South Med J 2002; 95:1140–1144.
5. Falanga V, Kapoor W. Cerebral cysticercosis: diagnostic value of subcutaneous nodules. J Am Acad Dermatol 1985; 12:304.
6. Vianna LG, Macedo V, Costa JM. Musculocutaneous and visceral cysticercosis: a rare disease? Rev Inst Med Trop Sao Paulo 1991; 33:129–136.
7. Rosenfeld E. Neurocysticercosis update. Pediatr Infec Dis J 2003; 22:181–182.
8. Okelo GBA. Hydatid disease: research and control in Turkana, III. Albendazole in the treatment of inoperable hydatid disease in Kenya – a report of 12 cases. Trans R Soc Trop Med 1986; 99:195–198.
9. Griffin MP, Tompkins KJ, Ryan MT. Cutaneous sparganosis. Am J Dermatopathol 1996; 18:70–72.

Chapter 10

Trematodes

Peter Leutscher and Pascal Magnussen

Synonyms:

- Schistosomiasis, bilharziasis
- Cercarial dermatitis, swimmer's itch, *Schistosoma* dermatitis, clam digger's itch
- Acute schistosomiasis syndrome, acute toxemic schistosomiasis, Katyama fever, snail fever
- Late cutaneous schistosomiasis, bilharziasis cutanea tarda

Key features:

- Infection takes place by skin contact with *Schistosoma* cercariae-infested water
- Three clinical stages with distinctive skin manifestations are successively related to the different stages of infection:
  - First stage (cercarial dermatitis): pruritic maculopapular rash at the site of penetration of the cercaria
  - Second stage (acute schistosomiasis syndrome): urticaria associated with migrating and maturing larva
  - Third stage (late cutaneous schistosomiasis): granulomatous cutaneous lesions in response to deposited eggs in the skin
- Diagnosis is confirmed by demonstration of *Schistosoma* eggs and/or by serology test
- Praziquantel is effective and well-tolerated for treatment of uncomplicated late cutaneous schistosomiasis

Introduction

Schistosomiasis is caused by blood flukes (trematodes) belonging to the genus *Schistosoma*. Humans are infected through contact with *Schistosoma*-infested water. A multitude of clinical manifestations are associated with *Schistosoma* infection in humans. The nature and severity of symptoms are determined by several factors, including the *Schistosoma* species, the stage and intensity of infection, and the immune status of the infected individual. The symptoms of urinary and gastrointestinal schistosomiasis are readily recognized, whereas ectopic forms, including the dermal schistosomiasis, often present a greater diagnostic challenge. Familiarity with the clinical manifestations of all stages and presentations of cutaneous schistosomiasis is essential for optimal therapeutic management.

History

The earliest evidence of schistosomiasis comes from calcified ova in ancient Egyptian mummies from 1220 BC.[1] In 1851, Theodor Bilharz discovered the parasitic blood fluke of the genus *Schistosoma* in postmortem studies in Cairo. Since then, five species of human schistosomiasis have been identified based on egg morphology and clinical features: *S. haematobium* in 1864, *S. mansoni* in 1902, *S. japonicum* in 1904, *S. intercalatum* in 1934, and *S. mekongi* in 1978. The existence of specific snail intermediate hosts for different species of *Schistosoma* was established by Leiper in 1915. *Schistosoma* cercariae were subsequently identified in 1926 as the cause of dermatitis in humans exposed to fresh water infested with schistosomes.[2]

Epidemiology

Human schistosomiasis is focally distributed in 76 countries located in the tropics and subtropics (Figs 10.1 and 10.2). An estimated 200 million people, most of whom live in sub-Saharan Africa, are infected by schistosomiasis.[3] *S. haematobium*, *S. mansoni*, and *S. japonicum* are numerically the most important *Schistosoma* species in humans. *S. haematobium* causes urogenital schistosomiasis and late cutaneous schistosomiasis, whereas *S. mansoni* and *S. japonicum* cause gastrointestinal schistosomiasis. Non-human *Schistosoma* species, in particular avian schistosomes, frequently cause cercarial dermatitis.

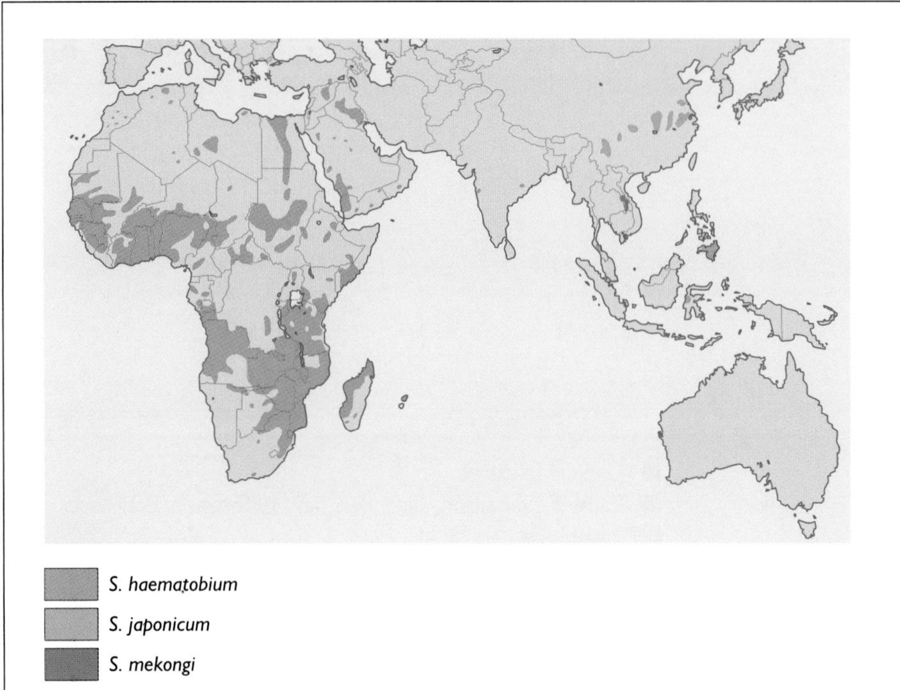

Figure 10.1 Distribution of *Schistosoma haematobium*, as the most common cause of late cutaneous schistosomiasis, and of *S. japonicum* and *S. mekongi*. (Courtesy of the World Health Organization.)

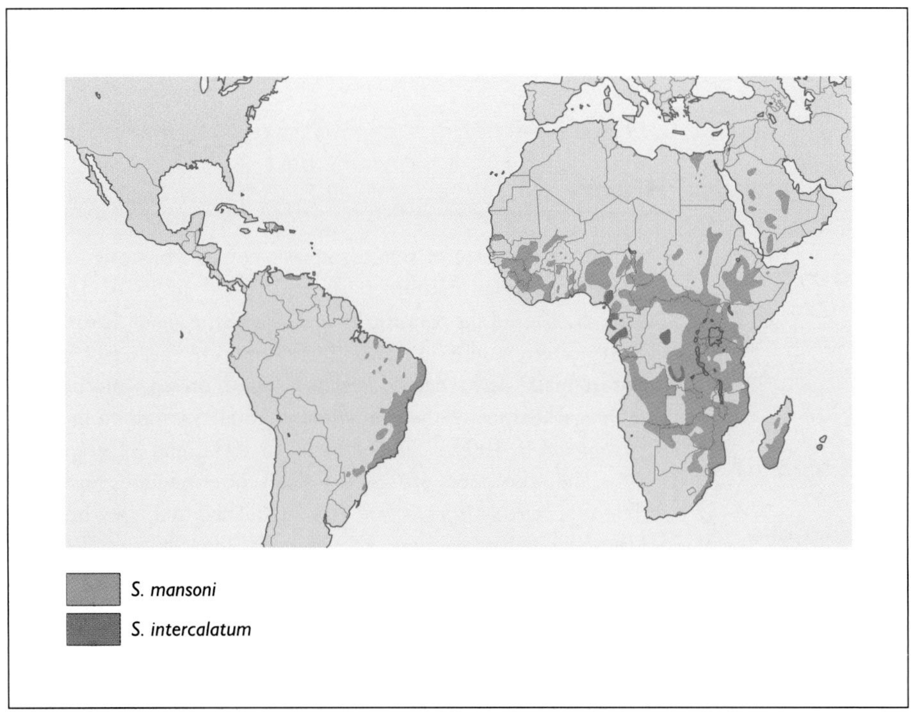

Figure 10.2 Distribution of *Schistosoma mansoni* and *S. intercalatum*. (Courtesy of the World Health Organization.)

The epidemiology of human schistosomiasis in a particular ecosystem is dependent on a complex interrelationship between people and their environment. Transmission of schistosomiasis requires human contact with water that is inhabited by the infected intermediate host snail. Human schistosomiasis is only transmitted in fresh water, whereas non-human schistosomiasis is also transmitted in salt water. When schistosome eggs, passed in urine or feces, come into contact with water, a miracidium hatches from the egg and searches for the specific snail host that is required to complete its life cycle (Fig. 10.3). After a variable period of weeks to months of asexual development in the snail, large numbers of microscopic infective larvae (cercariae) are produced and then leave the snail. The cercariae are free-swimming, colorless organisms about 0.7 mm in length.

Susceptibility to schistosomiasis infection is universal. Typically, water contact and exposure to *Schistosoma* infection begins early in life. The prevalence and intensity of infection increase during the first and second decade of life, with a peak around 15 years

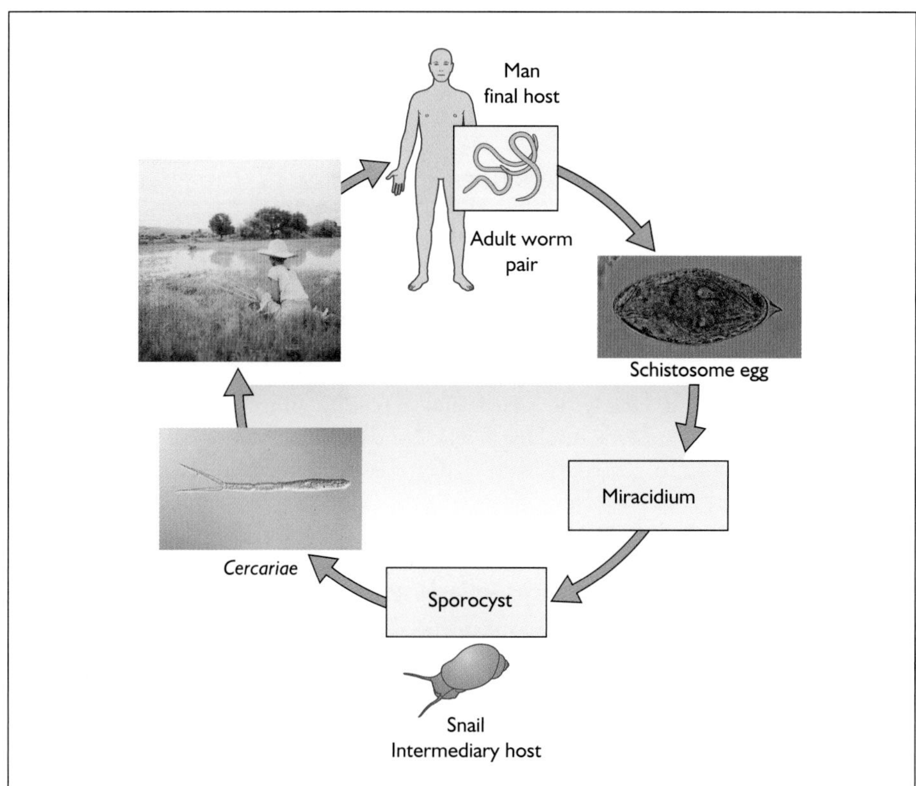

Figure 10.3 Life cycle of human schistosomes. (Courtesy of Peter Leutscher/Elsevier Science.)

of age, followed by a decline, especially in the intensity of infection in adulthood. This decline is partly due to the development of specific immunity and partly due to diminished exposure.[4] It is important to note that the foci for schistosomiasis transmission are increasing as a consequence of the development of irrigation systems and hydroelectrical projects. Migration is another important factor in the spread of schistosomiasis, either through the introduction of the parasite into previous schistosomiasis-free locations or by migration of non-infected individuals into endemic foci. Travelers engaging in recreational water activities in schistosomiasis-endemic areas are also at risk of infection. With increasing tourism in endemic areas, schistosomiasis is being encountered more frequently in returning travelers.[5,6]

The socioeconomic situation in most developing countries makes the eradication of schistosomiasis unlikely. Therefore, the strategy of schistosomiasis control tends to focus on the management of morbidity rather than on transmission. The main tools are anti-schistosomal treatment supported by an improvement in the sanitary conditions, and the provision of relevant health education.[3]

Pathogenesis and etiology

The symptoms of human schistosomiasis are primarily caused by the immune response against the invading and migrating larvae and later the parasite eggs deposited in the host tissue. Three distinctive clinical stages are associated with schistosomiasis infection: (1) cercarial dermatitis; (2) acute schistosomiasis; and (3) chronic schistosomiasis. Each stage, characterized by distinct pathological and clinical manifestations, is related to the different phases of the *Schistosoma* infection and to schistosomiasis-specific immunity (Table 10.1).

Table 10.1 Relative frequency of schistosomiasis-associated clinical manifestations in non-immune and indigenous persons by *Schistosoma* species

	S. haematobium		*S. mansoni*		*S. japonicum*		*Avian schistosoma*[a]	
	Non-immune	Indigenous	Non-immune	Indigenous	Non-immune	Indigenous	Non-immune	Indigenous
Cercarial dermatitis	+	–	+	–	+	–	+++	+++
Acute schistosomiasis syndrome	+	–	++	–	++	–	–	–
Late cutaneous schistosomiasis	+	++	(+)	+	(+)	+	–	–

[a]*S. trichobilharzia, S. gigantobilharzia, S. ornithobilharzia, S. microbilharzia.*

Cercarial dermatitis may develop soon after a person has been exposed to skin-invading cercariae.[7] When the human host comes into contact with infested water, the cercariae attach themselves to exposed skin surfaces by means of suckers and penetrate the dermal layers within 15 min. Observations of cercarial penetration suggest that the parasites can move easily between cells of the superficial layers of the epidermis without requiring enzymatic activity. However, when the cercariae reach the "spinous" layer of the middle part of the epidermis, they overcome cell–cell adhesions through proteolytic enzymes secreted by cercarial acetabular glands.[8] During the passage through the epidermis and dermis, the cercaria transforms into a schistosomulum. Cercarial dermatitis due to human *Schistosoma* species is most commonly observed in non-immune individuals and is rarely seen in people living in schistosomiasis-endemic areas. However, the high risk of developing cercarial dermatitis after exposure to avian schistosome cercariae does not differ between indigenous and non-indigenous people. In contrast to human schistosomes, where the cercariae mature into adult worms and thus give rise to systemic disease, non-human cercariae die shortly after penetration of the skin, thereby eliciting a marked, but self-limiting local inflammatory reaction. In this case, the symptoms of dermatitis are more intense than those observed in human schistosomiasis.

The clinical manifestations of the acute schistosomiasis syndrome comprise a severe, transient, systemic reaction, which resembles the acute serum sickness syndrome.[9] The acute schistosomiasis syndrome coincides with the migration of the juvenile worm in the blood stream and subsequently egg production, which triggers a type 3 immune reaction. This stage of acute schistosomiasis is often more severe in the case of *S. mansoni* and in *S. japonicum* infection than in *S. haematobium* infection. The syndrome is seen mostly in non-immune individuals, such as travelers, similar to the scenario observed with cercarial dermatitis caused by human schistosomiasis.

Following maturation and pairing of the worms in the liver, they migrate against the blood flow from the portal circulation to the venous plexus of the target organ, where egg excretion commences about 5–12 weeks after initial contact with infected water. Late cutaneous schistosomiasis is predominantly associated with *S. haematobium* infection, and less frequently with *S. mansoni* infection.[10,11] *S. haematobium* worms migrate within the distribution of the inferior vena cava mesenteric branches to the anorectal plexus and by various anastomoses to the venous plexus in the bladder, the internal and external genitals, the groin and the perineum. Several aberrant routes may be taken by the adult worms to various ectopic sites, for example, close to the skin. The worm pair lives for many years and the female worms are capable of producing up to hundreds of eggs per day. Approximately half of the eggs produced become trapped in adjacent tissues or are transported via the blood stream and lodge in the tissue elsewhere in the body. The pathological changes seen in chronic schistosomiasis infection are primarily due to the deposition of eggs in the tissue of the host. The deposited eggs evoke a delayed hypersensitivity granulomatous T-cell-mediated immune response, resulting in an accumulation of eosinophils, macrophages, and lymphocytes which form the classic *Schistosoma* granuloma.[12] Schistosome egg antigen (soluble egg antigen, SEA), originating from the secretory glands of the miracidia in the eggs, has been identified as an essential granuloma-inducing factor. The immune cells in the granuloma are gradually replaced by fibroblasts, which may lead to irreversible tissue changes in the affected organs.

Clinical features

Cercarial dermatitis

Cercarial dermatitis is an acute pruritic, papular rash at the cercarial penetration. A prickling sensation lasting a few hours may occur shortly after contact with infested water. Erythema or urticaria may be seen during this stage. After a period of 10–15 h, a clearly localized and intensely pruritic maculopapular rash appears, reaching a peak 2–3 days after exposure. The lesions begin to resolve after 5–7 days leaving a pigmented spot. Vesicles or pustules may form as a result of secondary infection caused by scratching.

Acute schistosomiasis syndrome

The symptoms of acute schistosomasis syndrome emerge 2–16 weeks after the initial cercarial invasion. The clinical manifestations depend on the immune status of the individual and the severity may vary considerably.[13] The most important clinical feature of the syndrome is persistent irregular fever with a gradual or sudden onset. Symptoms such as headache, fatigue, localized edema, cough, musculoskeletal pain, poor appetite, nausea, and diarrhea are also variably experienced by infected individuals. Hepato- and splenomegaly are often found on clinical examination. Normally the illness lasts 14–21 days.

Chronic visceral schistosomiasis

The key symptom related to *S. haematobium* infection, in particular in children living in endemic areas, is hematuria due to mucosal lesions in the urinary bladder. Painful and frequent urination is also commonly reported. After some years late-stage renal complications such as obstructive uropathy and hydronephrosis may occur. Urinary bladder involvement predisposes to the development of carcinoma. The main clinical manifestations of infection with *S. mansoni* and *S. japonicum* are abdominal discomfort and episodes of diarrhea with blood and mucus in the stool, but in general are non-specific. With time, liver fibrosis may develop, resulting in portal hypertension, ascites, and esophageal varices.

Late cutaneous schistosomiasis

Deposition of eggs in the dermis and subcutaneous tissues is usually seen months or even years after infection. The initial early-stage lesions are 2–3-mm firm, often pruritic, flesh-colored papules in a cluster formation. Later they may coalesce into lichenified plaques or nodular lesions, which may become pigmented.[10] The lesions are typically located in the anogenital area, the periumbilical area, the chest, and upper dorsal regions, where they may have a zosteriform distribution (Fig. 10.4). Involvement of the external genitals, particularly when seen in women, is an important clinical aspect of late cutaneous schistosomiasis. Female organ involvement is frequently localized to the labia majora, the clitoris, and the vulva.[14,15] Genital lesions present as a broad spectrum of abnormalities, ranging from papules and warts to polypoid growth and tumors (Fig. 10.5). Ulceration with risk of secondary bacterial

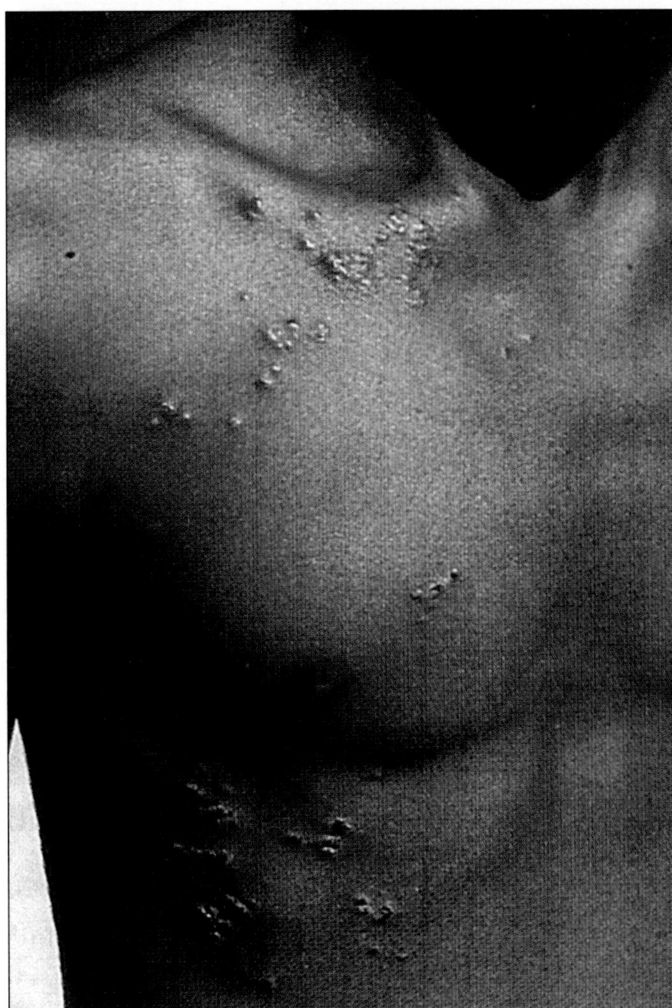

Figure 10.4 Late cutaneous schistosomiasis due to deposition of *Schistosoma* eggs in the dermis and the subcutaneous tissue. (Reproduced with permission from Grossetete G, Diabate I, Pichard E et al. Manifestations cutanées des bilharzioses. A propos de 24 observations au Mali. Bull Soc Pathol Exot 1989; 82:225–232.)

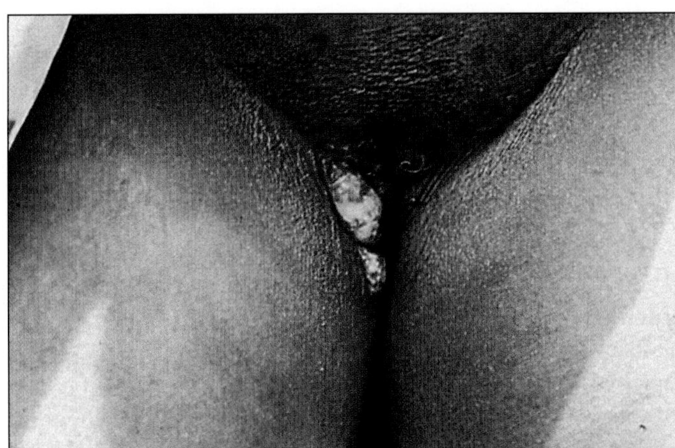

Figure 10.5 Polypoid growth in the genital area. The diagnosis of late cutaneous schistosomiasis was in this case based on identification of *Schistosoma haematobium* eggs in a tissue biopsy. (Reproduced with permission from Grossetete G, Diabate I, Pichard E et al. Manifestations cutanées des bilharzioses. A propos de 24 observations au Mali. Bull Soc Pathol Exot 1989; 82:225–232.)

infection may complicate the course. If the condition is left untreated, it may lead to irreversible damage of the tissue structure, including destruction of the clitoris and the formation of fistulae.

Patient evaluation, diagnosis, and differential diagnosis

Because the clinical presentation of schistosomiasis infection varies according to the stage of infection, different diagnostic procedures need to be applied in the assessment of the patient with presumed schistosomiasis infection (Table 10.2). The first step in the diagnostic process for such a patient should include a thorough history of exposure to cercarial-infested water in a schistosomiasis-endemic area.

Cercarial dermatitis

Complaints of a pruritic maculopapular rash, initially following skin contact with water, would strongly suggest cercarial dermatitis. The differential diagnosis to cercarial dermatitis includes flea bites, algae dermatitis, coelenterate stings, impetigo, chickenpox, herpes, and poison ivy. In contrast, sea bather eruption is an irritant or toxic transient reaction to the larval forms of marine coelenterates and only occurs on body parts covered by a swimming suit.

Acute schistosomiasis syndrome

This syndrome does not have the same acute expression of onset as cercarial dermatitis. This stage of infection may only manifest for 2–16 weeks after exposure and is characterized by several clinical and laboratory indicators. Acute schistosomiasis syndrome is difficult to identify because it is consistent with many other causes of febrile illness among residents or travelers in the tropics. The differential diagnosis must include malaria, typhoid fever, brucellosis, mononucleosis, invasive ankylostomiasis and strongyloidiasis, ascariasis, trichinosis, visceral larvae migrans, fascioliasis, trichinellosis, filariasis, and toxocariasis.[16] Clinical suspicion for acute schistosomiasis syndrome should be raised when the following differentiating conditions are observed: (1) exposure to fresh water in a schistosomiasis-endemic region within the last 2–3 months; (2) two or more of the following symptoms or signs: fever, dry cough, abdominal pain, diarrhea, weight loss, hepatomegaly, splenomegaly, musculoskeletal pain, urticaria, or swollen eyelids; (3) the presence of living eggs in feces or urine and/or positive schistosomiasis serology.[6] Regarding the last criterion, it may not be possible to detect eggs and serology may not yet be positive at this point of infection. If the initial tests are negative, they should be repeated later to confirm the diagnosis. Eosinophilia ($> 500/mm^3$) is in the meantime a strongly supportive indicator of infection.

Late cutaneous schistosomiasis

Late cutaneous schistosomiasis should be considered as a differential diagnosis of atypical skin lesions in a person with a history of residency or travel in a *S. haematobium*-endemic area. At this stage of infection, laboratory diagnosis is based on the demonstration of *Schistosoma* eggs in urine or in biopsy specimens. Urine sedimentation and filtration are used for the detection of *S. haematobium* eggs. Stool samples can be examined for the presence

Table 10.2 Diagnosis and treatment of schistosomiasis infection by stage of infection

	Diagnostic means					
	Signs/symptoms	Eosinophilia[a]	Serology[b]	Egg detection: Urine/feces[c]	Egg detection: Biopsy	Treatment
Cercarial dermatitis	+	–	–	–	–	Antipruritic cream (1% hydrocortisone), systemic antihistamine/steroid
Acute schistosomiasis syndrome	+	+	(+)	(+)	–	Systemic antihistamine/steroid
Late cutaneous schistosomiasis	+	(+)	+	(+)	+	Praziquantel (surgery)

[a] > 500/mm³.
[b]Depending on type of test.
[c]Yield outcome depends on intensity of infection, analysis technique, and number of specimens.

of the other human *Schistosoma* species' eggs. Day-to-day variation in egg excretion may necessitate repeated sampling on consecutive days, in particular in individuals from non-endemic areas with low infection intensity. The histological diagnosis of late cutaneous schistosomiasis is based on the finding of eggs and granulomas in a tissue biopsy by serial sections of the biopsy material, followed by staining with hematoxylin and eosin, or Ziehl–Neelsen. Gentle scraping of the skin lesions followed by microscopy, rather than by surgical biopsy or punch biopsy, may sometimes be sufficient to demonstrate the presence of eggs. Venereal diseases, tuberculosis, and cancer are the main differential diagnoses. Late cutaneous schistosomiasis localized to the anogenital area may easily be mistaken for a sexually transmitted infection such as primary syphilis, condylomata lata, genital warts, herpes simplex, and lymphogranuloma venereum. A tumor of the vulva may be interpreted as neoplasm. Lesions may also resemble lichen planus, subcutaneous tuberculosis, tuberculoid leprosy, or sarcoidosis.

Serology

Serological tests are important supplementary tools in the diagnosis of schistosomiasis. This is particularly true for travelers returning from visits to endemic areas. These patients typically present in the early stage of infection, when egg production has not yet started. In the chronic stage, egg excretion in urine or in stool may be very low due to sporadic exposure, resulting in a low-intensity infection which is therefore difficult to detect. Although there are a number of tests for detecting antibodies to infection, their use is limited to some extent since antibodies are not present until 6–12 weeks after exposure and they continue to be present even after successful pharmaceutical treatment.

Pathology

Late cutaneous schistosomiasis

Skin lesions observed in late cutaneous schistosomiasis are due to deposition of ova in the dermis. The lesions are characterized by a range of inflammatory reactions, including infiltrates with predominantly eosinophilic "microabscesses" to granulomatous giant cells and interstitial fibrosis. The presence of viable and calcified ova within the dermis and the epidermis, including the stratum corneum, suggests that transepithelial elimination of the eggs is part of the host response.[17] Hyperplasia of the epidermis and irregular expansion with downgrowth of the rete pegs (pseudoepitheliomatous hyperplasia) is another common histopathological feature (Fig. 10.6).

Treatment

Schistosomiasis infection can only be prevented by avoiding contact with cercariae-infested water. If water contact is unavoidable, clothes to cover skin exposed to contaminated water and/or a repellent may provide some protection. In addition, *N*,*N*-diethyl-*m*-toluamide (DEET) has shown promise as a topical agent for preventing skin penetration by *S. mansoni* cercariae, but this observation has yet to be confirmed in controlled studies.[18]

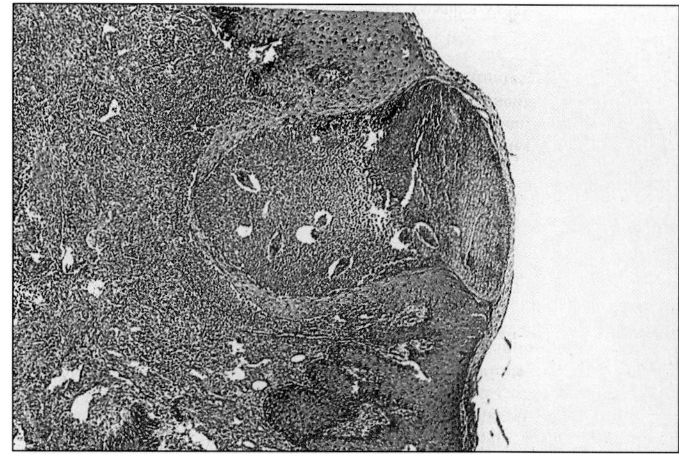

Figure 10.6 Pseudoepitheliomatous hyperplasia of the epidermis containing schistosomal eggs in granulomas characteristic for late cutaneous schistosomiasis. (Reproduced with permission from Grossetete G, Diabate I, Pichard E et al. Manifestations cutanées des bilharzioses. A propos de 24 observations au Mali. Bull Soc Pathol Exot 1989; 82:225–232.)

Treatment of cercarial dermatitis and the acute schistosomiasis syndrome is palliative (Table 10.2). Application of a 1% hydrocortisone cream combined with oral antihistamines is useful for relieving symptoms of cercarial dermatitis. Antibiotics are suggested in case secondary bacterial infection develops. It is recommended that acute schistosomaisis syndrome is only treated with systemic glucocorticoids, because early antischistosomal therapy may result in severe allergic reactions due to killing of the schistosome larvae and a subsequent strong antigen release.[19]

Currently, praziquantel is the most widely used antischistosomal drug for the treatment of chronic schistosomiasis. It is effective against all species of human schistosomes and it can be administered as a single dose (40 mg/kg), which increases compliance. Artemisine has also been shown to be effective for the treatment of schistosomiasis. The drug has the advantage of killing the schistosomule at an early stage of infection.[20] Excision of skin lesions may be required in cases where there is a poor response to initial antischistosomal treatment.

References

1. Ruffer MA. Note on the presence of *Bilharzia haematobia* in Egyptian mummies of the 20th dynasty 1220–1000 BC. Br Med J 1910; I:16.
2. Cort WW. *Schistosoma* dermatitis in the United States (Michigan). JAMA 1926; 90:1027–1029.
3. World Health Organization. Report of the WHO informal consultation on schistosomiasis control. WHO/CDS/CPC/SIP/99.2. Geneva:WHO; 1998.
4. Davis A. Schistosomiasis. In Robinson D, ed. Epidemiology and community control of disease in warm climate countries, 2nd edn. Edinburgh: Churchill Livingstone, 1985:389–412.
5. Istre GR, Fontaine RE, Tarr J et al. Acute schistosomiasis among Americans rafting the Omo River, Ethiopia. JAMA 1984; 251:508–510.
6. Visser LG, Polderman AM, Stuiver PC. Outbreak of schistosomiasis among travelers returning from Mali, West Africa. Clin Infect Dis 1995; 20:280–285.
7. Fitzpatrick TB, Johnson RA, Wolff K et al. Color atlas and synopsis of clinical dermatology. Common and serious diseases, 4th edn. London: McGraw-Hill; 2001.
8. McKerrow JH, Salter J. Invasion of skin by *Schistosoma cercariae*. Trends Parasitol 2002; 18:193–195.
9. Lawley TJ, Ottesen EA, Hiatt RA et al. Circulating immune complexes in acute schistosomiasis. Clin Exp Immunol 1979; 37:221–227.
10. Grossetete G, Diabate I, Pichard E et al. Manifestations cutanées des bilharzioses. A propos de 24 observations au Mali. Bull Soc Pathol Exot 1989; 82:225–232.
11. Ramos SF. Late cutaneous bilharziasis. South Afr Med J 1973; 47:2103–2108.
12. von Lichtenberg F. Consequences of infections with schistosomes. In Rollinson D, Simpson AJG, eds. The biology of schistosomes: from genes to latrines. London: Academic Press; 1987:185–232.
13. Stuiver PC. Acute schistosomiasis (Katayama fever). Br Med J 1984; 288:221–222.
14. Attili VR, Hira SK, Dube MK. Schistosomal genital granulomas: a report of 10 cases. Br J Venerol Dis 1983; 59:269–272.
15. Wright ED, Chiphangwi J, Hutt MSR. Schistosomiasis of the female genital tract: a histopathological study of 176 cases from Malawi. Trans R Soc Trop Med Hyg 1982; 76:822–829.
16. D'Acremont V, Burnand B, Ambresin AE et al. Practice guidelines for evaluation of fever in returning travelers or migrants. J Travel Med 2003; 10 (suppl.):25–52.
17. Ramdial PK. Transepithelial elimination of late cutaneous vulvar schistosomiasis. Int J Gynecol Pathol 2001; 20:166–172.
18. Salafsky B, Kalyanasundaram RE, Yi-Xum H et al. Evaluation of *N,N*-diethyl-*m*-toluamide (DEET) as a topical agent for preventing skin penetration by cercariae of *Schistosoma mansoni*. Am J Trop Med Hyg 1998; 58:828–834.
19. Harries AD, Cook GC. Acute schistosomiasis (Katayama fever): clinical deterioration after chemotherapy. J Infect Dis 1987; 14:159–161.
20. Utzinger J, Keiser J, Xiao SH et al. Combination chemotherapy of schistosomiasis in laboratory studies and clinical trials. Antimicrob Agents Chemother 2003; 47:1487–1495.

Chapter 11

HIV and HIV-associated disorders

Janek Maniar and Ratnakar Kamath

Introduction

The pandemic of human immunodeficiency/acquired immunodeficiency syndrome (HIV/AIDS) is proving to be a modern scourge. The sheer magnitude of the problem can be understood, to some extent, by a look at the figures in Tables 11.1 and 11.2.[1] There were an estimated 46 million individuals infected with HIV at the end of 2003, of whom almost 23 million were women and 3.2 million were children. There were an estimated 5.8 million new infections in 2003, while 3.5 million deaths occurred due to AIDS and AIDS-associated conditions.

It is also clear from Table 11.2 that the main problem rests in sub-Saharan Africa and Southeast Asia. These regions are part of the developing world and are densely populated. Thus, the onus of the battle against HIV/AIDS is shifting from the affluent nations of the developed world to the developing world, worsening the socioeconomic upheavals faced by these areas.

Table 11.1 Global summary of the human immunodeficiency virus (HIV)/acquired immunodeficiency syndrome (AIDS) epidemic, December 2003[1]

Number of people living with HIV/AIDS	Total	46 million
	Adults	42.8 million
	Women	23 million
	Children under 15 years	3.2 million
People newly infected with HIV in 2003	Total	5.8 million
	Adults	5.0 million
	Women	2.4 million
	Children under 15 years	800 000
AIDS deaths in 2003	Total	3.5 million
	Adults	2.9 million
	Women	1.2 million
	Children under 15 years	610 000

Table 11.2 Regional human immunodeficiency virus (HIV)/acquired immunodeficiency syndrome (AIDS) statistics and features, end of 2003[1]

	Epidemic started	Adults and children living with HIV/AIDS	Adults and children newly infected with HIV	Adult prevalence rate[a]	Percentage of HIV-positive adults who are women	Main mode(s) of transmission for those living with HIV/AIDS[b]
Sub-Saharan Africa	Late 1970s, early 1980s	29.4 million	3.6 million	8.8%	58%	Hetero
North Africa and Middle East	Late 1980s	730 000	83 000	0.3%	55%	Hetero, IDU
South and Southeast Asia	Late 1980s	8.2 million	1.2 million	0.6%	36%	Hetero, IDU
East Asia and Pacific	Late 1980s	1.2 million	270 000	0.1%	24%	IDU, hetero, MSM
Latin America	Late 1970s, early 1980s	1.9 million	180 000	0.6%	30%	MSM, IDU, hetero
Caribbean	Late 1970s, early 1980s	590 000	80 000	2.4%	50%	Hetero, MSM
Eastern Europe and Central Asia	Early 1990s	1.8 million	280 000	0.6%	27%	IDU
Western Europe	Late 1970s, early 1980s	680 000	40 000	0.3%	25%	MSM, IDU
North America	Late 1970s, early 1980s	1.2 million	54 000	0.6%	20%	MSM, IDU, hetero
Australia and New Zealand	Late 1970s, early 1980s	18 000	1000	0.1%	7%	MSM
Total		46 million	5 million	1.2%	50%	

[a]The proportion of adults (15–49 years of age) living with HIV/AIDS in 2002, using 2002 population numbers.
[b]Hetero, heterosexual transmission; IDU, transmission through injecting drug use; MSM, sexual transmission among men who have sex with men.

Modes of transmission of HIV[2]

HIV infection is transmitted in the following ways:

- By sexual contact, both homosexual and heterosexual.
- By transfusion of blood and blood products.
- From infected mother to infant, whether antepartum, perinatal, or via breast milk.

As yet, there is no evidence to prove that HIV is transmitted by casual contact or insect bite.

Sexual transmission

Unprotected sexual intercourse is the major cause of HIV transmission worldwide. In the tropics, including India and the African subcontinent, heterosexual transmission is the commonest mode of infection.[1]

- HIV has been demonstrated in semen, both within infected mononuclear cells and in the cell-free state.[3] The virus appears to concentrate in semen in inflammatory conditions such as urethritis and epididymitis, due to an increase in the number of mononuclear cells present. HIV has also been demonstrated in semen, and cervical and vaginal fluid.
- There is a strong association of HIV transmission with receptive anal sex.[4] The virus can also be transmitted to either partner through vaginal intercourse. A linear prospective study in the USA has shown that male-to-female transmission was approximately eight times more efficient than female-to-male transmission.[2,5]
- Sexually transmitted disease (STD), especially genital ulcer disease (GUD), is also a major risk factor, with regard to infectivity and susceptibility to infection.[2,6] Coinfection with syphilis, chancroid donovanosis, lymphogranuloma, or genital herpes, as well as non-ulcerative inflammation such as gonorrhea, non-gonococcal urethritis, trichomoniasis, bacterial vaginosis,[7] and reproductive tract inflammation such as vaginitis, cervicitis, and salpingitis have been linked to an increased risk of transmission.
- Lack of circumcision is also strongly associated with a higher risk.[8] This may be due to an increased susceptibility to ulcerative STDs and increased trauma.
- Oral sex is much less efficient in this regard. However, there are several documented cases of HIV transmission resulting solely from receptive fellatio and insertive cunnilingus.[2]

Transmission by blood and blood products

Persons who receive contaminated blood/blood products and organ transplants are also at risk. Intravenous drug users (IVDUs) are affected by sharing injection material such as needles and syringes. Subcutaneous (skin-popping) or intramuscular (muscling) injections can also transmit HIV. In IVDUs, the risk increases with the duration of the addiction and a large number of sharing partners.

Transfusions of whole blood, packed red blood cells, platelets, leukocytes, and plasma are also capable of transmitting HIV infection. In contrast, hyperimmune gamma globulin, hepatitis immune globulin, plasma-derived hepatitis B vaccine, and RhO immune globulin have not been associated with transmission of HIV infection. The procedures involved in their production either inactivate or remove the virus. Due to these risks, the screening of donated blood/blood products as well as of organ donors has been made mandatory worldwide.

There is also a small but definite occupational risk of HIV transmission in health care workers (HCWs), laboratory employees, and in individuals working with HIV-infected specimens, especially sharp objects.[9] The risk is increased with exposure involving a relatively large quantity of blood and/or a procedure that involves venesection or deep injury. The risk also increases with high concentration of the virus in the blood and with the presence of more virulent strains. The very occurrence of transmission of HIV, as well as hepatitis B and C, to and from HCWs in the workplace underscores the importance of the use of universal precautions when caring for all patients.

Mother-to-child transmission (MTCT)

This is an important form of transmission of HIV infection in developing countries. HIV can be transmitted from mother to fetus as early as the first or second trimester of pregnancy. However, maternal transmission to the fetus occurs mainly in the perinatal period.

Maternal factors[10] indicative of a high risk of transmission include:

- High levels of plasma viremia,[11] low CD4+ T-cell counts and anti-p24 antibody levels.
- Vitamin A deficiency, prolonged labor, chorioamnionitis at delivery or STDs during pregnancy, cigarette smoking and hard drug use during pregnancy, preterm labor.
- Obstetric procedures such as amniocentesis and amnioscopy.

Although MTCT occurs chiefly during pregnancy and at birth, breast-feeding may account for 5–15% of infants being infected after delivery.[12] High levels of HIV in breast milk, presence of mastitis, low maternal CD4+ T-cell counts and maternal vitamin A deficiency all increase the risk. The risk is highest in the early months prior to weaning, and with exclusive breast-feeding.

To summarize, the probability of HIV-1 infection per exposure can be assessed from Table 11.3.

Basic virology of HIV

HIV belongs to the subfamily Lentivirinae, which is a part of the family Retroviridae. There are two main groups of human retroviruses:

- Human T-lymphotropic virus (HTLV): there are two distinct transforming viruses, designated HTLV-I and HTLV-II respectively.
- HIV: these are designated HIV-1 and HIV-2.

Table 11.3 Infection rates for different modes of transmission of human immunodeficiency virus (HIV)/ acquired immunodeficiency syndrome (AIDS)

Mode of transmission	Infections per 100 exposures
Male to female, unprotected vaginal sex	0.05–0.5
Female to male, unprotected vaginal sex	0.033–0.1
Male to male or male to female, unprotected anal sex	0.5–10.0
Needlestick injury	0.3
Mother-to-child transmission	13–48
Exposure to contaminated blood products	90–100

HIV seroepidemiology

Molecular analyses of various HIV isolates reveal sequence variations in many parts of the viral genome, especially in the hypervariable region, e.g., the V3 region, which is a target for neutralizing antibodies and contains recognition sites for T-cell responses. There are three groups of HIV-1: (1) group M (major) which is responsible for most of the infections around the world; (2) group O (outlier) is a relatively rare form, found originally in Cameroon, Gabon, and France; and (3) group N was first identified in a Cameroonian woman with AIDS.[13]

The M group includes eight subtypes or clades, designated A, B, C, D, F, G, H, and J, as well as four major circulating recombinant forms (CRFs). These four CRFs are: (1) the AE virus, present in Southeast Asia; (2) AG from West and Central Africa; (3) AGI from Cyprus and Greece; and (4) AB from Russia. The pattern of HIV-1 variations worldwide may be a consequence of the sex trade.[2] Although subtype B predominates in the USA, Canada, certain South American countries, western Europe and Australia, the subtype C is the most common form worldwide. In Africa, more than 75% of strains recovered have been of subtypes A, C, and D, with C being the most common, while in Asia, HIV-1 isolates of subtypes E, C, or B predominate. Subtype E predominates in Southeast Asia, while subtype C is prevalent in India. Recombination among viruses of different clades occurs as a result of multiple infections in an infected individual with viruses of different clades, particularly in areas where clades overlap.

HIV-2 infection

HIV-2 was first isolated from AIDS patients from West Africa (Guinea-Bissale and Cape Verde) in 1986.[14,15] The genetic structure of HIV-2 is similar to HIV-1, although HIV-2 has a *vpx* gene instead of the *vpu* gene. The nucleotide and amino acid homology between the viruses is about 60% for the more conserved *gag* and *pol* genes, but only 30–40% for the other viral genes, including *env*.[16] The structure of the virion of HIV-2 is very similar to HIV-1. The difference in envelope and other proteins induces the host to form antibodies, which can be distinguished from HIV-1-induced antibodies. This forms the basis of the serological tests that differentiate between HIV-1 and HIV-2 infection. Sequencing

Table 11.4 Differences and similarities in the epidemiology of human immunodeficiency viruses HIV-1 and HIV-2[19]

	HIV-1	HIV-2
Mother-to-child transmission rate	20–30%	0–4%
Geographical spread	Worldwide	West Africa; with links to Portugal; India
Age peak	20–34 years	45–55 years
Excess mortality	10-fold	Twofold
Transmission routes	Heterosexual; homosexual; IVDU; BT; mother to child; needlestick	Heterosexual; homosexual; IVDU; BT; mother to child
Rural–urban difference	Higher prevalence in urban	Similar prevalence urban and rural
Trend	Prevalence rising in most countries	Stable prevalence in most countries

IVDU, intravenous drug use; BT, blood transfusion.

of *pol, env,* and *gag* genes has led to the distinction of six different HIV-2 subtypes.[17–19]

In the majority of individuals, HIV-2 single infection can be diagnosed confidently with serological assays in an appropriate algorithm. Dual seroreactivity is most suggestive of dual infection, although subsequent confirmation with sensitive genome detection techniques is required. In some cases, confirmation cannot be secured. Similar to HIV-1, HIV-2 also demonstrates molecular heterogeneity. There are six subtypes of HIV-2 virus, of which subtype A is the most common. Subtypes A and B are pathogenic; for the other subtypes (C, D, E, and F) pathogenicity is not known.

The lower transmissibility of HIV-2 by the heterosexual route[20,21] suggests that in a population where both viruses are being transmitted sexually, HIV-1 will competitively displace HIV-2 in the long term. The age peak of HIV-2 prevalence is distinctly higher than that of HIV-1 (HIV-1: 20–34 years, HIV-2: 35–45 years or 50–59 years). The higher peak age of HIV-2 may reflect several aspects of HIV-2 epidemiology, including lower heterosexual transmissibility, lower mortality, and cohort effect. Evidence for the classical transmission routes is strong for vertical and heterosexual transmission, good for blood transfusion, circumstantial for intravenous drug use and the homosexual route, and lacking for needlestick injuries (Table 11.4).

Biology of HIV[22]

The virus is an icosahedron, with a diameter of 100–120 nm (Fig. 11.1). It is surrounded by a lioprotein membrane in which are embedded 72 trimetric glycoprotein complexes composed of the external protein gp120 and the transmembrane gp41. These are important in viral attachment and entry. The icosahedron houses the conical nucleocapsid, which contains the matrix and the viral ribonucleic acid (RNA). The viral RNA is 9.7 kb long and contains genes that code for viral structural and regulatory proteins. These genes are the *gag* gene, which codes for the core; the *pol* gene, encoding the viral enzymes; and the *env* gene, encoding the membrane proteins. The regulatory and accessory genes are named *tat, rev, nef,* and *vpi, vpu, vpr,* and *vpx* respectively. They are important in transcription, translation, and maturation of viral proteins in the host cell. They also define the infectivity of the species.

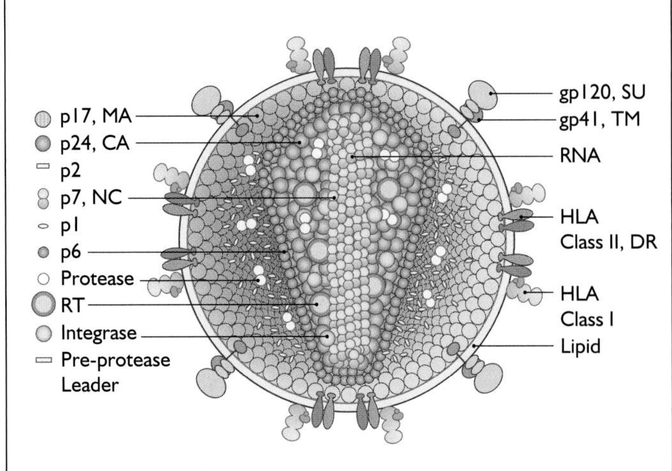

Figure 11.1 Structure of human immunodeficiency virus type 1 (HIV-1).

The viral life cycle[23]

The first event is attachment of the virion to the host cell (Fig. 11.2). The membrane protein gp120 expresses a binding site for the human CD4 receptor. The virus also utilizes two additional coreceptors, CCR5 and CXCR4, which are primary receptors for certain chemoattractant cytokines called chemokines. CCR5 is expressed on monocytes, macrophages, and lymphocytes while the CXCR4 receptor is expressed only on T lymphocytes. Certain strains of HIV utilize the CCR5 coreceptor (R5). These are usually macrophage-tropic, while those that use the CXCR4 coreceptor (X4) are T-cell tropic. However, many strains may be dual-tropic. R5 viruses are said to be non-syncytium-inducing (NSI), while the X4 strains are syncytium-inducing (SI). In reality, under ideal conditions, both R5 and X4 viruses are capable of syncytium formation in culture. The transmitting virus is almost invariably an R5 strain. However, in approximately 40% of individuals, there is a transition to the X4 strain later in the disease (the R5X4 switch), which is associated with an aggressive course and poorer prognosis.

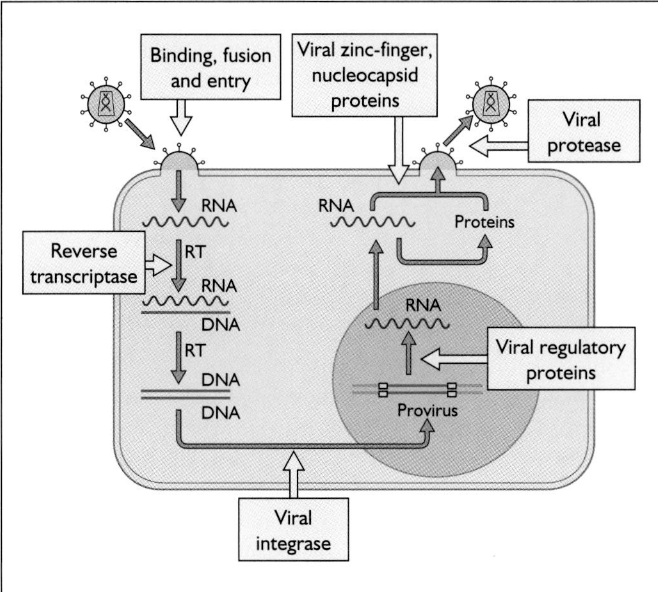

Figure 11.2 Life cycle of human immunodeficiency virus (HIV).

Attachment of gp120 to CD4 exposes gp41. This acts like a harpoon and facilitates viral fusion. Inside the cell, the virion is uncoated and the viral proteins are released. Reverse transcriptase (RT) has many functions: RNA-dependent DNA polymerization, DNA polymerization from a single-stranded DNA intermediate, and RNAseH activity that degrades the RNA intermediates. A copy of the viral genome is formed and transported to the host nucleus. This is integrated into the host DNA by the viral integrase. The provirus now controls the cell and reproduces itself. New molecules are cleaved by the viral protease, which results in infectious viral particles budding through the host membrane. In this process, various host cell proteins are incorporated into the lipid envelope. Reverse transcription is extremely error-prone. Combined with the high frequency of viral replication, this results in the formation of many closely related viral species in the same patient. These are called quasispecies. This infection is established in lymph nodes and other lymphoid organs, and persistent viral replication can be detected in these foci.

Latency[24]

Although attachment occurs, only limited reverse transcription occurs in the absence of a suitable stimulation. This is called pre-integration latency. Even after integration, the absence of cellular activation signals leads to latency, called postintegration latency. This pool of latently infected cells, mostly memory T cells, prevents the complete eradication of virus by antiretroviral drugs.

Viral dynamics[25]

The half-life of the circulating virion is approximately 30 min and that of a productively infected cell is 1 day. Given the relatively steady state of plasma viremia and of infected cells, it appears that extremely large numbers of virus (approximately 10^{10}) are produced and cleared from the circulation each day. Data also suggest that the minimum duration of the HIV-1 replication cycle in vivo averages 1.5 days. The steady-state level, called the viral set point, is attained after approximately 1 year. It has prognostic implications and the levels seem to correlate with the rapidity of disease progression.

CD4 lymphopenia

As a result of relentless viral replication, CD4 T-cell numbers and function are compromised. Infected T cells are destroyed, leading to depletion. This destruction may be a direct result of HIV attachment and multiplication, which cause decreased membrane integrity and interference with normal cellular events. Indirect mechanisms include syncytium formation, apoptosis, and the "bystander effect," in which uninfected cells are accidentally killed as a result of immune response directed to adjacent infected cells.

The immune response[26]

This has two components: the innate response and the adaptive response.

Innate immunity

This utilizes natural killer (NK) cells and macrophages. It is independent of cell-surface receptor/immunoglobulins, as well as of major histocompatibility complex (MHC) restriction. It also lacks memory. An early and vigorous non-specific protective response can prevent viral multiplication and spread. It also allows the adaptive system to mount an effective protective response.

Two cell-surface receptors on the innate immune cells play an important role. These are the Toll-like receptors, which interact with microorganisms and their products to generate interleukin-12 (IL-12), which in turn stimulates dendritic cells; and the heat-shock proteins, which bind to foreign antigens and enter the antigen-presenting cells (APCs). This facilitates the presentation of the antigens on the APC surface, and therefore to the cytotoxic T lymphocytes (CTLs), in conjunction with MHC class I molecules.

Adaptive immunity

Cellular immune responses, particularly specific anti-HIV perforin-secreting CTLs, are important in host response to HIV. Perforins are cytolytic "cell-killing" molecules. Besides direct cytolysis, CTLs also produce chemokines that compete with HIV-1 for the CCR5 receptor. However, HIV-1-infected patients demonstrate an impaired CTL response. This is because of a defective virus-specific Th1 response, as well as the development of CTL escape mutations in the infecting virus. Levels of CTLs are inversely related to the viral load. Thus, HIV-specific CTLs produce a full range of antiviral cytokines and chemokines on encounter with antigens, but are often characterized by low levels of perforins. This leads to ineffective target cell destruction. An antibody response is also noted. However, potent neutralizing antibodies are rarely formed in vivo and neutralization-resistant variants develop rapidly in chronic infection.

Thus, the various components[27] of the immune response to HIV can be tabulated as follows:

- Humoral immunity:
  - Binding antibodies
- Neutralizing antibodies:
  - Type-specific: generally directed to the V3 loop region, these antibodies are strain-specific and present in low titers
  - Group-specific: two forms, binding to specific amino acid regions of gp120 and gp41 respectively

- Antibodies participating in antibody-dependent cellular cytotoxicity (ADCC):
  - Protective: mediated by NK cells
  - Pathogenic: bystander killing
  - Enhancing antibodies: directed to gp41, which facilitate infection of cells through an Fc receptor-mediated mechanism
- Cell-mediated immunity:
  - Helper CD4+ T lymphocyte: a reverse correlation exists between the presence of these cells and levels of plasma viremia
  - Class I MHC restricted cytotoxic CD8+ T lymphocytes, through their HIV-specific receptors, bind and cause lytic destruction of target cells bearing identified MHC class I molecules associated with HIV antigen
  - CD8+T-cell-mediated inhibition (non-cytolytic): mediated by soluble factors inducing the CC-chemokines, viz. RANTES, MIP-1β and MIP-1α, which suppress HIV replication
  - ADCC
  - NK cells

Natural history of HIV infection

Within 2–3 weeks of viral transmission, the acute retroviral syndrome develops that lasts for about 2–3 weeks. It is followed by chronic HIV infection and, after an average period of 8 years, the patient develops symptomatic infection/AIDS-defining complex. The course of the disease from the time of initial infection to the development of full-blown AIDS is divided into the following stages.

Primary HIV infection[28]

Acute retroviral syndrome is the symptom complex that follows infection, and is experienced by 80–90% of HIV-infected patients, but this diagnosis is infrequently recognized. The time from the initial exposure to onset of symptoms is usually 2–4 weeks, but may be as long as 10 months in rare cases. The clinical symptoms include fever, lymphadenopathy, pharyngitis, erythematous maculopapular rash, arthralgia, myalgia, diarrhea, nausea, vomiting, headache, mucocutaneous ulceration involving mouth, esophagus, or genitals, hepatosplenomegaly, and thrush (Fig. 11.3). The neurological features include meningoencephalitis, peripheral neuropathy, facial palsy, Guillain–Barré syndrome, brachial neuritis, radiculopathy, cognitive impairment, and psychosis. The laboratory findings include lymphopenia followed by lymphocytosis with depletion of CD4 cells, CD8 lymphocytosis, and often, atypical lymphocytes. The transaminase levels may be elevated. The diagnosis is established by demonstrating quantitative plasma HIV RNA or qualitative HIV DNA and negative or indeterminate HIV serology. Complete clinical recovery with a reduction in plasma levels of HIV RNA follows. The preliminary studies indicate that aggressive antiretroviral therapy protects active HIV-specific CD4 cells from HIV infection to preserve a response analogous to the response seen in non-progressors. The observation emphasizes the importance of early recognition and aggressive antiretroviral therapy. The seroconversion with positive HIV serology generally takes place at an average of 3 weeks after transmission with the standard third-generation enzyme immunoassay (EIA). By using standard serological tests, it now appears that more than 95% of patients seroconvert within 5–8 months following transmission.

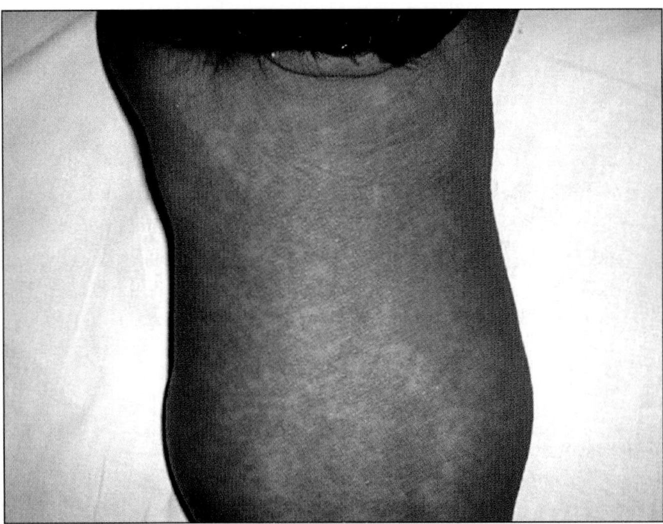

Figure 11.3 Viral exanthema due to human immunodeficiency virus type 1 (HIV-1) seroconversion.

Asymptomatic chronic infection, with or without persistent generalized lymphadenopathy (PGL)[29]

During this period, the patient is clinically asymptomatic and generally has no findings on physical examination, except in some cases for PGL; PGL is defined as enlarged lymph nodes involving at least two noncontiguous sites, other than inguinal nodes, persisting for more than 3 months. Detailed history-taking followed by thorough clinical examination is necessary. Incidental findings could be scars from previous genital ulcer disease (GUD) or herpes zoster, lymphadenopathy, oral hairy leukoplakia (OHL), and even asymptomatic dermatological manifestations. HIV screening of conjugal partners or relevant children after informed consent is essential. The baseline investigations to be undertaken include complete hemogram (including platelet count), erythrocyte sedimentation rate (ESR), serological tests for syphilis (STS), hepatitis B and C serology, liver function tests, urine examination, chest radiography, sonography of abdomen/pelvis, and Mantoux test. The evaluation of CD4/CD8 lymphocytes as well as estimation of HIV-1 viral load is optional in resource-poor setups, in the absence of a plan to initiate antiretroviral therapy. It may only help to decide regarding initiation of chemoprophylaxis against opportunistic infections (OI). It is important to offer counseling emphasizing maintenance of food and water hygiene, lifestyle modification, such as practicing safer sex, and refraining from organ donation (blood, semen, kidney, etc.). The periodic follow-ups (every 3–6 months), consisting of history taking, clinical examination, baseline investigations, and counseling, are of equal importance.

Symptomatic HIV infection[29]

During the symptomatic HIV infection previously known as AIDS-related complex (CD4 counts between 200 and 499 cells/mm^3, category B symptoms, CDC clinical classification), the skin and mucous membranes are predominantly involved. Widespread seborrheic dermatitis is the most common presentation. Other features include multidermatomal herpes zoster, molluscum contagiosum (MC) (Fig. 11.4), OHL, pruritic dermatitis, folliculitis, dermatophyte infection, recurrent vulvovaginal candidiasis, and oral candidiasis (Fig. 11.5). Upper and lower respiratory tract infections

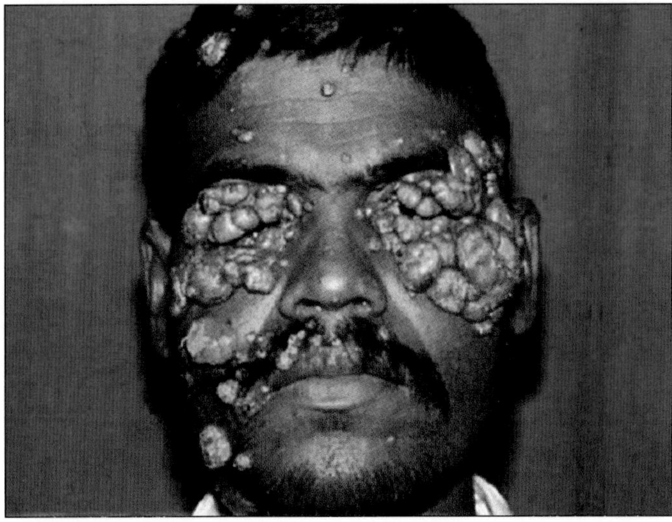
Figure 11.4 Molluscum contagiosum.

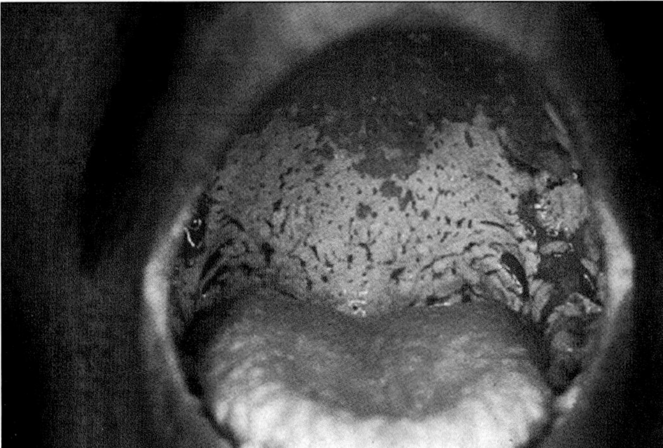
Figure 11.5 Oral candidiasis.

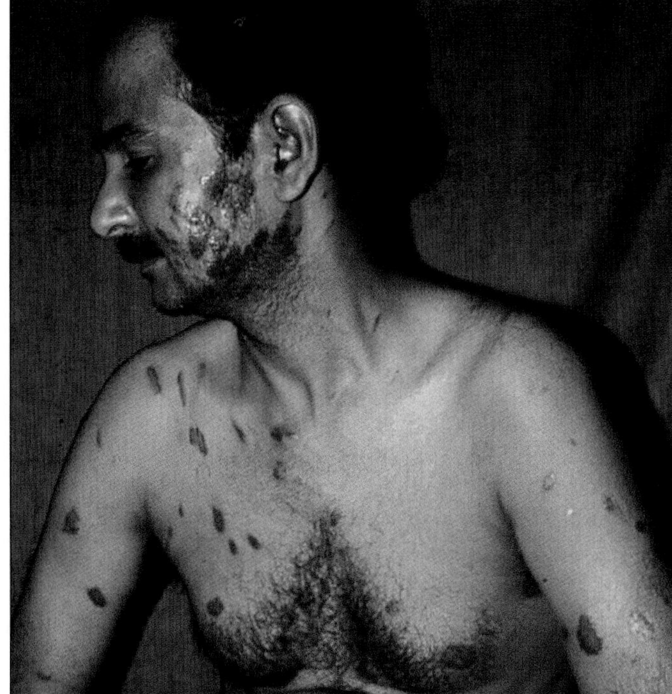
Figure 11.6 Kaposi's sarcoma.

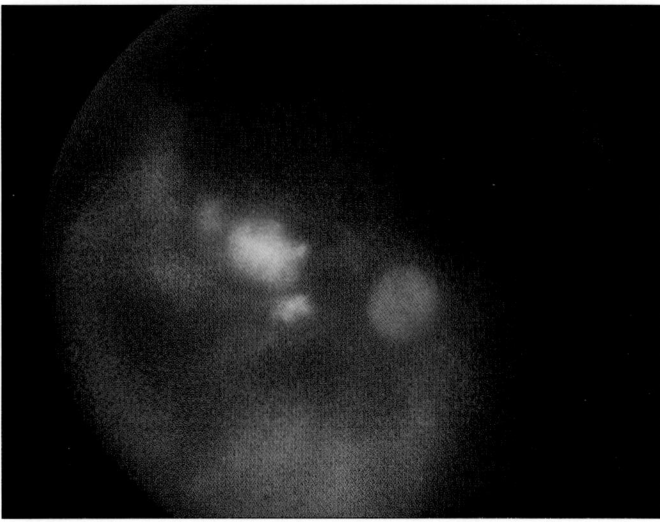
Figure 11.7 Cytomegalovirus (CMV) retinitis.

caused by *Streptococcus pneumoniae*, *Haemophilus influenzae*, and *Mycoplasma pneumoniae* may also occur. Other features during this stage include Kaposi's sarcoma (KS) (Fig. 11.6), pulmonary tuberculosis (TB), cervical dysplasia, and idiopathic thrombocytopenic purpura (ITP).

AIDS[29]

This stage (CD4 counts between 50 and 200 cells/mm^3, category C symptoms, CDC clinical classification) is characterized by opportunistic infection (OI) and malignancy. Other features are persistent and progressive constitutional symptoms, wasting disease, and neurological abnormalities.

Advanced HIV disease, characterized by CD4 cell counts of <50/mm^3[29]

As in the previous stage, advanced HIV disease is also characterized by AIDS-defining OIs and malignancy. Some of the infections are more frequently seen, like *M. avium* complex (MAC), cytomegalovirus (CMV) (Fig. 11.7), cryptococcal meningitis (Fig. 11.8), histoplasmosis (Fig. 11.9), slow virus disease, and cervical dysplasia. Central nervous system (CNS) involvement is also very prominent, and includes AIDS dementia complex, CNS lymphoma, and CMV infection. AIDS-wasting syndrome with a weight loss of >10% of ideal body weight is common.

The CDC has proposed the following clinical classification for HIV infection in adults and adolescents. It is based on three ranges of CD4 cell counts and three clinical categories, as given in Table 11.5.

Clinical features of HIV-2 infection

HIV-2 infection can also lead to CD4 decline, OIs, HIV-associated malignancies, and early death. The median time from infection to AIDS is longer than in HIV-1: cases with an incubation period of 14 years, and even 27 years, have been reported.[31] The clinical manifestations of symptomatic HIV-2 disease are broadly similar to those of HIV-1.[32] The only marked difference may be the lower frequency of KS among HIV-2 patients.[33] In a Gambian study, survival for HIV-2 patients with AIDS was three times longer than

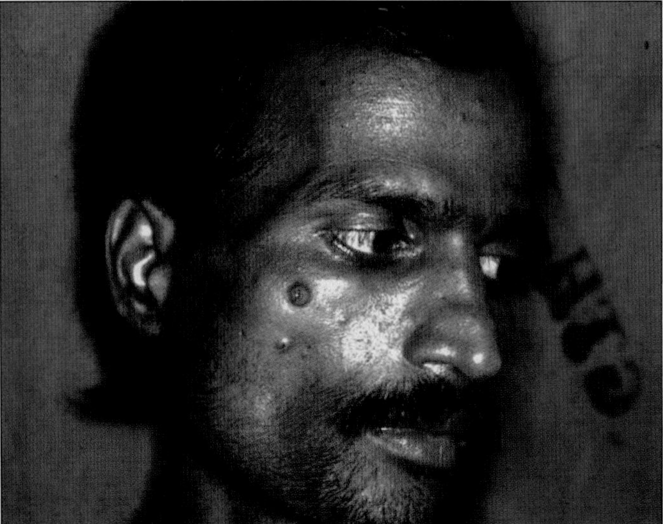

Figure 11.8 Cryptococcosis.

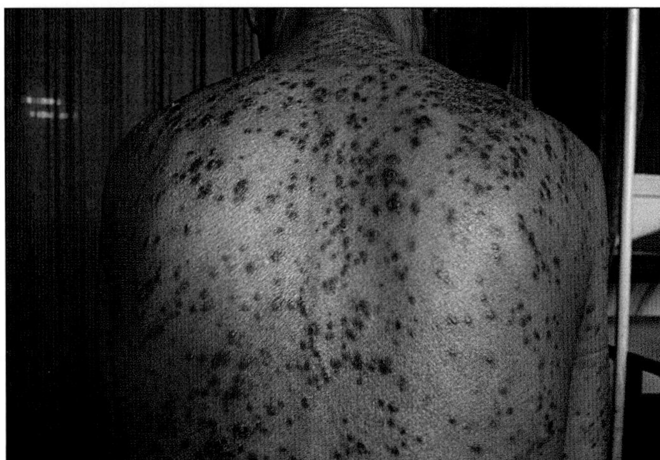

Figure 11.9 Histoplasmosis.

for HIV-1 AIDS patients.[34] Most studies demonstrated decreased CD4 cell percentage or CD4 cell count in HIV-2 subjects; also in those who are clinically asymptomatic,[35] the rate of decline was slower in HIV-2 patients.[36] The proviral load of the two infections did not differ in any stage of infection. The majority of HIV-2 patients are long-term non-progressors, who live in the community unnoticed by health services, and who have detectable provirus, stable CD4 cell percentage, no detectable plasma viral load, are asymptomatic, and have no increased mortality risk.

Long-term survivors and long-term non-progressors

Individuals who remain alive for 10–15 years after the initial infection are called "long-term survivors."[37] In such patients, the course is progressive and immunodeficiency is significant. In some of these individuals, CD4+T cells counts have decreased to <200/μl and many have suffered OIs. However the counts have remained stable for years at that level. The reasons are not defined, but highly active antiretroviral therapy (HAART) and prophylaxis against OI may play a role. In addition, certain viral and/or host determinants may play a role.

Table 11.5 Revised classification (1993) for human immunodeficiency virus (HIV) infection and the expanded acquired immunodeficiency syndrome (AIDS) surveillance definition for adolescents and adults[30]

CD4 count (per mm^3)	A	B	C
> 500	A1	B1	**C1**
200–500	A2	B2	**C2**
< 200	**A3**	**B3**	**C3**

The categories in bold type indicate the expanded AIDS surveillance case definition.
The conditions included in each category are given below:

A: This includes:
Acute retroviral syndrome
Persistent generalized lymphadenopathy
Asymptomatic disease

B: This includes:
Symptoms of AIDS-related complex
Bacillary angiomatosis (Fig. 11.10)
Candidiasis, mucosal (thrush, vulvovaginal: persistent, frequent or poorly responsive to therapy)
Cervical dysplasia (moderate or severe)/cervical carcinoma-in-situ
Constitutional symptoms, such as fever (38.5°C) or diarrhea lasting > 1 month
Herpes zoster (Fig. 11.11), recurrent and multidermatomal
Idiopathic thrombocytopenic purpura (ITP)
Listeriosis
Oral hairy leukoplakia (OHL)
Pelvic inflammatory disease, particularly tubo-ovarian abscess
Peripheral neuropathy

C: This includes:
AIDS-defining conditions
CD4 count < 200/mm^3
Candidiasis, pulmonary or esophageal
Cervical cancer, invasive
Coccidioidomycosis, disseminated or extrapulmonary
Cryptococcosis, extrapulmonary (Fig. 11.8)
Cryptosporidiosis, chronic intestinal (> 1 month)
Cytomegalovirus (CMV) infection (excluding liver, spleen, and lymph nodes) and retinitis (with loss of vision)
Herpes esophagitis, bronchitis, pneumonia or chronic cutaneous and/or oral ulcers (> 1 month)
HIV encephalopathy
Toxoplasmosis, disseminated or extrapulmonary
Isosporiasis, chronic intestinal (> 1 month)
Kaposi's sarcoma (Fig. 11.6)
Lymphoma, primary central nervous system or Burkitt's lymphoma
Mycobacterial disease (Figs 11.12–11.18)
Pneumocystis carinii infection, commonly pneumonia (PCP)
Pneumonia, recurrent bacterial
Progressive multifocal leukoencephalopathy (PML)
Salmonellosis
Wasting syndrome

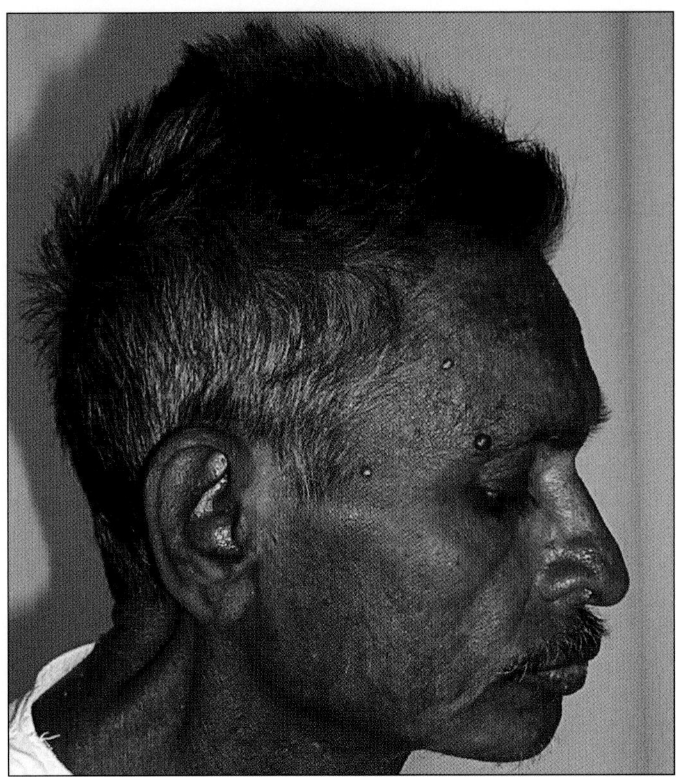

Figure 11.10 Bacillary angiomatosis.

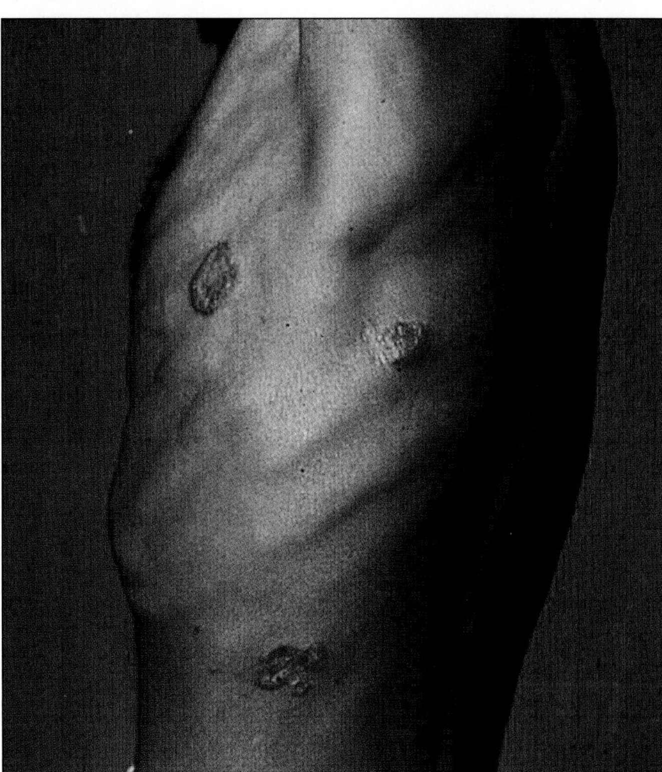

Figure 11.12 Hansen's disease (leprosy).

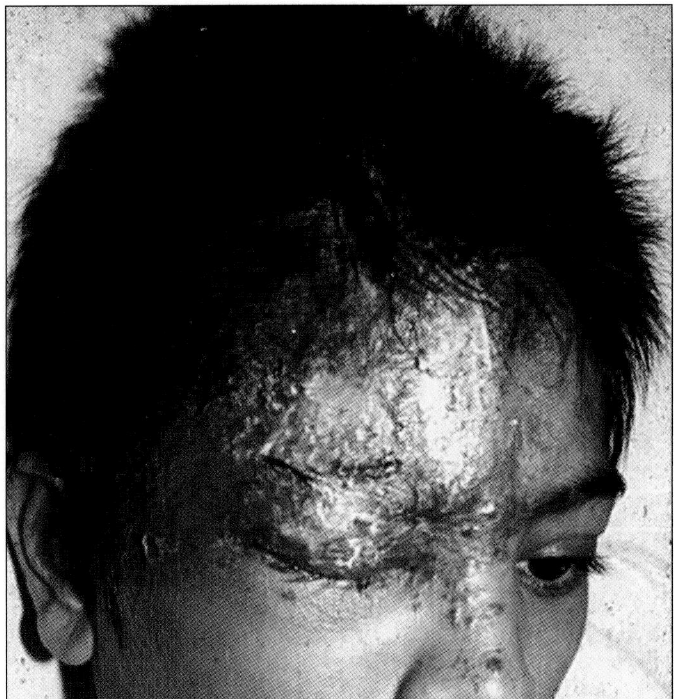

Figure 11.11 Herpes zoster.

Fewer than 5% of HIV-infected individuals are characterized as long-term non-progressors. These individuals have been infected with HIV for a long period (>10 years), but their CD4+ T cells counts are in the normal range, and they have remained stable over years despite not receiving antiretroviral therapy. These persons have extremely effective anti-HIV immune responses, both humoral and cell-mediated. Also some such individuals are infected with defective virus, e.g., with deletions in the *nef* gene[38] and other genome detects. Host factors[39] that contribute are heterozygosity[40] for the genes coding for the coreceptors, e.g., the CCR5-delta32 deletion or the CCR2-64I mutation.

Rapid progressors

Certain infected individuals develop low CD4+ T-cell counts and AIDS-defining illnesses within 2–3 years of infection.[41] They bear certain human leukocyte antigen (HLA) antigens, e.g., HLA-A1, -A24, -C7, etc., or are homozygous for the class I loci, or are usually infected with the X4 strains.[42]

Laboratory tests[2,43]

The diagnosis of HIV infection is based on the demonstration of antibodies to HIV/HIV antigens or the direct detection of viral antigens. These tests may be classified as:

1. Tests for HIV-specific antibodies in serum and plasma:
   (a) Screening tests:
      (i) Enzyme-linked immunosorbent assays (ELISA): the ELISA is the standard screening test used. It is a solid-phase assay in which the antibody is detected using the sandwich technique. It has a sensitivity of >99.5%, but the specificity is not optimal in low-risk cases. Also, a number of conditions may interfere with the test result and cause false-positive reactions.

   (ii) Rapid tests: these are visual tests in which a positive test appears as a dot on a tile or a comb, or as agglutination on a slide.
  (b) Supplemental tests:
   (i) Western blot assay: viral antigens are separated on the basis of their molecular weights and antibodies to each are detected as distinct bands. The test is considered positive if antibodies to at least two of the following are detected: p24, gp41, or gp120/160.
   (ii) Immunofluorescence tests.
2. Tests on saliva: although these kits are efficacious, there is some concern about how early following infection the antibody is detectable in saliva as compared to serum/plasma; as well as the minimum concentration of immunoglobulin G (IgG) at which each kit gives a correct result.
3. Confirmatory tests:
  (a) Virus isolation: this assay is 100% specific, but its sensitivity varies with the stage of HIV infection. In both adults and in children, the virus cannot be cultured from peripheral blood mononuclear cells (PBMCs) for approximately 6 weeks following the time of transmission. However, this procedure is labor-intensive and dangerous and only undertaken in specialized laboratories.
  (b) Detection of the p24 antigen: this test detects the unbound HIV p24 antigen in the serum. The test may be useful: (i) during the window period; (ii) during late disease when the patient is symptomatic; (iii) to detect HIV infection in the newborn because diagnosis is difficult due to presence of maternal antibodies; (iv) when neurologic involvement is suspected the test is performed with cerebrospinal fluid.
  (c) Detection of HIV RNA: three different techniques, namely RT polymerase chain reaction (RT-PCR), nucleic acid sequence-based amplification (NASBA) and branched DNA (bDNA) assay, have been employed to develop commercial kits.
4. Monitoring tests:
  (a) CD4+ T-cell counts: this is expressed as a product of the CD4 cell percentage, derived by flow cytometry, and the total lymphocyte count determined by the white blood cell counts. It is performed at diagnosis and every 3–6 months thereafter. Two determinations are usually performed before any decision to start or change HAART is taken.
  (b) Viral load: this is the same as detection of HIV RNA copies.
5. Surrogate tests: these include estimation of:
  (a) Circulating levels of neopterin, β_2-microglobulin, and soluble IL-2 receptors.
  (b) HIV IgA levels.
  (c) Levels of acid-labile endogenous interferon or tumor necrosis factor-α (TNF-α).

Opportunistic infections in AIDS[2,29]

Most OIs in AIDS occur when the CD4 count falls below 200 cells/mm^3. The spectrum of OIs in AIDS has been covered in the expanded CDC case definition. It can best be understood by studying the organ system involvement.

Systemic involvement in HIV infection

Disease of the respiratory system

TUBERCULOSIS (TB) In the tropics, the almost ubiquitous presence of *Mycobacterium tuberculosis* leads to the flare of hitherto quiescent lesions into active foci of infection, as a result of immunosuppression. TB is therefore the commonest presentation of HIV disease in the tropics. Over 15% of TB patients in India are likely to be HIV-positive. Extrapulmonary infections occur more commonly in advanced HIV disease (Figs 11.13–11.18). Pulmonary TB tends to be more occult and patients with advanced AIDS form poor granulomas and have large numbers of acid-fast bacilli in their sputum. They may be clinically and radiologically normal. However, radiologic evidence of diffuse, bilateral lower-lobe infiltrates is more common than the upper-lobe lesions seen in immunocompetent patients. Patients with HIV are highly prone to the development of active TB on exposure to bacilli in the community. Thus, TB in HIV patients may be as a result of new infections, rather than just reactivation of previous lesions. Approximately one-third of all AIDS-related deaths are due to TB. In AIDS patients, the clinical presentations can vary depending on the CD4 count. During the early phase with the CD4 count above 200 cells/mm^3, the disease has classic upper-lobe cavitatory changes, whereas in the late stage, it characteristically affects the middle and lower lobe and cavitatory changes are less frequently observed.

In summary, the global resurgence of TB is being accelerated by the spread of HIV, with TB already the leading cause of death among HIV-positive individuals. TB, along with AIDS, has overwhelmed health services and devastated urban populations in parts of Africa.

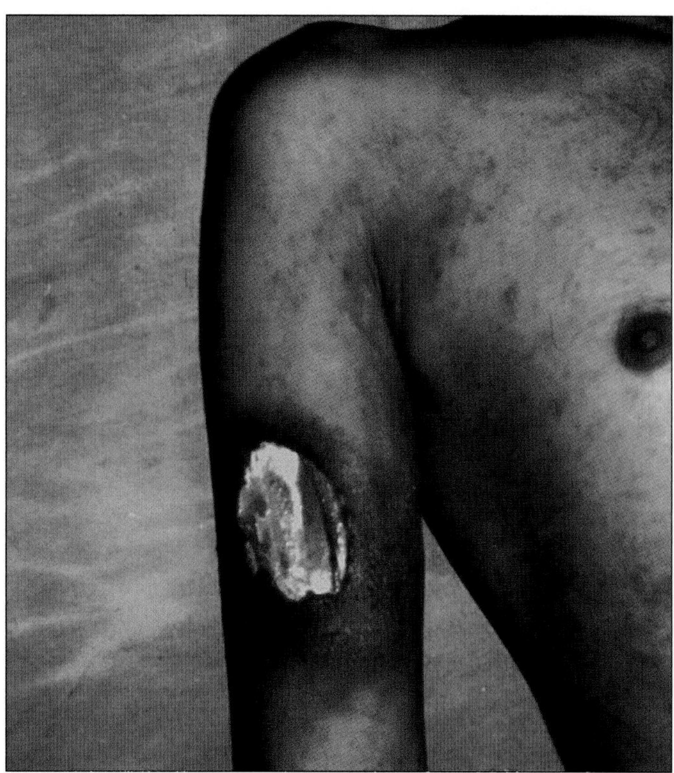

Figure 11.13 Cutaneous tuberculosis.

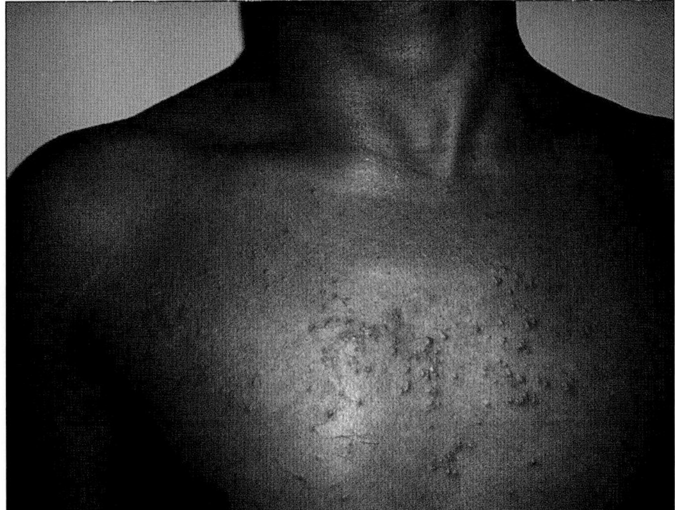

Figure 11.14 Tuberculids.

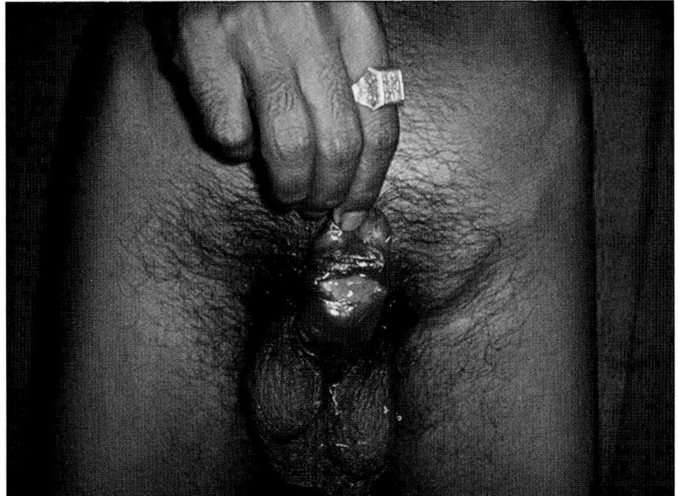

Figure 11.15 Penile tuberculosis.

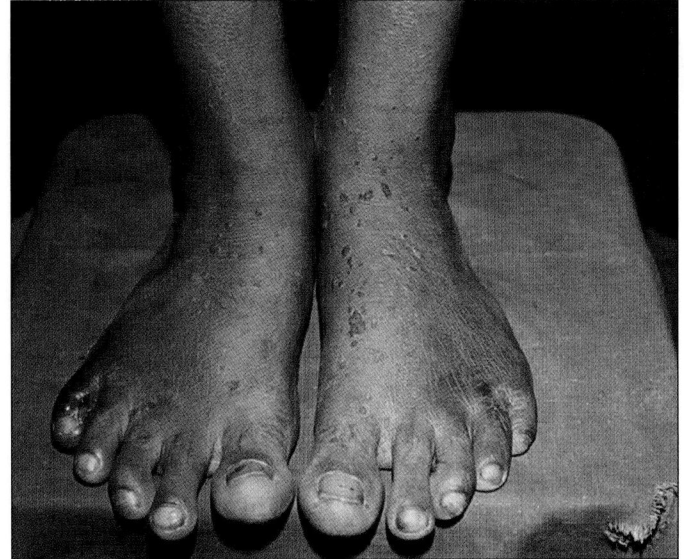

Figure 11.16 Tuberculous dactilytis right fifth toe with warts (HPV infection).

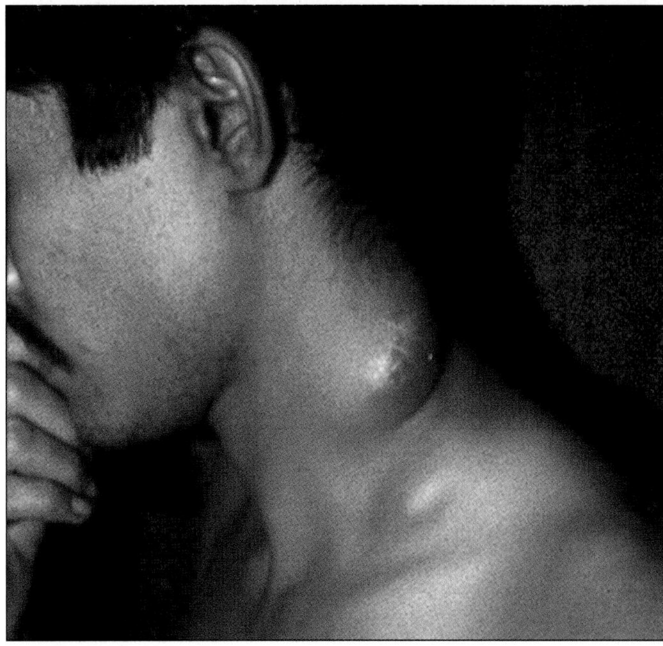

Figure 11.17 Tuberculosis of cervical lymph node.

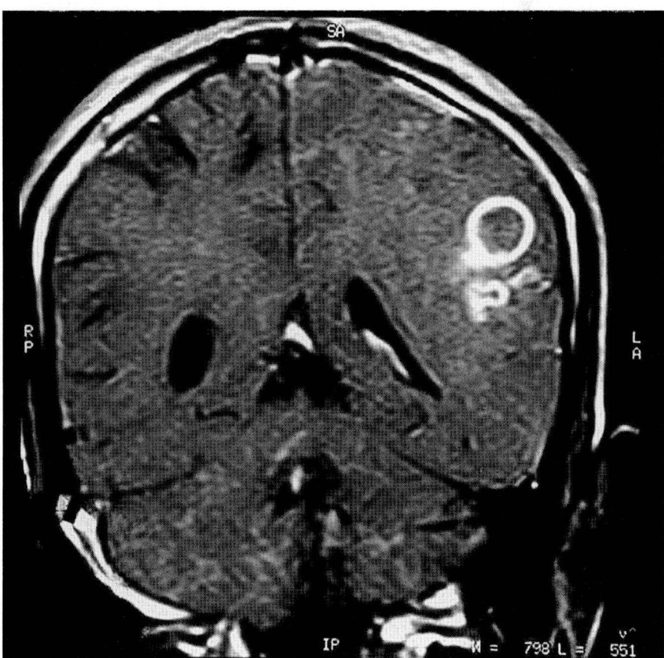

Figure 11.18 Tuberculoma.

Atypical mycobacterial infections are also seen in AIDS patients, especially with *M. avium*, *M. intracellulare* or MAC. MAC infection is usually a late occurrence when the CD4+ T cell count is <50 cell/mm^3. The most common presentation is disseminated disease with fever, weight loss, and night sweats. Other findings are abdominal pain, diarrhea, lower-lobe infiltrates suggestive of miliary spread; sometimes alveolar, nodular, hilar, or mediastinal adenopathy may occur.

OTHER RESPIRATORY TRACT INFECTIONS Acute bronchitis and maxillary sinusitis are quite common. The most common manifestation of pulmonary diseases is pneumonia. Both bacterial (pyogenic) and *Pneumocystis carinii* pneumonia (PCP) occur in AIDS. *P. carinii* is the most common life-threatening OI in most developed countries. The usual presentation is subacute, with malaise, fatigue, weight loss, characteristic retrosternal chest pain that is typically worse on inspiration, and non-productive cough. The chest radiograph may be normal or may show the classical finding of dense perihilar infiltrate. The arterial oxygen tension is usually low. The diagnosis is usually confirmed by direct demonstration of the trophozoite or the cyst in the sputum induced with hypertonic saline or in bronchial lavage obtained by fiberoptic bronchoscopy. Other causes of pulmonary infiltrate include mycobacterial infections, fungal infections, non-specific interstitial pneumonitis, KS, and lymphoma.

Pulmonary fungal infections, such as histoplasmosis, coccidioidomycosis, and aspergillosis, have been identified. Two forms of idiopathic interstitial pneumonia have been described – lymphoid interstitial pneumonitis (LIP) and non-specific interstitial pneumonitis (NIP).

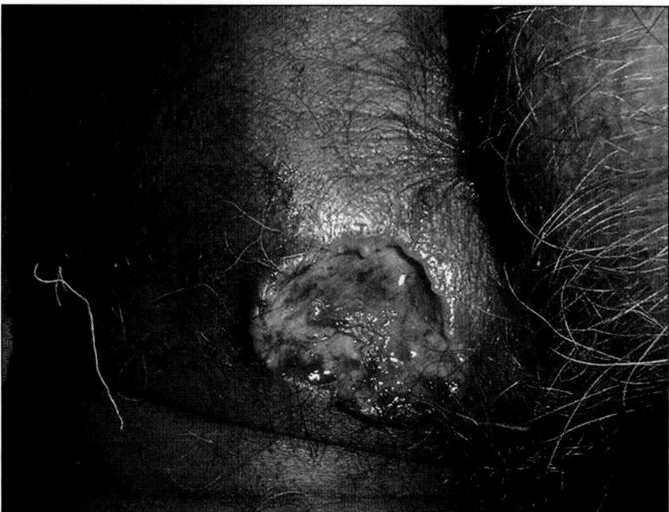

Figure 11.19 Amebiasis cutis.

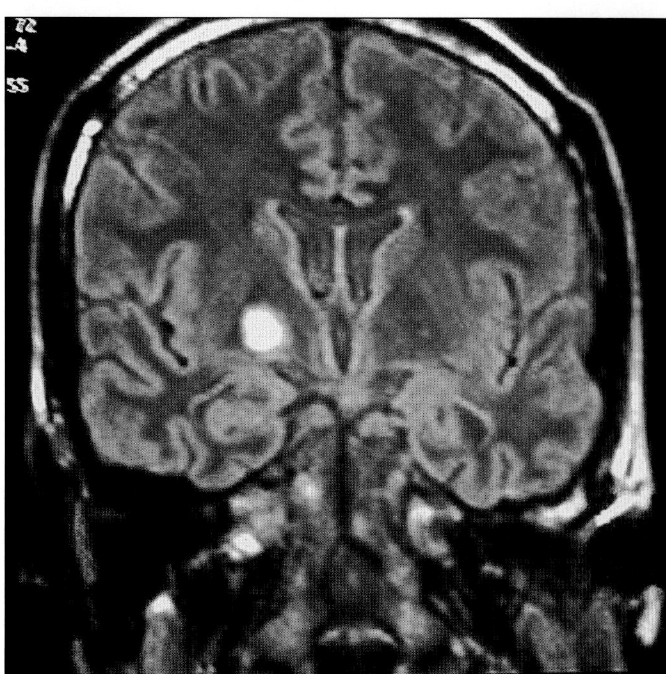

Figure 11.20 *Toxoplasmosis* of the brain.

Disease of the oropharynx and gastrointestinal tract (GIT)

Most oral, pharyngeal, and gastrointestinal diseases are due to secondary infection. The oral lesions are thrush, OHL and aphthous ulcers. Thrush is caused by *Candida albicans* and rarely by *C. krusei*. It appears as white cheesy exudates, often on an erythematous mucosa in the posterior oropharynx, soft palate, or along the gingival border (Fig. 11.5). OHL caused by Epstein–Barr virus (EBV) presents as white frond-like lesions, usually along the lateral borders of the tongue, but sometimes on the buccal mucosa. Thrush and OHL usually occur in patients with CD4+ T cell counts of $<200/cm^3$.

Oesophagitis can be caused by *Candida*, CMV, or herpes simplex virus (HSV). CMV infection is associated with a single large ulcer whereas herpetic infection presents with multiple small ulcers.

Infections of the small and large intestine with various bacteria, protozoa, and viruses can cause diarrhea and abdominal pain. *Cryptosporidium*, microsporidia, and *Isospora belli* are the most common opportunistic protozoa that infect the GIT and cause non-inflammatory diarrhea. *Giardia intestinalis* and *Entamoeba histolytica* infections are common in homosexual men (Fig. 11.19). Among the bacteria, *Salmonella*, *Shigella*, and *Campylobacter* are commonly isolated, especially in homosexuals. CMV colitis presents as non-bloody diarrhea, abdominal pain, weight loss, and anorexia. Endoscopic examination reveals multiple mucosal ulcerations and the biopsy shows characteristic intranuclear inclusion bodies. In advanced disease, MAC infection and various fungi like histoplasmosis and coccidioidomycosis may also cause diarrhea. Besides these secondary infections, HIV infection per se can cause AIDS enteropathy.

HIV and the nervous system

INFECTIONS Cerebral toxoplasmosis is the most frequent OI of the CNS. It usually results from reactivation of toxoplasma cyst in the brain, causing abscess formation (Fig. 11.20). The abscess can be unifocal or multifocal. Clinically, it presents with features of a space-occupying lesion (SOL). The computed tomography (CT) scan shows ring-enhancing lesions with surrounding edema.

Cryptococcal meningitis accounts for 5–10% of OIs in patients with HIV infection. The clinical presentation is subacute with headache, fever, and cranial nerve palsies. Neck stiffness is relatively rare. Cerebrospinal fluid analysis will demonstrate the yeast in 70% of the cases and antigen detection is positive in 100% of patients.

Progressive multifocal leukoencephalopathy (PML) is a demyelinating disease (slow virus disease) caused by JC virus. Clinically there may be focal deficits, ataxia, and personality changes.

HIV ENCEPHALOPATHY Patients with this disorder have a form of dementia known as AIDS-related cognitive–motor complex. In the early stages, there is impairment of memory and concentration. Later, motor signs appear, such as hyperreflexia, extensor plantar responses, incoordination, and ataxia.

Other neurological features in HIV infection are progressive vacuolar myelopathy (with spastic paraplegia, ataxia, and loss of sphincter control), transverse myelitis (due to varicella-zoster virus (VZV), HSV, and CMV infections), peripheral neuropathy, and psychiatric manifestations (acute psychosis, depression).

Disease of the liver, gallbladder, and pancreas

Liver involvement is usually in the form of coinfection with hepatitis B or C virus. This is covered in detail elsewhere in this chapter. Direct HIV infection of the liver may lead to functional defects, which may present as porphyria cutanea tarda (PCT). The liver is also affected as a result of drug administration, both HAART and therapy for OIs, especially antituberculous treatment.

Sclerosing cholangitis and papillary stenosis are reported in cryptosporidiosis, CMV infection, and KS. Pancreatitis usually occurs secondary to drug toxicity, mainly with didanosine.

Diseases of the kidney (HIV nephropathy)

The most common presentation is with nephritis and renal failure. Focal segmental glomerulosclerosis and mesangial proliferative glomerulonephritis account for most cases of HIV-associated nephropathy. Renal disease can also occur as a side-effect of therapy in HIV disease.

STDs and HIV/AIDS

The interaction between HIV transmission and STDs has already been dealt with earlier.[2,6]

- Syphilis:[44] HIV coinfection has been associated with higher titers of Venereal Disease Research Laboratory (VDRL), multiple primary chancres, florid secondary disease, faster progression to tertiary and ocular disease, lues maligna, slower resolution after therapy, a propensity to develop the Jarisch–Herxheimer reaction, and higher rates of relapse (Fig. 11.21). Coinfection may increase the frequency or accelerate the development of neurologic sequelae, such as aseptic meningitis or CNS gummata.
- The reactivation of genital/perianal HSV infection is common and its presence helps in the algorithmic clinical diagnosis of HIV/AIDS (Fig. 11.22). The dosage and duration of oral aciclovir therapy vary with the severity of disease.
- The incidence of malignant transformation of STDs, especially human papillomavirus (HPV) infection, viz. cervical intraepithelial neoplasia (CIN), cancer of the penis or vulva or perianal area, is higher in HIV-seropositive individuals (Figs 11.23 and 11.24).
- The occurrence of more than one STD at a given time carries higher positive predictive value for HIV/AIDS.

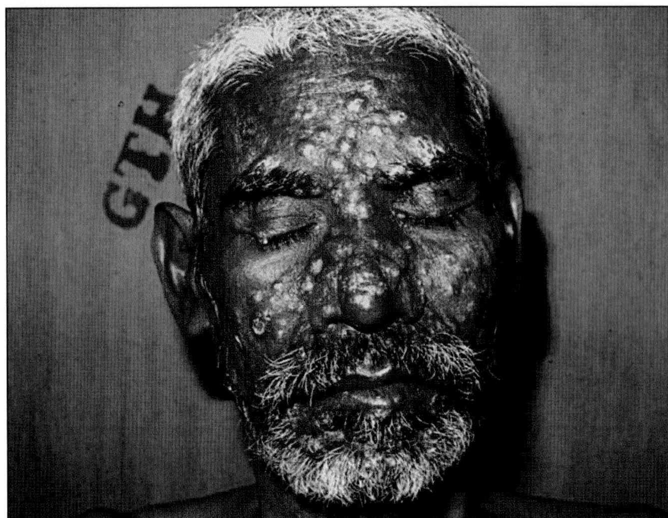

Figure 11.21 Secondary syphilis.

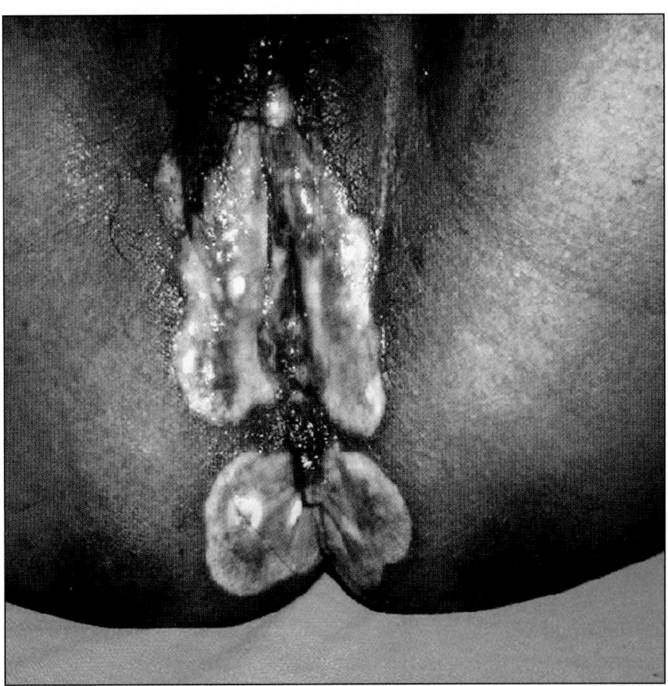

Figure 11.22 Anogenital herpes simplex.

HIV and tumors

Kaposi's sarcoma

This is dealt with in detail later in the chapter.

Non-Hodgkin's lymphoma[45]

At least 6% of all AIDS patients develop lymphomas at some point during their illness (Fig. 11.25). The initiation of HAART has no effect on the incidence. Most tumors are extralymphatic and histologically, they are high-grade, large-cell immunoblastic or non-cleaved small-cell tumors. Burkitt's lymphoma has also been reported. Their pathogenesis may be related to EBV and also to

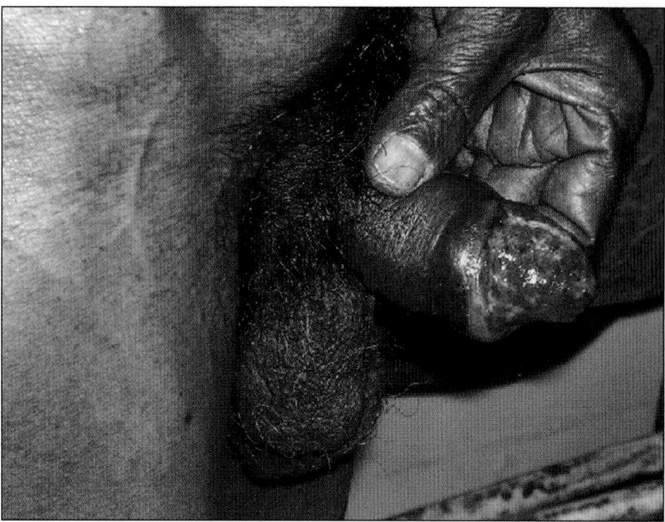

Figure 11.23 Carcinoma of the penis.

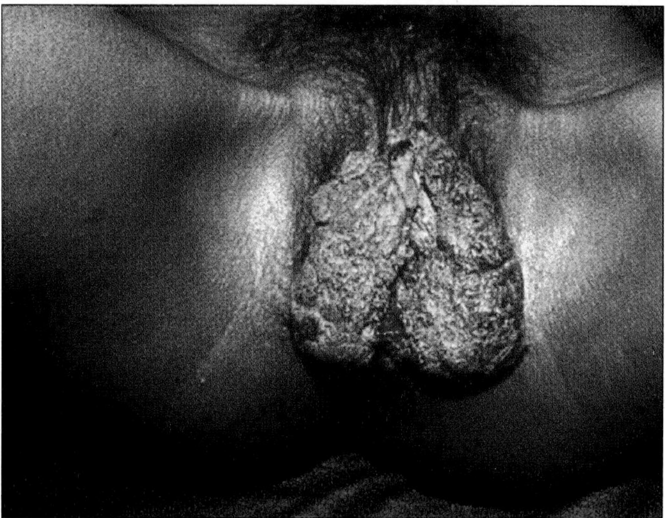

Figure 11.24 Giant condyloma accuminata on the vulva.

human herpesvirus 8 (HHV-8). The CNS is the most common site. Clinically, it presents with signs and symptoms of a SOL. Systemic lymphoma is seen at an earlier stage of infection. In addition to lymph node involvement, the bone marrow (leading to pancytopenia), liver, lung, and GIT (~25% patients) may be involved. Any site in the GIT may be involved. Patients may present with dysphagia and pain. Pulmonary disease may present as a mass lesion, multiple nodules, or an interstitial infiltrate. A variant called primary effusion lymphoma or body-cavity lymphoma has also been described. Lymphomatous pleural, pericardial, and/or peritoneal effusions, in the absence of discrete nodal or extranodal masses, are seen.

Other tumors that can occur in AIDS[46] are: Hodgkin's lymphoma, squamous cell carcinoma of the anus, especially in homosexual men, cervical cancer, adenocarcinoma, renal cell carcinoma, teratoma, and seminoma.

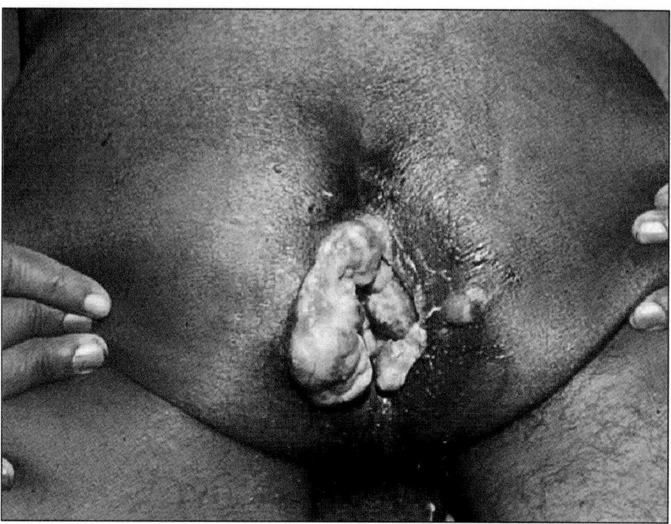

Figure 11.25 Non-Hodgkin's lymphoma.

HIV and hepatitis[2]

The HIV/AIDS and hepatitis coinfection is the current topic of interest globally. According to Fauci and Lane,[2] over 95% of HIV-infected individuals have evidence of infection with HBV; 5–40% are coinfected with hepatitis C virus and coinfection with hepatitis D, E, and/or G viruses is common. There is approximately a threefold increase in the development of persistent hepatitis B surface antigenemia. Patients coinfected with HIV and hepatitis B virus have a low incidence of inflammatory disease, presumably because of the antecedent immunosuppression. Severe hepatitis may develop due to immune reconstitution as a result of antiretroviral therapy. IFN-α is less successful as a treatment of hepatitis B virus and lamivudine is the drug of choice. Since it is also a potent antiretroviral drug, it should never be used as a single agent in the treatment of hepatitis B virus in HIV patients to prevent the development of resistant quasispecies.

In contrast, hepatitis C virus infection is more severe in patients with HIV and levels of hepatitis C virus are 10-fold higher than in the HIV-negative patient, as also is the incidence of liver failure. It is recommended that all HIV-positive individuals who have not experienced natural infection be immunized with hepatitis A and/or hepatitis B vaccines. End-stage liver disease is the commonest cause of mortality amongst such individuals, especially if not treated with HAART.

Dermatological disorders associated with HIV infection[47–51]

The cutaneous manifestations of HIV infection are as much a consequence of the altered immune response as of the immunosuppression.

HIV exanthemata

Acute primary HIV infection may present with an infectious mononucleosis-like transient, generalized, morbilliform eruption (Fig. 11.3). The exanthem is a pruritic, erythematous eruption of macules and papules involving the trunk, extremities, and the head and neck region. Individual lesions include round or oval erythematous macules and papules with or without desquamation, sometimes with a hemorrhagic or necrotic center. Histopathology reveals dermal edema and a perivascular lymphocytic papillary dermal infiltrate, often with associated focal degeneration of basal keratinocytes. Urticaria, enanthemata, perlèche, and oral ulcers have also been described.

In the early asymptomatic stage, no signs of infection other than lymphadenopathy are present. With the onset of immunosuppression, non-specific skin changes, such as treatment-resistant seborrheic dermatitis, and OHL are noted. Common disorders with atypical presentations, including extensive verrucae and recurrent herpes zoster, may also occur. As the immunity worsens, chronic HSV, MC, and CMV appear.

Mycobacterial infections and mucocutaneous candidiasis occur.

Physical

Cutaneous manifestations of HIV disease can be classified as neoplastic, infections and infestations, inflammatory, metabolic, and idiopathic.

Neoplastic

KAPOSI'S SARCOMA[52] KS was the first neoplasm reported in HIV disease (Fig. 11.6). It is usually seen in gay and bisexual men, and in women in Africa. The worldwide incidence of KS in patients with AIDS may approach 34%. KS occurs at all stages of HIV disease, and its severity is not strictly correlated with the degree of immunosuppression. KS is believed to be a proliferation of endothelial cells induced by HHV-8, acquired through sexual transmission.

The seroprevalence of HHV-8 has been studied in Malaysia, India, Sri Lanka, Thailand, Trinidad, and Jamaica, in both healthy individuals and those infected with HIV.[53] Seroprevalence was found to be low in these countries in both the healthy and the HIV-infected populations. This correlates with the fact that hardly any AIDS-related KS has been reported in these countries. In contrast, the African countries of Ghana, Uganda, and Zambia showed high seroprevalences in both healthy and HIV-infected populations. This suggests that HHV-8 may be either a recently introduced virus or one that has extremely low infectivity. The evidence reviewed shows that the causal virus, HHV-8, is prevalent in many African countries, including places where KS was almost unknown before HIV, and that it is as common in women as in men.[54] Therefore, the geographical distribution of KS in Africa before the spread of HIV and its predominance as a disease affecting men are not a simple reflection of the distribution of HHV-8. Since the epidemic of HIV in Africa, KS has become relatively more frequent in women, and the incidence has increased in countries where it was previously rare, but where HHV-8 is prevalent, as well as in countries where it was already common. These changes point to a role for other (as yet unknown) factors in the etiology of KS that may have the most effect in the absence of concurrent HIV infection.

India has more than 12 million people estimated to be living with HIV by end of the year 2002.[55] The major transmission is through the heterosexual route. The HIV epidemic is widespread in India: there are growing numbers of newly detected HIV patients below 25 years and above 50 years of age, a gender ratio (M:F) approaching 2:1, and a growing number of HIV-defining and HIV-associated malignancies. However the incidence of KS is negligible for unknown reasons.

About one-third of HIV-infected cases have a preponderance of tumors on the legs and feet. However, lesions may develop elsewhere on the skin, including the scalp, lips, hard palate, and gums. Lesions may occur singly or in groups. KS begins as pink, red, brown, or purple macules that disseminate and progress to violaceous plaques or nodules. They may easily be mistaken for bruises, purpurae, or nevi. Lesions may be symmetrical with smooth borders or asymmetrical with jagged edges. They darken and become scaly as they age. Involvement of internal organs and mucosa is common. As a rule, a patient has approximately one internal lesion for every five skin lesions. Gastrointestinal involvement is common and may result in hemorrhage or obstruction. The course of KS in HIV-infected patients is more aggressive than the other clinical types of KS. Overall mortality is approximately 41% with over 60% of patients alive at 1 year and 60% at 22 months. Overall survival is 18 months, with some exceptions.

For limited disease, local therapy with liquid nitrogen, alitretinoin, or intralesional vincristine may be effective. Surgery, radiotherapy, and systemic single-agent chemotherapy, usually with vinblastine, vincristine, bleomycin, doxorubicin, or etoposide, may be useful. However, systemic chemotherapy has not been shown to improve the long-term survival rates. Immune reconstitution after HAART may lead to remission of KS. Interferon (IFN)-α and IFN-β, photodynamic therapy and systemic hyperthermia have also been used. Cryotherapy, laser irradiation, and electrodesiccation can be useful for localized solitary lesions of KS.

OTHER HIV-ASSOCIATED MALIGNANCIES[45,46] Nodular B-cell non-Hodgkin lymphomas (NHL) tend to be more progressive and aggressive (Fig. 11.25). There have been occasional reports of multifocal and intraoral squamous cell carcinoma, Bowen's disease, and metastatic basal cell carcinoma. Malignant melanoma[56] appears to be more aggressive, with shorter disease-free and overall survival rates in patients with melanoma and HIV as compared with patients with melanoma without HIV. Pediatric patients are at a higher risk of developing leiomyosarcoma, although the tumor is very rare.

Infections and infestations

VIRAL INFECTIONS

- **HSV**[57] On the basis of serum antibody testing, latent HSV-1 and 2 infections have been reported to be prevalent in 66% and 77% of AIDS patients, respectively. Approximately two-thirds of such people have clinically apparent recurrences at any CD4 count (Fig. 11.22). They are more severe and prolonged in patients with CD4 counts <200 cells/μl. Recurrent oral and anogenital HSV may present as clusters of small vesicles or as multiple small or confluent large ulcers on the lips, nose, oral mucosa, buttocks, perineum, scrotum, vulva, or penis. Proctitis, presenting with rectal pain and tenesmus, is rare. Chronic ulcerations are also common. Chronic, ulcerative herpetic stomatitis is seen in infected children. Diagnosis is confirmed by culturing a swab taken from the base of the ulcer. Reduced response to acyclovir or acyclovir resistance generally only occurs in patients with advanced HIV (<100 CD4 cells/μl). Intravenous foscarnet and topical cidofovir or trifluridine are effective.

- **VZV**[58] Primary varicella infection with visceral dissemination may be seen in HIV-infected adults, but is rare. It may progress to chronic skin involvement. Disseminated and severe herpes zoster (shingles) infections are observed in advanced AIDS. Atypical manifestations, including hyperkeratotic papules, folliculitis, verrucous lesions, chronic ulcerations, disseminated ecthymatous lesions, and chronic VZV infection mimicking basal cell carcinoma have also been described. Herpes zoster ophthalmicus may involve the conjunctiva, cornea, anterior chamber, or the retina. Blindness is a complication of zoster retinitis (Fig. 11.11). Recurrent, multidermatomal or disseminated herpes zoster is an AIDS-defining illness. Acyclovir (or famciclovir or valacyclovir) is the treatment of choice for HSV/VZV diseases in these patients. This class of antivirals is activated by viral thymidine kinase. In some disseminated cases, the virus may develop resistance to acyclovir as a result of defective enzyme activity and prolonged/suboptimal dosage. In this scenario, the use of other drugs, including cidofovir, foscarnet, and vidarabine, may be necessary.
- **EBV**[59] EBV has been implicated in the pathogenesis of OHL. OHL is characterized by white, filiform, corrugated and feathery plaques on the sides of the tongue and sometimes on the oropharyngeal mucosa; these plaques may be mistaken for candidiasis. It has no malignant potential, but it may be the initial sign of progressive immunosuppression. Treatment is usually not necessary. If symptomatic, the patient may be prescribed systemic aciclovir (3200 mg/day), topical application of 25% podophyllum resin, ganciclovir, or foscarnet.
- **CMV infection**[60] Persistent perineal ulcers are the most common presentation of CMV infection in HIV-infected patients. Concurrent infection with other viruses, such as HSV, in the same lesions causes further confusion. HSV is proposed to be the initiating infection leading to ulcer formation, with CMV secondarily localizing in the granulation tissue. Most patients with CMV-induced ulcers also have intractable proctitis or colitis with diarrhea caused by enteric CMV infection, suggesting that these ulcers are the result of contiguous spread from the GIT.

  CMV is also associated with non-specific cutaneous lesions: generalized maculopapular or morbilliform rash, vesicular or bullous eruptions, a generalized bullous toxic epidermal necrolysis-like eruption, purpuric or petechial rash as a result of thrombocytopenia, hyperpigmented indurated cutaneous plaques and bluish-red cutaneous nodules in pediatric patients (blueberry-muffin lesions), which indicate extramedullary erythropoiesis.

  The etiologic diagnosis of cutaneous CMV infection in immunocompromised individuals is considered a poor prognostic sign. Foscarnet, cidofovir, and ganciclovir are the preferred treatments.
- **HPV infection** HIV-infected individuals may suffer from severe, extensive and recalcitrant verrucae, which may arise on the oral mucosa, the face, the perianal region, and the female genital tract (Fig. 11.24). Apart from the immunosuppression, a possible explanation for this is that the HIV TAT protein secreted from infected cells acts as a growth factor for HPV-infected cells.

  Extensive flat and filiform warts on the beard area, exuberant condylomata acuminata showing features of intraepithelial neoplasia, i.e., the Buschke–Loewenstein tumor, multiple and large hyperkeratotic warts on and around the fingers, large plantar warts caused by HPV-66[61] and an epidermodysplasia verruciformis (EDV)-like eruption[62] have also been reported. Bowenoid papulosis and anal/cervical carcinoma-in-situ (AIN/CIN) may be found in up to 50% of patients using exfoliative cytology.

  Therapy with imiquimod or IFN-α_{2b} is preferred. Ablation and curettage may be useful.
- **MC** In HIV infection, MC may be widespread and atypical. The lesions may be observed on extragenital sites,[63] such as the face, the neck, and the scalp; or they may show altered morphology and size (Fig. 11.4). Such unusual forms include solitary endophytic, aggregated, inflamed, and giant MCs. MCs mimicking sebaceous nevus of Jadassohn, ecthyma, and giant condylomata accuminata have been reported.[64] Topical cidofovir or imiquimod following ablation and curettage may be most useful.
- **Pityriasis rosea** In HIV infection, an atypical variant with prolonged fever and malaise, but with typical papulosquamous skin lesions, has been reported.
- **Other viral infections** Parvovirus B19, coxsackie and enteroviruses have been associated with morbilliform or vesicular exanthemata. An unusual palisaded granulomatous inflammatory dermatitis[65] has been reported. An adenovirus has been implicated in the etiology.

FUNGAL INFECTIONS[47–51]

Superficial fungal infections

- **Candidiasis** *Candida* generally causes mucosal disease: cutaneous, oropharyngeal, vulvovaginal, and esophageal. Recurrent and persistent mucocutaneous candidiasis is common in HIV-infected patients (Fig. 11.5). Clinically, it manifests as whitish, curd-like exudates on the dorsal or buccal mucosa that can be easily scraped away with a cotton swab, leaving behind a reddish friable surface that may be associated with a burning sensation – the so-called pseudomembranous candidiasis or thrush. Sometimes, only a beefy red, eroded surface can be seen (erosive candidiasis). Chronic atrophic candidiasis, presenting as angular cheilitis and candidial leukoplakia, is also noted. The symptoms include burning pain, altered taste sensation, and dysphagia, which is more prominent with esophageal candidiasis.

  Recurrent vulvovaginal candidiasis (RVVC) presents with a creamy-white vaginal discharge, with vaginal or vulvar pruritus, burning pain, and dyspareunia. The vaginal mucosa is inflamed and pseudomembranous plaques are often seen. Candidial balanitis, or balanoposthitis, intertrigo,[66] and chronic candidial paronychia are also common. Oral azole treatment, especially fluconazole, is preferred. Fluconazole-refractory disease is common in advanced AIDS. Higher doses of fluconazole, itraconazole, 5-fluorocytosine or amphotericin B may be required for treatment.
- **Dermatophytosis** Tinea capitis, typically caused by *Trichophyton rubrum* or *Microsporum canis*, as well as proximal subungual onychomycosis (PSO) is indicative of HIV infection (Fig. 11.26). Extensive dermatophytosis is also common.[67] It may be resistant to topical antifungal creams and may require systemic antifungal therapy with griseofulvin, fluconazole, ketoconazole, or terbinafine.
- **Malassezia furfur** Persistent and recurrent tinea versicolor has been reported (Fig. 11.27). Other conditions caused by the fungus are folliculitis, which presents as multiple erythematous, pruritic papules on the trunk, and confluent and reticulate papillomatosis. Oral fluconazole/ketoconazole and topical antifungal preparations are used for treatment.

Deep fungal infections

- **Cutaneous cryptococcosis** Disseminated cryptococcosis is by far the most common systemic mycosis in HIV disease; cutaneous involvement may be seen in 5–10 % of cases (Fig. 11.8). Skin lesions

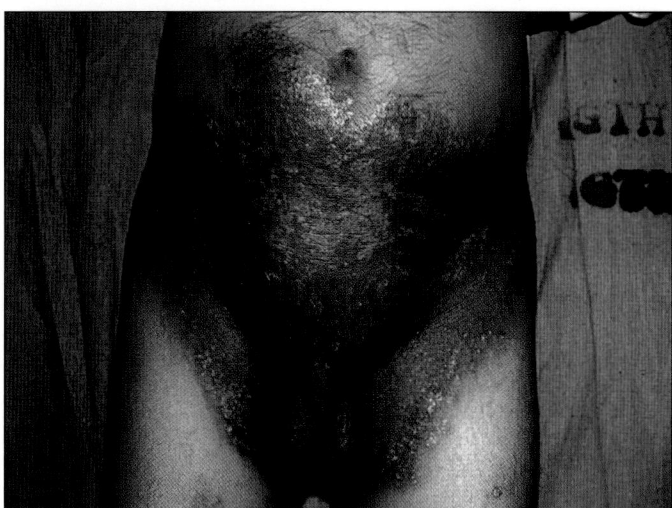

Figure 11.26 Dermatophytosis.

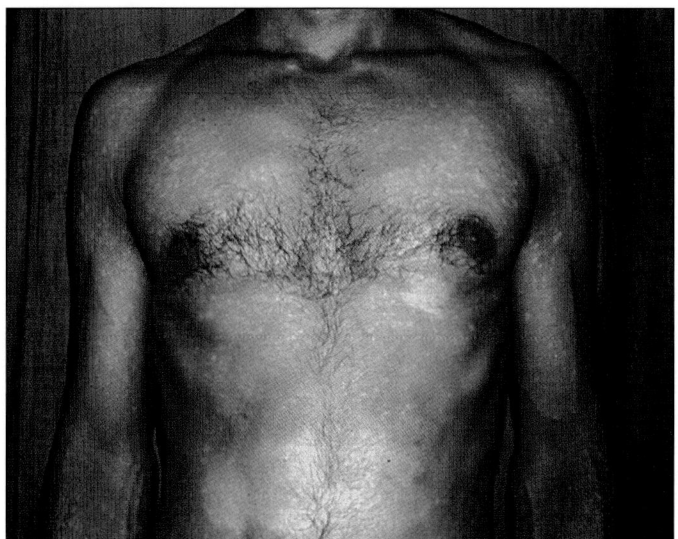

Figure 11.27 Tinea versicolor.

may be present for weeks or months before presentation, occurring most commonly on the head, face, and neck (78%), but may be widespread. The most common presentation is of translucent, dome-shaped, and umbilicated MC-like lesions (54%). Other presentations may include palpable purpura, pustules, vegetating plaques, ulcers, panniculitis, pyoderma gangrenosum-like lesions, or subcutaneous abscesses. Skin biopsy, followed by use of the mucicarmine stain, is diagnostic. A careful history and neurological examination may reveal subtle signs of meningitis or CNS disease in asymptomatic patients. In such cases, spinal fluid examination, including fungal culture, is indicated.

- **Cutaneous histoplasmosis**[68] The incidence of disseminated histoplasmosis in AIDS patients is approximately 10%. The patient may present with widespread and inflamed macules and papules, one or many indurated, erythematous, and vegetative plaques, a cellulitis-like eruption, ulcers, scattered acneiform lesions, pustules, panniculitis, or MC-like lesions (Fig. 11.9). Lesions occur most commonly on the face, followed by extremities and trunk. Oral mucosal lesions include nodules and vegetations; ulcers occur on the soft palate, oropharynx, epiglottis, and nasal vestibule. Hepatosplenomegaly and/or lymphadenopathy are common. In addition, cutaneous histoplasmosis has been demonstrated to exist in situ with other cutaneous disorders such as KS, psoriasis, and psoriasiform dermatitis.
- **Coccidioidomycosis** Systemic infection by *Coccidioides immitis* may spread to the skin, beginning as papules and evolving to pustules, plaques, or nodules with minimal surrounding erythema, MC-like lesions, abscesses, cellulitis, verrucous and hemorrhagic papules or nodules, and healing scars.
- **Sporotrichosis**[69] Hematogenous dissemination of *Sporothrix schenckii* to the skin may present as papules to nodules that become eroded, ulcerated, crusted, or hyperkeratotic, usually sparing the palms, soles, and oral mucosa. The classical lymphangitic form may also be observed. Skin biopsy shows the characteristic asteroid bodies.
- **Penicilliosis** *Penicillium marneffei* infection is the third most common OI in HIV/AIDS, in Southeast Asia. It is more common in the Chiang Mai province of north Thailand and in southern China. Cutaneous involvement is seen in up to 76% of cases. The most common skin lesions are umbilicated papules resembling MC, occurring most frequently on the face, pinnae, upper trunk, and arms (Fig. 11.28). Folliculitis, ecthyma-like lesions, subcutaneous nodules, genital ulcers, and morbilliform lesions have also been described. Skin biopsy is diagnostic.
- **Aspergillosis**[70] Invasive disease is rare, presenting as primary cutaneous infection, occurring under adhesive tape near central

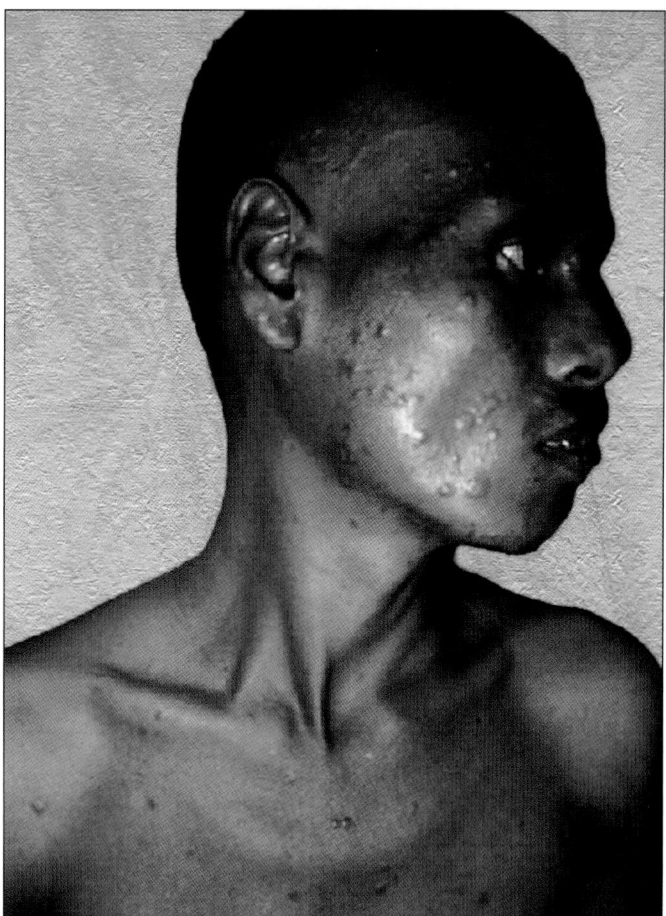

Figure 11.28 Penicilliosis.

venous catheters, or occurring as disseminated infection. Skin lesions appear as skin-colored to pink umbilicated papules resembling MC. Prognosis is poor, in spite of treatment.

- **North American blastomycosis** Is rare and may present as a disseminated maculopapular eruption. Amphotericin B/itraconazole are the mainstay of treatment, in deep mycoses in HIV; 5-fluorocytosine and liposomal amphotericin B may be used in resistant cases. Fluconazole is used in maintenance therapy in cases of cryptococcosis.

BACTERIAL INFECTIONS[47-51]

Impetigo, folliculitis, furuncles, and abscesses *Staphylococcus aureus* is the most common bacterial pathogen causing cutaneous and systemic infections in HIV disease. An increased prevalence of *S. aureus* carriage in the nares and the perineum has been noted in HIV-infected patients. Impetigo may be recurrent and persistent in pediatric HIV disease. It is commonly caused by coagulase-positive staphylococci and by beta-hemolytic streptococci. It occurs not only on the face, but also in axillary, inguinal, and other flexural locations (Fig. 11.29). Clinical presentation is usually typical, but therapeutic response may be delayed. It may frequently complicate HSV infection of the skin.

Adults do not suffer from any unique staphylococcal infections in HIV disease. A wide range of pyodermas and soft-tissue infections do occur (Fig. 11.30). Primary staphylococcal infections include impetigo, bullous impetigo, and ecthyma, furuncles and carbuncles, cellulitis, botryomycosis, and pyomyositis. Secondary infection of underlying dermatoses, sometimes leading to bacteremia or septicemia, may also occur. Disseminated folliculitis and furunculosis caused by *S. aureus* may be a presenting feature of HIV infection. Infections tend to be recurrent and management consists of treating the acute infection, eradication of the carrier state (mupirocin), and chronic oral prophylaxis (co-trimoxazole or rifampicin).

Pseudomonas aeruginosa causes ecthyma gangrenosum, infection of catheter sites, and secondary infection of underlying disorders such as KS in advanced HIV disease. It may lead to septicemia and death.

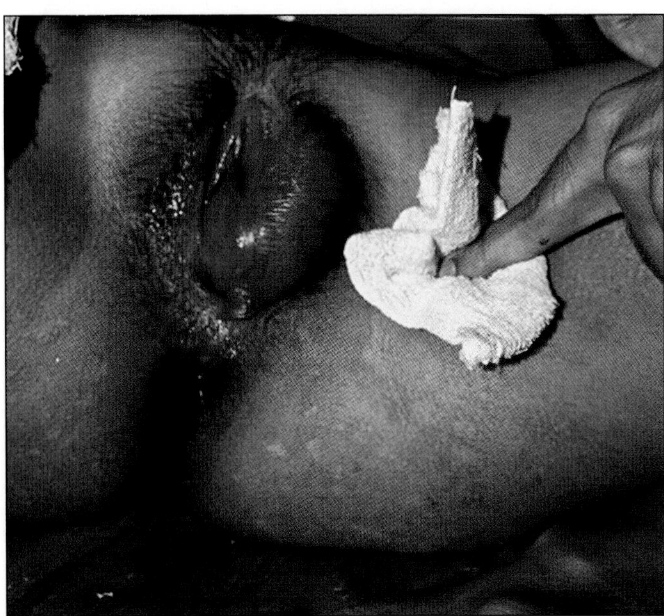

Figure 11.29 Bartholin gland abscess.

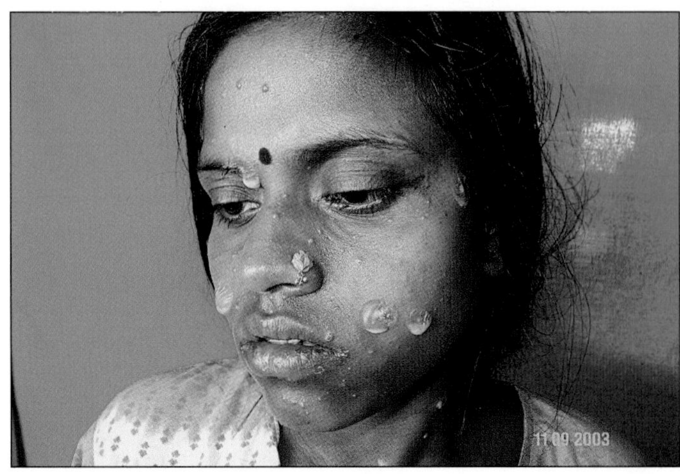

Figure 11.30 Pyoderma.

Helicobacter cinaedi causes a syndrome characterized by fever, bacteremia, and recurrent and/or chronic cellulitis (resembling erythema nodosum) in immunocompromised patients. The organism is carried as bowel flora in 10% of homosexual men.

Corynebacterium diphtheriae has been associated with a cutaneous infection leading to septicemia in an HIV-infected patient.

Bacillary angiomatosis (BA) and bacillary peliosis (BAP)[71] This condition, caused by *Bartonella henselae* and rarely by *B. quintana*, is characterized by angioproliferative lesions resembling cherry angiomas, pyogenic granulomas, and KS (Fig. 11.10). Clinically, the skin lesions are red to violaceous, dome-shaped papules, nodules, or plaques resembling KS, and ranging from a few millimeters up to 2–3 cm in size. Subcutaneous lesions are rare, but may occur. Lesions are soft or firm, but tender. The number varies from a few to hundreds. Any site, except the palms, soles, and oral cavity may be involved. Hematogenous or lymphatic dissemination to the bone marrow and other lymphoid organs may occur. The course is variable and the disease can recur. It is an AIDS-defining illness. Oral erythromycin (250–500 mg PO q.i.d.) or doxycycline (100 mg b.i.d.), continued until the lesions resolve (3–4 weeks), is usually effective. Secondary prophylaxis is recommended in patients with recurrent BA.

Nocardia spp. can cause brain abscesses and commonly infect the lung. Mycetomas resulting from *Nocardia* spp. can appear as nodules which suppurate and drain seropurulent material (Fig. 11.31).

MYCOBACTERIAL INFECTIONS

Mycobacterium tuberculosis In HIV disease, the incidence of extrapulmonary tuberculosis is 20–40%, which increases to 70% in advanced disease. Cutaneous tuberculosis, however, is relatively uncommon. Multifocal lupus vulgaris, tuberculous gummata, orofacial TB, scrofuloderma, and miliary abscesses may be seen (Figs 11.13–11.18). The hypersensitivity phenomena, papulonecrotic tuberculids and lichen scrofulosorum[72] also occur in HIV-infected individuals on treatment for pulmonary or extrapulmonary disease. Response to conventional treatment is usually satisfactory.

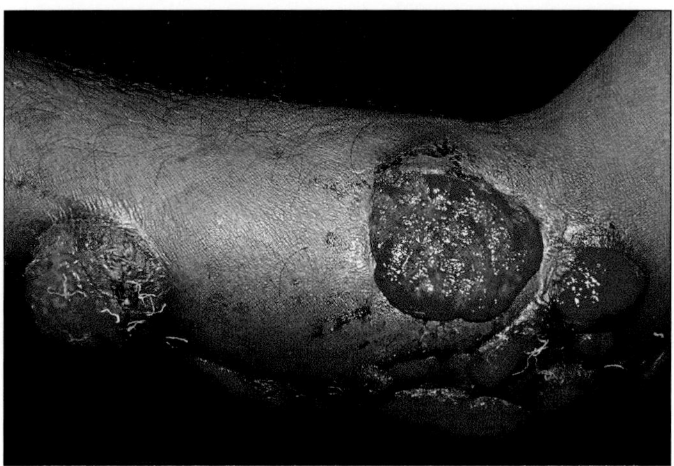

Figure 11.31 Nocardiosis.

Mycobacterium avium–intracellulare complex MAC usually manifests as disseminated disease involving the lung, lymph nodes, and GIT. Primary cutaneous infections with MAC are extremely rare. Most cutaneous lesions are caused by dissemination. Cutaneous manifestations thus far reported include scaling plaques, crusted ulcers, ecthyma-like lesions, verrucous ulcers, inflammatory nodules, panniculitis, pustular lesions, and draining sinuses. Localized, primary cutaneous MAC infection resembling sporotrichosis[73] is unusual, but was described in a patient with AIDS. Response to treatment with conventional antituberculous regimens is unsatisfactory, and addition of macrolides such as clarithromycin and azithromycin, minocycline, rifabutin, or clofazimine is necessary. The incidence of MAC infections has fallen with primary prophylaxis with azithromycin and, more recently, with HAART.

Mycobacterium kansasii Cutaneous infection with *M. kansasii* is rare. In HIV-infected individuals, the infection may present with acneiform papules and/or indurated, crusted plaques. Diagnosis is confirmed by smear and culture, and treatment is similar to the treatment of other atypical mycobacterial infections.

Mycobacterium haemophilum *M. haemophilum* can also present as violaceous, draining nodules and superficial ulcers on the extremities, the trunk, the head, and the genitalia. Diagnosis is confirmed by smear and culture, and treatment is similar to treatment of other atypical mycobacterial infections.

Mycobacterium leprae As a result of immunosuppression in HIV disease, it was thought that coinfection with leprosy may present as a downgrading of disease, multibacillary disease, and an increased incidence of lepra reactions (Fig. 11.12). However, a World Health Organization meeting in 1993 concluded that there was no convincing evidence of such an association. A case–control study conducted in South India in 1994 also supported this conclusion.[74]

PROTOZOAL INFECTIONS

Leishmania donovani[75] Visceral leishmaniasis (VL) is recognized with increasing frequency in HIV patients who live in or travel to endemic areas. VL promotes the development of AIDS-defining conditions and clinical progression, as well as diminishes the life expectancy of HIV-infected subjects. Conversely, HIV infection increases the risk of developing VL by 100–1000 times in endemic areas, reduces the probability of therapeutic response, and enhances the possibility of relapse. Extensive parasitic dissemination, atypical lesions, a chronic and relapsing course, poor response to standard therapy, and lack of anti-*Leishmania* antibodies characterize HIV-associated VL.

The clinical presentation is one of hepatosplenomegaly, fever, and other constitutional symptoms, lymphadenopathy, systemic involvement affecting the GIT, the kidneys, the lungs and rarely the skin, and hematologic abnormalities. Cutaneous involvement of VL is rare, but characteristic of HIV disease. It is seen in 2–12% of patients with coinfection (Fig. 11.32). The lesions can be papular, maculopapular, or nodular. Organisms may be isolated from cultures of bone marrow aspirates. Conventional therapy includes the pentavalent antimonials or liposomal amphotericin B. Allopurinol, IFN-γ, or imiquimod may be combined with antimonials in refractory cases, or in relapse.

Entamoeba histolytica Severe intestinal amebiasis may be associated with cutaneous involvement (Fig. 11.19). It commonly appears as one or more lesions on the buttocks, and these lesions may have a rapid and destructive course. The lesion may be a deeply invading ulcer or an ulcerated granuloma. The ulcers are 2–3 cm wide, serpiginous with distinct, indurated, and (may have) undermined edges with an erythematous rim. The floor shows hemopurulent exudate and necrotic slough. Penile amebiasis may occur in homosexual men. Invasive amebiasis is not especially common in HIV infection. Treatment consists of the nitroimidazoles, metronidazole or tinidazole, which may have to be given in a higher

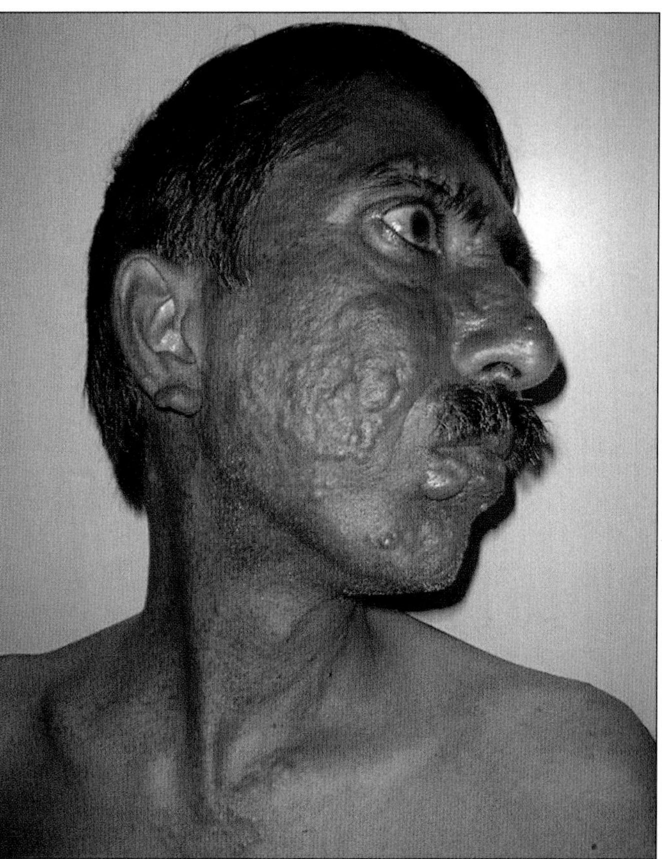

Figure 11.32 Leishmaniasis.

dosage, in combination with either diloxanide furoate and/or chloroquine.

***Acanthamoeba castellani*[76]** Infection usually causes progressive encephalitis, but skin lesions are quite common in AIDS. Pustules, deep nodules, and ulcers develop on the trunk and extremities, which may ulcerate. Diagnosis and treatment are difficult and systemic pentamidine, flucytosine, fluconazole, and sulfadiazine have been used.

Toxoplasma gondii Cutaneous involvement is rare, and manifests as an eruption of papules involving the trunk and extremities. Histology reveals a mixed cellular infiltrate with eosinophils. Treatment is the same as that of systemic disease.

Pneumocystis carinii Cutaneous pneumocystosis may be rarely observed. It presents with erythematous friable papules, usually in the region of the external ear. It may also present as molluscum-like papules, vascular lesions mimicking KS, as well as bluish ill-defined patches in the sternal region. Biopsy and cultures are often required for diagnosis. Sulfonamides (co-trimoxazole) or pentamidine are preferred treatments.

INFESTATIONS

Scabies Scabies is common in HIV-infected individuals. In cases with severe immunosuppression, crusted or Norwegian scabies, characterized by hyperkeratotic plaques on the palms, soles, trunk, or extremities has been reported. These lesions house millions of mites. A widespread and scaly maculopapular/papulosquamous eruption, resembling atopic dermatitis, and involvement of scalp and face in adults, resembling seborrheic dermatitis, have been reported. Secondary infection may be complicated by bacteremia and fatal septicemia.

Treatment is difficult and consists of application of topical antiscabetics, such as permethrin, gamma benzene hexachloride, or benzyl benzoate, in the recommended dosage. Treatment may have to be continued for a longer duration in cases of crusted scabies. Oral ivermectin (200 μg/kg) is also effective.

Demodicidosis Florid colonization by the *Demodex folliculorum* mites may result in a persistent, follicular eruption; which is characterized by widespread pruritic, reddish papules distributed on the face, trunk, and extremities. Scraping and skin biopsy demonstrate the mites. Topical 5% permethrin cream, benzyl benzoate, benzoyl peroxide, and oral ivermectin are effective. However, recurrences are common.

Helminthiasis Hyperinfective *Strongyloides stercoralis* infestation may disseminate and give rise to a rapidly migrating livedo reticularis-like cutaneous eruption, called larva currens, that may mimic generalized vasculitis or connective tissue disorders. Pruritus is common. Albendazole is the mainstay of therapy.

Inflammatory disorders

PAPULOSQUAMOUS DERMATOSES OF AIDS[77]

Seborrheic dermatitis This may be the initial cutaneous manifestation of HIV disease. The prevalence ranges from 7 to 80%. Its presence correlates inversely with decreasing CD4+ T-cell counts and thus, the incidence and severity in HIV-infected persons are closely related to the stage of HIV infection. Most cases have an ordinary clinical presentation. However, atypical features, such as thick greasy scales on the face and the scalp, and involvement of axillae, groin, and perianal areas, have been described. It may progress to erythroderma. Histologically, distinct features such as parakeratosis, keratinocyte necrosis, lymphoid clusters at the dermoepidermal junction, and a perivascular plasma cell infiltrate have been reported.

Seborrheic dermatitis occurs with increased frequency in patients with AIDS-associated dementia. A neurohormonal regulatory dysfunction leads to increased sebum production and consequent overgrowth of the yeast, *Malassezia furfur*. Treatment is difficult. Application of antifungal/corticosteroid creams separately or in combination is the treatment of choice. Treatment with coal tar, sulfur, and salicylic acid shampoos and topical tacrolimus may be effective.

Psoriasis Although the occurrence of psoriasis in HIV-infected persons is similar to that in the general population, there appears to be a strong correlation between the initial onset of psoriasis and HIV infection. The development of eruptive psoriasis or a sudden exacerbation of preexisting disease in a person at risk should suggest possible HIV infection. Psoriasis is more commonly noticed at some point after seroconversion. The severity increases with the degree of immunodeficiency.

Atypical lesions are common (Fig. 11.33). Guttate psoriasis and affection of the groin, axillae, scalp, palms, and soles may be seen. Severe palmoplantar keratoderma and nail involvement are common. Erythroderma may be precipitated. The prevalence of psoriatic arthritis is increased in HIV infection. Histopathology may differ from the classical picture. Less spongiosis and acanthosis is seen, as compared to that in similarly affected HIV-negative individuals, as are fewer Munro's microabscesses. The infiltrate is diffuse and consists of macrophages and plasma cells, but few T cells. T-cell stimulation and increased cytokine secretion, which increase the levels of neopterin, may play a role in the pathogenesis. Streptococcal infection may also influence the development of guttate psoriasis in HIV-infected patients.

Treatment for limited disease consists of moderately potent corticosteroid preparations applied twice or thrice daily. If response

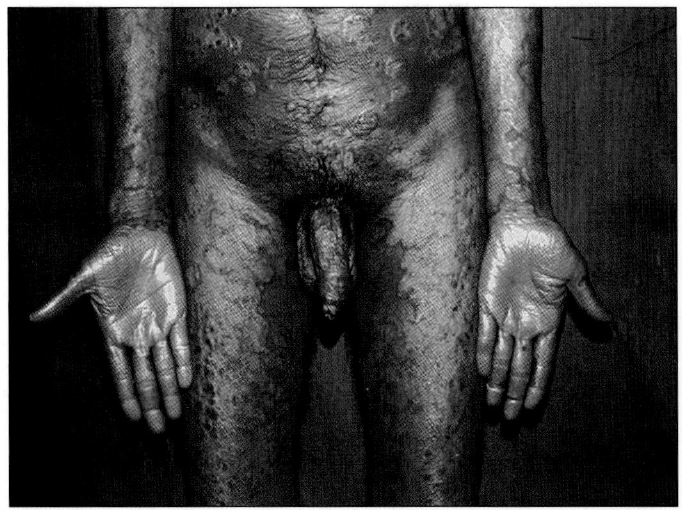

Figure 11.33 Psoriasis.

is unsatisfactory, other topical agents, such as coal tar, calcipotriol, and anthralin, may be tried. In widespread disease, use of phototherapy (either psoralens and long-wave ultraviolet light (PUVA) or ultraviolet B) is safe and effective. Systemic retinoids, such as etretinate (1 mg/kg per day) may be used alone or in combination with ultraviolet light. Immunosuppressive therapy is usually avoided. Zidovudine and HAART have been reported to be extremely effective.

Reiter's disease Reiter's disease is more prevalent among HIV-infected individuals, with a reported incidence ranging from 1.7% to 10%. The onset of disease may predate or be simultaneous with the appearance of symptoms of HIV infection. Articular symptoms may be the first to appear and manifest as severe and persistent oligoarticular arthritis, affecting the large joints of the lower limbs, or as sacroiliitis. The classical features of conjunctivitis/uveitis, circinate balanitis and keratoderma blenorrhagicum are also seen, albeit in a severe form (Fig. 11.34). Considerable overlap exists between Reiter's disease, psoriatic arthritis, and psoriasis. Treatment is similar to the treatment of psoriasis.

Pityriasis rubra pilaris Pitryiasis rubra pilaris occurs with increased frequency in HIV infection. The clinical features include follicular papules with elongated spines and comedo-like lesions. Nail involvement, palmoplantar keratoderma, and the presence of islands of normal skin are similar to classical disease. There may be progression to erythroderma. Simultaneous occurrence of severe nodulocystic acne is also observed. The lesions are located on the back, flanks, and proximal extremities. Histopathology reveals orthokeratotic plugs and perifollicular mucinous degeneration. Treatment is unsatisfactory. Retinoid (etretinate) therapy and HAART may be useful.[78]

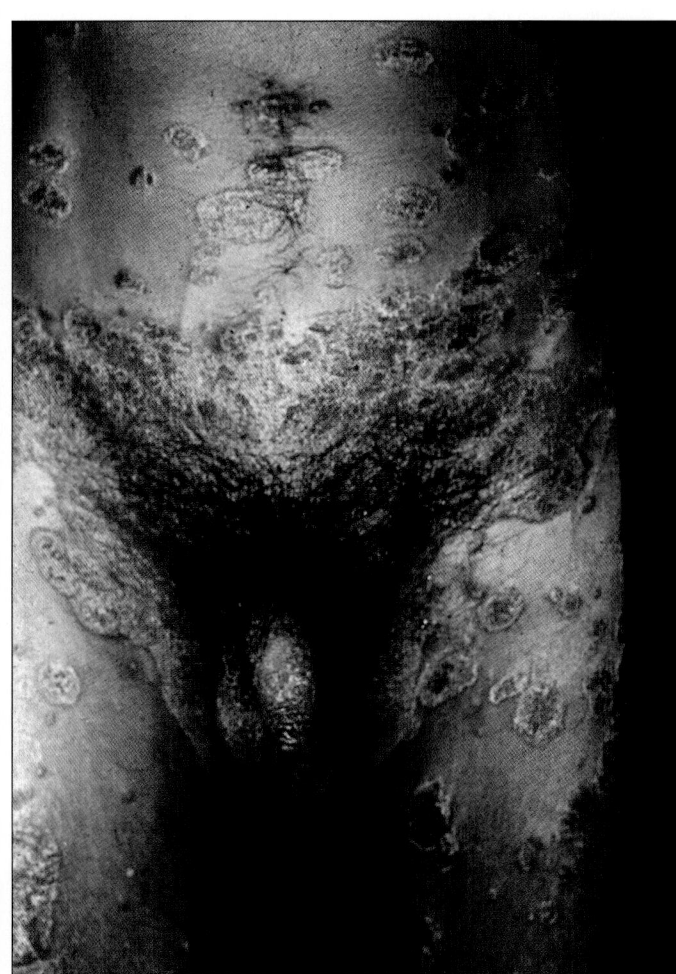

Figure 11.34 Reiter's disease.

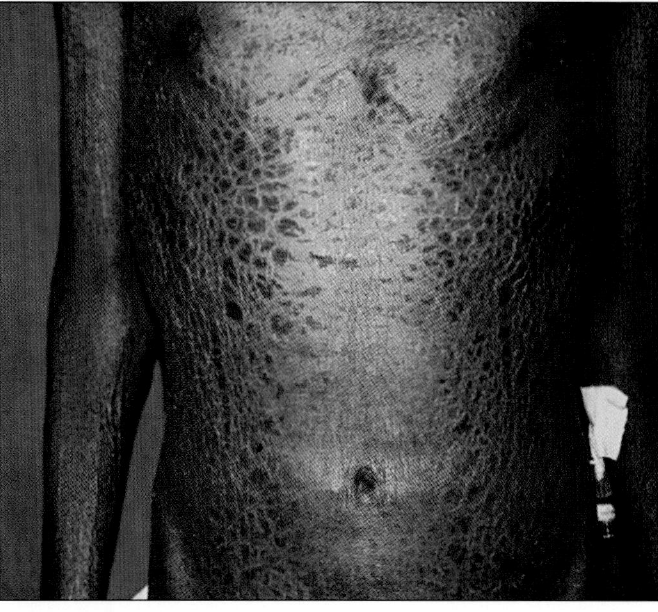

Figure 11.35 Ichthyosis.

Acquired ichthyosis Severe ichthyosis of the lower extremities has been reported in 23–30% of HIV-infected patients (Fig. 11.35). Causation is multifactorial with malnutrition, poor hygiene, chronic illness, and immunologic deficits playing a role. It may be a marker of concomitant infection with HIV-1 and HTLV-II in IVDUs.[79] The severity of ichthyosis is not directly related to the stage of immunosuppression. Treatment is symptomatic with the use of keratolytics such as salicylic acid, lactic acid, and urea, in conjunction with emollients.

Xerosis or generalized dry skin Dry and cracked skin, often leading to pruritus, has been reported in many series, as the initial clinical manifestation of AIDS. The extent of disease is not related to the stage of immunosuppression. Treatment consists of anti-histamines to control pruritus, and the liberal use of emollients, moisturizers, and humectants.

Eosinophilic folliculitis Eosinophilic folliculitis is a chronic, pruritic, culture-negative follicular eruption seen in patients with advanced HIV disease, usually when CD4+ cell counts are at or less than 250 cells/mm^3. It may also occur in the immune restoration syndrome.

It is postulated to be a TH2 immune response to an unknown antigen. Clinically, it presents as multiple symmetrical, pink to red, edematous, folliculocentric papules and sometimes pustules, 1–4 mm in diameter, which are scattered on the face, neck, proximal extremities, and the trunk above the level of the nipples (Fig. 11.36). The papules may coalesce to form plaques and

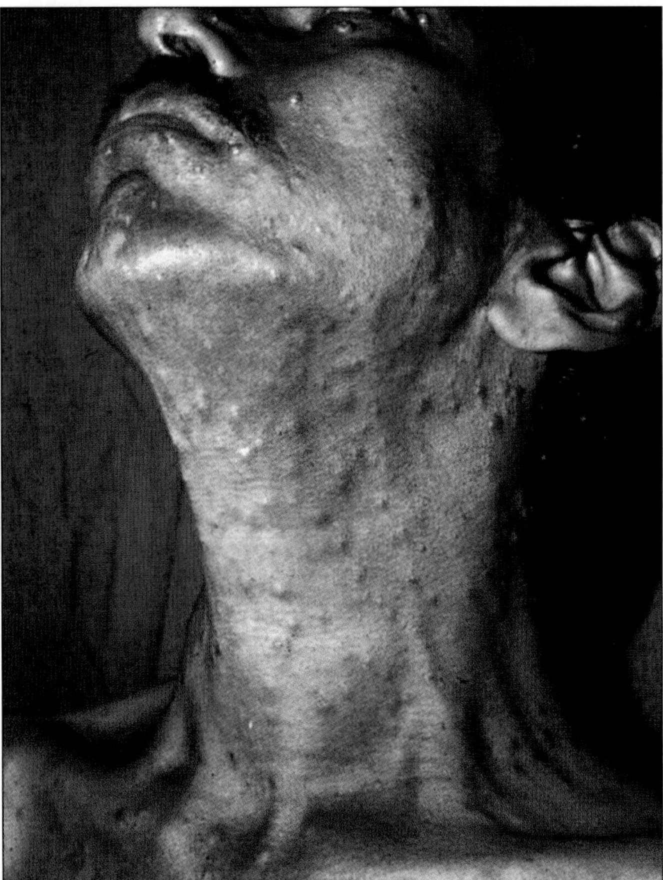

Figure 11.36 Eosinophilic folliculitis.

secondary changes such as excoriation, lichenification, and prurigo nodularis may occur. Postinflammatory hyperpigmentation is common in dark-skinned individuals. Resolution occurs after immune reconstitution, consequent to HAART. The main histologic feature is a neutrophilic and eosinophilic infiltrate around the hair follicle. The serum IgE level and blood eosinophil count may be increased.

The most effective therapy is systemic corticosteroids, which can be tapered every 7–14 days. Recurrences are common. Oral isotretinoin has been used, but causes hyperlipidemia and may compound that caused by PIs. Therefore, it should be used with caution. Phototherapy using PUVA/ultraviolet B[80] and high-potency topical steroids are also helpful. Topical tacrolimus and pimecrolimus are also effective, as is zidovudine/HAART.

Pruritic papular eruption[81] Various descriptions have been proposed for this entity. The etiology is obscure and no definite cause has been detected. Pruritic papular eruptions may present with different types of rashes. These include:

- Transient, maculopapular eruptions: occur most frequently on the face and trunk. They usually heal within 4–6 weeks. Histologically, a lymphoplasmacytic angiitis is repeatedly observed in many cases.
- A more chronic eruption has also been described in individuals with AIDS and AIDS-related complex: it consists of multiple discrete, 2–5-mm skin-colored papules distributed over the head, neck, and upper trunk. Histology is non-specific. No correlation has been found between disease severity and stage of HIV infection.
- A chronic, follicular eruption on the limbs and trunk: characterized histologically by a perifollicular neutrophilic infiltrate.

No pathogen has been detected in any of these conditions. The treatment is also empirical. Topical corticosteroids, phototherapy with PUVA and ultraviolet B, dapsone, topical 4% cromolyn sodium and pentoxifylline[82] have been reported to be effective.

DRUG ERUPTIONS The complete panorama of drug reactions, ranging from insignificant mild dermatitis to life-threatening Stevens–Johnson syndrome (SJS) and toxic epidermal necrolysis (TEN), has been reported in HIV infection (Fig. 11.37). In general, they resolve when the offending drug is discontinued. Severe reactions may require considerable supportive care, especially if there is extensive denudation and the risk of sepsis. The following drug reactions are the most commonly described.

Trimethoprim–sulfamethoxazole This drug can cause hypersensitivity reactions in up to 30% of cases. They may range from mild erythema with fever to an acute morbilliform reaction to SJS. In many cases, the rash does not recur on rechallenge. However, this should not be tried in patients who have had serious reactions such as erythema multiforme. Amprenavir, with a structural similarity to sulfones, may also cause a rash.

Zidovudine (AZT) Distinctive nail pigmentation, affecting the fingernails more than the toenails, has been reported. Discoloration is similar to that produced by chemotherapeutic agents such as doxorubicin; AZT also produces pigmentation of the buccal mucosa.

Non-nucleoside reverse transcriptase inhibitors (NNRTIs) Skin rash is common with NNRTIs, and most frequent and severe with nevirapine (Fig. 11.38). It occurs in the first 2–3 weeks after instituting HAART. Most reactions are mild and can be managed without drug interruption, with symptomatic antihistamines. Interestingly, cross-reactivity with other drugs of this class is not common.

Abacavir Mild erythema may be a component of the abacavir hypersensitivity syndrome.

Foscarnet Severe penile ulcerations, which are considerably worse in uncircumcised individuals, have been described. They resolve on stoppage of the drug.

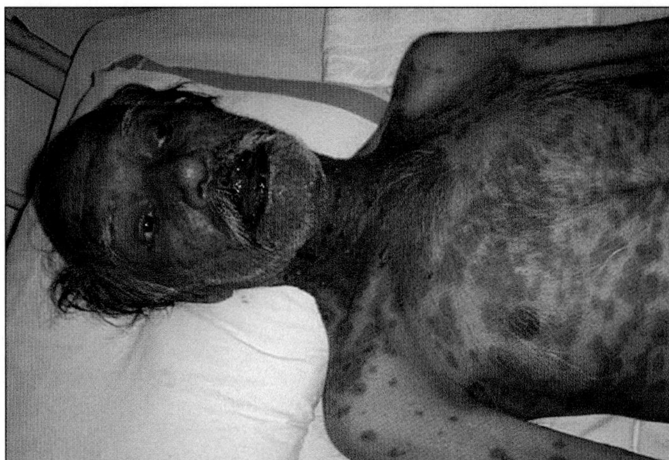

Figure 11.37 Stevens–Johnson syndrome.

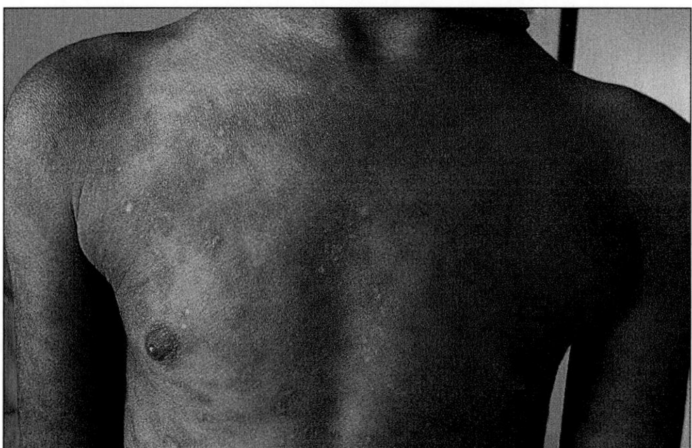

Figure 11.38 Drug reaction due to nevirapine.

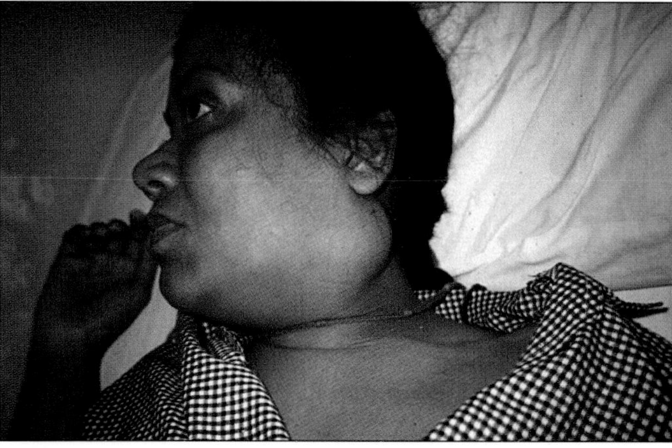

Figure 11.39 Parotid gland enlargement in sicca syndrome.

Glucan-induced keratoderma[83] Glucan is an oligosaccharide used as an immunostimulant. Keratoderma, presenting as thick, yellow hyperkeratosis of the palms and soles with fissures, which develop after 2–3 weeks of therapy, has been reported. The condition is symmetrical and resolves over 2–4 weeks after treatment. The mechanism is thought to be a reaction to the yeast, *Saccharomyces cerevisiae*.

Aphthosis

Recurrent and refractory aphthous stomatitis is considered an indication for HIV serotesting in individuals at risk. The clinical presentation in HIV infection is more severe, as compared to immunocompetent individuals. CMV infection should be ruled out in patients with chronic, refractory aphthae. Treatment is difficult. Tacrolimus and thalidomide[84] are reported to be effective in treatment.

HIV-associated autoimmune conditions[85]

The following conditions have been described:

- ITP: This is one of the most common autoimmune conditions associated with HIV disease. It may be the presenting sign of the disease. Bruising, non-palpable purpura, petechiae, and hemorrhage characterize it. The mechanism is different from that in HIV-negative patients. Platelet survival is however longer than that in seronegative patients with ITP. Diagnosis is difficult and consists of exclusion of other causes of thrombocytopenia. Treatment should be considered in patients with platelet counts $<20\,000/mm^3$. Immunoglobulin, HAART, and steroids, especially prednisolone, should be considered. In resistant or relapsed disease, IFN-α and even splenectomy may be required.
- Sicca syndrome: This entity has been reported in HIV infection. It is a part of the diffuse infiltrative lymphocytosis syndrome (DILS) described in HIV infection. Diagnosis is clinical with parotid gland enlargement (Fig. 11.39) and/or marked CD8 expansion in peripheral blood combined with a minor salivary gland biopsy. However, it differs from classical disease such that most cases are men with different HLA types, who have no antibodies and show inflammatory infiltrates of salivary glands. The glandular enlargement regresses to a significant degree with HAART. High-dose steroids and cytotoxic drugs may at times be necessary.
- Vitiligo: It is unclear whether this condition is caused by the polyclonal hypergammaglobulinemia as a result of HIV infection, or whether it is just an unrelated finding.
- Bullous pemphigoid: This condition has also been reported in HIV disease. Patients present with severe pruritus and antibodies to the basement membrane may be detected. The presentation and management of disease remain unchanged.
- Transient acantholytic dermatosis: Transient acantholytic dermatosis or Grover's disease is a widespread, pruritic, papular eruption characterized by scaly, crusted erythematous papules, usually distributed on the trunk and extremities. In immunocompetent persons, it usually develops in middle-aged or elderly individuals and is short-lived and self-limiting. In HIV infection, younger patients may manifest a more severe and persistent variant, which is difficult to treat. Histology reveals focal acantholytic dyskeratosis in the epidermis.

Other vesicobullous disorders have also been reported. Antinuclear antibodies and some features of systemic lupus erythematosus (SLE) have been described, but true SLE has not been proven. The management of these disorders is similar to that in HIV-negative patients, although immunosuppressive agents should be used with caution.

Atopic eczema

Atopic dermatitis may be exacerbated by HIV disease. There may be a reactivation of disease in HIV-infected individuals, in whom the disease was quiescent earlier. The severity of disease is more marked in children. Increased serum IgE levels have been reported, although no correlation with disease severity has been detected. Atopic disease associated with raised IgE levels has responded to zidovudine/HAART. Kaposi's varicelliform eruption has also been described in HIV-infected atopic individuals with concomitant HSV infection. Management of atopic dermatitis in HIV infection is similar to that in immunocompetent individuals.

Vasculitis

Extensive cutaneous leukocytoclastic vasculitis has been reported in HIV infection. It may be primary, in which case the HIV virus is the precipitating antigen, or secondary, in which drugs, infections

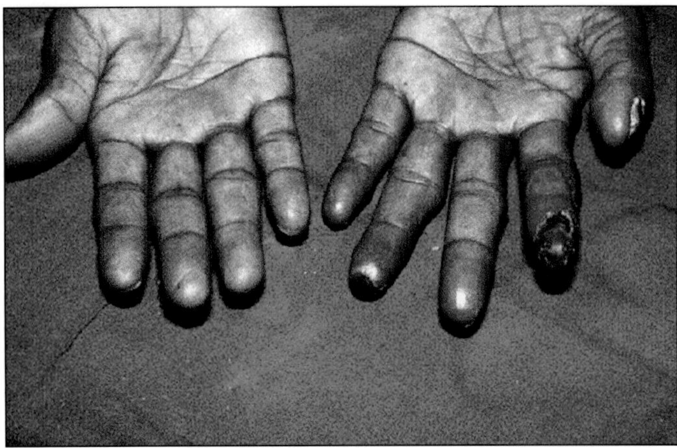

Figure 11.40 Immune complex vasculitis.

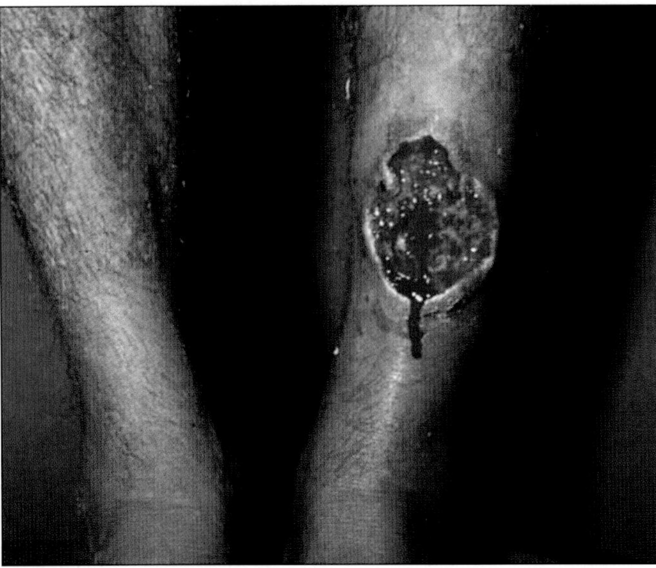

Figure 11.41 Vascular ulcer.

such as CMV, hepatitis B virus and parvovirus B19,[86] or autoimmune phenomena are the cause (Fig. 11.40). The eruption is polymorphic, and consists of petechiae, purpura, papules, pustules, bullae, and ulcers (Fig. 11.41).

Polyarteritis nodosa and erythema elevatum diutinum[87] have also been reported in HIV infection. Indinavir may also cause leukocytoclastic vasculitis.[88] Corticosteroids are the mainstay of treatment in most cases. Immunosuppressive agents such as cyclophosphamide, azathioprine, and cyclosporin, as well as immunoglobulin, are best avoided, but may be considered in unresponsive cases.

Urticaria

The eruption is a hypersensitivity reaction and presents as multiple, pruritic, erythematous, or pale, dome-shaped, evanescent papules or polycyclic plaques on the trunk and extremities. The eruption may be recurrent or persist for months. It may be poorly responsive to conventional therapies. Treatment consists of topical antipruritic medication such as menthol- or phenol-containing preparations, calamine and pramoxine. Systemic antihistamines, doxepin, and ultraviolet B can be used in refractory cases. Cold urticaria[89] has also been associated with HIV disease.

Erythroderma[90]

Exfoliative dermatitis/erythroderma in HIV disease is usually caused by an exacerbation of preexisting dermatoses such as atopic dermatitis, psoriasis vulgaris, photosensitivity dermatitis, the hypereosinophilic syndrome, coexisting HTLV-I infection, or cutaneous T-cell lymphoma. Drug hypersensitivity is also a major cause and should always be kept in mind. Treatment involves management of the primary dermatosis and supportive therapy such as maintenance of fluid/electrolyte balance and thermoregulation.

Metabolic

PORPHYRIA CUTANEA TARDA This is a rare condition, resulting from a decrease in hepatic uroporphyrinogen decarboxylase activity, with a consequent rise in metabolic precursors. Clinical presentation may occur before the diagnosis of HIV infection, or at any time in the course of the disease. The onset of skin involvement usually coincides with deterioration of immune function. The close temporal association between HIV infection and the onset of PCT suggests a cause-and-effect relation. Viral hepatitis (hepatitis B or C virus), alcohol intake, use of drugs such as estrogens or iron supplements, and altered estrogen metabolism also contribute to the process.

Clinically, photosensitivity is the principal symptom, along with facial hypertrichosis, generalized hyperpigmentation,[91] scarring, pseudosclerodermatous change, and milia formation. Lesions vary from skin-colored papules/plaques to fluid-filled vesicles and bullae that may erode and heal slowly.

Avoidance of ultraviolet light is essential and effective. Phlebotomy is effective, but undesirable in HIV-infected patients. Chloroquine and hydroxychloroquine are viable alternatives.

Idiopathic

PHOTOSENSITIVITY[92] Increased photosensitivity has been reported in patients with advanced HIV disease (Fig. 11.42). It may result in increased pigmentation, especially in black individuals, and may progress to erythroderma. Most likely, it represents a form of drug hypersensitivity and races with darker skin are disproportionately affected. Lichenoid photodermatitis has also been reported in HIV infection. Several photo-induced pathologic changes have also been described. Vin-Christian et al.[93] reported that patients with HIV were sensitive to ultraviolet B light and those most severely affected were sensitive to both ultraviolet B and light. It is speculated that an immune response to certain photoproducts may cause the generalized lesions described in these cases.

Treatment consists of discontinuation of the suspected offending medication, use of sunscreens, application of intermediate-strength topical corticosteroids, and possible photoexposure to graded intensities for the hardening of skin.

- **Hair disorders**: Numerous abnormalities of hair have been reported.
  - Diffuse alopecia affecting the scalp, in addition to telogen effluvium, is the most common abnormality observed. In some cases, an underlying inflammatory cell infiltrate has also been reported. Generalized alopecia has been reported in patients treated with indinavir.[93]

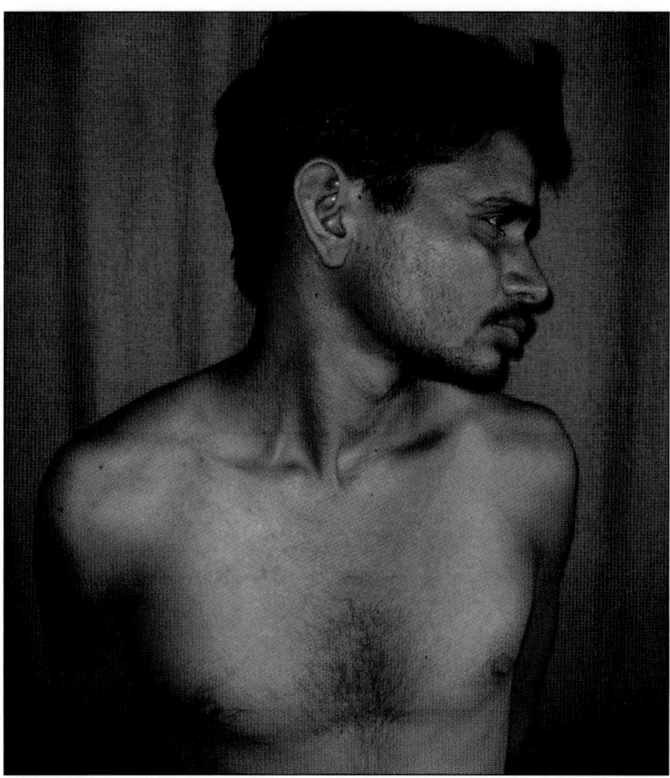

Figure 11.42 Photosensitivity.

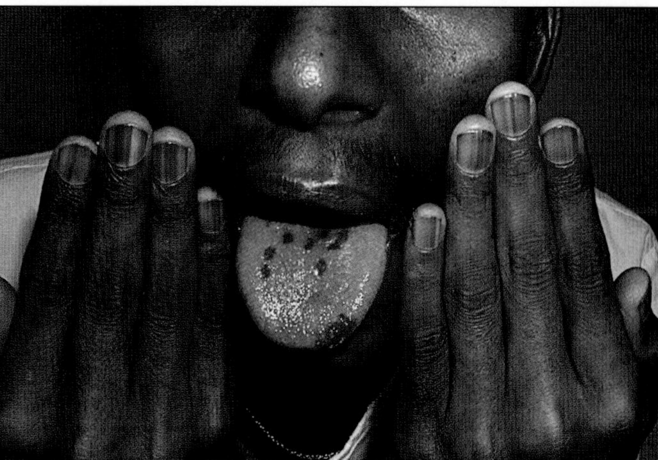

Figure 11.43 Addisonian pigmentation of tongue and nails.

- Hypertrichosis has also been reported in certain patients. It is also a feature of HIV-infected individuals with PCT.
- Loss of hair curls: a large number (~50%) of black patients may manifest this change.
- There may be sudden premature graying of hair.
- Elongation of the eyelashes: this may result from increased levels of prolactin, which may be a consequence of neurologic involvement.
- Necrotizing folliculitis:[94] this entity presents with erythematous papules on the trunk and extremities, resembling papulonecrotic tuberculid. Biopsy reveals fibrinoid necrosis in the hair follicle with a neutrophilic infiltrate. No organism can be isolated and biopsy findings suggest a vascular hypersensitivity reaction.

- **Nail changes**: Beau's lines, pallor of the nail beds, and pigmentation of the nail plates are the commonest abnormalities reported.
  - Longitudinal/transverse melanonychia[95] is common in HIV infection. As noted earlier, zidovudine/hydroxyurea administration is associated with diffuse grayish-brown or blue discoloration of the nail plate.
  - Yellow discoloration of the nails is reported among patients with AIDS and PCP pneumonia. The other features of the yellow-nail syndrome, such as the absence of cuticles and distinctive onychodystrophy, are not present. Many other conditions other than HIV infection, such as diabetes mellitus, drug reactions, and use of zidovudine and nail polish can cause yellow discoloration of the nail plate.
- **Pigmentation**:[96,97] Abnormalities of pigmentation are common in patients with HIV infection and AIDS.
  - Diffuse, blotchy hyperpigmentation of the face similar to melasma has been reported in patients with advanced AIDS. Patients usually also have associated xerosis.
  - Diffuse or localized pigmentation of the flexural skin as well as the oral mucosa, similar to Addisonian pigmentation, has also been reported (Fig. 11.43).
  - CMV adrenalitis may lead to an increased secretion of adrenocorticotropic hormone. This may produce an unusual "suntan" that has been observed in up to 56% of patients with CMV infection.
  - Postinflammatory hyper- or hypopigmentation is also common in addition to significant atrophic or hypertrophic scarring. This may lead to serious cosmetic disfigurement, especially if present on the visible sites. If dermatosis is chronic, the pigmentation may become persistent and progressive.
  - Zidovudine administration is associated with diffuse pigmentation of the nail beds with grayish-brown discoloration in longitudinal streaks, and similar macular pigmentation of the lip and buccal mucosa.
- **Interface dermatitis**: This is a histopathologic entity, characterized by vacuolization and necrosis of basal keratinocytes and an accompanying dense lymphohistiocytic infiltrate at the dermoepidermal junction. It is considered specific to HIV disease and clinically may manifest as a maculopapular eruption, erythroderma, blister formation, or erythema multiforme.
- **Granuloma annulare** (GA):[98] An increased incidence of GA has been reported in HIV infection. However, it is difficult to make a strong association because of its common nature. Both localized and generalized forms have been reported. Perforating GA and reactive perforating collagenosis (RPC) have also been reported. Evidence of severe cellular immune depletion, manifest as CD4 counts less than 100 cells/mm^3, has been cited. Some cases of generalized GA respond to therapy with AZT. Histology is similar to that in HIV-negative cases, showing focally altered collagen surrounded by a palisading granuloma. However, suppressor T cells are seen in AIDS-associated GA, in contrast to the helper T cell infiltrate in immunocompetent cases.
- **Calciphylaxis**: Widespread systemic and cutaneous calcification has been reported in HIV-infected patients with renal disease. Patients prone to develop this condition suffer from chronic renal insufficiency and secondary hyperparathyroidism, which sensitizes the tissues to a potential deposition of calcium. When any precipitating factor such as an infection/blood transfusion occurs, marked widespread precipitation of calcium and phosphorus salts occurs. Vessel wall involvement, with thrombosis and secondary ischemic necrosis, is also common. In the

skin, this manifests as widespread cutaneous infarcts that ulcerate and lead to fatal septicemia.

- **Hyperalgesic pseudothrombophlebitis**: This condition is characterized by induration, erythema, and edema of the calf, accompanied by severe pain and exquisite tenderness of the overlying skin. Investigations reveal no evidence of deep-vein thrombosis. A majority of these patients also have KS. Hence, whether this entity is a complication of KS or a drug reaction should be considered.
- **Secondary erythermalgia**[99]: Erythromelalgia or erythermalgia is characterized by the appearance of well-defined, tender, and erythematous plaques and nodules on the palms and soles, which worsen on exposure to warmth. An autoimmune cause has been proposed for the same.
- **Telangiectasia**: Widespread telangiectasia of the anterior chest, neck, and face has been reported. This usually manifests as reticulate erythematous areas on photoexposed areas of skin. The cause may be a circulating vascular proliferation factor, proposed since some patients have had coexisting KS. The clinical appearance is somewhat similar to the poikiloderma of Civatte.

Antiretroviral therapy[100]

There are two important enzymes in the life cycle of HIV, which are targeted by the antiretroviral agents. Reverse transcriptase (RT) is necessary for translating viral RNA into viral DNA before it can be incorporated into host DNA. The RT inhibitors act at this stage, and are of three classes:

1. Nucleoside reverse transcriptase inhibitors (NRTIs)
2. Non-nucleoside reverse transcriptase inhibitors (NNRTIs)
3. Nucleotide reverse transcriptase inhibitors (NtRTIs).

The second enzyme is the protease enzyme, which is necessary for maturation of the virions. Inhibitors of this enzyme are called protease inhibitors or PIs.

Based on these classes of drugs, there can be two kinds of approaches towards combination therapy for HIV:

1. Convergent approach: Using this approach a combination of drugs is given, which acts only on one enzyme (i.e., RT), for example, a combination of 3 NRTIs, or 2 NRTIs + 1 NNRTI.
2. Divergent therapy: This approach targets both enzymes, using a combination of 2 NRTIs + 1 PI.

Currently there are more than 20 antiretroviral drugs approved for use in HIV infection. Numerous combinations of three drugs can be designed using these drugs. The combination to use depends on numerous factors and treatment should be individualized according to patient characteristics.

The currently available antiretroviral drugs are given in Table 11.6.

There are three aims of antiretroviral therapy:

1. Prevention of vertical transmission of HIV
2. Clinical management of HIV-infected individuals
3. Post-exposure prophylaxis (PEP) for HCWs.

A dramatic decline in deaths and hospitalization due to AIDS has been reported from the developed world. This has been attributed to the widespread use of combination therapy using 2 NRTIs + 1 PI, popularly referred to as highly active antiretroviral therapy or HAART. Today, in the developed world, HIV infection is no longer considered as fatal, but as a chronic manageable illness.

The Multicenter AIDS Cohort Study (MACS), currently in progress at centers in Baltimore, Chicago, Pittsburgh, and Los Angeles, has demonstrated the importance of viral load and CD4 count as prognostic markers for disease progression.[101] Hence the goal of therapy is maximal and durable suppression of HIV replication. The durability of viral load suppression is greatest with triple-drug therapy, as opposed to monotherapy with zidovudine (introduced in 1987) or dual therapy (as practiced in 1994).

Table 11.6 Currently available antiretroviral drugs

Reverse transcriptase inhibitors	Protease inhibitors	Fusion inhibitor
Nucleoside analogs (NRTIs)	Saquinavir (SQV)	Enfuvirtide (T-20)
Zidovudine (AZT)	Indinavir (IDV)	
Stavudine (d4T)	Ritonavir (RTV)	
Lamivudine (3TC)	Nelfinavir (NFV)	
Zalcitabine (ddC)	Amprenavir	
Didanosine (ddI)	Fosamprenavir	
Abacavir (ABC)	Atazanavir	
Emtricitabine	Kaletra (Lopinavir + Ritonavir)	
Trizivir (AZT /3TC/ABC)	Ritonavir-boosted regimens (RTV + other PIs)	
Combivir (AZT/3TC)		
Non -nucleoside analogs (NNRTIs)		
Nevirapine (NVP)		
Delaverdine (DLV)		
Efavirenz (EFV)		
Nucleotide analogs (NtRTIs)		
Tenofovir		

Triple therapy helps prevent the development of resistance over a period of time and thus ensures a durable response.

If a patient is failing on his/her first regimen, it is important to switch his/her therapy to a second-line regimen early, as this is associated with a better response. Thus, when prescribing a first-line regimen, second- and third-line strategies should be formulated, keeping in mind the high-level cross-resistance seen amongst the same class of drugs. Indiscriminate use of the drugs will lead to minimal options for the future.

The most important considerations when choosing therapy include:

1. The potency of the combination
2. The adverse effect profile
3. The durability of response
4. Patient convenience
5. Cost and availability
6. Future options.

The most widely tested regimens are 2 NRTIs + 1 PI combinations; however, a large amount of evidence is available suggesting the efficacy of 2 NRTIs + 1 NNRTI. Current PI-based regimens lack a balance between potency, tolerability, and convenience. Although these regimens are potent, they are associated with long-term side-effects (such as lipodystrophy, insulin resistance, hypercholesterolemia, hypertriglyceridemia, and osteoporosis), and have a high pill burden and demanding feed/fasting requirements.

The current strategy is to individualize therapy on a case-by-case basis. Various factors, such as baseline viral load, CD4 count, side-effect profile, previous exposure to drugs, and concomitant rifampicin use influence this choice. When initiating HAART, all drugs should be started simultaneously rather than sequentially. If initial tolerance to the drugs is poor, then all drugs should be discontinued simultaneously, except for NNRTI-based regimens where the 2 NRTIs are discontinued a week after discontinuation of NNRTI; considering the long half-life of NNRTIs.

Finally, it is essential to choose a regimen which has some drugs that penetrate the blood–brain barrier and ensure activity inside the CNS. The CNS is an important reservoir of HIV infection where local replication occurs.

It is important to discuss the following points with the patient prior to initiating HAART:

1. Therapy is not curative.
2. It is lifelong and expensive.
3. Long-term adverse events may occur.
4. Drugs, particularly rifampicin, interact with PIs and NNRTIs; TB is the commonest manifestation of HIV/AIDS in the tropics.
5. Pill burden is high.
6. Adherence is critical, otherwise the virus develops resistance.

HAART should only be initiated when the patient has understood these issues and is ready for long-term treatment.

Clinical outcomes of HAART

1. Decreased incidence of OIs, due to improved CD4 counts. If improvement is consistent and durable, chemoprophylaxis for OIs can also be discontinued.
2. Clinical improvement of refractory infections: for example, PML or *Cryptosporidium* diarrhea, which do not have specific treatments, spontaneously improve.
3. Improved quality of life: There is a reduction in morbidity and hospitalization.
4. Immune reconstitution syndrome: This subject will be discussed later in the chapter.

When to initiate antiretroviral therapy

Current evidence suggests that it is possible to reconstitute the immune system even when HAART is initiated in advanced disease. As long as treatment is begun before the CD4 cell counts fall to very low levels or the viral load is not very high, response to HAART is satisfactory. Optimal viral suppression in all persons starting therapy is probably the most important criterion in determining the success of first-line regimens, rather than when therapy is started. Hence, rather than "Hit early, hit hard," it is more prudent to "Hit any time, but hit hard." HAART is also indicated during acute infection or within the first 6 months of seroconversion, although there are few trials which establish the efficacy of early treatment.

Structured treatment interruption (STI), structured intermittent treatment (SIT), and drug holidays were popular concepts, postulated to reduce the pill burden, increase patient compliance, and also allow multiplication of sensitive strains. However, development of drug resistance, a sudden spurt in the viral load, and decreased CD4 counts have demonstrated these concepts to be counterproductive. Thus, the achievement of a fine balance is paramount.

Adverse events[102]

Side-effects on HAART are so common that treatment involves achieving a fine balance between the benefits of durable HIV suppression and the risks of drug toxicities. More than 50% of patients stop or change therapy within a few weeks because of the side-effects. Patients need to be counseled in detail about these reactions, so that they can recognize them and consult the treating doctor in time.

The main cause of adverse effects in patients on HAART is mitochondrial toxicity. Inhibition of mitochondrial DNA polymerase gamma by NRTIs and NtRTIs results in impaired synthesis of mitochondrial enzymes that generate adenosine triphosphate by oxidative phosphorylation. The major toxicities, particularly over the medium and long term, include myopathy (AZT), neuropathy (d4T, ddI, ddC), hepatic steatosis and lactic acidosis (ddI, d4T, AZT) and possibly also peripheral lipoatrophy (all NRTIs, predominantly d4T), and pancreatitis (ddI). Some toxicities, such as peripheral neuropathy and renal tubular acidosis, may worsen for several weeks after drug stoppage (the "coasting" phenomenon). The various toxicities of HAART may be described as:

1. Gastrointestinal side-effects: These are the most common side-effects of almost all the antiretroviral drugs (NRTIs, NNRTIs, and PIs), and occur during the early stages of therapy. Typical symptoms include abdominal discomfort, loss of appetite, diarrhea, nausea, and vomiting. Heartburn, meteorism, and constipation may also occur. Nausea is common with AZT-containing regimens, while diarrhea occurs frequently with AZT, ddI, and all PIs, especially nelfinavir.

Management is mainly symptomatic and involves taking drugs with meals or with suitable food or an empty stomach if required. Antimotility drugs are also helpful, in addition to calcium (in nelfinavir diarrhea), oatbran tablets, and psyllium.

2. CNS effects: In up to 40% of patients, treatment with efavirenz leads to neurologic effects such as dizziness, insomnia, nightmares, and even mood changes. These are seen in the early days of therapy. Lorazepam and haloperidol are beneficial, but patient information is a must.
3. Peripheral nervous system effects: Peripheral neuropathy is caused mostly by the NRTIs, zalcitabine (ddC), didanosine (ddI), and stavudine (d4T). It presents as a bilaterally symmetrical distal sensorimotor paralysis; with pain and paresthesias in hands and feet after several months of therapy. Alcoholism, diabetes mellitus, and vitamin deficiency add to the risk. Treatment is difficult and mainly symptomatic. Alternative treatments such as acupuncture and electrical nerve stimulation have met with variable success. Tight shoes and prolonged standing are best avoided.
4. Renal effects: Nephrolithiasis develops in approximately 10% of patients on indinavir, as a result of indinavir crystals in urine. It may cause acute colic as well as lower abdominal/back pain, and also hematuria. Management is the same as in HIV-negative individuals. Prophylaxis involves a daily intake of at least 1.5 l of water, and avoidance of risk factors such as alcohol, quinolones, ampicillin, non-steroidal antiinflammatory drugs, and allopurinol.
5. Hepatotoxicity: It occurs in 2–18% of patients on HAART, independent of the drug class used. Severe hepatotoxicity and liver failure have been reported with nevirapine and the PIs, indinavir and ritonavir. Coinfection with hepatitis B or C virus may complicate the picture as a result of immune reconstitution, with increased cytolytic activity against the viruses. Frequent monitoring, such as liver function tests and ultrasonography of the abdomen or abdominal ultrasound, is necessary. Treatment is mainly supportive.
6. Hematologic effects:
   (a) Anemia/leukopenia/thrombocytopenia: 5–10% of patients on AZT develop anemia. Preexisting myelosuppression and chemotherapy are added risk factors. If severe, AZT should be stopped and blood transfusion may be indicated. Anemia is less frequent with stavudine, lamivudine, and abacavir. Leukopenia may occur with indinavir, abacavir, and tenofovir.
   (b) Increased bleeding episodes are noted in HIV patients with hemophilia A or B, on treatment with PIs. The joints, soft tissues, and rarely the brain or the GIT may be involved.
7. Allergy/hypersensitivity: Allergies occur approximately 100 times more frequently in HIV-infected individuals than in the general population. They occur with all the NNRTIs as well as with the NRTI, abacavir and the PI, amprenavir. A genetic predisposition (HLA B57) may be present in certain cases.
   (a) NNRTI allergy: This reversible systemic reaction presents as an erythematous, maculopapular, and confluent pruritic rash, distributed mainly over the trunk and arms. Fever may precede the rash and myalgia, fatigue, and mucosal ulceration may ensue. SJS and TEN are rare. Approximately 50% of reactions resolve despite continuation of drug. Antihistamines may be helpful.
   (b) Abacavir hypersensitivity reaction: The rash is discrete and fever is common. Also, patients suffer from malaise and gastrointestinal side-effects such as nausea, vomiting, diarrhea, and abdominal pain. Changes in blood cell counts and elevated liver enzymes are also common. The rash begins within the first 6 weeks of treatment. If the drug is discontinued, the hypersensitivity reaction is reversible. If a hypersensitivity reaction is not diagnosed and treated, death may occur. Rechallenge is contraindicated.
8. Pancreatic effects: Pancreatitis is caused mainly by didanosine, and occasionally by stavudine, lamivudine, and zalcitabine. Alcohol and pentamidine treatment are added risk factors. The symptoms and signs and management are the same as in pancreatitis of any other etiology.
9. Metabolic effects:
   (a) Lactic acidosis: This occurs most frequently with stavudine and didanosine. Obesity, female sex, and pregnancy are risk factors. Clinical presentation is non-specific, with fatigue, nausea, and vomiting, weight loss, and dyspnea. In such patients, serum lactate levels are monitored. Treatment with various drugs has met with limited success. Vitamin B complex, coenzyme Q10, vitamin C, and L-carnitine have been tried, alone and in combination. Normalization of lactate levels takes an average of at least 8 weeks after discontinuation of therapy.
   (b) Hyperglycemia and diabetes mellitus: The mechanism is probably a treatment-related impairment of glucose transport, and/or influence on intracellular phosphorylation of glucose. Hyperglycemia occurs on PI treatment, especially indinavir and less frequently with NRTIs. Risk factors include old age, obesity, and altered lipid levels. Blood glucose levels decrease once therapy has been discontinued.
   (c) Lipodystrophy/dyslipidemia: HIV-related lipodystrophy is a terminology used to describe the abnormal physical and metabolic changes in individuals taking HAART. Abnormal physical changes include lipohypertrophy (dorsocervical fat enlargement, central visceral obesity, breast enlargement) and lipoatrophy (fat wasting in arms, legs, face, buttocks) (Figs 11.44 and 11.45). Abnormal metabolic changes include those due to altered lipid metabolism (increased triglycerides, total cholesterol, and low-density lipoprotein cholesterol) and altered glucose metabolism (insulin resistance, impaired glucose tolerance, and diabetes mellitus). The cause of this syndrome is multifactorial. The most appropriate management of lipodystrophy has not yet been determined.
10. Bone changes:
   (a) Avascular necrosis: This occurs in approximately 0.4% of HIV patients. An unsubstantiated association with PIs has been postulated. Risk factors are alcoholism, hyperlipidemia, steroid treatment, hypercoagulability, hemoglobinopathy, trauma, nicotine abuse, and chronic pancreatitis. The most common site is the femoral head, followed by the head of the humerus. Patients complain

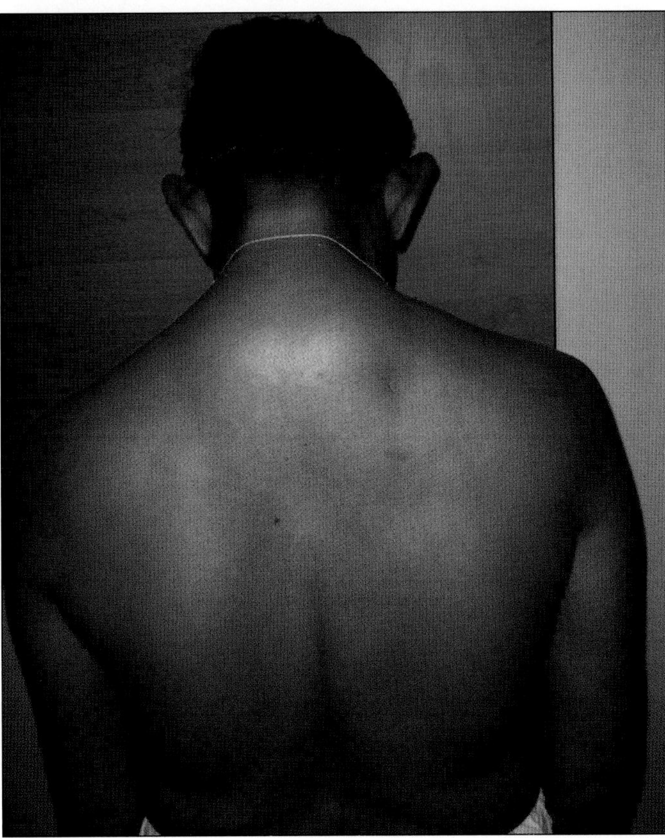

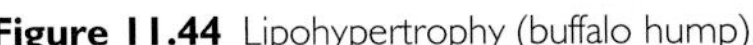
Figure 11.44 Lipohypertrophy (buffalo hump).

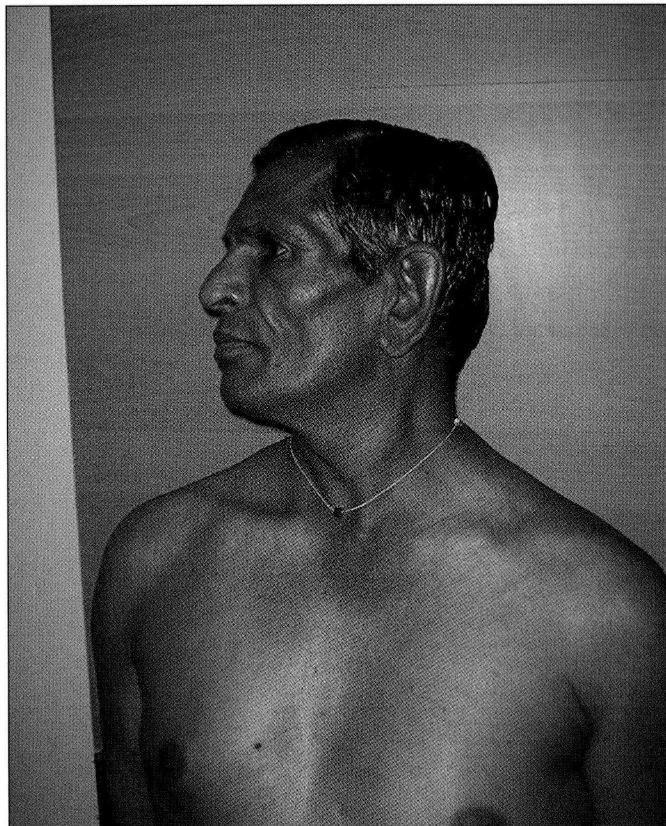

Figure 11.45 Lipoatrophy of the face.

of pain on weight-bearing, which worsens over time. Severe bone pain and reduced mobility may occur. Treatment depends on disease localization and severity. Surgical decompression and osteotomy or a total endoprosthesis may be necessary. Non-steroidal antiinflammatory drugs and physiotherapy are recommended for the pain.

(b) Osteopenia/osteoporosis: HIV-infected individuals have a lower bone density than uninfected individuals. Other factors, such as malnutrition, diminished fat tissue, steroid treatment, immobilization, and treatment with PIs and NRTIs are also implicated. Usually asymptomatic, the effects are mainly seen in the vertebrae, hips, and lower arms. Vitamin D supplements (1000 IE daily) and calcium-rich diet/supplements with a dose of 1200 mg/day are recommended. Exercise is essential, and alcohol and nicotine abuse should be stopped. In osteoporosis, aminobiphosphonates may be added.

Drug interactions

Induction of the cytochrome P450 coenzymes by HAART may lead to interaction between rifampicin and PIs or NNRTIs. Usually, an initial intensive phase of TB therapy is completed and then HAART is added with an ethambutol-based antituberculous regimen for the maintenance phase. Alternatively efavirenz, ritonavir, ritonavir/ saquinavir-based regimens can be used along with rifampicin. Interactions with anticonvulsants, antipsychotics, and other drugs should also be considered.

Newer and investigational drugs

- NRTIs: amdoxovir is a guanine analog.
- NNRTIs: capravirine, emivirine, TMC 125, and DPC 083 are in various stages of development.
- PIs: tipranavir and mozenavir are being studied.
- Fusion and entry inhibitors: T-1249, which binds to viral gp41, shows promise.
- Coreceptor antagonists: SCH-C and Pro-140 (CCR5) and AMD-3100 and T-22 (CXCR4) are under investigation.

Immune reconstitution syndrome

This is also called "immune restoration syndrome" or reversal phenomenon. It occurs following HAART. The incubation period for its development varies. It could involve any system of the body and is difficult to recognize. The various clinical manifestations are herpes zoster, reactivation of leprosy, tuberculosis (lymphadenopathy, pneumonitic patch, tuberculoma of brain or liver), PCP, hepatitis reactivation, CMV retinitis, fever, and cryptococcosis. The management of immune reconstitution syndrome-related illnesses is challenging.

Summary

The epidemic of HIV infection has hit every corner of the world but has had devastating consequences on non-industrialized countries which are generally located in tropical areas. Every organ system is affected by HIV, but cutaneous manifestations are seen in over 90% of infected persons. These manifestations, however, may differ both qualitatively and quantitatively in tropical and temperate countries depending on the availability of HAART, and the type of OIs in the area. Whereas HAART has markedly reduced morbidity and mortality from HIV in industrialized counties, 99% of HIV-positive persons in the world cannot afford the cost of these medications (e.g., US$ 20 000/year). Most importantly, HAART does not provide a cure for HIV. Therefore, public health measures must be emphasized to reduce the transmission of HIV. It is hoped that in the future a vaccine will become available which can prevent HIV infection and that it will be used in conjunction with these public health interventions.

References

1. Joint United Nations programme on HIV/AIDS (UNAIDS). Report on the global HIV/AIDS epidemic. Geneva: WHO; 2003.
2. Fauci AS, Lane HC. Human immunodeficiency virus (HIV) disease. In: Braunwald E, Fauci AS, Kasper DL, eds. Harrison's principles of internal medicine, 15th edn. New York: McGraw-Hill; 2001:1852–1913.
3. Fauci AS. Host factors and the pathogenesis of HIV-induced disease. Nature 1996; 384:529.
4. Vittinghoff E, Douglas J, Judson F et al. Per-contact risk of human immunodeficiency virus transmission between male sexual partners. Am J Epidemiol 1999; 150:306.
5. Padian NS, Shiboski SC, Glass SO et al. Heterosexual transmission of human immunodeficiency virus (HIV) in northern California: results from a ten-year study. Am J Epidemiol 1997; 146:350.
6. Centers for Disease Control and Prevention. HIV/AIDS surveillance report, 1999; 11(No. 2):1. Atlanta, GA: US Department of Health and Human Services, Public Health Service, National Center for HIV, STD and TB prevention; 2000.
7. Sewankambo N, Gray RH, Wawer MJ et al. HIV-1 infection associated with abnormal vaginal flora morphology and bacterial vaginosis. Lancet 1997; 350:546.
8. Halperin DT, Bailey RC. Male circumcision and HIV infection: 10 years and counting. Lancet 1999; 354:1813.
9. Centers for Disease Control and Prevention. Public Health Service guidelines for the management of health-care worker exposures to HIV and recommendations for postexposure prophylaxis. MMWR 1998; 47(RR-7):1.
10. Landesman SH, Kalish LA, Burns DN et al. Obstetrical factors and the transmission of human immunodeficiency virus type 1 from mother to child. N Engl J Med 1996; 334:1617.
11. Garcia PM, Kalish LA, Pitt J et al. Maternal level of plasma human immunodeficiency virus type 1 RNA and the risk of perinatal transmission. N Engl J Med 1999; 341:394.
12. Miotti PG, Taha TE, Kumwenda NI et al. HIV transmission through breast-feeding: a study in Malawi. JAMA 1999; 212:744.
13. Simon F, Mauclere P, Roques P et al. Identification of a new human immunodeficiency virus type distinct from group M and group O. Nat Med 1998; 4:1032.
14. Clavel F, Guetard D. Brun-Vezinet F et al. Isolation of a new human retrovirus from West African patients with AIDS. Science 1986 ; 233:343–346.
15. Brun-Vezinet F, Rey MA, Katlama C et al. Lymphadenopathy associated virus type 2 in AIDS and AIDS-related complex: clinical and virological features in four patients. Lancet 1987; 1:128–132.
16. Guyader M, Emerman M, Sonigo P et al. Genome organization and transactivation of the human immunodeficiency virus type 2. Nature 1987; 326:662–669.
17. Gao F, Yue L, Robertson DL et al. Genetic diversity of human immunodeficiency virus type 2: evidence for distinct sequence subtypes with differences in virus biology. J Virol 1994; 68:7433–7447.
18. Chen Z, Luckay A, Sodora DL et al. Human immunodeficiency virus type 2 (HIV-2) seroprevalence and characterization of a distinct HIV-2 genetic subtype from the natural range of simian immunodeficiency virus infected sooty mangabeys. J Virol 1997; 71:3953–3960.
19. Schim van der Loeff MF, Aaby P. Towards a better understanding of the epidemiology of HIV-2. AIDS 1999; 13 (suppl. a):S69–S84.
20. De Cock KM, Adjorlolo G, Ekpini E et al. Epidemiology and transmission of HIV-2. Why there is no HIV-2 pandemic. JAMA 1993; 270:2083–2086.
21. Kanki PJ, De Cock KM. Epidemiology and natural history of HIV-2. AIDS 1994; 8:S85–S93.
22. Essex M, Kanki PJ, Marlink R et al. Antigenic characterization of the human immunodeficiency viruses. J Am Acad Dermatol 1990; 22:1206–1210.
23. Fauci AS, Panteleo G, Stanley S et al. Immunopathogenic mechanisms of HIV infection. Ann Intern Med 1996; 124:654.
24. Chun TW, Fauci AS. Latent reservoirs of HIV: obstacles to the eradication of the virus. Proc Natl Acad Sci USA 1999; 96:10958.
25. Perelson AS, Neumann U, Markowitz M et al. HIV-1 dynamics in vivo: virion clearance rate, infected cell life span, and viral generation time. Science 1996; 271:1582.
26. Kandil H, Stebbing J, Gazzard B et al. Innate and adaptive immunological insights into HIV pathogenesis. Intl J STD AIDS 2003; 14:652–655.
27. Cohen OJ. The immunology of human immunodeficiency virus infection. In: Mandell GL, Bennett JE, Dolin R, eds. Principles and practice of infectious diseases, 5th edn. Philadelphia, PA: Churchill Livingstone; 2000:1374–1397.
28. Kahn JO, Walker BD. Acute human immunodeficiency virus type 1 infection. N Engl J Med 1998; 339:33.
29. Maniar JK. Clinical presentation of HIV infection. In: Sharma VK, ed. Sexually transmitted diseases and AIDS. New Delhi, India: Viva Books; 2003:77–86.
30. Centers for Disease Control and Prevention. 1993 Revised classification for HIV infection and expanded AIDS surveillance case definition for adolescents and adults. MMWR 1992 ; 42(RR-17).
31. Mota-Miranda A, Gomes MH, Serrao MR et al. Long term nonprogressive HIV-2 infection. XI International Conference on AIDS, Vancouver, 1996 (abstract We.C.3469).

32. Greeberg AE, Kadio A, Grant AD et al. Clinical manifestations of advanced HIV disease using hospital surveillance, clinical and autopsy data in Abidjan, Cote d'Ivoire. 12th World AIDS Conference Geneva, 1998 (abstract 12146). Marathon Multimedia.
33. Ariyoshi K, Schim van der Loeff M, Cook P et al. Kaposi's sarcoma in The Gambia, West Africa is less frequent in human immunodeficiency virus type 2 than in human immunodeficiency virus type 1 infection despite a high prevalence of human herpes virus 8. J Hum Virol 1998; 1:193–199.
34. Whittle H, Morris J, Todd J et al. HIV-2 infected patients survive longer than HIV-1 infected patients. AIDS 1994; 8:1617–1620.
35. Whittle H, Egboga A, Todd J et al. Immunological responses of Gambians in relation to clinical stage of HIV-2 disease. Clin Exp Immunol 1993; 93:45–50.
36. Jaffar S, Wilkins A, Ngom PT et al. Rate of decline of percentage CD4+ cells is faster in HIV-1 than in HIV-2 infection. J AIDS Hum Retroviral 1997; 16:327–332.
37. Cao Y, Qin L, Zhang L et al. Virologic and immunologic characterization of long-term survivors of human immunodeficiency virus type-1 infection. N Engl J Med 1995; 332:201.
38. Kirchhoff F, Greenbough TC, Brettler DB et al. Brief report: absence of intact *nef* sequences in a long-term survivor with nonprogressive HIV-1 infection. N Engl J Med 1995; 332:228.
39. Balotta C, Bagnarellli P, Corvasce S et al. Identification of two distinct subsets of long-term nonprogressors with divergent viral activity by stromal-derived factor-1 chemokine gene polymorphism analysis. J Infect Dis 1999; 180:285.
40. Carrington M, Nelson GW, Martin MP et al. HLA and HIV-1: heterozygote advantage and B*35-cw*04 disadvantage. Science 1999; 283:1.
41. Faure S, Meyer L, Costagliola D et al. Rapid progression to AIDS in HIV+ individuals with a structural variant of the chemokine receptor CX3CR1. Science 2000; 287:2274.
42. Kaslow RA, Carrington M, Apple R et al. Influence of combinations of human major histocompatibility complex genes on the course of HIV-1 infection. Nat Med 1996; 2:405.
43. Powderley WG. Acute HIV infection. In: Powderley WG, ed. Manual of HIV therapeutics, 2nd edn. Philadelphia, PA: Lippincott/Williams and Wilkins; 2001:6–13.
44. Kassutto S, Sax PE. HIV and syphilis coinfection: trends and interactions. AIDS Clin Care 2003; 15:9–15.
45. Myskowski PL, Straus DJ, Safai B. Lymphoma and other HIV-associated malignancies. J Am Acad Dermatol 1990; 22:1253–1260.
46. Goedert JJ, Cote TR, Virgo P et al. Spectrum of AIDS-associated malignant disorders. Lancet 1998; 351:1833.
47. Cockerell CJ, Friedman-Kien AE. Cutaneous signs of HIV infection. In: Broder S, Merigan TC Jr, Bolognesi D, eds. Textbook of AIDS medicine. Baltimore, MD: Williams and Wilkins; 1994:507–524.
48. Safai B. Dermatologic complications of HIV infection. In: DeVita VT Jr, Hellman S, Rosenberg SA, eds. AIDS: biology, diagnosis, treatment and prevention, 4th edn. Philadelphia, PA: Lippincott-Raven; 1997:393–400.
49. Johnson RA. Cutaneous manifestations of human immunodeficiency virus disease. In: Fitzpatrick TB, Eisen AZ, Wolff K et al., eds. Dermatology in internal medicine, 6th edn. New York: McGraw Hill, 2003:2138–2150.
50. Powderley WG. Dermatologic manifestations of human immunodeficiency virus infection. In: Powderley WG, ed. Manual of HIV therapeutics, 2nd edn. Philadelphia, PA: Lippincott/Williams and Wilkins; 2001:107–112.
51. Calikoglu E, Zalewska A. Cutaneous manifestations of HIV disease. In: Shear N, Butler DF, Joyce Rico M, eds. eMedicine. 2003. Available online at: www.eMedicine.com (accessed August 16, 2004).
52. Antman K, Chang Y. Kaposi's sarcoma. N Engl J Med 2000; 342:1027.
53. D'Ablashi L, Chatlynne H, Cooper D et al. Seroprevalence of human herpesvirus-8 (HHV-8) in countries of Southeast Asia compared to the USA, the Caribbean and Africa. Br J Cancer 1999; 81:893–897.
54. Dedicoat M, Newton R. Review of the distribution of Kaposi's sarcoma-associated herpesvirus (KSHV) in Africa in relation to the incidence of Kaposi's sarcoma. Br J Cancer 2003; 88:1–3.
55. Maniar JK. Health care systems in transition III. India, Part II. The current status of HIV-AIDS in India. J Public Health Med 2002; 22:33–37.
56. Aboulafia DM. Malignant melanoma in an HIV-infected man: a case report and literature review. Cancer Invest 1998; 16:217–224.
57. Severson JL, Tyring SK. Relation between herpes simplex viruses and human immunodeficiency virus infections. Arch Dermatol 1999; 135:1393–1397.
58. Gulick RM, Heath-Chiozzi M, Crumpacker CS. Varicella-zoster virus disease in patients with human immunodeficiency virus infection. Arch Dermatol 1990; 126:1086–1088.
59. Resnick L, Herbst JS, Raab-Traub N. Oral hairy leukoplakia. J Am Acad Dermatol 1990; 22:1278–1282.
60. Nico MM, Cymbalista NC, Hurtado YC et al. Perianal cytomegalovirus ulcer in an HIV infected patient: case report and review of literature. J Dermatol 2000; 27:99–105.
61. Davis MD, Gostout BS, McGovern RM et al. Large plantar wart caused by human papillomavirus-66 and resolution by topical cidofovir therapy. J Am Acad Dermatol 2000; 43:340–343.
62. Barzegar C, Paul C, Saiag P et al. Epidermodysplasia verruciformis-like eruption complicating human immunodeficiency virus infection. Br J Dermatol 1998; 139:122–127.
63. Kolokotronis A, Antoniades D, Katsoulidis E et al. Facial and perioral molluscum contagiosum as a manifestation of HIV infection. Aust Dent J 2000; 45:49–52.
64. Itin PH, Gilli L. Molluscum contagiosum mimicking sebaceous nevus of Jadassohn, ecthyma and giant condylomata acuminata in HIV-infected patients. Dermatology 1994; 189:396–398.
65. Cockerell CJ. Cutaneous manifestations of HIV infection other than Kaposi's sarcoma: clinical and histologic aspects. J Am Acad Dermatol 1990; 22:1260–1269.
66. Calikoglu E, Soravia-Dunand VA, Perriard J et al. Acute genitocrural intertrigo: a sign of primary human immunodeficiency virus type 1 infection. Dermatology 2001; 203:171–173.

67. Bournerias I, De Chauvin MF, Datry A et al. Unusual *Microsporum canis* infections in adult HIV patients. J Am Acad Dermatol 1996; 35:808–810.
68. Ramdial P, Mosam A, Dlova NC. Disseminated cutaneous histoplasmosis in patients infected with human immunodeficiency virus. J Cutan Pathol 2002; 29:215–225.
69. Lipstein-Kresch E, Isenberg HD, Singer C et al. Disseminated *Sporothrix schenckii* infection with arthritis in a patient with acquired immunodeficiency syndrome. J Rheumatol 1985; 12:805–808.
70. Stanford D, Boyle M, Gillespie R. Human immunodeficiency virus-related primary cutaneous aspergillosis. Australas J Dermatol 2000; 41:112–116.
71. Plettenberg A, van Dyk U, Stoehr A et al. Increased risk for opportunistic infections during chemotherapy in HIV-infected patients with Kaposi's sarcoma. Dermatology 1997; 194:234–237.
72. Arianayagam AV, Ash S, Jones RR. Lichen scrofulosorum in a patient with AIDS. Clin Exp Dermatol 1994; 19:74–76.
73. Kayal JD, McCall CO. Sporotrichoid cutaneous *Mycobacterium avium* complex infection. J Am Acad Dermatol 2002; 47 (suppl.):S249–S250.
74. Sekar B, Jayasheela M, Chattopadhya D et al. Prevalence of HIV infection and high-risk characteristics among leprosy patients of south India; a case-control study. Int J Lepr Other Mycobact Dis (US) 1994; 62:527–531.
75. Paredes R, Munoz J, Diaz I et al. Leishmaniasis in HIV infection. J Postgrad Med 2003; 49:39–49.
76. Torno MS Jr, Babapour R, Gurevitch A et al. Cutaneous acanthamoebiasis in AIDS. J Am Acad Dermatol 2000; 42:351–354.
77. Sadick NS, McNutt NS, Kaplan MH. Papulosquamous dermatoses of AIDS. J Am Acad Dermatol 1990; 22:1270–1277.
78. Gonzalez-Lopez A, Velasco E, Pozo T et al. HIV-associated pityriasis rubra pilaris responsive to triple antiretroviral therapy. Br J Dermatol 1999; 140:931–934.
79. Kaplan MH, Sadick NS, McNutt NS et al. Acquired ichthyosis in concomitant HIV-1 and HTLV-II infection: a new association with intravenous drug abuse. J Am Acad Dermatol 1993; 29:701–708.
80. Misago N, Narisawa Y, Matsubara S et al. HIV-associated eosinophilic pustular folliculitis: successful treatment of a Japanese patient with UVB phototherapy. J Dermatol 1998; 25:178–184.
81. Boonchai W, Laohasrisakul R, Manonukul J et al. Pruritic papular eruption in HIV seropositive patients: a cutaneous marker for immunosuppression. Int J Dermatol 1999; 38:348–350.
82. Berman B, Flores F, Burke G 3rd. Efficacy of pentoxifylline in the treatment of pruritic papular eruption of HIV-infected persons. J Am Acad Dermatol 1998; 38:955–959.
83. Duvic M, Reisman M, Finley V et al. Glucan-induced keratoderma in acquired immunodeficiency syndrome. Arch Dermatol 1987; 123:751–756.
84. Jacobson JM, Greenspan JS, Spritzler J et al. Thalidomide for the treatment of oral aphthous ulcers in patients with human immunodeficiency virus infection. N Engl J Med 1997; 336:1487.
85. Sekigawa I, Ogasawara H, Kaneko H et al. Retroviruses and autoimmunity. Intern Med 2001; 40:80–86.
86. Martinelli C, Azzi A, Buffini G et al. Cutaneous vasculitis due to human parvovirus B19 in an HIV-infected patient: report of a case. AIDS 1997; 11:1891–1893.
87. Muratori S, Carrera C, Gorani A et al. Erythema elevatum diutinum and HIV infection: a report of five cases. Br J Dermatol 1999; 141:335–338.
88. Rachline A, Lariven S, Descamps V et al. Leucocytoclastic vasculitis and indinavir. Br J Dermatol 2000; 143:1112–1113.
89. Yu RC, Evans B, Cream JJ. Cold urticaria, raised IgE and HIV infection. J R Soc Med 88(5):294P-295P, 1995.
90. Herman LE, Kurban AK. Erythroderma as a manifestation of the AIDS-related complex. J Am Acad Dermatol 1987; 17:507–508.
91. Pascual C, Garcia-Patos V, Bartralot R et al. Cutaneous pigmentation, only manifestation of porphyria cutanea tarda in a HIV-1 positive patient. Ann Dermatol Venereol 1996; 123:262–264.
92. Vin-Christian K, Epstein JH, Maurer TA et al. Photosensitivity in HIV-infected individuals. J Dermatol 2000; 27:361–369.
93. Harry TC, Matthews M, Salvary I. Indinavir use: associated reversible hair loss and mood disturbance. Int J STD AIDS 2000; 11:474–476.
94. Barclow RJ, Schulz EJ. Necrotizing folliculitis in AIDS-related complex. Br J Dermatol 1987; 116:581–584.
95. Hira SK, Wadhawan D, Kamanga J et al. Cutaneous manifestations of human immunodeficiency virus in Lusaka, Zambia. J Am Acad Dermatol 1988; 19:451–457.
96. Granel F, Truchetet F, Grandidier M. Diffuse pigmentation (nail, mouth and skin) associated with HIV infection. Ann Dermatol Venereol 1997; 124:460–462.
97. Molinero J, Vilata JJ, Nagore E et al. Ashy dermatosis in an HIV antibody-positive patient. Acta Dermatol Venereol 2000; 80:78–79.
98. Toro JR, Chu P, Yen TS et al. Granuloma annulare and human immunodeficiency virus infection. Arch Dermatol 1999; 135:1341–1346.
99. Dolan CK, Hall MA, Turlansky GW. Secondary erythermalgia in an HIV-1-positive patient. AIDS Read 2003; 13:91–93.
100. Hoffmann C. Overview of antiretroviral drugs. In: Hoffmann C, Kamps BS, eds. HIV medicine 2003. Paris: Flying Publisher; 2003:59–116.
101. Mellors JW, Munoz A, Giorgi JV et al. Plasma viral load and CD4+ lymphocytes as prognostic markers in HIV-1 infection. Ann Intern Med 1997; 126:946–954.
102. Carr A, Cooper DA. Adverse effects of antiretroviral therapy. Lancet 2000; 356:1423–1430.

Chapter 12

Hemorrhagic fevers

- **Old-World hemorrhagic fevers** ▪ *Omar Lupi and Stephen K. Tyring*
- **New-World hemorrhagic fevers** ▪ *Omar Lupi and Ivan Semenovitch*
- **Dengue** ▪ *Omar Lupi, Gustavo Kouri and Maria G. Guzman*
- **Yellow fever** ▪ *Omar Lupi and Leticia Spinelli*

Introduction

Viruses are important pathogens in the tropical areas, most of them producing several mucocutaneous manifestations, especially among the tropical hemorrhagic fevers. More than any other kind of pathogen, viruses have a greater possibility for wide spread since they have a higher degree of mutations than bacteria, can easily cross species barriers, and infect both humans and animals in habitats with a great biodiversity. The tropical habitats have also been submitted to major ecological changes in the last few decades, exposing these viruses to direct contact with humans, and transforming new emergent viruses such as Ebola virus fever (filoviruses), hemorrhagic fevers due to arenaviruses, and hantavirus infections – all major threats to public health.

The dissemination of some vectors, especially mosquitoes with a broad ecological range, due to the collapse of eradication programs in many countries or even because of a population increase and ecological modifications, has led to the wide spread of dengue and yellow fever to large portions of the world. Viruses previously restricted to some geographic areas, such as Rift Valley fever, Crimean–Congo hemorrhagic fever, and West Nile fever, are now affecting new countries and populations. Dermatological lesions are present in all these diseases and can lead to an early diagnosis, controlling the dissemination of the illness and helping to prevent possible outbreaks.

Old-World hemorrhagic fevers

Omar Lupi and Stephen K. Tyring

Synonyms: Lassa fever: arenaviruses
hemorrhagic fever with renal syndrome (HFRS): hantaviruses
Ebola and Marburg fever: filoviruses
Rift Valley fever (RVF) and Crimean–Congo hemorrhagic fever (CCHF): bunyaviruses

Key features:

- These are systemic viral diseases caused mainly by arenaviruses and hantaviruses and have a worldwide distribution
- Hemorrhagic fevers caused by bunyaviruses and filoviruses are mainly restricted to tropical parts of Africa and Asia
- Hantavirus/arenavirus is shed in the infected rodent's saliva, urine, and feces. No vector or host has been established for filoviruses
- Old-World hemorrhagic fevers are characterized by severe hemorrhagic fever with purpura, gingival bleeding, and disseminated non-palpable petechiae on the skin
- Hantaviruses may cause HFRS with a characteristic facial flushing, and usually a petechial rash. The hemorrhagic manifestations also include skin hemorrhages with petechiae, purpura, ecchymoses, gingival and nasal bleeding, and hematuria

Introduction

Tropical hemorrhagic viruses with dermatological manifestations are common in many tropical countries from the Old World. In the past, most of these viruses were restricted to very specific geographic areas where the viruses, their hosts and vectors coevolved for long periods of time. There are, however, some situations in which the tropical virus is disseminated to areas that were previously free from the pathogen. A common situation involves the accidental contamination of a traveler, tourist, or worker who comes into contact with a tropical virus and spreads the disease.[1] A contaminated animal can also act as a vector of the disease to new areas or countries.[2] Rodents, common mammals in the Old World, with a close phylogenetic relation with humans and a long history of geographical contact (Africa and Asia), are very efficient vectors for this kind of dissemination, as a study of arenavirus and hantavirus infection easily shows.

Another common theme in the story of these tropical viruses is that humans enter new areas where viruses are circulating, rodents carrying the viruses enter ecologically disturbed areas to carry infection to humans, and viruses may then spread to larger geographical areas.[1] This is the main pattern of distribution in filovirus, hantavirus, and arenavirus infections, some of the most deadly causes of hemorrhagic fevers.

Arenaviruses

Arenaviruses are generally associated with benign infection in restricted rodent hosts but cause a severe, often lethal, disseminated disease in humans.[2] These viruses are pleomorphic enveloped RNA viruses with cellular ribosomes incorporated into the virion.[1] Most of the general characteristics and properties of the Arenaviridae family are discussed in depth in the section on New-World hemorrhagic fevers, below, as the South American complex is associated with most cases of arenavirus infection. However, it is important to discuss two important arenaviruses from the Old World: Lassa virus and lymphocytic choriomeningitis (LCM) virus.

The arenavirus genome consists of two distinct single-stranded viral RNA species, called L and S[2]. The arenaviruses have ambisense genomes: the 3′ half is antisense, whereas the 5′ half is positive-sense.[3] The envelope that surrounds the virion contains two major glycoprotein (GP) components (GP1, GP2) that appear as spikelike or clublike projections with variable spacing along the virus envelope.[1,2]

History and epidemiology

In 1934, the prototypic arenavirus, LCM virus, was first isolated during serial monkey passage of human material that was obtained from a fatal infection in the first documented epidemic of St. Louis encephalitis, a totally unrelated virus.[1] LCM virus was the first recognized cause of aseptic meningitis in humans.[1] Arenaviruses have been divided into two groups based on whether the virus is found in the Old World (eastern hemisphere) or the New World (western hemisphere).[1,2] Of the 15 arenaviruses known to infect animals, all living in tropical regions, two are related to human infection in the Old World and only Lassa virus is related to dermatological findings.[1] LCM virus is the only arenavirus to exist in both areas but it is classified as an Old World virus[1,2] (Table 12.1).

LCM and Lassa viruses are associated with Old-World rats and mice (family Muridae, subfamily Murinae)[3]. The restricted areas affected by Lassa virus in West Africa may reflect the geographic distribution of their natural host.[4] The endemic regions are near forests and still have a low population density.[1,2] The progressive occupation of previous wild areas will expose humans to new cases of Lassa fever. In recent years, significant numbers of LCM infections have been attributed to silently infected pet hamsters and field mice (*Mus musculus*) in biomedical laboratory colonies, explaining the different distribution of LCM virus.[2]

Pathogenesis and etiology

Knowledge of the multiplication of arenaviruses is fragmentary. Most of what is known comes from studies with LCM virus.[2] LCM virus replicates in a wide variety of cell types.[1,2] Although the virus receptor has not been identified, it must be highly conserved and widely distributed. Transcription of the genome and replication are confined to the cytoplasm. The small RNA in the virion encodes in the negative sense a nucleoprotein, and in the positive or message sense a precursor GP, which is cleaved into two virion GPs (GP1 and GP2).[1,5] The large RNA in the virion encodes in the negative sense an RNA-dependent RNA polymerase, and in the positive sense a zinc-binding protein which binds to the ribonucleoprotein complex.[1,5] The virus buds from the plasma membrane, incorporating host lipids into the virus membrane.[1,6]

The onset of the hemorrhagic fevers caused by Lassa virus may be insidious: the disease may present 7–14 days after infection simply as pyrexia, headache, sore throat, and myalgia.[1] Lassa virus can be recovered from the blood and serum for up to 3 weeks after onset of the infection, and from the urine for up to 5 weeks.[1] Hemorrhagic phenomena, heralded by unremitting high fever, can begin after day 5 of illness and are followed by dehydration and hemoconcentration, shock, hemorrhagic manifestations, and cardiovascular collapse.[7]

Compared with the dramatic clinical course and mortality, the gross pathology is unimpressive and of little help in constructing a pathogenetic scheme.[7] Complete autopsies have not been performed on patients with Lassa fever;[6] however, autopsies performed on patients with Argentine hemorrhagic fever show a lack of deposited immunoglobulin and complement component C3 in the kidneys and small blood vessels.[7] Mediators released from infected cells have a potential role in the pathogenesis of dysfunction of some target organs.[7] Although LCM virus can produce severe human disease, characterized by prominent neurologic manifestations, pathologic lesions have not been studied extensively.[6] However, in the mouse model the immune response against LCM virus (specifically in the T-cell compartment) is central to the development of fatal neurologic disease.[7] Furthermore, mice infected with a lethal dose of this virus can invariably be saved by treatment with antibody to interferon-α/β, raising the possibility that endogenous interferon-α/β enhances the immunopathology.[2,6,7]

Antibodies develop following overt human infection with arenaviruses and are detectable by enzyme-linked immunosorbent assay (ELISA), complement fixation, neutralization, and fluorescent antibody techniques.[3] The humoral response is exceptionally slow, but ultimately a long-lasting and vigorous production of antibodies occurs.[3] Usually, antibodies demonstrable by immunofluorescence

Table 12.1 Old-World arenaviruses

Arenavirus	Rodent	Location	Habitat	Human contact
Lymphocytic choriomeningitis (LCM) virus	*Mus musculus*, *M. domesticus* (house mouse), *Mesocricetus auratus* (Syrian hamster)	Europe, Asia, and the Americas	Peridomestic, grasslands	Primarily within households
Lassa virus	*Mastomys natalensis*	West Africa	Savanna, forest clearing	Primarily within houses

are the first to appear, followed by complement-fixing antibodies. The complement-fixing antibodies are short-lived, with titers diminishing rapidly 5–12 months after onset. In contrast, neutralizing antibodies remain detectable for many years.[3] Cell-mediated immunity is important in arenavirus infections of experimental animals; it is sometimes harmful, but is probably beneficial in human infections, at least for Lassa fever.[6] In Lassa fever passive transfer of early-convalescent-phase human antibodies does not protect monkeys or guinea pigs, whereas late antibodies neutralize virus and are protective.[1,4] All evidence suggests that viral clearance in humans is complete and that chronic infection is not established. Reinfection with Lassa virus is possible, but appears to be uncommon.

Clinical features

The incubation period is around 2 weeks.[6] Disease onset usually begins with insidious progression of general malaise and fever over a 5-day period. In clinical illness the onset is gradual, with fever, malaise, headache, sore throat, cough, nausea, vomiting, diarrhea, myalgia, and chest and abdominal pain.[6] The fever may be either constant or intermittent with spikes. Inflammation of the throat and eyes is commonly observed.[1]

Progression beyond this stage is not common for Lassa fever.[1] In severe cases, hypotension or shock, pleural effusion (fluid in the lung cavity), hemorrhage, seizures, encephalopathy, and swelling of the face and neck are frequent. Approximately 15% of hospitalized patients die. The disease is more severe in pregnancy, and fetal loss occurs in more than 80% of cases.[1]

Hemorrhages, neurological signs and symptoms, leukopenia and thrombocytopenia are commonly present. Hair loss and loss of coordination may occur in convalescence. In addition, deafness occurs in 25% of patients, with only half recovering some hearing function after 1–3 months.[1,6] Immunity to reinfection occurs following infection, but the length of this period of protection is unknown.[1]

Other hemorrhagic fevers of viral origin, such as Ebola infection and hemorrhagic Dengue, should be considered in the differential diagnosis. Meningococcemia and other diseases leading to sepsis, with disseminated intravascular coagulation and shock, can be confused with the Latin American hemorrhagic fever complex.

Diagnosis and differential diagnosis

Lassa virus can be isolated by inoculation of Vero cells. All arenaviruses appear to share antigenic determinants in the ribonucleoproteins, as well as antigenically distinct determinants in their outer GPs.[2] Positive immunofluorescent staining of acetone-fixed infected cells is definitive for more than just family identification, since Old World arenaviruses can be readily distinguished from New World viruses with limiting dilutions of antibody.[2] Arenavirus species may be identified by their unique surface GPs and infectivity neutralization.[2] Most cases, however, are diagnosed by the epidemiological and clinical data. Lassa fever must be suspected if arenaviruses are prevalent in geographic areas where infections have occurred and in regions known to harbor reservoir rodent species.

Treatment and prophylaxis

Although several classes of antiviral compounds have been found with specific in vitro activity against arenaviruses, only ribavirin has been proven to be effective against Lassa fever.[1] It may be used at any point in the illness, as well as for postexposure prophylaxis.[1] The adult dose for Lassa fever (with hepatitis and/or hemorrhagic manifestations) is 2 g (30 mg/kg) IV initially; 1 g (15 mg/kg) IV q 6 h for 4 days, and then 500 mg (7.5 mg/kg) IV q 8 h for 6 days.[4,6] The suggested prophylactic dose is 600 mg PO q.i.d. for 10 days. Ribavirin is contraindicated in pregnancy. Systemic ribavirin use causes dose-related anemia and hyperbilirubinemia related to extravascular hemolysis, and at higher doses, bone marrow suppression of the erythroid elements may occur.[8]

Vaccines are under development.[6] A Lassa virus GP gene has been cloned and expressed in vaccinia virus. This vaccine has offered a high degree of protection against disease and death in monkeys challenged with the intact Lassa virus.[6] Use of plasma is not yet indicated for patients with Lassa fever.[6] At least seven serologically distinct strains of Lassa virus have been isolated; animal studies suggest that effective therapy should involve geographic matching of immune plasma and virus strain. In view of the frequency of Lassa virus transmission from person to person in a hospital setting, strict measures must be taken to isolate patients who have or are suspected of having the disease.[4,6] Isolation of patients with the other pathogenic arenaviruses is desirable.

Filoviruses

Filoviruses are filamentous, enveloped particles with a negative-sense, single-stranded RNA genome, approximately 19 kbp long. Genes are defined by conserved transcriptional start and termination signals and arranged linearly.[9] A single GP forms the spikes on the virion surface. The nucleocapsid contains the RNA and four viral structural proteins, including the virus-encoded polymerase.[9,10] Within the Filoviridae there is a single genus, *Filovirus*, and a separation into two genotypes, Marburg and Ebola. Ebola is subdivided into three subtypes: Zaire, Sudan, and Reston.[10] They are similar in morphology, density, and electrophoresis profile, with a close serological relationship among them. According to electron microscopy, Filoviridae virions are pleomorphic, usually b-shaped, containing a nucleocapsid (20 nm in diameter) surrounded by a helical capsid (50 nm in diameter).[9,10] Transcription of the virions takes place in the cytoplasm of the infected cells but the mechanism of virus entry is still unknown.[9]

History and epidemiology

This family is indigenous to Africa. Marburg and Ebola both cause severe hemorrhagic fevers. Marburg virus was first recognized in laboratory workers exposed to tissues and blood from African green monkeys (*Cercopithecus aethiops*) in Marburg, Germany, in 1967.[1] Since then, sporadic, virologically confirmed Marburg disease cases have occurred in Zimbabwe, South Africa, and Kenya.[11,12] Ebola virus first emerged in two major disease outbreaks, with mortality rates of 88%, in Zaire and Sudan in 1976.[1] Sporadic cases and minor outbreaks occurred again in the same locations previously affected and also in Gabon,[1] the Ivory Coast and Uganda, after 1977.[1]

The Ebola Reston virus was first discovered in 1989 in monkeys imported from the Philippines, which had died in a holding facility in Reston, Virginia, just outside Washington, DC.[13] While monkeys suffer a severe disease, often leading to death, the limited information available indicates that humans may not become clinically ill. However, this is only based on the isolation of Reston virus from one asymptomatically infected animal handler identified during the original outbreak and a few seroconversions that were not associated with clinical disease.[13] A formal quarantine procedure for imported monkeys was developed following the original Reston episode and it is this system that apparently identified the current cases.[13] The Ebola Reston virus has also been isolated from two non-human primates (*Cynomolgus*) held at a quarantine facility in Texas, USA.[1] The monkeys had also been imported from the Philippines.

Serological studies suggest filoviruses are endemic in many countries of the central African region.[14,15] Although serological data based on ELISA are only of limited reliability, they at least suggest the possible occurrence of subclinical infections caused by known or unknown filoviruses.[14,15] The mode of primary infection in any natural setting is unknown for Marburg and Ebola viruses.[14] All secondary cases, however, were due to intimate contact with infected patients.[4,16,17] After hospitalization of an infected person, the disease spreads rapidly via contaminated needles and contact with blood, which seems to be the most important route of contamination.[16] In each Ebola outbreak in Africa, the initial patient spread the disease to close family members through intimate contact with the patient.[1] The natural reservoir of these two viruses remains unknown. However, on the basis of available evidence and the nature of similar viruses, they must be zoonotic and normally maintained in an animal host that is native to the African continent. The infected monkeys were not considered to be the natural host since they also died with hemorrhagic symptoms.[16,17]

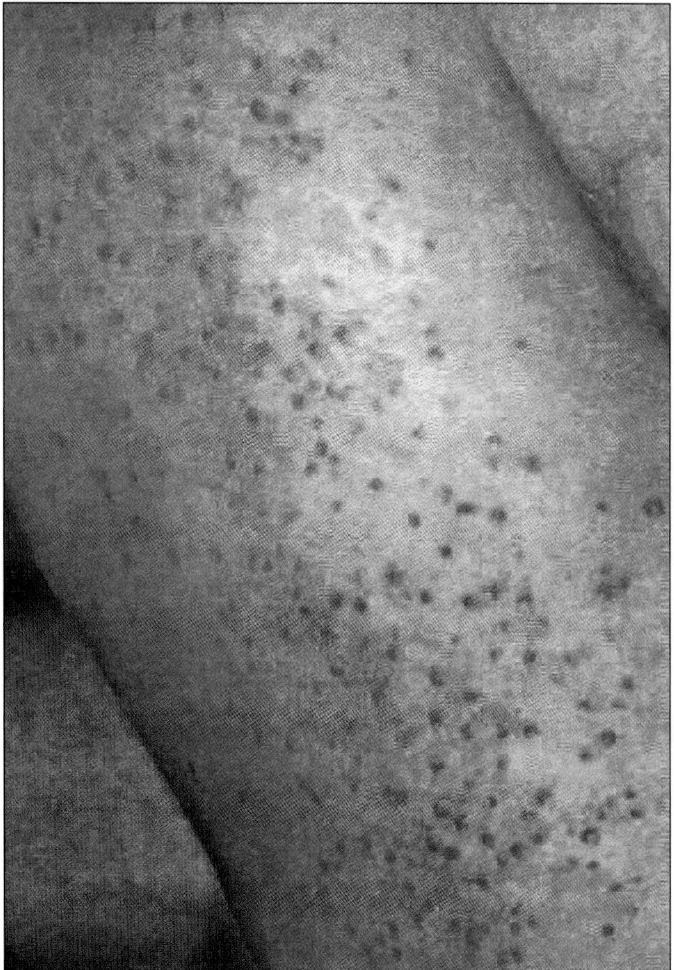

Figure 12.1 Macular, papular centripetal rash of Ebola infection.

Pathogenesis and etiology

Filoviridae viruses are usually recovered from acute-phase sera and have also been found in throat washes, urine, soft-tissues effusions, semen, and anterior eye fluid.[1,12] It has also been regularly isolated from autopsy material, such as spleen, lymph nodes, liver, and kidney.[1] Clinical and biochemical findings support anatomical observations of extensive liver involvement, renal damage, changes in vascular permeability, and activation of the clotting cascade.[17] Visceral organ necrosis is the consequence of virus replication in parenchymal cells. However, no organ is sufficiently damaged to cause death. Fluid distribution problems and platelet abnormalities indicate dysfunction of endothelial cells and platelets.[7,12] The shock syndrome in severe and fatal cases seems to be mediated by virus-induced release of humoral factors such as cytokines.[12,16,17] Filovirus GPs carry a presumably immunosuppressive domain, and immunosuppression has been observed in infected monkeys.[12]

Clinical features

Filoviruses cause a severe hemorrhagic fever in both human and non-human primates.[7] Following an incubation period of 4–15 days, onset is sudden, marked by high fever, fatigue, headache, erythematous transient rashes, and myalgia.[1] Abdominal pain, sore throat, nausea, vomiting, cough, arthralgia, diarrhea, and pharyngeal and conjunctival vasodilatation[18] may follow these symptoms. Patients are dehydrated, apathetic, and disoriented. They may develop a characteristic, nonpruritic, maculopapular centripetal rash (Fig. 12.1) associated with varying degrees of erythema, which desquamates by day 5 or 7 of the illness.[18]

Hemorrhagic manifestations develop at the peak of the illness, and are of prognostic value. Bleeding into the gastrointestinal tract is the most prominent, besides petechiae and hemorrhages from puncture wounds and mucous membranes.[18] Most patients develop severe hemorrhagic manifestations in the next few days, with bleeding from multiple sites such as the gastrointestinal tract, oropharynx, and lungs.[18] The skin and mucous membranes are also affected with echymoses, disseminated non-palpable petechiae, and massive gingival bleeding that usually herald a fatal outcome.[18]

Diagnosis and differential diagnosis

Laboratory parameters are less characteristic, but the following are associated with the disease: leukopenia (as low as 1000/μl), left shift with atypical lymphocytes; thrombocytopenia (50 000–100 000/μl); markedly elevated serum transaminase levels (typically aspartate aminotransaminase exceeding alanine aminotransferase); hyperproteinemia; and proteinuria.[18] Prothrombin and partial thromboplastin times are prolonged, and fibrin split products are detectable. At a later stage, secondary bacterial infection may lead to elevated white blood counts. There is fever in patients, who eventually recover in about 5–9 days.[18] In cases ending in death, clinical signs occur at an early stage and the patient dies between day 6 and 16, from hemorrhage and hypovolemic shock. The mortality rate is between 30 and 90%, depending on the virus, and the highest rate has been reported for Ebola Zaire.[14,15] Ebola Reston seems to possess a very low pathogenicity for humans or may even be apathogenic.[14] Convalescence is prolonged and sometimes associated with myelitis, recurrent hepatitis, psychosis, or uveitis. An increased risk of abortion exists for pregnant women, and clinical observations indicate a high death rate for children of infected mothers.[14,15,18]

In tropical settings, filoviral hemorrhagic fever may be difficult to identify, since the most common causes of severe, acute, febrile disease are malaria and typhoid fever. The differential diagnosis should also include other viral hemorrhagic fevers, such as yellow fever, Dengue infection, or arenavirus hemorrhagic fevers, as well as meningococcemia, leptospirosis, and idiopathic thrombocytopenic purpura.[1] Travel, treatment in local hospitals, and contact with sick persons or wild and domestic monkeys are useful historical features in returning travelers, especially in those from Africa. Diagnosis of single cases is extremely difficult, but occurrence of clusters of cases with prodromal fever followed by cases of hemorrhagic diatheses and person-to-person transmission are suggestive of viral hemorrhagic fever, and containment procedures must be initiated. In filoviral hemorrhagic fever prostration, lethargy, wasting, and diarrhea are usually more severe than is observed with other viral hemorrhagic fever patients. The rash is characteristic and extremely useful in the differential diagnosis.[1]

Laboratory diagnosis can be achieved in two different ways: by measuring the host-specific immunological response to the infection and by detecting viral antigen and genomic RNA in the infected host. The most commonly used assays to detect antibodies to filoviruses are the indirect immunofluorescence assay (IFA), immunoblot, and ELISA (direct immunoglobulin G (IgG) and IgM ELISA, and IgM capture assay).[17,19] Direct detection of viral particles, viral antigen, and genomic RNA can be achieved by electron microscopy (negative contrast, thin-section), immunohistochemistry, immunofluorescence on impression smears of tissues, antigen detection ELISA, and reverse transcriptase PCR (RT-PCR).[14]

Attempts to isolate the virus from serum and/or other clinical material should be performed using Vero or MA-104 cells (monkey kidney cells).[19] However, most filoviruses do not cause extensive cytopathogenic effects on primary isolation. The most useful animal system, besides non-human primates, is guinea pigs which develop fever within 10 days upon primary infection.[19]

Treatment and prophylaxis

There is no standard treatment for Ebola and Marburg infection and virus-specific treatment does not exist.[20] Supportive therapy should be directed towards maintaining effective blood volume and electrolyte balance.[18] Shock, cerebral edema, renal failure, coagulation disorders, and secondary bacterial infection must be managed. Heparin treatment should only be considered when there is clear evidence of disseminated intravascular coagulopathy.[20] Filoviruses are resistant to the antiviral effects of interferon, and interferon administration to monkeys has failed to increase survival rate or to reduce virus titer.[10,20] Ribavirin does not affect filoviruses in vitro and thus is probably not of clinical value, in contrast to its efficacy against other viral hemorrhagic fevers.[20] Isolation of patients is recommended, and protection of medical and nursing staff is required. Monkeys caught in the wild are an important source of the introduction of filoviruses. Quarantine of imported non-human primates and professional handling of animals will help prevent introduction into humans.[10]

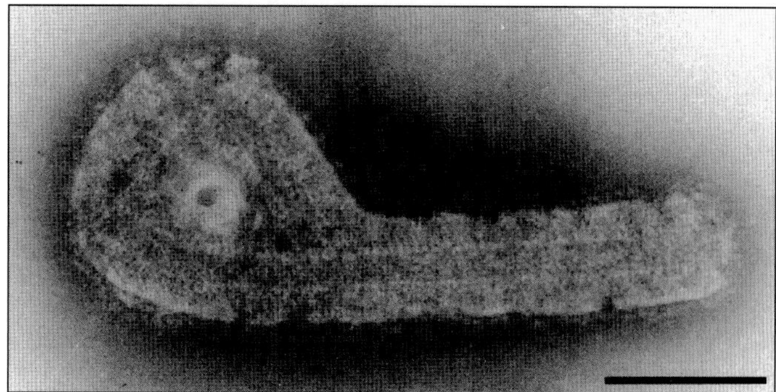

Figure 12.2 Marburg virus. (Courtesy of Professor H. Klenk.)

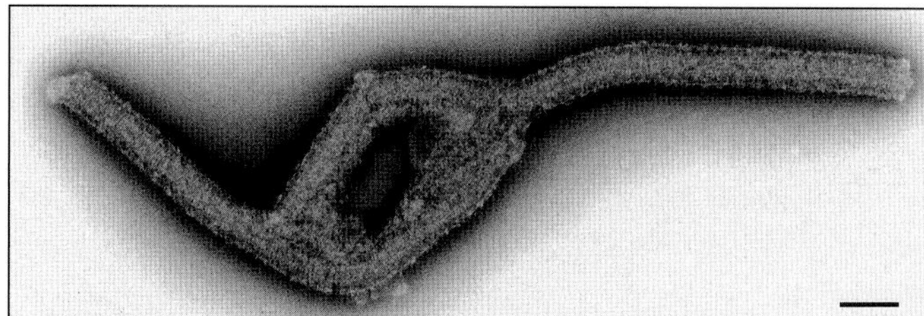

Figure 12.3 Ebola virus. (Courtesy of Professor H. Klenk.)

Even though filoviral hemorrhagic fever outbreaks have been rare and were mainly restricted to a small number of cases, vaccines would be of value for both medical personnel in Africa and for laboratory personnel.[17] Cross-protection among different Ebola subtypes in experimental animal systems has been reported, suggesting a general value of vaccines.[10] Inactivated vaccines have been developed by treatment with formalin or heat of cell culture-propagated Marburg (Fig. 12.2) and Ebola (Fig. 12.3) subtypes Sudan and Zaire.[17,18,20] Protection, however, has only been achieved by carefully balancing the challenge dose and virulence. Because of the biohazardous nature of the agents, recombinant vaccines would be an attractive approach in the future.[20]

Bunyaviruses

The Bunyaviridae family encompasses about 300 different viruses, two of them associated with severe hemorrhagic fevers and mucocutaneous manifestations in humans: RVF and CCHF.[1,21]

History and epidemiology

Although primarily a zoonosis, sporadic cases and outbreaks of CCHF affecting humans do occur.[22] The disease is endemic in many countries in Africa, Europe, and Asia, and, during 2001, cases or outbreaks were recorded in Albania, Iran, Kosovo, Pakistan, and South Africa.[23] CCHF was first described in the Crimea (Central Asia) in 1944 and given the name Crimean hemorrhagic fever.[21,22] In 1969 it was recognized that the pathogen causing Crimean hemorrhagic fever was the same as that responsible for an illness identified in 1956 in the Congo, and linkage of the two place names resulted in the current name for the disease and the virus.[21,22] CCHF is a severe disease in humans, with a high mortality rate.[22] Fortunately, human illness occurs infrequently, although animal infection may be more common. The CCHF virus may infect a wide range of domestic and wild animals. Many birds are resistant to infection, but ostriches are susceptible and may show a high prevalence of infection in endemic areas.[23] Animals become infected with CCHF from the bite of infected ticks. The most efficient and common vectors for CCHF appear to be members of the *Hyalomma* genus.[24,25] Humans who become infected with CCHF acquire the virus from direct contact with blood or other infected tissues from livestock, or they may become infected from a tick bite. The majority of cases have occurred in those involved with the livestock industry, such as agricultural workers, slaughterhouse workers, and veterinarians.[25]

RVF virus was first isolated near Lake Naivasha in Kenya in 1931.[21,22] Since then, the virus has been shown to be widespread in sub-Saharan Africa and Egypt.[26,27] Major epidemics/epizootics occurred in Egypt in 1977[27] (200 000 human infections with 600 deaths) and 1993, in Mauritania in 1987 (200 human deaths),[28] Madagascar in 1991, and in eastern Africa (89 000 infections and more than 500 deaths reported so far), with outbreaks in 1997–1998 in Kenya, Tanzania, and Somalia.[26] In 2000, the Ministries of Health of Yemen and Saudi Arabia received reports of unexplained hemorrhagic fever in humans and associated animal deaths on the first confirmed occurrence of RVF outside Africa.[29] More than 315 persons with suspected severe RVF have been reported from primary health care centers and hospitals and at least 66 (21%) patients have died with hemorrhagic manifestations.[29] The epidemiology of RVF consists in both epizootic and interepizootic cycles. Epizootics of RVF in Africa often occurred when unusually heavy rainfall was observed. During an epizootic, virus circulates among infected arthropod vectors and mammalian hosts, particularly cattle and sheep, which represent the most significant livestock amplifiers of RVF virus.[28,30] The interepizootic survival of RVF virus is believed to depend on transovarial transmission of virus in floodwater *Aedes* mosquitoes.[21,22] Virus can persist in mosquito eggs until the next period of heavy rainfall, when they hatch and yield RVF virus-infected mosquitoes.[21,22] Although RVF has a more circumscribed distribution than CCHF, the disease presents a greater potential of dissemination because of the more widespread vector. Field populations of *Aedes canadensis*, *A. cantator*, *A. excrucians*, *A. sollicitans*, *A. taeniorhynchus*, *A. triseriatus*, *Anopheles bradleyi-crucians*, *Culex salinarius*, *C. tarsalis*, and *C. territans* perorally exposed to 10 (6.2)–10 (7.2) plaque-forming units (PFU) of RVF virus readily became infected.[31,32] Infection rates ranged from 51% (65/127) for *C. salinarius* to 96% (64/67) for *Aedes canadensis*. Disseminated infection rates were generally greater at 14 days than at 7 days after the infectious blood meal and, with the exception of *Anopholes bradleyi-crucians*, they were not significantly different from the pooled rate of 59% for each species tested. For most species, about half of the mosquitoes with a disseminated infection transmitted an infectious dose of virus to hamsters.[31] While all species, with the exception of *A. bradleyi-crucians*, transmitted virus, *Aedes canadensis*, *A. taeniorhynchus*, and *Culex tarsalis* had the highest vector potential of the species tested. Following inoculation of approximately 10 (1.6) PFU of virus, 100% of the mosquitoes of each species became infected.[32] For most species, transmission rates were similar for inoculated individuals and those that developed a disseminated infection following peroral infection. Viral titers of transmitting and non-transmitting disseminated individuals were similar for all species tested.

Clinical features

The clinical presentation of both diseases is quite similar. The incubation period is about 6 days, with a documented maximum of 13 days.[23] Onset of symptoms is sudden, with fever, myalgia, dizziness, neck pain and stiffness, backache, headache, sore eyes, and photophobia. There may be nausea, vomiting, and sore throat early on, which may be accompanied by diarrhea and generalized abdominal pain. Over the next few days, the patient may experience sharp mood swings, and may become confused and aggressive.[26,33] After 2–4 days, the agitation may be replaced by sleepiness, depression, and lassitude, and the abdominal pain may localize to the right upper quadrant, with detectable hepatomegaly. Other clinical signs that emerge include tachycardia, lymphadenopathy, and a petechial rash both on internal mucosal surfaces, such as in the mouth and throat, and on the skin.[26,33] The petechiae may give way to ecchymoses and other hemorrhagic phenomena such as melena, hematuria, epistaxis, and bleeding from the gums. There is usually evidence of hepatitis. The severely ill may develop hepatorenal and pulmonary failure after the fifth day of illness.[24,33]

The mortality rate from CCHF is approximately 30%, with death occurring in the second week of illness. In those patients who recover, improvement generally begins on the ninth or 10th day after the onset of illness. RVF presents a more benign course, with severe eye disease (2%), meningoencephalitis, and hemorrhagic fever syndrome in 1% of patients.[24,33]

Diagnosis and treatment

Diagnosis of suspected CCHF and RVF is performed in especially equipped, high-biosafety-level laboratories.[23,25,33] IgG and IgM antibodies may be detected in serum by ELISA from about day 6 of illness.[23,34] IgM remains detectable for up to 4 months, and IgG levels decline but remain detectable for up to 5 years.[25] General supportive therapy is the mainstay of patient management in both diseases. Intensive monitoring to guide volume and blood component replacement is required. Ribavirin has been used in the treatment of established CCHF infection, with apparent benefit.[34,35] Both oral and intravenous formulations seem to be effective.[35] The value of immune plasma from recovered patients for therapeutic purposes has not been demonstrated, although it has been employed on several occasions.

There is no safe and effective vaccine widely available for human use against both viruses.[22] Persons living in endemic areas should use personal protective measures that include avoidance of areas where tick vectors and mosquitoes are located. When patients with CCHF are admitted to the hospital, there is a risk of nosocomial spread of infection. In the past, serious outbreaks have occurred in this way and it is imperative that adequate infection control measures be observed to prevent this outcome.[35] Patients with suspected or confirmed CCHF should be isolated and cared for using a barrier nursing technique.[34,35] Specimens of blood or tissues taken for diagnostic purposes should be collected and handled using universal precautions. Sharps (needles and other penetrating surgical instruments) and body wastes should be safely disposed of using appropriate decontamination procedures.[34]

Hantaviruses

Hantaviruses are discussed in depth in the section on New-World hemorrhagic fever (below) because of the emergence of sin nombre virus (SNV) in the USA in the recent past.[1] However, the geographic scope of hantaviruses is far more disseminated in the Old World than in the Americas, and the disease has been recognized as a hemorrhagic fever with great morbidity and mortality for many years.

Epidemiology

Hantaviruses are endemic in most parts of the Old World, affecting some regions of Southeast Asia and southeast Europe that have a mild tropical climate (Table 12.2). However, the distribution of the natural reservoir has a great impact on the geographic distribution of a disease that can reach remote areas of Scandinavia, western Russia and even far-east Russia (Table 12.2).[1,36,37]

Hantaviruses are transmitted by aerosols of rodent excreta, saliva, and urine. The most common mode of transmission is inhalation of dust or dried particles that carry dried saliva or waste products of an infected rodent.[36]

Pathogenesis and etiology

Once infected, a rodent experiences a brief viremia that lasts 5–10 days. Following this stage, the viral antigens remain present in many major organs for weeks to months. In spite of the antibody presence in the rodent's serum, infectious virus is shed in the rodent's saliva, urine, and feces, possibly for the rest of its life. Mice appear to be most infectious 40 days after their infection with the virus.[36–38] No arthropod vector has been established for hantaviruses.

In general, there are two seasonal peaks for almost all outbreaks of hantavirus diseases: a small one in spring, and a large one in fall.[38] It is suspected that this corresponds to seasonal increases in the infection rate of the rodents, and with farming cycles, during which farmers are exposed to rodents in the fields during planting and harvest periods.[38] Unusually high rainfall in dry parts of the country results in increased food sources for rodents, and subsequently increased rodent populations. Fall/winter outbreaks, such as those in Greece,[37] correspond to the movement of rodents from the fields into artificial structures.

Clinical features

Symptoms of HFRS associated with hantaviruses of the Old World usually occur about 5–6 weeks after exposure to the virus. Initial onset is marked by non-specific flu-like symptoms: fever, myalgia, headache, abdominal pain, nausea, and vomiting.[36,38] There is a characteristic facial flushing, and usually a petechial rash (usually limited to the axilla, or armpit).[36] Sudden and extreme albuminuria occurs about day 4; this is characteristic of severe HFRS.[38] The hemorrhagic manifestations also include skin hemorrhages with petechiae, purpura, ecchymoses, gingival and nasal bleeding, and hematuria. Gastrointestinal bleeding is very common, with hematemesis and melena, and increased menstrual flow.[36,38] Additional symptoms may include hypotension, respiratory distress and/or failure, and renal impairment and/or failure.[38]

Diagnosis and treatment

Upon examination, peripheral blood smears of patients with HFRS are found to have thrombocytopenia, increased immature granulocytes, and large immunoblastoid lymphocytes, accompanied by an elevated white blood cell count.[39,40] While coagulopathy is not common, increased partial thromboplastin and prothrombin times are observed. In addition, several enzymes are elevated, including serum lactate, lactate dehydrogenase, aspartate aminotransferase, and alanine aminotransferase. Chest radiographs of hantavirus pulmonary syndrome (HPS) patients show diffuse interstitial pulmonary infiltrates, advancing to alveolar edema with severe bilateral involvement. Severe infections may have pulmonary secretions with a total protein ratio of edema fluid/serum greater than 80%. Pleural effusions may be seen in the radiograph, along with peribronchial cuffing.[39,40]

Serologic assay will detect the presence of serum IgG and/or IgM to hantavirus strains Seoul, Hantaan, Puumala, and Dobrava, which are the most clinically important strains in the Old World.[40,41] Geographic distribution of rodent hosts, as well as clinical manifestations of the infection, can aid in further identification since individual strains cannot be distinguished in this assay due to antigenic similarities between the hantavirus strains.[40,41]

The crude mortality rate is approximately 40–50%. The patients need intensive cardiopulmonary support. Ribavirin given IV has been shown to be effective during the early phase of the HFRS illness.

Table 12.2 Most common Old-World hantaviruses

Virus	Natural reservoir	Distribution
Hantaan virus	Striped field mouse (*Apodemus agrarius*)	Asia, mainly Korea
Seoul virus	Domestic rat (*Rattus norvegicus* and *R. rattus*)	Asia and sea ports worldwide
Puumala virus	Bank vole (*Clethrionomys glareolus*)	Scandinavia and western Russia
Dobrava virus	Yellow-necked mouse (*Apodemus flavicollis*)	Eastern Europe, mainly Greece
Khabarovsk virus	*Microtus fortis*	Far-east Russia

References

1. Lupi O, Tyring S. Tropical dermatology: viral tropical diseases. J Am Acad Dermatol 2003; 49:975–1000.
2. Albarino CG, Posik DM, Ghiringhelli PD et al. Arenavirus phylogeny: a new insight. Virus Genes 1998; 16:39–46.
3. Oldstone MB, Lewicki H, Homman D et al. Common antiviral cytotoxic T-lymphocyte epitope for diverse arenaviruses. J Virol 2001; 75:6273–6278.
4. Salazar-Bravo J, Ruedas LA, Yates TL. Mammalian reservoirs of arenaviruses. Curr Top Microbiol Immunol 2002; 262:25–63.
5. Bowen MD, Rolin PE, Ksiazek TG et al. Genetic diversity among Lassa virus strains. J Virol 2000; 74:6992–7004.
6. McCormick JB. Lassa, Junin, Machupo and guanarito viruses. In: Webster RG, Granoff A, eds. Encyclopedia of virology. San Diego: Academic Press; 1994:776–837.
7. Peters CJ, Zaki SR. Role of the endothelium in viral hemorrhagic fevers. Crit Care Med 2002; 30 (Suppl. 5):S268–S273.
8. Kilgore PE, Ksiazek TG, Rollin PE et al. Treatment of Bolivian hemorrhagic fever with intravenous ribavirin. Clin Infect Dis 1997; 24:718–722.
9. Ikegami T, Calaor AB, Miranda ME et al. Genome structure of Ebola virus subtype Reston: differences among Ebola subtypes. Arch Virol 2001; 146:2021–2027.
10. Casillas AM, Nyamathi AM, Sosa A et al. A current review of Ebola virus: pathogenesis, clinical presentation, and diagnostic assessment. Biol Res Nurs 2003; 4:268–275.
11. Sleuczka WG. The Marburg virus outbreak of 1967 and subsequent episodes. Curr Trop Microbiol Immunol 1999; 235:49–75.
12. Takada A, Kawaoka Y. The pathogenesis of Ebola hemorrhagic fever. Trends Microbiol 2001; 9:506–511.
13. Ikegami T, Miranda ME, Calaor AB et al. Histopathology of natural Ebola virus subtype Reston infection in cynomolgus macaques during the Philippine outbreak in 1996. Exp Anim 2002; 51:447–455.
14. Freed EO. Virology. Rafting with Ebola. Science 2002; 296:279.
15. Portela Camara F. Epidemiology of the Ebola virus: facts and hypotheses. Braz J Infect Dis 1998; 2:265–268.
16. Mwanatambwe M, Yamada N, Arai S et al. Ebola hemorrhagic fever: mechanism of transmission and pathogenicity. J Nippon Med Sch 2001; 68:370–375.
17. Leroy EM, Baize S, Debre P et al. Early immune responses accompanying human asymptomatic Ebola. Clin Exp Immunol 2001; 124:453–460.
18. Rowe AK, Bertolli J, Khan AS et al. Clinical, virologic, and immunologic follow-up of convalescent Ebola hemorrhagic fever patients and their household contacts, Kikwit, Democratic Republic of the Congo. J Infect Dis 1999; 179:S28–S35.
19. Morikawa S. Ebola virus and Marburg virus. Nippon Rinsho 2003; 61 (Suppl. 3):544–549.
20. Bray M, Paragas J. Experimental therapy of filovirus infections. Antiviral Res 2002; 54:1–17.
21. Sidwell RW, Smee DF. Viruses of the Bunya- and Togaviridae families: potential as bioterrorism agents and means of control. Antiviral Res 2003; 57:101–111.
22. Zeller H, Bouloy M. Infections by viruses of the families Bunyaviridae and Filoviridae. Rev Sci Tech 2000; 19:79–91.
23. Burt FJ, Leman PA, Abbott JC et al. Serodiagnosis of Crimean-Congo haemorrhagic fever. Epidemiol Infect 1994; 113:551–562.
24. Yashina L, Vyshemirskii O, Seregin S et al. Genetic analysis of Crimean-Congo hemorrhagic fever virus in Russia. J Clin Microbiol 2003; 41:860–862.
25. Burt FJ, Swanepoel R, Braack LE. Enzyme-linked immunosorbent assays for the detection of antibody to Crimean-Congo hemorrhagic fever virus in the sera of livestock and wild vertebrates. Epidemiol Infect 1993; 111:547–557.
26. Gerdes GH. Rift valley fever. Vet Clin North Am Food Anim Pract 2002; 18:549–555.
27. Abd el-Rahim IH, Abd el-Hakim U, Hussein M. An epizootic of Rift Valley fever in Egypt in 1997. Rev Sci Tech 1999; 18:741–748.
28. Nabeth P, Kane Y, Abdalahi MO et al. Rift Valley fever outbreak, Mauritania, 1998: seroepidemiologic, virologic, entomologic, and zoologic investigations. Emerg Infect Dis 2001; 7:1052–1054.
29. Balkhy HH, Memish ZA. Rift Valley fever: an uninvited zoonosis in the Arabian peninsula. Int J Antimicrob Agents 2003; 21:153–157.
30. Digoutte JP. Present status of an arbovirus infection: yellow fever, its natural history of hemorrhagic fever, Rift Valley fever. Bull Soc Pathol Exot 1999; 92:343–348.
31. Gargan TP, Clark GG, Dohm DJ et al. Vector potential of selected North American mosquito species for Rift Valley fever virus. Am J Trop Med Hyg 1988; 38:440–446.
32. Turell MJ, Bailey CL, Beaman JR. Vector competence of a Houston, Texas strain of *Aedes albopictus* for Rift Valley fever virus. J Am Mosq Control Assoc 1988; 4:94–96.
33. Shawky S. Rift Valley fever. Saudi Med J 2000; 21:1109–1115.
34. Drosten C, Gottig S, Schilling S et al. Rapid detection and quantification of RNA of Ebola and Marburg viruses, Lassa virus, CCHF virus, Rift Valley fever virus, dengue virus, and yellow fever virus by real-time PCR. J Clin Microbiol 2002; 40:2323–2330.
35. Bangash SA, Khan EA. Treatment and prophylaxis with ribavirin for Crimean-Congo hemorrhagic fever – is it effective? J Pak Med Assoc 2003; 53:39–41.
36. Clement JP. Hantavirus. Antiviral Res 2003; 57:121–127.
37. Nemirov K, Vapalahti O, Papa A et al. Genetic characterization of new Dobrava hantavirus isolate from Greece. J Med Virol 2003; 69:408–416.
38. Lednicky JA. Hantaviruses. A short review. Arch Pathol Lab Med 2003; 127:30–35.
39. Khaiboullina SF, St Jeor SC. Hantavirus immunology. Viral Immunol 2002; 15:609–625.
40. Hujakka H, Koistinen V, Kuronen I et al. Diagnostic rapid tests for acute hantavirus infections: specific tests for Hantaan, Dobrava and Puumala viruses versus a hantavirus combination test. J Virol Methods 2003; 108:117–122.
41. Araki K, Yoshimatsu K, Ogino M et al. Truncated hantavirus nucleocapsid proteins for serotyping Hantaan, Seoul, and Dobrava hantavirus infections. J Clin Microbiol 2001; 39:2397–2404.

New-World hemorrhagic fevers

Omar Lupi and Ivan Semenovitch

Synonyms: Machupo fever, Junin fever, Guanarito fever, Sabia fever: arenaviruses
Hantavirus pulmonary syndrome (HPS): hantaviruses

Key features:

- The New-World hemorrhagic fevers are systemic viral diseases caused mainly by arenaviruses and hantaviruses and with a worldwide distribution
- Virus is shed in the infected rodent's saliva, urine, and feces. No arthropod vector has been established
- Arenaviruses are characterized by severe hemorrhagic fever with purpura, gingival bleeding, and disseminated non-palpable petechiae on the skin
- HPS, caused mainly by SNV (hantavirus), is primarily a lung infection; the kidneys and the skin are largely unaffected

Introduction

Viruses are important pathogens worldwide, most of them producing several mucocutaneous manifestations, especially among the tropical hemorrhagic fevers. The tropical habitats, still common in most of the Americas, have undergone major ecological changes in the last few decades, exposing these viruses to direct contact with humans, and transforming emergent viruses such as Junin and Machupo virus (arenavirus), and SNV (hantavirus) as major threats to public health. The emergent New-World hemorrhagic fevers are mainly due to arenaviruses and hantaviruses, both transmitted by contaminated rodents and with a widespread distribution in the Americas. Yellow fever and dengue, important flaviviruses that are also associated with hemorrhagic features, will be discussed in a subsequent section.

Arenaviruses (New-World Complex)

The Arenaviridae are a family of viruses whose members are generally associated with benign infection in restricted rodent hosts but cause a severe disease in humans.[1] Arenaviruses are enveloped RNA viruses, 110–130 nm in diameter. During morphogenesis, sandy-appearing granules are found within new virions.[1,2] These particles give arenaviruses their name ("arena" is the Latin word for sand).

Epidemiology

In every case in which a human arenavirus disease has been studied, an interface between humans and rodents has been described; the one common characteristic of these zoonotic infection patterns is human contact with rodent excreta.[3] The most common situations are the exposure of agricultural workers to rodents during crop harvesting or the incidental infection of hunters who are in contact with rodents in forests.[3,4] The fact that only a specific species of rodent is infected in each geographic area and the severe diseases that arenaviruses cause in all other species, including other rodents, suggests that the benign infection in restricted rodent hosts is an important measure developed by these animals to survive.[4] They probably adopted this symbiotic relationship with these viruses in order to eliminate competition for food and shelter in the local ecology.[3,4] The infection of human beings is incidental to the natural cycle of the viruses.[1]

Five arenaviruses pathogenic to humans are associated with severe hemorrhagic fever with a mortality of about 15% among hospitalized patients. Lassa virus (West Africa), Junin virus (Argentine pampas), Machupo virus (Bolivia lowlands), Guanarito virus (Venezuela), and Sabia virus (southeast province of Brazil) affect very specific geographic regions of South America and Africa.[1,2] The sixth pathogenic arenavirus is LCM virus, the only one that is more widely distributed, but that causes only milder neurologic infection. LCM and Lassa viruses are associated with the Old-World rats and mice (family Muridae, subfamily Murinae), while the Latin American viruses, also known as the Tacaribe complex viruses, are associated with the New-World rodents (family Muridae, subfamily Sigmodontinae).[1–3]

Two arenaviruses were also described as causing human casualties in the USA (Fig. 12.4); Tamiami virus regularly infected *Sigmodon hispidus* (cotton rat) in Florida and the Whitewater Arroyo virus is prevalent among *Neotoma albigula* (white-throated wood rat) and infected three individuals in California in 1999.[1] All three patients had acute respiratory distress syndrome and two developed liver failure and hemorrhagic manifestations.[1,2] A few other arenaviruses infecting *Oryzomys* genus (Parana virus in Paraguay, Amapari and Flexal virus in Brazil) may cause isolated infection in humans.[1,2]

Pathogenesis and etiology

Suitable conditions for transmission occur in areas where humans come into contact with rodent urine containing virus.[1] These viruses are transmitted from mother rodents to their offspring during pregnancy, and thus remain in the rodent population generation after generation.[1–3] Persistent viremia and viruria in rodents result from a slow or insufficient immune response when immunologically immature rodent fetuses or neonates are infected.[3] The disease in humans is acute.

Although aerosol and respiratory spread, as well as cuts and abrasions in the skin, are suspected, the portal of entry of arenaviruses is still unknown. Most infections are asymptomatic, but about 30% of infected patients may present a more severe clinical course.[1] The infection presents such a wide spectrum of manifestations that a typical case is difficult to characterize. Nevertheless, headache, photophobia, apathy, and confusion are very common. This infection can be temporarily debilitating but is rarely fatal and complete recovery is the general rule.[1,2]

Clinical features

The clinical presentation of all these South American hemorrhagic fever diseases is similar in several ways. The incubation period is around 2 weeks. Disease onset usually begins with insidious progression of general malaise and fever over a 5-day period.[2] Hemorrhaging, neurological signs and symptoms, as well as leukopenia and thrombocytopenia are commonly present.[1,2] Dehydration and unremitting high fever are followed by hemoconcentration,

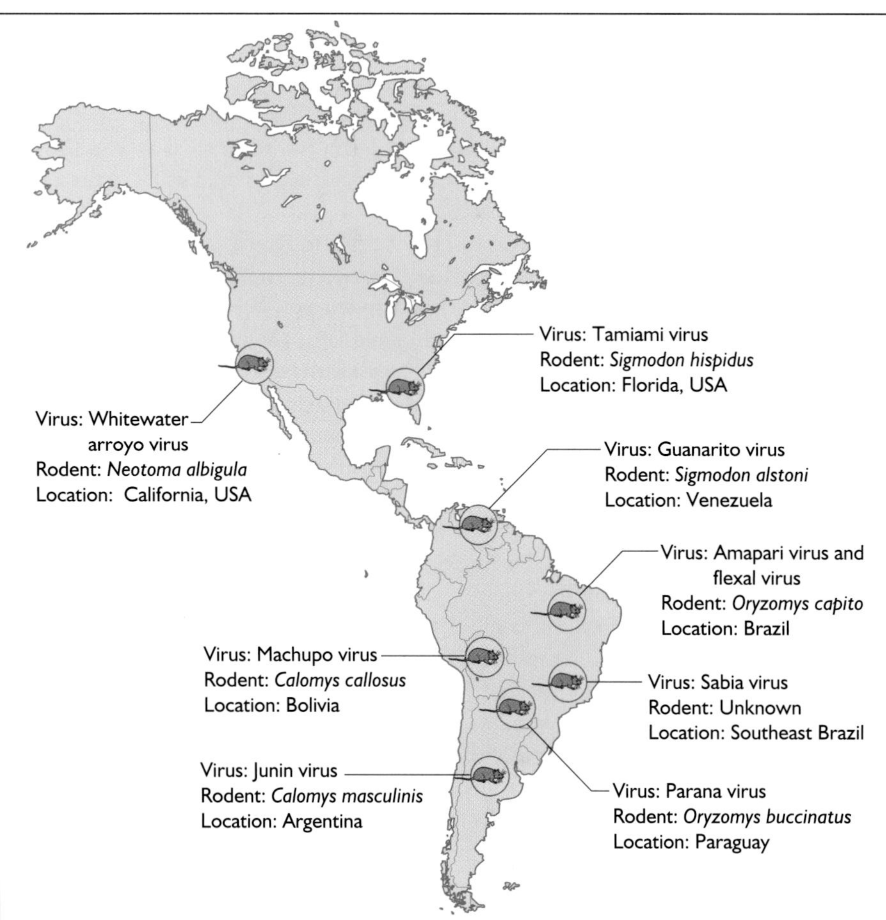
Virus: Tamiami virus
Rodent: Sigmodon hispidus
Location: Florida, USA
Virus: Whitewater arroyo virus
Rodent: Neotoma albigula
Location: California, USA
Virus: Guanarito virus
Rodent: Sigmodon alstoni
Location: Venezuela
Virus: Amapari virus and flexal virus
Rodent: Oryzomys capito
Location: Brazil
Virus: Machupo virus
Rodent: Calomys callosus
Location: Bolivia
Virus: Sabia virus
Rodent: Unknown
Location: Southeast Brazil
Virus: Junin virus
Rodent: Calomys masculinis
Location: Argentina
Virus: Parana virus
Rodent: Oryzomys buccinatus
Location: Paraguay

Figure 12.4 Distribution of New-World arenaviruses.

shock syndrome, hemorrhagic manifestations on skin and mucous membranes, and cardiovascular collapse. Purpura, minor gingival bleeding, and disseminated non-palpable petechiae on the skin are commonly seen (Fig. 12.5).[1,2,5] The pantropic nature of these viruses is revealed by their presence in various affected organs.[1]

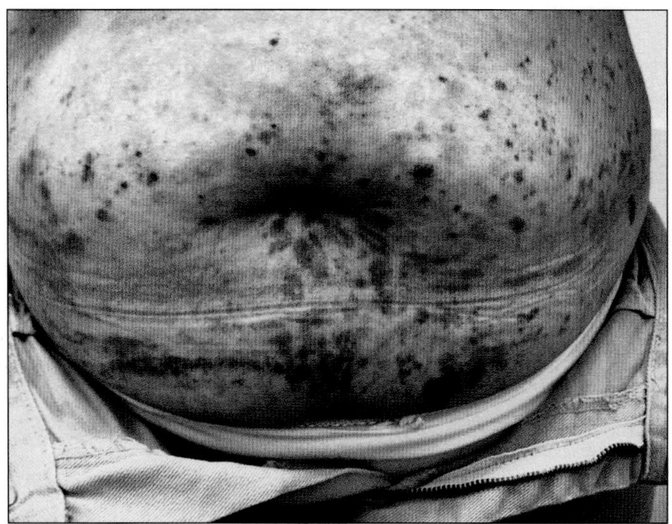

Figure 12.5 Palpable purpura of the skin associated with Brazilian hemorrhagic fever. (Courtesy of Dr. A. M. Peixoto.)

Diagnosis and differential diagnosis

Junin and Machupo viruses are isolated by intracerebral inoculation of newborn hamsters. All arenaviruses share some antigenic determinants detected by ELISA. Most of the cases, however, are diagnosed by the epidemiological and clinical data. Other hemorrhagic fevers from viral origin, such as Ebola infection and hemorrhagic dengue, should be considered in the differential diagnosis. Meningococcemia and other diseases leading to sepsis, with disseminated intravascular coagulation and shock, can be confused with arenaviruses.

Treatment and prophylaxis

Although several classes of antiviral compounds have been found with specific in vitro activity against arenaviruses, only ribavirin has been proven to be effective against Machupo and Junin virus.[1,5] The efficacy of this drug against the other members of the family has not yet been established. Vaccines are under development.

The only measure that has already proved to be safe and effective is a successful rodent-control program in areas affected by these viruses. The Bolivian savannas in Beni province were a endemic region of Machupo virus with hundreds of patients affected each year and dozens of deaths in the 1980s: after implementation of the rodent-control program the incidence was drastically reduced and only a few cases have been described in the last decade.[5]

Hantaviruses

Hantaviruses are single-stranded, negative-sense RNA viruses that encompass 25 antigenically distinguishable viral species.[6] They are enveloped virus particles, measuring 80–115 nm in diameter, and belong to the family Bunyaviridae.

History

Hantavirus was first identified during the Korean war in the early 1950s when about 3000 US and United Nations forces were infected.[6] The virus was named Hantaan, in recognition of the Hantaan river, which flows through Korea, and the major clinical manifestations were HFRS.[6]

Hantaviruses have been causing outbreaks of hemorrhagic fevers in Russia (1913), Manchuria and Scandinavia (1932–1935), and Finland (1945), but the Hantaan virus was only isolated in 1976, in Korea, from the rodent *Apodemus agrarius* (striped field mouse).[6–8] HPS, first recognized in 1993, is caused by several related viruses in the genus *Hantavirus*.[6]

Epidemiology

Hantaviruses are found worldwide and appear to be host-specific to rodent genus and possibly rodent species (Fig. 12.6).[7,8]

A hantavirus affected the USA in 1993 when several young Navajo Indians died in the Four Corners region.[9] The primary reservoir of this new hantavirus, SNV, is the deer mouse, *Peromyscus maniculatus*. Deer mice adapt to a variety of habitats and are found across most of the USA;[7,9] their presence in and around homes has been implicated as a risk factor for HPS. Hantavirus infection prevalence in deer mice in and around urban and rural homes was 27.5–32.5%.[9] Initial cases were identified in southwest USA, affecting Arizona, California, and New Mexico. Now HPS has been identified in 31 states and Canada, with an incidence of 280 cases since 1993.[9]

Other hantaviruses have been described in the Americas. Black Creek canal virus and Bayou virus infect the cotton rat (*Sigmondon hispidus*) and the rice rat (*Oryzomys palustris*) in most areas of southeast USA, while New York virus is regularly isolated from the white-footed mouse (*Peromyscus leucopus*) in New York (Fig. 12.6).[1,2]

Pathogenesis and etiology

Hantaviruses are transmitted by aerosols of rodent excreta, saliva, and urine.[6] The most common mode of transmission is inhalation of dust or dried particles that carry dried saliva or waste products of an infected rodent. Once infected, hantavirus is shed in the rodent's saliva, urine, and feces, possibly for the rest of its life. Mice appear to be at their most infectious 40 days after their infection with the virus.[6] No arthropod vector has been established for hantaviruses.

Clinical features

Symptoms of HFRS are rare in the western hemisphere but usually occur between 1 and 6 weeks after exposure to the virus. Initial onset is marked by fever, myalgia, headache, and abdominal pain.[6,7] The hemorrhagic manifestations also include skin hemorrhages with petechiae, purpura, ecchymoses, and hematuria.[10] Gastrointestinal bleeding is common, with hematemesis, melena, and hematochezia.[1,11] Additional symptoms may include hypotension and shock.[6,10]

HPS, caused mainly by SNV, is primarily a lung infection; the kidneys and the skin are largely unaffected. HPS is characterized

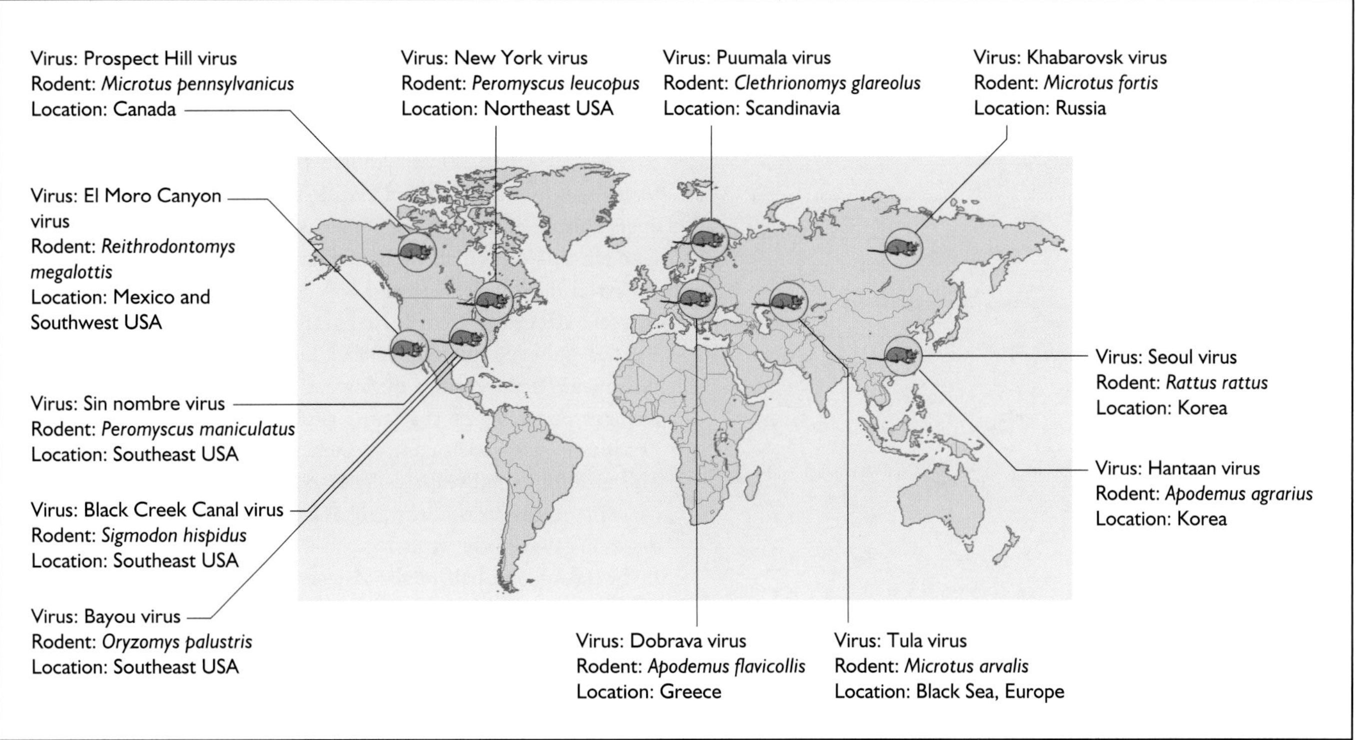

Figure 12.6 Distribution of hantaviruses worldwide.

by flu-like symptoms: fever, myalgia, headache, and cough.[9,11] Subsequent symptoms include coughing and shortness of breath, tachypnea, tachycardia, dizziness, arthralgia, sweating, and back or chest pain. Further symptoms can include thrombocytopenia and hypoxemia. Eventually, the patient experiences hypotension, shock, and respiratory distress.[9,10]

Diagnosis and differential diagnosis

Upon examination, peripheral blood smears of patients with both HPS and HFRS are found to have thrombocytopenia. While coagulopathy is not common, increased partial thromboplastin and prothrombin times are observed. Chest radiographs of HPS patients show diffuse interstitial pulmonary infiltrates, advancing to alveolar edema with severe bilateral involvement. Severe infections may have pulmonary secretions with a total protein ratio of edema fluid/serum greater than 80%.[6,11]

Serologic assay will detect the presence of serum IgG and/or IgM to hantavirus strains Seoul, Hantaan, Puumala, Dobrava, and SNV, which are the most clinically important strains.[7,11] Individual strains cannot be distinguished in this assay due to antigenic similarities between the hantavirus strains; however, geographic distribution of rodent hosts, as well as clinical manifestations of the infection can aid in further identification.[6,7,11] Differential diagnosis should also be performed with other hemorrhagic fevers such as Ebola fever, yellow fever, and dengue hemorrhagic fever (DHF).

Treatment

The illness progresses rapidly to severe respiratory failure and shock. The crude mortality rate is approximately 40–50%. The patients usually need intensive cardiopulmonary support with invasive hemodynamic monitoring. Ribavirin given IV has been shown to be effective during the early phase of the HFRS illness; it has not shown any effectiveness for HPS to date.[6,11]

References

1. Charrel RN, Lamballerie X. Arenaviruses other than Lassa virus. Antiviral Res 2003; 57:89–100.
2. Peters CJ. Human infection with arenaviruses in the Americas. Curr Top Microbiol Immunol 2002; 262:65–74.
3. Fritz CL, Fulhorst CF, Enge B et al. Exposure to rodents and rodent-borne viruses among persons with elevated occupational risk. J Occup Environ Med 2002; 44:962–967.
4. Salazar-Bravo J, Ruedas LA, Yates TL. Mammalian reservoirs of arenaviruses. Curr Top Microbiol Immunol 2002; 262:25–63.
5. Centers for Disease Control. Bolivian hemorrhagic fever – El Beni Department, Bolivia, 1994. JAMA 1995; 273:194–196.
6. Hawes S, Seabolt JP. Hantavirus. Clin Lab Sci 2003; 16:39–42.
7. Schmaljohn C, Hjelle B. Hantaviruses: a global disease problem. Emerg Infect Dis 1997; 3:95–104.
8. Lednicky JA. Hantaviruses. a short review. Arch Pathol Lab Med 2003; 127:30–35.
9. Botten J, Mirowsky K, Kusewitt D et al. Persistent Sin Nombre virus infection in the deer mouse (*Peromyscus maniculatus*) model: sites of replication and strand-specific expression. J Virol 2003; 77:1540–1550.
10. Bausch DG, Ksiazek TG. Viral hemorrhagic fevers including hantavirus pulmonary syndrome in the Americas. Clin Lab Med 2002; 22:981–1020.
11. Lupi O, Tyring S. Tropical dermatology: viral tropical diseases. J Am Acad Dermatol 2003; 49:975–1000.

Dengue

Omar Lupi, Gustavo Kouri and Maria G. Guzman

Synonyms:

- Dengue
- Breakbone fever

Key features:

- Systemic viral disease
- Dengue virus is in the genus *Flavivirus* of the family *Flaviviridae* (group B arbovirus)
- *Aedes aegypti* is the major vector and the true reservoir for the virus
- Classical Dengue fever lasts for 2-5 days, with severe headache, intense myalgia, arthralgia and retroorbital pain
- Cutaneous findings include a diffuse morbilliform rash that may be pruritic and heals with desquamation
- Diffuse capillary leakage of plasma is responsible for the hemoconcentration and thrombocytopenia that characterize Dengue hemorrhagic fever (DHF)

Introduction

The *Flavivirus* genus comprises more than 68 arthropod-transmitted viruses, of which 30 are known to cause human disease.[1] The flaviviral infections include Dengue, yellow fever, as well as Japanese encephalitis, and tick-borne encephalitis.[1,2] The clinical picture of Dengue was described by Benjamin Rush during an epidemic that occurred in Philadelphia in 1778. Later, during the 19th Century, several outbreaks were reported in tropical regions around the world.

It is believed that the global Dengue pandemic began in the Asian and Pacific regions during and after World War II. Ecological changes occurring at that time probably favoured the geographic expansion of the vector and its increase in density. The high number of susceptible individuals (local populations, soldiers) and their movement due to the war probably created the conditions for the dissemination of the virus.[3]

In the second half of the last century a severe disease, Dengue hemorrhagic fever/Dengue shock syndrome (DHF/DSS) was recognized as a clinical syndrome of Dengue infection and the first cases were described by Hammon in Manila and Bangkok during the 50's.[4] Since then, the number of cases has steadily increased worldwide and DHF/DSS emerged in new areas of the world, such as the American region, where the first devastating epidemic was

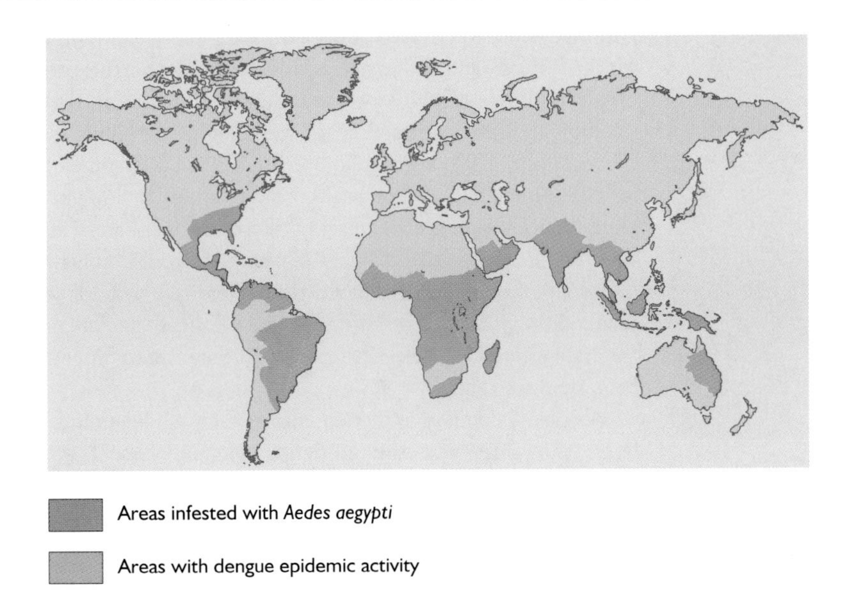

Figure 12.7 Dengue distribution worldwide.

reported in 1981.[5] Dengue is a mosquito-borne endemo-epidemic viral disease, caused by any one of the four Dengue serotypes (DEN 1,2,3,4). Currently, it is the most important arthropod-borne viral disease in terms of morbidity and mortality.

The pathophysiology of dengue was largely inferred from vaccine studies in rhesus monkeys using the attenuated vaccines.[1] After inoculation in rhesus monkeys, the virus replicated initially in local lymph nodes, followed by blood-borne spread and subsequent replication, mostly occurring in regional lymph tissue, spleen, and bone marrow, followed by the liver, lung, and adrenal glands.[3]

Epidemiology

Dengue transmission has increased geographically during the past few decades.[6] Epidemics have been reported in tropical and subtropical regions of Asia and Africa and more recently in the American region. Successive introduction of new serotypes into the Carribean, Central and South America has occurred since 1977[6–8] (Fig. 12.7). A DHF epidemic was first reported in Cuba in 1981 and was followed eight years later by the second DHF epidemic in Venezuela. Since then, epidemics have occurred in many other Latin American countries.[5,6]

According to the World Health Organization (WHO), 2.5 billion people live in areas at risk of Dengue,[1] 50–100 million Dengue infections and around 25 0000 DHF/DSS cases are estimated to occur yearly.[9]

In 2002 alone, there were more than 1 million reported cases of Dengue in the Americas, of which 14 374 cases were classified as DHF/DSS.[6,7] This is more than double the number of Dengue cases, which were recorded in the same region in 1995. Not only are the number of cases increasing as the disease is spreading to new areas, but explosive outbreaks are occuring.[6] In 2002, Brazil reported over 700 000 cases including more than 2500 DHF/DSS cases.

Complex and different factors play a causative role in the emergence and re-emergence of this disease, in particular population growth and unscheduled urbanization, resulting in substandard housing and inadequate water supply, sewage and waste management systems. This is worsened by air travel, migration and deteriorated health programs. However, poverty and health inequities are behind almost all of these factors.[10,11]

The transmission dynamics of Dengue viruses are determined by the interaction of the environment, the agent, the host population and the vector.[12]

The macro-determinants of transmission include environmental factors such as latitude (35°N to 35°S), elevation (<2200m), ambient temperature range (15–40°C), relative humidity (moderate to high) and the social factors mentioned above (population density, settlement patterns, unscheduled urbanization, inadequate water supply and waste management) and insufficient knowledge about the disease. The micro-determinants of Dengue transmission include host factors (gender, age, immune status, occupation), Dengue virulence factors (serotype, level of viremia) and vector factors (abundance and types of mosquito production sites, density of adult females, age of females, host preference, frequency of feeding, etc.).[12,13]

Aedes aegypti is the main vector although *Aedes albopictus* has been described as an important vector in some epidemics in Southeast Asia. *Aedes aegypti* is a domestic mosquito, which lives in the human environment, mainly anthropophilic, bites during daylight and usually breeds in clean water. Once the vector bites a person during the viremic phase, the virus multiplies within the mosquito (extrinsic incubation period) and within a few days, usually 7-11, it can transmit the virus to another person. After 3-7 days (intrinsic incubation period) the infected individual begins to show symptoms of the disease. *Aedes aegypti* transmits Dengue (horizontal transmission) and can also pass the virus via infected eggs to its offspring (vertical transmission).[1,14] Therefore, the mosquito is the true reservoir and the vector for Dengue disease. This vector, flourishing in urban and suburban environments, has disseminated the disease to many parts of the world (Fig. 12.8).

Pathogenesis

Secondary infection by a different Dengue serotype has been recognized as a major DHF/DSS risk factor since the 1950's.

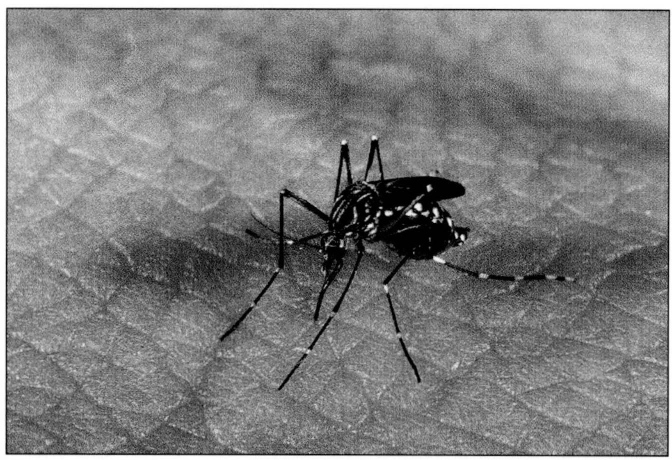

Figure 12.8 *Aedes aegypti*. (Courtesy of Dr. Genilton Vieira, FIOCRUZ/RJ.)

Severe disease was observed mainly in children experiencing secondary Dengue virus and infants born to dengue-immune mothers who experienced their first infection. Seroepidemiologic studies first performed in Thailand and later in Cuba suggested that the presence of heterotypic antibodies from primary Dengue infection is a risk factor for developing DHF/DSS.[15–17]

It is accepted that the infection with one Dengue serotype produces lifelong immunity to re-infection with the same serotype, but only temporal and partial protection to the other serotypes.

Neutralizing antibodies could attenuate the severity of the disease: the presence of low amounts of heterotypic neutralizing antibodies could prevent severe disease; in contrast, non-neutralizing, cross-reactive antibodies can augment Dengue virus infection of Fcγ receptor-positive cells such as monocytes and macrophages. This phenomenon termed antibody-dependent enhancement (ADE) of infection has been hypothesized to occur in vivo during secondary infections.[18]

It has been demonstrated that following primary infection, the Dengue virus-specific memory T lymphocyte population is composed predominantly of serotype cross-reactive T lymphocyte clones. This observation has led to a new integrated hypothesis arguing that during secondary infection, non-neutralizing antibodies can increase the number of Dengue-infected monocytes via ADE. In addition, serotype cross-reative CD8+ and CD4+ T lymphocytes are activated and produce high levels of lymphokines. Marked T cell and monocyte activation results in the production of higher levels of cytokines and chemical mediators that consequently induce malfunction of vascular endothelial cells and derangement of blood coagulation with the final outcome of plasma leakage, shock and hemorrhagic manifestations.[19,20] Massive complement activation is also present.[21] Recently, it has been suggested that an inappropriate "T cell" response could contribute to immunopathology while doing little to clear the virus. T cells with relatively low affinity for the serotype of the secondary infection and high affinity for those that produced the primary infection have been demonstrated.[21]

Besides secondary infection, other factors depending on the host, the virus and the epidemiological/ecological conditions contribute to the development of DHF, both in individuals and in epidemics. These have been identified in Figure 12.9.[22] Age (children have a higher risk of developing DHF/DSS), chronic diseases such as intrinsic asthma, diabetes mellitus, sickle cell anemia, ethnicity (higher risk in Whites than Blacks) and the genetic background of the individual represent host factors for severe disease.[22–24]

Four viruses have been associated with DHF/DSS epidemics. However, serotypes 2 and 3 and some particular genotypes are the most frequently reported. Several mutations that are associated with changes in virulence have been identified in the genome of Dengue 2 virus belonging to the Asian genotype; a decreased ability to replicate in human monocyte-derived macrophages of American strains has also been observed.[25–26]

Clinical features

The spectrum of the disease is broad. Most of the infections are asymptomatic or very mild, characterized by undifferentiated fever with or without rash mainly in infants and young children. Studies performed in Cuba provide evidence that for each clinically reported case at least 10 sub-clinical or asymptomatic infections may occur.[5] Given limited access to medical services in many countries, it is conceivable that this relation could be higher.

Classic dengue fever is a febrile viral syndrome of sudden onset, characterized by fever for 2–5 days, severe headache, intense myalgia, arthralgia, retroorbital pain and, sometimes, a diffuse morbilliform rash that may be pruritic and heals with desquamation

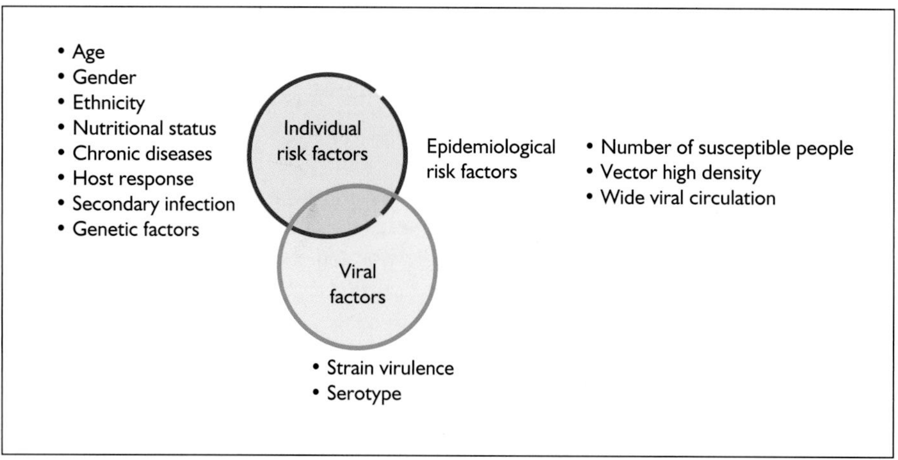

Figure 12.9 Risk Factors for DHF/DSS: and integral hypothesis.

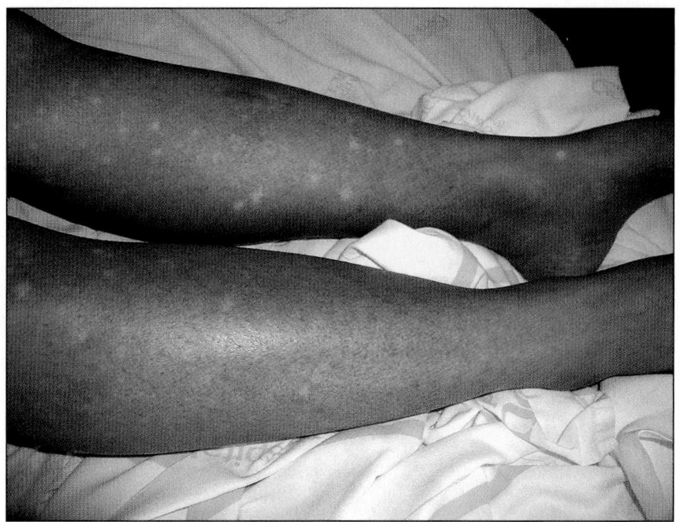

Figure 12.10 Diffuse morbiliforum rash affecting the lower limbs. (Courtesy of Dr. Ivo Castello Branco.)

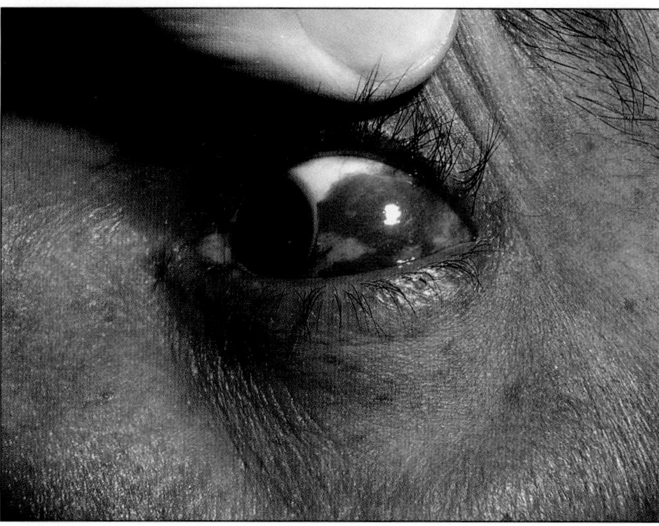

Figure 12.11 Minor hemorrhagic ocular lesions. (Courtesy of Dr. Ivo Castello Branco.)

(Fig. 12.10).[1] Skin hemorrhage and petechiae are frequently observed. Leukopenia and thrombocytopenia may be observed. Recovery is slow, characterized by massive fatigue and severe depression, especially in adults. In some epidemics unusual bleeding has been described.[1,12]

DHF is characterized by high fever, hemorrhagic phenomena[7,12,27,28] —often with enlargement of the liver — and circulatory failure. Thrombocytopenia (below 100 000/mm^3) and hemoconcentration (hematocrit > = 20% or associated signs of plasma leakage such as pleural effusion, ascites, hypoproteinemia) are regularly present. Plasma leakage is the major pathophysiological alteration that determines the severity of the disease in DHF and differentiates it from Dengue fever.

DHF is more likely to develop if an individual previously infected with one serotype is later infected with a different viral serotype.[15] It is primarily recognized in children less than 15 years and has a more severe course, including vomiting, facial flushing and circumoral cyanosis, and weakness.[1] Minor bleeding phenomena such as epistaxis, petechiae, and gingival bleeding may occur at any time but major bleeding phenomena such as menorrhagia and gastrointestinal hemorrhage are poor prognostic indicators[1] (Fig. 12.9–12.13).

Diffuse capillary leakage of plasma is responsible for the hemoconcentration. In the presence of hemoconcentration and thrombocytopenia, the patient is considered to have DHF as classified according to the World Health Organization (Table 12.3).[12] DHF is a potentially deadly complication that is characterized by high fever, hemorrhagic phenomena – often with enlargement of the liver – and, in severe cases, circulatory failure.[12] The illness commonly begins with a sudden rise in temperature accompanied by facial flush and other non-specific constitutional symptoms of dengue fever. The fever usually continues for 2–7 days and can be as high as 40–41°C, possibly with febrile convulsions and hemorrhagic phenomena.[12] In moderate DHF cases, all signs and symptoms abate after the fever subsides (grades I and II). In severe cases, the patient's condition may suddenly deteriorate after a few days of fever; the temperature drops, followed by signs of circulatory failure, and the patient may rapidly go into a critical state of shock and die within 12–24 h (dengue shock syndrome: DSS).[12] The case-fatality of DHF/DSS is 10% or higher if untreated. With supportive treatment, fewer than 1% of such cases succumb.

Warning signs are valuable as early predictors of DHF/DSS. Intensive and ongoing abdominal pain, intense vomiting, sudden

Table 12.3 World Health Organization classification of dengue hemorrhagic fever

	Signs and symptoms
Grade I	Thrombocytopenia + hemoconcentration. Absence of spontaneous bleeding
Grade II	Thrombocytopenia + hemoconcentration. Presence of spontaneous bleeding
Grade III	Thrombocytopenia + hemoconcentration. Hemodynamic instability: filiform pulse, narrowing of the pulse pressure (< 20 mmHg), cold extremities, and mental confusion
Grade IV	Thrombocytopenia + hemoconcentration. Declared shock, patient pulseless and with arterial blood pressure = 0 mmHg (dengue shock syndrome: DSS)

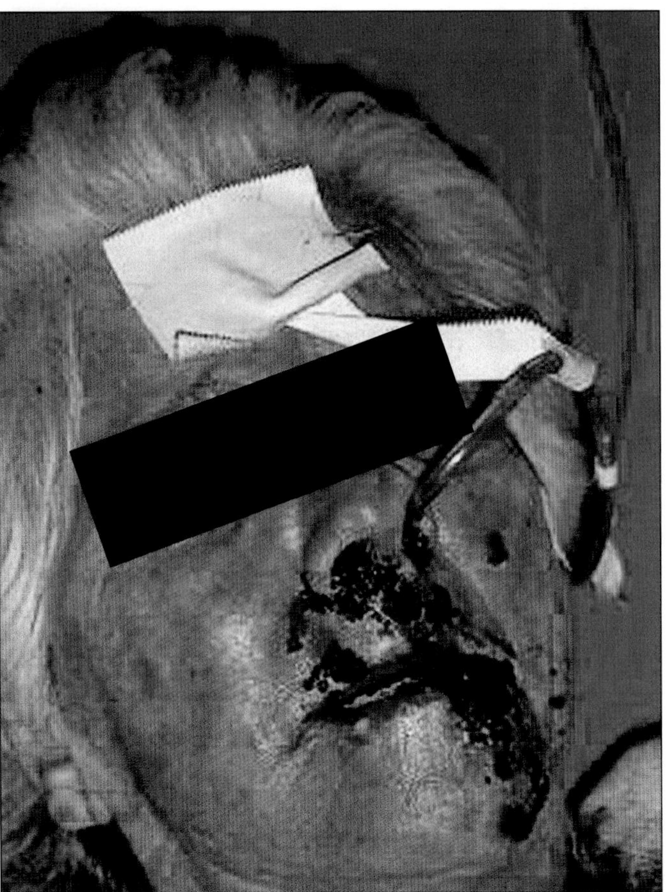

Figure 12.12 Dengue hemorrhagic fever grade III, with gastrointestinal hemorrhage, thrombocytopenia, hemodynamic instability, and mental confusion.

decrease of temperature, irritability, depression lethargy, or ultrasound evidence of plasma leakage indicate that a rapid and appropiate treatment must be administered.[12,28]

Diagnosis and differential diagnosis

The differential diagnosis in the early phase of Dengue is difficult. Meningococcaemia, leptospirosis, malaria, typhus, yellow fever, other hemorrhagic viral fevers, influenza, rubella and other diseases producing rash, must be considered.[1,6,28]

Confirmation of the suspected diagnosis can be done by serological studies and by virus detection. Dengue IgM detection is routinely used as a serological marker of recent infection. 5-6 days after the onset of fever, dengue IgM can be detected by IgM ELISA. This assay is 95% sensitive and is widely employed. The determination of IgG antibodies in paired sera provides serological confirmation. A fourfold increase in anti-Dengue IgG titer is confirmatory. Viral isolation mainly in mosquito cell lines followed by identification using immunofluorescence techniques with specific Dengue antibodies and genome detection using the polymerase chain reaction (PCR) represent methods for virus detection. The virus can be recovered from acute serum samples collected in the first days after onset of fever and in tissues (liver, spleen, lymph nodes and others) in fatal cases.[29,30]

Serotype determination should be done by PCR and virus isolation. At present, the neutralization test is the only serological assay for serotype determination.

Treatment

Treatment of dengue is non-specific and supportive. For patients with severe bleeding and shock syndrome, measures to correct hypovolemia, hypoxia, and shock can reduce complications and death. The use of high doses of corticosteroids has not been shown to alter mortality rates in this situation.[1,7] Specific chemotherapies under investigation include interferon and ribavirin.[31] When interferon is administered to monkeys within 8 h of infection, mortality is reduced; however, interferon is ineffective when given at 24 h.[31] The use of interferon in combination with other immune-enhancing drugs is continuing to be researched. Ribavirin, although effective in vitro, has not been proven effective in vivo because of an inability to achieve sufficient concentrations in the blood.[31]

An effective vaccine against dengue is a difficult task since the different serotypes of the dengue virus are present in most countries, and a future infection with other serotypes can predispose to DHF.[7]

Prophylaxis

Prevention and control of the arthropod vector rely on insecticides, barrier measures, protective clothing, bed netting, and insect repellents.[1,8] In Asia and the Americas, *Aedes aegypti* breeds primarily in artificial containers like earthenware jars, metal drums, and concrete cisterns used for domestic water storage, as well as discarded plastic food containers, used automobile tires, and other items that collect rainwater. In Africa it also breeds extensively in natural habitats such as tree holes and leaf axils. In recent years, *A. albopictus*, a secondary dengue vector in Asia, has become established in the USA, several Latin American and Caribbean countries, and in parts of Europe.[8] The rapid geographic spread of this species has been largely attributed to the international trade in used tires.[8]

Vector control is implemented using environmental management and chemical methods. Proper solid waste disposal and improved water storage practices, including covering containers to prevent access by egg-laying female mosquitoes, are among the methods that are encouraged through community-based programs.[8,12] The application of appropriate insecticides to larval habitats, particularly those that are considered useful by householders, e.g., water storage vessels, prevent mosquito breeding for several weeks but must be reapplied periodically.[8,12] Biocontrol efforts include the use of predatory fish to reduce larvae populations. These methods are interesting option for the long-term control of the infection in endemic areas.[8]

A Dengue vaccine must confer long-lasting protective immunity against the four Dengue serotypes in order to avoid the ADE phenomenon and sensitization to future Dengue infections and consequently DHF/DSS. Six vaccine candidates are currently under study.[32–34] Two attenuated live and four live chimeric vaccine candidates, the former generated by passaging each of the four dengue viruses in non-human tissue cultures and the last generated by introducing prM and E genes from Dengue virus into the full length cDNA of attenuated yellow fever or Dengue vaccine viruses constitute new windows of opportunity.[32–34]

Four principles are crucial for Dengue control: political will (financial support, human resources); improvement of public health infrastructure and vector control programmes as well as, intersectorial coordination (partnerships among donors, the public sector, civil society, non-government organizations and private as well as commercial sectors); active community participation; and reinforcement of health legislation.[35] Currently, new initiatives for Dengue management are being conducted by international organizations in order to supply endemic countries with affordable tools for Dengue control. Integrated Dengue monitoring and control, insecticide-treated curtains, improved formulations of larvicides, the implementation of the Dengue/Net, a global system for standardized epidemiological and virological surveillance and the COMBI approach (Communication for Behavioral Impact) will assist planners in developing sustained community action plans for Dengue prevention and control.[36]

References

1. Halstead SB. Dengue. Curr Opin Infect Dis 2002;15:471–476.
2. Mahe A, Lamaury I, Strobel M. Mucocutaneous manifestations of dengue. Presse Med 1998; 27:1909–1913.
3. Gubler DJ. Dengue and dengue hemorrhagic fever: Its history and resurgence as a global public health problem. In: Gubler DJ, Kuno G (eds.), Cab International, New York: 1997;1–22.
4. Hammon WM, Rudnick A, Sather G, et al. New hemorrhagic fevers of children in the Philippines and Thailand. Trans Assoc Am Physicians 1960; 73:140–155.
5. Kouri GP, Guzman MG, Bravo JR, et al. Dengue haemorrhagic fever/dengue shock syndrome: lessons from the Cuban epidemic, 1981. Bull World Health Organ 1989; 67:375–380.
6. Isturiz RE, Gubler DJ, Brea del Castillo J. Dengue and dengue hemorrhagic fever in Latin America and Caribbean. Infect Dis Clin North Am 2000; 14: 121–140.
7. Guzman MG, Kouri G. Dengue: an update. Lancet Infect Dis 2002; 2:33–42.
8. Guzman MG, Kouri G. Dengue and dengue hemorrhagic fever in the Americas: lessons and challenges. J Clin Virol 2003; 27:1–13.
9. World Health Organization. Scientific Working Group on Dengue. Meeting Report, Geneva, Switzerland, 3-5 April 2000.
10. Farmer P. Social inequalities and emerging infectious diseases. Emerg Infect Dis 1996; 2:259–269.
11. Gubler DJ. The changing epidemiology of yellow fever and dengue, 1900 to 2003: full circle? Comp Immunol Microbiol Infect Dis 2004; 27:319–330.
12. Pan American Health Organization. Dengue and dengue hemorrhagic fever in the Americas: Guidelines for prevention and control. Scientific publication No. 548, 1994.
13. Kuno G. Factors influencing the transmission of dengue viruses. In: Gubler DJ, Kuno G (eds.). Cab International, New York, 1997: 61–88.
14. Lindback H, Lindback J, Tegnell A, et al. Dengue Fever in travelers to the tropics, 1998 and 1999. Emerg Infect Dis 2003; 9: 438–442.
15. Halstead SB. The Alexander D. Langmuir Lecture. The pathogenesis of dengue. Molecular epidemiology in infectious disease. Am J Epidemiol 1981; 114:632–648.
16. Sangkawibha N, Rojanasuphot S, Ahandrik S, et al. Risk factors in dengue shock syndrome: a prospective epidemiologic study in Rayong, Thailand. I. The 1980 outbreak. Am J Epidemiol 1984; 120:653–669.
17. Guzman MG, Kouri G, Valdes L, et al. Epidemiologic studies on Dengue in Santiago de Cuba, 1997. Am J Epidemiol 2000; 152:793–799; discussion 804.
18. Halstead SB. Antibody, macrophages, dengue virus infection, shock, and hemorrhage: a pathogenetic cascade. Rev Infect Dis 1989;11: (Suppl 4):S830–S839.
19. Kurane I, Takasaki T. Dengue fever and dengue haemorrhagic fever: challenges of controlling an enemy still at large. Rev Med Virol 2001; 11:301–311.
20. Rothman AL. Dengue: defining protective versus pathologic immunity. J Clin Invest 2004; 113:946–951.
21. Mongkolsapaya J, Dejnirattisai W, Xu XN, et al. Original antigenic sin and apoptosis in the pathogenesis of dengue hemorrhagic fever. Nat Med 2003; 9:921–927.
22. Kouri GP, Guzman MG, Bravo JR. Why dengue haemorrhagic fever in Cuba? 2. An integral analysis. Trans R Soc Trop Med Hyg 1987; 81:821-823.
23. Bravo JR, Guzman MG, Kouri GP. Why dengue haemorrhagic fever in Cuba? 1. Individual risk factors for dengue haemorrhagic fever/dengue shock syndrome (DHF/DSS). Trans R Soc Trop Med Hyg 1987; 81:816–820.
24. Guzman MG, Kouri GP, Bravo J, et al. Effect of age on outcome of secondary dengue 2 infections. Int J Infect Dis 2002; 6:118–124.
25. Leitmeyer KC, Vaughn DW, Watts DM, et al. Dengue virus structural differences that correlate with pathogenesis. J Virol 1999; 73:4738–4747.
26. Cologna R, Rico-Hesse R. American genotype structures decrease dengue virus output from human monocytes and dendritic cells. J Virol 2003; 77:3929–3938.
27. John TJ. Dengue fever and dengue hemorrhagic fever. Lancet 2003; 361:181–182.
28. Martinez E. Dengue hemorrágico en criancas. Editorial Jose Marti, La Habana, 1992: 1–180.
29. Guzman MG, Kouri G. Dengue diagnosis, advances and challenges. Int J Infect Dis 2004; 8:69–80.
30. Guzman MG, Kouri G. Advances in dengue diagnosis. Clin Diagn Lab Immunol 1996; 3:621–627.
31. Crance JM, Scaramozzino N, Jouan A, et al. Interferon, ribavirin, 6-azauridine and glycyrrhizin: antiviral compounds active against pathogenic flaviviruses. Antiviral Res 2003; 58:73–79.
32. Jacobs M, Young P. Dengue vaccines: preparing to roll back dengue. Curr Opin Investig Drugs 2003; 4:168–171.
33. Halstead SB, Deen J. The future of dengue vaccines. Lancet 2002; 360:1243–1245.
34. Pang T. Vaccines for the prevention of neglected diseases—dengue fever. Curr Opin Biotechnol 2003; 14:332–336.
35. Kroeger A, Nathan M, Hombach J, et al. Dengue. Nat Rev Microbiol 2004; 2:360–361.
36. Guzman MG, Kouri G, Diaz M, et al. Dengue, one of the great emerging health challenges of the 21st century. Expert Rev Vaccines 2004; 3:511–520.

Yellow fever

Omar Lupi and Leticia Spinelli

Introduction

Yellow fever, the original viral hemorrhagic fever, has caused large epidemics in Africa and the Americas. It can be recognized from historic texts stretching back 400 years. Infection causes a wide spectrum of disease, from mild symptoms to severe illness and death. The "yellow" in the name is explained by the jaundice that affects some patients. Although an effective vaccine has been available for 60 years, the number of people infected over the last two decades has increased and yellow fever is now a serious public health issue again. Today the disease still affects as many as 200 000 persons annually in tropical regions of Africa and South America.[1,2]

History

Yellow fever was first recognized in an outbreak occurring in the New World in 1648. Slave-trading vessels infested with *Aedes aegypti* (mosquito) most likely introduced the yellow fever virus from West Africa, with similar outbreaks occurring in port cities in the New World and in Europe. Sanitation measures, such as piped water, greatly diminished the transmission of the disease.

The viral cause of yellow fever was not discovered until after 1928, which led to Theiler's discovery of the attenuated 17D vaccine strain in the 1930s that earned him a Nobel prize.[1,2]

Epidemiology

Humans and monkeys are the principal animals to be infected. The virus is carried from one animal to another (horizontal transmission) by a biting mosquito (the vector). The mosquito can also pass the virus via infected eggs to its offspring (vertical transmission). The eggs produced are resistant to drying and lie dormant through dry conditions, hatching when the rainy season begins. Therefore, the mosquito is the true reservoir of the virus, ensuring transmission from one year to the next.[3,4]

Several different species of the *Aedes* and *Haemogogus* (South America only) mosquitoes transmit the yellow fever virus (Fig. 12.13). These mosquitoes are either domestic (i.e., they breed around houses), wild (they breed in the jungle), or semidomestic types (they display a mixture of habits). Any region populated with these mosquitoes can potentially harbor the disease. Control programs successfully eradicated mosquito habitats in the past, especially in South America. However, these programs have lapsed over the last 30 years and mosquito populations have increased. This favors epidemics of yellow fever.[5]

There are three types of transmission cycles for yellow fever: sylvatic, intermediate, and urban. All three cycles exist in Africa, but in South America only sylvatic and urban yellow fever occur.[5]

Sylvatic (or jungle) yellow fever

In tropical rain forests, yellow fever occurs in monkeys that are infected by wild mosquitoes. The infected monkeys can then pass the virus on to other mosquitoes that feed on them. These infected wild mosquitoes bite humans entering the forest, resulting in sporadic cases of yellow fever. The majority of cases are young men working in the forest (logging, etc.). On occasion, the virus spreads beyond the affected individual.[5]

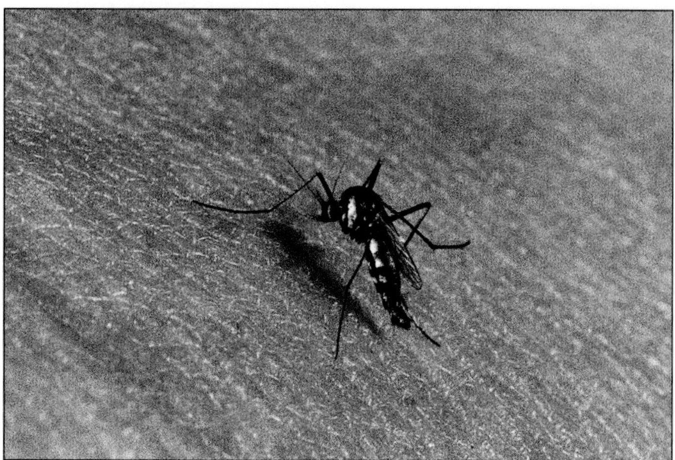

Figure 12.13 *Haemogogus* mosquito bite. (Courtesy of Dr.Genilton Vieira, FIOCRUZ/RJ.)

Intermediate yellow fever

In humid or semihumid savannas of Africa, small-scale epidemics occur. These behave differently from urban epidemics; many separate villages in an area suffer cases simultaneously, but fewer people die from infection. Semidomestic mosquitoes infect both monkey and human hosts. This area is often called the "zone of emergence," where increased contact between humans and infected mosquitoes leads to disease. This is the most common type of outbreak seen in recent decades in Africa. It can shift to a more severe urban-type epidemic if the infection is carried into a suitable environment (with the presence of domestic mosquitoes and unvaccinated humans).[5]

Urban yellow fever

Large epidemics can occur when migrants introduce the virus into areas with high human population density. Domestic mosquitoes (of one species, *Aedes aegypti*) carry the virus from person to person; no monkeys are involved in transmission (Fig. 12.14).

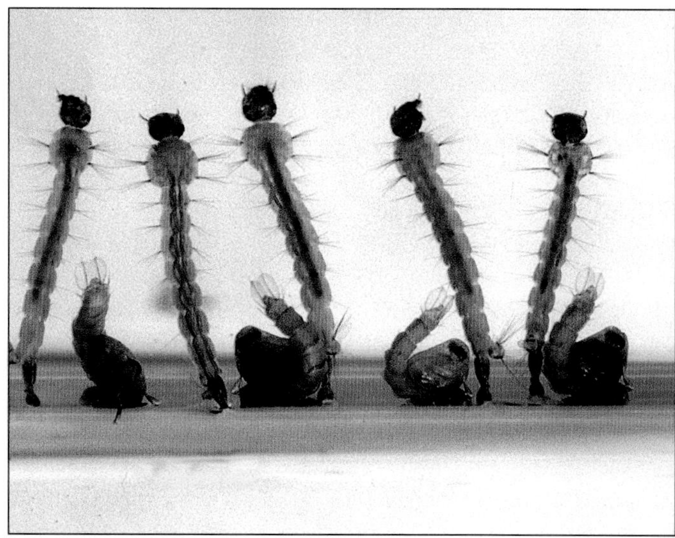

Figure 12.14 *Aedes aegypti* larvae. (Courtesy of Dr.Genilton Vieira, FIOCRUZ/RJ.)

These outbreaks tend to spread outwards from one source to cover a wide area.[4]

Yellow fever transmission predominantly occurs in areas of sub-Saharan Africa and South America 15° north and 10° south of the Equator. It has never been documented in Asia.[5]

Yellow fever epidemics were dominant in Africa from 1986 to 1991, with close to 20 000 cases and 6000 deaths. This is considered to be grossly underestimated because of underreporting. These epidemics commonly include 30–1000 cases and have fatality ratios of 20–50%. In areas of West Africa, 200 000 endemic cases may occur annually. In South America, an annual mean of 100 cases has been reported for the last 25 years. These cases predominate from January to March among males aged 15–45 years who work outdoors in agriculture and forestry. The last outbreak in the western hemisphere occurred in 1954 in Trinidad.[5]

The last epidemic of yellow fever in North America occurred in New Orleans in 1905: in this epidemic more than 3000 cases were met with 452 deaths. Because *A. aegypti* has now reinfested the southeastern USA, autochthonous transmission in the USA is possible.[5]

Yellow fever's range continues to expand, now including areas in which it was previously believed to be eradicated (e.g., eastern and southern African countries).

The virus is constantly present with low levels of infection (i.e., endemic) in some tropical areas of Africa and the Americas. This viral presence can amplify into regular epidemics. Until the start of this century, yellow fever outbreaks also occurred in Europe, the Caribbean islands, and Central and North America. Even though the virus is not felt to be present in these areas now, they must still be considered at risk for yellow fever epidemics.[1,5]

Pathogenesis and etiology

Yellow fever virus is in the genus *Flavivirus* of the family Flaviviridae (group B arbovirus). The *Flavivirus* genus is comprised of more than 68 arthropod-transmitted viruses, of which 30 are known to cause human disease. Other flaviviral infections include dengue, Japanese encephalitis, St. Louis encephalitis, and tick-borne encephalitis.[5]

The virus can be isolated in mosquitoes, arthropods, and vertebrate tissue cultures; baby mice; and several monkey species. Rhesus monkeys regularly succumb following experimental inoculation, and their disease mimics severe human disease.[3,5]

The pathophysiology of yellow fever infection was largely inferred from vaccine studies in rhesus monkeys using the attenuated 17D vaccine. After inoculation in rhesus monkeys, the virus replicated initially in local lymph nodes, followed by blood-borne spread and subsequent replication, mostly occurring in regional lymph tissue, spleen, and bone marrow, followed by the liver, lung, and adrenal glands.[1,5]

The liver and kidneys demonstrate the greatest degree of pathologic changes. Hemorrhage and erosion of the gastric mucosa lead to hematemesis, popularly known as "black vomit." Hepatocellular damage is characterized by lobular necrosis with the subsequent formation of Councilman bodies. Albuminuria and renal insufficiency evolve secondary to the prerenal component of yellow fever, ultimately leading to acute tubular necrosis with advanced disease. Fatty infiltration of the myocardium, including the conduction system, can lead to myocarditis and arrhythmias.[5]

Central nervous system findings can be attributed to cerebral edema and hemorrhages compounded on metabolic disturbances. The bleeding diathesis of this disease can be attributed to reduced hepatic synthesis of clotting factors, thrombocytopenia, and platelet dysfunction. The terminal event of shock can be attributed to a combination of direct parenchymal damage and a systemic inflammatory response.[2]

Clinical features

The skin is icteric, and there may be multiple hemorrhages or petechiae of the skin, mucous membranes, and multiple organs.

The virus remains silent in the body during an incubation period of 3–6 days.

There are then two disease phases. The first, acute phase is normally characterized by fever, muscle pain (with prominent backache), headache, shivers, loss of appetite, nausea, and/or vomiting. Often, the high fever is paradoxically associated with a slow pulse. After 3–4 days most patients improve and their symptoms disappear.[5]

However, 15% enter a toxic phase within 24 h. Fever reappears and several body systems are affected. The patient rapidly develops jaundice and complains of abdominal pain with vomiting (Fig. 12.15). Bleeding can occur from the mouth, nose, eyes, and/or stomach. Once this happens, blood appears in the vomit and feces. Kidney function deteriorates; this can range from abnormal protein levels in the urine (albuminuria) to complete kidney failure with no urine production (anuria). Half of the patients in the toxic phase die within 10–14 days. The remainder recover without significant organ damage. Convalescence with symptoms of weakness and fatigue may last up to 3 months. Convalescence with symptoms of weakness and fatigue may last up to 3 months.[4,5]

Diagnosis and differential diagnosis

To arrive at a diagnosis, consider the patient's clinical features and his or her places and dates of travel, including the epidemiological history of the places visited, immunizations, and activities.

Specific diagnosis depends on isolation of virus from blood, demonstration of viral antigen in serum by ELISA or of viral RNA by PCR during the period of infection. Serologic diagnosis includes

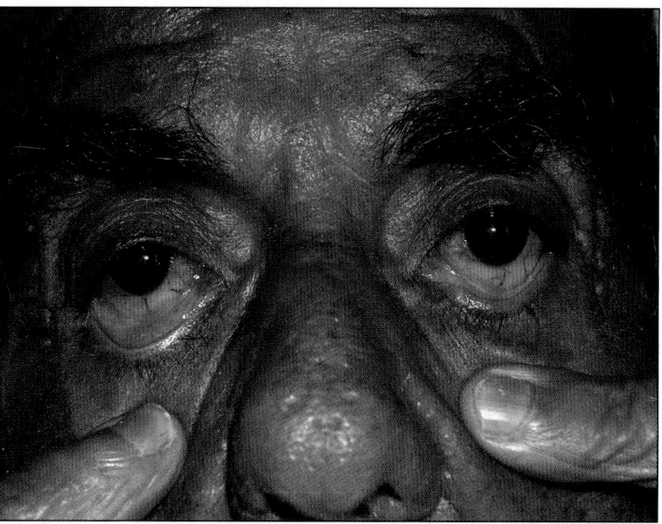

Figure 12.15 Jaundice due to yellow fever.

IgM antibody-capture ELISA, hemagglutination inhibition (HI), complement fixation (CF), or neutralization (N) tests.[5] It is important to consider that IgM, HI, and N antibodies appear within 5–7 days and CF antibodies within 7–14 days of onset. Thus, paired acute and convalescent sera should be tested (at an interval of 14 days). IgM testing by ELISA is the preferred method of testing. This assay is 95% sensitive when serum specimens are collected 7–10 days after the onset of illness.[5]

Liver biopsy confirms the diagnosis by isolation of virus (direct immunofluorescence or DNA hybridization), but it is absolutely contraindicated because of the bleeding diathesis. Pathologic examination of the liver may suggest, but not assure, a postmortem diagnosis.[5]

Yellow fever is difficult to recognize, especially during the early stages. The mild form of yellow fever is not distinguishable from other tropical fevers. Severe yellow fever simulates viral hepatitis, dengue fever, leptospirosis, and malignant malaria.[2,5]

Laboratory findings include: leukopenia and neutropenia; a very low erythrocyte sedimentation rate, with values approaching 0; thrombocytopenia; increase in serum bilirubin (predominantly direct); possibly presence of fibrin degradation products; marked increase in serum transaminase levels; alkaline phosphatase levels are generally normal; increased blood urea nitrogen and serum creatinine (second phase of disease); hypoglycemia (second phase of disease), albuminuria (300–500 mg%), bilirubinuria; prolonged time of coagulation; normal cerebrospinal fluid.[2,5]

Pathology

The lesions of yellow fever involve primarily the liver, heart, kidneys, and lymphoid tissues. Histologic findings are often characteristic in patients who die before the ninth day of illness, but the lesions are not always pathognomononic. The most striking lesion is the eosinophilic degeneration and coagulation of hepatocytes (Councilman's bodies). Intranuclear eosinophilic granular inclusions or enlarged nucleoli (Torres bodies) are also described.[3]

Treatment

Patients should be protected from mosquito bites to avoid spread of the infection and blood and needle precautions should be instituted. No specific antiviral therapy is available for yellow fever. Specific chemotherapies under investigation include interferon and ribavirin.[5]

Treatment aims basically for relief of symptoms and support of the patient. Adjunctive measures include non-hepatotoxic antipyretics to reduce fever and pain and an H_2-receptor antagonist to prevent gastric bleeding. Use of heparin for documented cases of disseminated intravascular coagulation is controversial.[5]

Avoid drugs that act centrally, including phenothiazines, barbiturates, and benzodiazepines because they may precipitate or aggravate encephalopathy. Avoid drugs dependent on hepatic metabolism, and, in cases of reduced renal function, medications should be renally dosed. Electrolyte imbalance should be corrected.[1]

References

1. Monath TP. Yellow fever: an update. Lancet Infect Dis 2001; 1:11–20.
2. Monath TP. Flaviviruses. In: Mandell GL, Bennett JE, Dolin R. Mandell Douglas and Bennett's principles and practice of infectious diseases, 4th edn. New York: Churchill-Livingstone; 1995.
3. Shope RE. Hemorrhagic fever viruses. In: Goldman L, Bennett JC. Cecil textbook of medicine, 21st edn. Philadelphia, PA: WB Saunders; 2000.
4. World Health Organization. Viral hemorrhagic fevers. Geneva: WHO; 2001.
5. Lupi O, Tyring S. Tropical dermatology: viral tropical diseases. J Am Acad Dermatol 2003; 49:975–1000.

Chapter 13

Poxviruses

Joachim Richter, Karl Heinz Richter* and Dieter Häussinger

Introduction

Since the last natural smallpox infection, reported in Somalia in 1977, human poxvirus infections (other than molluscum contagiosum) have only been observed sporadically either after vaccination with *Poxvirus officinale* (vaccinia), or due to zoonotic poxviruses, such as monkeypox, catpox, or tanapoxvirus. As it is highly lethal and infectious, smallpox virus is feared for its potential use by bioterrorists.[1]

History

Smallpox epidemics have decimated whole populations since antiquity. Smallpox has been demonstrated in Egyptian mummies. Indian (Shitala) and African/Afro–American (Shapanan) divinities share the characteristics of both deadly disease and protection of the person who has already survived the disease.[2] In 1798, Edward Jenner made use of the observation that milkers who had contracted cowpox did not suffer from smallpox. This was the beginning of vaccination, i.e., the inoculation of cowpox virus in order to protect against smallpox (Latin: vacca = cow). Smallpox eradication is the greatest success story of the World Health Organization (WHO). Once eradication was declared by the WHO in May 1980, compulsory vaccination was generally abandoned. Monkeypox was initially recognized in 1958 in captive primates. The first human cases were reported in 1970 in the Congo. Since then, monkeypox has been reported sporadically in humans in Africa but not outside Africa until 2003, when the infection first appeared in the USA.[3]

Tanapox virus was first recognized in 1957 after an outbreak among schoolchildren in Kenya, in a village of the Tana river valley.[4] Indications for smallpox vaccination have been newly established in order to prepare for bioterroristic attacks as well as to prevent monkeypox, as this has been imported into the USA.

Epidemiology

Poxviruses which can affect humans comprise four main genera:[5] orthopox, yatapox, parapox, and molluscipox virus (Table 13.1). Orthopox viridae are endemic in many animals throughout the world. The natural hosts of poxviruses are usually rodents, which can occasionally transmit the virus to humans. Monkeypox is a zoonotic poxvirus infection endemic in Africa; it was imported from Ghana to the USA in 2003 by infected Gambia giant rats and transmitted to prairie dogs and humans.[3] Although human-to-human transmission of monkeypox may occur, further spread among humans is limited. Other zoonotic poxvirus infections occur sporadically, e.g., cowpox or catpox.[6–8] These orthopox viruses usually cause self-limited infections, but may become life-threatening in immunocompromised patients or subjects suffering from a predisposing skin disease. This also applies to the virus used for vaccination against smallpox, *P. officinale* (vaccinia virus). This virus may sometimes be inadvertently transmitted from a smallpox vaccinee to another individual.

Non-orthopox viruses comprise pseudocowpox (milker's nodules) and yatapox viruses, including tanapox virus.[4] Human tanapox occurs sporadically in Africa or in individuals handling laboratory animals.[5,6,9,10] Tanapox is acquired by direct contact with infected non-human primates, and the infection cycle appears to be maintained between primates and mosquitoes.

For molluscipox virus causing molluscum contagiosum, the distribution is worldwide, and it is not considered to be a tropical disease.

*This chapter is dedicated to the memory of our coauthor Professor Emeritus Karl Heinz Richter, who was a distinguished smallpox specialist and who has managed three smallpox outbreaks in Germany. He died during the writing of this chapter.

Table 13.1 Poxviruses that may cause disease in humans

Genus and species	Primary reservoir	Other hosts	Geographic region	Mode of transmission	Protection provided by vaccinia vaccination
Orthopoxvirus (OPV)					
Smallpox (variola major-virus), alastrim (variola minor-virus)	High-security laboratories in Russia and USA		Declared eradicated in 1980 Maintained in high-security laboratories in USA and Russia	Direct contact, respiratory droplets	Yes
Vaccinia (*OPV officinale*)[a]	Laboratories producing dermovaccine			Direct contact, inoculation	
Cowpox/catpox (*OPV bovis*)	Rodents	Ungulates, cats	Europe, Africa, central and northern Asia	Direct contact	Yes
Monkeypox (*OPV simiae*)	Rodents	Monkeys, apes, prairie dogs, other mammals (?)	Central and West Africa	Direct contact, respiratory droplets	Yes
Other OPV	Rodents	Mammals (ungulates, camels, elephants, raccoons, voles, dogs, cats), birds	Worldwide?	Direct contact	Yes
Yatapoxvirus (YPV)					
Tanapox	Non-human primates		Central and East Africa	Direct contact	No
Yabapox	Non-human primates		Central Africa	Direct contact	No
Parapoxvirus (PPV)					
Pseudocowpox (milkers nodules and paravaccinia)	Ungulates		Worldwide	Direct contact	No
Bovine papular stomatitis	Ungulates		North America, Africa, Australia, New Zealand, Europe	Direct contact	No
Orf	Ungulates		North America, New Zealand, Europe	Direct contact	No
Sealpox	Seals		Atlantic and Pacific Ocean, North Sea	Direct contact	No
Molluscipoxvirus					
Molluscipox (molluscum contagiosum)	Humans		Worldwide	Direct contact	No

[a]It is not clear if the modified orthopoxvirus cultured for smallpox vaccination originates from a cowpox- or an equine orthopoxvirus

Pathogenesis and etiology

Poxvirus penetrates into the organism by virus-containing material coming into contact with the skin or with the respiratory tract (smallpox and monkeypox). Smallpox virus replicates at the site of contact and in the local lymph nodes. Subsequently, primary viremia develops, followed by multiplication of the virus in the reticulo-endothelial system during the incubation period. Secondary viremia is accompanied by fever and the cutaneous eruptions appear.

Clinical features

Poxviruses typically produce skin lesions, initially presenting as maculae or papules which evolve to become vesicles and pustules, which eventually dry up, forming a crust. The multifaceted clinical pictures due to poxviruses and the clinical course of smallpox are shown in Figure 13.1 and Tables 13.2–13.3. Complications after smallpox vaccination also share features with smallpox eruptions. When the infection is acquired by inoculation either by inadvertent

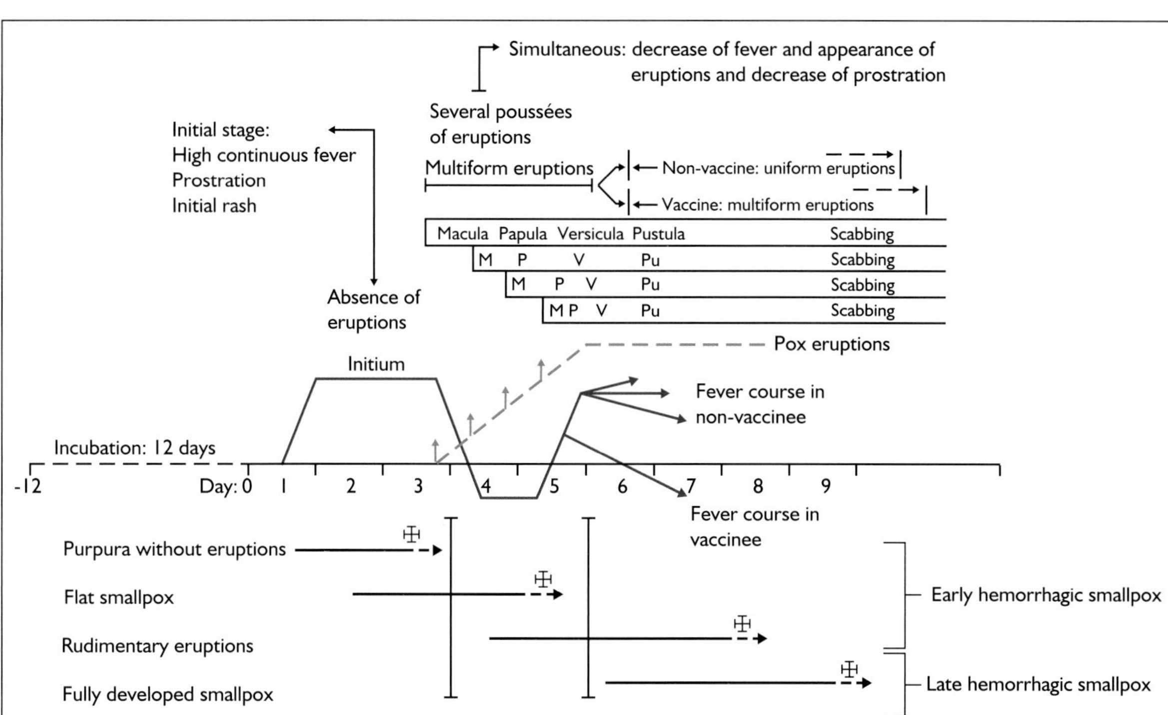

Figure 13.1 Clinical evolution of smallpox.

Table 13.2 Clinical presentations of poxvirus infections

Smallpox	Alastrim (variola minor) Smallpox in a vaccinee (variolois) Smallpox (variola major) Non-complicated smallpox Complicated smallpox Flat (hyporeactive) smallpox Early hemorrhagic smallpox (purpura variolosa) Late hemorrhagic smallpox (variola haemorrhagica)
Vaccinia	Allergic erythema multiforme after vaccinia inoculation Bacterial super infection (auto-)inoculation Vaccinia keratitis Eczema vaccinatum Generalized vaccinia Progressive vaccinia Post vaccinial encephalitis Fetal vaccinia Myocardial damage (?)
Monkeypox and other zoonotic orthopoxvirus infections	Non-complicated orthopoxvirus infection Complicated orthopoxvirus infection
Milker's nodule and paravaccinia Tanapox	Multiple stages: usually resolve within 6 weeks

contamination of a preexisting skin injury or by vaccination, a primary lesion appears on the respective site.

For smallpox surveillance the Center for Disease Control (CDC) and Prevention has established a case definition and various probability categories for smallpox[11,12] (Table 13.4). Monkeypox eruptions resemble those due to smallpox, but the clinical picture is usually less severe (Figs 13.2–13.4). In immunocompromised hosts, small children and infants, monkeypox is life-threatening. As with smallpox, monkeypox may present as a primarily hemorrhagic infection.[3,13–15] The reported lethality in Africa reaches 15% and more; breast-fed infants of monkeypox-infected mothers and malnourished children are at particular risk.[14] Also as with smallpox, generalized eruptions only appear after 2–3 days of febrile illness (Fig. 13.3). In other zoonotic poxvirus infections, a primary lesion appears at the inoculation site, and the clinical course is mild if the patient is immunocompetent.[5–8]

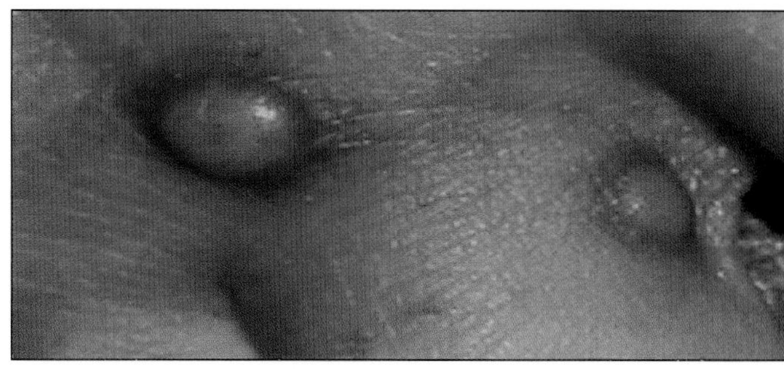

Figure 13.2 Pustules of monkeypox on the hand of a child in Wisconsin after handling an infected prairie dog. (Countesy of Dr. J. Melski.)

Table 13.3 Clinical courses and outcomes of smallpox

Date	Stage	Skin eruptions	Skin eruptions indicating complications	Contagiousness	Figures
−12 (−7 to −17) to 0 days	Incubation			None	
0–2	Initial/prodromal stage	High continuous fever and prostration Initial morbilliform rash and enanthem (mouth), easily overlooked	Early hemorrhagic smallpox (purpura variolosa), leading to death	Yes	Flat smallpox Purpura variolosa
2–3		M		High	Macular eruption
4–5	Eruptive stage: multiform eruptions	Different generations of M, P, V Fever recrudescence	Flat-type (rudimentary) pustules, (semi-)confluent eruptions, leading to death	High	Multiform early eruptions
6–10	Uniform appearance and pustulation[a]	Pu	Flat eruptions, leading to death Hemorrhage into eruptions (late hemorrhagic smallpox), leading to death	Highest	Uniform vesicles Uniform pustules Hemorrhagic vesicles (late hemorrhagic smallpox)
11–	Desiccation of eruptions	C and scarring		After scabs have fallen off, patients are no longer contagious	Crust

[a]In vaccines multiform eruptions persist.
M, macule; P, papule; V, vesicle (cental umbilication); Pu, pustule; C, crust.

Tanapox virus infection is usually a mild self-limiting disease which shares the febrile prodromal stage with other poxvirus infections. In tanapox, the prodrome is mild and may be accompanied by headache and myalgia.[3,6,7] Towards the end of the febrile phase, a mostly solitary erythematous macule appears. As the fever wanes, a papule appears and this expands to a diameter of approximately 1 cm. The center may become umbilicated, develop a necrotic crust, or deepen and form a nodule. On light skins the expanding nodule is surrounded by a reddish halo (Fig. 13.4). Regional lymphadenopathy appears 4–5 days after the appearance of the papule. The lesion can be extremely tender, and it may also be pruritic. The maximal diameter (approximately 2 cm) is reached at the end of the second week. From this point the lesion slowly involutes with the whole evolution–involution taking 6 weeks, leaving a small scar.

Patient evaluation, diagnosis, and differential diagnosis

Smallpox is likely to be initially misdiagnosed because clinicians are no longer familiar with the features of these infections. Because of the high lethality and infectivity of smallpox, it is necessary to differentiate smallpox as soon as possible from other diseases with vesicular eruptions, especially chickenpox. The CDC has therefore provided an algorithm for the probability of smallpox and for the differential diagnosis of papulovesicular eruptions:[11,12] a highly suspicious smallpox case is defined by an illness characterized by acute onset of fever (38.8°C/101°F) followed 1–4 days later by a centrifugal rash with firm deep-seated vesicles or pustules in the same stage of development without other apparent cause (Table 13.4; Fig. 13.5). The occurrence of a febrile prodrome before generalized eruption is an equally important criterion for monkeypox and catpox/cowpox. The suspicion of zoonotic poxvirus infections is raised by contact with animals, e.g., prairie dogs, cats, or other animals which can transmit poxviruses (Table 13.5).[3,12–15] The potentially transmitting animal must be traced and investigated for symptoms of poxvirus infection. Unique clinical features of tanapox are the nodular nature of tender lesions, the paucity of lesions, the lack of pustulation, the benign course of the disease, and the prolonged resolution of the rash.[3–6] Vaccinia (disease due to inoculation of the smallpox dermovaccine) is suspected when a smallpox vaccination has been administered or when the patient was in contact with a smallpox vaccinee within less than 21 days (inadvertent inoculation).[14] For differential diagnosis of poxvirus infection versus other papulovesicular eruptions, see Table 13.6 and Figures 13.5–13.18.

Other differential diagnoses comprise generalized herpes simplex or herpes zoster, impetigo, drug eruptions, and erythema multiforme. In rickettsialpox, an eschar (inoculation site with a black scar) is seen; this may sometimes be difficult to distinguish from an inoculation site of a poxvirus infection. Rickettsialpox rapidly responds to doxycycline.[16] The typical symptom of scabies is intense itching, especially at night, whereas pox eruptions are painful and lesions are tender to palpate. Scabies and molluscum contagiosum are not accompanied by fever. Early (flat) hemorrhagic smallpox (Figs 13.13–13.16) and hemorrhagic monkeypox

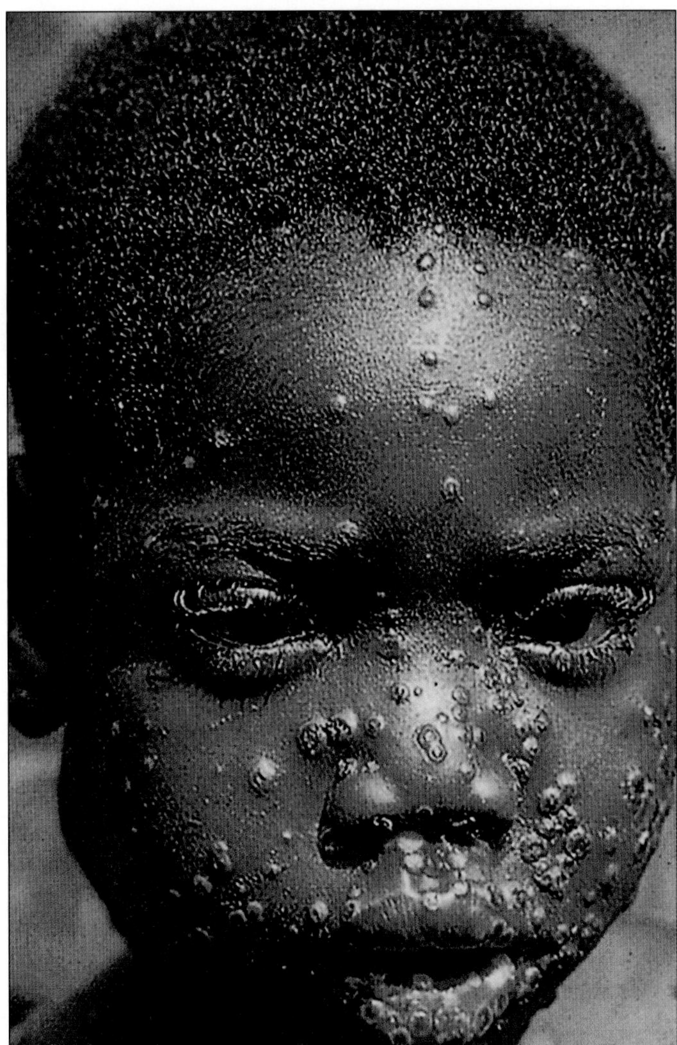

Figure 13.3 Monkeypox is a zoonotic infection, caused by an orthopox virus morphologically indistinguishable from that of smallpox, produces a relatively benign infection in humans in parts of the tropical rain forest areas of West and Central Africa. This girl from Zaire showed large numbers of papules and pustules on the trunk, head, extremities and external genitalia. Infection is acquired by handling or eating infected monkeys. (Reproduced from Peters W and Pasvol G (eds). Tropical Medicine and Parasitology, 5th edition, Mosby, London 2002: image 826.)

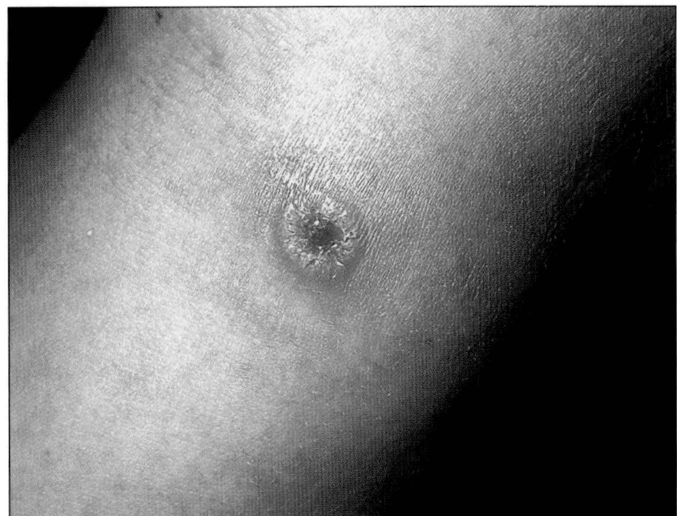

Figure 13.4 Nodule of tanapox surrounded by red halo on the arm of a student after contact with chimpanzees near the Tana river. (Courtesy of Dr. S. Klaus.)

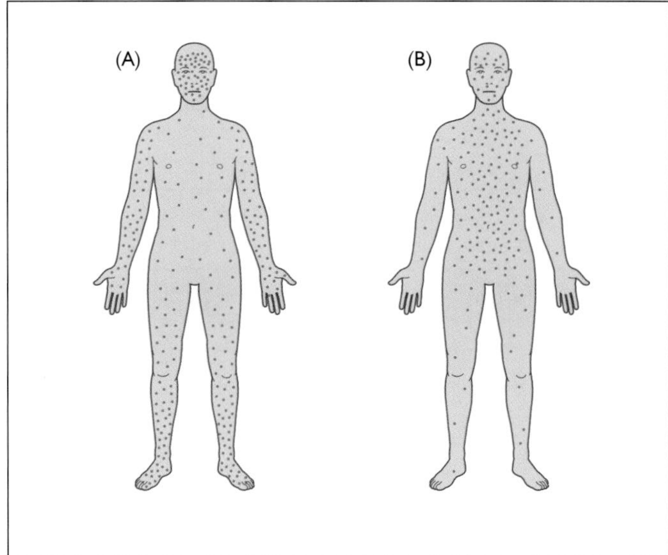

Figure 13.5 Distributions of eruptions in (A) smallpox and (B) chickenpox. (Courtesy of World Health Organization.)

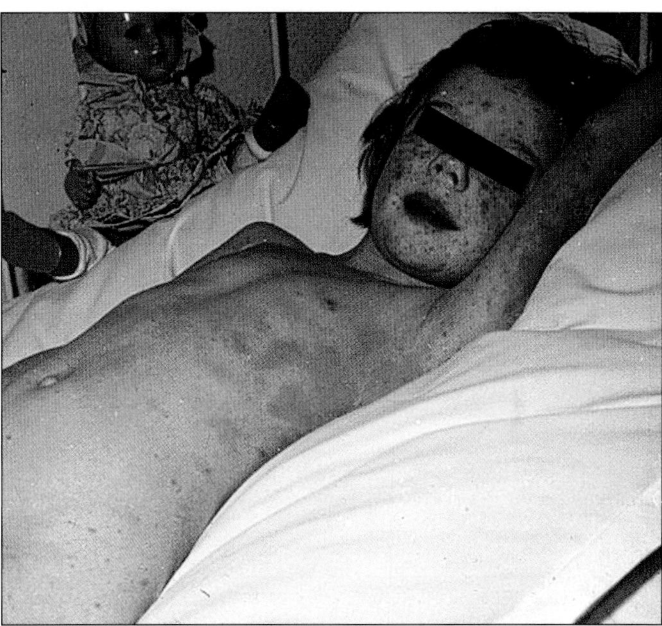

Figure 13.6 Smallpox: initial rash.

must be differentiated from fulminant meningitis, viral hemorrhagic fevers, and acquired immunodeficiency syndrome (AIDS) with thrombocytopenia and disseminated herpes virus infections.[11,12]

Smallpox-vaccine-associated adverse events may be due to the vaccinia virus itself or to autoimmune processes induced by the virus, or may represent non-specific allergic side-effects to other vaccine components (erythema multiforme major/Lyell/syndrome), or may be a bacterial superinfection (Table 13.2). The suspicion is raised by the history of smallpox vaccination of the individual or a contact person, because inoculation of vaccinia virus may occur inadvertently from a vaccinee to another individual.[14]

Laboratory diagnosis

Laboratory investigation must be performed in high-security laboratories. Security criteria for vaccinia virus, monkeypox virus

Table 13.4 Smallpox criteria

CDC smallpox case definition	
	An illness characterized by an acute onset of fever (38.3°C/101°F) followed 1–4 days later by a rash with firm deep-seated vesicles or pustules in the same stage of development without other apparent cause[a]
	High probability is defined by a febrile prodrome **and** classical smallpox lesions **and** uniformity of lesions (lesions at the same stage of development)
	Moderate probability of smallpox is defined by a febrile prodrome and either one other major smallpox criterion or four minor smallpox criteria
	Low probability of smallpox is defined by the presence of fewer than four smallpox criteria, whether or not preceded by a febrile prodrome
Major smallpox criteria	
	Febrile prodrome occurring 1–4 days before rash onset, fever ≥ 38.3°C (101°F) and at least one of the following: prostration, headache, backache, chills, vomiting, or severe abdominal pain
	Classic smallpox lesions: deep-seated firm, hard, round well-circumscribed vesicles or pustules; as they evolve, lesions become umbilicated or confluent
	Lesions in the same stage of development: on any part of the body (e.g., the face or arm); all the lesions are in the same stage of development (i.e., all are vesicles, or all are pustules)[a]
Minor smallpox criteria	
	Centrifugal distribution, greater concentration of lesions on the face and on distal extremities
	First lesions on the mucosal palate, face, or forearms
	Patient appears septic or moribund
	Slow evolution: lesions evolve from vesicles to papules–pustules over days (each stage lasts 1–2 days)
	Lesions on the palms and soles
CDC laboratory criteria for confirmation	
	Polymerase chain reaction (PCR) identification of variola DNA in clinical specimen or
	Isolation of smallpox (variola) virus from a clinical specimen (World Health Organization smallpox reference laboratory or laboratory with appropriate reference capabilities) **with** variola PCR confirmation

[a]Authors' note: it must be emphasized that at the beginning of a rash the lesions are not yet uniform but become so after 2 days. In vaccinees the multiform picture may persist for the whole course of the disease.
CDC, Centers for Disease Control.

and smallpox virus have been defined by the CDC.[14,17] Suitable material for diagnostic examinations includes vesicle fluid from the eruptions and tissue samples. Orthopox virus belongs to the largest viruses in nature (Fig. 13.19). They are visible even with an optical microscope. Electronmicroscopically, orthopox viruses are brick-shaped. All orthopox viruses have a similar appearance and are not morphologically distinguishable. Polymerase chain reaction (PCR) assay is performed in specialized centers. Tissue samples may be inoculated onto primary and continuous cell lines, including rhesus-monkey kidney cells, rabbit kidney cells, VERO cells, and other cells. Cytopathic changes are observed in those cell lines within 1–4 days. Samples may also be inoculated onto rabbit skin. A PCR assay that amplifies a conserved segment of the DNA polymerase gene (E9L) which is present in all Old-World orthopox viruses except variola allows the differentiation between monkeypox and smallpox viruses. Further combined PCR tests allow the characterization of orthopox virus species, and, for example, in monkeypox the subclassification of monkeypox virus strains.[12] Tests for antibodies against poxviruses do not allow the differentiation between antibodies against vaccinia virus in vaccinees or between monkeypox virus and smallpox virus infection.

Pathology

Eruptions are initially due to hyperemia and capillary congestion, surrounded by lymphoplasmacellular and histiocytic inflammation. Epithelial cells swell and form small confluent vacuoles. The vesicle

Table 13.5 Centers for Disease Control case definition for human monkeypox

Clinical criteria

- Rash (macular, papular, vesicular, or pustular; generalized or localized; discrete or confluent)
- Fever (subjective or measured temperature ≥ 37.4°C (≥ 99.3°F))
- Other symptoms: chills and/or sweats, headache, backache, lymphadenopathy, sore throat, cough, shortness of breath

Epidemiologic criteria

- Exposure[a] to an exotic or wild mammalian pet[b]
- With clinical signs of illness (e.g., conjunctivitis, respiratory symptoms and/or rash), **and/or** has been in contact with either a mammalian pet[c] or a human with monkeypox
- Exposure[d] to a suspect, probable, or confirmed human case of monkeypox

Laboratory criteria

- Isolation of monkeypox virus in culture
- Demonstration of monkeypox virus DNA by polymerase chain reaction testing of a clinical specimen
- Demonstration of virus morphologically consistent with an orthopoxvirus by electron microscopy in the absence of exposure to another orthopoxvirus
- Demonstration of presence of orthopoxvirus in tissue using immunohistochemical testing methods in the absence of exposure to another orthopoxvirus

Case classification

Suspect case

- Meets one of the epidemiological criteria

and

- Fever or unexplained rash **and** two other signs or symptoms with onset of first sign or symptom ≤ 21 days after last exposure meeting epidemiologic criteria

Probable case

- Meets one of the epidemiological criteria

and

- Fever **and** vesicular–pustular rash with onset of first sign or symptom ≤ 21 days after last exposure meeting epidemiologic criteria

Confirmed case

- Meets one of the laboratory criteria

Exclusion criteria

A case may be excluded as a suspect or probable monkeypox case if:

- An alternative diagnosis can fully explain the illness[e]
- The case was reported on the basis of primary or secondary exposure to an exotic or wild mammalian pet or a human (see epidemiologic criteria) subsequently determined not to have monkeypox, provided other possible epidemiologic exposure criteria are not present **or**
- A case without a rash does not develop a rash within 10 days of onset of clinical symptoms consistent with monkeypox[f]
- The case is determined to be negative for a non-variola generic orthopoxvirus by polymerase chain reaction testing of a well-sampled lesion following the approved Laboratory Response Network (LRN) protocol

[a]Includes living in a household, petting or handling, or visiting a pet-holding facility (e.g., pet store, veterinary clinic, pet distributor).
[b]Includes prairie dogs, Gambian giant rats, and rope squirrels. Exposure to other exotic or non-exotic mammalian pets will be considered on a case-by-case basis; assessment should include the likelihood of contact with a mammal with monkeypox and the compatibility of clinical illness with monkeypox.
[c]Includes living in a household, or originating from the same pet-holding facility as another animal with monkeypox.
[d]Includes skin-to-skin or face-to-face contact.
[e]Factors that might be considered in assigning alternate diagnoses include the strength of the epidemiologic exposure criteria for monkeypox, the specificity of the diagnostic test, and the compatibility of the clinical presentation and course of illness for the alternative diagnosis.
[f]If possible, obtain reconvalescent-phase serum specimen from these patients. See specimen collection guidelines (www.cdc.gov/ncidod/monkeypox/lab.htm) for details on collecting serum for convalescence evaluation.
Modified from Centers for Disease Control. Updated interim case definition for human monkeypox. CDC, 2003.

represents a chambered cavity originating from the rupture of these swollen cells. Leukocytes and necrotic tissue transform the vesicle into a pustule, which eventually dries up, forming a scab. When deep parts of the skin are affected, scarring occurs.

Histological skin and mucosal specimens show characteristic cytoplasmic eosinophilic inclusions in the perinuclear regions (Guarneri bodies).

Treatment and prevention

Smallpox vaccination with the dermovaccine

Orthopox virus infections may be prevented by a smallpox vaccine. At present, smallpox vaccination is performed by inoculating an attenuated orthopox virus (dermovaccine with vaccinia virus). If an appropriate skin reaction follows vaccine inoculation, protection

Table 13.6 Differential diagnosis between chickenpox and orthopoxvirus infections

	Chickenpox	Smallpox	Smallpox in a vaccinee (variolois)	Monkeypox
Medical history	Contact with other individual with chickenpox	Contact with individual with smallpox Laboratory worker Suspicion of bioterrorism		Contact with pet prairie dogs or Gambia rats Close contact with humans with monkeypox
Appearance of lesions	At fever peaks; prodrome, if present, mild	2–3 days after onset of fever, when fever decreases		Possibly inoculation site: first lesion with lymph node swelling Generalization, 1–3 days after onset of fever
Picture of rash	Multiform rash ("starry sky") Development of lesions, each evolving without synchronization	Transient multiform rash for 2–3 days M-P-V-Pu-C with subsequent synchronization and uniform rash	Persistent multiform rash M-P-V-Pu-C	Uniform evolution of lesions (M-)P-V-Pu-C
Morphology of vesicles	Not chambered vesicle: "dew drop on a rose petal"	Chambered deep-seated umbilicated vesicle (vesicle with "belly bottom")	Chambered but abortive	Chambered umbilicated vesicle
Distribution of lesions	Centripetal = maximum density of lesions: trunk Rarely on palms and soles	Always centrifugal distribution of lesions Maximum density of lesions: extremities, head Lesions also appear on palms and soles	In many but not all patients there is centrifugal distribution of lesions Maximum density of lesions: extremities, head Lesions also appear on palms and soles	Centrifugal generalized rash, maximum density of lesions: extremities + lesion at inoculation site Lesions may appear on palms and soles
Evolution of lesions	More rapid (from vesicle to crust even within 24 h)	Slow (each stage lasts 1–2 days)		Slow (each stage lasts 1–2 days)

M, macule; P, papule; V, vesicle; Pu, pustule; C, crust.

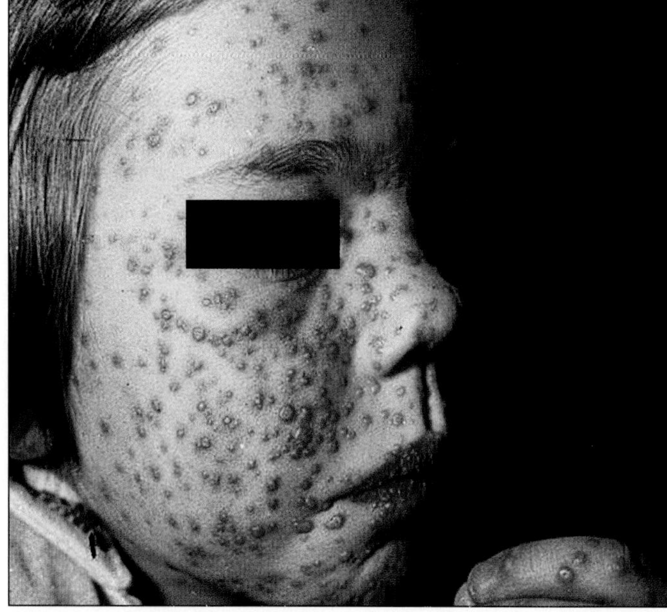

Figure 13.7 Smallpox: day 3 (vesicles).

against smallpox is achieved (Fig. 13.20) in more than 95% of individuals for at least 3–5 years; partial protection lasts longer. The vaccine protects against other orthopox viruses in at least 85% of vaccinees who have developed an appropriate skin reaction.[14,18] A more attenuated vaccine with modified vaccinia virus Ankara (MVA) was developed in Germany shortly before the eradication of the epidemic of smallpox.[8] Currently, the MVA vaccine is being further developed and it may play a role in the future, especially in patients with contraindications to the dermovaccine.

The dermovaccine is administered using a bifurcated needle that is dipped into the vaccine solution. The needle retains a droplet of the vaccine. The needle is used to prick the skin 15 times in a few seconds, usually in the upper arm. Immunization by the vaccine is evaluated by observing the evolution of the characteristic skin reaction at the vaccination site: a papule develops within 4 days. The papule develops to a vesicle and pustule within 1 week; it dries up and forms a scab within 2–3 weeks.

Since incubation is relatively long (12 days), the smallpox vaccine given during this period may prevent the disease when given within 3 days after exposure (Figs 13.21 and 13.22). Even when given on days 4–7 after exposure, life-threatening complications of smallpox (up to day 14 in monkeypox) can be prevented, provided a reaction to the smallpox vaccine develops.[18] Care must be taken to avoid inadvertent autoinoculation or infection of another individual with this live vaccinia virus until the scab has fallen off.

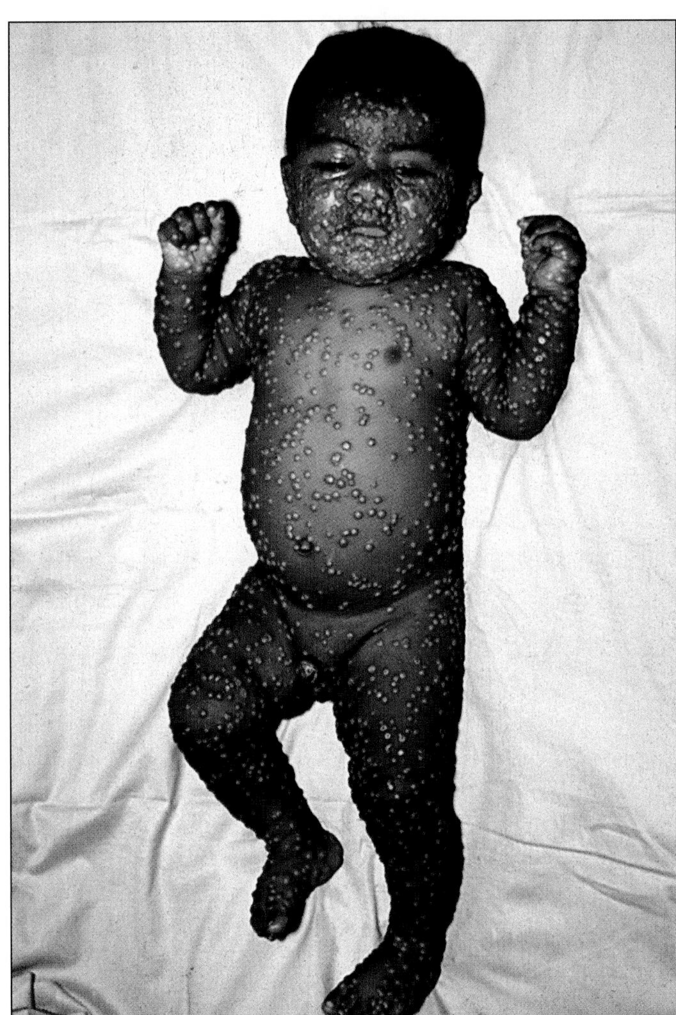

Figure 13.8 Smallpox: uniform vesicular eruption; distribution: eruption more concentrated on the face and extremities as compared to the trunk.

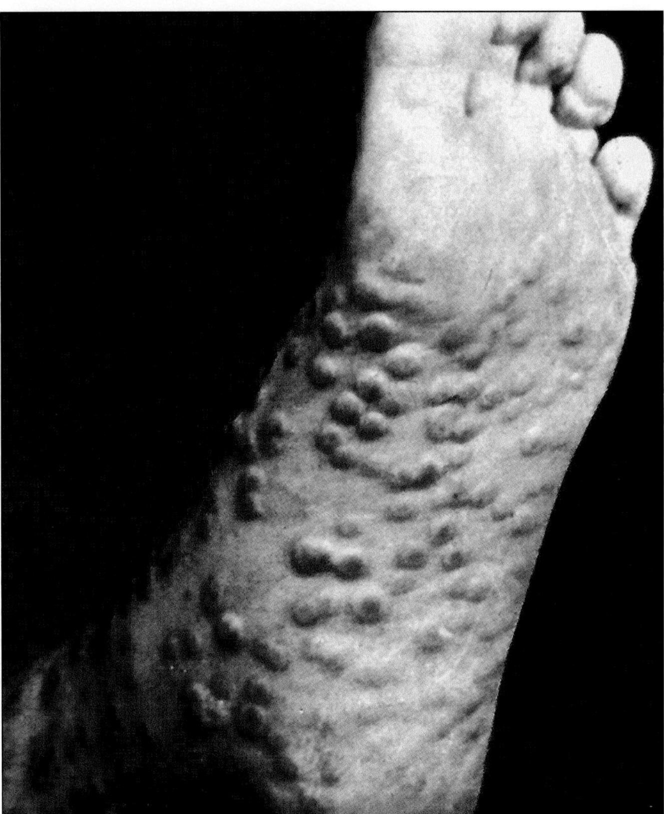

Figure 13.9 Smallpox: vesicular umbilicated lesions on the sole.

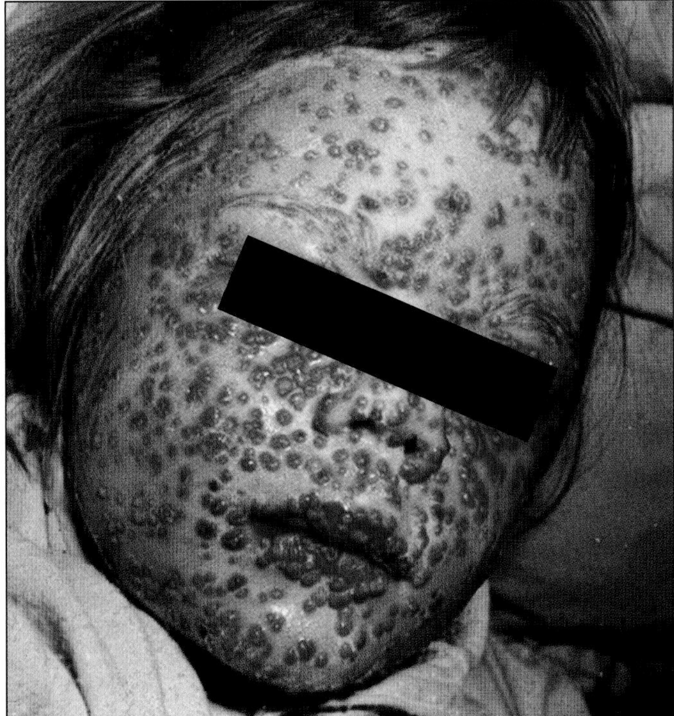

Figure 13.10 Smallpox: Day 5; uniform pustular eruption.

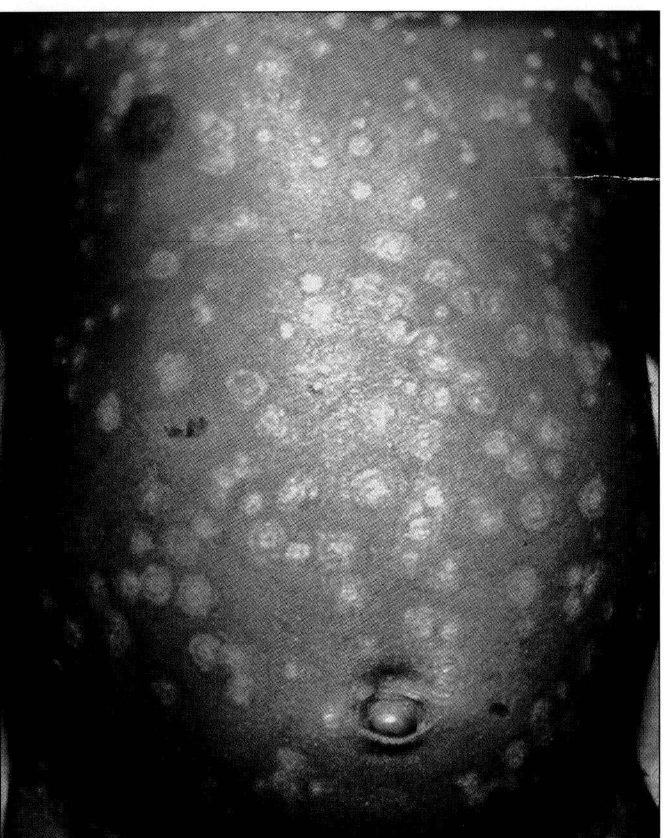

Figure 13.11 Smallpox: depigmented scars after loss of crusts.

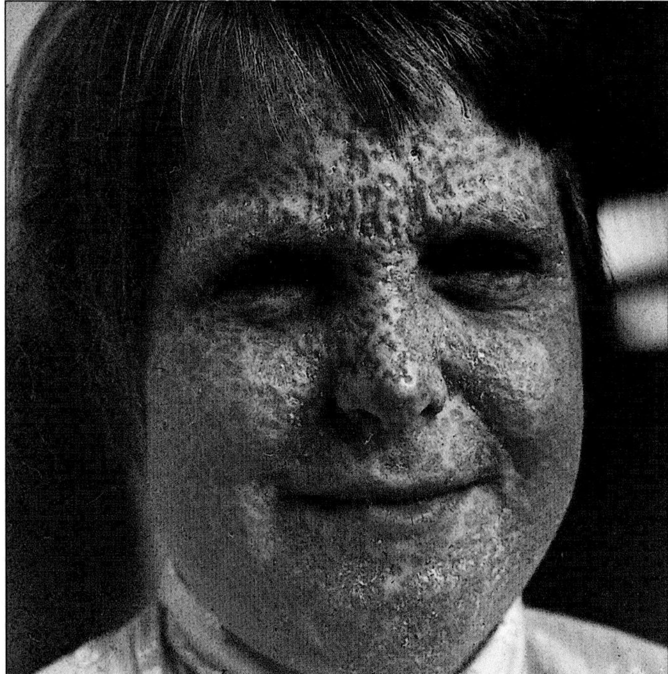

Figure 13.12 Smallpox: scarring after convalescence.

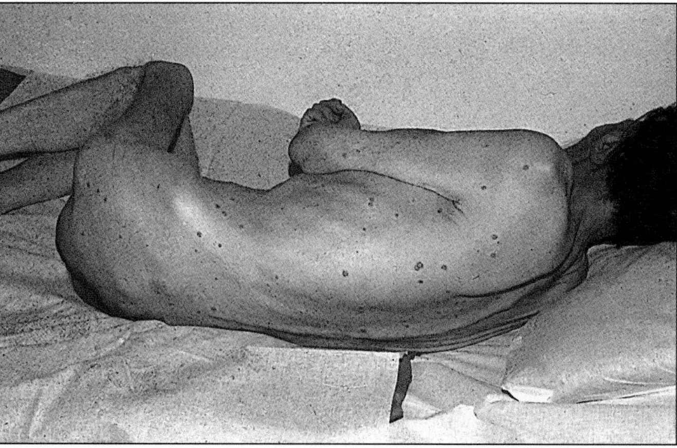

Figure 13.13 Complicated smallpox: flat hyporeactive smallpox in a 70 year old man.

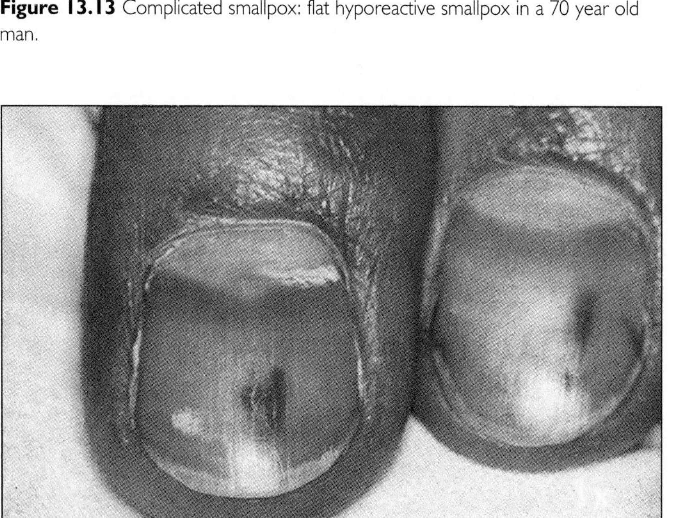

Figure 13.14 Complicated smallpox: early hemorrhagic smallpox, subungeal hemorrhage.

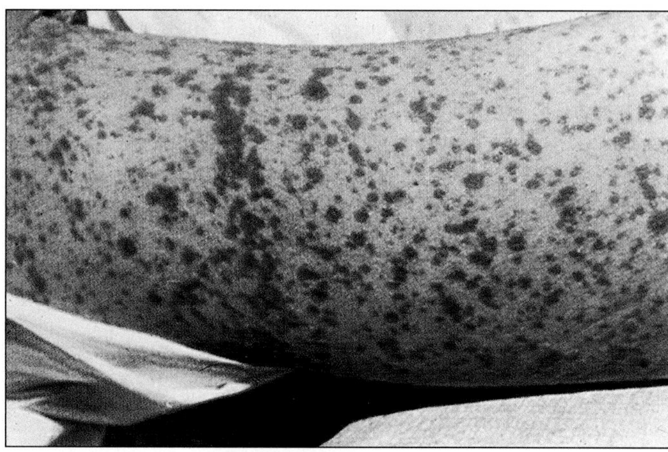

Figure 13.15 Complicated smallpox: early hemorrhagic smallpox.

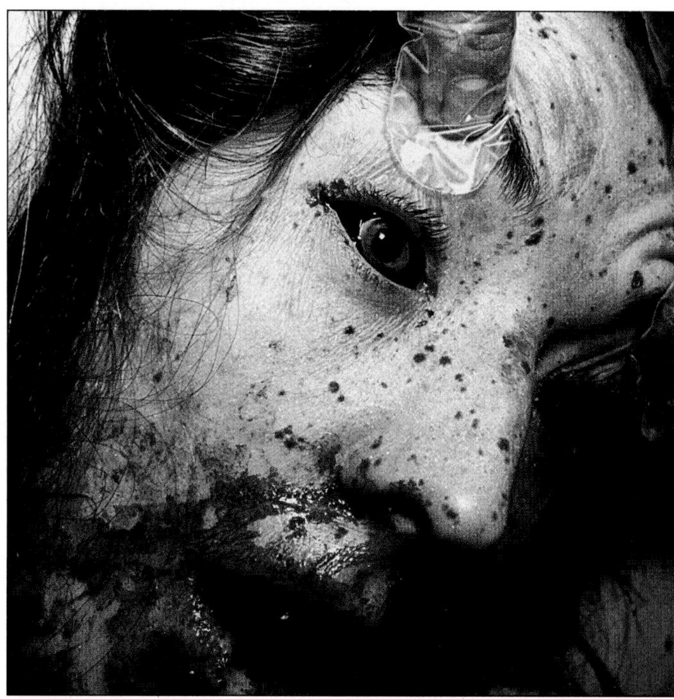

Figure 13.16 Complicated smallpox: early hemorrhagic smallpox, profuse conjunctival and mucosal bleeding.

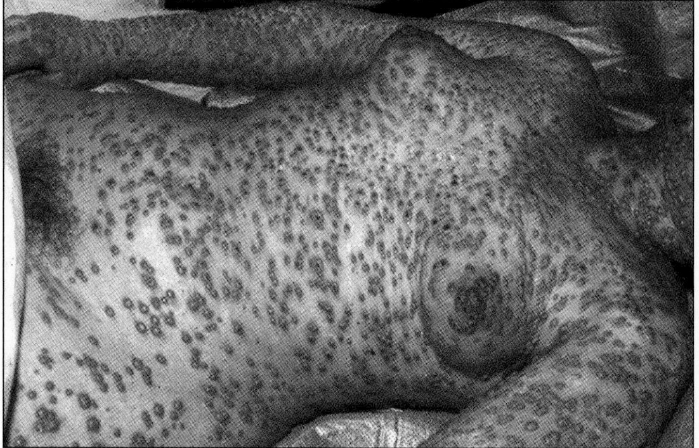

Figure 13.17 Complicated smallpox: late hemorrhagic smallpox, bleeding into pre-existing smallpox.

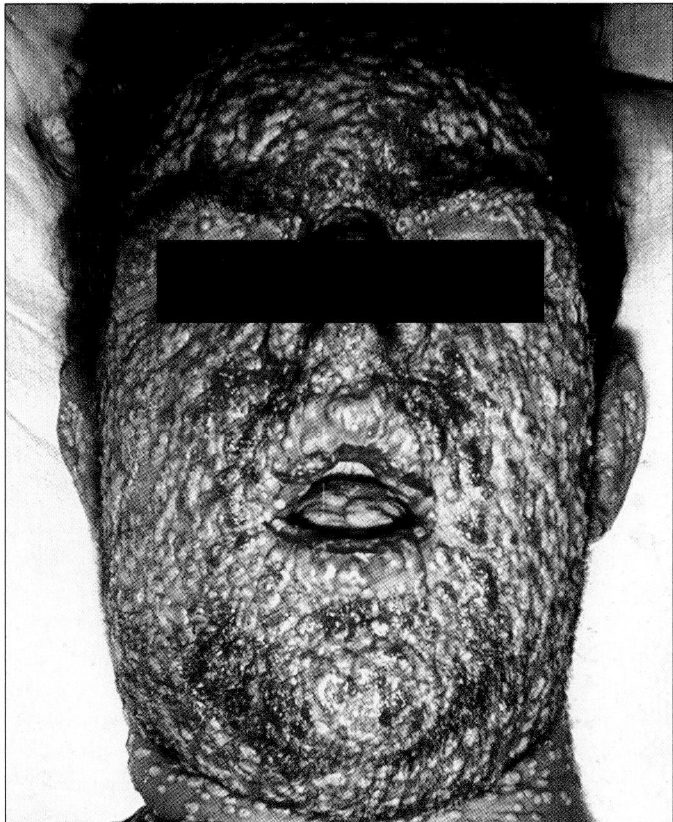

Figure 13.18 Complicated smallpox: massive excretion of poxviruses.

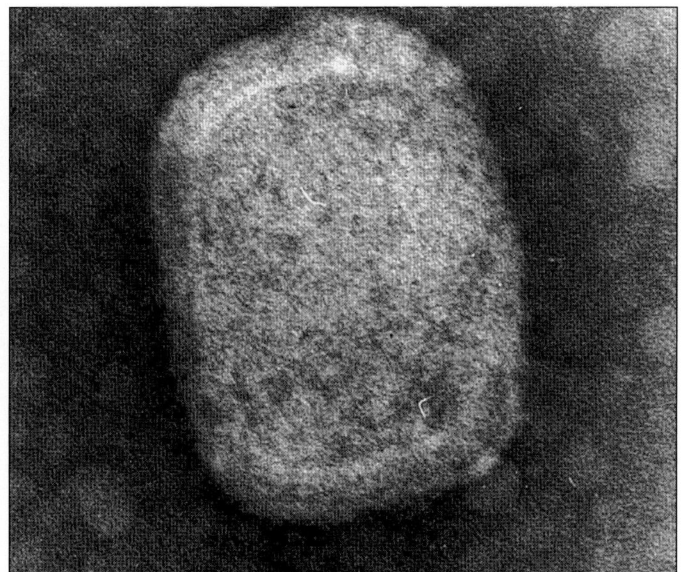

Figure 13.19 Electron microscopy of an orthopoxvirus (*vaccinia* virus).

Adverse events associated with smallpox vaccination and contraindications to the smallpox vaccine

In the past, the smallpox vaccine was associated with serious side-effects (Table 13.2) in 1/1000–1/5000 vaccinees and 1–2/1 000 000 vaccinees may die as a result of vaccination. Therefore, the indications must be weighed against contraindications in an

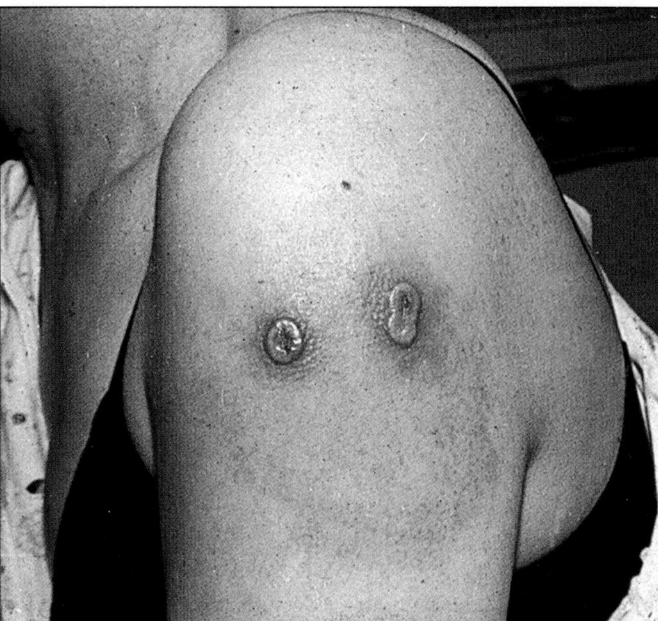

Figure 13.20 Positive reaction at vaccine in occulation site.

epidemiological and individual context, taking into account the probability of poxvirus exposure and of a severe poxvirus infection. Subjects at risk for adverse events include: individuals who have or have had, even once, certain skin conditions, especially eczema or atopic dermatitis; and immunocompromised patients (human immunodeficiency virus (HIV) infection, congenital immune defects, cancer, leukemia, immunosuppressive therapy). Immunocompromised patients should usually not receive the vaccine, unless the risk of a life-threatening poxvirus infection is higher than the risk of life-threatening adverse events due to the smallpox vaccine. Individuals using steroid-containing eye drops should, if possible, interrupt this medication. Subjects with ongoing skin diseases, including burns, chickenpox, shingles, impetigo, herpes, severe acne, or psoriasis should not receive the vaccine. Adolescents and children younger than 18 years should only receive the vaccine in an emergency. Smallpox vaccine is contraindicated in children younger than 12 months, pregnant (risk of fetal vaccinia), and breast-feeding women. During vaccinations of military personnel and civilians in the USA in 2001–2003, some cases of mild to life-threatening perimyocarditis have been observed. Therefore, current heart disease or previous myocardial infarction or cerebral ischemic attacks are contraindications to smallpox vaccine until more information on the clinical and statistical significance of myocardial adverse events is available. Relative contraindications include risk factors for coronary heart disease, such as hypercholesterolemia, diabetes, arterial hypertension, or a first-degree relative with cardiac disease before the age of 50 years.

Smallpox vaccination to prevent monkeypox infection is indicated in individuals investigating monkeypox outbreaks or involved in the care of patients with monkeypox. Smallpox vaccination is indicated in individuals who have had intimate contact with monkeypox-infected patients or animals.[8,19,20] Smallpox vaccination is contraindicated when the risk of severe adverse events is higher than the risk of serious complications of monkeypox infection.

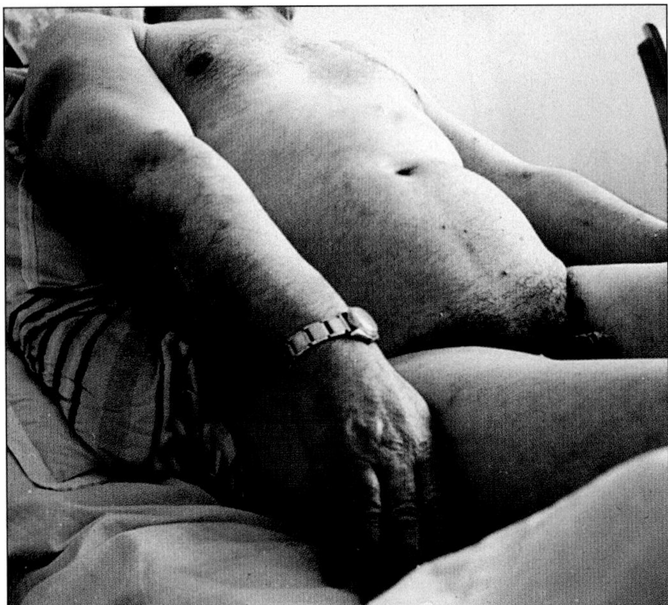

Figure 13.21 Abortive smallpox after vaccination during incubation; note exacerbated immune reaction at the vaccine site.

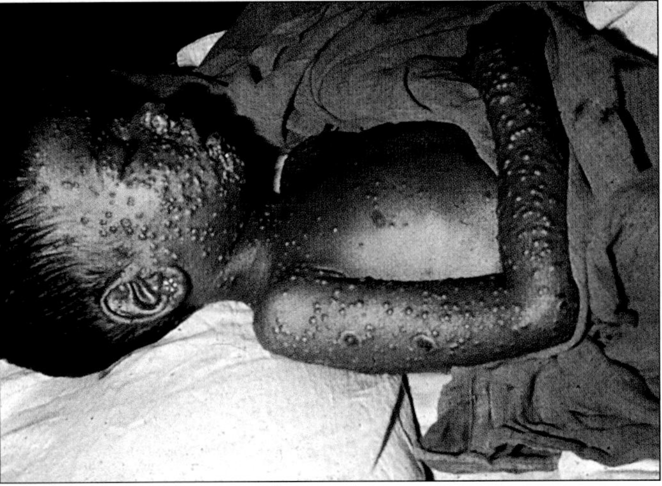

Figure 13.22 Exacerbated reaction to smallpox vaccination given during incubation in an Indian child.

Smallpox vaccination is not effective in preventing infections with non-orthopox viruses (Table 13.1).

Allergic reactions

Some adverse events after dermovaccination are due to a hypersensitivity reaction to components of the vaccine but not to the vaccinia virus itself. Allergic erythema multiforme and other allergic conditions have been reported. Individuals who have had life-threatening allergies to latex, smallpox vaccine, or any of its components (polymyxin, streptomycin, chlortetracycline, neomycin) are therefore excluded from smallpox vaccination. Inadvertently inoculated patients with such conditions, should be treated for allergic reactions but therapy must also take into account the possible increase of vaccinia virus virulence when immunosuppressive therapy is given.

Inadvertent inoculation/vaccinia keratitis

Inadvertent inoculation may occur in the same individual or, less frequently, from one individual to another when the vaccinia virus spreads from the inoculation site to the skin, especially when predisposing skin lesions (eczema, wounds) are present. Inadvertent inoculation is favored by the fact that the florid vaccination site contains high concentrations of vaccinia virus and that it is at the same time pruritic. Inadvertent inoculation is one of the most common adverse events following smallpox vaccination. Children and adolescents are at risk because of their tendency to scratch the itching vaccination site. Usually, inadvertent inoculation results in a normal primary smallpox vaccination after an incubation of approximately 10 days, but may become severe in subjects with contraindications to the vaccine.

When vaccinia virus is inoculated into the eye, e.g., by a contaminated hand or fingers, periorbital, conjunctival, and corneal lesions may occur. Periorbital and conjunctival lesions follow the typical skin evolution at the vaccination site, whereas corneal infection results in ulceration. Vaccinia keratitis may result in blindness. Fortunately, it is a relatively rare adverse event. Individuals with preexisting eye disease are particularly susceptible to inadvertent inoculation. Caretakers who handle or bathe vaccinated children are at particular risk for infection. Vaccinia keratitis is best recognized with slit-lamp examination.

In most cases of inadvertent inoculation, no treatment is required. Treatment of patients who develop complications is described below. Vaccinia keratitis is a contraindication to vaccinia immune globulin (VIG; see below), because this may accentuate an antigen–antibody reaction. Topical antiviral agents, such as acyclovir, vidarabine, and trifluridine, possibly in combination with interferon, have been used. Inadvertent inoculation is prevented by careful instructions to vaccinees. When children are vaccinated, the vaccination site may be covered by a loose dressing and parents are instructed about proper care.

Eczema vaccinatum

Eczema vaccinatum (Fig. 13.23) is a serious, potentially life-threatening condition, characterized by a rash caused by widespread infection of the skin in individuals with predisposing skin diseases such as atopic dermatitis. Distribution of eruptions typically follows that of atopic dermatitis, e.g., the antecubital and politeal fossa. This permits differentiation from bacterial superinfection. At first, lesions appear identical to the evolution of the primary vaccination site, but subsequently evolve into large contiguous patches. Confluent lesions may cover the face and other areas of the body as a result of contiguous spread or due to subsequent viremia. Death may result from severe systemic involvement resembling septic shock. Diagnosis relies on the history of smallpox vaccination in an individual with a preexisting skin disorder. In contact cases diagnosis may be especially difficult, when a history of contact with a vaccinee has not been appreciated. Laboratory investigation may be helpful for the differential diagnosis of generalized herpes and the diagnosis of bacterial and/or fungal superinfection. Mortality is prevented in patients treated promptly with VIG at an initial dose of 0.6–1.0 ml/kg body weight. In severe cases up to

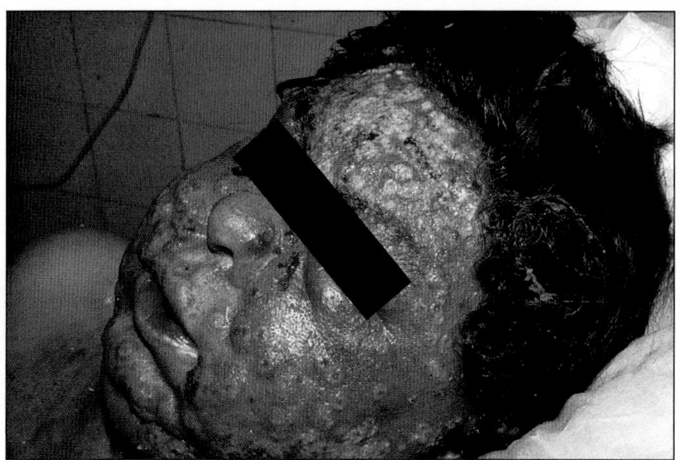

Figure 13.23 Eczema vaccinatum in a grandmother (with atopic dermatitis) of a smallpox-vaccinated child.

5–10 ml/kg may be given divided into multiple doses over several days. Potentially severe cases receive all supportive measures available in the intensive care unit.

Generalized vaccinia

Although generalized vaccinia resulting from systemic viral spread is usually a benign self-limited complication of smallpox vaccination, it may become life-threatening in immunocompromised individuals. Children with an ill-defined immunological immaturity or disorder of immune response are most likely to be affected. Fortunately, intact cell-mediated immunity usually prevents a severe or lethal outcome. Within a week of the onset of the reaction to vaccination, lesions similar to the primary inoculation site, but smaller in size, will appear. Lesions may be seen everywhere, most frequently on the trunk and abdomen, but also on palms and soles. In single cases, these lesions may recur at 4–6-week intervals for up to 1 year. The lesions differ from erythema multiforme and generalized chickenpox by their typical umbilicated aspect (in chickenpox, lesions are superficial, with a typical dewdrop aspect). In generalized vaccinia, in contrast to eczema vaccinatum, lesions are not concentrated on typical sites of atopic dermatitis. Unlike early progressive vaccinia, the primary vaccination site presents with normal evolution without inflammation. Generalized vaccinia is difficult to differentiate from smallpox, when the latter is attenuated due to a postexposure vaccine (variolois). Here, virologic diagnosis is mandatory.

Generalized vaccinia does not usually require specific therapy. In cases with extensive lesions or in recurring cases, one course of VIG at a dose of 0.6 ml/kg body weight IM is usually sufficient. Cidofovir is also a potentially effective therapy.

Progressive vaccinia

Progressive vaccinia is a life-threatening condition, also called vaccinia gangrenosa, vaccinia necrosum, and disseminated vaccinia. Its incidence will probably increase nowadays upon vaccination because of the increasing number of immunosuppressed individuals (patients with symptomatic HIV infection, and because of iatrogenic immunosuppression, e.g., with cancer and autoimmune disease). Although these conditions are contraindications to the dermovaccine, inadvertent inoculation after contact with a vaccinee may occur. Due to the impaired immune response of the host, the virus multiplies by cell-to-cell spread at the inoculation site, and the lesion expands circumferentially. Centrally the lesion becomes necrotic, whereas the edges advance. The virus may gain access to the blood at an early stage, and secondary skin lesions, which follow the same evolution as the inoculation site, may appear. Bacteria may infect the ulcerated, necrotic lesions. Coalescent lesions may cover large portions of the body with extensive tissue destruction. In contrast, neither lymphadenopathy nor splenomegaly are usually present as a consequence of the underlying immunodeficiency. Virological diagnosis is helpful when a virulent poxvirus infection is concurrently endemic. Opportunistic fungal, protozoal, or bacterial infections and the vaccinia itself may lead to septic shock and disseminated intravascular coagulation. Apart from treating opportunistic infections, immediate highly active antiretroviral therapy (HAART) in HIV patients and withdrawal of immunosuppressive therapy accompanied by aggressive administration of VIG are mandatory to save the patient's life. Intensive care and supportive treatment are required. VIG is given at up to 10 ml/kg body weight. Surgical removal of massive necrotic lesions may be necessary in order to prevent graft-versus-host disease in organ-transplanted patients, in whom immunosuppressive therapy would otherwise have to be discontinued to allow healing of the wound. In some cases, exchange transfusions have been performed in order to supply immunologic factors and plasma from recently vaccinated donors. Among antiviral substances, cidofovir showed some effect in preliminary studies.

For prevention, a thorough assessment of contraindications during vaccination campaigns and prevention of inadvertent inoculation by smallpox vaccinees are mandatory.

Postvaccinial encephalitis

The pathogenesis of postvaccinial (meningo)encephalitis is not well understood. Observations in the past suggest that it is not due to the vaccinia virus itself, but most probably to an autoimmune process induced by the virus. The incidence of this severe complication has been reported to range between 1/1000 and 1/20 000 vaccinees. Encephalitis occurs 10–14 days after inoculation, presenting with non-specific symptoms, e.g., fever, vomiting, drowsiness, and fever. In more severe cases, symptoms progress to focal neurological defects, paralysis, urinary incontinence or retention, and convulsions. Death usually occurs within 1 week of the onset of symptoms.

Non-specific findings include increases in cerebrospinal fluid (CSF) pressure, CSF lymphocytosis, and CSF protein. Among the cases reported, 25% were fatal and 25% of the survivors suffered from a residual neurologic defect.

Diagnosis relies on the history of inoculation 10–14 days before and the exclusion of other causes of encephalitis. Since VIG is not recommended, as it may exacerbate encephalitis, therapy relies on surveillance in an intensive care unit and appropriate supportive measures.

Congenital vaccinia

Congenital vaccinia is an infection of the fetus during the last trimester of pregnancy, with symptoms of the disease in the newborn. Vaccination in the first two trimesters may possibly result in intrauterine fetal death, but congenital abnormalities have never been proven in early pregnancy after vaccination. In the past, in large-scale campaigns, inadvertent vaccination of pregnant women must undoubtedly have occurred, but fewer than 50 cases of congenital disease have been reported in the literature. Treatment with VIG is indicated.

Myocardial damage

Sudden cardiac arrest and perimyocarditis have been observed during vaccination campaigns in American troops and civilians after September 11, 2001. The significance of this observation is not yet clear. In subjects with a history of cardiac disease, therefore, primary vaccination is contraindicated except in an emergency.

Vaccinia immune globulin

VIG is obtained from subjects who have recently been vaccinated against smallpox. Most VIG was obtained in the 1960s. Availability and safety are therefore limited. Recent vaccination campaigns in American troops will allow larger quantities of VIG to be obtained and processed according to current manufacturing standards. No data are available on the effectiveness of VIG in monkeypox. It has no proven benefit in complicated smallpox. VIG can be considered for prophylactic use in individuals with contraindications to the dermovaccine.

Antiviral treatment with cidofovir

Cidofovir has proven antimonkeypox viral activity in vitro and in animals.[19] No data are available on the effectiveness of cidofovir in zoonotic poxvirus infections. Since cidofovir is toxic, its use should be restricted to severe infection.

Prevention

Smallpox is a highly lethal and highly infectious disease. Immediate isolation and the use of high-performance respirators by personnel need to be established. If possible, personnel vaccinated against smallpox less than 3 years before should be selected for patients' care and specimen handling. When a respirator mask is not available, a surgical mask and protective eye glasses are mandatory. Laboratory material must be handled very cautiously and processed in reference laboratories.[14,17] Uncomplicated monkeypox cases have also been isolated at home; this is preferable to hospital settings because of the risk of nosocomial spread. Updated guidelines for the prevention of transmission of smallpox by animals to humans are available from the CDC.[20]

References

1. Gani R, Leach S. Transmission potential of smallpox in contemporary populations. Nature 2001; 414:748–751.
2. Verger P. Orisha. Les dieux Yorouba en Afrique et au nouveau monde [in French]. Paris: Editions AM Métailié; 1982:210–233.
3. Reed KD, Melski JW, Graham MB et al. The detection of monkeypox in humans in the western hemisphere. N Engl J Med 2004; 350:342–350.
4. Downie AW, Taylor-Robinson CH, Caunt AE et al. Tanapox: a new disease caused by a poxvirus. Br Med J 1971; 1:363–368.
5. Frey SE, Belshe R. Poxvirus zoonoses – putting pocks into context. N Engl J Med 2004; 350:324–327.
6. Stich A, Meyer H, Kohler B et al. Tanapox: first report in a European traveller and identification by PCR. Trans R Soc Trop Med Hyg 2002; 96:178–179.
7. Dhar AD, Werchniak AE, Li Y et al. Tanapox infection in a college student. N Engl J Med 2004; 350:361–365.
8. Mayr A. Danger for humans and animals by poxvirus-infected cats. Dtsch Ärtzebl 1993; 90:C817–C820.
9. Vestey JP, Yirrell DL, Aldridge RD. Cowpox/catpox infection. Br J Dermatol 1991; 124:74–78.
10. Steinborn A, Essbauer S, Marsch WCh. Human cowpox/catpox infection. A potentially unrecognized disease [in German]. Dtsch Med Wochenschr 2003; 128:607–610.
11. Centers for Disease Control. Evaluating patients with acute generalized vesicular or pustuler rash illnesses. From the training course: Smallpox; disease, prevention, and intervention. 2003. Available online at: www.bt.cdc.gov/agent/smallpox/training/overview (accessed August 31, 2004).
12. Centers for Disease Control. Emergency preparedness. Smallpox. CDC, 2003; December; Available online at: www.bt.cdc.gov/agent/smallpox/response-plan (accessed August 31, 2004).
13. Meyer A, Esposito JJ, Gras F et al. First appearance of monkeypox in human beings in Gabon [in French]. Med Trop (Marseille) 1991; 51:53–57.
14. Jezek Z, Szczeniowski M, Paluku KM et al. Human monkeypox: clinical features of 282 patients. J Infect Dis 1987; 156:293–298.
15. Centers for Disease Control. Updated interim case definition for human monkeypox. CDC, 2003. Available online at: www.cdc.gov/ncidod/monkeypox (accessed August 31, 2004).
16. Krusell A, Comer JA, Sexton DJ. Rickettsialpox in North Carolina: a case report. Emerg Infect Dis 2002; 8:727–728.
17. Centers for Disease Control. Interim biosafety guidelines for laboratory personnal of human and animal specimens for monkeypox testing. CDC, 2003. Available online at: www.cdc.gov/ncidod/monkeypox/lab.htm (accessed August 31, 2004).
18. Centers for Disease Control. Questions and answers: smallpox vaccine and monkeypox. CDC, 2003. Available online at: www.cdc.gov/ncidod/monkeypox/vaccineqa.htm (accessed August 31, 2004).
19. Centers for Disease Control. Updated interim CDC guidance for use of smallpox vaccine, cidofovir and vaccinia immune globuline (VIG) for prevention and treatment in the setting of an outbreak of monkeypox infections. CDC, 2003; June 12. Available online at: www.cdc.gov/ncidod/monkeypox/treatmentguidelines.htm (accessed August 31, 2004).
20. Centers for Disease Control. Monkeypox infections in animals: interim guidance for veterinarians. CDC, 2003; June 12. Available online at: www.cdc.gov/ncidod/monkeypox/animalguidance.htm (accessed August 31, 2004).

Chapter 14

Measles

Beatriz Meza-Valencia and Denise M. Demers

Synonyms: Measles, rubeola, rougeole (French), rosolia (Italian), sarampión (Spanish)

Key features:

- Measles is the leading cause of vaccine-preventable childhood morbidity and mortality worldwide
- Although measles is no longer endemic in the USA, sporadic cases still occur
- Measles is a clinical diagnosis made by recognizing the pathognomonic prodrome of fever, coryza, cough, conjunctivitis, and the classic course from oral enanthem to erythematous maculopapular rash
- Measles mortality is due to respiratory and neurologic complications
- Treatment with vitamin A can significantly decrease measles morbidity and mortality in malnourished populations
- Measles vaccine is very effective in preventing the disease when given in a two-dose schedule

Introduction

Measles can be accurately diagnosed clinically by its typical course and its pathognomonic dermatological findings. It is a highly infectious disease that causes 800 000 child deaths per year worldwide and is responsible for 10% of the mortality in children less than 5 years. Most of the complications from measles are currently seen in malnourished and immunocompromised populations of developing nations. The industrialized countries that have benefitted from successful vaccination campaigns face the continuous threat of measles outbreaks imported from less fortunate areas. Complacency towards diseases not frequently seen and fear of vaccine side-effects, both real and imagined, may decrease vaccination and increase outbreaks in areas previously protected.[1] While new therapies have proven useful in decreasing measles morbidity and mortality, worldwide vaccine campaigns have repeatedly been shown to be the best prevention.[2]

History

Measles epidemics have been documented for more than 1000 years. Nearly 500 years ago, European explorers brought measles to the Americas, resulting in significant destruction of the Native American population. The epidemiology and infectious properties of measles were first studied during a large outbreak in the Faroe Islands in 1846. Over 100 years later, Enders and Peebles isolated the measles virus, marking the beginning of the search for a measles vaccine. In 1963, Enders developed the live attenuated measles vaccine used today.[3]

Epidemiology

Measles remains a leading cause of childhood morbidity and mortality worldwide. The virus is highly contagious, causing disease in 90% of exposed susceptible contacts. In the prevaccination era, measles epidemics cycled every 2–3 years and caused more than 3 million deaths per year. The peak age of incidence was 5–10 years and most adults were immune due to prior disease. Since the measles vaccine was introduced in the 1960s, the incidence of disease has dropped by nearly 99% in the Americas. This decrease has occurred even as surveillance systems and reporting mechanisms have improved.[4]

In the USA the introduction of the one-dose live attenuated measles vaccine was very successful in reducing the incidence of measles. However, it did not prevent the 1985–1988 measles resurgence documented in teenagers and infants. This is thought to be due to a 5% primary vaccine failure rate, and to decreased vaccination rates in children less than 2 years old. In response, in 1989, the Advisory Committee on Immunizations Practices

Subcommittee on Measles Prevention, in conjunction with the American Academy of Pediatrics Committee on Infectious Disease, recommended the implementation of a two-dose vaccine series. The measles vaccine is now routinely given to all children at 12 months and 4–6 years. In the USA it is given in a combination vaccine with mumps and rubella. Since this change, epidemiological data suggest that measles is no longer endemic in the USA. However there are still more than 80 cases of measles per year, most of which are importation-related.[5]

Transplacental immunity provides protection against disease but also interferes with the anamnestic response to vaccination. Mothers with a history of the disease provide their child with protective antibodies that can last up to 9–12 months. In contrast, most mothers in the USA gain immunity to measles via vaccination and have lower immunoglobulin G (IgG) titers. The protective immunity afforded their infants is thought to be shorter in duration, thus putting the older infant at increased risk of disease.

Measles eradication campaigns throughout the Americas have proved to be very successful. In 1994, the Pan American Sanitary Conference set a goal to eliminate measles from North and South America by the year 2000. Although not completely realized, 2001 saw a record low of 537 cases, a decrease of 99% in 10 years. In 2002, only Venezuela and Colombia reported cases.[4]

In the rest of the world, measles continues to be endemic. Vaccination campaigns and surveillance systems have not been as successful in containing transmission of the disease, despite achieving close to 80% vaccine coverage.[6] Measles eradication requires that greater than 95% of susceptible individuals be vaccinated with the current two-dose vaccine strategy.[5,6.]

Lessons learned from what has been achieved in the Americas have been useful in guiding efforts to reduce the incidence in other nations, and include: (1) fixed health facilities with outreach vaccination programs; (2) measles surveillance programs; and (3) quick response to outbreaks.[7]

Pathogenesis and etiology

The measles virus is a large pleomorphic virus belonging to the family Paramyxoviridae and the genus *Morbillivirus*. The envelope is made up of an outer lipid bilayer and three viral proteins essential in measles pathogenesis. The matrix (M) protein forms the inner lining of the envelope surrounding the single-stranded RNA–nucleoprotein core. The other two proteins, called hemagglutinin (H) and fusion (F), project outward from the envelope.[8] The H protein facilitates viral attachment to the host cell receptors CD46 and CD150. The F protein allows for fusion between the envelope and the cell membrane, providing access of the viral genome into the host cell. The M protein then helps with viral replication and assembly of new virus particles released by budding.

Measles can easily be transmitted via air-borne droplets beginning 1–2 days before the onset of symptoms until 3–4 days after the onset of the rash. The virus can survive up to 2 h outside the body. Humans and primates are the only known natural hosts, with no known long-asymptomatic carrier states or animal reservoirs. The virus enters via the mucosal surfaces of the nasopharynx or conjunctiva, replicates throughout the respiratory tree, and spreads to local lymph nodes and the blood stream, causing a primary viremia. Replication in several regional lymph nodes eventually results in a generalized infection throughout the reticuloendothelial system and a secondary viremia 10–12 days after exposure. The virus spreads to multiple tissues, including the skin, gastrointestinal tract, respiratory tree, central nervous system, and thymus. Reticuloendothelial cells infected by the virus fuse and form multinucleated giant cells called Warthin–Finkeldey cells.

Recovery from measles, as in most viral infections, requires humoral and cell-mediated immunity. The antibody reduces the viral load and prevents future reinfection. Cytotoxic T lymphocytes stop replication by destroying the infected host cells. It is the interaction of T cells and viral antigen in the buccal mucosa that produces the pathognomonic enanthem in the early prodrome phase and heralds the delayed-type hypersensitivity reaction that occurs subsequently in the skin and other organs. Viral replication occurs in the epithelial and endothelial vessels of all target organs. Infected capillary endothelial cells with T-cell infiltrates are seen on biopsy of the morbilliform rash. IgM antibody levels peak 7 days after onset of the rash and IgG levels are highest 4 weeks after onset of disease. Although the humoral response is thought to be the most important in preventing reinfection, survival of acute measles infection is due to the cellular response, as demonstrated by the uneventful recovery of infected agammaglobulinemic patients.

Measles complications arise from the transient immunodeficiency that accompanies acute disease. After the immune system controls the viral illness, there is a loss of delayed-type hypersensitivity, making the host susceptible to opportunistic infections. Response to skin testing with a purified protein derivative is blunted and reactivation of latent tuberculosis disease after measles has been documented. Increased susceptibility to secondary bacterial infections is thought to be due to measles virus disruption of the mucosal barrier and differences in Th2 versus Th1 stimulation. Changes in host immunocompetence are not fully understood but may last for months or years.

Clinical features

The measles prodrome is well recognized as a triad of cough, coryza, and conjunctivitis. In uncomplicated classic measles cases, the immunocompetent patient develops these symptoms with low-grade fever and malaise after an 8–12-day incubation period. The pathognomonic enanthem, called Koplik spots, occurs 2 days before the rash. Although they may present anywhere in the mouth, characteristically these 1–2-mm blue-white macules appear alongside the second molars which gradually coalesce and fade after 12–72 h (Fig. 14.1).

The distinguishing rash (Fig. 14.2) appears 14 days after initial exposure and 2–4 days into the prodrome, accompanied by conjunctivitis (Fig. 14.3) and an increase in fever and severity of respiratory symptoms. It starts as a salmon-pink maculopapular rash on the head and neck that is non-pruritic. Over the next 3 days, it spreads from the face to the trunk and extremities, eventually becoming confluent on the head and upper extremities. The extent of confluency of the rash is proportional to the severity of illness. Resolution of the rash begins 4 days after onset, fading into a copper discoloration with brawny desquamation in the same cephalocaudal

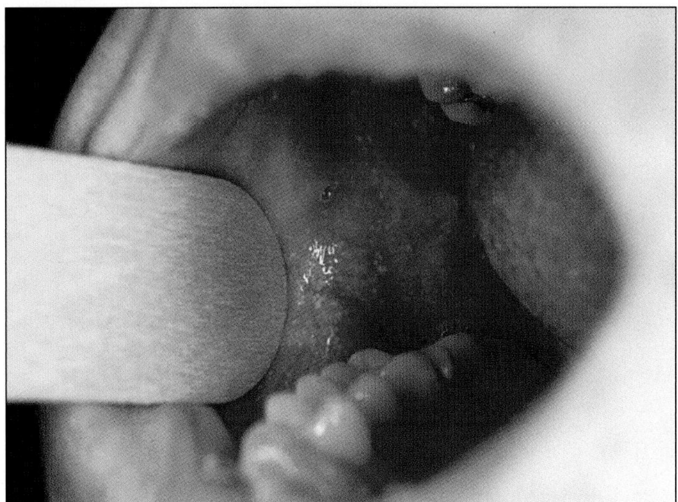

Figure 14.1 Koplik spots. (Courtesy of Donald A. Person.)

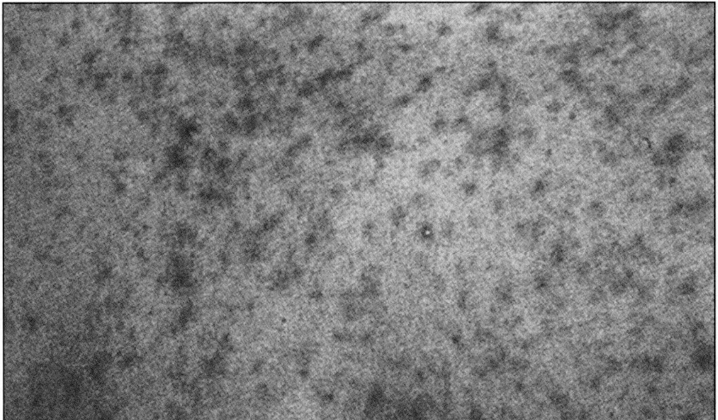

Figure 14.2 Exanthem associated with measles. (Courtesy of Donald A. Person.)

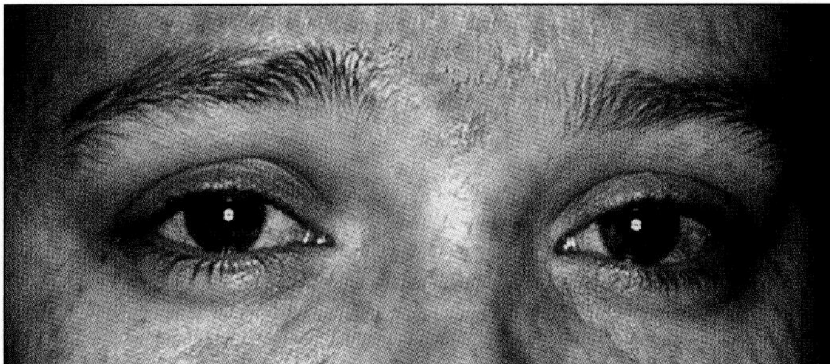

Figure 14.3 Measles conjunctivitis. (Courtesy of Donald A. Person.)

orientation. The fever resolves gradually as the exanthem fades. Other associated symptoms include pharyngitis, diarrhea, vomiting, abdominal pain, splenomegaly, and posterior cervical lymph adenopathy. Laboratory findings are usually non-specific and include leukopenia, relative lymphocytosis, thrombocytopenia, and mild elevation of liver enzymes.

Hemorrhagic (black) measles is associated with bleeding from multiple mucous membranes, pneumonitis, and disseminated intravascular coagulation. Onset is abrupt and characterized by high fever, seizures, and mental status changes.

Measles infection may not cause the characteristic symptoms in patients who are less than 1 year of age and in those who have been previously treated with exogenous immunoglobulin. Due to their preexisting partial immunity from maternal antibodies or an exogenous source, the incubation period is longer, while the prodrome duration is shorter. The symptoms are overall less severe, the rash does not become confluent, and the Koplik spots are usually absent.

Atypical measles may occur in individuals who received inactivated measles vaccine that was available in the USA from 1963 to 1967. The formalin inactivation reduced antigenicity of the fusion protein, allowing viral transmission among host cells. Those exposed to wild measles after receiving the killed-virus vaccine develop more severe symptoms with an atypical rash. The incubation period is unchanged but Koplik spots are rarely seen. The rash starts on the hands and feet, spreading to the proximal extremities and trunk with a hemorragic, petechial, and vesicular appearance. This commonly results in confusion with rickettsial diseases. Interstitial pneumonia, pleural effusions, hyperesthesia, urticaria, and edema of the hands and feet are common.[9] Despite the increase in severity, atypical measles usually resolves without complications.

In patients with human immunodeficiency virus (HIV), compromised T-cell immunity results in little or no rash and in continued prolonged measles virus replication and shedding. Also, immunity is depressed further as a direct result of measles infection, potentially leading to an increased risk of serious complications (pneumonitis and encephalitis) or hastening the progression to acquired immunodeficiency syndrome (AIDS). Measles vaccination prior to immune suppression may protect against fatal disease. Vaccine failure is more common in this population, requiring multiple doses of the vaccine to achieve seroconversion.[10]

Complications of measles are uncommon in immunocompetent and well-nourished hosts. Although measles virus may directly cause giant-cell pneumonitis and encephalopathy, the most common complications are due to bacterial superinfection of the compromised respiratory epithelium. Pathogens include *Streptococcus pneumoniae*, *Haemophilus influenzae*, *Staphylococcus aureus*, and enteric Gram-negative bacilli. Bacterial pneumonia is the most common fatal complication,[11] accounting for most of the 700 000 deaths in children with measles worldwide.

Central nervous system complications occur as the interaction of the measles virus and the host's immune system deviates from normal. The three identified complications include: (1) acute post-infectious measles encephalomyelitis (APME), an autoimmune phenomenon occurring in 1/1000 measles cases; (2) measles inclusion body encephalitis/subacute measles encephalitis (MIBE) that only occurs in those who are immunocompromised; and (3) subacute sclerosing panencephalitis (SSPE), a rare fatal complication thought to be due to persistent virus in the central nervous system.

Patient evaluation, diagnosis, and differential diagnosis

Measles follows a characteristic clinical course and until recently the diagnosis was made without laboratory confirmation in most countries endemic for the disease (Fig. 14.4). But the successful

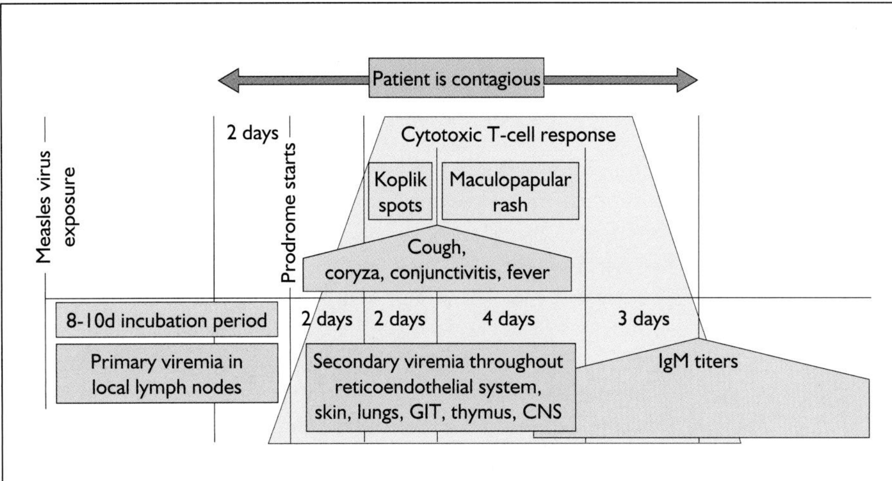

Figure 14.4 Timeline illustrating the appearance of clinical findings and immune response.

eradication from many regions has made surveillance dependent on accurate diagnosis as well as genotyping for strain characterization. Culturing the virus from secretions (urine, blood, and nasopharygeal (NP)) has low sensitivity and is difficult to perform. Currently, serologic IgM enzyme immunoassay detection is the most widely available diagnostic test and should be paired with an NP or urine sample for virus isolation. The IgM serologic test is most sensitive (83–89%) and specific (95–100%) just after the first week of rash onset. Specimens taken before or after this time are less reliable than paired acute and convalescent IgG comparison titers. Polymerase chain reaction, perhaps employing oral fluid samples or filter paper blood spots, is soon likely to become the standard in detecting viral RNA.[12]

Other diagnoses that may resemble the measles morbilliform rash include: exanthem subitum, rubella, enteroviral or adenoviral infection, scarlet fever, rickettsial diseases, Kawasaki syndrome, drug eruptions, and serum sickness.

Treatment

Supportive care and monitoring for complications are key to recovery from measles. Much controversy surrounds the use of prophylactic antibiotics to reduce secondary bacterial infections, although all agree on the need for aggressive treatment if they occur.

Since the 1930s vitamin A has been associated with decreased morbidity and mortality in measles cases. Vitamin A enhances protection and immunity against measles complications. It strengthens the mucosal barrier in the respiratory and gastrointestinal tract and enhances the humoral and cellular immune response. In developing nations, where there are large populations of malnourished children, administration of vitamin A to children with measles has been shown to decrease the mortality by 30%. This benefit is measles-specific and more pronounced in infants and malnourished populations where xerophthalmia from vitamin A deficiency is common.[13]

Interventions are available to stop the occurrence of measles in a susceptible individual after exposure. A live virus vaccine has been shown to ameliorate or stop symptom development if given within 72 h of exposure. Immune serum globulin is recommended for those individuals who cannot be immunized or who are at risk of severe disease or complications. Those less than 1 year of age, pregnant, or exposed more than 72 h previously may be given 0.25 ml/kg IM up to 6 days postexposure.[14] Immunocompromised patients may receive 0.5 ml/kg up to a maximum of 15 ml.

References

1. McBrien J, Murphy J, Gill D et al. Measles outbreak in Dublin, 2000. Pediatr Infect Dis 2003; 22:580–584.
2. Olive JM, Aylward RB, Melgaard B. Disease eradication as a public health strategy: is measles next? World Health Stat Q 1997; 50:185–187.
3. Griffin DE, Ward BJ, Esolen LM. Pathogenesis of measles virus infection: an hypothesis for altered immune responses. J Infect Dis 1994; 170 (suppl. 1):S24–S33.
4. de Quadros CA, Izurieta H, Carrasco P et al. Progress toward measles eradication in the region of the Americas: evolving strategies. J Infect Dis 2003; 187:224–229.
5. Centers for Disease Control. Measles – United States, 2000. MMWR 2002; 51:120–123.
6. Strebel P, Cochi S, Grabowsky M.et al. The unfinished measles immunization agenda. J Infect Dis 2003; 187 (suppl. 1):S1–S7.
7. Centers for Disease Control. Accelerated measles control – Cambodia, 1999–2002. MMWR 2003; 52:4–6.
8. Hilleman MR. Current overview of the pathogenesis and prophylaxis of measles with focus on practical implications. Vaccine 2001; 20:651–665.
9. Martin DB, Weiner LB, Nieburg PI et al. Atypical measles in adolescents and young adults. Ann Intern Med 1979; 90:877–881.
10. Duke T, Mgone CS. Measles: not just another viral exanthem. Lancet 2003; 361:763–773.
11. Makhene MK, Diaz PS. Clinical presentations and complications of suspected measles in hospitalized children. Pediatr Infect Dis J 1993; 12:836–840.

12. Bellini WJ, Helfand RF. The challenges and strategies for laboratory diagnosis of measles in an international setting. J Infect Dis 2003; 187 (suppl. 1):S283–S290.
13. Villamor E, Fawzi WW. Vitamin A supplementation: implications for morbidity and mortality in children. J Infect Dis 2000; 182 (suppl. 1):S122–S133.
14. Pickering LK (ed.) Red book 2003. Report of the Committee on Infectious Diseases, 26th edn. Elk Grove Village, IL: American Academy of Pediatrics; 2003:422.

Chapter 15

HTLV-1

Jennifer Aranda and Maria L. Turner

- Introduction
- History and epidemiology
- Clinical features
- Diagnosis
- Differential diagnosis
- Pathology
- Prevention
- Treatment

Introduction

Human T-cell lymphotropic virus type 1 (HTLV-1) is an enveloped, single-stranded RNA, type C retrovirus, in the subfamily Oncovirinae.[1]

In the host, the virus preferably infects the CD4 T cells. After infection, cells increase the interleukin-2 receptor (IL-2R; CD25) on their surface. As disease progresses the cells become less dependent on IL-2 for cell growth.[2]

Synonyms:

- Human T-cell lymphotropic virus (HTLV-1), human T-cell leukemia virus, adult T-cell leukemia retrovirus
- Adult T-cell leukemia, lymphoma (ATLL), adult T-cell leukemia (ATL)
- HTLV-1-associated myelopathy (HAM), tropical spastic paraparesis (TSP)

Key features:

- This retrovirus infection is endemic in certain areas of Japan, Africa, South America, the Caribbean, the Middle East, and Southeastern USA
- It is most commonly associated with ATLL and HAM/TSP
- The ATLL course may vary from indolent to rapidly fatal
- Cutaneous involvement usually occurs as a manifestation of ATLL or infective dermatitis in children
- The ATLL skin manifestations are similar to those of other cutaneous T-cell lymphomas (CTCLs), in particular mycosis fungoides

History and epidemiology

The first two isolates of HTLV-1 were reported in 1980, and were obtained from two adult patients diagnosed as having mycosis fungoides and Sézary's leukemia.[3]

HTLV-1 transmission occurs through intravenous drug use, blood transfusions, solid organ transplants, breast-feeding, and sexual contact.

The virus is estimated to infect between 15 and 25 million people worldwide. HTLV-1 is endemic in sub-Saharan Africa, southern Japan, the Caribbean basin, South America, the Middle East, and Southeastern USA.

Clinical features

Adult T-cell leukemia/lymphoma

ATLL was first recognized in Japan in 1973 and internationally acknowledged in 1977.[4,5] Most cases have been associated with HTLV-1. Approximately 5% of people with HTLV-1 antibodies eventually develop ATLL after a latent infection that lasts on average 10–30 years.[1]

The clinical picture of ATLL varies and typically presents with malaise, fever, lymphadenopathy (LAD), hepatosplenomegaly, and signs of other organ involvement. It is characterized by atypical peripheral blood cells with indented nuclei, referred to as "flower cells." Laboratory abnormalities usually include hypercalcemia, increased lactate dehydrogenase (LDH) levels, increased β_2-microglobulin and increased IL-2R α chain (CD25, Tac).

Based on clinical and prognostic features, ATLL has been divided into four major subgroups. These are classically referred to as acute, chronic, lymphoma, and smouldering types (Table 15.1).[6]

Others have further subdivided the smouldering type with skin manifestations into those with deep and those with superficial skin infiltration. This additional subclassification has been suggested based on prognostic differences.[7]

Patients often develop opportunistic infections, most commonly *Pneumocystis carinii* pneumonia, cytomegalovirus, disseminated zoster, and fungal infections. There is an increased incidence of the severe form of strongyloidiasis and crusted (Norwegian) scabies.

Cutaneous involvement occurs in up to 50% of patients with ATLL and there is no pathognomonic presentation. Different

Table 15.1 Diagnostic criteria for clinical subtypes of adult T-cell leukemia

	Smouldering	Chronic	Lymphoma	Acute
Lymphocyte (× 10^9/l)	<4	<4[a]	<4	*
Abnormal T lymphocytes	= 5%	+[b]	= 1%	+[b]
Flower cells	Occasional	Occasional	No	Yes
Lactate dehydrogenase	= 1.5N	= 2N	*	*
Corrected Ca (mmol/l)	<2.74	<2.74	*	*
Histology-proven lymphadenopathy (LAD)	No	*	Yes	*
Tumor lesion				
Skin	**	*	*	*
Lung	**	*	*	*
Lymph node	No	*	Yes	*
Liver	No	*	*	*
Spleen	No	*	*	*
Central nervous system	No	No	*	*
Bone	No	No	*	*
Ascites	No	No	*	*
Pleural effusion	No	No	*	*
Gastrointestinal tract	No	No	*	*

N, normal upper limit.
[a]Accompanied by T lymphocytosis = 3.5 × 10/l.
[b]If abnormal T lymphocytes are <5%, histology-proven tumor lesion is required.
*No essential qualification except terms required for other subtypes.
**No essential qualification if other terms are fulfilled, but histology-proven malignant lesion is required if T lymphocytes <5%.
Adapted from Shimoyama M and members of the Lymphoma Study Group (1984–1987). Diagnostic criteria and classification of clinical subtypes of adult T-cell leukemia-lymphoma. Br J Haematol 1991; 79:428–437.

morphologic types of skin lesions have been described and they may be indistinguishable from those of mycosis fungoides and Sézary syndrome (Fig. 15.1).

Patients may have lesions that resemble those of lepromatous leprosy, Kaposi's sarcoma, or pruritic vesicles of the hands that are indistinguishable from pompholyx[8] (Fig. 15.2).

A report consisting of eight patients illustrated the heterogeneity of disease presentations. One case had erythematous plaques over the eyelids that appeared granulomatous, while another patient with pompholyx-like lesions also had skin-colored papules on the eyelids, ears, and perioral region. Seven of these patients presented with cutaneous disease, of whom five subsequently developed leukemia.[9]

The clinical spectrum should include generalized follicular papules and vesicles or bullae, keloid-like plaques on the face, dorsal hands, elbows, inframammary, and intergluteal area, and hypopigmented plaques.[10,11]

Infective dermatitis

Infective dermatitis was originally reported in 1966 in Jamaican children and further defined in 1967.[12,13] The association with HTLV-1 was made in 1990[14] and has been reported in several endemic areas, including Japan, Columbia, Barbados, Trinidad and Tobago, and among Haitian immigrants in Miami.

Children generally acquire the virus through breast-feeding. On average, they present with clinical disease by 2 years of age,[12] but only a minority of those infected show clinical disease.

The disease usually presents as an eczematous dermatitis of the scalp, ears, eyelids, neck, groin, and axillae, along with eventual development of a generalized fine papular rash. Children usually have an accompanying chronic rhinorrhea. The nasal discharge and/or skin most commonly grow *Staphylococcus aureus* or β-haemolytic streptococci.[13] Criteria for diagnosis have been well defined (Table 15.2).[15]

Complications include crusted scabies, corneal opacities, chronic bronchiectasis, glomerulonephritis, strongyloidiasis, and other parasitic worm infestations. They are also at increased risk for future development of HAM/TSP and ATLL.

HTLV-1 associated myelopathy/tropical spastic paraparesis

TSP was first described in Jamaica as a neuropathy of unknown etiology. It was in 1985 that HTLV-1 was linked to TSP and a

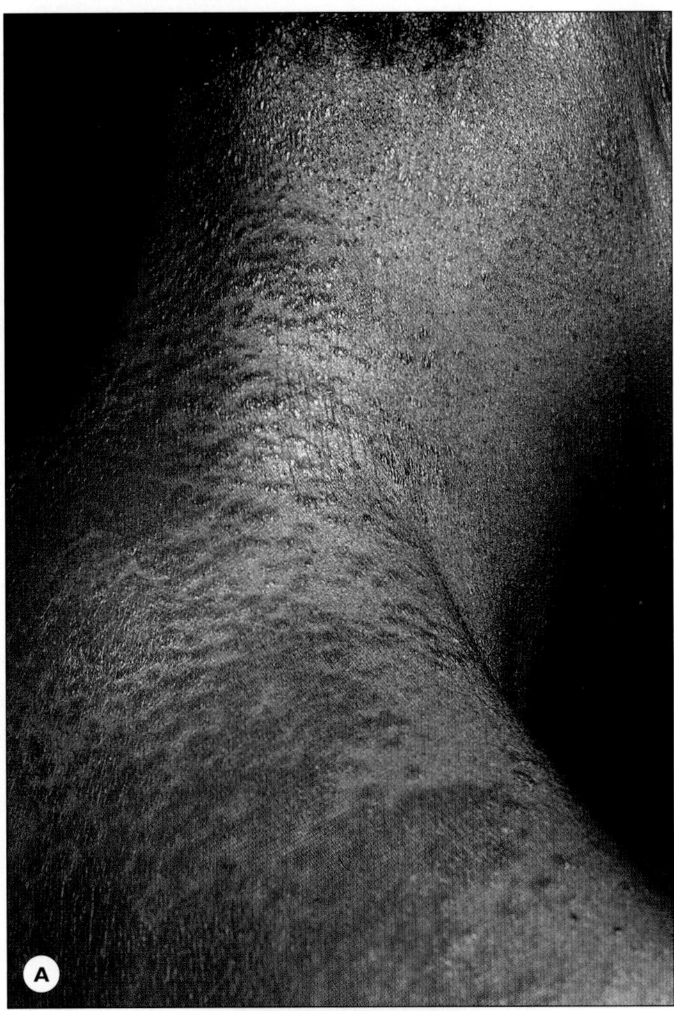

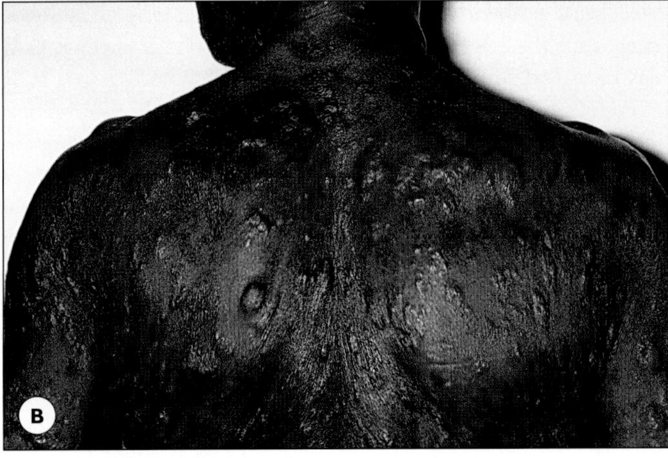

Figure 15.1 (A) Homogeneous-looking flat, smooth papules confluent over the upper back and posterior aspect of the neck as seen in the dermal form of ATLL. (B) Combination of tumors and hyperpigmented plaques simulating appearance of mycosis fungoides.

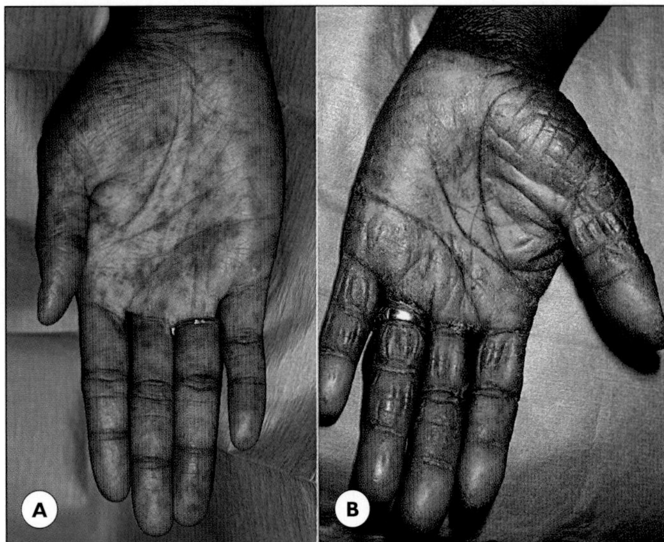

Figure 15.2 (A) Acute pompholyx-like palmar vesicles; (B) crusted papules from dried up pompholyx-like vesicles.

Table 15.2 Criteria for diagnosis of infective dermatitis

Major criteria (need 4 of 5 and must include numbers 1, 2, and 5)
1. Eczema of scalp, axillae, and groin, external ear and retroauricular areas, eyelid margins, paranasal skin, and/or neck (at least two sites)
2. Chronic watery nasal discharge without other signs of rhinitis and/or crusting of the anterior nares
3. Chronic relapsing dermatitis with a prompt response to antibiotics and recurrence on withdrawal
4. Onset in early childhood
5. HTLV-1 antibody seropositivity
Minor criteria
Positive cultures for *Staphylococcus aureus* and/or β-hemolytic streptococci from the skin or anterior nares
Generalized fine papular rash (in most severe cases)
Generalized lymphadenopathy with dermatopathic lymphadenitis
Anemia
Elevated erythrocyte sedimentation rate
Hyperimmunoglobulinemia (IgD and IgE)
Elevated CD4 count, CD8 count, and CD4/CD8 ratio
HTLV-1, human T-lymphotropic virus-1; IgD, immunoglobulin D.
Adapted from La Grenade L, Manns A, Fletcher V et al. Clinical, pathologic, and immunologic features of human T-lymphotophic virus type I-associated infective dermatitis in children. Arch Dermatol 1998; 134:439–444.

similar condition was described in 1986 under the name of HTLV-1-associated myelopathy (HAM).[16,17] In 1988, a World Health Organization (WHO) group decided that both conditions were the same.[18]

The lifetime risk of HAM/TSP is estimated at less than 2%.[1] Clinically, the disease is characterized by a progressive spastic weakness, paresthesiae of the legs, and hyperreflexia, along with lower back pain, impotence, and urinary frequency or incontinence.

In a recent report on HAM/TSP, cutaneous findings including xerosis, cutaneous candidiasis, and palmar erythema were observed. More importantly, in this group of patients, 25% of those who had skin biopsies were shown to have histologic findings consistent with CTCL. On clinical grounds, of these eight patients whose biopsy findings were consistent with CTCL, seven were thought to have xerosis or chronic eczema and one was thought to have erythroderma.[19]

Other diseases associated with HTLV-1

HTLV-1 has been implicated in the pathogenesis of other diseases, including uveitis, polymyositis, arthropathy, bronchopneumonopathy, and Sjögren's syndrome.

Diagnosis

Antibodies are initially detected through enzyme-linked immunosorbent assay (ELISA), with repeat positives confirmed by Western blot or polymerase chain reaction (PCR). The Western blot technique and PCR can help to make the distinction between HTLV-1 and HTLV-2.

Finally, in order to distinguish ATLL from the carrier state, detection of a monoclonal integration of the virus should be confirmed by Southern blot analysis or inverse PCR.

Differential diagnosis

Cutaneous forms of ATLL are frequently indistinguishable clinically and histopathologically from other forms of CTCL, in particular mycosis fungoides.

Infective dermatitis may be difficult to distinguish from seborrheic eczema. It is also important to rule out dermatophyte scalp infections.

Pathology

The histopathologic features of ATLL are variable and usually reveal a perivascular infiltrate in the upper dermis, consisting of neoplastic pleomorphic cells that are typically CD4+, CD25+, and CD30– (Fig. 15.3). Occasional CD8+ variants occur. The presence of epidermotropism and Pautrier's microabscesses may make ATLL indistinguishable from mycosis fungoides on routine histology and there may be a role for the use of in situ hybridization to aid in differentiating between cutaneous ATLL and other forms of CTCL.

Prevention

The main mode of prevention is through public health measures. Educational programs, both on safer sexual practices, as well as avoidance of mother-to-child transmission need to be instituted.

Blood donor screening is already being done in several countries and there is promise for the development of a vaccine in the future.

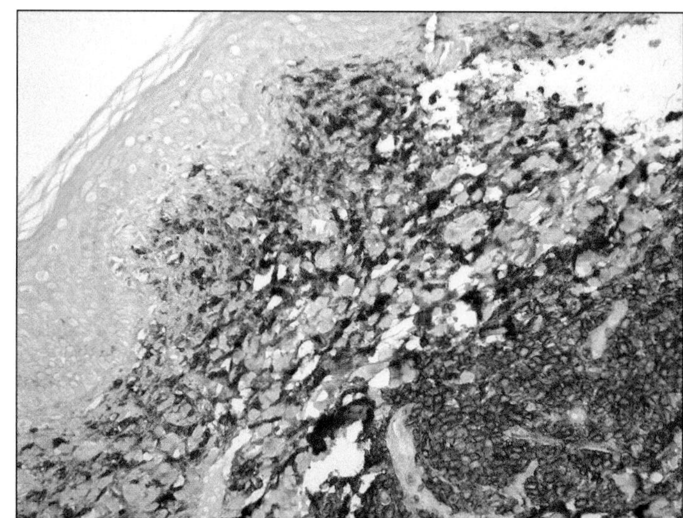

Figure 15.3 CD25-positive infiltrate of atypical lymphocytes in the upper dermis from a patient with the dermal form of adult T-cell leukemia.

Treatment

Treatment of ATLL with combination chemotherapy has not been shown to improve survival.

A combination of zidovudine or retinoids with interferon-α has been successful in several patients and the use of all three agents simultaneously has also been described.[20]

Most recently, emphasis has been placed on IL-2R-directed therapy, since these receptors have been found to play a key role in the proliferation of the leukemic cells and are not found on normal resting cells. This treatment modality includes anti-Tac (CD25, IL-2Rα chain) antibodies and has induced remission in some patients. To enhance the effect of these humanized anti-Tac antibodies, they may be armed with α- and β-emitting radionuclides.[2]

Infective dermatitis responds well to systemic antibiotics, antihistamines, and mild topical steroids. Keratolytic shampoos may be used for scalp involvement.

HAM/TSP treatment usually consists of intrathecal corticosteroids or systemic steroids. Anti-Tac has also shown clinical benefit.[2]

References

1. Manns A, Hisada M, La Grenada L. Human T-lymphotropic virus type I infection. Lancet 1999; 353:1951–1958.
2. Waldmann TA. The promiscuous IL-2/IL-15 receptor: a target for immunotherapy of HTLV-I-associated disorders. J AIDS Hum Retrovirol 1996; 13:S179–S185.
3. Poiesz BJ, Ruscetti FW, Reitz MS et al. Isolation of a new type C retrovirus (HTLV) in primary uncultured cells of a patient with Sezary T-cell leukemia. Nature 1981; 294:268–271.
4. Yodoi J, Takatsuki K, Masuda T. Two cases of T-cell chronic lymphocytic leukemia in Japan. N Engl J Med 1974; 290:572–573.
5. Takatsuki K, Uchiyama T, Sagawa K et al. Adult T-cell leukemia

in Japan. In: Seno S, Takaku F, Irino S, eds. Topics in hematology. Amsterdam: Excerpta Medica; 1977:73–77.

6. Shimoyama M. Diagnostic criteria and classification of clinical subtypes of adult T-cell leukaemia-lymphoma. A report from the Lymphoma Study Group (1984–87). Br J Haematol 1991; 79:428–437.
7. Setoyama M, Katahira Y, Kansaki T. Clinicopathologic analysis of 124 cases of adult T-cell leukemia/lymphoma with cutaneous manifestations: the smouldering type with skin manifestations has a poorer prognosis than previously thought. J Dermatol 1999; 26:785–790.
8. Chan HL, Su I, Kuo T et al. Cutaneous manifestations of adult T cell leukemia/lymphoma. J Am Acad Dermatol 1985; 13:213–219.
9. Whittaker SJ, Ng YL, Rustin M et al. HTLV-1-associated cutaneous disease: a clinicopathological and molecular study of patients from the UK. Br J Dermatol 1993; 128:483–492.
10. Michael EJ, Shaffer JJ, Collins HE et al. Bullous adult T-cell lymphoma/leukemia and human T-cell lymphotropic virus-1 associated myelopathy in a 60-year-old man. J Am Acad Dermatol 2002; 46:S137–S141.
11. DiCaudo DJ, Perniciaro C, Worrell JT et al. Clinical and histologic spectrum of human T-cell lymphotropic virus type I-associated lymphoma involving the skin. J Am Acad Dermatol 1996; 34:69–76.
12. Sweet RD. A pattern of eczema in Jamaica. Br J Dermatol 1996; 78:93–100.
13. Walshe MM. Infective dermatitis in Jamaican children. Br J Dermatol 1967; 79:229–236.
14. La Grenade L, Hanchard B, Fletcher V et al. Infective dermatitis of Jamaican children: a marker for HTLV-I infection. Lancet 1990; 336:1345–1347.
15. La Grenade L, Manns A, Fletcher V et al. Clinical, pathologic, and immunologic features of human T-lymphotophic virus type I-associated infective dermatitis in children. Arch Dermatol 1998; 134:439–444.
16. Gessain A, Barin F, Vernant JC et al. Antibodies to human T-lymphotropic virus type I in patients with tropical spastic paraparesis. Lancet 1985; 2:407–410.
17. Osame M, Usuku K, Izumo S et al. HTLV-1-associated myelopathy: a new clinical entity. Lancet 1986; 1:1031–1032.
18. Report from the scientific group on HTLV-1 infection and its associated diseases, convened by the regional office for the Western Pacific of the World Health Organization in Karoshima, Japan, 10–15 December 1988. Wkly Epidemiol Rc 1989; 49:382–383.
19. Lenzi ME, Cuzzi-Maya T, Oliveira AL et al. Dermatological findings of human T lymphotropic virus type 1 (HTLV-I)-associated myelopathy/tropical spastic paraparesis. Clin Infect Dis 2003; 36:507–513.
20. Chan EF, Dowdy YG, Lee B et al. A novel chemotherapeutic regimen (interferon alpha, zidovudine, and etretinate) for adult T-cell lymphoma resulting in rapid tumor destruction. J Am Acad Dermatol 1999; 40:116–121.

Chapter 16

Tropical manifestations of common viral infections

Jashin J. Wu, Katie R. Pang, David B. Huang and Stephen K. Tyring

Introduction

Common viruses that are widespread in tropical countries tend to have distinct manifestations compared to the manifestations seen in industrialized nations. We will discuss these manifestations for Epstein–Barr virus (EBV), human papillomavirus (HPV), and human herpesvirus 8 (HHV-8).

Epstein–Barr virus

Epidemiology

In 1964, EBV was first identified by Epstein, Achong, and Barr from a cultured African Burkitt's lymphoma using electron microscopy. Dr. Denis Burkitt, an English surgeon, was the first to report endemic Burkitt's lymphoma (eBL). He felt that the cancer was associated with an unknown infectious disease, and he sent tissue materials to Dr. Epstein's laboratory. Within several years, the new herpesvirus was discovered and was named EBV.

More than 90% of adults in the world have been infected with EBV and carry the virus as a lifelong persistent infection. This population has latent infection of B lymphocytes and virus production in saliva. In the majority of cases, primary infection occurs subclinically during childhood, often by spread between family members via salivary contact.

In low socioeconomic groups, EBV seroconversion occurs early in non-industrialized countries. Many tropical countries tend to be non-industrialized with large low-socioeconomic populations. In Thailand, the seroprevalence of anti-EBV immunoglobulin G (IgG) antibody in previously healthy hospitalized children aged 0–15 years was studied.[1] Of 589 cases, the seroprevalence of EBV infection was 50.4, 72.8, 92.3, 96.6, and 97.6% in children at the age range of 0–2, 3–5, 6–8, 9–11, and 12–14 years, respectively. Excluding infants below 6 months of age, the total seroprevalence rate was 68.4%. Children who were reared at home had lower seroprevalence rates, further suggesting that EBV is more easily spread in crowded conditions. A similar study of 425 volunteers aged 6 months to 15 years demonstrated a total seropositivity rate of 72.7%.[2]

A seroepidemiological study in Bangladesh was conducted on 502 patients between 15 days and 90 years.[3] The overall prevalence of EBV infection in the group was 81.3%. By the age of 1 year, 42.4% of infants had antibodies to EBV. There was a significant rise in the percentage of seropositives between 0–1- and 1–2-year-old children, demonstrating a high rate of primary infection at these ages. The prevalence of IgG antibody to EBV was 87.9% in the 2–10-years age group, and from 10 years of age and upward, the prevalence was sustained at over 85%.

In Turkey, a seroepidemiological study of 540 subjects found seropositivity to be 99.4%.[4] Increased IgG levels are directly correlated with age, exposure in public places, living in crowded families, and low income ($P < 0.05$). However, no relationship between the levels of IgG antibody and blood transfusion, educational status, or sex was found ($P > 0.05$).

In affluent industrialized nations, seroconversion may be delayed until adolescence, when infectious mononucleosis (IM) occurs in between 50% and 74% of cases. Those who remain uninfected throughout childhood may become infected during the teenage years through kissing, and consequently IM is often called the "kissing disease." However, there are reports of EBV detection in male and female genital secretions, suggesting the possibility of sexual transmission. A seroepidemiological study on university students adds support to this theory by showing strong correlations of both EBV seropositivity and history of IM with sexual intercourse and increasing numbers of sexual partners.[5] However, this study did not differentiate between spread by kissing versus direct transmission in genital secretions.

Transplanted organs with EBV infection into a previously seronegative recipient can cause infection, which is a risk factor for posttransplant lymphoproliferative disease (PTLD). The blood of healthy donors with latent EBV infection is another potential route of transmission.

Pathogenesis

EBV enters through the oropharyngeal passage and infects resting B cells and/or epithelial cells. In the productive primary phase, virus is released to infect B cells circulating in the oropharynx, resulting in a latent infection. The infected B cells induce an enormous expansion of virus-specific and non-specific T cells that cause the symptoms of IM. This antiviral T-cell response results in the regression of the infected B cells, which evade the immune system by limiting viral antigen expression of latent membrane protein 2 (LMP-2) and EBV-encoded RNA (EBERs). EBV then persists for the lifetime of the individual, periodically reactivating to shed virions and spreading the virus to new hosts.

There are two kinds of EBV (1 and 2 or A and B) circulating in the world, based on the polymorphism within the gene loci expressing Epstein–Barr nuclear antigen (EBNA) 2, 3A, 3B, and 3C proteins. The main difference is the reduced transformation capacity and thus the lower clinical aggressiveness of the type 2 virus. There is no specific disease association, but type 1 is more prevalent in the west, and types 1 and 2 are equally prevalent in Africa and Papua New Guinea. Further, different EBV isolates can be differentiated by varying lengths of genomic repeat sequences, which have been used to track individual isolates in organ donor/recipient pairs and through families.

Like the others in the herpesvirus family, EBV can establish either a lytic or latent infection in host cells. The EBV-infected tumor cells contain one of the three types of latent EBV infection, and expression of the latent EBV gene products is adequate for immortalization of B cells in vitro. The latent virus is replicated once per cell cycle as an episome using the host cell DNA polymerase, the viral oriP replication origin, and the viral EBNA-1 protein.

The role of EBV in oncology is thought to correlate with different types of viral latency and associated histology. Type I latency occurs when viral gene expression is limited to the EBNA-1 protein and BARF0. Burkitt's lymphoma typically exhibits type I latency. In type II latency, the cells express EBNA-1, LMP-1, LMP-2, and BARF0 (which is transcribed but possibly not translated). Hodgkin's lymphoma and nasopharyngeal carcinoma (NPC) are the characteristic cancers associated with type II latency. Type III latency is associated with expression of all latency-associated proteins (EBNA-1, 2A, 2B, 3A, 3B, 3C, LP, BARF0) and the two viral membrane proteins LMP-1 and LMP-2. Posttransplant-type lymphomas, lymphoproliferative disease in immunocompromised, and lymphoblastoid B-cell lines typify type III latency.

Infectious mononucleosis

In industrialized nations, IM, or glandular fever, is one of the common causes of prolonged illness in adolescents and young adults. The incubation period may last between 4 and 7 weeks, after which the patient may experience fever, sore throat, lymphadenopathy, splenomegaly, and hepatocellular dysfunction with possible jaundice. A rash, such as macular erythema, petechiae, and urticaria, occurs in only about 3% of cases, but concomitant administration of ampicillin or related antibiotics results in rash in about 90% of cases. Hypersomnia, prolonged fatigue, and short-term depressive disorders are common after IM.

Serological testing is the most common method of diagnosis confirmation. Although often absent in young children, heterophile antibody is present in 85% of adolescents and adults with IM.[6] The Monospot is a quick slide test for the detection of heterophile antibodies, but false-positives may occur in systemic lupus erythematosus, human immunodeficiency virus (HIV), lymphoma, rubella, parvovirus, and other viral infections. A more sensitive and specific test is IgM to the EB viral capsid antigen (VCA), which may persist for 1–2 months. IgG to early antigens in the acute phase or EBNAs, which are associated with convalescence, may be useful in some cases.

Although high-dose acyclovir reduces virus production in the throat, it does not significantly alter the duration of individual symptoms. The symptoms of IM are due to secretion of cytokines by the large numbers of activated cytotoxic (CD8) T lymphocytes rather than due to virus infection of B cells, explaining the lack of efficacy of acyclovir. These T cells attack lytic, and to a lesser extent latent, viral epitopes, and are thought to control the acute infection by killing infected B lymphoblasts.

Chronic active EBV (CAEBV) infection

CAEBV infection is a rare but serious condition that occurs in a previously healthy person after documented primary EBV infection. The peripheral blood has a significant increase of EBV load with infection of T and/or natural killer cells. The acute IM antibody pattern remains, including failure to produce antibodies to EBNA1, high IgG anti-VCA and early antigen, and sometimes persistence of anti-VCA IgM. Vital organ involvement often occurs, such as bone marrow hypoplasia, hepatitis interstitial pneumonia, and splenomegaly. CAEBV has a high morbidity and mortality rate due to hemophagocytic syndrome, hepatic failure, lymphoma, or sepsis. This condition is hard to treat, but adoptive immunotherapy[7] or bone marrow transplantation[8] has been reported to be useful.

Oral hairy leukoplakia

First reported in 1984, oral hairy leukoplakia was described in young male homosexuals who were immunosuppressed. It is now well-documented to occur in all risk groups for HIV, including HIV-2,[9] as well as in transplant patients[10] and drug-induced immunosuppression.[11] The prevalence has been estimated between 7.5% and 25% of AIDS patients.[12]

It is characterized by bilateral, elevated white patches with a verrucous or filiform, irregular surface that cannot be scraped off on the lateral borders and dorsum of the tongue (Fig. 16.1). These asymptomatic, non-malignant lesions have also been found on the ventral surfaces of the tongue, buccal mucosa, floor of the mouth, palatal mucosa, and oropharynx. The presence of koilocytes in the superficial epithelial layers is the histologic pathognomonic sign. Other unique histopathological features include a lack of a notable inflammatory infiltrate in the associated submucosa and profound acanthosis, often with koilocytic changes.

Oral hairy leukoplakia is the only EBV-related chronic disease where the virus replicates profusely. The amount of viral replication

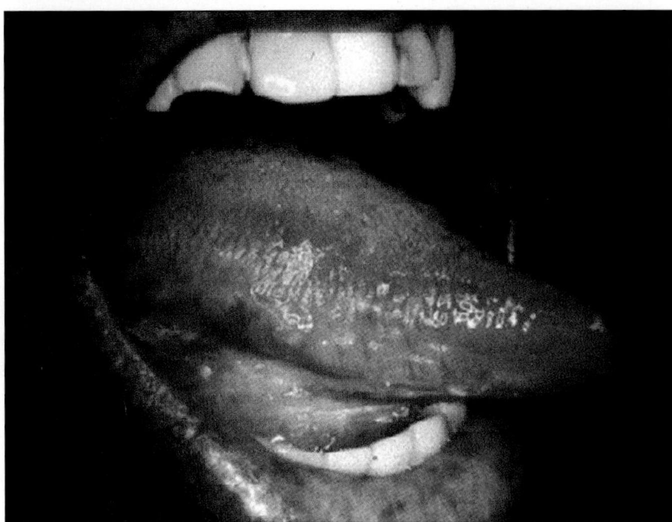

Figure 16.1 Oral hairy leukoplakia in an acquired immunodeficiency syndrome (AIDS) patient in India. (Courtesy of Dr. J.K. Maniar.)

is directly proportional to the degree of keratinocyte differentiation. For example, massive levels of EBV may be detected in the upper layers of the affected epithelium. Interestingly, there may be multiple EBV strains that extensively undergo inter- and intrastrain recombination. Further, in permissive herpesvirus infections where abundant virus production results in cell lysis, the epithelial cells housing this replicative activity remain intact.

Whether oral hairy leukoplakia develops after EBV reactivation from latency or by superinfection is not clear. Further, although its frequent association with HIV usually motivates the search for immunosuppression, oral hairy leukoplakia and its link with HIV in direct lesion development have not been determined. It has been related to a high HIV viral load and a low CD4 count. Oral hairy leukoplakia may develop secondary to EBV reactivation. The presence of EBV DNA in basal and parabasal lingual cells suggests that oral hairy leukoplakia in HIV patients might represent a reactivation of latent lingual infection. However, hematogenous superinfection of the tongue with EBV of HIV-positive individuals may precede or lead to the development of oral hairy leukoplakia. EBV strains replicating in the oral hairy leukoplakia lesion are different from those shed into the oral cavity, which had been hematogenously carried to the lingual epidermis. It has been demonstrated that different EBV strains in different body compartments can occur in simian immunodeficiency virus-infected rhesus monkeys[13] and HIV patients.[14]

Since the prevalence of HIV in Africa is so high, several studies have attempted to determine whether the prevalence of oral hairy leukoplakia is also elevated. In Kenya, only 4.9% of 61 HIV-positive patients had oral hairy leukoplakia.[15] Of 270 HIV-patients in Lesotho, 12% had oral hairy leukoplakia.[16] In two South African studies, 19.7% of 600 HIV-positive patients[17] and 26.6% of 772 HIV-positive patients[18] developed the lesion. Of 186 HIV-positive patients in Tanzania, 36% had oral hairy leukoplakia.[19] Thus, it appears that the prevalence of oral hairy leukoplakia found in Africa is similar to the prevalence found in the USA. In other parts of the world, the prevalence of oral hairy leukoplakia in HIV-positive patients varies in India (3%), Singapore (5%), Hong Kong (11%), Thailand (7–26%), Cambodia (35.6%), and Australia (45.2%).

Since it is a benign lesion with low morbidity, oral hairy leukoplakia does not require specific treatment in every case. However, the patient may wish to reduce symptoms such as discomfort, mild pain, and paresthesiae, or to treat the lesion for cosmetic reasons. To be effective, acyclovir has to be prescribed at a higher dose (800 mg five times a day). However, treatment failures with acyclovir occur commonly, especially in the immunocompromised patient. One study showed that valacyclovir appears to be a safe and effective treatment for oral hairy leukoplakia in HIV-positive patients.[20]

Cancers

EBV is one of the most diversely oncogenic viruses known. We will describe some of the cancers most commonly associated with EBV.

Breast cancer

The link between EBV and breast cancer is controversial. Breast cancer from 509 patients was studied in areas with varying risks of NPC.[21] High-risk areas are Algeria and Tunisia in North Africa. An intermediate-risk area is Marseilles in southern France. Low-risk areas are northern France, the Netherlands, and Denmark. Polymerase chain reaction (PCR) demonstrated that 31.8% of the tumors contained the EBV genome, and EBV type 1 was the predominant strain. No significant differences were observed among the geographical areas. However, using in situ hybridization with protein localization via immunohistochemistry, researchers did not find any EBV viral gene products in 43 female breast cancers.[22] Studies of 48 invasive breast cancers[23] and 60 invasive breast cancers,[24] using in situ hybridization and immunohistochemical studies, concluded that there was no significant role for EBV in the pathogenesis of breast carcinoma.

Gastric carcinoma

In 1992, it was first reported that EBV could be found in a small percentage of gastric carcinomas. Tumor cells had a uniform presence of EBER, but the surrounding normal tissue did not. Multiple studies have shown that approximately 6–18% of all gastric carcinomas are associated with EBV. Seven percent of all gastric carcinomas are associated with EBV in Japan, the nation with the highest incidence of gastric cancer. Other areas of the world show the following proportions of EBV-associated gastric carcinoma: India 5%, Korea 5.6%, northern China 6%, southern China 9%, Mexico 8.2%, Russia 8.7%, Colombia 11.1%, the USA 16%, Chile 16%, and Germany 18%. It has been suggested that areas with a low incidence of gastric cancer have relatively high proportions of EBV-associated gastric carcinoma.

EBV-associated gastric carcinoma is a result of inappropriately regulated gastric immune response to the infection. Disturbance in the level and activity of interleukin (IL)-10 and tumor necrosis factor (TNF)-α has been reported as a key modulating factor in EBV-related malignancies. One study of 30 patients with EBV-associated gastric carcinoma examined the distribution of IL-10 and TNF-α polymorphisms with that in 220 control subjects.[25] It was found that the high-producer allele –308A of the TNF-α gene was positively associated with EBV-associated gastric carcinoma and that the high-producer allele –1082G of the IL-10 gene was related to an increased risk of EBV-negative gastric carcinoma.

Nasopharyngeal carcinoma

In 1966, sera from NPC patients were found to have precipitating antibodies against EBV. In 1970, nucleic acid hybridization was used to show that EBV DNA was present in African NPC. Single clonal populations of EBV were found in NPCs, demonstrating that this malignancy derives from expansions of single progenitor cells infected by EBV.

The primary tumor of NPC is typically asymptomatic, and the disease frequently presents with metastases to lymph nodes in the head and neck (Fig. 16.2).[26]

In Caucasians of North America and Northern Europe, the age-adjusted incidence rate of NPC is less than 1/100 000.[27] In New Zealand, the incidence rate of NPC is also less than 1/100 000, which may be due to the high (80%) percentage of Caucasians of European descent.[28] However, in southern China and Hong Kong, NPC accounts for 18% of all cancers,[29] and the age-adjusted incidence rate is between 25.6 and 54.7/100 000 in Hong Kong.[27] In North Africa and the Mediterranean, the incidence rate is 8–12/100 000.[30] In India, one study showed that EBV was detected in 28 of 40 NPCs (70%).[31]

In some parts of central Africa, both eBL and NPC appear to coexist with relatively high frequency, and there is a greater geographic overlap between eBL and NPC than is currently recognized. In Kenya, a high incidence of NPC as well as eBL was documented. In contrast to the general belief that NPC is mainly a disease found in Asia, it was found that over a 10-year period (1961–1970), 434 patients, or 9% of all hospital admissions for malignancy in Nairobi, had NPC.[32] In the cancer registry in Nairobi between 1986 and 1990, NPC was the sixth most common cancer, with 234 cases.[33]

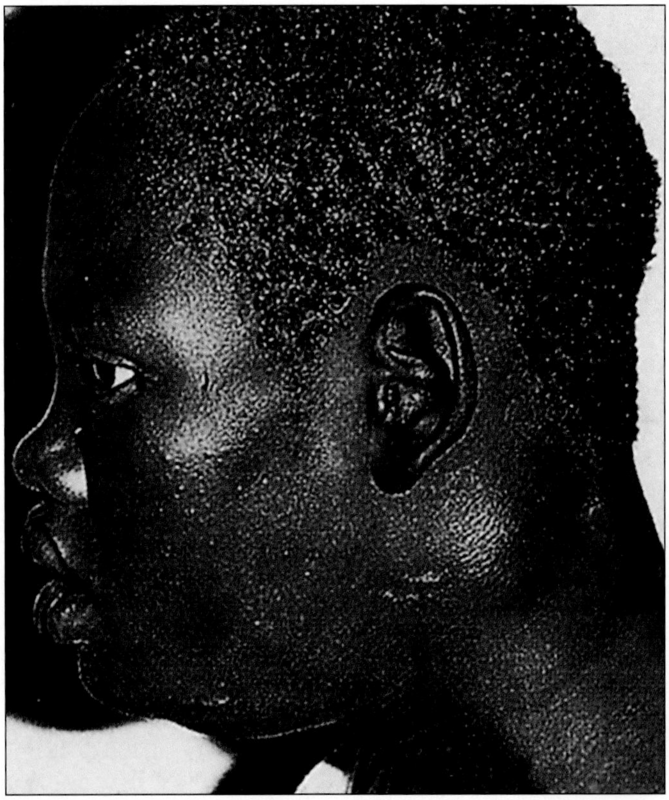

There is an interesting relationship between altitude and disease and the inverse correlation between eBL and NPC. In high areas of Kenya (over 1800 m), only NPC occurred; in areas at medium altitude (1000–1800 m), both NPC and eBL were prevalent; and below 1000 m, only eBL was found.[33]

Figure 16.2 Nasopharyngeal carcinoma in a patient from Sudan. (Reproduced from Peters W and Pasvol G (eds). Tropical Medicine and Parasitology, 5th edition, Mosby, London 2002, image 1032).

Burkitt's lymphoma

Burkitt's lymphoma is a small non-cleaved-cell lymphoma with vast geographic differences in incidence and character. African, or endemic, Burkitt's lymphoma usually arises in lymphoid tissue associated with the oropharyngeal mucosa or gastrointestinal tract and may manifest in salivary glands or submandibular lymph nodes (Fig. 16.3).[26] In equatorial Africa, it is about 50% of all childhood cancers, with an incidence of 100 per 1 million children under 15 years of age. This is in contrast to an incidence of 2 per million under 15 years of age in North America. Over 96% of eBL in central Africa is associated with EBV.

Only 20% of Burkitt's lymphoma in the USA (sporadic Burkitt's lymphoma) has this association. Burkitt's lymphoma in the USA and western Europe is morphologically and cytogenetically indistinguishable from eBL. eBL differs from sporadic Burkitt's lymphoma by its stronger association with EBV, its disposition for the jaw, and a different preferential breakpoint location within the *c-myc* gene on chromosome 8.

Malaria is thought to be a cofactor in the occurrence of eBL. This theory is based on a similar geographical distribution of both diseases, the increased numbers of EBV-infected cells in patients with malaria, and the occurrence of polyclonal B-cell proliferation. Other epidemiologic factors include the reduction of Burkitt's lymphoma with malaria prophylaxis and the fact that the peak age incidence for malaria is closely followed by the peak age incidence for Burkitt's lymphoma.

Recent studies suggest that the prevalence of eBL is declining in central Africa. In the Ibadan Cancer Registry between 1991 and

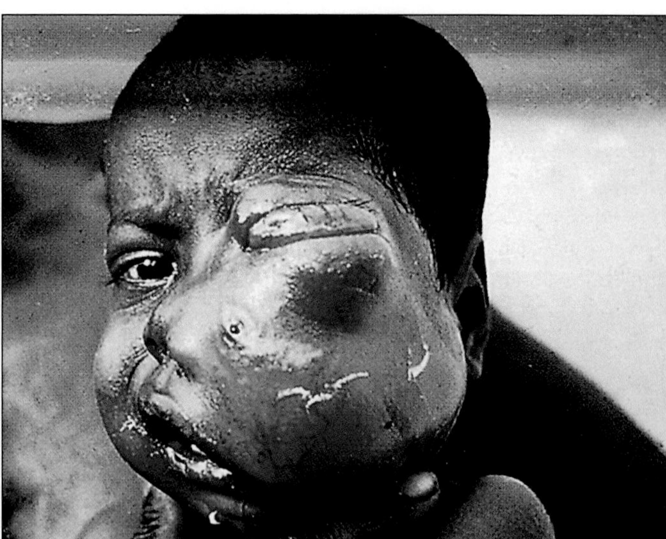

Figure 16.3 Burkitt's lymphoma of the maxilla in an African child. (Reproduced from Peters W and Pasvol G (eds). Tropical Medicine and Parasitology, 5th edition, Mosby, London 2002, image 1028.)

1999, 665 cases of childhood malignancy were reported. Burkitt's lymphoma (19.4%) and retinoblastoma (17.9%) remained the two most common specific childhood malignancies.[34] Similar surveys for the periods 1960–1972 and 1973–1990 show that Burkitt's lymphoma accounted for 51.5 and 37.1%, respectively. A real decline in the incidence of Burkitt's lymphoma might be partly ascribed to improved living conditions and greater control of malaria.

Outside Africa, the high association of EBV with Burkitt's lymphoma is found in other areas of the world such as New Guinea, which has similar climatic conditions to Africa. Bahia, a region in northeast Brazil, is between 9° and 17° south of the Equator and has climatic and socioeconomic conditions similar to central Africa. Eighty-seven percent of Burkitt's lymphoma in Bahia expressed EBER, and EBV type A and type I latency are predominant.[35] Burkitt's lymphoma in Bahia has a higher frequency of EBV association compared with southeast Brazil[36] and Argentina. Bahia is very similar to North Africa, which is intermediate between the frequency of eBL and sporadic Burkitt's lymphoma. Northeast Brazilian Burkitt's lymphoma has preferential abdominal localization rather than jaw distribution, which is similar to North African cases. Bahia has endemic parasitic diseases such as leishmaniasis and schistosomiasis that cause polyclonal B-cell proliferation and immunosuppression at an early age. This would be analogous to malaria in central Africa. Further, the intestinal wall is the most common site of *Schistosoma mansoni* egg deposition, which is also the preferential site of northeast Brazilian Burkitt's lymphoma.

India also appears to be an intermediate-risk area for Burkitt's lymphoma. In 25 cases of Burkitt's lymphoma, 80% were EBER-positive.[37] EBV typing using EBNA-3C primers showed a predominance of type A in India (13 of 16). The abdomen was the most common, while jaw involvement was rare.

Hodgkin's disease

In 1978, serological studies showed that EBV infection was associated with Hodgkin's lymphoma. Years later, hybridization blotting techniques showed the presence of the virus in Hodgkin's lymphoma, and in situ hybridization localized EBV to Hodgkin and Reed–Sternberg cells. Hodgkin's lymphoma may manifest primarily with palpable lymphadenopathy, especially in the cervical and submandibular lymph nodes.[26]

The relationship between EBV and Hodgkin's disease is well documented. IM increases the risk of Hodgkin's disease. Prior to the diagnosis of Hodgkin's disease, EBV titers are increased. LMP-1 is expressed in all neoplastic cells in EBV positive Hodgkin's disease.

Children in non-industrialized nations have a strong correlation of age of peak incidence with Hodgkin's lymphoma and EBV infection. These countries include Mexico (65%), Brazil (77%), Malaysia (93%), China (100%), Honduras (100%), Kenya (100%), and Peru (100%). This is in contrast to Hodgkin's lymphoma in industrialized nations where the bimodal peak is in early adulthood and in the elderly, with less association with EBV infection. Hodgkin's lymphoma associated with EBV occurred in 56% of American cases,[38] 50% of English cases,[39] and 59% of Japanese cases.[40]

The histological subtype of Hodgkin's lymphoma also appears to have an association with EBV. The mixed cellularity subtype has a strong association with EBV. In non-industrialized nations, the EBV incidence in the nodular sclerosing subtype is between 45 and 100%,[41] and in industrialized nations, the EBV incidence is between 20 and 33%.[42] Male children are also more likely to have EBV-associated Hodgkin's lymphoma.

Mucocutaneous lymphomas

Several mucocutaneous lymphomas have also been associated with EBV. The most common cutaneous manifestation is subcutaneous lymphadenopathy secondary to invasion of, or metastases to, pre-existing lymph nodes.[26] EBV-associated lymphoproliferation may less commonly involve the skin and subcutaneous tissues directly.

A Japanese review described four distinct types for EBV-associated cutaneous lymphoproliferative disorders: (1) angiocentric cutaneous lymphoma; (2) subcutaneous lymphoma; (3) histiocytoid lymphoma; and (4) vesiculopapular lesions of the face.[43] Angiocentric cutaneous T-cell lymphoma is an unusual type of T-cell lymphomas that presents with a papular or vesicular eruption mimicking hydroa vacciniforme.[44,45] Most patients have been children from Latin America and Asia. Most cases have a considerable number of phagocytosing cells, so-called beanbag cells. Between 42%[46] and 75%[47] of cases have been found to be associated with EBV. One study in Peru found all six of six cases to be EBV-associated.[48] EBV expression is less likely to be found when an angiocentric lymphoma primarily affects the skin. This has been suggested to be related to the histopathologic grade of the lesions. Infiltrates with more atypical cells have a higher grade and a worse prognosis. Grade I or II angiocentric lymphomas, which are the most likely to affect the skin, will have lower amounts of EBV. Grade III angiocentric lymphomas are more likely to be EBV-positive, suggesting that EBV may transform low-grade angiocentric lymphomas into more aggressive and systemic lymphomas.

Subcutaneous lymphoma is characterized by atypical lymphocyte infiltration into subcutaneous tissue and fatty tissue, and it is associated with hemophagocytosis. There are many case reports of subcutaneous panniculitis-like T-cell lymphoma associated with EBV. Individual reports were from Costa Rica, Taiwan,[45] and Korea, while there are many studies from Japan.[49] In three studies in the western hemisphere, the subcutaneous T-cell lymphoma was found to have EBV RNA in 0% of cases.[50]

However, in a Chinese study, five of 17 cases of subcutaneous panniculitis-like T-cell lymphoma (29.4%) were found to have EBV-EBER1 and 2.[51] In a Japanese study, three of three cases demonstrated an EBV-association.[52] Similar to angiocentric cutaneous T-cell lymphoma, many of these cases also have beanbag cells, which is another histological hallmark suggestive of EBV infection.[52] It is interesting that many cases of EBV-positive subcutaneous lymphomas have been reported in Asia. This is reminiscent of the discrepancy between non-endemic Burkitt's lymphoma, which is unrelated to EBV infection, and endemic African Burkitt's lymphoma, which is closely related to EBV infection.

Histiocytoid lymphoma presents with papules with necrosis, and it is also associated with hemophagocytosis. It is characterized by a diffuse infiltration of the skin with phagocytosing histiocytoid cells and atypical lymphoid cells.

Vesiculopapular lesions of the face, which mimics hydroa vacciniforme, presents as vesiculopapular eruptions or subcutaneous nodules only in children. It is described as dermal angiocentric infiltration of atypical lymphoid cells with dermal necrosis. It is not initially malignant, but it may eventually evolve into malignancy.

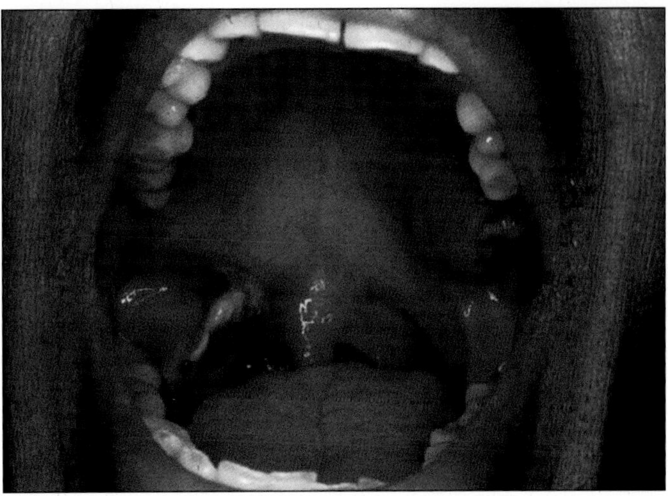

Figure 16.4 B-cell lymphoma in an acquired immunodeficiency syndrome (AIDS) patient in India. (Courtesy of Dr. J.K. Maniar.)

Primary cutaneous B-cell lymphoma is also associated with EBV. In acquired immunodeficiency syndrome (AIDS) patients, both T-cell and B-cell lymphomas can occur in the oral cavity, presenting with swelling and ulcerations of the tongue, gingivae, or hard palate (Fig. 16.4). In iatrogenically immunosuppressed patients secondary to solid organ transplantation, patients may present with multiple ulcerative cutaneous nodules without internal organ involvement or peripheral lymphadenopathy.

The role of EBV in cutaneous T-cell lymphoma (CTCL) is controversial. Some studies report that there is no significant role,[53] whereas two case reports involving three patients and three studies showed that 19.7%,[54] 32%,[55] and 41.7%[56] of CTCL have association with EBV. A study of CTCL in Pakistan showed that 50% of all cases were positive for EBV.[57] The clinical manifestations include multiple violaceous plaques, bullae, nodules, papules, chronic ulcers, and subcutaneous tumors on the trunk and extremities.[26] A history of hypersensitivity to mosquito bites, such as fever, hepatitis, and erythematous swelling and skin ulceration, was reported for some patients with EBV-associated lymphoproliferative disease.

Potential therapies for specific EBV-associated cancers

The continued growth of most, if not all, EBV-associated lymphomas may require persistent expression of certain EBV-encoded gene products.[58] There is a possibility of treating some EBV-associated lymphomas by inducing loss of the EBV episome or by inhibiting the expression of EBV-encoded oncogenes. EBV-dependent promoters and replication origins to express toxic genes within EBV-positive tumor cells are actively being researched. Another novel strategy is induction of the lytic form of EBV replication in tumor cells, using the virus itself to kill tumor cells in conjunction with the prodrug ganciclovir, which is converted into its cytotoxic form in lytically infected cells. Another approach is to enhance the host immune response to EBV proteins.

Human papillomavirus

Introduction

There are about 100 genotypes of HPVs, which are DNA tumor viruses that infect the epithelial cells of skin and mucosa and commonly cause warts, or benign papillomas.[59] Skin and anogenital warts can be disfiguring and a serious recurrent problem for patients. Additionally there are some types of HPV that are considered high-risk, including types 16 and 18, because they are the primary etiologic agent for cervical cancer, some anogenital cancers, and a few upper aerodigestive tract and skin cancers.[60] HPV is a major concern in the tropics because HPV infections, especially cervical lesions, have a greater tendency to persist and a higher risk of malignant transformation in immunocompromised patients such as patients with AIDS, and in many tropical countries, HIV is not well controlled due to the decreased availability of highly active antiretroviral therapy (HAART).[61] Also some tropical areas have a higher incidence of malignant anogenital lesions that is thought to be due to higher oncogenic activity in the HPV variants endemic to those areas.[62] In order to prevent cervical HPV infection, there are current trials evaluating vaccines based on virus-like particles (VPL), and research continues to determine which HPV types need to be included in the vaccines.[63]

Epidemiology

Among sexually active women, infection with HPV is common, with an incidence of 15–40%.[64] Risk factors for infection include sexual intercourse at an early age, high number of sexual partners, and low socioeconomic status.[65] Greater than 25 types of HPV can infect the oral and anogenital mucosa. The HPV types are distinguished by the relatedness of their DNA sequences, which can be determined by PCR.[66] The frequency of high-risk types varies with geographic, demographic, and clinical–pathologic factors.[67] The International Association for Research in Cancer (IARC) conducted an international study that found that the most common high-risk HPV types that infect the cervix are HPV-16 (53%), HPV-18 (15%), HPV-45 (9%), HPV-31 (6%), and HPV-33 (3%).[68] In one study done in Brazil, the HPV types in women presenting with abnormal cytological results in Pap smears were identified, and the prevalence of types was found to be 43.8% HPV-16, 12.5% HPV-58, 10% HPV-31, 6.3% HPV-53, 3.8% HPV-18, and 3.8% HPV-33.[69] The incidence of cervical cancers is higher in tropical areas, such as Kyadondo county in Uganda, where it is the commonest cancer in women, with an age-standardized incidence rate of 16.25 cases per 100 000 women, which represents about 20% of all cancers in women.[70] In one study, expression levels of the ligase chain reaction region of HPV-16 isolates from Ugandan patients and the isolates E6 and E7 transformation activity suggested a higher oncogenic activity that could explain the higher incidence and more rapid progression to advanced lesions seen in Ugandan cervical and penile cancers.[71]

The prevalence of cervical intraepithelial neoplasia (CIN) is higher in HIV-positive women than in HIV-negative women.[72] One study comparing rates of CIN in HIV-positive and HIV-negative women showed that 7% of about 400 HIV-positive women had high-grade CIN versus 1% of about 300 HIV-negative women, but HIV-positive women were not found to have an increased risk of invasive cervical cancer.[72] Being HIV-positive is a strong risk factor for CIN, and those with CD4+ counts less than 200×10^6/l have the greatest risk.[72] HIV-positive women also have 16 times higher incidence of all lower genital tract lesions, excluding cervical, when compared with HIV-negative women (Fig. 16.5).[73] It has also been shown that HIV-positive women are more likely to be infected with high-risk types of HPV, to be infected with multiple types

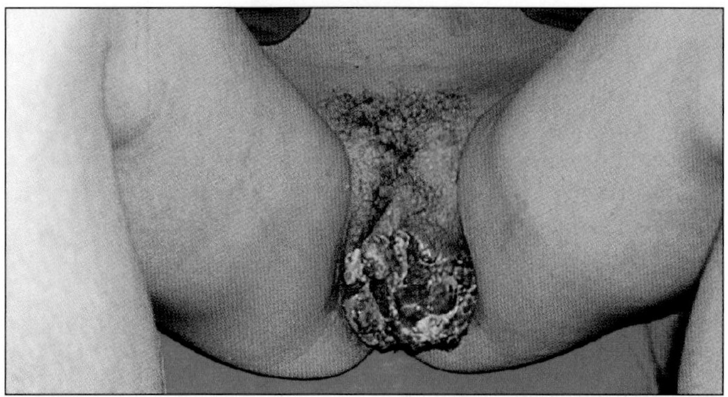

Figure 16.5 Vulvar squamous cell carcinoma. (Courtesy of Dr. J.K. Maniar.)

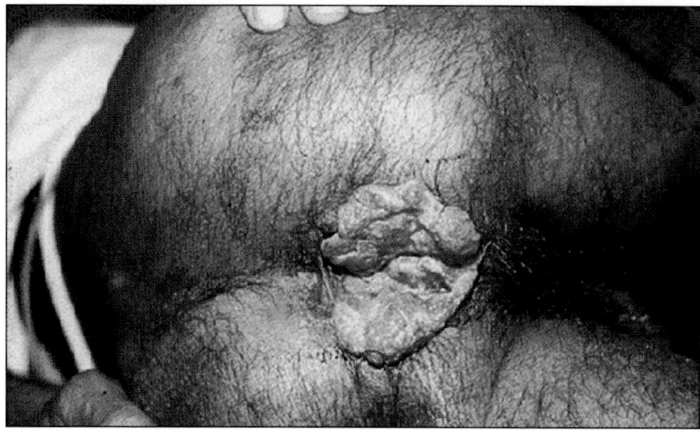

Figure 16.7 Anal squamous cell carcinoma. (Courtesy of Dr. J.K. Maniar.)

of HPV, and more likely to have persistent HPV infection, which is correlated with low CD4+ counts and higher HIV plasma RNA loads.[74] In addition, HIV-2-positive women are more likely to have high-grade CIN than HIV-1-positive women.[75]

The prevalence of oral HPV infection is not known, but there is evidence that HPV is involved in the pathogenesis of oral cancers.[76] The infections can be transmitted sexually by digit or oral–genital contact. In a study comparing the prevalence of HPV in HIV-negative and HIV-positive patients, high-risk HPV types were found in 2.1% of tonsil and 6.3% of oral-rinse specimens: HPV-16 was the most common high-risk type, and the prevalence of oral high-risk HPV types was greater in HIV-positive patients than in HIV-negative individuals (13.7% versus 4.5%).[77]

Similar to CIN, anal squamous intraepithelial lesions (SIL) and penile cancers (Fig. 16.6) are associated with HPV infection.[71,78] Anal HPV infection and SIL (Fig. 16.7) are more common in HIV-positive men who have sex with men (MSM) than in HIV-negative MSM, and the prevalence and incidence of anal HPV infection and SIL increase with decreasing CD4+ counts.[79] HAART does not seem to affect the rates of anal HPV and SIL. In a cross-sectional study, the prevalence of anal HPV infection and SIL was not found to differ between HIV-seropositive patients who had received HAART for a median of 32 months and those who had not received HAART.[80] Another prospective study demonstrated that there was no significant regression of anal SIL after 6 months of HAART and minimal effect on detection of HPV.[81] This suggests that if HAART does not change the incidence or progression of anal SIL, in the future there could be an increased incidence of anal cancer as anal HPV infections and SIL have more time to progress to cancer, with more HIV-seropositive patients living longer due to HAART. Penile cancer is more common in the tropics and, since the 1950s, has been the most diagnosed cancer in Ugandan men, with an incidence of 41% in the Bunyoro district.[82]

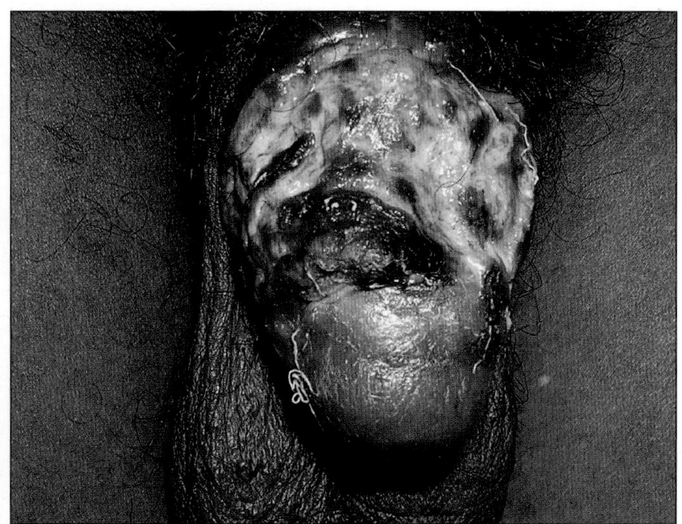

Figure 16.6 Penile squamous cell carcinoma. (Courtesy of Dr. J.K. Maniar.)

Epidermodysplasia verruciformis (EV) is a genetic disease associated with increased susceptibility to infection with specific HPV types, which are called EV-HPV types and include HPV 5, 8, 9, 12, 14, 15, 17, 19–25, 36–38, 47, and 49.[83] In about half of patients, and usually in those over 30 years old, the lesions can transform into carcinomas, primarily squamous cell carcinomas (SCC).

Pathogenesis

Infection with HPV begins with the breakdown of the epithelium that exposes basal cells to the virus, and viral binding and entry require viral capsid proteins L1 and L2.[84] Then the covalently closed circular DNA genome establishes in the nuclei of basal cells, and if stem cells are infected, persistent infection can follow.[85] Products of two genes of the early region, E6 and E7, are central to the cellular immortalization and transformation caused by HPV.[64] Individual types of HPV have varied activity of E6 and E7 genes, accounting for the difference in oncogenicity of the different types.[60]

HPV infection is necessary for the development of CIN and cervical cancer, but other factors, including accumulation of other mutations and integration of viral DNA into the host genome, must also be present for the infection to be persistent and progress to CIN or cancer.[59] A factor studied under the Ludwig–McGill HPV Natural History Study in Brazil is nutritional status. It was found that there is a decreased risk of persistent HPV infection in women who had high intake of β-cryptoxanthin, lutein/zeaxanthin, vitamin C, and papaya.[86] Another factor may be a genetic susceptibility to cervical lesions, and in another study done in Brazil, there was evidence that different polymorphic human leukocyte antigen (HLA) genes are involved in the maintenance and clearance of HPV infection and that the homozygous codon 72 p53-Arg gene allele is associated with increased susceptibility to cervical cancer.[64]

The host control of HPV infection is primarily due to cell-mediated responses. It follows that HIV-induced immunosuppression and inability to control the expression of high-risk types of HPV are likely the reason why HIV infection increases the risk of developing CIN.[75] Also, since HIV-2-seropositive women have a slower decrease in CD4+ cell count, and are immunosuppressed for longer periods, it is hypothesized that they have a decreased ability to control HPV infections and longer exposure to HPV oncoproteins, which may explain why they are at higher risk for developing high-grade CIN or invasive cervical cancer than women infected with HIV-1.[75]

In one model of the pathogenesis of anal SIL in HIV-seropositive patients, anal SIL is rare early in the course of HIV as HPV is controlled by the host's immune response.[87] While CD4+ counts decrease, HPV-specific immunity decreases, and there is a corresponding increase in levels of HPV infection, expression of HPV proteins like E6 and E7, and development and progression of anal SIL. It is not clear what role immunosuppression plays in the progression of anal SIL to cancer, and host genomic mutations may also be involved. If these mutations, which may be due to the high levels of expression of HPV proteins, drive the progression to cancer, this may explain why the restoration of HPV-specific immunity seen with HAART does not affect the natural history of anal SIL.[88]

Clinical and pathologic features

HPV infections are divided into two groups, those that affect the skin and the mucosa. Manifestations depend on the HPV type, immune status of the host, and the area involved. Cervical warts, or condyloma lata, may be difficult to visualize by examination without application of acetic acid, which causes subclinical lesions to become white. The histologic lesions are described as CIN, and there are grading systems to assess the degree of neoplasia. The characteristic features include abnormal kertinocyte maturation, nuclear pleomorphism, and dyskeratosis.[89]

Patients with EV have widespread cutaneous lesions that are chronic pityriasis versicolor-like macules and flat wart-like papules. The SCC occur on areas that are sun-exposed in most patients, and nearly all the SCC contain specific oncogenic EV-HPV types, predominantly HPV 5 and sometimes HPV 8, 14, 17, 20, or 47, in high copy numbers in episomal form.[83] It is hypothesized that, in addition to the role played by oncogenic EV-HPV types, ultraviolet radiation, especially the chronic exposure found in the tropics, can explain the promotion of skin cancers in EV patients.

Treatment

There is no curative therapy for HPV infections. The aim of current treatments is physically to destroy the lesions, with agents such as trichloroacetic acid, or to modulate the host's immune response against infected cells, with imiquimod. There are efforts to prevent genital HPV infections with prophylactic vaccines, which have been created using recombinant DNA technology and consist of viral capsid proteins that self-assemble into empty viral capsids called VLP. These VLP resemble native virions and carry neutralization epitopes on their surface but do not have viral DNA. The recent development of an in vitro culture system for HPV has improved the environment for vaccine research.[90] There are currently clinical trials on HPV-16 L1 VPL and other subtypes, and recently a double-blind, placebo-controlled study on the HPV-16 vaccine showed a reduced incidence of HPV-16 infections and CIN at a median follow-up of 17 months when the vaccine was given to HPV-16-negative women.[91] In patients with HIV infection, studies have suggested that HAART reduces the progression and increases regression of some cases of CIN.[92] However it is not known what effect HAART has on CIN since other studies have shown no significant reduction in the prevalence of CIN after a mean of 15 months of HAART, and no decrease in the prevalence of cervical HPV infection after HAART.[93]

Human herpesvirus 8

Introduction

HHV-8, or Kaposi sarcoma-associated herpesvirus (KSHV), was identified in 1994 and is considered to be the etiologic agent for all forms of Kaposi sarcoma (KS), including classic KS, African endemic KS (Fig. 16.8), iatrogenic immunosuppression-related KS, and AIDS epidemic KS.[94] KS is a tumor that involves blood and lymphatic vessels, and while each type of KS is clinically distinct, the histopathological characteristics are similar.

Epidemiology

There are several subtypes of HHV-8, including subtypes A, B, C, and D. These subtypes have a geographical distribution, with subtypes A and C common in Europe, subtype B found in Africa, and the rare subtype D found in aborigines in Polynesia and Australia.[95] The highest prevalence of KS is in sub-Saharan Africa, where endemic KS is found. In children living in endemic areas, the seroprevalence ranges from 13% in Cameroon to 47% in Zambia, and in adults, from 22% in central Africa to 87% in the Congo and Botswana.[96] KS accounts for 15–20% of malignancies in Nigeria, which is endemic for HHV-8, and about 9% of all reported cancers in equatorial Africa.[97] It is not known why there is a high prevalence of HHV-8 in Africa or why there is a male predominance in adults with KS.[98] There is evidence that HHV-8 can be transmitted by blood and sexual contact, which is the route of transmission in AIDS-related epidemic KS and the primary mode of transmission in industrialized countries, with most cases detected in homosexual men.[99] Studies have reported significant associations between

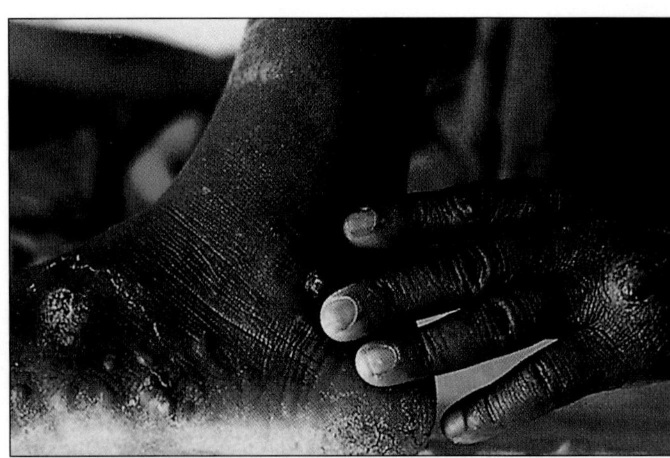

Figure 16.8 African endemic Kaposi's sarcoma. (Reproduced from Peters W and Pasvol G (eds). Tropical Medicine and Parasitology, 5th edition, Mosby, London 2002.)

HHV-8 seropositivity and multiple sexual partners and a history of sexually transmitted infections in adults in Nigeria and Kenya.[100,101] In Uganda, HHV-8 infection is common among blood donors, and the risk of transmission through transfusion is the same as the 1-year cumulative risk of infection from community sources.[102] Transmission through exposure to blood is also supported by the association between injection drug use and HHV-8 infection.[103] Evidence also suggests that HHV-8 can be transmitted by close contact between family members, crowded living conditions, and poor hygiene and sanitation, which are likely the commonest methods of transmission in endemic areas.[104] In endemic populations, like Brazilian Amerindian tribes, HHV-8 transmission is thought to occur from mother to child, between siblings, and between young children by premastication of food or bites,[105] and associations have been found between the serostatus of children living in Guyana and Tanzania and their parents and siblings.[106] Other evidence of non-sexual transmission is seen in the high prevalence of seropositivity in children before the onset of sexual activity and the higher frequency of HHV-8 in saliva compared with semen.[107]

After the onset of the AIDS epidemic, the incidence of KS has increased in areas of equatorial Africa, including in women and children, and it is the most common AIDS-associated malignancy worldwide.[108] In Uganda, KS was rare before the spread of HIV but is now the most common cancer in men and the second most common cancer in women, after cervical cancer.[109] With the spread of AIDS, there has also been an increase in aggressive, disseminated oral and facial cutaneous pediatric KS seen in Central African countries and progressive immunodeficiency, leading to increased susceptibility to, and morbidity with, HHV-8 infection.[110] With the spread of HIV-1 between 1987 and 1995 in Zimbabwe, the incidence of KS has increased more than 40 times in Zimbabwean men and more than 200 times in Zimbabwean women.[111]

Pathogenesis

HHV-8 likely infects a B-lymphoid precursor or KS precursor cell, which is endothelial, but it is not known if it is vascular, lymphatic, or both. HHV-8 integrates into the cells and becomes latent until reactivation through immunosuppression or genetic, endocrine, metabolic, microbiologic, and social stimuli.[112] With reactivation, HHV-8 genes are transcribed, and the lesions result from cytokine-driven autocrine and paracrine stimulation of KS cells.[112]

Because HHV-8 seropositivity does not always translate into KS, there have been studies to identify risk factors, including a case–control study analyzing 50 potential risk factors in HIV-seronegative adults in Uganda. The prevalence of anti-HHV-8 antibodies was found to increase with age and to be equal in both genders, which suggested that the male predominance of KS is not explained by differences in seroprevalence between the genders but may be related to other cofactors, such as income, tribe, age of leaving home, pig or goat ownership, and going barefoot, all of which were found to be associated with KS.[113] Barefoot walking exposes the skin of the feet to iron oxide-rich volcanic clays which are hypothesized to cause dermal lymphatic damage and impaired local immunity.[97]

Many associations have been noted between HHV-8, KS, and HIV, including the suggestion that AIDS-epidemic KS pathogenesis is related to HHV-8 lytic replication. As seen with other herpesviruses, HHV-8 has both latent and lytic patterns of gene expression,[114] and in most cases of non-AIDS-epidemic KS, KS-cell HHV-8 gene expression has evidence of only latent replication, but in AIDS-epidemic KS, HHV-8-infected peripheral blood mononuclear cells show the lytic pattern of gene expression.[115,116] The use of antivirals that inhibit HHV-8 lytic replication in cell culture has decreased the risk of KS development in persons at high risk for KS and has induced regression of established cases of KS.[117] In HIV-1-seropositive patients, the risk of KS is increased after the development of new HHV-8 infection.[118] Also since patients with AIDS-KS have a higher level of HHV-8 viremia than patients with non-AIDS-epidemic KS, and the use of antiretrovirals to treat AIDS-KS is associated with reduced HHV-8 viremia, it is suggested that HIV-1 infection augments HHV-8 replication.[119] Whether this is due to decreased control of HHV-8 replication from HIV-1-induced immunosuppression or activation of HHV-8 activation through HIV-infected cell production of cytokines or other factors like tat protein is not known.[120,121] Tat has been found to induce KS-cell expression and activation of metalloproteinase-2, which is necessary for angiogenesis and tumor invasion, and to have an antiapoptotic role through activation of KS cell phophatidylinositol 3-kinase/Akt-dependent survival pathways.[122,123]

Clinical and histopathologic features

Classic KS is mostly a chronic skin disease of elderly Mediterranean, east European, or Jewish men and presents as multiple firm purple-red plaques and nodules on the lower extremities.[124] African endemic KS, generally an indolent tumor in HIV-seronegative adults, has the following four clinical subtypes: (1) benign cutaneous nodular disease that is similar to classic KS, seen mostly in young adults, and that runs a mean duration of 5–8 years; (2) aggressive infiltrative cutaneous disease that invades the dermis, subcutaneous tissue, muscle, and bone and usually becomes fatal in 5–7 years; (3) florid disseminated visceral and mucocutaneous disease, in which an extensive number of cutaneous lesions involves one or more extremities; and (4) fulminant lymphadenopathic disease without cutaneous manifestations that disseminates to lymph nodes and multiple organs and is found in children.[125] The lymphadenopathic form is mostly found in prepubertal children, most commonly in Bantu children of South Africa, presents with local or general lymphadenopathy, and can rapidly disseminate and become fatal.[126] Asymptomatic gastrointestinal involvement is found at autopsy in 90% of patients with African endemic KS. Immunosuppression-related KS clinically resembles classic KS and is associated with the use of posttransplant drugs. AIDS-related epidemic KS usually affects HIV-positive patients with CD4+ counts less than 500 cells/mm^3.[127] The clinical features may vary from single cutaneous macules, papules or plaques on the trunk or midface, to disseminated cutaneous lesions like coalescing and constricting papules and plaques that can ulcerate and become secondarily infected or cause lymphedema and impairment of the movement of extremities.[128] Diagnosis is made clinically and confirmed by biopsy. The histopathologic appearance between the four types is similar and is characterized by dilated blood vessels surrounded by spindle-shaped cells, slit-like vascular spaces, and hemorrhage.

Treatment

In general, patients with classic KS respond to local therapy, like excision, alitretinoin, and intralesional chemotherapy, and endemic

KS to systemic therapies, like chemotherapy with vinca alkaloids or paclitaxel and interferon-α.[129] Immunosuppression-related KS usually regresses after decreasing or discontinuing the immunosuppressive drugs.[128] There is no curative therapy for AIDS-related KS, but highly active antiretroviral therapy can prevent and treat the lesions.[128] In those HIV-seropositive patients already receiving HAART, KS has a less aggressive presentation but its natural history and outcome are not affected.[130]

Summary

Viruses commonly found in temperate climates may have different clinical presentations in tropical parts of the world due to genetics and lack of early interventions. In the tropics, the high rate of HIV changes the clinical presentations of all opportunistic infections both quantitatively and qualitatively. In the case of measles (Chapter 14), the presentation is affected by lack of vaccines and by malnutrition. Cervical cancer is prevalent in the tropics due to lack of regular Pap smears, in addition to high rates of HPV/HIV coinfection. Likewise, the clinical presentations of herpesviruses, poxviruses, human T-lymphotropic virus-1 (HTLV-1), and hepatitis viruses may be affected in the tropics by coinfections, lack of therapy, environment, genetics, and nutrition.

References

1. Pancharoen C, Bhatrarakosol P, Thisyakorn U. Seroprevalence of Epstein–Barr virus infection in Thai children. J Med Assoc Thai 2001; 84:850–854.
2. Pancharoen C, Mekmullica J, Chinratanapisit S et al. Seroprevalence of Epstein–Barr virus antibody among children in various age groups in Bangkok, Thailand. Asian Pac J Allergy Immunol 2001; 19:135–137.
3. Haque T, Iliadou P, Hossain A et al. Seroepidemiological study of Epstein–Barr virus infection in Bangladesh. J Med Virol 1996; 48:17–21.
4. Ozkan A, Kilic SS, Kalkan A et al. Seropositivity of Epstein–Barr virus in Eastern Anatolian region of Turkey. Asian Pac J Allergy Immunol 2003; 21:49–53.
5. Crawford DH, Swerdlow AJ, Higgins C et al. Sexual history and Epstein–Barr virus infection. J Infect Dis 2002; 186:731–736.
6. Evans AS. Infectious mononucleosis and related syndromes. Am J Med Sci 1978; 276:325–339.
7. Kuzushima K, Yamamoto M, Kimura H et al. Establishment of anti-Epstein–Barr virus (EBV) cellular immunity by adoptive transfer of virus-specific cytotoxic T lymphocytes from an HLA-matched sibling to a patient with severe chronic active EBV infection. Clin Exp Immunol 1996; 103:192–198.
8. Okamura T, Hatsukawa Y, Arai H et al. Blood stem-cell transplantation for chronic active Epstein–Barr virus with lymphoproliferation. Lancet 2000; 356:223–224.
9. Labandeira J, Peteiro C, Toribio J. Hairy leucoplakia and HIV-2: a case report and review of the literature. Clin Exp Dermatol 1994; 19:335–340.
10. Greenspan D, Greenspan JS, de Souza Y et al. Oral hairy leukoplakia in an HIV-negative renal transplant recipient. J Oral Pathol Med 1989; 18:32–34.
11. Fluckiger R, Laifer G, Itin P et al. Oral hairy leukoplakia in a patient with ulcerative colitis. Gastroenterology 1994; 106:506–508.
12. Smith KJ, Skelton HG, Yeager J et al. Cutaneous findings in HIV-1-positive patients: a 42-month prospective study. Military Medical Consortium for the Advancement of Retroviral Research (MMCARR). J Am Acad Dermatol 1994; 31:746–754.
13. Baskin GB, Roberts ED, Kuebler D et al. Squamous epithelial proliferative lesions associated with rhesus Epstein–Barr virus in simian immunodeficiency virus-infected rhesus monkeys. J Infect Dis 1995; 172:535–539.
14. Triantos D, Boulter AW, Leao JC et al. Diversity of naturally occurring Epstein–Barr virus revealed by nucleotide sequence polymorphism in hypervariable domains in the BamHI K and N subgenomic regions. J Gen Virol 1998; 79:2809–2817.
15. Butt FM, Chindia ML, Vaghela VP et al. Oral manifestations of HIV/AIDS in a Kenyan provincial hospital. East Afr Med J 2001; 78:398–401.
16. Kamiru HN, Naidoo S. Oral HIV lesions and oral health behaviour of HIV-positive patients attending the Queen Elizabeth II Hospital, Maseru, Lesotho. S Afr Dent J 2002; 57:479–482.
17. Arendorf TM, Bredekamp B, Cloete CA et al. Oral manifestations of HIV infection in 600 South African patients. J Oral Pathol Med 1998; 27:176–179.
18. Badri M, Maartens G, Wood R. Predictors and prognostic value of oral hairy leukoplakia and oral candidiasis in South African HIV-infected patients. S Afr Dent J 2001; 56:592–596.
19. Schiodt M, Bakilana PB, Hiza JF et al. Oral candidiasis and hairy leukoplakia correlate with HIV infection in Tanzania. Oral Surg Oral Med Oral Pathol 1990; 69:591–596.
20. Walling DM, Flaitz CM, Nichols CM. Epstein–Barr virus replication in oral hairy leukoplakia: response, persistence, and resistance to treatment with valacyclovir. J Infect Dis 2003; 188:883–890.
21. Fina F, Romain S, Ouafik L et al. Frequency and genome load of Epstein–Barr virus in 509 breast cancers from different geographical areas. Br J Cancer 2001; 84:783–790.
22. Deshpande CG, Badve S, Kidwai N et al. Lack of expression of the Epstein–Barr virus (EBV) gene products, EBERs, EBNA1, LMP1, and LMP2A, in breast cancer cells. Lab Invest 2002; 82:1193–1199.
23. Chu PG, Chang KL, Chen YY et al. No significant association of Epstein–Barr virus infection with invasive breast carcinoma. Am J Pathol 2001; 159:571–578.
24. Chu JS, Chen CC, Chang KJ. In situ detection of Epstein–Barr virus in breast cancer. Cancer Lett 1998; 124:53–57.
25. Wu MS, Huang SP, Chang YT et al. Tumor necrosis factor-alpha and interleukin-10 promoter polymorphisms in Epstein–Barr virus-associated gastric carcinoma. J Infect Dis 2002; 185:106–109.
26. Walling DM, Yen-Moore A, Hudnall SD. Epstein–Barr virus. In: Tyring SK, ed. Mucocutaneous manifestations of viral diseases, 1st edn. New York, NY: Marcel Dekker; 2002:145–171.

27. Liebowitz D. Nasopharyngeal carcinoma: the Epstein–Barr virus association. Semin Oncol 1994; 21:376–381.
28. Popat SR, Liavaag PG, Morton R et al. Epstein–Barr virus genome in nasopharyngeal carcinomas from New Zealand. Head Neck 2000; 22:505–508.
29. Frank DK, Cheron F, Cho H et al. Nonnasopharyngeal lymphoepitheliomas (undifferentiated carcinomas) of the upper aerodigestive tract. Ann Otol Rhinol Laryngol 1995; 104:305–310.
30. Cvitkovic E, Bachouchi M, Armand JP. Nasopharyngeal carcinoma. Biology, natural history, and therapeutic implications. Hematol Oncol Clin North Am 1991; 5:821–838.
31. Rathaur RG, Chitale AR, Banerjee K. Epstein–Barr virus in nasopharyngeal carcinoma in Indian patients. Ind J Cancer 1999; 36:80–90.
32. Clifford P. Carcinogens in the nose and throat: nasopharyngeal carcinoma in Kenya. Proc R Soc Med 1972; 65:682–686.
33. Xue SA, Labrecque LG, Lu QL et al. Promiscuous expression of Epstein–Barr virus genes in Burkitt's lymphoma from the central African country Malawi. Int J Cancer 2002; 99:635–643.
34. Ojesina AI, Akang EE, Ojemakinde KO. Decline in the frequency of Burkitt's lymphoma relative to other childhood malignancies in Ibadan, Nigeria. Ann Trop Paediatr 2002; 22:159–163.
35. Araujo I, Foss HD, Bittencourt A et al. Expression of Epstein–Barr virus-gene products in Burkitt's lymphoma in Northeast Brazil. Blood 1996; 87:5279–5286.
36. Klumb CE, Hassan R, DeOliveira DE et al. Geographic variation in Epstein–Barr virus-associated Burkitt's lymphoma in children from Brazil. Int J Cancer 2004; 108:66–70.
37. Rao CR, Gutierrez MI, Bhatia K et al. Association of Burkitt's lymphoma with the Epstein–Barr virus in two developing countries. Leuk Lymphoma 2000; 39:329–337.
38. Ambinder RF, Browning PJ, Lorenzana I et al. Epstein–Barr virus and childhood Hodgkin's disease in Honduras and the United States. Blood 1993; 81:462–467.
39. Weinreb M, Day PJ, Murray PG et al. Epstein–Barr virus (EBV) and Hodgkin's disease in children: incidence of EBV latent membrane protein in malignant cells. J Pathol 1992; 168:365–369.
40. Kusuda M, Toriyama K, Kamidigo NO et al. A comparison of epidemiologic, histologic, and virologic studies on Hodgkin's disease in western Kenya and Nagasaki, Japan. Am J Trop Med Hyg 1998; 59:801–807.
41. Zarate-Osorno A, Roman LN, Kingma DW et al. Hodgkin's disease in Mexico. Prevalence of Epstein–Barr virus sequences and correlations with histologic subtype. Cancer 1995; 75:1360–1366.
42. Pallesen G, Hamilton-Dutoit SJ, Zhou X. The association of Epstein–Barr virus (EBV) with T-cell lymphoproliferations and Hodgkin's disease: two new developments in the EBV field. Adv Cancer Res 1993; 62:179–239.
43. Iwatsuki K, Ohtsuka M, Harada H et al. Clinicopathologic manifestations of Epstein–Barr virus-associated cutaneous lymphoproliferative disorders. Arch Dermatol 1997; 133:1081–1086.
44. Tsai TF, Su IJ, Lu YC et al. Cutaneous angiocentric T-cell lymphoma associated with Epstein–Barr virus. J Am Acad Dermatol 1992; 26:31–38.
45. Su IJ, Tsai TF, Cheng AL et al. Cutaneous manifestations of Epstein–Barr virus-associated T-cell lymphoma. J Am Acad Dermatol 1993; 29:685–692.
46. Medeiros LJ, Jaffe ES, Chen YY et al. Localization of Epstein–Barr viral genomes in angiocentric immunoproliferative lesions. Am J Surg Pathol 1992; 16:439–447.
47. Magana M, Sangueza P, Gil-Beristain J et al. Angiocentric cutaneous T-cell lymphoma of childhood (hydroa-like lymphoma): a distinctive type of cutaneous T-cell lymphoma. J Am Acad Dermatol 1998; 38:574–579.
48. Barrionuevo C, Anderson VM, Zevallos-Giampietri E et al. Hydroa-like cutaneous T-cell lymphoma: a clinicopathologic and molecular genetic study of 16 pediatric cases from Peru. Appl Immunohistochem Mol Morphol 2002; 10:7–14.
49. Kunisada M, Adachi A, Matsumoto S et al. Nasal-type natural killer cell lymphoma preceded by benign panniculitis arising in an asymptomatic HTLV-1 carrier. Int J Dermatol 2003; 42:710–714.
50. Hoque SR, Child FJ, Whittaker SJ et al. Subcutaneous panniculitis-like T-cell lymphoma: a clinicopathological, immunophenotypic and molecular analysis of six patients. Br J Dermatol 2003; 148:516–525.
51. Wang L, Yang Y, Liu W et al. Subcutaneous panniculitis-like T-cell lymphoma: expression of cytotoxic-granule-associated protein TIA-1 and its relation with Epstein–Barr virus infection. Zhonghua Bing Li Xue Za Zhi 2000; 29:103–106.
52. Iwatsuki K, Harada H, Ohtsuka M et al. Latent Epstein–Barr virus infection is frequently detected in subcutaneous lymphoma associated with hemophagocytosis but not in non-fatal cytophagic histiocytic panniculitis. Arch Dermatol 1997; 133:787–788.
53. Angel CA, Slater DN, Royds JA et al. Absence of Epstein–Barr viral encoded RNA (EBER) in primary cutaneous T-cell lymphoma. J Pathol 1996; 178:173–175.
54. Anagnostopoulos I, Hummel M, Kaudewitz P et al. Low incidence of Epstein–Barr virus presence in primary cutaneous T-cell lymphoproliferations. Br J Dermatol 1996; 134:276–281.
55. Dreno B, Celerier P, Fleischmann M et al. Presence of Epstein–Barr virus in cutaneous lesions of mycosis fungoides and Sezary syndrome. Acta Derm Venereol 1994; 74:355–357.
56. Park CK, Ko YH. Detection of EBER nuclear RNA in T-cell lymphomas involving the skin – an in situ hybridization study. Br J Dermatol 1996; 134:488–493.
57. Noorali S, Yaqoob N, Nasir MI et al. Prevalence of mycosis fungoides and its association with EBV and HTLV-1 in Pakistanian patients. Pathol Oncol Res 2002; 8:194–199.
58. Israel BF, Kenney SC. Virally targeted therapies for EBV-associated malignancies. Oncogene 2003; 22:5122–5130.
59. Shah KV, Howley PM. Papillomaviruses. In: Fields BN, Knipe DM, Howley PM, eds. Fields virology. Philadelphia, PA: Lippincott-Raven; 1996:2077–2109.
60. zur Hausen H. Papillomavirus infection – a major cause of human cancers. Biochem Biophys Acta 1996; 1288:F55–F78.
61. Folkers G. Increased risk of cervical abnormalities among HIV-infected African women. NIAID AIDS Agenda 1996; 9–11.

62. Buonaguro FM, Tornesello ML, Salatiello I et al. The Uganda study on HPV variants and genital cancers. J Clin Virol 2000; 19:31–41.
63. Walraven G. Prevention of cervical cancer in Africa: a daunting task? Afr J Reprod Health 2003; 7:7–12.
64. Savio de Araujo Souza P, Lina Villa L. Genetic susceptibility to infection with human papillomavirus and development of cervical cancer in women in Brazil. Mutat Res 2003; 544:375–383.
65. Centers for Disease Control. Prevention of genital HPV infection and sequelae: report of an external consultant's meeting. Atlanta: Department of Health and Human Services; 1999.
66. de Villiers EM. Papillomavirus and HPV typing. Clin Dermatol 1997; 15:199–206.
67. Lo KW, Cheung TH, Chung TK et al. Clinical and prognostic significance of human papillomavirus in a Chinese population of cervical cancers. Gyn Obst Invest 2001; 51:202–207.
68. Munoz N. Human papillomavirus and cancer: the epidemiological evidence. J Clin Virol 2000; 19:1–5.
69. Camara GN, Cerqueira DM, Oliveira AP et al. Prevalence of human papillomavirus types in women with preneoplastic and neoplastic cervical lesions in the Federal District of Brazil. Mem Inst Oswaldo Cruz 2003; 98:879–883.
70. IARC. Cancer incidence in five continents. In: IARC scientific publications no. 143. Lyon: IARC Scientific Publications; 1997.
71. Buonaguro FM, Tornesello ML, Salatiello I et al. The Uganda study on HPV variants and genital cancers. J Clin Virol 2000; 19:31–41.
72. Wright TC Jr, Ellerbrock TV, Chiasson MA et al. Cervical intraepithelial neoplasia in women infected with human immunodeficiency virus: prevalence, risk factors, and validity of Papanicolaou smears. New York Cervical Disease Study. Obstet Gynecol 1994; 84:591–597.
73. Conley LJ, Ellerbrock TV, Bush TJ et al. HIV-1 infection and risk of vulvovaginal and perianal condylomata acuminata and intraepithelial neoplasia: a prospective cohort study. Lancet 2002; 359:108–113.
74. Sun XW, Kuhn L, Ellerbrock TV et al. Human papillomavirus infection in women infected with the human immunodeficiency virus. N Engl J Med 1997; 337:1343–1349.
75. Hawes SE, Critchlow CW, Niang MAF et al. Increased risk of high-grade cervical squamous intraepithelial lesions and invasive cervical cancer among African women with human immunodefiency virus type 1 and 2 infections. J Infect Dis 2003; 188:555–563.
76. Kreimer AR, Alberg AJ, Daniel R et al. Oral human papillomavirus infection in adults is associated with sexual behavior and HIV serostatus. J Infect Dis 2004; 189:686–698.
77. Kreimer AR, Alberg AJ, Daniel R et al. Oral human papillomavirus infection in adults is associated with sexual behavior and HIV serostatus. J Infect Dis 2004; 189:686–698.
78. Palefsky JM, Holly EA, Gonzales J et al. Detection of human papillomavirus DNA in anal intraepithelial neoplasia and anal cancer. Cancer Res 1991; 51:1014–1019.
79. Palefsky JM, Holly EA, Ralston ML et al. High incidence of anal high-grade squamous intra-epithelial lesions among HIV-positive and HIV-negative homosexual and bisexual men. AIDS 1998; 12:495–503.
80. Piketty C, Darragh TM, Heard I et al. High prevalence of anal squamous intraepithelial lesions in HIV-positive men despite the use of highly active antiretroviral therapy. Sex Transm Dis 2004; 31:96–99.
81. Palefsky JM, Holly EA, Ralston ML et al. Effect of highly active antiretroviral therapy on the natural history of anal squamous intraepithelial lesions and anal human papillomavirus infection. J AIDS 2001; 28:422–428.
82. Tornesello ML, Buonaguro FM, Beth-Giraldo E et al. Sequence variations and viral genomic state of human papillomavirus type 16 in penile carcinomas from Ugandan patients. J Gen Virol 1997; 1997:2199–2208.
83. Majewski S, Jablonska S. Epidermodysplasia verruciformis as a model of human papillomavirus-induced genetic cancer of the skin. Arch Dermatol 1995; 131:1312–1318.
84. Kawana Y, Kawana K, Yoshikawa H et al. Human papillomavirus type 16 minor capsid protein L2 N-terminal region containing a common neutralization epitope binds the cell surface and enters the cytoplasm. J Virol 2001; 75:2331–2336.
85. Law MF, Lowy DR, Dvoretzky I et al. Mouse cells transformed by bovine papillomavirus contain only extrachromosomal viral DNA sequences. Proc Natl Acad Sci USA 1981; 78:2727–2731.
86. Giuliano AR, Siegel EM, Roe DJ et al. Dietary intake and risk of persistent human papillomavirus (HPV) infection: the Ludwig-McGill HPV natural history study. J Infect Dis 2003; 188:1508–1516.
87. Chin-Hong PV, Palefsky JM. Natural history and clinical management of anal human papillomavirus disease in men and women infected with human immunodeficiency virus. Clin Infect Dis 2002; 35:1127–1134.
88. Palefsky JM, Holly E. Molecular virology and epidemiology of human papillomavirus and cervical cancer. Cancer Epidemiol Biomarkers Prev 1995; 4:415–428.
89. Lever WF, Elder DE. Lever's histopathology of the skin. Philadelphia, PA: Lippincott-Raven; 1997.
90. The Jordan report: accelerated development of vaccines. Bethesda, MD: National Institute of Allergy and Infectious Diseases; 1998.
91. Koutsky LA, Ault KA, Wheeler CM et al. A controlled trial of a human papillomavirus type 16 vaccine. N Engl J Med 2002; 347:1645–1651.
92. Minkoff H, Ahdieh L, Massad LS et al. The effect of highly active antiretroviral therapy on cervical cytologic changes associated with oncogenic HPV among HIV-infected women. AIDS 2001; 15:2157–2164.
93. Lillo FB, Ferrari D, Veglia F et al. Human papillomavirus infection and associated cervical disease in human immunodeficiency virus-infected women: effect of highly active antiretroviral therapy. J Infect Dis 2001; 184:547–551.
94. Cesarman E, Chang Y, Moore PS et al. Kaposi's sarcoma-associated herpesvirus-like DNA sequences in AIDS-related body-cavity-based lymphomas. N Engl J Med 1995; 332:1186–1191.
95. Lacoste V, Kadyrova E, Chistiakova I et al. Molecular characterization of Kaposi's sarcoma-associated herpesvirus/human

herpesvirus-8 strains from Russia. J Gen Virol 2000; 81:1217–1222.

96. Engels EA, Sinclair MD, Biggar RJ et al. Latent class analysis of human herpesvirus B assay performance and infection prevalence in sub-saharan Africa. Int J Cancer 2000; 88:1003–1008.
97. Ziegler JL. Endemic Kaposi's sarcoma in Africa and local volcanic soils. Lancet 1993; 342:1348–1351.
98. Amir H, Kaaya EE, Kwesigbo G et al. Kaposi's sarcoma before and during the HIV epidemic in Tanzania: a study of cancer registry data 1968–95. Int J Oncol 1997; 11:1363–1366.
99. Schultz TF. Kaposi's sarcoma-associated herpesvirus (human herpesvirus-8). J Gen Virol 1998; 79:1573–1591.
100. Eltom MA, Mbulaiteye SM, Dada AJ et al. Transmission of human herpesvirus 8 by sexual activity among adults in Lagos, Nigeria. AIDS 2002; 16:2473–2478.
101. Lavreys L, Chohan BH, Ashley R et al. Human herpesvirus 8: seroprevalence and correlates in prostitutes in Mombasa, Kenya. J Infect Dis 2003; 187:359–363.
102. Mbulaiteye SM, Biggar RJ, Bakaki PM et al. Human herpesvirus 8 infection and transfusion history in children with sickle-cell disease in Uganda. J Natl Cancer Inst 2003; 95:1330–1335.
103. Atkinson J, Edlin BR, Engels EA et al. Seroprevalence of human herpesvirus 8 among injection drug users in San Francisco. J Infect Dis 2003; 187:974–981.
104. Davidovici B, Karakis I, Bourboulia D et al. Seroepidemiology and molecular epidemiology of Kaposi's sarcoma-associated herpesvirus among Jewish population groups in Israel. J Natl Cancer Inst 2001; 93:194–202.
105. Biggar RJ, Whitby D, Marshall V et al. Human herpesvirus 8 in Brazilian Amerindians: a hyperendemic population with a new subtype. J Infect Dis 2000; 181:1562–1568.
106. Mbulaiteye SM, Pfeiffer RM, Whitby D et al. Human herpesvirus 8 infection within families in rural Tanzania. J Infect Dis 2003; 187:1780–1785.
107. Pauk J, Huang ML, Brodie SJ et al. Mucosal shedding of human herpesvirus 8 in men. N Engl J Med 2000; 343:1369–1377.
108. He J, Bhat G, Kankasa C et al. Seroprevalence of human herpesvirus 8 among Zambian women of childbearing age without Kaposi's sarcoma (KS) and mother-child pairs with KS. J Infect Dis 1998; 178:1787–1790.
109. Wabinga H, Parkin DM, Wabwire-Mangen F et al. Cancer in Kampala, Uganda, in 1989–91: changes in incidence in the era of AIDS. Int J Cancer 1993; 1993:26–36.
110. Amir H, Kaaya EE, Manji KP et al. Kaposi's sarcoma before and during a human immunodeficiency virus epidemic in Tanzanian children. Pediatr Infect Dis J 2001; 20:518–521.
111. Chokunonga E, Levy LM, Bassett MT et al. AIDS and cancer in Africa: the evolving epidemic in Zimbabwe. AIDS 1999; 13:2583–2588.
112. Sturzi M, Zietz C, Monini P et al. Human herpesvirus-8 and Kaposi's sarcoma: relationship with the multistep concept of tumorigenesis. Adv Cancer Res 2001; 81:125–159.
113. Ziegler J, Newton R, Bourboulia D et al. Risk factors for Kaposi's sarcoma: a case-control study of HIV-seronegative people in Uganda. Int J Cancer 2003; 103:233–240.
114. Sarid R, Flore O, Bohenzky RA et al. Transcription mapping of the Kaposi's sarcoma-associated herpesvirus (human herpesvirus 8) genome in a body cavity-based lymphoma cell line (BC-1). J Virol 1998; 72:1005–1012.
115. Staskus KA, Zong W, Gebhard K et al. Kaposi's sarcoma-associated herpesvirus gene expression in endothelial (spindle) tumor cells. J Virol 1997; 71:715–719.
116. Decker LL, Shankar P, Khan G et al. The Kaposi's sarcoma-associated herpesvirus (KSHV) is present as an intact latent genome in KS tissue but replicates in the peripheral blood mononuclear cells of KS patients. J Exp Med 1996; 184:283–288.
117. Mazzi R, Giuseppe P, Sarmati L et al. Efficacy of cidofovir on human herpesvirus 8 viraemia and Kaposi's sarcoma progression in two patients with AIDS. AIDS 2001; 15:2061–2062.
118. Jacobson LP, Jenkins FJ, Springer G et al. Interaction of human immunodeficiency virus type 1 and human herpesvirus 8 infections on the incidence of Kaposi's sarcoma. J Infect Dis 2000; 181:1940–1949.
119. Campbell TB, Borok M, White IE et al. Relationship of Kaposi sarcoma (KS)-associated herpesvirus viremia and KS disease in Zimbabwe. Clin Infect Dis 2003; 36:1144–1151.
120. Harrington W Jr, Sieczkowski L, Sosa C et al. Activation of HHV-8 by HIV-1 *tat*. Lancet 1997; 349:774–775.
121. Chang J, Renne R, Dittmer D et al. Inflammatory cytokines and the reactivation of Kaposi's sarcoma-associated herpesvirus lytic replication. Virology 2000; 266:17–25.
122. Toschi E, Barillari G, Sgadari C et al. Activation of matrix-metalloproteinase-2 and membrane-type-1-matrix-metalloproteinase in endothelial cells and induction of vascular permeability in vivo by human immunodeficiency virus-1 Tat protein and basic fibroblast growth factor. Mol Biol Cell 2001; 12:2934–2946.
123. Deregibus MC, Cantaluppi V, Doublier S et al. HIV-1-Tat protein activates phosphatidylinositol 3-kinase/AKT-dependent survival pathways in Kaposi's sarcoma cells. J Biol Chem 2002; 277:25195–25202.
124. Friedman-Birnbaum R, Weltfriend S, Katz I. Kaposi's sarcoma: retrospective study of 67 cases with the classical form. Dermatologica 1990; 180:13–17.
125. Wabinga HR, Parkin DM, Wabwire-Mangen F et al. Trends in cancer incidence in Kyadondo County, Uganda. Br J Cancer 2000; 82:1585–1592.
126. Cook-Mozaffari P, Newton R, Beral V et al. The geographical distribution of Kaposi's sarcoma and of lymphomas in Africa before the AIDS epidemic. Br J Cancer 1998; 78:1521–1528.
127. Tappero JW, Conant MA, Wolfe SF et al. Kaposi's sarcoma. Epidemiology, pathogenesis, histology, clinical spectrum, staging criteria, and therapy. J Am Acad Dermatol 1993; 28:371–395.
128. Martinelli PT, Tyring SK. Human herpesvirus 8. Dermatol Clin 2002; 20:307–314.
129. Toschi E, Sgadari C, Monini P et al. Treatment of Kaposi's sarcoma – an update. Anticancer Drugs 2002; 13:977–987.
130. Nasti G, Martellotta F, Berretta M et al. Impact of highly active antiretroviral therapy on the presenting features and outcome of patients with acquired immunodeficiency syndrome-related Kaposi sarcoma. Cancer 2003; 98:2440–2446.

Chapter 17

Superficial mycoses and dermatophytes

Seema Patel, Jeffery A. Meixner, Michael B. Smith and Michael R. McGinnis

Introduction

Fungal disease involving human keratinized tissue may be caused by dermatophytes, non-dermatophytic fungi, or a combination of both. Superficial disease caused by non-dermatophytes is limited to the stratum corneum, hair, or both. When fungi grow on the host, there is little to no host immune response. Cutaneous disease involves the epidermis and dermis and there is an inflammatory reaction similar to contact dermatitis. Because the stratum corneum, hair, and nail are non-viable, disease caused by these fungi is simply colonization of the host and not an infection. Infection occurs when a fungus grows and replicates in sterile viable tissue or body fluids.

The dermatophytes are a phylogenetically related group of filamentous ascomycetes classified in the genera *Epidermophyton*, *Microsporum*, and *Trichophyton*. These molds have keratinases which allow them to grow in keratinized tissues on the host. Fungi that are able to use the protein keratin for growth are referred to as keratinophilic fungi. Not all keratinophilic fungi are dermatophytes, whereas all dermatophytes are keratinophilic. The distinction between the two groups relates to the fact that dermatophytes grow on the living host whereas the other fungi do not.

Historically, mycoses involving skin, nail, and hair have been classified based upon their clinical presentation and body site of involvement (Table 17.1). Clinically descriptive terms such as black piedra and tinea nigra have been used for some of these diseases when dematiaceous fungi are the etiologic agents, and the term tinea versicolor has been used for the lipophilic yeast genus *Malassezia*. To maintain the integrity of the clinical term tinea for dermatophyte, tinea should be restricted to dermatophyte-caused disease, and other well-established terms like pheohyphomycosis, hyalohyphomycosis,[1,2] and pityriasis versicolor should be used for diseases caused by non-dermatophytes. Hyalohyphomycosis is a companion term to pheohyphomycosis and includes non-dematiaceous fungi, whereas pityriasis versicolor is caused by yeast, even though hyphae may be present in the lesions.

Superficial mycoses

Superficial pheohyphomycosis caused by *Piedraia*

Key features:

- Black nodules adhering to hair shaft
- Ascospores in potassium hydroxide mount
- Culture not necessary
- Management with haircut
- Etiologic agent is *Piedraia hortae*

Introduction

Black piedra is a disease of hair in which the ascomycete *Piedraia hortae* forms ascostromata containing asci and ascospores. The disease is primarily found on people living in Africa, Asia, and Central America. Hair involvement is least among children, and both sexes are equally involved.

Pathogenesis and etiology

As the fungus grows on the hair, it destroys the cuticular layers of the hair. The fungus then penetrates deeply into the cortex. Around the hair, the ascomycetous fruiting body contains locules that have asci and ascospores are formed. These structures are black, hard, and remain attached to the hair when the hair is pulled between two fingers. Management consists of a hair cut. The use of antifungal agents is not necessary, nor is there a need to culture the fungus in the laboratory. The diagnosis is made by the clinical presentation and direct examination of the black nodules in 10–15% potassium hydroxide.

Table 17.1 Superficial mycoses and their clinical manifestations

Disease	Body area	Primary clinical symptoms
Pityriasis versicolor	Trunk, arms	Branny discoloration or depigmentation
Pheohyphomycosis		
Black piedra	Hair	Carbonaceous black nodules
Superficial	Palms, dorsum of foot	Non-scaly, sharply marginated, brown-black macules
Tinea barbae	Beard	Scaling, red patches on face and neck
Tinea capitis	Scalp	Scaling, fissures, erythema, burning
Tinea corporis	Body	Scaling, alopecia, inflammation, secondary bacterial infection
Tinea cruris	Groin	Erythema, papules, well-demarcated lesions
Tinea pedis	Foot	Erythema, scaling, maceration, interdigital spaces
Tinea unguium and onychomycosis	Nail	Opaque, yellow, thickened nail

Superficial pheohyphomycosis caused by *Hortaea*

Synonyms: Tinea nigra, tinea nigra palmaris, keratomycosis nigricans, cladosporiosis epidemica, pityriasis nigra, microsporosis nigra

Key features:

- Asymptomatic development of a light-brown macule, usually on the palmar surface of the hand and fingers (synonym: tinea nigra palmaris). Lesions may be observed on the plantar surface of the foot (synonym: tinea nigra plantaris), neck, and thorax. The light-brown macules spread centrifugally and darken to brown-black owing to the presence of the dematiaceous fungus
- Color is mottled, with deeper pigmentation seen on the periphery of the involved tissue
- The etiologic agent is *Hortaea werneckii* (synonym: *Cladosporium werneckii, Exophiala werneckii, Phaeoannellomyces werneckii*)
- The condition is endemic in tropical and subtropical coastal regions of the Caribbean, Asia, Africa, South and Central America. Cases have been reported in southeastern US coastal regions[1] and Europe. The etiologic agent possesses a high tolerance for salt

Introduction

The disease is painless and characterized by single, sharply demarcated non-scaly macules found on the palm of the hand and fingers. Lesions may also occur on the sole of the foot and other skin surfaces such as the neck and thorax. The lesion gradually enlarges, with the darkest pigmentation being at the periphery. The disease typically does not elicit an inflammatory response. This disease has been often been misdiagnosed as other hyperpigmentation processes such as malignant melanomas.

The first authentic description of the disease was made by Alexandra Cerqueira (1891) in Bahai, Brazil. He gave it the clinical name keratomycosis nigricans palmaris. It was not until 1916 that Alexandra Cerqueira's son, Castro Cerqueira-Pinto, published findings for eight other cases. For the disease seen in Asia, Castellani described the etiologic agent *Cladosporium mansoni*. It was not until 1921 that Horta described the etiologic agent as C. *werneckii*. McGinnis and Schell showed that C. *werneckii* and C. *mansoni* were the same species and then renamed the fungus *Phaeoannellomyces werneckii*. Nishimura and Miyaji subsequently renamed the same fungus as *Hortaea werneckii*. Owing to the fact that Nishimura and Miyaji named the fungus first, *H. werneckii* is the correct name.

With increased travel by many individuals, the disease has been found in tropical and non-tropical areas. For example, 15 cases of tinea nigra were described in North Carolina. With increased awareness of the disease, more cases have since been reported in the USA and Europe. People living in coastal regions of the Caribbean, Asia, Africa, South and Central America, and the southeastern USA coastal regions[3] and Europe most frequently develop superficial pheohyphomycosis caused by *Hortaea*. This may be related to the high tolerance the fungus has for salt. Children and young adults are more often affected, as well as non-immunocompromised individuals. In most studies, females are affected more frequently then males. There appears to be no genetic predisposition to this disease.

Pathogenesis and etiology

The fungus is confined to the stratum corneum and does not normally elicit an inflammatory response. A second fungus, known as *Stenella araguata*, has been described as a rare etiologic agent of this disease. A slightly abnormal thickening of the stratum corneum may be observed because of the large amount of fungal elements that can be present. Branched, brown hyphae (Fig. 17.1) appear in the stratum corneum: the stratum lucidum is spared. Biopsies show small areas of abnormality in the horny layer of the skin, which result in disturbance of keratinization. A small amount of perivascular infiltrate can also be seen.

The disease is asymptomatic in most cases but may be associated with pruritus. It is characterized by the formation of a single, sharply demarcated non-scaly macule that may resemble a silver nitrate

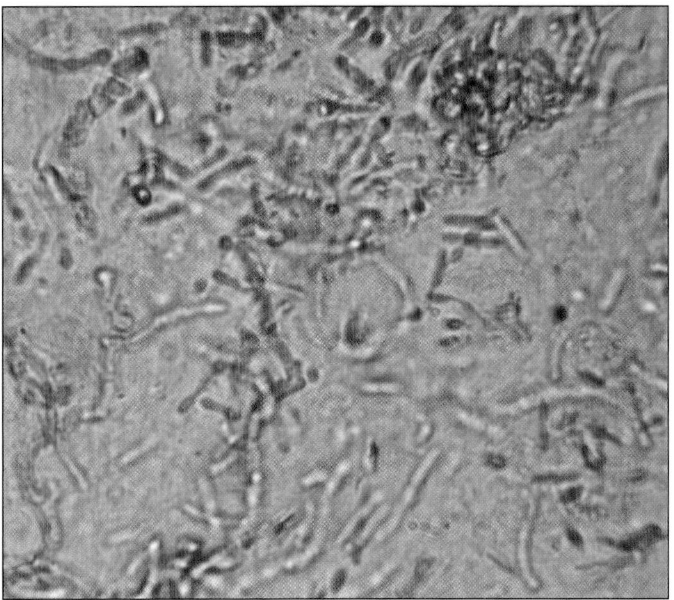

Figure 17.1 Dematiaceous hyphae and yeast cells of *Hortaea werneckii* in stratum corneum. Potassium hydroxide preparation. (Courtesy of Julius Kane, D.Sci.)

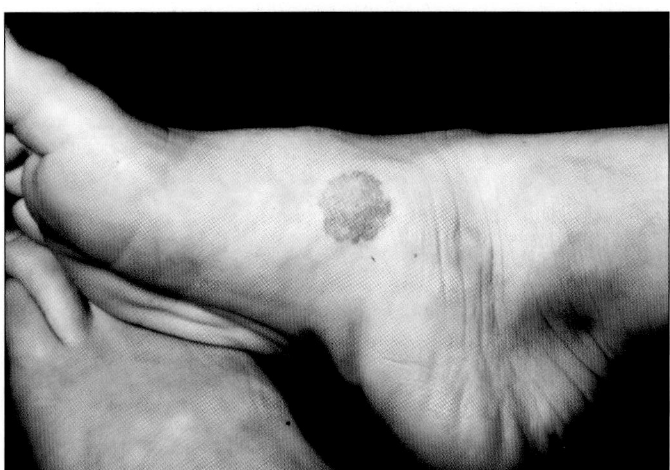

Figure 17.2 Superficial pheohyphomycosis caused by *Hortaea werneckii*. (Courtesy of Dr. Carlyn Halde.)

stain (Fig. 17.2). Lesions enlarge (1 mm to 1.5 cm) gradually and the darkest pigmentation can be seen at the periphery. The dark color of the lesion is due to the melanin in the cell walls of the etiologic agent.

Patient evaluation, diagnosis, and differential diagnosis

Diagnosis of the infection can be done by a simple epidermal scraping from the lesion. Examination of skin scrapings reveals brown to olive, septate, branching hyphae measuring 1.5–5 μm in diameter. Elongate, two-celled, budding yeast cells, 3 × 10 μm, are also typically seen in skin scrapings. The budding cells may be in clusters or along the length of dark hyphae. Older growth may appear twisted, with numerous septa and thickening of the cell walls, which become deeply pigmented. *H. werneckii* is a black yeast because of the presence of melanin in its yeast cell walls, which contributes to the pheoid color of its yeast-like colonies.

Skin scrapings can be inoculated on to potato glucose agar, mold-inhibitory agar, or Sabouraud glucose agar. After 5–7 days of incubation at 30 °C, slow-growing mucoid colonies develop that become olive to greenish-black in color. As the colonies mature, aerial mycelium develops.

Macules showing an uneven rate of spread, coalescence, or both raise the suspicion of melanomas, melanocytic nevi, or junctional nevi. Other differential diagnoses include pigmentation of Addison's disease, melanosis from syphilis, postinflammatory melanosis, palmoplantar pigmentation, and stains from chemicals or dyes.

Treatment

Spontaneous resolution of the condition is rare. Whitfield's ointment, salicylic acid preparations, and tincture of iodine and other keratolytic agents have been successful to various degrees.[4] The topical use of 10% tiabendazole, an antiparasitic drug, or azoles such as miconazole, clotrimazole, ketoconazole, and itraconazole have been used. Oral griseofulvin is ineffective in the treatment of this disease.

Pityriasis versicolor

Synonyms: Tinea versicolor, tinea alba, dermatomycosis furfuracea, tinea flava, achromia parasitica, malasseziasis, liver spots

Key features:

- Pityriasis versicolor is a chronic, asymptomatic to mild disease of the stratum corneum.
- Lesions are bran-like to furfuraceous in consistency. They are discrete or joined together, discolored or depigmented areas of skin. The lesions appear mainly on the upper trunk, neck, and upper arms
- The etiologic agent is the lipophilic yeast *Malassezia furfur*, formerly known as *Pityrosporium orbiculare* or *P. ovale*. *M. symptodialis* is also associated with humans. *M. pachydermatis* is less frequently seen in humans but is common in certain animals. Six different species of *Malassezia* have been described
- It is a common condition in temperate climates and is very prevalent in the tropics and subtropics, sometimes occurring in up to 60% of the population. It has been reported in Mexico, Samoa, South and Central America, India, parts of Africa, Cuba, regions of the Mediterranean, and the West Indies

Introduction

Pityriasis versicolor is a mild to chronic colonization of the stratum corneum by the lipophilic fungus *Malassezia furfur*. The clinical manifestation is characterized by scaly hypopigmented or hyperpigmented lesions that are usually on the trunk of the body (Fig. 17.3). *M. furfur* is a human and animal colonizer whilst *M. pachydermatis* is most commonly found in animals such as dogs. *M. furfur* is most commonly identified with human infections, followed by *M. pachydermatis*. The role of *M. symptodialis* as an etiologic agent of human disease has not been extensively studied. Some case reports suggest that this lipophilic yeast may be involved

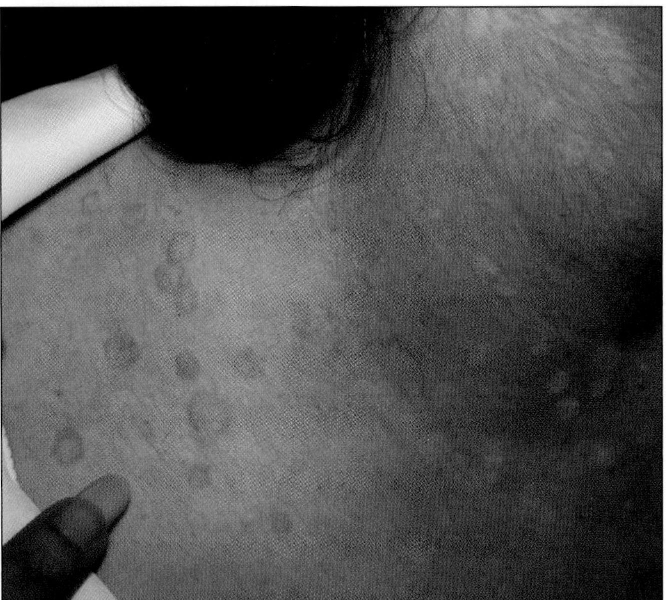

Figure 17.3 *Malassezia furfur* in stratum corneum. (Courtesy of Dr. Carlyn Halde.)

with human disease. It appears that *M. furfur* is universally present as part of the normal human flora of the skin.

A lesion may consist of one continuous scaling sheet at the affected area. In contrast, other lesions may present as patches of fawn, yellow-brown, or dark-brown-colored processes. Owing to the characteristics of the lesions, tinea corporis, secondary syphilis, pinta, melanoma, seborrheic keratoses, acanthosis nigricans, melasma, diabetic dermopathy, reticulated papillomatosis of Gougerot–Carteaud syndrome, and postinflammatory hyperpigmentation or hypopigmentation after trauma, skin irritation, or dermatoses must be considered in the differential diagnosis.[5,6]

In 1846, Eickstedt, and later Sluyter in 1847, observed the fungal etiology of the disease and named it pityriasis versicolor. In 1853, Robin named the etiologic agent *Microsporum furfur*, because he thought that it was related to the dermatophyte *Microsporum audouinii*. He changed the disease epithet to tinea versicolor because he thought it was related to the other ringworm infections. Baillon changed the name in 1889 when he concluded that the two fungi were not related. He created the monotype genus *Malassezia* and named the fungus *M. furfur*. Morris Gordon first isolated the fungus in culture and named it *Pityrosporium orbiculare*,[7] which is now considered a synonym of *Malassezia*. Based on molecular data, the genus *Malassezia* has recently been revised and several new species have been added.[8,9]

Epidemiology

Malassezia species are saprophytic yeasts that grow on normal skin of the trunk, head, and neck, where there tends to be large quantities of lipids. It is a disease that classically affects young people of either sex. Typically, the disease occurs in individuals prior to puberty. It is thought that the composition of sebum from the sebaceous glands influences the frequency of pityriasis versicolor in different age groups. This may be due to the hormonal changes, malnutrition, oral contraceptives, and hyperhidrosis. Rarely, pityriasis versicolor may occur in immunocompromised individuals such as those with Cushing's syndrome. Transitory fungemia has been observed in infants who received intravenous lipid-containing formulations. This problem does not require antifungal agents, but the catheter must be replaced. Pityriasis versicolor occurs in patients living in all climates, but its prevalence in the tropics is very high, sometimes with 60% of the population showing clinical signs of the disease.

Pathogenesis and etiology

There are at least eight species in the genus *Malassezia*. The most common and well-characterized species causing pityriasis versicolor are *M. furfur* and *M. pachydermatis*. *M. globosa* and other species of *Malassezia* may be associated with this disease. Members of this genus are considered one of the factors that initiate seborrheic dermatitis.[10,11]

The yeast is a basidiomycetous fungus that forms bottle-shaped cells having a small collarette. The yeast cells occur in clusters with the presence of septate hyphae that appear truncate (Fig. 17.4). In stratum corneum, the fungus may occur only as yeast cells, yeast cells with hyphae, or only hyphae.

Treatment

Topical and oral therapies are effective in treating this disease, even though relapse is common. Selenium sulfide, propylene glycol, sulfur with salicylic acid, and benzoyl peroxide – chemical agents that remove the stratum corneum and that are not active against the yeast – are effective therapeutic modalities. Clotrimazole, miconazole, ketoconazole, and fluconazole, the latter two replacing the other azoles, are effective in 2% creams and shampoos, or as foaming gels.

Terbinafine as a 1% solution, a cream, a gel, and a spray is effective. Ketoconazole, itraconazole, and fluconazole have been shown to be effective when taken orally by patients with large or multiple lesions.[6]

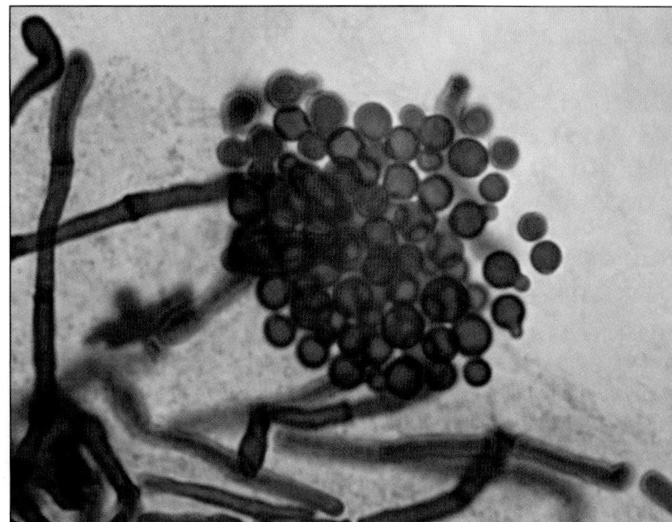

Figure 17.4 *Malassezia furfur* in stratum corneum, periodic acid–Schiff stain.

Dermatophytes

Tinea capitis

Synonyms: Ringworm of the scalp, eyebrows, and eyelashes, tinea tonsurans

Key features:

- Inflammation and pain, red scaling areas, alopecia, brittle hair leading to hair loss and formation of black dots, boggy ulcerated skin lesions
- Broad range of clinical presentation
- Griseofulvin, itraconazole, terbinafine, ketoconazole, and fluconazole are effective treatments
- Oral therapy is necessary to penetrate the hair shaft and clear scalp disease

Introduction

Historically, *Microsporum audouinii* has been one of the major etiologic agents of tinea capitis throughout the world (Fig. 17.5). *M. audouinii* is an anthropophilic species that is commonly spread from person to person. With the widespread use of griseofulvin, this species has become nearly extinct. *M. canis*, originating from pet dogs and cats, and *Trichophyton verrucosum*, from cattle, are important zoophilic etiologic agents of this disease.

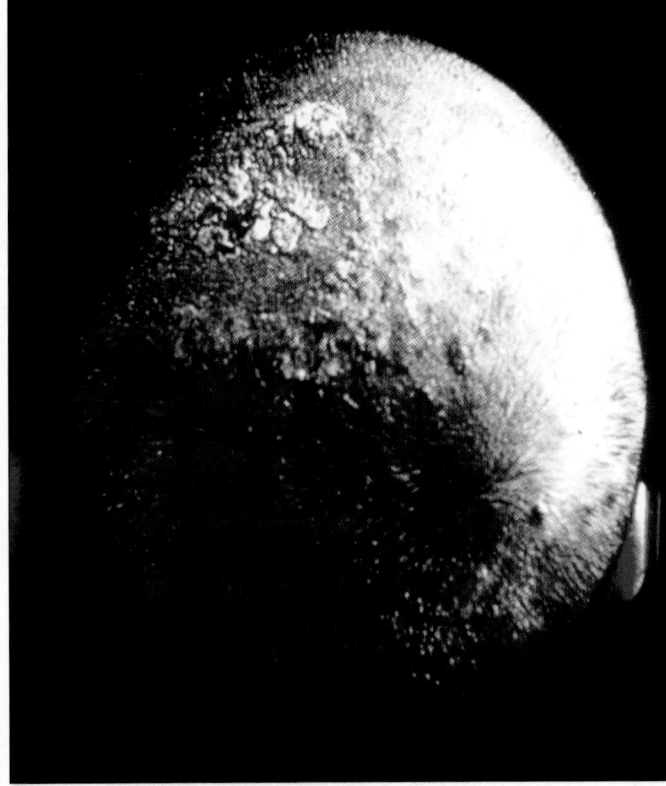

Figure 17.5 Tinea capitis caused by *Microsporum audouinii*. (Courtesy of Dr. Libero Ajello.)

Epidemiology

Tinea capitis is seen primarily in infants, children, and young adolescents.[12] The etiologic agents spread from person to person (anthropophilic, i.e. people-loving fungi), from soil to person (geophilic, i.e. soil-loving fungi), and from animal to person (zoophilic, i.e. animal-loving fungi). Overall, the most common cause of this disease is the anthropophilic dermatophyte *T. tonsurans*. Other important etiologic agents of tinea capitis include *T. soudanense* and *T. violaceum*.

Pathogenesis and etiology

Arthroconidia are important propagules for the dissemination of dermatophytes. These conidia have been demonstrated to be more virulent in animal models than hyphae or microconidia. The infective propagule arrives on the scalp where it grows and then invades the stratum corneum. If the hyphae grow into a hair follicle, the fungus then penetrates the non-living portion of the hair. As the fungus grows within the hair shaft, three potential outcomes may occur. If arthroconidia are formed only within the hair and the hair's cuticle remains intact, the invasion is endothrix. This is most commonly seen in *T. tonsurans* disease. When the fungus produces arthroconidia inside and along the outside of the hair shaft, ectothrix invasion has occurred. In ectothrix hair invasion, the hair cuticle is destroyed. *M. canis* (Fig. 17.6) and *M. audouinii* are examples of ectothrix causing dermatophytes. When the hyphae simply grow within the hair shaft and no conidia are made, a special situation occurs that is referred to as favic hair invasion. The diagnosis of this type of hair invasion by *T. schoenleinii* (Fig. 17.7) is made by immediately observing the hair with a microscope when it is first placed in potassium hydroxide mounting medium. Air bubbles can be seen racing through the hyphae within the hair.

In some instances, hyphal aggregates (Fig. 17.8) may form in the subcutaneous tissue and these resemble the sclerotia seen in mycetoma. The hyphal aggregates are apparently expelled into the adjacent tissue from ruptured hair follicles. The aggregates are present in non-viable tissue. Hence the process is not a mycetoma, as suggested by some.[13]

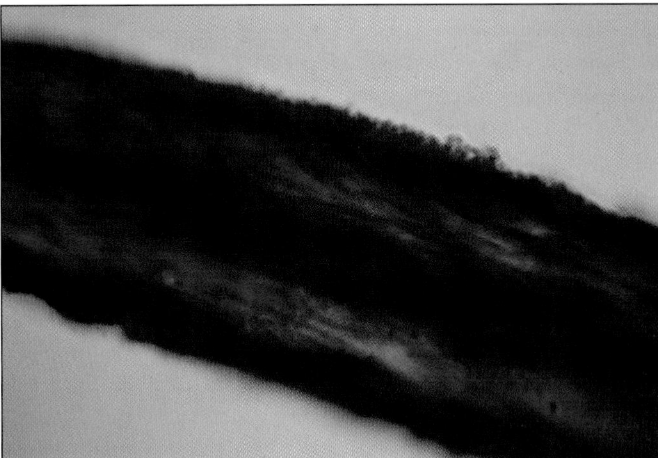

Figure 17.6 Ectothrix hair invasion by *Microsporum canis*. Arthroconidia can be seen within and around the hair shaft. Periodic acid–Schiff stain.

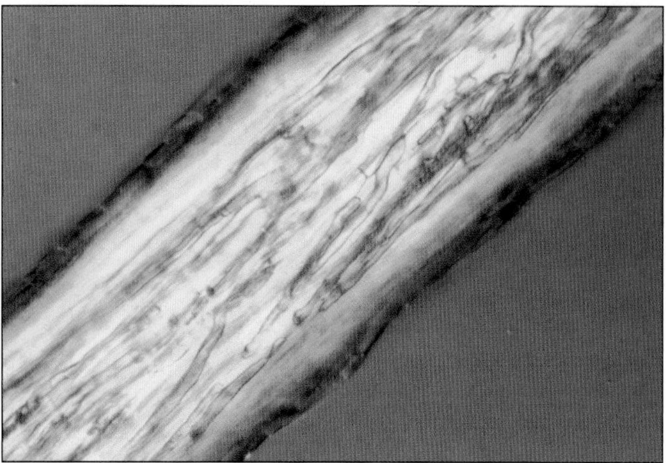

Figure 17.7 Favic hair invasion caused by *Trichophyton schoenleinii*. Differential interference contrast microscopy.

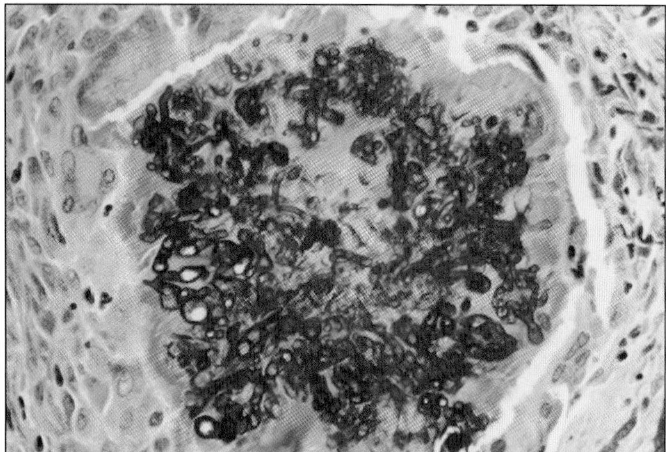

Figure 17.8 Hyphal aggregate of *Microsporum canis* in scalp tissue. Periodic acid–Schiff stain.

Clinical features

Tinea capitis is a fungal disease involving the scalp, eyebrows, and eyelashes. Primary lesions may be papules, pustules, plaques, or nodules with or without alopecia. Scaling, erythema, and alopecia are common. If hairs are broken at the surface of the scalp, black-dot alopecia and scaling may be present. An increased cell-mediated immune response can lead to kerion formation with exudative, nodular, boggy lesions, and alopecia.[14–15]

Disease caused by *M. canis* is called "gray-patch" ringworm because there are circular patches of alopecia with scaling. Infection by *T. tonsurans* and *T. violaceum* causes black-dot ringworm, in which diffuse broken hair shafts within areas of alopecia resemble black dots. *T. verrucosum* and *T. mentagrophytes* are zoophilic species that can cause a severe inflammatory response that tends to resolve itself more rapidly than non-zoophilic species. Anthropophilic isolates of *T. mentagrophytes* result in less inflammatory lesions. The endothrix-type hair invasion by *T. violaceum* results in a persistent infection.

Patient evaluation, diagnosis, and differential diagnosis

Diagnosis is made by microscopically observing hyphae in the stratum corneum, endothrix, ectothrix, or favic hair invasion, or with a Wood's lamp if the infection is caused by a *Microsporum* spp. Greenish fluorescence of hairs invaded by species such as *M. audouinii* (Fig. 17.9) can be selectively examined microscopically or placed on to an isolation medium. Skin scales are best collected with a brush or as skin scrapings.

Tinea capitis may be confused with seborrheic dermatitis, atopic dermatitis, abscesses, neoplasias, psoriasis, lupus, erythematosus, alopecia areata, pseudopelade, impetigo, trichotillomania, pyoderma, bacterial folliculitis, decalvans, and secondary syphilis.

Treatment

Tinea capitis is treated with oral antifungal agents to insure that the fungus in hair and hair follicles is eradicated. Griseofulvin at 10 mg/kg per day for 8–10 weeks is more effective when taken with fatty foods. Shorter treatment periods can be achieved with itraconazole at a dosage of 5 mg/kg per day for 1–4 weeks taken without food. Fluconazole is another effective azole antifungal agent. Tinea capitis can be effectively treated with terbinafine; if the patient is under 20 kg, the suggested dose is 62.5 mg/day; 20–40 kg patients should receive 125 mg/day; and patients over 40 kg should receive 250 mg/day. These doses should be taken for 4 weeks. In conjunction with oral therapy, creams containing azoles and shampoos containing selenium sulfide can be used topically as a means of reducing the risk of disease progression.[10,11,14–16]

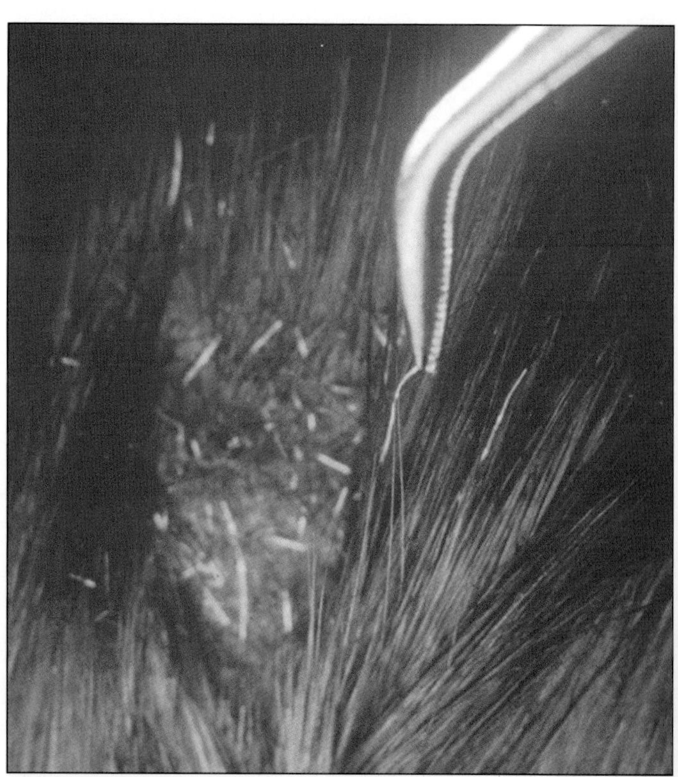

Figure 17.9 Fluorescence of hair invaded by *Microsporum audouinii*. (Courtesy of Dr. Libero Ajello.)

Tinea corporis

Synonym: Ringworm of the body

Key features:

- Infection of the stratum corneum in the glabrous skin
- Tends to resolve spontaneously
- Griseofulvin, fluconazole, itraconazole, and terbinafine are treatments

Introduction

Tinea corporis is a dermatophyte disease of the glabrous skin, excluding the scalp, beard, face, hands, feet, and groin. The fungus grows in the stratum corneum of the epidermis and does not grow in viable tissue. Fungal metabolites are believed to cause toxic and allergenic responses. Tinea corporis is ubiquitous, but most prevalent in the tropics.

Pathogenesis and etiology

All of the dermatophytes can cause this disease, but the most prevalent species are *Trichophyton rubrum* (Fig. 17.10) and *T. mentagrophytes* (Fig. 17.11). The fungi causing tinea corporis can be transmitted by scales, hyphae, or arthroconidia; either through direct contact or through fomites such as sheets.

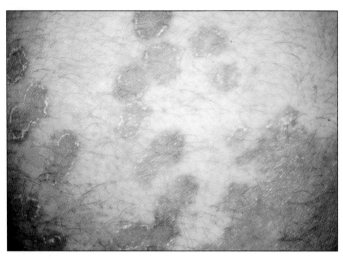

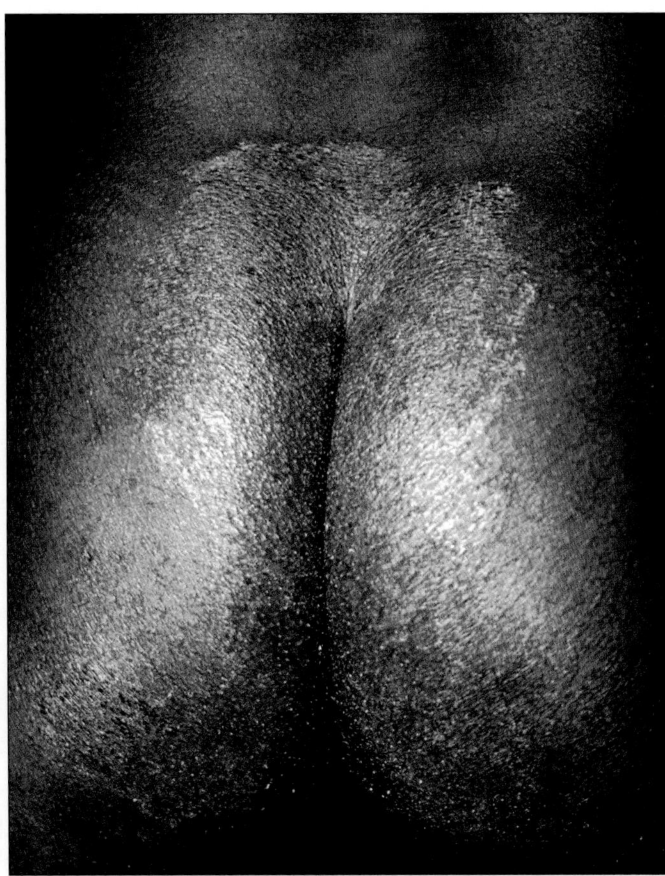

Figure 17.10 Tinea corporis caused by *Trichophyton rubrum*. (Courtesy of Dr. Benjamin Smith.)

Figure 17.11 Tinea corporis caused by *Trichophyton mentagrophytes*. (Courtesy of Dr. Earl Jones.)

Clinical features

Tinea corporis may appear as annular lesions, bullous lesions, Majocchi's granuloma, pustular lesions, psoriasiform plaques, or verrucous lesions.[17] The lesions usually appear as single or multiple, annular, scaly processes with central clearing, a slightly elevated, reddened edge, and sharp margination. The border of the lesion may contain pustules or follicular papules. Each lesion may have one or several concentric rings with red papules or plaques in the center. As the lesion progresses, the center may clear, leaving postinflammatory hypopigmentation or hyperpigmentation. Active growth of the dermatophyte is at the edge of the lesion. *Trichophyton* spp. antigens can elicit both immediate (type 1) and delayed-type (type 4) hypersensitivity skin test reactions. Immediate hypersensitivity reaction occurs in individuals who have chronic recurrent infections characterized by low-grade inflammatory lesions and immunoglobulin E (IgE) antibodies. Delayed hypersensitivity occurs in individuals who have highly inflamed lesions that spontaneously resolve and are resistant to reinfection. Cell-mediated immune responses are more effective in resolving and to some degree preventing *Trichophyton* disease. In immunocompromised individuals, *T. rubrum* has been observed to penetrate beyond the superficial keratinized epithelium of the skin and nail to dermal invasion.

Patient evaluation, diagnosis, and differential diagnosis

Treatment with topical corticosteroids can alter the appearance of the lesions and may be a factor in the development of Majocchi's granuloma.

Scrapings from the active edge of the lesion or the top of blisters is examined in 10% potassium hydroxide for the presence of septate, hyaline, branching hyphae with or without arthroconidia. The addition of calcofluor white to the potassium hydroxide is an excellent dye to see the florescent hyphae in clinical specimens. This technique requires the use of a fluorescent microscope.

Tinea corporis can be confused with seborrheic dermatitis, contact dermatitis, psoriasis, pityriasis rosea, pityriasis versicolor, lichen planus, fixed drug eruption, candidiasis, nummular eczema, erythema annulare, granuloma annulare, Lyme disease, and annular secondary syphilis.

Treatment

Treatment consists of drying the involved skin and the use of topical antifungals. Rarely, widespread infections may require systemic therapy. Antifungal agents for the management of tinea corporis include griseofulvin 500 mg once daily for 4–6 weeks, fluconazole 150 mg once daily for 4–6 weeks, itraconazole 100 mg daily for 1–2 weeks, or terbinafine 250 mg daily for 2–4 weeks.

Tinea cruris

Synonyms: Jock itch, ringworm of the groin

Key features:

- Infection of the upper thighs and buttocks
- Ubiquitous but prevalent in tropical areas
- Griseofulvin, fluconazole, itraconazole, terbinafine, and ketoconazole are treatments

Introduction

Tinea cruris is an acute or chronic infection of the genitalia, pubic area, and perineal and perianal skin. It is an anatomic variety of tinea corporis.

The disease is normally seen in young males, but rarely seen in women. It occurs throughout the world but is more prevalent in tropical areas owing to temperature and humidity. The etiological agent can be spread by direct contact or through inanimate objects such as fabric. The primary etiological agents are *Epidermophyton floccosum*, *T. mentagrophytes*, and *T. rubrum*, the last of which causes a chronic disease.

Clinical features

The skin appears red, itchy, and inflamed and blisters may form. A discharge of watery exudate produces crusting and scaling.

Patient evaluation, diagnosis, and differential diagnosis

Tinea cruris can be misdiagnosed as candidiasis (intertrigo), seborrheic dermatitis, psoriasis, contact dermatitis, lichen simplex, or erythrasma.

Treatment

Medicated powders and creams are normally sufficient for therapy, but in cases of widespread or severe disease the following oral agents are recommended: griseofulvin 500 mg once daily for 4–6 weeks, fluconazole 150 mg once daily for 4–6 weeks, itraconazole 100 mg daily for 1–2 weeks, terbinafine 250 mg daily for 2–4 weeks. Relief of many of the symptoms is seen within 3 days when treated with griseofulvin. This is most likely due to detoxification or antiinflammatory side-effects of the drug and not to the eradication of the infectious agent. Therapy should be continued until the organism can no longer be cultured.

Tinea imbricata

Synonyms: Oriental, scaly, Tokelau, Burmese, Chinese, or Indian ringworm, herpes desquamans, Malabar itch, tinea circinata tropical, gogo, lofa tokelau, tinea tropicalis

Key features:

- Imbricate or concentric circular skin lesions
- Form of tinea corporis
- Etiological agent is *Trichophyton concentricum*
- Griseofulvin or terbinafine is the treatment

Introduction

Tinea imbricata is a form of tinea corporis caused by *Trichophyton concentricum*. It can be recognized by concentric circular lesions (imbricate rings) which can cover most of the body (Fig. 17.12). These lesions permeate from the initial site of infection. The geographical distribution of patients is the Pacific, Southeast Asia, and Central and South America. Inherited autosomal-recessive susceptibility may play a part in determining the epidemiology of tinea imbricata.[18] Patients with this disease often have a negative delayed-type hypersensitivity to *T. concentricum* cytoplasmic antigen and T-lymphocyte hyporeactivity.

Clinical features

Initially, brown maculopapules appear that increase in size. Layers of the stratum corneum become detached, producing a region of concentric circular lesions (imbricate rings) that can cover most of the body.

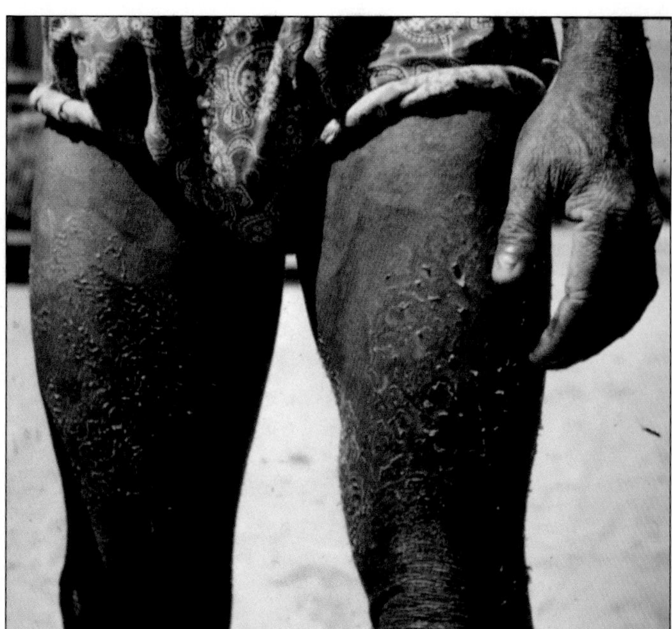

Figure 17.12 Tinea imbricata is a form of tinea corporis caused by *Trichophyton concentricum*. (Courtesy of Dr. Carlyn Halde.)

Patient evaluation, diagnosis, and differential diagnosis

The presence of widespread, annular, erythematosus concentric rings of scaling devoid of erythema is distinctive of tinea imbricata. Similar lesions have been described in tinea corporis caused by *T. mentagrophytes* and *T. tonsurans*.[19,20]

Treatment

Griseofulvin 500 mg twice daily for 4 weeks and terbinafine 250 mg daily for 4 weeks are effective in treating tinea imbricata.[21]

Tinea pedis

Synonyms: Athlete's foot, ringworm of the foot

Key features:

- Dermatophyte infection of the feet
- The lesions are of varying types, mild, chronic, and acute. In the acute form the lesions can be exfoliative, pustular, bullous, or both
- Organisms commonly involved are *Trichophyton rubrum*, *T. mentagrophytes*, and *Epidermophyton floccosum*
- It is more common among men than women; it is generally uncommon among children

Introduction

Tinea pedis is one of the most common fungal diseases of humans and is among the most prevalent of all infectious diseases.[1] The disease can be classified into three categories: (1) interdigital; (2) scaling hyperkeratotic moccasin-type of the plantar surface of the foot; and (3) highly inflammatory vesiculobullous eruptions. In interdigital disease there is an ecological interplay between dermatophytes and bacteria. The scaling process is a result of the dermatophyte invading the stratum corneum. As the tissue becomes macerated, secondary colonization by bacteria such as Gram-negative species occurs and this contributes to the odor associated with tinea pedis. Although very rare, *Candida* species may also be involved in interdigital tinea pedis.

A common clinical manifestation of athlete's foot is the intertriginous form where maceration, peeling, and fissuring of the interdigital web spaces of the fourth and fifth toe are typically involved. Another presentation of the disease is the chronic form, the squamous, hyperkeratotic type, in which fine silvery scales cover the pinkish skin of the soles, heel, and side of the foot (moccasin foot). An acute inflammatory type, which is characterized by the formation of vesicles, pustules, and at times bullae, is caused by *T. mentagrophytes*. The chronic agents of athlete's foot are *T. rubrum*, *T. mentagrophytes* var. *interdigitale*, and *E. floccosum*. Tinea pedis is thought to be a modern disease and has become prevalent owing to the wearing of shoes. The occlusive nature of shoes is thought to increase the incidence of tinea pedis, which correlates with the disease being more commonly seen during the summer months and in tropical climates.

History

The first recognized case of tinea pedis was recorded by Pellizzari in 1888. Raymond Sabouraud classified the dermatophytes into four genera: *Archorion*, *Epidermophyton*, *Microsporum*, and *Trichophyton*. In 1934 Chester Emmons modernized the taxonomic interpretation of Sabouraud and others and established the current classification of the dermatophytes on the basis of conidial morphology and accessory organs. In his classification, Emmons discarded the genus *Archorion* and only recognized three genera. Nutritional and physiological studies conducted by Lucile Georg and Libero Ajello led to the reduction of the number of species of dermatophytes, thus simplifying the identification of this group of fungi.

Epidemiology

Tinea pedis is one of the most common superficial fungal diseases. It affects at least 10% of the world's population at any given time. Tinea pedis is seen in men more commonly than in women, and it is uncommon in prepubertal children, although a few investigators have documented the occurrence of tinea pedis in children. Individuals with immune deficiency disorders such as human immunodeficiency virus (HIV) infection are prone to develop tinea pedis. Patients with a history of atopic dermatitis have an increased incidence of tinea pedis.

Pathogenesis and etiology

Organisms involved are *Trichophyton rubrum*, *T. mentagrophytes*, and *Epidermophyton floccosum*. Non-dermatophytic molds such as *Scytalidium dimidiatum* are known to cause tinea pedis. The yeast *Candida albicans* and the bacterium *Corynebacterium minutissimum* may also be involved.

Clinical features

Interdigital disease is by far the most common form of tinea pedis (Fig. 17.13), and may be chronic. Fissuring, scaling, and maceration of the interdigital spaces, particularly between the fourth and fifth toe, are involved. The fungus can spread to the sole of the foot. In some cases the third to fourth interdigital space may be affected. A whitish buildup of scales, with weepy red erosions, may be present. Along with this hyperhidrosis, pruritus, and a foul odor may be present. Some studies have implicated the interaction of the dermatophytes *T. rubrum* and *T. mentagrophytes* with various bacterial species as important in the pathogenesis of interdigital tinea pedis. Dermatophytosis simplex is a term used to describe uncomplicated interdigital tinea pedis. A severe form of the disease can leave the patient disabled and may involve the overgrowth of bacteria, which may manifest as lesions that are inflamed and macerated.

Tinea pedis with a papulosquamous pattern (moccasin-like) affects the soles and the lateral portions of the foot. The disease resembles someone wearing a moccasin. This type of tinea pedis is predominantly caused by *T. rubrum*. Moderate to severe presentations of moccasin-type tinea pedis may manifest with cracked and inflamed skin, and odor. In some instances it may develop into onychomycosis and the nail may become a reservoir for dermatophytes.

Vesicobullous tinea pedis is the least common form of the disease. *T. mentagrophytes* is the most common organism involved in this form of tinea pedis. The mildest form of vesicobullous tinea pedis may present as small, isolated vesicles filled with clear

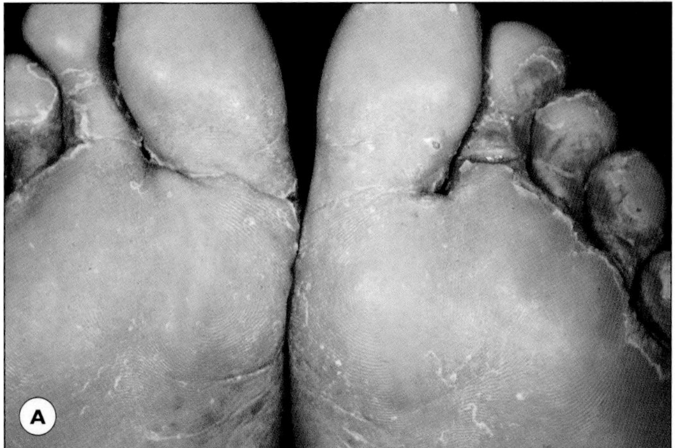

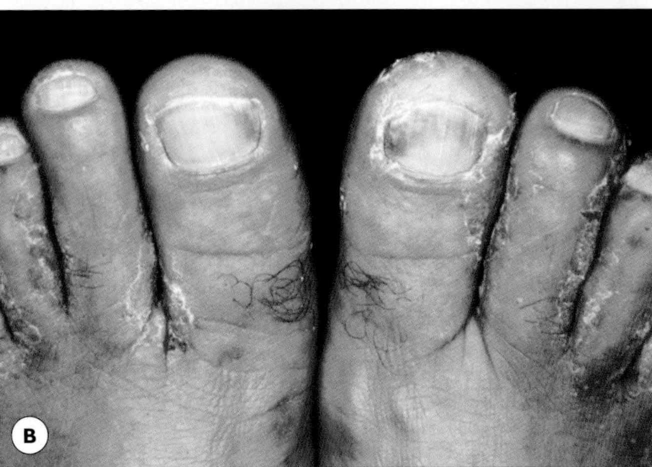

Figure 17.13 Tinea pedis. (Courtesy of Dr. Carlyn Halde.)

liquid. The vesicles may rupture independently and the disease may disappear spontaneously. However, the probability of recurrence is high. The instep may be affected, with the fungus spreading over the entire sole of the foot. If the disease is allowed to spread, the vesicles may become large, acute, pruritic, ulcerative erosive bullae.

Patient evaluation, diagnosis, and differential diagnosis

Tinea pedis may be difficult to diagnose when it is severe. Overgrowth of secondary bacteria may force the dermatophytes into the deeper layers of the stratum corneum, thus masking the presence of fungal elements. Staphylococci and streptococci can cause inflammation and odor without the presence of the dermatophytes. These organisms can cause foot infection in the absence of tinea pedis.

Scrapings from the active borders of the lesions, or the roof of a vesicle, are mounted in 10% potassium hydroxide and gently heated to assist in dissolving the epidermal cells. Examination with a microscope should reveal the presence of branched hyphae and arthroconidia in the stratum corneum.

Treatment

Topical antifungal therapy can be used to treat mild, non-inflammatory infections of tinea pedis. Systemic therapy is useful in treating hyperkeratotic areas such as the soles of the feet. Terbinafine and itraconazole have been proven to be effective.

Tinea unguium and onychomycosis

Synonyms: Ringworm of the nail, dermatophytic onychomycosis, onychomycosis

Key features:

- Invasive dermatophytic onychomycosis
- Two main types of nail involvement: invasive subungual and superficial white mycotic infection (leukonychia trichohytica)
- The dermatophytes commonly associated with tinea unguium are *Trichophyton rubrum* and *T. mentagrophytes*

Introduction

There is a trend to use the term onychomycosis for fungal nail disease, regardless of whether the etiologic agent is a dermatophyte, non-dermatophyte mold, or yeast. Historically, tinea unguium refers to nail disease caused by a dermatophyte, whereas onychomycosis included diseases caused by non-dermatophytic fungi. A major controversy centers on the role of non-dermatophytic molds as primary invaders of nail. With the exception of a few fungi, like *Scopulariopsis*, *Scytalidium*, and *Onychocola*, many reported mold infections most likely represent instances where the fungus is a secondary colonizer, or a contaminant.

Fusarium, *Scopulariopsis*, *Scytalidium*, *Onychocola*, and a few other molds cause approximately 1.5–6% of nail disease. In contrast, dermatophytes such as *T. mentagrophytes* and *T. rubrum* account for approximately 90% of toenail fungal disease and 50% of fingernail disease. *Candida* spp. are the primary cause of fingernail paronychia (Fig. 17.14), 1–32% toenail, and 51–70% of toenail disease. Interestingly, *Candida* is often found in association with dermatophytes and non-dermatophytic molds.[22,23]

Clinical features

Opaque, yellow, thickened nails are associated with fungal disease of the nails. Pain may be present, patients may experience problems conducting some daily activities, and they may suffer embarrassment.[10] Predisposing conditions include diabetes, HIV or

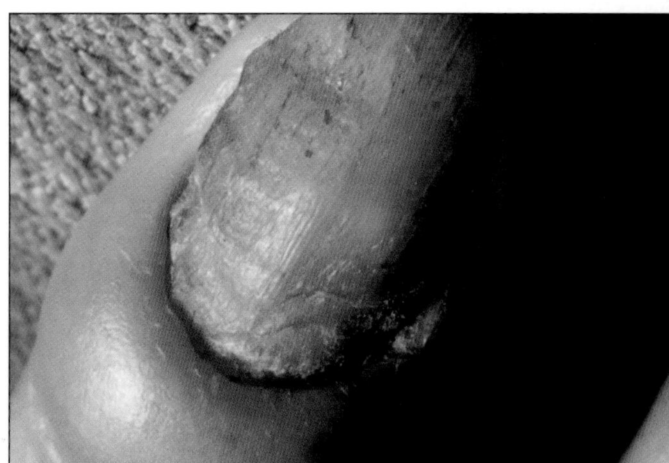

Figure 17.14 Fingernail-associated paronychia caused by *Candida albicans*. (Courtesy of Dr. Carlyn Halde.)

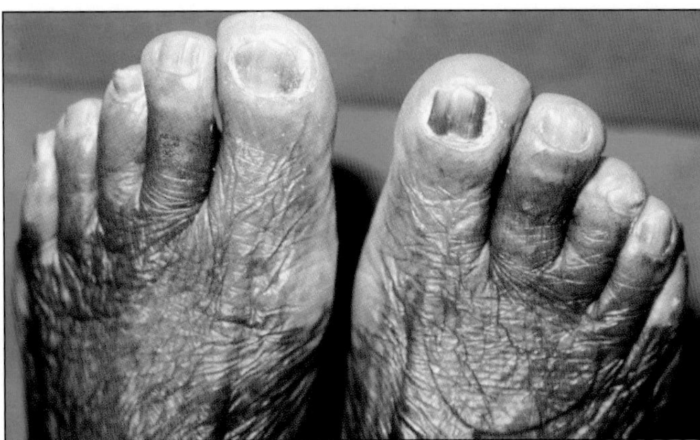

Figure 17.15 *Scytalidium dimidiatum* causing onychomycosis. (Courtesy of Dr. John Rippon.)

acquired immunodeficiency syndrome (AIDS), atopic conditions, compromised immune systems, over 60 years in age, psoriasis-caused nail damage, trauma, hyperhidrosis, and concomitant tinea pedis.

Distal and lateral subungual onychomycosis is the most common presentation. *Trichophyton rubrum* is the most common dermatophyte encountered in this disease. Other fungi, such as *Scytalidium dimidiatum*, *Fusarium oxysporum*, and *S. brevicaulis* have been associated with this problem. Onycholysis and paronychia of the fingernails are often associated with non-dermatophytic molds such as *S. dimidiatum* (Fig. 17.15). Superficial white onychomycosis is primarily caused by *T. mentagrophytes*. Proximal white superficial tinea unguium is often seen in AIDS patients (Fig. 17.16). *Aspergillus terreus*, *F. oxysporum*, *C. albicans*, and other fungi may cause this type of disease. Proximal subungual onychomycosis is uncommon and caused by *Trichophyton* species. *Candida* onychomycosis (Fig. 17.17) occurs, with the extreme being exhibited in patients with chronic mucocutaneous candidiasis (Fig. 17.16). Endonyx onychomycosis differs from distal and lateral subungual onychomycosis by having the hyphae directly invading the nail plate. White patches form without subungual hyperkeratosis or onycholysis being present. *T. soudanense* and *T. violaceum* are known causes of this disease.[22]

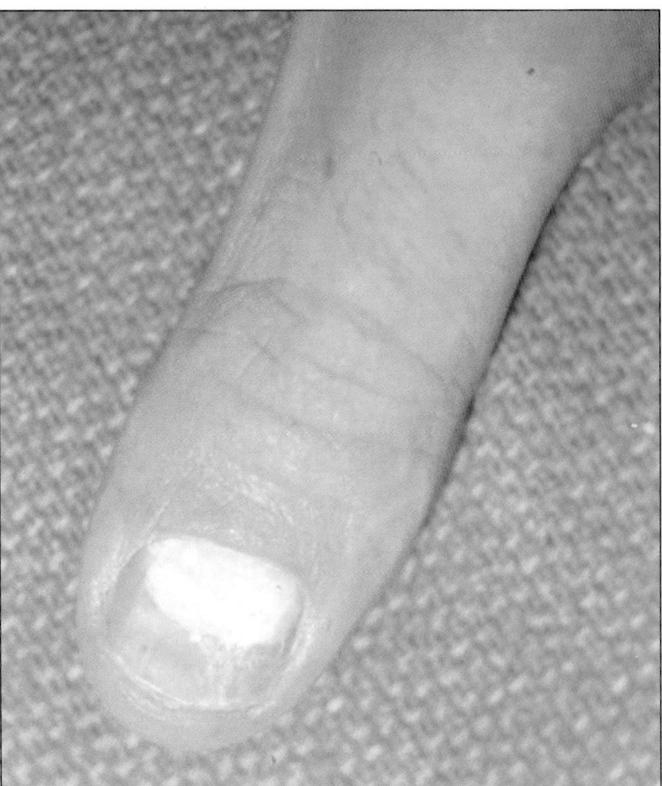

Figure 17.16 Proximal white superficial tinea unguium in an acquired immunodeficiency syndrome (AIDS) patient. (Courtesy of Dr. Raza Aly.)

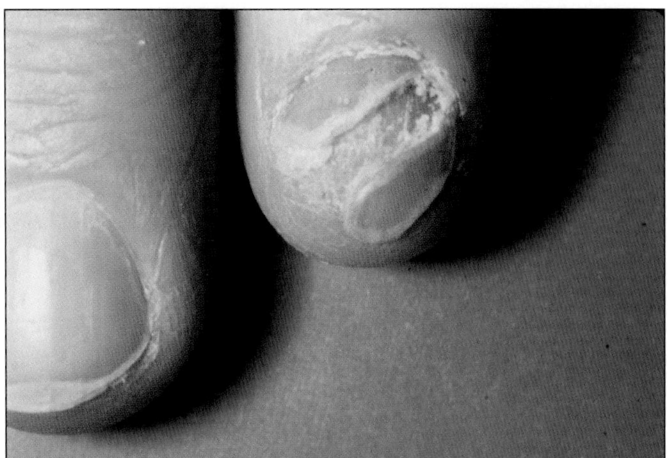

Figure 17.17 Onychomycosis caused by *Candida albicans*. (Courtesy of Dr. Carlyn Halde.)

Patient evaluation, diagnosis, and differential diagnosis

Fungal elements seen in potassium hydroxide preparations of nail material must be compatible with the recovered fungus. Melanized hyphae in nail specimens correlate with a dematiaceous fungus like *Scytalidium* and pseudohyphae are compatible with *Candida*. The isolation of a dermatophyte indicates that it is the etiologic agent of the disease, whereas the confirmation that a non-dermatophytic mold is the etiologic agent requires the isolation of the same fungus on two or more separate occasions and the absence of a dermatophyte being recovered. If a dermatophyte is present, the possibility of two etiologic agents must be considered. This also holds true for the isolation of a yeast like *C. albicans*.

Historically, a medium containing cycloheximide has been used to recover dermatophytes and exclude non-dermatophytic fungi. Nail specimens must be inoculated to media with and without cycloheximide to insure that all potential pathogens are recovered. Clinically, non-dermatophytic mold is often associated with one or two infected nails in the absence of tinea pedis, a history of trauma to the nails prior to nail dystrophy, and the absence of response to azoles and terbinafine.

Treatment

The correct identification of the etiologic agent is important because non-dermatophytic molds often respond poorly to therapy. Success in treating onychomycosis has been described with terbinafine, itraconazole, and fluconazole. Even though griseofulvin has a higher relapse rate, it can be effective for dermatophytes. It is not effective against *Candida* or non-dermatophytic molds.

Most cases of tinea unguium do not respond to topical treatment because of poor penetration of the treatment agent to the nail bed. Terbinafine is given at 250 mg every day for 6 weeks for fingernails and 12 weeks for toenails. Itraconazole as pulsed therapy is given at 400 mg each day for 1 week, and then repeated in 1 month for fingernails. It is continued for 3–4 months for toenail involvement. Fluconazole pulsed therapy is 150–300 mg once a week for 3–6 months when fingernails are being treated, and 6–12 months for toenails. Treatment may be required for additional periods of time until normal growth has replaced the infected nails.[10] Meta-analysis of the published worldwide literature indicates that terbinafine is significantly more effective than itraconazole in achieving mycologic cure of toenail disease.[24] Combined drug therapy is an option to be considered.[25]

References

1. McGinnis MR, Ajello L. Conceptual basis for hyalohyphomycosis. In: Ajello L, Hay R, eds. Topley and Wilson's microbiology and microbial infections, vol. 4, 9th edn. London: Arnold; 1998:499–502.
2. McGinnis MR. Chromoblastomycosis and phaeohyphomycosis: new concepts, diagnosis, and mycology. J Am Acad Dermatol 1983; 8:1–16.
3. McGinnis MR, Schell WA, Carson J. *Phaeoannellomyces* and the Phaeococcomycetaceae, new dematiaceous blastomycete taxa. Sabouraudia 1985; 23:179–188.
4. Gupta AK, Chaudhry M, Elewski B. Tinea corporis, tinea cruris, tinea nigra, and piedra. Dermatol Clin 2003; 21:395–400.
5. Stulberg DL, Clark N, Tovey D. Common hyperpigmentation disorders in adults: part II. Melanoma, seborrheic keratoses, acanthosis nigricans, melasma, diabetic dermopathy, tinea versicolor, and postinflammatory hyperpigmentation. Am Family Phys 2003; 68:1963–1968.
6. Gupta AK, Batra R, Bluhm R et al. Pityriasis versicolor. Dermatol Clin 2003; 21:413–429.
7. Rippon JW. Medical mycology, the pathogenic fungi and the pathogenic Actinomycetes. Philadelphia, PA: WB Saunders; 1984.
8. Gueho E, Midgley G, Guillot J. The genus *Malassezia* with description of four new species. Antonie van Leeuwenhoek 1996; 69:337–355.
9. Sugita T, Takashima M, Kodama M et al. Description of a new yeast species, *Malassezia japonica*, and its detection in patients with atopic dermatitis and healthy subjects. J Clin Microbiol 2003; 41:4695–4699.
10. Vander Straten MR, Hossain MA, Ghannoum MA. Cutaneous infections dermatophytosis, onychomycosis, and tinea versicolor. Infect Dis Clin North Am 2003; 17:87–112.
11. Gupta AK, Ryder JE, Nicol K et al. Superficial fungal infections: an update on pityriasis versicolor, seborrheic dermatitis, tinea capitis, and onychomycosis. Clin Dermatol 2003; 21:417–425.
12. Patterson TF, McGinnis MR. Tinea capitis and tinea favosa. Doctor fungus. Available online at: http://www.doctorfungus.org/mycoses/human/other/tinea_capitis_favosa.htm (accessed 5 August, 2004).
13. McGinnis MR. Mycetoma. Dermatol Clin 1996; 14:97–104.
14. Vander Straten MR, Hossain MA, Ghannoum MA. Cutaneous infections: dermatophytosis, onychomycosis, and tinea versicolor. Infect Dis Clin North Am 2003; 17:87–112.
15. Fuller LC, Child FJ, Midgley G et al. Diagnosis and management of scalp ringworm. Br Med J 2003; 326:539–541.
16. Pomeranz AJ, Sabnis SS. Tinea capitis: epidemiology, diagnosis and management strategies. Paediatr Drugs 2002; 4:779–783.
17. Elewski BE. Superficial mycoses, dermatophytosis, and selected dermatomycosis. In: Elewski BE, ed. Cutaneous fungal infections. Tokyo: Igaku-Shoin; 1992:12–59.
18. Hay RJ. Genetic susceptibility to dermatophytosis. Eur J Epidemiol 1992; 8:346–349.
19. Batta K, Ramlogan D, Smith AG et al. 'Tinea indecisiva' may mimic the concentric rings of tinea imbricata. Br J Dermatol 2002; 147:384.
20. Lim SP, Smith AG. "Tinea pseudoimbricata": tinea corporis in a renal transplant recipient mimicking the concentric rings of tinea imbricata. Clin Exp Dermatol 2003; 28:332–333.
21. Wingfield AB, Fernandez-Obregon AC, Wignall FS et al. Treatment of tinea imbricata: a randomized clinical trial using griseofulvin, terbinafine, itraconazole and fluconazole. Br J Dermatol 2004; 150:119–126.
22. Gupta AK, Ryder JE, Baran R et al. Non-dermatophyte onychomycosis. Dermatol Clin 2003: 21:257–268.
23. Ellis DH, Watson AB, Marley JE et al. Non-dermatophytes in onychomycosis of the toenails. Br J Dermatol 1997; 136: 490–493.
24. Krob AH, Fleischer AB Jr, D'Agostino R Jr et al. Terbinafine is more effective than itraconazole in treating toenail onychomycosis: results from a meta-analysis of randomized controlled trials. J Cutan Med Surg 2003; 7:306–311.
25. Olafsson JH, Sigurgeirsson B, Baran R. Combination therapy for onychomycosis. Br J Dermatol. 2003; 149 (suppl. 65):15–18.

Chapter 18

Subcutaneous mycoses

Introduction

Subcutaneous mycoses are a group of fungal diseases produced by a heterogeneous group of fungi that infect the skin, subcutaneous tissue, and in some cases the underlying tissues and organs. The causative agents are commonly found in the soil, leaves, and organic material, and introduced by traumatic injury of the skin. The diseases usually remain localized and slowly spread to the surrounding tissue; symptoms are usually minimal or absent. In rare occasions, lymphatic and hematogenous spreading of the infection can occur.

Most of the causative organisms of subcutaneous mycoses have been cultured from the affected tissues, and identified by histopathological examination. One of them, *Lacazia loboi*, has not been cultivated in vitro. *Rhinosporidium seeberi* causing rhinosporidiosis has been reclassified as a protist. Mycetoma can also be produced by bacteria belonging to the aerobic actinomycetes group, which causes more than 50% of the total cases reported worldwide; in some geographic areas they are the predominant causative agents of this disease.

The fungi producing sporotrichosis and cutaneous mucormycosis are also found worldwide. Other organisms, like those causing chromomycosis and mycetoma – eumycetoma and actinomycetoma – are mainly found in tropical and subtropical regions.

Rhinosporidiosis, entomopthoromycosis, and Lobo's disease are limited to some areas in Central and South America as well as Africa. Rhinosporidiosis has been reported in India, the Americas, Africa, Asia, and occasionally in Europe.

The clinical picture varies among the different diseases, but the appearance of a localized nodule, verrucous plaques, ulcerations; granulomatous tissue, subcutaneous tumors with abscesses, and fistulae should alert the clinician to the diagnosis of a subcutaneous mycosis. It is important to consider the places where the patient has lived or traveled, and the geographic epidemiology of fungal and aerobic actinomycete infections in those areas. The differential diagnosis is generally made with mycobacterial infections, other bacterial, parasitic, and fungal infections, as well as neoplasms. The diagnosis is based on the demonstration of the causative agents either by direct observation of the fungal structures in the material from the lesions with potassium hydroxide or by histopathological studies with specific stains such as periodic acid–Schiff (PAS) or Gomori–Groccott. The isolation of the etiological agent by culture, when possible, confirms the diagnosis and allows the clinician to select the proper treatment.

Mycetoma

Antônio Carlos Francescone do Valle, Olivera Welsh and Luciano Vera-Cabrera

Synonyms: Madura foot, maduromycosis

Key features:

- Mycetoma is an infectious disease caused by fungi or aerobic actinomycetes and characterized by an increased volume of involved area with fibrosis, abscesses, and fistulae
- It is mainly found in farmers of tropical and subtropical regions of the Americas, India, and Africa
- The causative agents are identified by direct examination, histopathology, and culture
- Treatment of actinomycetoma includes sulfamethoxazole, trimethoprim, and amikacin
- Therapy of eumycetoma includes itraconazole, terbinafine, and surgical resection of the lesions

Introduction

Mycetoma is a non-contagious chronic infection of the skin and subcutaneous tissue which can involve deeper structures like the

Table 18.1 Clinical entities involving formation of grains

Clinical entity	Infection sites	Sources	Etiologic agents
Mycetoma	Subcutaneous	Exogenous (traumatic inoculum)	Filamentous fungi or aerobic actinomycetes
Actinomycosis	Cervicofacial, pulmonary, abdominal, and pelvic	Endogenous (microbiota of the digestive and genital tracts)[a]	Anaerobic filamentous bacteria[b]
Botryomycosis	Subcutaneous and visceral	Microbiota of the skin and digestive tract[a]	Cocci and bacilli[c]

[a]Principal sources of infection.
[b]*Actinomyces israelii*, [c]*Staphylococcus aureus* (most frequent agents).

fasciae, muscles, and bones; it is acquired by traumatic inoculation of the etiologic agent. Clinically it is characterized by an increased volume of the affected area, fibrosis, tumefaction, and the formation of abscesses that drain pus-containing grains through fistulae. The grains represent an aggregate of hyphae produced by some species of fungi – eumycotic mycetoma – or bacterial filaments from aerobic actinomycetes – actinomycotic mycetoma.[1]

There is considerable confusion in the medical literature between mycetoma and other clinical entities presenting grains. To facilitate understanding, Table 18.1 presents the basic differences between these diseases. This confusion is further aggravated by the fact that various etiologic agents of eumycetoma can also cause pheohyphomycosis, chromoblastomycosis, and hyalohyphomycosis, for example, *Exophiala jeanselmei* and *Pseudallescheria boydii* (*Scedosporium apiospermum*).

Mycetomas are probably much more frequent than the cases published in the literature would lead us to believe, and early diagnosis and proper treatments are crucial for avoiding complications and extensive, mutilating surgeries.

History

Mycetoma was first described by Gill in 1842 with the term "Madura foot," in the district of Madura, India, and in 1860 Carter introduced the term mycetoma to designate all tumors produced by fungi. Later, Pinoy introduced the term actinomycetoma to designate those cases produced by aerobic actinomycetes, and eumycetoma for those caused by true fungi.

Epidemiology

This infection is more commonly found in young to middle-aged males from rural areas (ratio 3:1), probably reflecting occupational contact with the causative agents. These microorganisms live saprophytically in nature, in soil and plants, deriving nutrition from organic material in decomposition. Some species have a worldwide distribution, while others are limited to some regions. The ecological environment determines the presence and prevalence of different agents. The infection is more common in tropical and subtropical areas, and is endemic in India and various countries in Africa and the Americas. However, both forms of mycetoma have been reported in areas with a temperate climate, such as the USA.[1,2]

Pathogenesis and etiology

Saprophytic fungi or bacteria from the soil or plants penetrate the skin and subcutaneous tissue by traumatic implantation. The infection evolves slowly by contiguity and can invade deeper structures like fasciae, muscles, tendons, bones, and exceptionally adjacent organs. Nutritional factors and repeated trauma can contribute to the development of mycetoma.

Approximately half of the cases are caused by fungi, amongst which the most frequently isolated are *Madurella mycetomatis* and

Table 18.2 Principal etiologic agents of mycetoma and the different color of grains produced by them

Red-colored actinomycotic grains
Actinomadura pelletieri
White-colored actinomycotic grains
Actinomadura madurae
Nocardia brasiliensis
Nocardia asteroides
Nocardia otitidis caviarum (= *N. caviae*)
Streptomyces somaliensis
White-colored eumycotic grains
Pseudallescheria boydii (*Scedosporium apiospermum*)
Acremonium kiliense, *A. falciforme*, *A. recifei*
Neotestudina rosatii
Fusarium moniliforme
Aspergillus nidulans (*Eumericella nidulans*), *A. flavus*
Black-colored eumycotic grains
Madurella mycetomatis, *M. grisea*
Exophiala jeanselmei
Pyrenochaeta romeroi
Leptosphaeria senegalensis, *L. tompkinsii*
Curvularia lunata, *C. geniculata*

M. grisea and, less frequently, *Pseudallescheria boydii* (*Scedosporium apiospermum*), species of *Acremonium* (*kiliense*, *falciforme*, and *recifei*), *Exophiala jeanselmei*, and *Leptosphaeria senegalensis*. Many other species of fungal agents of mycetoma have been (and continue to be) described.[1,3]

The most frequently reported agents of actinomycetoma are species of *Nocardia*, especially *N. brasiliensis*, which is the most frequent agent in many countries of the Americas. The literature reports several cases involving *Actinomadura madurae* and sporadic cases from *Streptomyces somaliensis* and *A. pelletieri* (Table 18.2).

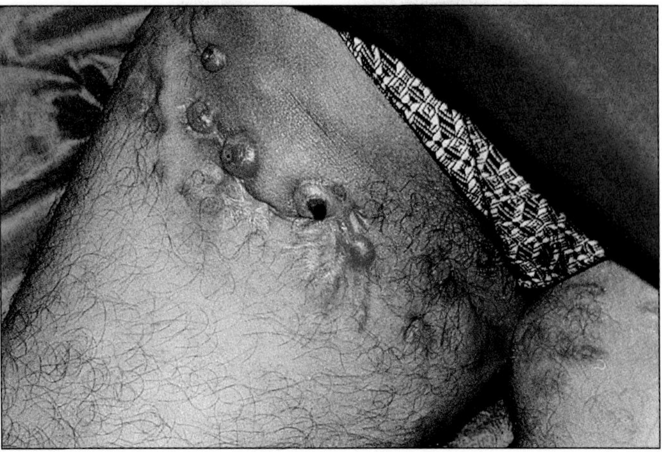

Figure 18.2 Lesion on posterior thigh with gummata, fistulae, and secretion containing black *Madurella mycetomatis* grains.

Clinical features

At the inoculation site, after a variable incubation period (weeks or months), a nodule appears, generally painless, which suppurates and drains a serosanguineous or seropurulent secretion through fistulae. Contiguous and similar lesions appear, and after a period of one to several years, the affected area presents an increased volume, with numerous fistulae draining secretion with grains (Figs 18.1 and 18.2). Bones and ligaments may also be affected, with osteomyelitis, the extension of which depends on the time of evolution of the disease and the pathogen's aggressiveness. Later stages involve skin hyperpigmentation, fibrosis, and local deformity. The presence of a secondary infection helps aggravate the inflammatory process. Actinomycetoma are usually more inflammatory and suppurative, while fibrosis and less secretion predominate in eumycetoma. Although they can affect an entire body segment, mycetoma are usually localized and unilateral.[4,5]

Patient evaluation, diagnosis, and differential diagnosis

When mycetoma is suspected, one should investigate: (1) history of trauma; (2) presence of an increased volume of the affected area, formation of nodules, abscesses, fistulae, and drainage of grains; (3) the color and size of the grains, as well as their microscopic characteristics (10% potassium hydroxide fresh mount) will help to classify the agent as either a fungus or filamentous bacteria, and in some organisms even suggest the specific etiologic agent; (4) histopathology of the lesion; (5) culture for isolation and identification of the agent; (6) an imaging study to evaluate the degree and extension of the lesion, with conventional X-ray, computed tomography, and magnetic resonance studies for detecting bone lesions and alterations in soft tissues.[6]

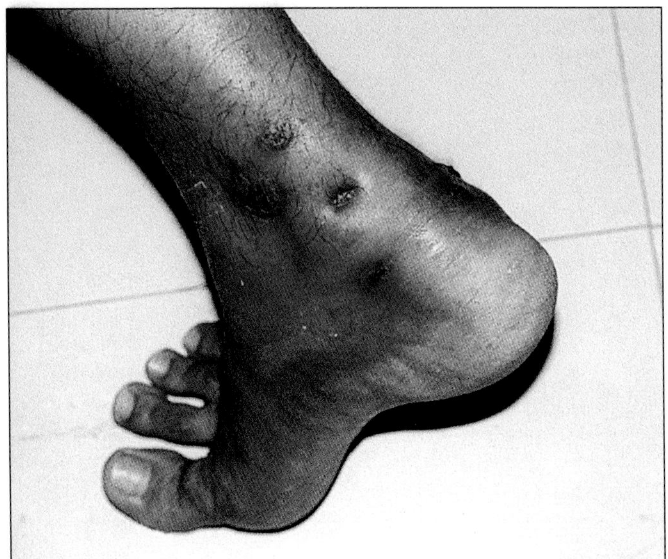

Figure 18.1 Lesion on right heel showing increased volume and multiple fistulae (*Nocardia brasiliensis*).

Clinical differential diagnoses include botryomycosis and actinomycosis, which also form grains, and in some cases with chronic osteomyelitis. Cutaneous tuberculosis, other fungal subcutaneous diseases, and tumors must also be considered.

Pathology

In histological sections stained with hematoxylin and eosin (H&E), the grains are frequently observed surrounded by an eosinophilic material (Splendore–Hoeppli phenomenon), an accumulation of polymorphonuclear neutrophils producing microabscesses, chronic inflammatory infiltrate, and granulation tissue containing epitheloid and giant cells. By using H&E it is possible to identify *A. pelletieri*, *A. madurae*, and *S. somaliensis* grains based on their color, size, and morphology (Fig. 18.3A and B). *Nocardia* granules are small, oval or lobular, and appear homogeneously stained with H&E; they may have peripheral clubs. In order to differentiate *Nocardia* from *Actinomyces*, different staining techniques for bacteria can be used, such as Gram, Brown–Brenn (both are Gram-positive), and Kinyoun; in general, *Nocardia* species are partially acid-fast.

In eumycetoma it is possible to identify *M. mycetomatis* grains in sections stained with H&E. Other fungal agents require further investigation using PAS and Grocott staining, showing the hyphae (Fig. 18.4). In both actinomycetoma and eumycetoma, precise identification of the agent requires isolation in culture and subsequent identification using complementary techniques.[1]

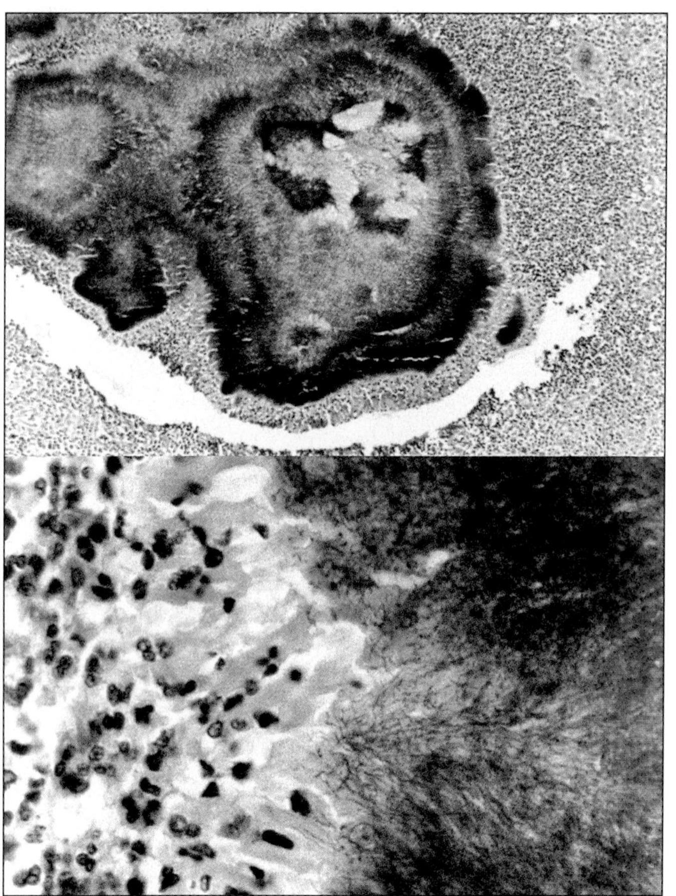

Figure 18.3 (A) Hematoxylin and eosin (H&E)-stained histopathology of skin with *Actinomadura madurae* grains (10×); (B) H&E-stained histopathology of skin with *A. madurae* grains (1000×).

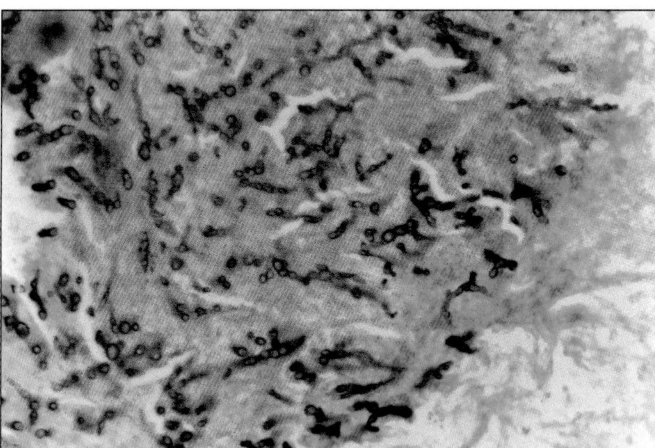

Figure 18.4 Grocott-stained histopathology of skin with *Madurella mycetomatis* grains (40×).

Treatment

In the treatment of mycetoma it is extremely important to characterize the etiologic agent (or at least to determine the nature of the infection, whether bacterial or fungal) and to evaluate the extent of tissue invasion.

Actinomycetoma with *Nocardia* are treated successfully with a combination of sulfamethoxazole (1200 mg) and trimethoprim (240 mg) (SXT) b.i.d., and occasionally dapsone at a dose of 100–300 mg/day for 24–36 months. Oxytetracycline 1.5–2 g/day and minocycline 200 mg/day for 1–2 years are used to treat *N. brasiliensis*, *N. asteroides*, *A. madura*, and *A. pelletieri*. Amoxicillin (500 mg) and clavulanic acid (125 mg) t.i.d. for 6 months for *N. brasiliensis* and amikacin (500 mg 12/12 h) for 3 weeks followed by 2 weeks of rest has been reported to be useful in some cases. Amikacin in combination with SXT is the best treatment for those cases caused by *N. brasiliensis* and *Actinomadura* that are unresponsive to the conventional antimicrobials, or those with potential dissemination to underlying organs. The medication is given in cycles of 5 weeks consisting of 15 mg/kg per day of amikacin for 3 weeks, and 5 weeks of sulfamethoxazole–trimethoprim 80:40 mg/kg per day. Creatinine clearance and audiometry must be performed periodically every cycle – 1 to 4 – in order to detect aminoglycoside's side-effects.[7]

Treatment response in eumycotic mycetoma is variable, and in many cases shows poor results. The drugs of choice are itraconazole (200–300 mg/day) or ketoconazole (400 mg/day) for 1 or 2 years or even for longer periods; amphotericin B IV or intralesional (total dose 2.0–4.0 g) can be used in some cases. Treatment failure could be due to the intense fibrosis, and the low sensitivity of certain etiologic agents to current antifungals. Corticosteroids can be combined with antifungals for a short period to improve the inflammatory process. A combination of surgery and drug therapy is the best option.[1,7]

Sporotrichosis

Iphis Campbell

Synonyms: Schenck's disease, rose gardener's disease

Key features:

- Worldwide infection caused by the dimorphic fungus *Sporothrix schenckii* is mainly found in temperate warm and tropical areas
- After cutaneous inoculation, ulcers and verrucous plaques with or without lymphangitic spread occur in immunocompetent individuals
- Pulmonary and disseminated disease can occur by conidia inhalation associated with immunosuppression
- The *S. schenckii* infection is confirmed by immunohistochemical techniques and culture
- Treatment includes the use of saturated solution of potassium iodide, and in pulmonary and disseminated cases itraconazole and amphotericin B are indicated

Introduction

Sporotrichosis is caused by the thermal dimorphic fungus *Sporothrix schenckii*, largely found as a saprophyte in nature. The usual mode of infection is by cutaneous inoculation of the organism, and in most cases the disease is localized in the skin and subcutaneous tissues.

Pulmonary and disseminated forms of the disease, although uncommon, can occur when *S. schenckii* conidia are inhaled. Dissemination is rare and appears to occur more often in patients who have a history of alcoholism, diabetes mellitus, hematological malignancies, chronic obstructive pulmonary disease, long-term treatment with corticosteroids, in transplant recipients, and in patients with acquired immunodeficiency syndrome (AIDS).

History

The first report of sporotrichosis was made in 1898 by Schenck, a medical student at the Johns Hopkins Hospital in Baltimore, Maryland, USA.

Less than 5 years later, Beurman and Gougerot in France used potassium iodine to treat sporotrichosis and it remains a satisfactory therapy today.[8]

In 1908 in Brazil, Splendore described the asteroid bodies in human tissues obtained from patients with sporotrichosis. These structures remain very useful in the histological diagnosis of sporotrichosis and other diseases.[8]

Epidemiology

Sporotrichosis is worldwide in distribution, but it is mainly found in temperate, warm, and tropical areas.

S. schenckii has been found in nature as a saprophyte and the main sources of infection are living or decaying vegetation, animal excreta, and soil.[8] Temperature between 26 and 27°C, humidity of 92–100%, and presence of organic material are the ecological factors that promote growth and viability of the fungus.[9] Although *S. schenckii* has a definite association with plants, it has never been proved to be a plant pathogen.[8] Rodents and insects are passive vectors.[10]

Occupations that predispose persons to infection include gardening, farming, masonry, floral work, outdoor labor, and other activities involving exposure to contaminated soil or vegetation such as sphagnum moss, salt marsh hay, prairie hay, or roses.[8]

In contrast to the occupational risk reported in severe outbreaks, sporotrichosis has not been associated with specific occupations in the endemic areas.[9]

The disease has been reported in various domestic and wild animals, including horses, cats, mules, camels, rats, fowl, donkeys, swine, armadillos, and cattle.[8,9]

Usually patients with the cutaneous form of sporotrichosis are otherwise healthy young adults and children and the number of males and females are approximately equal.

Reported cases of patients with pulmonary, osteoarticular, or hematogenous sporotrichosis show a marked male predominance in widely scattered geographical areas.[8]

Sporotrichin skin test surveys of randomized populations have been a productive method for determining endemic regions.

At the beginning of the twentieth century in France, sporotrichosis was a common disease. In the USA there were fewer cases reported before 1932, but the incidence has been rising since then.[8] Between 1941 and 1944 in the gold mines of Witwatersrand, South Africa, the largest outbreak recorded in any area occurred, with 3000 workers infected.[8] Sporotrichosis has been diagnosed in a wide range of climatic and geographical conditions, such as those existing in Mexico, Brazil, Peru, India, and Japan.[9] At present the largest number of reported cases comes from the American continent.

Pathogenesis and etiology

S. schenckii is a thermal dimorphic pathogenic fungus. It usually enters the body though traumatic implantation or by inhalation of the conidia, causing clinical manifestations similar to those of other thermal dimorphic pathogenic fungi. The different clinical manifestations appear to result from the portal of inoculation of the fungus and from fungus and host's inherent factors. Subcutaneous disease, without systemic symptoms, results from cutaneous inoculation; on the other hand, systemic disease is usually associated with conidia inhalation in an immunodeficient patient.

There are no differences in thermotolerance among isolates that could explain the different clinical presentations such as lymphocutaneous, fixed cutaneous, or cutaneous disseminated.[9]

S. schenckii's melanin protects it from being killed by ultraviolet solar irradiation, and during infection it affects host defense mechanisms by reducing phagocytosis.[11] Rhamnomannan polysaccharide, a cell-wall component, plays a role in *S. schenckii* virulence.[12] CD4+ T lymphocytes and macrophages are required for the development of cellular immunity against *S. schenkii.*[13]

Many predisposing conditions of the host, such as alcoholism, diabetes, hematological malignancies, chronic obstructive pulmonary disease, aging, long-term treatment with corticosteroids, transplant recipients, and AIDS, increase the probability of hematogenous dissemination of infection to the skin and other organs, as occurs in opportunistic mycosis.

Clinical features

The most common type of sporotrichosis in endemic and non-endemic regions is the lymphocutaneous form, which follows the implantation of spores in a wound. A nodule or pustule forms and this may break down into a small ulcer (the inoculation chancre) that enlarges over days or weeks, evolving to produce subsequent nodular lesions spreading along proximal lymphangitic channels (Fig. 18.5 A and B). These nodular or ulcerative gummatous lesions remain relatively painless and infrequently involve the regional lymph nodes. The preferential localizations are the upper and lower extremities; in children the face is generally affected.[8,10]

The fixed cutaneous presentation of sporotrichosis appears at sites of trauma, remains as a single chronic lesion, and commonly affects the face, trunk, arm, hands or feet. It can vary in appearance from erythematous papules or plaques that tend to become ulcerated, to verrucous, abscess-like lesions, found especially on children's faces. The dermoepidermis is characterized by violaceous plaques that follow the superficial lymphatics. Multiple chancres constitute the mycetomatoid form which is more frequently seen in the foot.[8,10]

It has not yet been clearly defined why some individuals develop lymphocutaneous sporotrichosis and others develop the fixed

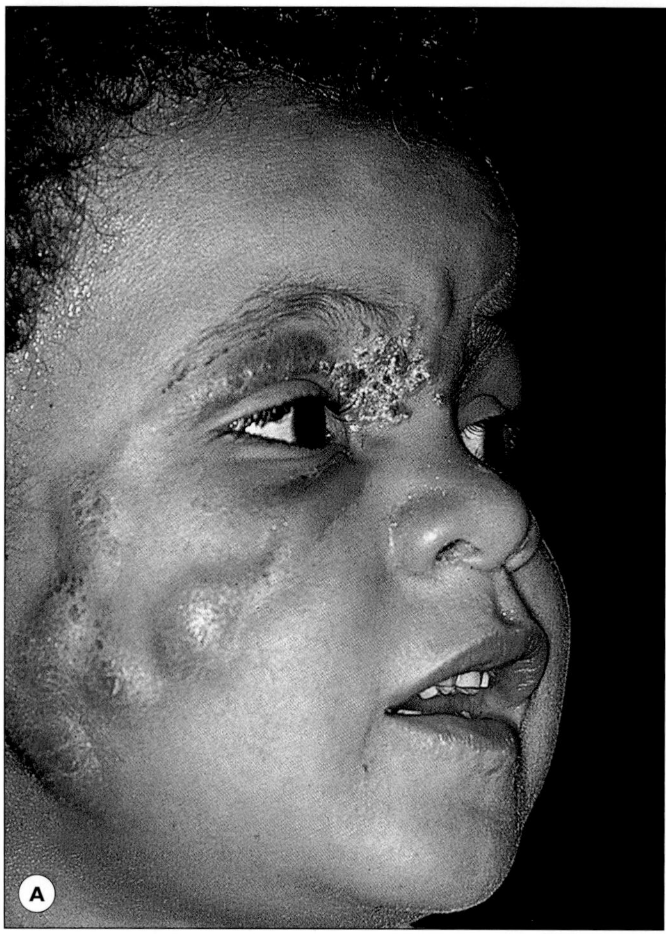

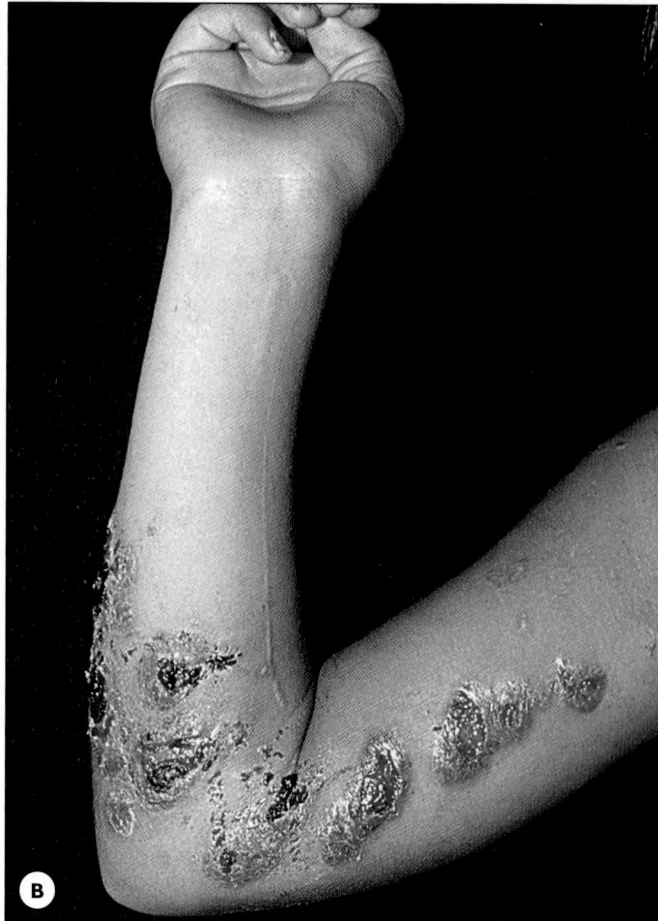

Figure 18.5 (A, B) Sporotrichosis: fixed cutaneous form.

cutaneous form of the disease.[9] The two forms can even appear in the same patient.

Occasionally, patients with pulmonary sporotrichosis present with dissemination to other organs, particularly skin or bones.[8]

The osteoarticular sporotrichosis is the most frequent mycotic arthropathy that usually starts with an indolent onset of stiffness and pain in a large joint, most commonly knee, elbow, ankle, or wrist. There are multiple lytic lesions on the bone with a predilection for the tibia.[8]

In the cutaneous disseminated form of sporotrichosis patients may present with multiple skin lesions from hematogenous spread, with or without lung or bone lesions. Ulcerated nodules, ulcers, or verrucous plaques may also be seen. Patients with AIDS and several other immunosuppressed states are very prone to develop multiple and widespread cutaneous ulcers with or without a phagedenic border predominantly in the scrotal area, face, and lower extremities.[14]

Other rare clinical presentations of the disease may occur by hematogenous spread, such as endophthalmitis, brain abscesses, and chronic meningitis. Internal organs are affected less frequently.

Pathology

There is epidermal hyperplasia and sometimes pseudoepitheliomatous hyperplasia. The inflammatory response to *S. schenckii* is characteristically pyogranulomatous, exhibiting small collections of neutrophils with large surrounding areas of epitheloid cells, lymphocytes, and multinucleated giant cells. The biopsy is not diagnostic unless the presence of a fungal cell typical of *S. schenckii* can be demonstrated. Asteroid bodies (yeasts surrounded by radiating eosinophilic material) may be observed (Fig. 18.6). The fungal cells stain poorly with H&E, and are better visualized with PAS and Gomori methenamine silver (GMS) stains.[8]

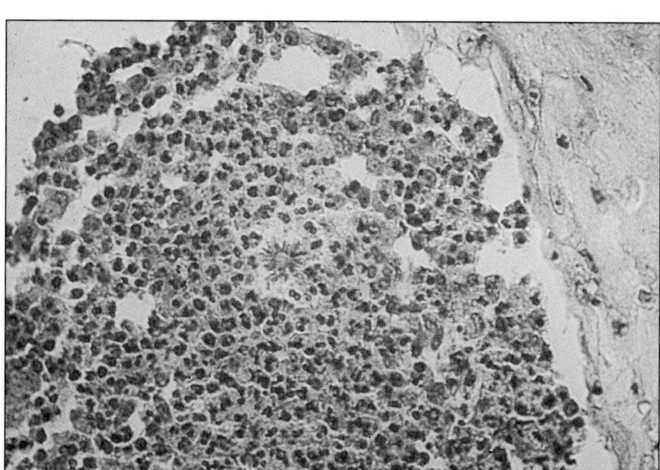

Figure 18.6 Asteroid body within a microabscess. Periodic acid–Schiff (×200).

Patient evaluation, diagnosis, and differential diagnosis

Confirmation of the diagnosis is based on isolation of the fungus by culture of the exudates, skin biopsy, joint aspirate, or sputum.[8]

The main differential diagnosis of the fixed cutaneous form includes paracoccidioidomycosis, leishmaniasis, chromoblastomycosis, tuberculosis, mycetoma (mainly in Central and South America), psoriasis, foreign-body granuloma, Majocchi's granuloma and squamous cell carcinoma. Lesions of the fixed form on the face, especially in children, may be mistaken for abscesses and chronic staphylococcal ecthyma, when ulcerated.

The cutaneous lymphatic form must be distinguished from mycobacteriosis and leishmaniasis with lymphangitic spread. The differential diagnosis of pulmonary sporotrichosis is broad, and includes chronic pulmonary paracoccidioidomycosis, histoplasmosis, tuberculosis, and coccidioidomycosis.

The diagnosis of sporotrichosis is based on the culture which is the best, most rapid, and cheapest diagnostic method widely available.

Isolates of *S. schenckii* grow well on most mycology media at 25–30 °C after a few days. The colonies are white to cream-colored, and then, within 10–15 days, they turn brown to black. The agar slide culture shows dark or hyaline conidia arranged in a bouquet on a long conidiophore (Fig. 18.7).

Although the yeast form may be seen occasionally in a Gram-stained smear, a wet mount from pus or a biopsy specimen, direct examination of such material is often not helpful because of the paucity of fungal cells. Fluorescent antibodies can be applied to tissue sections to aid in the diagnosis, but they are neither readily available nor standardized.[8]

Histopathological examination of tissues stained with conventional H&E lacks sensitivity. The type of inflammatory response and the appearance of the fungus are factors on which experienced pathologists base their diagnosis, but the variable morphologic features of the tissue form can be misleading.[8]

Immunohistochemical staining techniques can reach 83% sensitivity.[15]

Serological tests for the diagnosis of subcutaneous sporotrichosis have not been adequately evaluated. In recent studies, an antigenic fraction of the cell wall of *S. schenckii* showed high reactivity with sera from patients with sporotrichosis without significant cross-reactivity.[9] This antigenic fraction is not available commercially.

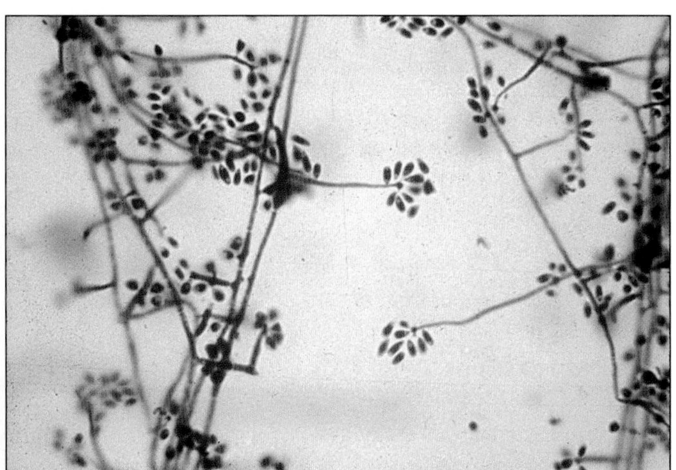

Figure 18.7 *Sporotrix schenckii*: hyaline conidia arranged in a bouquet on a long conidiophore.

Treatment

Despite the lack of clinical trials, it is accepted that potassium iodine is an effective and inexpensive therapy. It is the treatment of choice for the fixed cutaneous and lymphocutaneous forms of sporotrichosis. In adults, the orally saturated solution of potassium iodine (SSKI) t.i.d. 3–6 g/day is given for 2–3 months or for 1 month after the clinical and mycological cure is achieved. Children are treated with 50% of the dose used in adults.

Topical potassium iodine 10% in a cream or ointment is very effective for treating ulcerated cutaneous lesions, especially from the fixed form.

Side-effects of oral SSKI include a bitter taste, nausea, rumbling stomach, sialorrhea, and acneiform eruption. SSKI is better tolerated if the initial dose is small and then gradually increased. Pregnant women should not receive SSKI because of its toxicity for the fetal thyroid. Oral itraconazole, 100–200 mg given daily for several months, has been proved successful in small numbers of patients with cutaneous sporotrichosis.[8]

Patients with the disseminated cutaneous form with multiple skin lesions from hematogenous spread usually have an underlying disease and immunosuppression. In these patients the rate of response to SSKI is poor and treatment with amphotericin B or itraconazole is required.

Patients with pulmonary sporotrichosis respond poorly to treatment. Severe infections require therapy with amphotericin B; mild or moderate infection may be treated with itraconazole.[16]

The preferred treatment for osteoarticular sporotrichosis is itraconazole, and the therapy must be given for at least 12 months.[16]

Meningeal sporotrichosis is rare and usually requires treatment with amphotericin B.[15]

Patients with AIDS or with other severely immunosuppressed states have an increased risk for dissemination of the infection to the skin and other sites. Despite antifungal therapy, the outcome for patients with AIDS is usually poor, although a few cases of sustained remission have been reported. Amphotericin B, alone or in combination with other antifungal drugs, is the therapy of choice; itraconazole can be used for lifelong maintenance therapy.[16]

Chromoblastomycosis

Arival Cardoso de Brito

Synonyms: Chromomycosis, Lane's mycosis, Pedroso's disease

Key features:

- Chromoblastomycosis is a chronic cutaneous and subcutaneous fungal infection which predominates in exposed areas and is caused by several dematiaceous fungi implanted by traumatic injury

- It is found worldwide but predominates in tropical climates of Central and South America, and Madagascar
- Skin lesions are characterized by papules, nodules, plaques, verrucoid, and papillomatous slow-growing lesions
- Thick-walled septated brown cells (muriform cells) located inside multinucleated cells and extracellularly are present in the granulomatous tissue
- Treatment includes surgery, cryosurgery, carbon dioxide laser excision, topical heat application, amphotericin B, itraconazole, and terbinafine

Introduction

Dematiaceous fungi can produce a wide variety of clinicopathological infections, including chromoblastomycosis (muriform cells), pheohyphomycosis (septated brown hyphae or pseudohyphae-like elements), and mycetoma (tumor-like growth and black-grained). According to McGinnis,[17] chromomycosis is a term that has been rejected for mycosis caused by dematiaceous agents.

Chromoblastomycosis is a localized chronic, suppurative, granulomatous cutaneous and subcutaneous infection of the skin caused by pigmented fungi, inducing typical warty cutaneous lesions. The causative agents are worldwide saprophytes, common in soil enriched with organic waste and in decaying wood and vegetation. This disease has been reported with increasing frequency from most parts of the world, especially in tropical and subtropical zones, and usually with a history of trauma followed by a slow-growing skin lesion, often for several weeks or years before presentation.

History

The first cases of chromoblastomycosis in the world were described by Rudolph[18] in 1914 in Brazil, in the state of Minas Gerais: Rudolph emphasized the clinicopathological features of the disease. In 1922, Terra et al.[19] coined the term chromoblastomycosis and Moore and Almeida, in 1935,[20] proposed the new name chromomycosis to replace that term. In 1915, Medlar[21] and Lane[22] reported the first US case and Thaxter created the name *Phialophora verrucosa* for the etiologic agent. Pedroso and Gomes, in 1920,[23] published a Brazilian case which had been observed in 1911 (São Paulo, Brazil).

Epidemiology

Chromoblastomycosis has been recorded on all continents (Americas, Africa, Asia, Europe, Oceania), and most cases have been described in tropical and subtropical regions, mostly in Madagascar, Gabon, Mexico, Brazil, Costa Rica, Puerto Rico, Venezuela, Cuba, Dominican Republic, India, and Australia. In Europe, the disease has been diagnosed in several countries. In Japan, Fukushiro in 1983,[24] reported 290 cases between 1955 and 1980, with 275 strains of dematiaceous fungi isolated. In 249 cases of the disease, *Fonsecaea pedrosoi* was present in the overwhelming majority (215 strains). Esterre et al.[25] studied retrospectively 1343 confirmed cases of chromoblastomycosis in Madagascar from 1955 through 1994, of which *F. pedrosoi* was identified from 61.8% of the fungal strains. Madagascar is probably the most important focus in the world. Silva et al.[26] reported a retrospective study of 325 cases of the mycosis diagnosed in the previous 55 years in the Amazon region, Brazil, in the state of Para. In 2001, Bonifaz et al.[27] studied 51 cases of chromoblastomycosis detected in a 17-year period: most were males (36/51) and the principal agent was *F. pedrosoi* (90%).

The great majority of patients are inhabitants of rural areas (farmers, wood cutters, latex gatherers), between 35 and 50 years of age. Men are more affected than women and the lesions are usually on the lower limbs. There is no ethnic predominance as all races seem to be susceptible. Spontaneous chromoblastomycosis in the marine toad (*Bufo marinus*) has been reported.

Pathogenesis and etiology

The black molds live as saprophytes in soil, vegetable matter, wood, and timber, and inoculation in humans occurs via minor traumas. Chromoblastomycosis is produced by a group of genetically closely related dematiaceous fungi that have only one single-tissue form, characterized by round, thick-walled muriform cells – sclerotic bodies. Five principal etiologic agents have been recognized worldwide:

1. *Phialophora verrucosa*[28] produces brownish-gray to dark-olive-gray colonies on Sabouraud's agar at 25–30 °C, and typical phialides with cup-shaped collarettes.
2. *Fonsecaea pedrosoi*[29] produces dark-brown, dark-olive or black colonies on Sabouraud's agar. There are three types of sporulation: *Cladosporium*, *Rhinocladiella*, and *Phialophora*.
3. *Fonsecaea compacta*[30–32] produces olivish-black colonies and the same type of sporulation as *F. pedrosoi*.
4. *Cladosporium carrionii*[33] colonies are velvety to wooly, dark-olivish or nearly black on Sabouraud's agar, with oval conidia. They are usually uniform in size in the same conidial chain.
5. *Rhinocladiella aquaspersa* (Borelli)[34] are wooly colonies, dark to olive-gray in color, with erect conidiophores, and cylindrical, thick-walled, one-celled conidia, elliptical to club-shaped, and pale brown.

Some pigmented fungi such as *Exophiala spinifera*[35,36] and *Exophiala jeanselmei*[37,38] have been recognized as agents of chromoblastomycosis. On the other hand, *F. pedrosoi* and *P. verrucosa* may produce pheohyphomycosis.[17] Ajello et al. (1975) coined the term pheohyphomycosis to include a heterogeneous group of infections caused by dematiaceous fungi in which the agents are present in tissue as yeasts, hyphae, or pseudohyphae-like elements.[17]

Clinical features

The human chronic infection begins with one or more nodules at the traumatized area. Many patients do not recall an injury. The lesions gradually grow to form an erythematous plaque with a well-defined border, which subsequently expands to form irregular

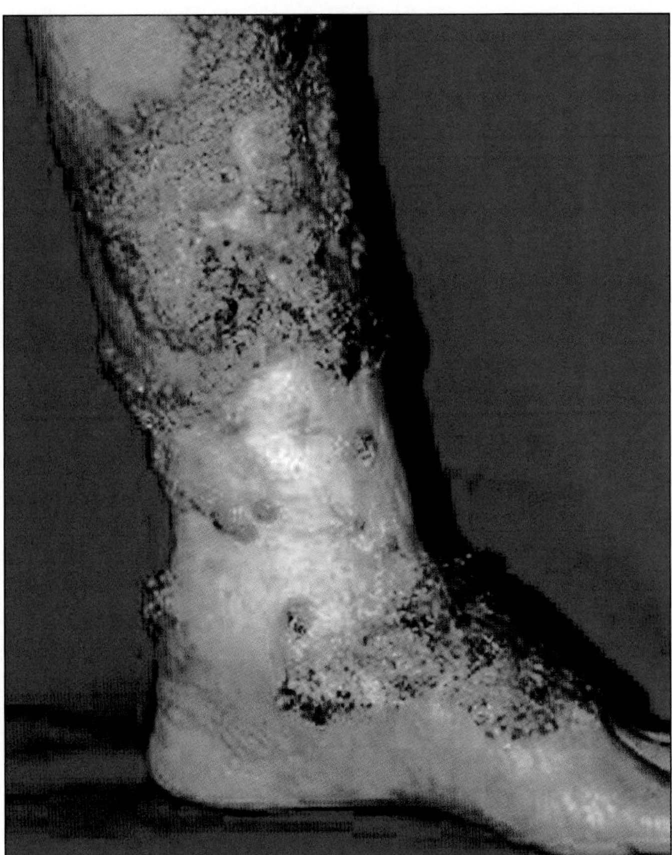

Figure 18.8 Verrucous and cicatricial lesions of chromoblastomycosis on the lower limb.

verrucous or papillomatous lesions that are isolated or coalescent (Fig. 18.8), often with superimposed ulceration. Multiple lesions may occur following lymphatic and perhaps hematogenous dissemination. The infection shows a greatly varied morphology of the lesions, among them keloid-like, cauliflower, pedunculated, ulcerated, and cicatricial, by expanding centrifugally. Rarely, psoriasis-like lesions can be observed in some patients. Lymphadenopathy is due to secondary bacterial infections and, in advanced disease, lymphostasis may resemble elephantiasis. Lesions are mostly seen on the lower extremities (feet, knee, legs), followed by those located on the upper extremities (hands, wrist, forearms). Other sites of lesions may include face, neck, dorsum, buttocks, and rarely, on mucous membranes. Some patients complain of pruritus and pain. Despite the protracted course of the disease, dissemination of the mycosis is rare. Complications such secondary infections, elephantiasis, and carcinomatous degeneration may occur in chromoblastomycosis.

Patient evaluation and differential diagnosis

Direct examination of potassium hydroxide preparations, from crusts or exudates, obtained by scraping, curettage, or applying a piece of clear tape, usually shows the typical fungal muriform cells. The material is cultured for isolation of the fungus on Sabouraud's medium containing antibacterial antibiotics and incubated at room temperature or at 25–30°C. Colonies will develop within 2–4 weeks of incubation.

Serology is not used routinely to diagnose the infection.

Chromoblastomycosis must be differentiated from pheohyphomycosis, blastomycosis, lobomycosis, paracoccidioidomycosis, sporotrichosis, protothecosis, lupus vulgaris, tuberculosis verrucosa cutis, leishmaniasis, leprosy, tertiary syphilis, sarcoidosis, keloids, squamous cell carcinoma, and keratoacanthoma. Direct examination and biopsy can easily distinguish these clinical entities from other conditions.

Pathology

Examination of biopsy specimens shows pseudoepitheliomatous hyperplasia of the epidermis with hyperparakeratosis, spongiosis, and occasionally abscesses. In the dermis, a characteristic granulomatous reaction is observed with lymphocytes, plasma cells, neutrophils, eosinophils, macrophages, and multinucleated giant cells and abscesses. Fibrosis is prominent in older cases. Muriform cells, 4–12 μm in diameter, are found alone or in clusters (Fig. 18.9), either extracellularly or inside multinucleated giant cells in microabscesses present in the dermis or epidermis. Gomori–Grocott methenamine silver and PAS stains may be employed in a few cases.

Treatment

Chromoblastomycosis is a disease that is often unresponsive to many antifungal and surgical procedures. In early localized lesions a wide and deep excision is recommended. Therapeutic approaches include amphotericin B and triazole derivatives such as itraconazole and fluconazole.[39] Terbinafine has been successfully used in a few cases.[40,41] Cryosurgery, Mohs's micrographic surgery, carbon dioxide laser, and topical heat applications have been used with variable success. Treatment in advanced cases is difficult and frequently requires extensive surgery combined with antifungal and physical therapy.

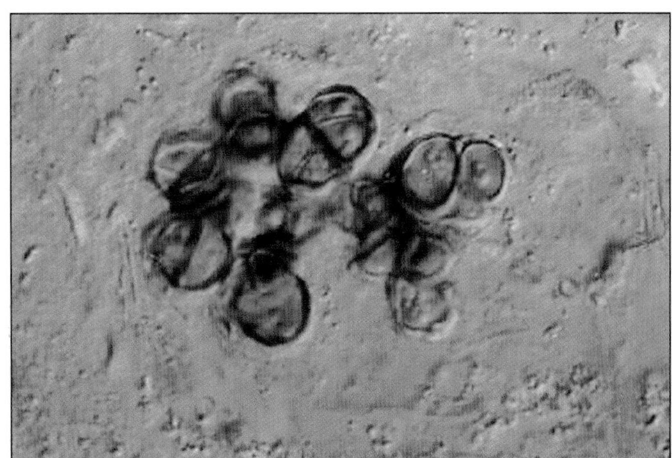

Figure 18.9 Cluster of muriform cells of chromoblastomycosis.

Rhinosporidiosis

Iphis Campbell

Key features:

- Rhinosporidiosis is a chronic infection caused by the protist *Rhinosporidium seeberi*
- Polyps affect the mucosal surfaces, mainly the nose and ocular conjunctivae
- Skin lesions and disseminated infection are rare
- Diagnosis is made by histopathology
- Surgical removal is the treatment of choice

Introduction

Rhinosporidiosis is a chronic infective disease characterized by slow-growing polypoid masses, usually of nasal mucosa or ocular conjunctiva of humans and animals. Occasionally lesions occur in more than one mucous membrane, in the skin, and rarely disseminate to subcutaneous sites, bones, and viscera.[42] The disease occurs throughout the world, with cases reported from the Americas, Europe, Africa, and Asia. It is most common in the tropics, with the highest prevalence in southern India and Sri Lanka.[42]

The etiologic agent, *R. seeberi,* is a protist , belonging to a novel group of fish parasites.[43]

The diagnosis is established by the characteristic of the organism in tissues biopsies.[42]

History

In 1900, Guillermo Seeber described an apparent protozoan parasite in a nasal polyp from an agricultural worker in Argentina. At that time he believed that its causative agent was a protist close to the coccidia, and his teacher, Wernicke, named the organism *Coccidium seeberia.*[44] In 1923, Ashworth described the life cycle of the parasite, concluded that it was a fungus, and renamed it *Rhinosporidium seeberi.*[45] Although the systematic position of *R. seeberi* was inconclusive, the organism was considered to be a fungus and remained a taxonomic mystery for about 100 years. In 2000, Fredricks et al. confirmed the protistan nature of *R. seeberi.*[43]

Epidemiology

Although the disease is distributed worldwide, almost 90% of reported cases are from southern India and Sri Lanka. The next highest prevalence rates are in South America and Africa.[42]

The disease affects mainly males, most often between 15 and 40 years of age.[42]

The observation that nose and eyes are the most common sites of the disease suggests that the natural reservoirs could be water, mud, dust, and soil.[42]

Since *R. seeberi* belongs to a clade of aquatic parasites, this generates a testable hypothesis: the natural hosts are fishes or other aquatic animals, and humans acquire the infection when they come into contact with water.[43]

R. seeberi has not been found anywhere other than in infected tissues of humans and animals such as horses, mules, cattle, goats, dogs, wild ducks, and geese.[42]

Pathogenesis and etiology

R. seeberi had been classified as a fungus on the basis of morphologic and histochemical characteristics.

Using polymerase chain reaction (PCR), a portion of the *R. seeberi* 18S rRNA gene was directly amplified from infected tissue. Phylogenetic analysis suggests that *R. seeberi* is the first known human pathogen from a novel clade of aquatic protistan parasites affecting fishes.[43]

Originally, this group of pathogens was identified as the DRIP clade, an acronym derived from *Dermocystidium,* rosette agent, *Ichthyophonus,* and *Psorospermium.*[46] With the addition of *R. seeberi* to the group, however, the DRIP acronym is no longer appropriate (Table 18.3).

The life cycle of *R. seeberi* has several stages. In its earliest stage, it is a 5–10-μm sphere with a very thin membrane. It begins to grow as it penetrates the tissue. When it reaches 50–100 μm, it acquires a double membrane and one pore. Then it turns into a cyst

Table 18.3 Current taxonomic distribution of the class Mesomycetozoea including DRIP and *Rhinosporidium seeberi*

Kingdom	Protozoa[a]
Subkingdom	Neozoa
Infrakingdom	Neomonada
Phylum	Neomonada
Subphylum	Choanozoa
Class	Mesomycetozoea[b]
Order	Dermocystida
	Dermocystidium spp.
	Rhinosporidium seeberi
	Rosette agent
Order	Ichthyophonida
	Ichthyophonus spp.
	Psorospermium spp.

DRIP, *Dermocystidium*, rosette agent, *Ichthyophonus*, and *Psorospermium*.
Adapted from Mendoza L, Ajello L, Taylor JW. The taxonomic status of *Lacazia loboi* and *Rhinosporidium seeberi* has been finally resolved with the use of molecular tools. Rev Iberoam Micol 2001; 18:95–98.
[a]Cavalier-Smith T. Neomonada and the origin of fungi. In: Coombs GH, Vickerman K, Sleigh MA et al., eds. Evolutionary relationships among protozoa. Dordrecht: Kluwer; 1998:375–407.
[b]Ajello L, Mendoza L. The phylogeny of *Rhinosporidium seeberi*. 14th Meeting of the International Society for Human and Animal Mycology. Buenos Aires, Argentina: 2000:78.

of 300 μm or larger, undergoes nuclear division, and forms up to 20 000 trophozoites. The mature cyst expels the trophozoites, restarting the parasitic cycle.[45]

Clinical features

Rhinosporidiosis is a chronic infection primarily of the mucous membranes of humans and animals, characterized by the formation of friable, red-to-purple, soft, vascular, lobulated polyp lesions. Tiny white dots, corresponding to mature cysts, may be seen underneath the epithelium.[42]

Infection usually presents in the nasal mucosa (Fig. 18.10). Unilateral nasal obstruction or epistaxis is the usual presenting symptom. A thin mucoid nasal discharge is often noted. Blood tinges in the mucus and frank epistaxis may occur.[42]

The conjunctiva is the next most common site. The palpebral conjunctiva is the usual site, with the bulbar conjunctiva, corneal limbus, lacrimal caruncle, and canthus less often involved. The lesion is more often seen than felt, but the sensation of a foreign body may be noted.

Occasionally, it affects the lips, palate, uvula, maxillary antrum, conjunctiva, lacrimal sac, epiglottis, larynx, trachea, bronchus, ear, scalp, vulva, rectum, vagina, penis, or skin.

The infection is usually limited to surface epithelium, but sometimes there is wide dissemination with visceral involvement. Generalized involvement of the skin is extremely uncommon.[47]

Patient evaluation, diagnosis, and differential diagnosis

Diagnosis is easily made by histopathological study of the excised specimen, even without special stains (Fig. 18.11).

Nasal lesions may be mistaken for polyps of allergic origin but the characteristic appearance of the lesion with the soft, vascular, red-to-purple aspect and the tiny white dots is very helpful in diagnosis.[42]

Vaginal or penile lesions resemble condylomata. Rectal lesions may look like a prolapsed internal hemorrhoid.

In the extremely uncommon generalized involvement of the skin, the lesions resemble warts, granuloma pyogenicum, or verrucous tuberculosis.[47]

Pathology

The most striking histopathological feature is the conspicuous sharply defined globular cysts in various maturation states in the subepithelial connective tissue. Some cysts releasing trophozoites may be found (Fig. 18.11).[42]

Treatment

Complete surgical excision with electrodesiccation of the tumor base is used to prevent recurrence.[42]

Lobomycosis

Arival Cardoso de Brito

Synonyms: Jorge Lobo's disease, Lobo's mycosis, keloidal blastomycosis, Amazonian blastomycosis

Key features:

- Lobomycosis is a chronic granulomatous localized subcutaneous mycosis caused by *Lacazia loboi*
- It is characterized by variably sized nodular (keloid-like) plaques, verrucoid and ulcerative skin lesions
- It commonly develops on the ears, face, and extremities of humans with no visceral dissemination
- Diagnosis is made by observing globose yeast-like fungal cells in the histological study of the lesions. Culture is not available
- Wide and deep excision for localized lesions is the treatment of choice

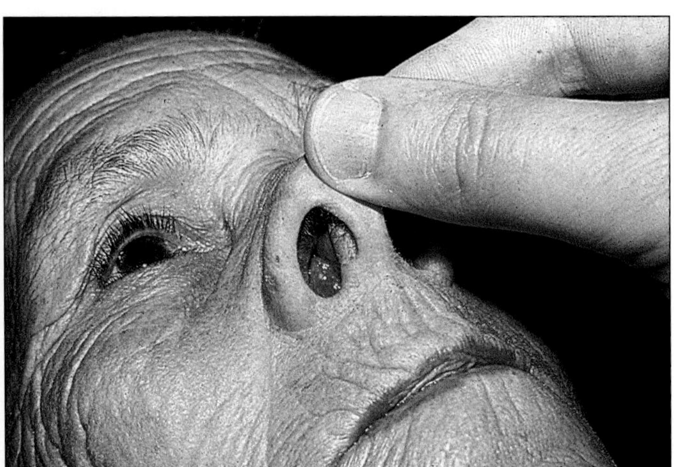

Figure 18.10 Red-to-purple, soft, vascular, and lobulated lesion with tiny white dots in the nose.

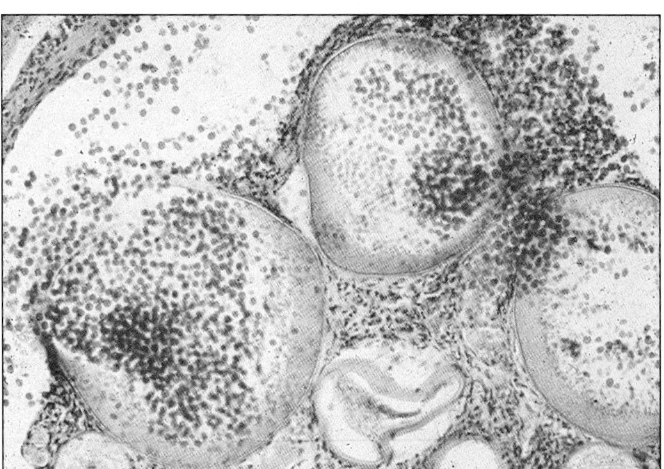

Figure 18.11 Rhinosporidiosis. Cysts releasing trophozoites through an opening in the wall. Periodic acid–Schiff (×200).

Introduction

Lobomycosis in humans is a chronic subcutaneous infection, which occurs predominantly in several countries of Central and South America, particularly the Amazon valley. The disease affects mostly young adults, and has been reported among the Caiabi tribe in the state of Mato Grosso (Central Brazil), the Amorua tribe (Colombia), in bush negroes (Surinam), in Europe (Gulf of Gascony), and in the USA, and has been demonstrated in two species of dolphins.

History

This mycosis was originally described by Jorge Lobo in 1931 in Recife (Pernambuco), Brazil.[48] The patient, a 52-year-old-man from the Brazilian Amazon region, had keloid-like nodules and plaques of 19 years' duration on the lumbosacral area. Microscopic examination revealed budding cells with morphologic features resembling those of *Paracoccidioides brasiliensis*. Based on this feature, Lobo termed the disease keloidal blastomycosis. Fialho in 1938 described the second case and proposed the name Lobo's disease.

Epidemiology

Lobomycosis occurs in tropical and subtropical climates where compact forests and numerous rivers keep the weather usually hot and humid (annual mean temperature 24–28°C and annual rainfall over 2000 mm). The majority of the patients come from the Amazonian region and adjoining countries. Special attention must be drawn to the high occurrence among Caiabi Indians living in Central Brazil, where 61 cases of the disease have been diagnosed.[49]

Lobomycosis mainly affects adults who work as farmers, fishers, hunters, gold or diamond seekers (prospecting), rubber workers, and other jungle activities. Males are predominantly affected, and the age of onset of the disease is between 1 and 70 years with an average range from 21 to 45 years. Among the Caiabi tribe, prevalence in women represents 32% of the general population. There is no racial difference.

The human disease has been reported in several countries of Latin America and there has been one case in Europe.[49] In 2000, Burns et al.[50] described the first and only human case in the USA: a 42-year-old white male, resident in Georgia, who 7 years earlier had had a pustule on the skin of his right chest wall and developed a nodule. There was a history of travel to Angel Falls (Venezuela).

Up until 2003, 307 lobomycosis cases have been identified and documented in Brazil, including 61 Caiabi Indians. Until March 2003, 477 cases of lobomycosis have been reported worldwide, including: 307 in Brazil; 50 in Colombia; 34 in Surinam; 23 in Venezuela; 16 in French Guiana; 21 in Costa Rica; 13 in Panama; 3 in Bolivia; 3 in Peru; 2 in Ecuador; 2 in Guyana; 1 in Mexico; 1 in Europe, and 1 in the USA.

Pathogenesis and etiology

The prevalence of lobomycosis in tropical climates suggests that the fungus is distributed in soil and vegetation, and infection is acquired by single or multiple skin traumas in animals (dolphins, monkeys) and humans. However the ecological distribution of the fungus has not yet been confirmed since, despite many attempts, *L. loboi* has never been cultured.

Several names have been given to the etiologic agent of lobomycosis: *Glenosporella loboi*;[51,52] *Paracoccidioides loboi*;[53–55] *Lobomyces loboi* Borelli, 1958. In 1999 Taborda et al. proposed a new genus, *Lacazia*, to accommodate this pathogen.[56]

In infected tissues, *Lacazia loboi* is observed as globose or subglobose lemon-shaped cells, 8–12 μm in diameter, which reproduce by single or multiple budding, forming a bead-like pattern of 2–10 cells connected by narrow tubes. The cell wall is 1 μm thick, doubly refractive, and contains constitutive melanin demonstrated by the Fontana–Masson stain. This pigment is absent in the cell walls of *Paracoccidioides brasiliensis*.

In 2001, Herr et al.[57] reported the nucleotide sequence analysis of *L. loboi*'s 18S small-subunit ribosomal DNA (SSU rDNA), and a 600-bp fragment of the chitin synthase-2 (CHS-2) gene (*CHS2*). According to this phylogenetic analysis, *L. loboi* is related to *Paracoccidioides brasiliensis*, and both species belong to the order Onygenales.

Clinical features

Lobomycosis is a fungal infection characterized by polymorphous lesions on exposed areas of the body. The lesions are more frequently observed in the lower extremities (44:42.72%), ears (28:27.18%), upper extremities (11:10.67%), face (5:4.85%), chest (3:2.91%) and, in some cases, the infection is disseminated (12:11.65%). No cases have been reported in mucosal membranes.

The onset is insidious and the lesion starts as an asymptomatic papule or dermal nodule (Fig. 18.12) that grows slowly and tends to expand and recur. Sometimes large cutaneous areas can be involved (Fig. 18.13). New satellite-like lesions or remote locations can appear on rare occasions. Silva and De Brito[58] have proposed a classification that includes the types: infiltrated, keloidal, gummatous, ulcerative, and verrucoid. The most frequent clinical feature observed is the keloid-like lesion, isolated or in plaques, characterized by an atrophic, smooth, shiny epidermis, with hypo- or hyperchromic changes, and telangiectasias. The verrucoid type is mainly found in the lower extremities; ulcerative lesions can develop in some cases. Patients may complain of minor pruritus, a burning sensation, hypoesthesia, and anesthesia. The infection may be spread by autoinoculation, contiguity, or by lymphatics, and it is mainly observed in lesions of the limbs.

Secondary bacterial infection is a common complication. In occasional cases with long evolution, squamous cell carcinoma has been reported.

Lobomycosis can be associated with chromoblastomycosis, leishmaniasis, paracoccidioidomycosis, superficial mycosis, AIDS, and leprosy.

Patient evaluation and differential diagnosis

The diagnosis is established by the clinical and microscopic identification of the fungus. Direct examination of potassium hydroxide

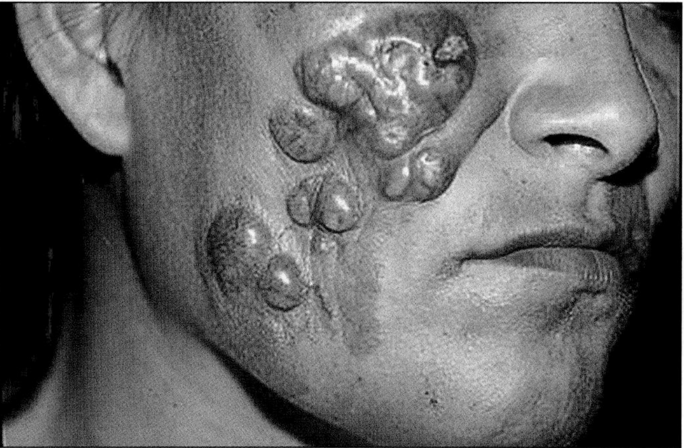

Figure 18.12 Infiltrated and keloidal lesions of lobomycosis.

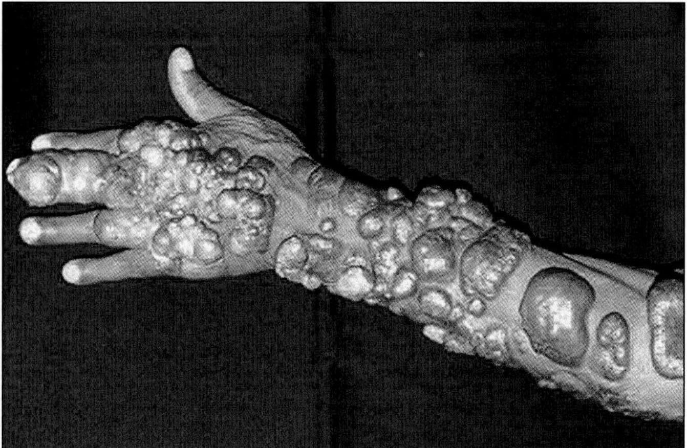

Figure 18.13 Lobomycosis. Keloid-like skin lesions over the upper limb.

preparations from material obtained by scraping, curettage, or applying a piece of clear tape shows a great number of yeast-like globose cells singly or in a chain: this is also observed on histological study.

Lobomycosis must be differentiated from lepromatous leprosy, anergic diffuse cutaneous leishmaniasis, paracoccidioidomycosis, chromoblastomycosis, sporotrichosis, lupus vulgaris, keloids, dermatofibrosarcoma protuberans, squamous cell carcinoma, melanoma, lymphomas, leukemias, Kaposi's sarcoma, and cutaneous metastasis of malignant neoplasms.

Pathology

The histological examination exhibits a massive and diffuse granulomatous infiltrate of foamy macrophages and multinucleated giant cells, which contain abundant fungal cells. Granulomas in the dermis can cause destruction of the nerves and cutaneous appendages, and are almost invariably separated from the epidermis by a Grenz zone of normal collagen. In some cases granulomas extend into the subcutaneous fat. There are clusters of foamy macrophages that resemble Gaucher's cells and asteroid bodies may be detected in giant cells. The epidermis is usually atrophic but may exhibit pseudoepitheliomatous hyperplasia or ulceration. The pathogen is clearly demonstrated by GMS (Fig. 18.14) or PAS stain.

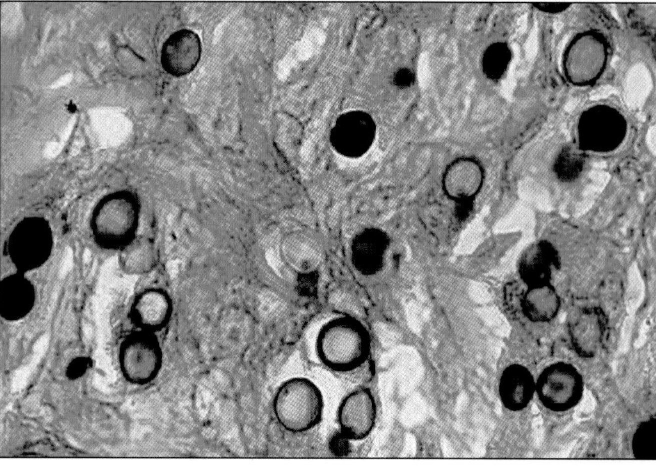

Figure 18.14 *Lacazia loboi* (Gomori's methenamine silver, 400×). Chains of rounded and hyaline cells with a double and birefringent membrane.

Diniz et al.[59] report that under the scanning electron microscope the fungus often presented buds attached to the mother cell at more than one point as well as scars in the budding regions.

Treatment

The most reliable therapeutic modality for early localized lesions is wide and deep excision. Relapse may occur in some cases. Systemic therapy with azoles (ketoconazole, itraconazole, fluconazole) or clofazimine is generally not helpful in disseminated lobomycosis and the experience is based on anecdotal case reports.

Zygomycosis

Clarisse Zaitz

Synonym: Phycomycosis

Key features:

- Zygomycosis includes two different mycoses: mucormycosis and entomophthoromycosis
- Mucormycosis is a worldwide-distributed mycosis associated with immunosuppression, while entomophthoromycosis is a rare subcutaneous and mucocutaneus mycosis observed in normal immunocompetent hosts
- Diagnosis is made by identification of the causative agent by histopathology and culture
- In mucormycosis the treatment is amphotericin B, debridement of the necrotic tissue, and improvement of the immunological status
- In entomophthoromycosis the treatment is potassium iodide

Introduction

Zygomycosis is an infection caused by fungi of the class Zygomycetes and includes two different entities: mucormycosis and entomophthoromycosis. The first is a rare opportunistic fungal infection caused by Zygomycetes of the order Mucorales.[60] *Rhyzopus* spp., *Rhyzomucor* spp., *Absidia* spp., and *Mucor* spp. from the family Mucoraceae are the organisms most commonly isolated from clinical specimens. The number of species causing mucormycosis as well as the numbers of cases of disease have increased in recent years due to of a greater number of immunocompromised patients. Mucormycosis represents the third leading cause of invasive fungal infection, following those caused by *Aspergillus* spp. and *Candida* spp. The clinical importance of the disease is underlined by its high mortality and morbidity rates. Pulmonary, rhinocerebral, gastrointestinal, cutaneous, and disseminated forms commonly occur in patients with cancer, hematological malignancies, neutropenia, uncontrolled diabetes, transplant recipients, and patients receiving immunosuppressive therapy.[61] Entomophthoromycosis is a rare subcutaneous and mucocutaneus mycosis caused by Zygomycetes of the order Entomophthorales.[62] The name is derived from the Greek word "entomon," meaning insect, reflecting their original identification as parasites infecting insects. The human pathogens in this taxonomic order include *Basidiobolus ranarum*, agent of basidiobolomycosis, and *Conidiobolus* spp., agents of conidiobolomycosis. Despite the worldwide environmental distribution of these fungi, human disease is concentrated in tropical and subtropical regions. Entomophthoromycosis occurs predominantly in immunocompetent individuals and most infections result from traumatic implantation of the fungus.[62]

History

The earliest report of pulmonary mucormycosis is from Furbringer, who described, in 1876, a patient who died of cancer and in whom the right lung showed a hemorrhagic infarct with fungal hyphae and a few sporangia. Platauf published the first case of disseminated mucormycosis in a cancer patient, in 1885.[60]

Basidiobolomycosis was first reported by Lie-Kian-Joe et al. in 1956 in an Indonesian patient.[1] In 1965, Bras et al. reported the first case of conidiobolomycosis in a patient from the West Indies.[62]

Epidemiology

Fungi of the order Mucorales have a wide geographic distribution. Because mucormycosis is an opportunistic infection, the distribution of the various clinical forms is based on predisposing factors rather than age, sex, race, or geography. Members of the order Mucorales are found in air, soil, and food. Their spores become airborne and are encountered as common laboratory contaminants.[60]

Basidiobolomycosis occurs predominantly in childhood and adolescence. Males are more affected than females. The disease occurs most frequently in tropical Africa and Southeast Asia, but has been identified in other tropical countries, including Brazil. *B. ranarum* is found in decaying vegetation, soil, and the gastrointestinal tract of reptiles, fishes, amphibians, and bats.[62]

Conidiobolomycosis is restricted to the region between the tropics of Cancer and Capricorn, mainly in areas of tropical rain forest from Africa and the Americas. The disease occurs predominantly in males over 15 years of age. *Conidiobolus coronatus* is the species that is most commonly isolated, and it is found in decaying vegetation, soil, insects, and the gastrointestinal tract of lizards and toads.[62]

Pathogenesis and etiology

Mucorales are saprophytic aerobic fungi that have a special predilection for the nasal sinuses and lungs. Rhinocerebral and pulmonary mucormycosis is acquired by inhaling spores. Several nosocomial cutaneous infections originate at the skin site of catheters, adhesive tapes, and surgical wounds. Ingestion of meals contaminated by fungal spores is believed to be the source of primary gastrointestinal mucormycosis.[60,61,63] Mucorales have a high affinity for invading blood vessels. The invasion causes ischemia, arterial thrombosis, tissue infarction, and necrosis. When veins are affected, hemorrhages can occur.[60,61,63] Mucormycosis is a disease of immunocompromised hosts, although it is rarely seen in AIDS patients.[63] The most commonly isolated fungi are *Rhyzopus* spp., *Rhyzomucor* spp., *Absidia* spp., and *Mucor* spp. from the Mucoraceae family; however, many other organisms belonging to others families and genera from the order Mucorales may also cause this disease (Table 18.4).

Most cases of entomophthoromycosis occur mainly as a result of implantation via minor trauma and insect bites in immunocompetent patients.[61] The human pathogens of entomophthoromycosis include organisms of the order Entomophthorales, including *B. ranarum*, the agent of basidiobolomycosis and *Conidiobolus* spp., agents of conidiobolomycosis.

Clinical features

Different clinical pictures are observed in mucormycosis. The rhinocerebral form occurs mainly in patients with diabetes, particularly those with ketoacidosis. Orbital involvement results in cellulitis, ophthalmoplegia, proptosis, and chemosis and may form a frontal lobe abscess in the brain (Fig. 18.15). Black necrotic tissue may be seen in the oral mucosa. Imaging studies are helpful when planning surgery for the lesion rather than establishing the diagnosis.[63]

Pulmonary mucormycosis commonly affects the upper lobes. The endobronchial form is mainly found in patients with diabetes, presenting bronchial obstruction and hemoptysis. The cutaneous form is usually related to trauma or is part of the disseminated form of the disease.[63]

The clinical syndromes caused by individual genera of Mucorales were reviewed by Yeung et al. in 2001, in a Medline literature search. The conclusion was that the main underlying risk factors for mucormycosis included hematological malignancy, diabetes mellitus, solid organ transplant recipients, and chronic renal failure.[63]

Conidiobolomycosis begins in the submucosa of the nose, and sinusitis is the most common initial manifestation. Epistaxis and rhinorrhea may occur. The infection slowly extends to the skin of the nose, glabella, cheek, upper lip, paranasal sinus, and pharynx. Hematogenous spread is rare.[62]

Table 18.4 Taxonomic organization of the Zygomycetes

	Phylum Zygomycota	
Order Mucorales	Class Zygomycetes	Order Entomophthorales
Mucoraceae	Cunninghamellaceae	Ancylistaceae
Absidia	*Cunninghamella*	*Conidiobolus*
A. corymbifera	*C. bertholletiae*	*C. coronatus*
Apophysomyces	Mortierellaceae	*C. incongruous*
A. elegans	*Mortierella (animal pathogen)*	*Conidiobolus spp.*
Mucor	Saksenaceae	*C. lamprauges* (animal pathogen)
M. circinelloides	*Saksenaea*	Basidiobolaceae
M. hiemalis	*S. vasiformis*	*Basidiobolus*
M. racemosus	Syncephalastraceae	*B. ranarum*
M. ramosissimus	*Syncephalastrum*	
M. rouxianus	*S. racemosum*	
Rhizomucor		
R. pusillus		
R. miehei (animal pathogen)		
Rhizopus		
R. arrhizus		
R. azygosporus		
R. microsporus		
var. microsporus		
var. oligosporus		
var. rhizopodiformismis		
R. schipperae		
R. stolonifer		

Adapted from Ribes JA, Vanover-Sams CL, Baker DJ. Zygomycetes in Human Disease. Clin Microbiol Rev 2000; 13:236–301.

Basidiobolomycosis presents as a single, painless, sharply circumscribed and hard subcutaneous mass, mainly in the arm or lower leg (Fig. 18.16). Infection spreads along contiguous subcutaneous tissue and hematogenous spread is virtually unknown.[62]

Patient evaluation, diagnosis, and differential diagnosis

Mucormycosis is rarely suspected on the basis of clinical presentation. In most patients with the pulmonary form, the presumed diagnosis is invasive aspergillosis and frequently the correct diagnosis is only made postmortem.[4] The rhinocerebral form is easily suspected clinically.

The definitive way to diagnose mucormycosis is to visualize the characteristic broad irregular coenocytic hyphae, with right-angled branching in materials such as sputum, exudates, scrapings, and tissue (Fig. 18. 17).

A positive culture is highly suggestive of infection in relevant clinical settings, although it is not diagnostic since these fungi are normally present in the environment. A study of the zygospore production allows the differentiation between the genera and species.[60,63]

The microbiological diagnosis has a low sensitivity and most cases still reported today rely on the morphologic tissue findings.

The clinical differential diagnosis of basidiobolomycosis includes diseases such as: sporotrichosis, mycetomas, filariasis, onchocercosis, Burkitt's lymphoma, bacterial cellulitis, and others.[62]

Conidiobolomycosis must be distinguished from midline granuloma, Wegener's granulomatosis, paracoccidioidomycosis, and leishmaniasis.[62]

In the direct examination, broad, non-septated or sparsely septated hyphae with granular inclusions are seen. Growth of dirty-white colonies of Entomophthorales with radial folds occurs in 2–5 days. *B. ranarum* produces sporangia, chlamydospores, hyaline zygospores, and capillospores. *Conidiobolus coronatus* produces primary and secondary conidia and villose conidia.[64]

Pathology

Demonstration of tissue invasion by hyphae in a biopsy specimen is the gold standard for the diagnosis of mucormycosis. The broad, non-septate hyphae, with right-angle branching and angioinvasive, suggest infection with a fungus belonging to the order Mucorales. The invasion of blood vessels determines thrombosis, tissue necrosis, acute inflammation, and dissemination[61] (Fig. 18.17). The most characteristic feature of entomophthoromycosis is the presence of large, non-septated or sparsely septated hyphae surrounded by eosinophilic hyalin Splendore–Hoeppli material within a subcutaneous granuloma.[62]

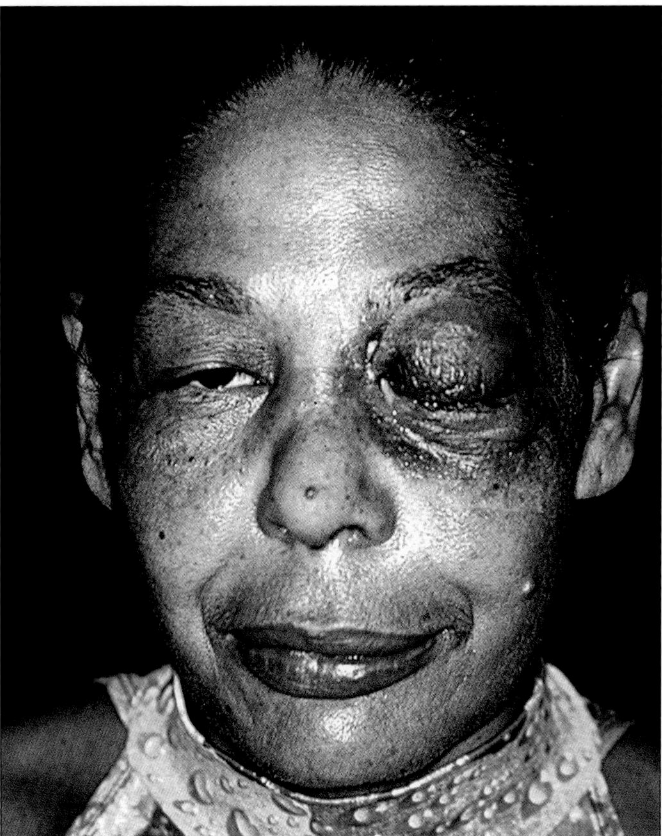

Figure 18.15 Zygomycosis: mucormycosis, rhinocerebral form.

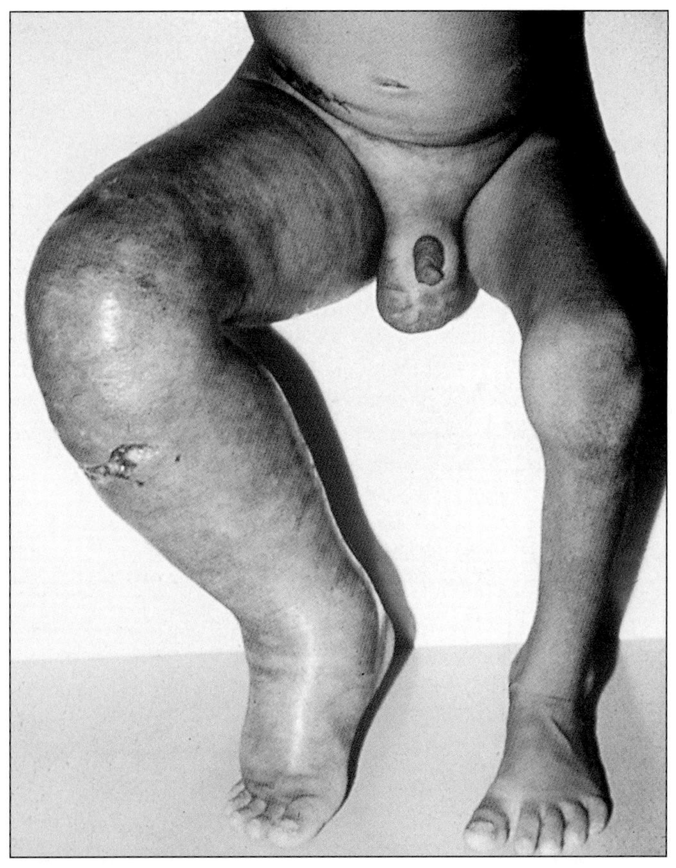

Figure 18.16 Zygomycosis: entomophthoromycosis, basidiobolomycosis. (Courtesy of Dr. Jorge Gouvea.)

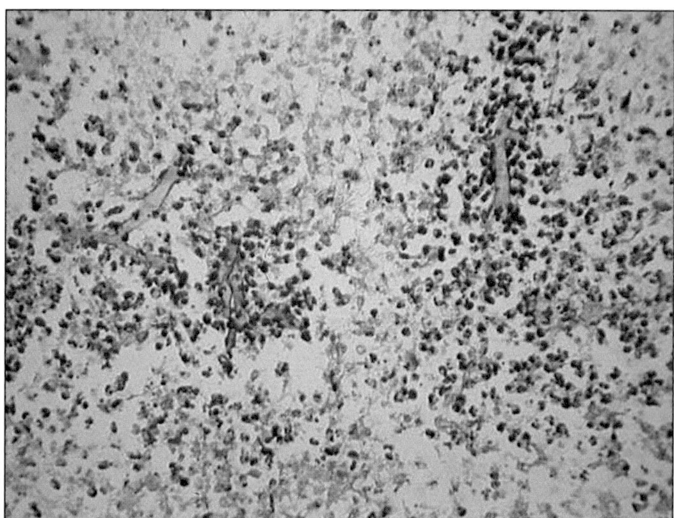

Figure 18.17 Zygomycosis: mucormycosis. Broad, non-septate with right-angle-branching hyphae. Periodic acid–Schiff.

Treatment

Mucormycosis survival is associated with early diagnosis. Correcting or controlling the underlying predisposing condition is very important. A combination of surgical intervention with effective antifungal agents is the indicated treatment. Amphotericin B is clinically effective in a dose of 1–1.5 mg/kg per day for 3–6 weeks, at a total dose of 2.0–4.0 g. Liposomal amphotericin B (3–5 mg/kg per day) has less nephrotoxic effect.[61,63]

In the era of newer antifungal agents, potassium iodide is very effective and now, as before, is considered to be the gold standard in the treatment of entomophthoromycosis. Oral potassium iodide 40 mg/kg per day is continued for 4–6 weeks after clinical cure. The drug has a direct antifungal effect, and also enhances the proteolytic and myeloperoxidase activities of phagocytes.[64]

References

1. Rippon J. Mycetoma. In: Rippon J, ed. Medical mycology: the pathogenic fungi and the pathogenic actinomycetes, 3rd edn. Philadelphia, PA: WB Saunders; 1988:325–352.
2. Kwon Chung KJ, Bennett JE. Mycetoma. In: Kwon Chung KJ, Bennett JE, eds. Medical mycology, 1st edn. Philadelphia, PA: Lea & Febiger; 1992:560–593.
3. Padhye AA, McGinnis MR. Fungi causing eumycetomic mycetoma. In: Murray PR, Baron EJ, Pfaller MA, eds. Manual of clinical microbiology. Washington, DC: ASM Press; 1999:1318–1326.
4. Brito AC. Micetoma. In: Talhari S, Neves RG, eds. Dermatologia tropical. São Paulo: MEDSI; 1997; 203–217.
5. McGinnis MR. Mycetoma. Dermatol Clin 1996; 14:97–104.
6. Palestine FR, Rogers RS. Diagnosis and treatment of mycetoma. J Am Acad Dermatol 1982; 6:107–111.
7. Welsh O. Mycetoma. Current concepts in treatment. Int J Dermatol 1991; 30:387–398.

8. Kwon-Chung KJ, Bennett JE. Sporotrichosis. In: Medical mycology, 1st edn. Philadelphia, PA: Lea & Fabiger; 1992:707–729.
9. Bustamante B, Campos PE. Endemic sporotrichosis. Curr Opin Infect Dis 2001; 14:145–149.
10. Arenas R. Sporotrichosis. In: Arenas R, Estrada R, eds. Tropical dermatology. Georgetown: Landes Bioscience; 2001:63–67.
11. Romero-Martínez R, Wheeler M, Guerrero-Plata A et al. Biosynthesis and functions of melanin in *Sporothrix schenckii*. Infect Immun 2000; 68:3696–3703.
12. Fernandes KS, Mathews HL, Lopes Bezerra LM. Differences in virulence of *Sporothrix schenckii* conidia related to culture conditions and cell-wall components. J Med Microbiol 1999; 48:195–203.
13. Tachibana T, Matsuyama T, Mitsuyama M. Involvement of CD4+ T cells and macrophages in acquired protection against infection with *Sporothrix schenckii* in mice. Med Mycol 1999; 37:397–404.
14. Rocha MM, Dassin T, Lira R et al. Sporotrichosis in patient with AIDS: report of a case and review. Rev Iberoam Micol 2001; 18:133–136.
15. Marquez MEA, Coelho KIR, Sotto MN et al. Comparison between histochemical and immunohistochemical methods for diagnosis of sporotrichosis. J Clin Pathol 1992; 45:1089–1093.
16. Kauffman CA, Hajjeh R, Chapman SW. Practice guidelines for the management of patients with sporotrichosis. Clin Infect Dis 2000; 30:684–687.
17. McGinnis MR. Chromoblastomycosis and phaeohyphomycosis: new concepts, diagnosis, and mycology. J Am Acad Dermatol 1983, 8:1–16.
18. Rudolph MW. Über die brasilanishe "Figueira." Arch Schiffs Tropen-Hygien 1914; 18:498.
19. Terra F, Torres M, da Fonseca O et al. Novo typo de dermatite verrucosa mycose por *Acrotheca* com associação de leishmaniose. Brazil-Méd 1922; 2:363–368.
20. Moore M, de Almeida F. Etiologic agents of chromomycosis (chromoblastomycosis of Terra, Torres, Fonseca and Leão, 1922) of North and South America. Rev Biol Hyg (S Paulo) 1935; 6:94–97.
21. Medlar EM. A cutaneous infection caused by a new fungus, *Phialophora verrucosa*, with a study of the fungus. J Med Res 1915; 32:507–521.
22. Lane CG. A cutaneous lesion caused by a new fungus (*Phialophora verrucosa*). J Cut Dis 1915; 33:840–846.
23. Pedroso A, Gomes JM. Sobre quarto casos de dermatite verrucosa produzida pela *Phialophora verrucosa*. Anais Paul Med Cirurg 1920; 11:53–61.
24. Fukushiro R. Chromomycosis in Japan. Int J Dermatol 1983; 22:221–229.
25. Esterre P, Andriantsimahavandy A, Ramarcel ER et al. Forty years of chromoblastomycosis in Madagascar: a review. Am J Trop Med Hyg 1996; 55:45–47.
26. Silva JP, de Souza W, Rozental S. Chromoblastomycosis: a retrospective study of 325 cases on Amazonic region (Brazil). Mycopathologia 1998–1999; 143:171–175.
27. Bonifaz A, Carrasco-Gerard E, Saul A. Chromoblastomycosis: clinical and mycologic experience of 51 cases. Mycoses 2001; 44:1–7.
28. Medlar EM. A cutaneous infection caused by a new fungus, *Phialophora verrucosa*, with a study of the fungus. J Med Res 1915; 32:507–521.
29. Negroni P. Estudio micológico del primer caso argentino de cromomicosis Fonsecaea (n.g.) pedrosoi (Brumpt, 1921). Rev Inst Bacteriol Malbrán 1936; 7:419–426.
30. Carrión AL. Chromoblastomycosis: preliminary report on a new clinical type of the disease caused by *Hormodendrum compactum*, nov. sp. Public Health Trop Med 1935; 10:543–545.
31. Carrión AL. Chromoblastomycosis: a new clinical type caused by *Hormodendrum compactum*. Public Health Trop Med 1936; 11:663–682.
32. Carrión AL. Chromoblastomycosis. Mycologia 1942; 34:424–441.
33. Trejos A. *Cladosporium carrionii* n. sp. and the problem of Cladosporia isolated from chromoblastomycosis. Rev Biol Trop 1954; 2:75–112.
34. Schell WA, McGinnis MR, Borelli D. *Rhinocladiella aquaspersa*, a new combination for *Acrotheca aquaspersa*. Mycotaxonomy 1983; 17:341–348.
35. Barba-Gomez JF, Mayorga J, McGinnis MR et al. Chromoblastomycosis caused by *Exophiala spinifera*. J Am Acad Dermatol 1992; 26:367–370.
36. Padhye AA, Hampton AA, Hampton MT et al. Chromoblastomycosis caused by *Exophiala spinifera*. Clin Infect Dis 1996; 22:331–335.
37. Naka W, Harada T, Nishikawa T et al. A case of chromoblastomycosis: with special reference to the mycology of the isolated *Exophiala jeanselmei*. Mykosen 1986; 29:445–452.
38. Kinkead S, Jancic V, Stasko T et al. Chromoblastomycosis in a patient with a cardiac transplant. Cutis 1996; 58:367–370.
39. Restrepo A. Treatment of tropical mycosis. J Am Acad Dermatol 1994; 31:S91–S102.
40. Esterre P, Andriantsimahavandy A, Raharisolo C. Histoire naturelle des chromoblastomycoses à Madagascar et dans l'Océan indien. Bull Soc Pathol Exot 1997; 90:312–317.
41. Hay RJ. Therapeutic potential of terbinafine in subcutaneous and systemic mycoses. Br J Dermatol 1999; 141 (suppl. 156): 36–40.
42. Kwon-Chung KJ, Bennett JE. Rhinosporidiosis. In: Kwon-Chung KJ, Bennett JE, eds. Medical mycology, 1st edn. Philadelphia, PA: Lea & Febiger; 1992:695–706.
43. Fredricks DN, Jolley JA, Lepp PW et al. *Rhinosporidium seeberi*: a human pathogen from a novel group of aquatic protistan parasites. Emerg Infect Dis 2000; 6:273–282.
44. Seeber G. Un nuevo esporozoario parásito del hombre: dos casos encontrados en pólipos nasales. Thesis. Buenos Aires: Universidad Nacional de Buenos Aires; 1900.
45. Ashworth JH. On *Rhinosporidium seeberi* with special reference to its sporulation and affinities. Trans R Soc Edinb 1923; 53:302–342.
46. Mendoza L, Ajello L, Taylor JW. The taxonomic status of *Lacazia loboi* and *Rhinosporidium seeberi* has been finally resolved with the use of molecular tools. Rev Iberoam Micol 2001; 18:95–98.
47. Thappa DM, Venkatesan S, Sirka CS et al. Disseminated cutaneous rhinosporidiosis. J Dermatol 1998; 25:527–532.
48. Lobo J. Um caso de blastomicose produzido por uma espécie nova, encontrada em Recife. Rev Med Pernambuco 1931; 1:763–775.

49. Pradinaud R. *Loboa loboi*. In: Collier L, Balows A, Sussman M, eds. Topley and Wilson's microbiology and microbial infections. New York: Oxford University Press; 1998:585–594.
50. Burns RS, Roy JS, Woods C et al. Report of the first human case of lobomycosis in the United States. J Clin Microbiol 2000; 38:1283–1285.
51. Fonseca Filho O, Arêa Leão AE. Contribuição para o conhecimento das graunulomatoses blastomycoides. O agente etiológico da doença de Jorge Lobo. Rev Med Cirurg Brasil 1940; 48:147–158.
52. Fonseca Filho O, Arêa Leão AE. Contribuição para o conhecimento das graunulomatoses blastomycoides. O agente etiológico da doença de Jorge Lobo. Bol Acad Nac Med (Rio de Janeiro) 1940; 112:42–53.
53. Almeida FP, Lacaz CS. Blastomicíase "tipo Jorge Lobo". Rev Paul Med 1948; 32:161–162.
54. Almeida FP, Lacaz CS. Blastomicose "tipo Jorge Lobo". Anais Fac Med S Paulo 1948–1949; 24:5–37.
55. Lacaz CS, Porto E, Martins JEC et al. Tratado de micología médica de Lacaz, 9th edn. São Paulo, Brazil: Sarvier; 2002:462–478.
56. Taborda PR, Taborda VA, McGinnis MR. *Lacazia loboi* gen. nov., comb. nov., the etiologic agent of lobomycosis. J Clin Microbiol 1999; 37:2031–2033.
57. Herr RA, Tarcha EJ, Taborda PR et al. Phylogenetic analysis of *Lacazia loboi* places this previously uncharacterized pathogen within the dimorphic Onygenales. J Clin Microbiol 2001; 39:309–314.
58. Silva D, De Brito A. Formas clinicas não usuais de micose de Lobo. Anais Bras Dermatol 1994; 69 :133–136.
59. Diniz JAP, Teixeira CEC, Soares MCP et al. Ultrastructural aspects of *Lacazia loboi*. Acta microscópica. In: Yacaman MJ, ed. Proceedings of the XVIII Congress of the Brazilian Society for Microscopy and Microanalysis. São Paulo, Brazil: Águas de Lindoia ; 2001:103–104.
60. Kwon-Chung KJ, Bennett JE. Mucormycosis. In: Kwon-Chung KJ, Bennett JE, eds. Medical mycology, 1st edn. Philadelphia, PA: Lea & Febiger; 1992:524–559.
61. Eucker J, Sezer O, Graf B et al. Mucormycosis. Mycoses 2001; 44:254–260.
62. Kwon-Chung KJ, Bennett JE. Entomophthoromycosis. In: Kwon-Chung KJ, Bennett JE, eds. Medical mycology, 1st edn. Philadelphia, PA: Lea & Febiger; 1992:447–463.
63. Yeung CK, Cheng VCC, Lie AKW et al. Invasive disease due to mucorales: a case report and review of the literature. Hong Kong Med J 2001; 7:180–188.
64. Krishnan SGS, Sentamilselvi G, Kamalam A et al. Entomophthoromycosis in Índia – a 4 year study. Mycosis 1998; 41:55–58.

Chapter 19

Systemic fungal infections

- **Histoplasmosis** ▪ *Clarisse Zaitz*
- **Coccidioidomycosis** ▪ *Michael B. Smith, Seema Patel, Jeffery A. Meixner and Michael R. McGinnis*
- **Blastomycosis** ▪ *Jeffery A. Meixner, Seema Patel, Michael B. Smith and Michael R. McGinnis*
- **Paracoccidioidomycosis (South American blastomycosis)** ▪ *Sebastião A.P. Sampaio*
- **Penicilliosis marneffei** ▪ *Michael B. Smith, Seema Patel, Jeffery A. Meixner and Michael R. McGinnis*

Introduction

Without any doubt systemic fungal infections constitute public health and economic problems. Nowhere is this clearer than in tropical countries where these diseases are endemic, or at least, have a high incidence. The World Health Organization has acknowledged the importance of systemic tropical mycoses and urged countries to recognize their impact and morbidity, and improve mycological awareness and capabilities.

Dermatologists from all over the world should be prepared to recognize and diagnose systemic tropical mycoses since these diseases occur worldwide. Most of these diseases are endemic in specific regions of the world, such as paracoccidiodomycosis in South America, penicilliosis in Southeast Asia, and blastomycosis, mainly restricted to North America. Others are, however, more widespread in their distribution, such as histoplasmosis, described in every continent, and coccidiodomycosis, affecting many countries of the western hemisphere.

It is important to point out that the mode of transmission for these fungal infections is inhalation of the fungus. The incubation period can be as short as a few weeks for penicilliosis or can last for years, as in paracoccidioidomycosis. People who have traveled to endemic areas can develop skin lesions and clinical manifestations even without any kind of traumatic inoculation of the pathogen through the skin. It is critical for the diagnosis to recognize the clinical pattern of lesions that can be restricted to the skin and mucous surfaces or even present a visceral dissemination.

Histoplasmosis

Clarisse Zaitz

Synonyms: Darling's disease, reticuloendothelial cytomycosis, Ohio valley disease

Key features:

- Histoplasmosis is a respiratory and systemic mycosis caused by a thermally dimorphic fungus *Histoplasma capsulatum*
- Histoplasmosis infection occurs in immunocompetent individuals, and rarely causes significant clinical symptoms
- Histoplasmosis manifests as a progressive, disseminated disease that can be fatal if not treated promptly in individuals with an impairment in the immune system

Introduction

Histoplasmosis, a respiratory and systemic infection, is caused by a thermally dimorphic fungus *Histoplasma capsulatum*.

H. capsulatum is found globally in soil, but displays some relative variations in geographic and environmental distribution.

It has been associated with rich soil containing high concentrations of bird or bat guano.

In highly endemic areas, most of the human population has been infected by inhalation of this fungus, as reflected in specific skin test reactivity. It is believed that, even in cases of subclinical disease, the fungus is not cleared from the body and establishes persistent capacity to cause reactivation of the disease.

There is increased risk of clinically significant primary infection or for reactivation of the disease in patients with acquired immunodeficiency syndrome (AIDS) or other immunosuppressive disease.[1]

Primary infection occurs in the lungs, but dissemination through the mononuclear phagocytic system can result in systemic disease.

Skin lesions are uncommon in US cases, but occur frequently in cases reported from Latin America. Genetic differences among strains of *H. capsulatum* may alter the pathogenesis and clinical manifestations of histoplasmosis.[2]

History

In 1904 Samuel Taylor Darling observed a fatal case of disseminated histoplasmosis in Panama. The autopsy showed that the organism was intracellular, similar to *Leishmania*, but without kinetoplasts. Darling concluded that the organism was a new protozoan, which he named *H. capsulatum*.[1]

In 1913 Rocha-Lima, a Brazilian studying in Hamburg, was the first to suggest that Darling's microorganism was a yeast instead of a protozoan.[1]

De Monbreun, in 1934, discovered the dimorphism of *H. capsulatum* and concluded that the saprophytic form probably exists in nature.[1]

Duncan, in 1943, was the first to isolate the etiologic agent of African histoplasmosis. In 1952, Vanbreuseghem described the agent as a new species: *H. duboisii*.[1]

Epidemiology

H. capsulatum var. *capsulatum* is endemic in certain areas of North and Latin America, but cases have also been reported from Europe and Asia (it has been diagnosed in at least 60 countries). In the USA, most cases have occurred within the Ohio and Mississippi river valleys.[1]

H. capsulatum var. *duboisii* is endemic in tropical areas of Africa between 20°N and 20°S of the Equator. The distribution lies between the Sahara and Kalahari deserts.[1]

H. capsulatum var. *farciminosum* causes epizootic lymphangitis in horses and mules.[1]

Histoplasmin skin test surveys of a randomized population have been a productive method of determining endemic regions, although there may be cross-reactivity with *Coccidioides immitis*, *Paracoccidioides brasiliensis*, and *Blastomyces dermatitides*.[1]

Children from endemic areas become skin test-positive by the age of 10–15 years. No significant differences in racial susceptibility for acute pulmonary histoplasmosis have been documented, while chronic pulmonary disease is predominantly found among Caucasian adult males. Disseminated histoplasmosis occurs in all age groups, with the highest incidence in those who are immunosuppressed. Histoplasmosis is rarely transmitted from person to person.[1]

Moderate climate, humidity, and soil characteristics may be some of the reasons for this endemic distribution pattern. Bird and bat excrement enhances the growth of the organism in soil by accelerating sporulation and explains in part the localization of histoplasmosis in microfoci. Activities that disturb such sites are associated with exposure to *H. capsulatum*. Air currents carry spores for many kilometers, exposing individuals who were unaware of contact with the contaminated site.[1]

Pathogenesis and etiology

The dimorphic fungus *H. capsulatum* grows in the environment (25°C) in a differentiated mold form and shifts to an undifferentiated yeast form in the mammalian host (37°C).[1]

After inhalation of spores, regulatory mechanisms that use temperature, yeast phase-specific (*yps*) genes and other environmental factors are essential to the mold-to-yeast shift and successful adaptation of the organism, as an effective intracellular pathogenic yeast of humans macrophages.[3,4]

Kasuga et al.,[5] after evaluation of *H. capsulatum* DNA sequences, identified six different species instead of the three known varieties, *capsulatum*, *duboisii*, and *farciminosum*.

Class 1: North American *H. capsulatum* var. *capsulatum* (mostly found in patients with AIDS)
Class 2: North American *H. capsulatum* var. *capsulatum* (found in patients with and without AIDS)
Class 3: Central American *H. capsulatum* var. *capsulatum*
Class 4: South American *H. capsulatum* var. *capsulatum* group A
Class 5: South American *H. capsulatum* var. *capsulatum* group B
Class 6: *H. capsulatum* var. *duboisii* (found in tropical Africa).

Histoplasma capsulatum var. *farciminosum* was found within the South American *H. capsulatum* var. *capsulatum* group A.[5]

Clinical features

Severity of illness after inhalation exposure to *H. capsulatum* varies, depending on the intensity of exposure and the immunity of the host.[6,7] Histoplasmosis causes a broad spectrum of clinical findings.

Asymptomatic infection or acute pulmonary disease follows low-intensity exposures in healthy individuals and the course is self-limited.[6,7]

Heavy exposure may cause severe diffuse acute pulmonary infection (Fig. 19.1), causing respiratory distress and even death.[6,7]

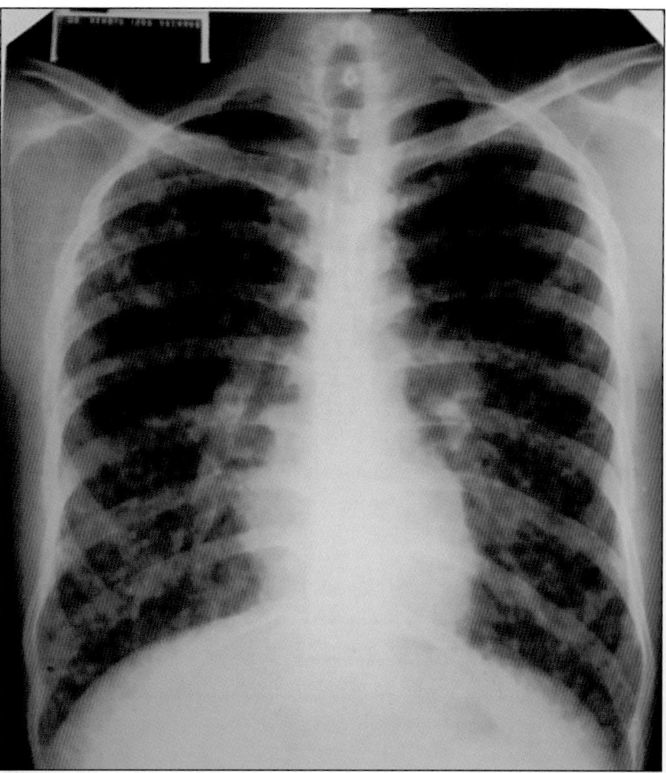

Figure 19.1 Histoplasmosis: multiple nodules disseminated in both lungs. (Courtesy of Dr. Jorge Ethel.)

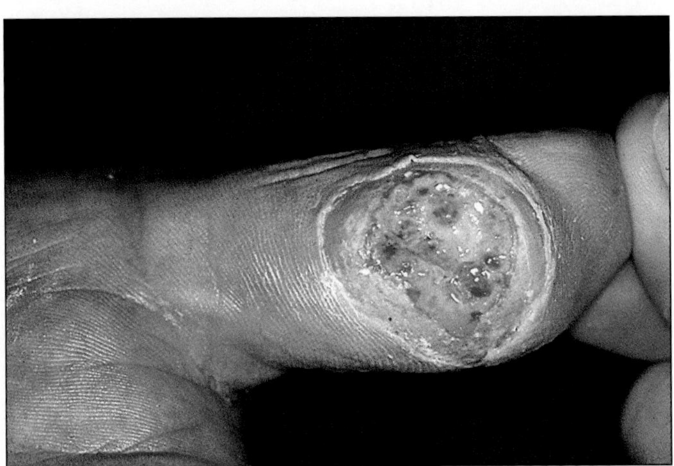

Figure 19.2 Histoplasmosis: reactivation disease with dissemination to skin in a corticodependent patient.

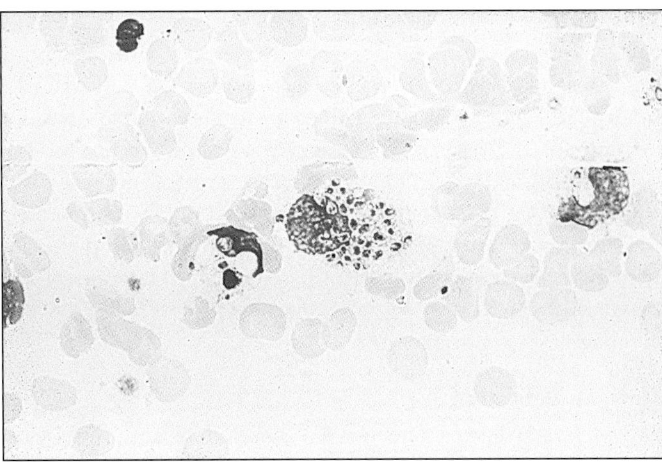

Figure 19.3 Histoplasmosis: demonstration of yeast cells of *Histoplasma capsulatum* in the cerebrospinal fluid.

Hematogenous dissemination from the lungs to other tissues probably occurs in all infected individuals during the first 2 weeks of infection before specific immunity has developed, but it is non-progressive in most cases, and leads to the development of calcified granulomas in the liver and/or spleen.[6,7]

About 10–20% of patients may experience chronic complications, including progressive chronic pulmonary infection and disseminated disease. Progressive dissemination occurs primarily in those with underlying immunosuppressive disorders or those at the extremes of age.[6,7]

Skin lesions are uncommon in US cases, but occur frequently in cases reported from Latin America[2] (Fig. 19.2).

Histoplasmosis can be classified based in the clinical manifestations:

- Histoplasmosis infection
- Asymptomatic
- Acute pulmonary (self-limited)
- Histoplasmosis disease
- Diffuse acute pulmonary
- Chronic pulmonary
- Disseminated (in AIDS or in non-AIDS).

A variety of other acute and chronic manifestations of histoplasmosis appear to result from unusual inflammatory or fibrotic responses to infection: rheumatologic syndromes, pericarditis, chronic mediastinal inflammation or fibrosis, histoplasmoma, broncholithiasis, and enlarging parenchymal granulomas.[6]

Patient evaluation, diagnosis, and differential diagnosis

The diagnosis may be missed or delayed because histoplasmosis is not considered in the differential diagnosis. The disease should be suspected when several patients develop a respiratory illness about 2 weeks after a common outdoor exposure.[1] The main differential diagnosis is with pneumonia, tuberculosis, paracoccidioidomycosis, coccidioidomycosis, and blastomycosis.

The diagnosis of histoplasmosis is based on direct examination, culture, histopathology, measurement of antibodies or antigen detection and polymerase chain reaction (PCR). Each of these approaches has advantages and limitations.

Direct examination

Demonstration of yeast cells of *H. capsulatum* in sputum, urine, cerebrospinal fluid (CSF), or blood is only easy in AIDS patients, where the organisms tend to be abundant. The yeast cells appear oval in shape and may be seen within monocytes or macrophages (Fig. 19.3). The yeast cells of the var. *duboisii* are larger and show prominent bud scars.[1]

Culture

White, tan, or light-brown colonies with smooth margins grow on Sabouraud's agar after 4 weeks at 30°C. A colony with lobulated margins grows on Sabouraud's agar after 4 weeks at 25°C. Cultures may be false-negative. Agar slide culture shows characteristic macroconidias with finger-like projections (Fig. 19.4).[1]

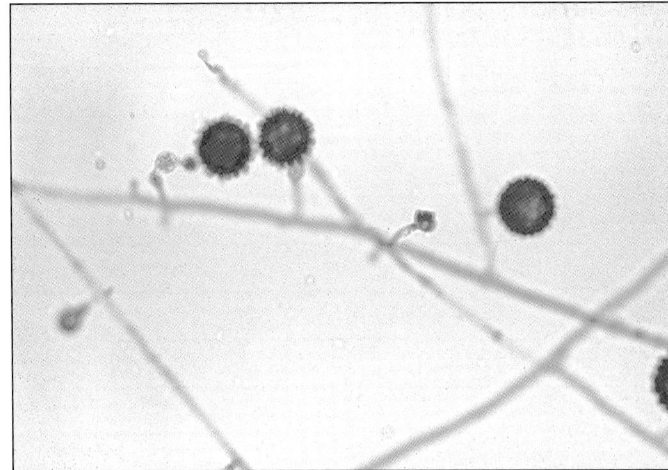

Figure 19.4 Histoplasmosis: agar slide culture. Characteristic macroconidia with finger-like projections.

Measurement of antibodies

Serological tests may be false-negative in acute disease or in immunosuppressive disorders and false-positive in patients with other fungal and mycobacterial disease.[8] Antibody-based detection systems for the diagnosis of histoplasmosis with highly purified and well-characterized immunodominant antigens deriving from the application of recombinant techniques (94 kDa glycoprotein M antigen and 120 kDa glycoprotein H antigen), in combination with more advanced assay systems (enzyme-linked immunosorbent assay: ELISA), offer improvements in reproducibility and specificity.[9]

Antigen detection

H. capsulatum antigen detection has proven to be a useful method for rapid diagnosis in patients with disseminated or acute pulmonary histoplasmosis (high sensitivity and specificity using polyclonal antibodies and sandwich enzyme immunoassay: EIA) and for monitoring the effect of treatment.[8] Urine, serum, bronchoalveolar lavage fluid, and CSF should be tested. Antigen clears from the blood and urine with effective therapy and levels rise with relapse.[8]

Histopathology

The inflammatory response varies in the different clinical forms, from one organ to another and from different areas in the same organ. *H. capsulatum* cells can be seen in macrophages of the lesion with periodic acid–Schiff (PAS) or silver staining, but the sensitivity is low.[1]

Rapid PCR-based diagnosis

PCR assays amplifying sequences of *H. capsulatum* genes have been successfully introduced into the armamentarium for diagnosis of invasive histoplasmosis.[9,10]

The 18S rDNA is a commonly and highly sensitive target used for diagnostic PCR assays; however it does result in a high number of unspecific amplifications.[10]

PCR targeting a gene encoding a 100-kDa-like protein, essential for the survival of *H. capsulatum* in human cells, specifically indicates the pathogen.[10]

Treatment

Treatment recommendations vary with severity of illness and immune competency of the host. Three decisions must be made: (1) to treat or to observe? (2) to use amphotericin B formulation or itraconazole? and (3) the duration of therapy[7] (Table 19.1).

Treatment is not required for the acute self-limited pulmonary syndrome. Patients with pericardial and rheumatic manifestations recover without antifungal treatment. Other chronic and sequel forms of disease, such as broncholithiasis and histoplasmoma, are unresponsive to pharmacologic treatment. The therapy of fibrosing mediastinitis is controversial and probably ineffective. Presumed ocular histoplasmosis does not represent active infection and antifungal therapy is not recommended.[6,7]

Treatment is appropriate in patients with diffuse acute pulmonary infection, chronic pulmonary infection, disseminated infections, or mediastinal granuloma causing obstruction of important structures.[6,7]

For severe histoplasmosis or for patients who require hospitalization, amphotericin B (0.7–1 mg/kg per day; 35 mg/kg total) or liposomal amphotericin B (3–5 mg/kg per day) can be recommended as initial treatment. Itraconazole (200 mg twice daily) is recommended for patients who can be treated at home, those who have milder illness, or to those who need to complete treatment after response to amphotericin B. Fluconazole 800 mg/day is used in cases of meningitis[7] (Table 19.1).

Recently, newer antifungal agents have been evaluated in animal models of histoplasmosis. Of these new triazoles, posaconazole appears the most promising. Intravenous formulation of itraconazole may be an alternative to amphotericin B, but more studies are required.[7]

References

1. Kwon-Chung KJ, Bennett JE. Histoplasmosis. In: Kwon-Chung KJ, Bennett JE, eds. Medical mycology. Philadelphia, PA: Lea & Febiger; 1992:464–513.

Table 19.1 Summary of antifungal treatment recommendation for histoplasmosis

Type	Severe manifestation	Moderate manifestation
Diffuse acute pulmonary	Amphotericin B with corticosteroids followed by itraconazole for 12 weeks	None in usual cases or itraconazole for 6–12 weeks in those with persistent symptoms > 4 weeks
Chronic pulmonary	Amphotericin B followed by itraconazole for 12–24 months	Itraconazole for 12–24 months
Disseminated in non-AIDS	Amphotericin B followed by itraconazole for 6–18 months	Itraconazole for 6–18 months
Disseminated in AIDS	AmBisome followed by itraconazole for life	Itraconazole for life
Meningitis	AmBisome for 3 months followed by fluconazole for 12 months	AmBisome for 3 months followed by fluconazole for 12 months
Mediastinal granuloma	Amphotericin B followed by itraconazole for 6–12 months	Itraconazole for 6–12 months

AIDS, acquired immunodeficiency syndrome.
Adapted from Mocherla S, Wheat LJ. Treatment of histoplasmosis. Semin Resp Infect 2001; 16:141–148.

2. Karimi K, Wheat LJ, Connolly P et al. Differences in histoplasmosis in patients with acquired immunodeficiency syndrome in the United States and Brazil. J Infect Dis 2002; 186:1655–1660.
3. Retallack DM, Woods JP. Molecular epidemiology, pathogenesis, and genetics of the dimorphic fungus *Histoplasma capsulatum*. Microb Infect 1999; 1:817–825.
4. Woods JP. *Histoplasma capsulatum* molecular genetics, pathogenesis, and responsiveness to its environment. Fungal Genet Biol 2002; 35:81–97.
5. Kasuga T, Taylor JW, White TJ. Phylogenetic relationships of varieties and geographical groups of human pathogenic fungus *Histoplasma capsulatum* Darling. J Clin Microb 1999; 37:653–663.
6. Wheat J, Sarosi G, McKinsey D et al. Practice guidelines for the management of patients with histoplasmosis. Clin Infect Dis 2000; 30:688–695.
7. Mocherla S, Wheat LJ. Treatment of histoplasmosis. Semin Resp Infect 2001; 16:141–148.
8. Wheat LJ, Garringer T, Brizendine ED et al. Diagnosis of histoplasmosis by antigen detection based upon experience at the histoplasmosis reference laboratory. Diagn Microbiol Infect Dis 2002; 43:29–37.
9. Reiss E, Obayashi T, Orle K et al. Non-culture based diagnostic tests for mycotic infections. Med Mycol 2000; 38:147–159.
10. Bialek R, Feucht A, Aepinus C et al. Evaluation of two nested PCR assays for detection of *Histoplasma capsulatum* DNA in human tissue. J Clin Microbiol 2002; 40:1644–1647.

Coccidioidomycosis

Michael B. Smith, Seema Patel, Jeffery A. Meixner and Michael R. McGinnis

Synonyms: Valley fever, Posadas' disease, desert rheumatism

Key features:

- *Coccidioides immitis*
- *Coccidioides posadasii*
- Respiratory infection
- It occurs in arid southwestern USA and other portions of the Americas
- Liposomal amphotericin B, fluconazole, ketoconazole, voriconazole, posaconazole, itraconazole, and caspofungin are treatments

Introduction

Coccidioidomycosis is an infectious disease caused by the dimorphic fungi *Coccidioides immitis* and *C. posadasii*. These fungi live in sandy soil located in the arid portions of the western hemisphere, primarily the Lower Sonoran Life Zone of the southwestern USA, Mexico, Central and South America. Infection has been documented in patients who have traveled through an endemic area, or were occupationally exposed to the fungus when it was transported in agricultural commodities such as cotton. Because these two species represent distinct monophyletic genetic populations that are phenotypically identical, and cause identical disease that is managed in the same manner, *C. immitis* will be used as the name for the etiologic agent of coccidioidomycosis in this section. Even though they have been distinguished from one another by numerous DNA polymorphisms, there does not appear to be a need to recognize them as two separate species clinically.

C. immitis can cause disease either following the inhalation of arthroconidia in dust, or rarely through cutaneous inoculation of contaminated soil. One-half to two-thirds of the estimated 100 000 new infections per year are subclinical, but severe and life-threatening infections can develop in some patients. Approximately 0.5% of cases develop serious disseminated disease that is often fatal. Most people who have been infected enjoy immunity from subsequent infection when exposed to the fungus at a later date.[1]

History

In 1892, an Argentine soldier by the name of Domingo Ezcurra became the first described case of coccidioidomycosis. Alejandro Posadas described the infection and proposed the name *C. immitis* for the etiologic agent. Posadas believed that *C. immitis* was a protozoan. The recently described and newly proposed species *C. posadasii* was named to honor Posadas and his original work in describing this important infection.[2]

Epidemiology

Occupations involving agricultural and construction work increase the risk of exposure. In endemic areas, the arthroconidia are readily aerosolized during agitation of soil containing the fungus by wind and work activities. The dissemination potential of the fungus is affected by gender, age, ethnicity, and immune status. People of African–American descent, especially males, as well as people of Filipino descent are more prone to develop disseminated disease. Similarly, human immunodeficiency virus (HIV)-positive individuals, solid organ recipients, diabetics, and women in their third trimester of pregnancy have an increased risk of disseminated disease. The incidence of coccidioidomycosis in a population is associated with the number of air-borne dispersed arthroconidia present in the environment. The concentration of arthroconidia in the air has been shown to correlate with periodic cyclic weather patterns involving the amount of rainfall and length of drought preceding epidemics.[3] Genetic analysis of the fungus suggests that it may have migrated, possibly with humans or other animals, to South America from a North American central location in Texas during the Pleistocene epoch.

Pathogenesis and etiology

Inhaled arthroconidia evade normal host defense mechanisms such as filtration of the respiratory tract, mucociliary transport, and inhibition by chemicals in the mucus. Within 2 days, the arthroconidia increase in size and begin to develop into spherules. An initial polymorphonuclear leukocyte response changes to a mononuclear cell infiltration, eventually followed by granulomata formation. A Th-1 type immune response is important for the control of the infection and the protective immunity seen in this disease after initial infection and recovery. A Th-2 type response with elevated antibody production has been associated with disease that is increasing in severity.

During systemic infections, erythema multiforme or erythema nodosum (Fig. 19.5) may be present, as well as fatigue, weakness, and anorexia. The skin (Figs 19.6 and 19.7) is the most common site of dissemination where plaques, superficial abscesses, pustules, and granulomatous lesions may develop.[4] Primary cutaneous lesions are rare, being associated with localized trauma to the skin.

Within tissue, spherules serve as the reproductive form of the fungus. Spherules are sac-like cells that give rise to endospores, which are subsequently released into the adjacent tissue. Endospores may increase in size and then become new spherules, forming additional endospores. If endospores enter blood vessels, hematogenous dissemination is likely to occur. In some patients, hyphae may form; arthroconidia may develop, and then evolve into spherules, producing typical endospores. Spherules containing endospores in tissue are diagnostic for this infection (Fig. 19.8).

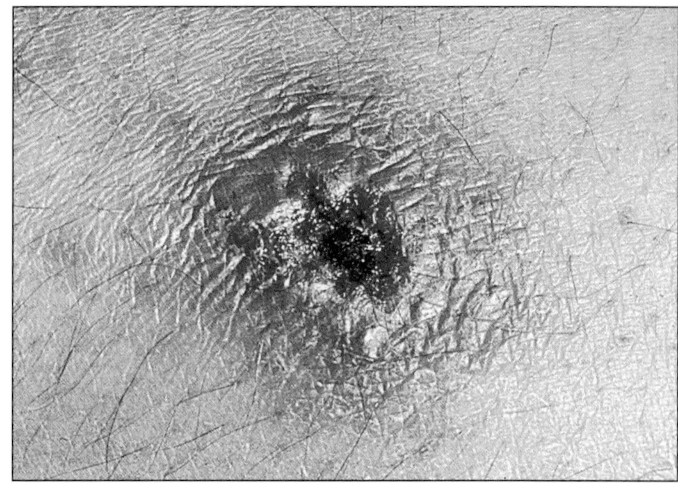

Figure 19.6 Cutaneous lesion following hematogenous dissemination of *Coccidioides immitis*. (Courtesy of Dr. Richard Graybill.)

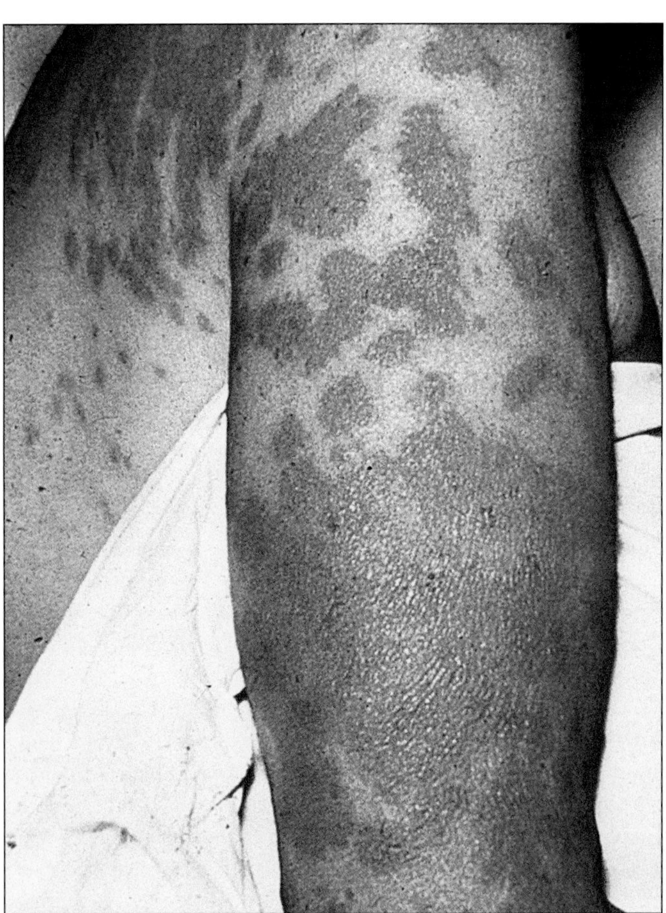

Figure 19.5 Erythema nodosum in a female. (Courtesy of Dr. Carlyn Halde.)

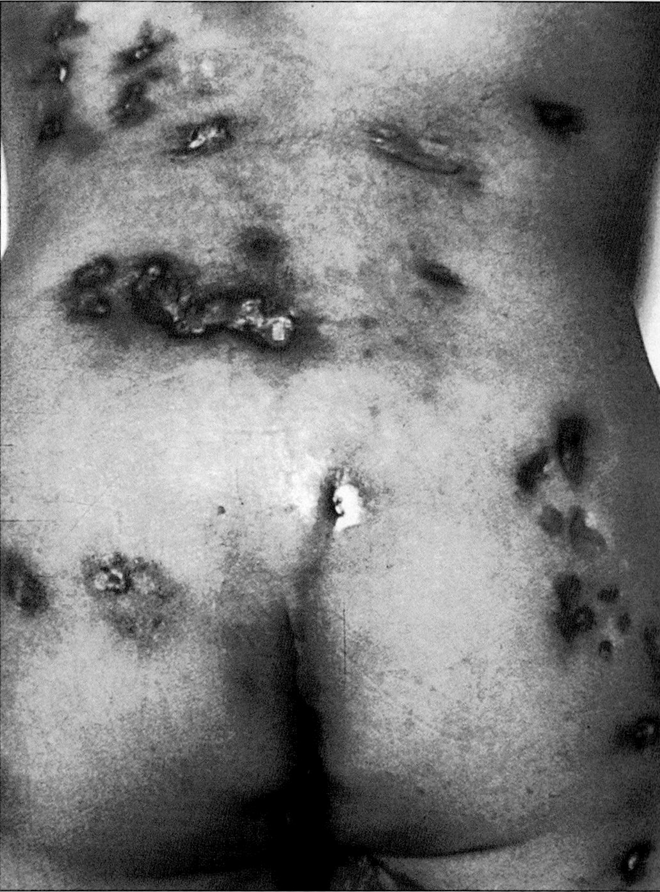

Figure 19.7 Cutaneous lesions of coccidioidomycosis. (Courtesy of Dr. Carlyn Hal

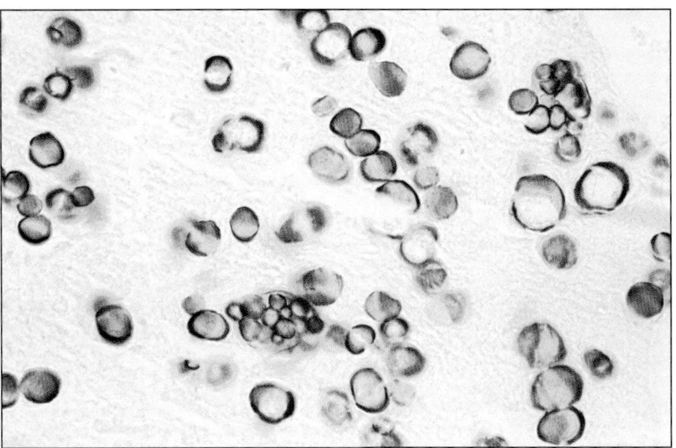

Figure 19.8 Spherules and endospores of *Coccidioides immitis* in lung tissue. 400×, Gomori methenamine silver stain.

Clinical features

Coccidioidomycosis typically manifests itself as a primary pulmonary infection: approximately 40% of patients experience influenza-like symptoms such as cough, fever with night sweats, or pleuritic chest pain with arthralgias and myalgias. In symptomatic patients, who represent about 50% of all patients, abnormal radiographs show infiltrates associated with ipsilateral hilar adenopathy. Most symptoms disappear in 2–3 weeks, but months may pass before fatigue disappears. Approximately 5% of patients will develop extrapulmonary or disseminated disease. Bone, joint, eye, larynx, thyroid, peritoneum, genitourinary system, meninges, and central nervous system disease may be involved. C. *immitis* can cause a diffuse pneumonia either early or late in the infection. Nodules and cavitations may develop in a few patients. Patients with solitary nodules are typically asymptomatic. Cavities may develop in approximately 5% of patients with acute pneumonia.[4]

As noted, the skin is the most common site for dissemination, and is usually present as papules and verrucous lesions. Typically there is minor acute inflammation. Even though spherules can be seen in biopsy specimens, isolation of the fungus may prove more helpful in making a diagnosis of disseminated coccidioidomycosis.

Patient evaluation, diagnosis, and differential diagnosis

Coccidioidomycosis can be mistaken for influenza, primary atypical pneumonia, bronchitis, bronchial pneumonia, colds, tuberculosis, neoplasias, syphilis, tularemia, glanders, osteomyelitis, and other mycotic infections. The fungus is easily cultivated in the laboratory on routine media; however, the mold form is highly infectious and must be handled in a safe manner to avoid laboratory-acquired infection. Biopsy and other tissue specimens typically contain the parasitic form of the fungus. The presence of spherules containing endospores allow for a tissue diagnosis. Tube precipitin-reacting (immunoglobulin M: IgM) and complement-fixing (IgG) antibodies are useful for the serodiagnosis of coccidioidomycosis. Skin testing is a useful tool for epidemiological studies or as a diagnostic tool when there is a previously known negative skin test that allows for determining when the exposure occurred. A positive skin test that becomes negative is a poor prognostic indicator.

Pathology

Identification of *Coccidioides* species in tissue is by observation of the characteristic spherules containing endospores. Visualization on routine hematoxylin and eosin (H&E) can be accomplished; however, the Gomori methenamine silver (GMS) stain facilitates identification, particularly if spherules are infrequent or the small endospores or collapsed spherules predominate. Spherules measure from 20 to 200 μm in size, while endospores are typically 2–5 μm in diameter. In many, if not most infections, varying stages of the developmental cycle are seen in tissue, ranging from endospores to immature spherules without endospores, to mature spherules containing endospores, and finally, to collapsed spherules which have discharged their endospores.

Overall, the tissue reaction in *Coccidioides* infection is characterized by a mixed suppurative–granulomatous response, but the histological manifestations of infection in a given case are somewhat dependent on the stage of infection and immune status of the patient. Early pulmonary infection in the non-immunocompromised patient shows a predominance of granulomas, usually without caseation. Non-caseous necrosis may be present, and as the initial inflammatory reaction to newly released endospores involves a predominance of neurophils, microabscesses can be seen. Tissue eosinophilia is an infrequent but unique manifestation of this mycosis. In immunocompromised patients, the granulomatous response can be poor or non-existent. Prolonged infection in the lung results in fibrogranulomatous nodules, and caseous-type necrosis may be present. Dissemination beyond the pulmonary entry point to distant sites, especially the skin, can occur, and the inflammatory reaction is usually an identical mixed suppurative–granulomatous response. In prolonged infection of the skin, pseudoepitheliomatous hyperplasia of the epidermis occurs over infected sites.

Treatment

Practice guidelines for the treatment of coccidioidomycosis have been modified from the National Guideline Clearinghouse (NGC).[5] Management of primary respiratory infections caused by C. *immitis* is controversial. Some authorities propose treatment of all symptomatic patients. Underlying disorders such as HIV infection, organ transplant, high doses of corticosteroids, or severe infection should be treated. Diagnosis of primary infection during the third trimester of pregnancy or immediately in the postpartum period should raise consideration for treatment. During pregnancy, amphotericin B is the treatment of choice because fluconazole and possibly other azole antifungals are teratogenic.

The severity of an acute infection can be determined using indicators such as weight loss of >10%, intense night sweats persisting for >3 weeks, infiltrates involving more than one-half of one lung or portions of both lungs, prominent or persistent hilar adenopathy, complement fixing antibody titer of >1:16, failure to develop dermal hypersensitivity to coccidioidal antigens, inability to work, or symptoms that persist for >2 months.

When bilateral reticulonodular or miliary infiltrates are present, there is probably an underlying immunodeficiency. Therapy usually starts with amphotericin B. Several weeks of therapy are often required to produce improvement. During convalescence, amphotericin B may be discontinued and replaced with oral azole antifungal therapy. The total length of therapy is approximately 1 year or longer. For patients with severe immunodeficiency, oral azole therapy should be continued as secondary prophylaxis. Because diffuse pneumonia due to C. *immitis* is usually a manifestation of fungemia, patients should be evaluated for other extrapulmonary lesions that may also require attention.

When a solitary nodule is found by non-invasive means or by fine-needle aspiration, antifungal therapy or resection is unnecessary. Similarly, in the absence of significant immunosuppression, antifungal therapy is not recommended if the lesion is completely resected and the diagnosis is determined by examination of the excised tissue.

Many cavities caused by C. *immitis* are benign and do not require intervention. Such cavities contain viable fungus. Most authorities do not consider asymptomatic cavities sufficient reason to initiate treatment. With the passage of time, some cavities disappear, obviating the need for intervention. Although indefinite follow-up without intervention is appropriate for many patients, eventual resection from 1 to several years after the cavity is identified may be necessary to avoid future complications, especially if the cavity is still detectable after 2 years, if it shows progressive enlargement, or if it is immediately adjacent to the pleura.

Complications of coccidioidal cavities are local discomfort, superinfection with other fungi, possibly bacteria, or hemoptysis. Should these complications occur, oral therapy with azole antifungals may result in improvement, although recurrence of symptoms, at least in some patients, occurs upon cessation of therapy. Where the surgical risks are not unusually high, resection of localized cavities will probably resolve the problem and may be recommended as an alternative approach to chronic or intermittent therapy.

Rupture of a coccidioidal cavity into the pleural space, resulting in pyopneumothorax, is an infrequent but well-recognized complication. For young, otherwise healthy patients, surgical closure by lobectomy with decortication is the preferred management. Antifungal therapy is recommended for coverage, particularly in acute cases with active disease, delay of diagnosis, or coexistent diseases.

Initial treatment of chronic fibrocavitary pneumonia is with oral azole antifungals. If the patient's condition improves sufficiently, therapy should be continued for at least 1 year. If therapy is not satisfactory, alternatives are switching to an alternative azole antifungal, raising the dose of fluconazole if it was the oral azole initially selected, and administering amphotericin B. Surgical resection may be a useful option for refractory lesions that are well localized or where significant hemoptysis has occurred.

Therapy[6] is usually initiated with oral azole antifungals. Clinical trials have used 400 mg/day of ketoconazole, itraconazole, or fluconazole. Some experts recommend higher dosages of fluconazole. Amphotericin B is alternative therapy, especially if lesions are appearing to worsen rapidly and are in particularly critical locations such as the vertebral column. The dosage of amphotericin B is similar to that for treatment of diffuse coccidioidal pneumonia, although the duration may be longer. Surgical debridement or stabilization is an occasionally important, if not critical, adjunctive measure.

Therapy with oral fluconazole is currently preferred for meningitis. The dosage used in some clinical trials was 400 mg/day. Some physicians begin therapy with 800 or 1000 mg/day of fluconazole. Dosages of itraconazole of 400–600 mg/day have also been reported to be comparably effective. Some physicians initiate therapy with intrathecal amphotericin B in addition to an azole on the basis of their belief that responses are more prompt with this approach. The dose and duration of intrathecal amphotericin B in this circumstance have not been defined. Patients who respond to azole therapy should continue this treatment indefinitely.

Hydrocephalus nearly always requires a shunt for decompression. Hydrocephalus may develop regardless of the therapy used, and switching to alternative therapy is not required. Patients who do not respond to fluconazole or itraconazole are candidates for intrathecal amphotericin B therapy with or without continuation of azole treatment. The intrathecal dose of amphotericin B normally ranges from 0.01 to 1.5 mg; it is administered at intervals ranging from daily to weekly, beginning at a low dose and increasing until patient intolerance appears.

References

1. Galgiani JN, Ampel NM, Catanzaro A et al. Practice guidelines of the treatment of coccidioidomycosis. Clin Infect Dis 2000; 30:658–661.
2. Fisher MC, Koenig GL, White TJ et al. Molecular and phenotypic descriptions of *Coccidioides posadasii* sp. nov., previously recognized as the non-California population of *Coccidioides immitis*. Mycologia 2002; 94:73–84.
3. Kolivras KN, Comrie AC. Modeling valley fever (coccidioidomycosis) incidence on the basis of climate. Int J Biometeorol 2003; 47:87–101.
4. Chiller TM, Galgiani JN, Stevens DA. Coccidioidomycosis. Infect Dis Clin North Am 2003; 17:41–57.
5. Department of Health and Human Services USA. Practice guidelines for the treatment of coccidioidomycosis. Available online at: http://www.guidelines.gov/summary/summary.aspx?doc_id=2674&nbr=1900&string=coccidioidomycosis (accessed 5 August, 2004).
6. Yamada H, Kotaki H, Takahashi T. Recommendations for the treatment of fungal pneumonias. Expert Opin Pharmacother 2003; 4:1241–1258.

Blastomycosis

Jeffery A. Meixner, Seema Patel, Michael B. Smith and Michael R. McGinnis

Synonyms: Chicago disease, Gilchrist's disease, North American blastomycosis

Key features:

- Pulmonary with potential cutaneous dissemination
- Dimorphic fungus
- Formally thought to be restricted to the North American continent, the disease has been described in some parts of Africa, South Africa, Congo, Morocco, Tanzania, Uganda, and Madagascar
- Treatment includes itraconazole, amphotericin B, and ketoconazole

Introduction

The thermally dimorphic fungus *Blastomyces dermatitidis* causes blastomycosis. *B. dermatitidis* is the imperfect stage or asexual form of the ascomycete *Ajellomyces dermatitidis*.[1] Historically, it was assumed that there were two distinct forms of blastomycosis – pulmonary and cutaneous. It was hypothesized that all forms of blastomycosis begin as a pulmonary infection and that cutaneous lesions were a manifestation of disseminated disease. Essentially all infections are acquired by inhalation of conidia of *B. dermatitidis*. Even though primary cutaneous infections have been described, they are very rare.[2]

History

Initially, Gilchrist thought the disease was caused by a parasite, even though he observed yeast cells in tissue that were morphologically similar to what he believed was *Cryptococcus neoformans*. After studying a second case, he cultured the fungus and studied it in animals. Gilchrist and Stokes named the fungus *B. dermatitidis* in 1898.

Epidemiology

Blastomycosis is endemic in the regions of the USA along the Mississippi and Ohio rivers. Formerly thought to be restricted to North America, the disease has been described in patients living in parts of Africa, South Africa, Congo, Morocco, Tanzania, Uganda, and Madagascar. Prevalence of the disease is higher in males than in females, which is probably related to exposure while involved in outdoor activities.

Pathogenesis and etiology

B. dermatitidis is the sole etiologic agent of blastomycosis. The fungus has been isolated from decomposing wood,[3] where it is believed that it produces mycelium and air-borne conidia. Various environmental studies indicate that the fungus does not grow in soil. The fungus has a sexual stage that has been classified in the genus *Ajellomyces* as *A. dermatitidis*.

Clinical features

Beginning with the 1896 Gilchrist case, it was thought that blastomycosis had two distinctive clinical forms, pulmonary and cutaneous (Figs 19.9–19.11). We now know that virtually all infections originate in the lungs where the extracellular yeast form can proliferate. The clinical spectrum of blastomycosis is varied, including acute or chronic pneumonia, asymptomatic infection, and disseminated disease.[4] Asymptomatic infection occurs in approximately 50% of all cases. Symptomatic disease appears to develop after 30–45 days of incubation. The disease can mimic bacterial

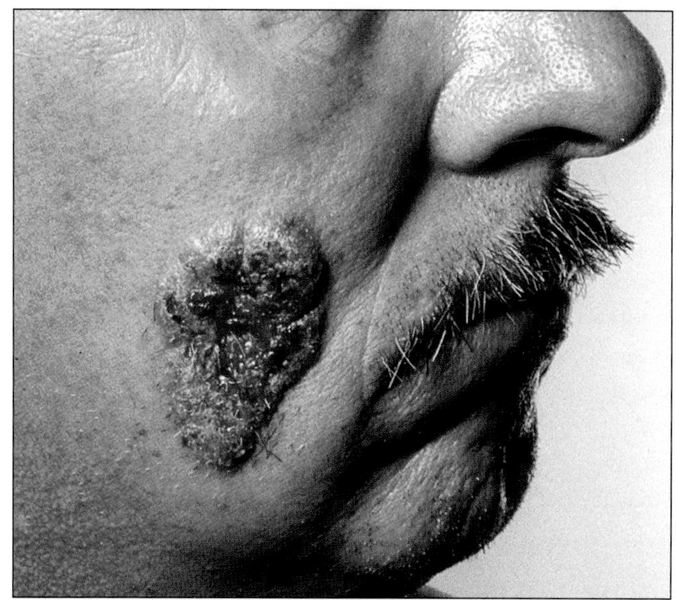

Figure 19.9 Cutaneous lesion of blastomycosis following hematogenous dissemination of the fungus. (Courtesy of Dr. Richard Graybill.)

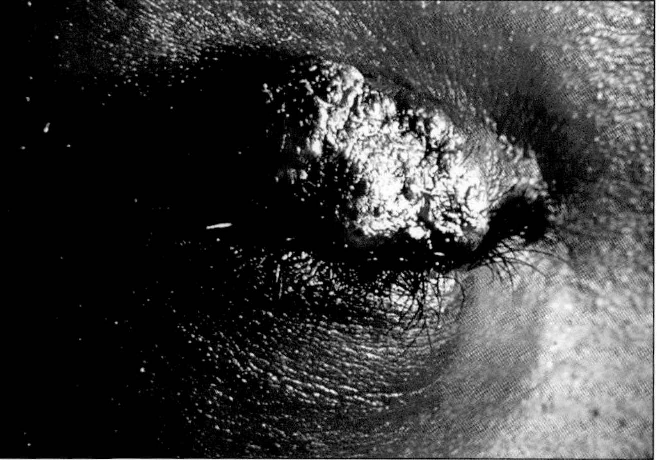

Figure 19.10 Blastomycosis on an eyelid. (Courtesy of Dr. Libero Ajello.)

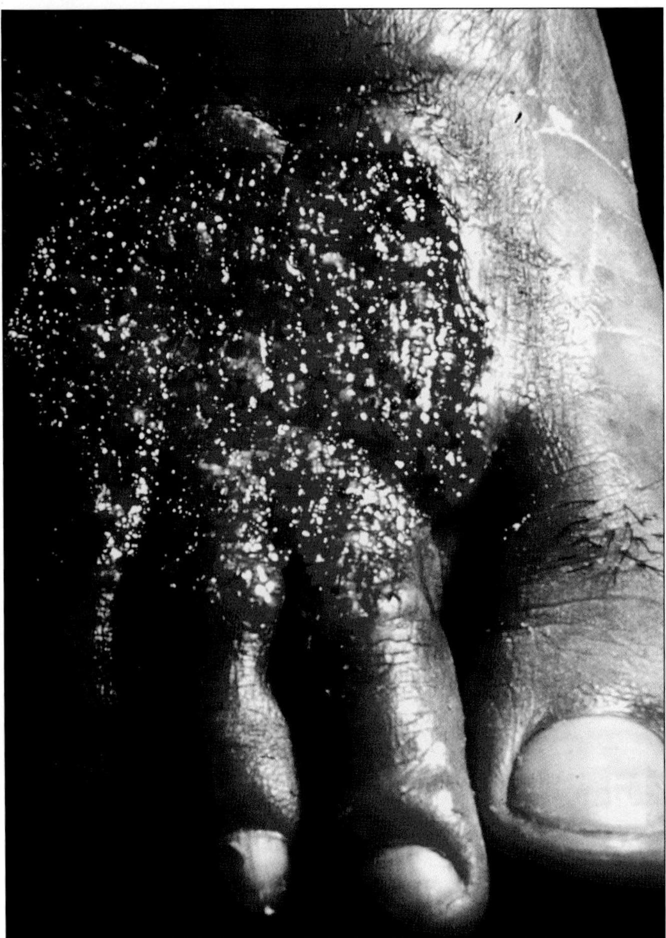

Figure 19.11 Cutaneous lesion following dissemination of *Blastomyces dermatitidis*. (Courtesy of Dr. Carlyn Halde.)

pneumonia, influenza, tuberculosis, and other fungal infections, as well as cancer.[1] Most patients diagnosed with blastomycosis have the onset of chronic pneumonia. In three recent clinical studies, extrapulmonary disease was found in 25–40% of patients studied. The sites of extrapulmonary infection included skin, bone, kidneys, and the urogenital system. In addition, infection has involved the central nervous system, eyes, larynx, paranasal sinuses, tongue, adrenal glands, gastrointestinal tract, liver, and spleen. Approximately 40% of AIDS patients with blastomycosis have an associated central nervous system disease. This is manifested as either mass lesions or meningitis.[1]

Patient evaluation, diagnosis, and differential diagnosis

Growth of *B. dermatitidis* in culture from a suspected case is one of the most reliable diagnostic approaches because serologic testing is unreliable. Visualization of the budding yeast in clinical specimens (Fig. 19.12) or tissue sections is an indication of blastomycosis. In the cutaneous form of the disease, material from the pustules at the outer edge of the lesion or the pus from an open lesion can be examined in a 10–20% potassium hydroxide solution. The yeast consists of thick-walled round cells, 8–15 μm in diameter,

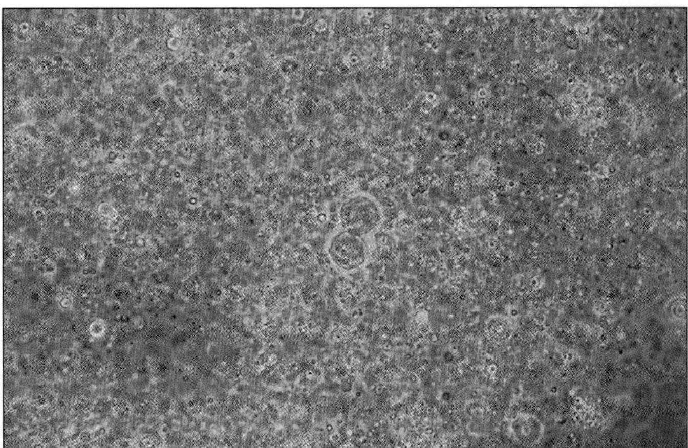

Figure 19.12 Potassium hydroxide preparation of lung tissue containing a round, broadly attached daughter cell. 400×.

that may become as large as 30 μm in diameter. The blastoconidium formed by the parent cell has a broad base of attachment. This is a key feature that allows *B. dermatitidis* to be distinguished from organisms such as *Paracoccidioides brasiliensis* and *Histoplasma capsulatum*. Occasionally, hyphae maybe seen in clinical material collected from sites such as the ear where the body temperature is lower. In pulmonary cases the first morning sputum should be examined for the presence of yeast cells. Researchers are currently working on developing a non-culture-based ELISA.[5]

Pathology

B. dermatitidis infection produces a mixed suppurative–granulomatous inflammatory reaction in the immune-competent patient, with a neutrophilic infiltrate and abscesses predominating in early lesions, and often a predominance of granulomas in older lesions. The granulomas almost always have a microabscess in the center, and it is in this location that the characteristic yeasts are often seen. They can be demonstrated on routine hematoxylin and eosin (H&E) stain, although the GMS is more sensitive, particularly in older lesions where the yeast may be rare. The round yeast ranges from 2 to 30 μm, but most often is 6–15 μm. The thick, refractile cell wall and the broad-based budding are diagnostic. A definitive identification can be rendered on tissue biopsy with confidence when these features are seen.

In the skin, the characteristic abscesses seen early after dissemination from the lung give way to granulomas and chronic inflammation, although, as noted above, small microabscesses are usually present, even in older lesions. Subcutaneous abscesses, which drain to the surface, can be present. The hyperplastic skin lesions, so characteristic of chronic infection and which can be clinically confused with neoplasia, demonstrate marked pseudoepitheliomatous hyperplasia of the epidermis and the exuberant proliferation of the squamous epithelium over and around the infection that can result in intraepidermal abscesses. As noted above, yeasts can be infrequent in chronic skin lesions and examination of multiple sections with a GMS stain may be necessary to arrive at the diagnosis.

Treatment

Practice guidelines for the treatment of blastomycosis have been modified from the NGC.[6] Spontaneous cure has been well documented for non-immunocompromised patients with acute pulmonary infection. All immunocompromised patients and patients with progressive pulmonary infection should be treated. Complicating this management decision, some patients present with serious extrapulmonary disease after the resolution of pulmonary infection. Patients must be carefully evaluated for extrapulmonary disease before a decision is made to withhold therapy.

Patients with life-threatening disease, such as acute respiratory distress syndrome, should be treated[7] with amphotericin B (0.7–1 mg/kg per day; total dose 1.5–2.5 g). Therapy for some patients may be switched to itraconazole (200–400 mg/day) after clinical stabilization with an initial course of amphotericin B, usually a minimum dose of 500 mg.

Patients with mild to moderate disease should be treated with itraconazole at a dosage of 200–400 mg/day for a minimum of 6 months. An alternative to itraconazole includes 6 months of either ketoconazole at a dosage of 400–800 mg/day or fluconazole at a dosage of 400–800 mg/day. For patients who are unable to tolerate an azole or whose disease progresses during azole treatment, therapy should be changed to amphotericin B (0.5–0.7 mg/kg per day; total dose 1.5–2.5 g).

All patients with disseminated disease require treatment. The presence or absence of central nervous system infection is the critical factor for determining therapy. Patients with central nervous system disease should receive a dosage of amphotericin B of 0.7–1 mg/kg per day (total dose at least 2 g). The use of lipid formulations of amphotericin B has not been reported for central nervous system blastomycosis, but this treatment may be an alternative for patients unable to tolerate amphotericin B because of toxicity. Azoles should not be considered for primary treatment of patients with central nervous system blastomycosis. However, fluconazole, because of its excellent cerebrospinal fluid penetration, could be considered at higher dosages (minimum 800 mg/day) in special circumstances.

Patients with life-threatening disseminated disease should be treated with amphotericin B (0.7–1 mg/kg per day; total dose 1.5–2.5 g). Therapy for some patients may be switched to itraconazole after clinical stabilization using amphotericin B. Patients with mild to moderate disseminated blastomycosis that does not involve the central nervous system should be treated with itraconazole (200–400 mg/day) for at least 6 months. Ketoconazole and fluconazole, both at dosages of 400–800 mg/day, are alternatives to itraconazole. Bone disease is more difficult to treat and more likely to relapse. Therefore, patients with blastomycotic osteomyelitis should receive at least 1 year of treatment with an azole. For patients whose disease progresses during treatment with an azole or who are unable to tolerate an azole because of toxicity, amphotericin B (0.5–0.7 mg/kg per day; total dose 1.5–2.5 g) is recommended.

Blastomyces dermatitidis may infrequently act as an opportunistic pathogen, notably in patients who are in the late stages of AIDS, transplant recipients, and patients treated with immunosuppressive or cytotoxic chemotherapy. Disease in these patients is more aggressive and is more often fatal than in the normal host. Pulmonary disease is more likely to present with diffuse pulmonary infiltrates and respiratory failure. Dissemination to multiple organs, including the central nervous system, also occurs more frequently. Mortality rates of 30–40% have been reported, and most deaths attributed to blastomycosis occur during the first few weeks of therapy. Thus, early and aggressive treatment with amphotericin B (0.7–1 mg/kg per day) is indicated for blastomycosis in the immunocompromised patient. Most experts recommend a total dose of 1.5–2.5 g, although treatment for selected patients without central nervous system infection may be switched to itraconazole after clinical stabilization with amphotericin B (usually a minimum dose of 1 g).

Despite amphotericin B treatment, frequent relapses occur in patients with AIDS and in those who have immunosuppressive therapy. Some authorities recommend chronic suppressive therapy with an azole, preferably itraconazole, for those patients who respond to a primary course of amphotericin B treatment. Fluconazole treatment may be given special consideration for selected patients who have had central nervous system disease or patients unable to tolerate itraconazole owing to toxicity or drug interactions.

Amphotericin B is the drug of choice for treating blastomycosis in pregnant women. The azoles should never be used as treatment for this patient cohort because of their embryotoxic and teratogenic potential. Although blastomycosis is less commonly described in children, the clinical spectrum of disease is similar to that described in adults. However, a recent report has indicated that the diagnosis of blastomycosis in children, compared with adults, is more difficult to establish and that the response to oral azoles in children is less than satisfactory. Children with life-threatening or central nervous system disease should be treated with amphotericin B. Itraconazole, at a dosage of 5–7 mg/kg per day, has been used successfully as treatment of a limited number of pediatric patients with non-life-threatening non-central nervous system disease.

References

1. Patterson TF, McGinnis MR. Blastomycosis. Doctor fungus. Available online at: http://www.doctorfungus.org/mycoses/human/blasto/blastomycosis.htm (accessed August 5, 2004).
2. Rippon JW. Medical mycology: the pathogenic fungi and the pathogenic actinomycetes, 2nd edn. Philadelphia, PA: WB Saunders; 1982.
3. Baumgardner DJ, Paretsky DP. The in vitro isolation of *Blastomyces dermatitidis* from a woodpile in north central Wisconsin, USA. Med Mycol 1999; 37:163–168.
4. Chapman SW, Bradsher RW, Campbell DG et al. Practice guidelines for the management of patients with blastomycosis. Clin Infect Dis 2000; 30:679–683.
5. Roomiany PL, Axtell RC, Scalarone GM. Comparison of seven *Blastomyces dermatitidis* antigens for the detection of antibodies in humans with occupationally acquired blastomycosis. Mycoses 2002; 45:282–286.
6. Department of Health and Human Services USA. Practice guidelines for the treatment of coccidioidomycosis. Available online at: http://www.guidelines.gov/summary/summary.aspx?doc_id=2669&nbr=1895&string=blastomycosis (accessed August 5, 2004).

7. Yamada H, Kotaki H, Takahashi T. Recommendations for the treatment of fungal pneumonias. Expert Opin Pharmacother 2003; 4:1241–1258.

Paracoccidioidomycosis (South American blastomycosis)

Sebastião A.P. Sampaio

Introduction

Paracoccidioido mycosis is caused by a dimorphic fungus. *Paracoccidioides brasiliensis* is a systemic granulomatous progressive infection that can affect any tissue of the body, mainly lungs, lymph nodes, oropharyngeal mucosa, and skin. It is an important fungus disease occurring in rural areas.

History

Paracoccidioimycosis was described in São Paulo, Brazil, by Lutz[1] in 1906 and later in other South American countries. The parasite was initially considered to be related to the agent of coccidiomycosis but Almeida[2] in 1930 demonstrated to be a different fungus, which was given the name *Paracoccidioides brasiliensis*.

Epidemiology

The disease occurs in all South American countries except Chile but most cases are found in Argentina, Brazil, Colombia, and Venezuela. It has been reported in Mexico and Central America but does not occur in the Caribbean islands or the USA. Sporadic cases reported in other countries are in patients who have lived in endemic areas with a latency period from a few to 60 years. The prevalence of the paracoccidoidomycosis is related to tropical and subtropical vegetation, acid soil, temperature between 12 and 30°C, 150–1500 m of altitude, and 1000–2500 mm of pluvial annual index.

The disease is found in agricultural workers or persons who lived in the endemic areas. It is more frequent in men than women but this may be due to greater exposure or female protection by 17β-estradiol. It occurs in any age but the highest incidence is between 20 and 60 years of age.

P. brasiliensis lives in the soil or vegetables, probably in an infectious saprobic form. Human infection is by aspiration or direct penetration of the fungus. Direct transmission from the patient to other people does not occur.

The fungus has been isolated from the soil and in the feces of bats (*Artibeus lituratus*), penguins (*Pygoscelis adeliae*), and simian (*Saimiri sciureus*) visceras. There are many reports of the infection in one species of armadillo (*Dasypus novemcinctus*) and recently one case of infection in a dog was described.

The prevalence of paracoccidioidomycosis infection in endemic areas is available from paracoccidioidin tests. Culture tests are currently performed with a polysaccharide of *P. brasiliensis*, according to Fava Netto.[3]

The index of positivity is 6.7–87.0% in different endemic areas. It has been described as a paracoccidioidin test using a specific glycoprotein of 43 kDa (gp43). The paracoccidioidin test could be positive in patients infected with histoplasmosis.

Etiology

P. brasiliensis is a dimorphic fungus, with a cottony mycelial phase in culture at room temperature and creamy or cerebriform phase with yeast-like cells in culture at 37°C. The yeast-like forms appear as spherical cells with a refringent wall, with single or multiple buds (Fig. 19.13). The mycelial phase can be changed to a yeast-like phase using the brain–heart infusion agar (BHIA).

P. brasiliensis can be successfully inoculated in animal species as hamster, albino rat, guinea pig, camondongo (mouse), and in the chorioallantoic membrane of embryonate eggs. It is a eukaryotic fungus which hydrolyzes urea and has glycoproteins, glycopeptides, lipids, and polysaccharides including the α-1–3-glucan which is related to fungus virulence. The antigenic structure of the fungus is complex, with common antigens to *Paracoccidioides loboi* and *Blastomyces dermatitis*. The glycoprotein gp43 is considered to be specific for *P. brasiliensis*. In clinical specimens small round forms, protoplasts, occur and these may be invasive forms.

Clinical features

Paracoccidioimycosis infection

This is a primary infection occurring in endemic areas which may evolve to cure, latency, or disease. Diagnosis is available by a paracoccidioidin test.

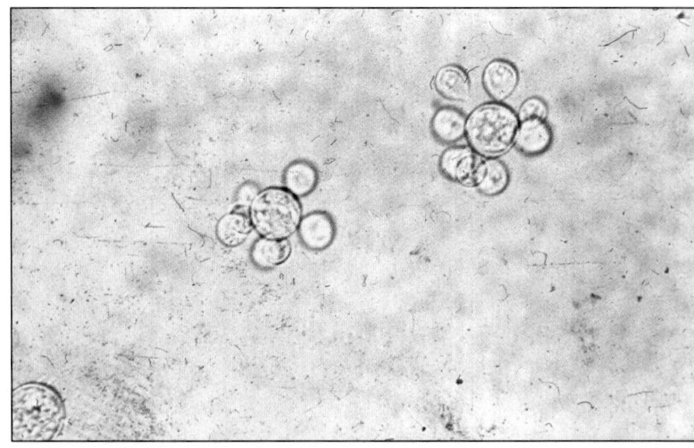

Figure 19.13 *Paracoccidioides brasiliensis* in a yeast-like form, appearing as spherical cells with a refringent wall, with multiple buds.

Paracoccidioidomycosis disease
Acute or subacute forms
Chronic forms

Acute or subacute forms (juvenile paracoccidioidomycosis). It is mainly found in children or adolescents and can be an evolution of primary infection. It is characterized by disseminated adenopathy (Figs 19.14 and 19.15), hepatosplenomegaly, cutaneous ulcerative lesions, and in general absence of oropharyngeal and lung lesions. Both sexes are equally affected.

Chronic forms. Chronic forms may originate from reactivation of the primary focus or occur by inhalation or direct penetration of the fungus. The most frequent route of invasion is through the lungs, followed by oropharyngeal mucosa, gastrointestinal tract, and skin.

Mucocutaneous forms

The lesions are found in the mouth, gingiva, tongue, nose, pharynx, and larynx. The lesions are initially superficial ulcerations and with progression become vegetating, infiltrated ulcerations. Thin granulations on the surface, with hemorrhagic points are characteristic, referred to as moriform stomatitis (Fig. 19.16). Cheilitis and macrocheilitis are frequent, with constant sialorrhea. The presence of hoarseness indicates the involvement of the larynx.

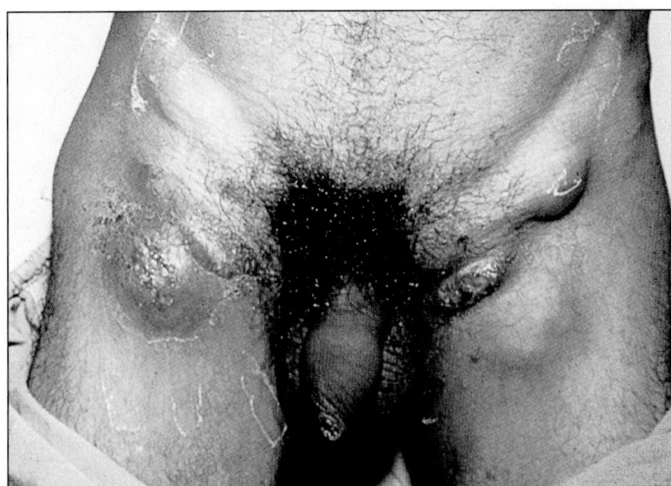

Figure 19.14 Disseminated adenopathy.

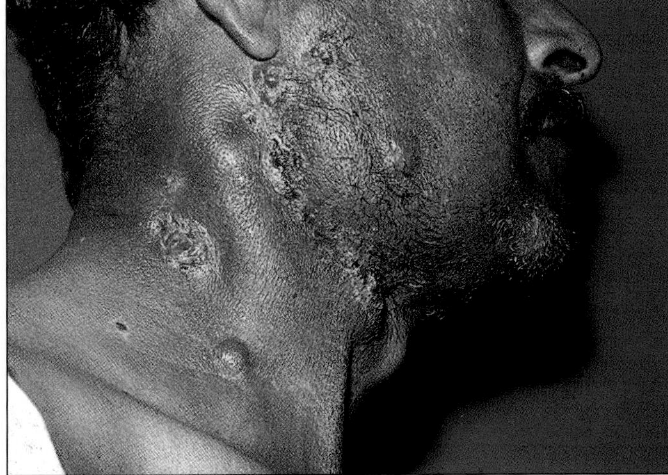

Figure 19.15 Paracoccidioidomycosis with cervical disseminated adenopathy.

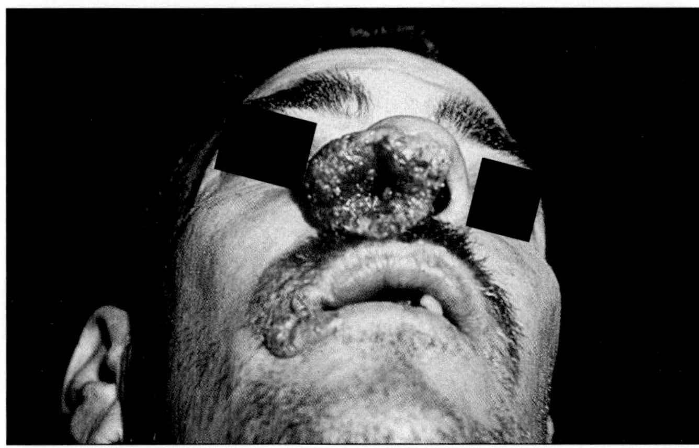

Figure 19.16 Moriform stomatitis and verrucous lesions.

With progression the infection extends to the labial and nasal areas. There is always involvement of the regional lymph nodes and frequently of the lungs.

The skin lesions are single or multiple. A single lesion is seen in the site of penetration of the parasite; it is initially a papule or nodule which evolves to an ulcerative crusty lesion.

Multiple lesions indicate hematogenous dissemination. In varying stages with papules and nodules, ulcerating, vegetating, and verrucous lesions are due to successive disseminations (Figs 19.17 and 19.18).

Lymph nodular forms

The initial manifestation is cervical adenopathy due to penetration of the parasite through the oropharyngeal or respiratory tract. Initially the adenopathy is painless or slightly tender, but with progression the lymph nodes become voluminous and can suppurate and drain. Other aspects of the lymph nodular form occur when the parasite penetrates through the gastrointestinal mucosa, sometimes with extensive intraabdominal adenopathy.

Pulmonary forms

Involvement of the lungs by inhalation or hematogenous spread occurs in 50–80% of patients. In most cases it is asymptomatic or with minimal symptoms and for this reason a chest radiograph is necessary in all patients. The pulmonary lesions are usually bilateral and mainly on the lower two-thirds of the lungs. Pleural involvement is uncommon.

Gastrointestinal forms

Penetration of the parasite through the intestinal mucosa causes a variable symptomatology according to the site of penetration and the involvement of lymph nodes. Intestinal hemorrhage or intestinal obstruction, hepatosplenomegaly, intraabdominal lymph node masses, ascites, and jaundice may occur. Pulmonary involvement is rare.

Disseminated forms

From the primary focus the fungus can reach any tissue of the organism by hematogenous dissemination with varied manifestations. Generalized adenopathy, multiple skin lesions, bone lesions, and hepatosplenomegaly are found. The adrenal glands are frequently involved with the picture of Addison's disease. Nervous

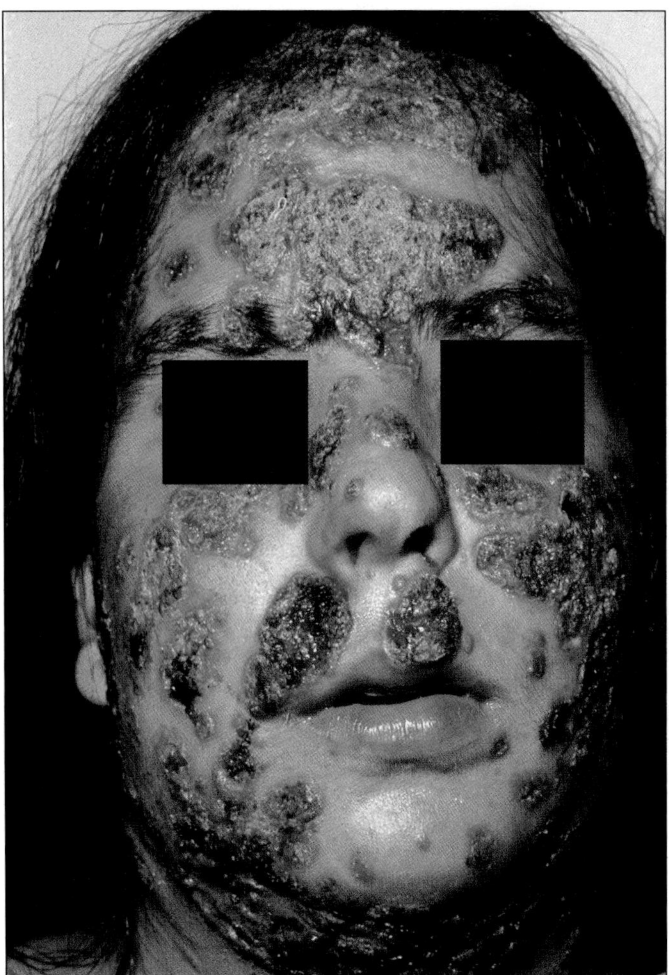

Figure 19.17 Massive dissemination of paracoccidiodomycosis.

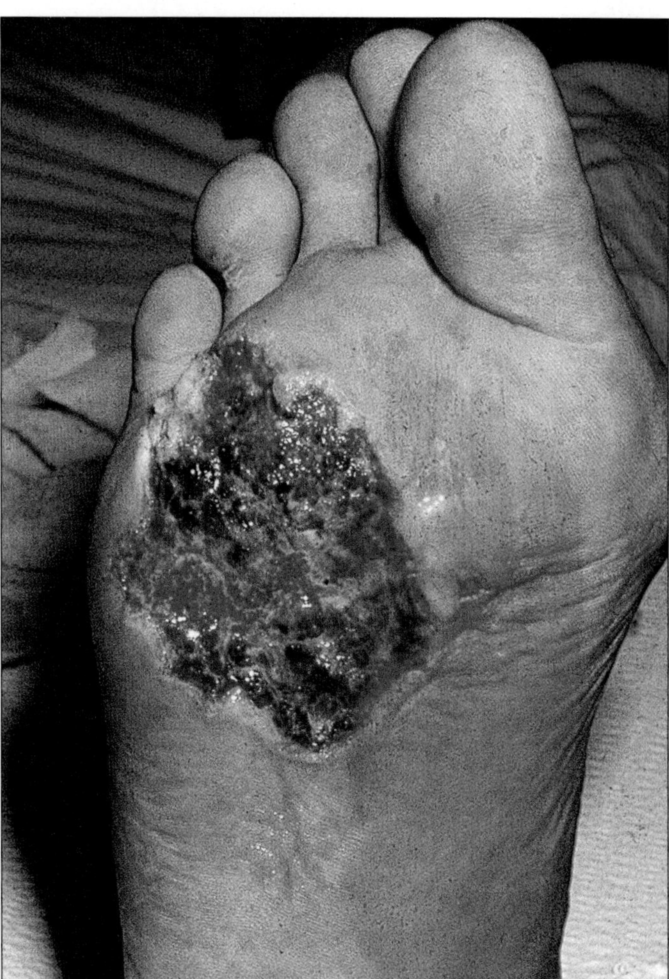

Figure 19.18 Hematogenous dissemination with a verrucous lesion of the foot.

system involvement is also very frequent and for this reason the cerebrospinal fluid must be examined in all cases of the disease.

Differential diagnosis

The clinical picture of paracoccidioidomycosis is very suggestive. The most frequent differential diagnosis with mucosal lesions is with leishmaniasis and occasionally tuberculosis, syphilis, and neoplasia. The cutaneous lesions may be differentiated from leishmaniasis, sporotrichosis, tuberculosis, and syphilis. The lymph nodular form may be distinguished from tuberculosis and Hodgkin's disease.

The juvenile paracoccidioidomycosis must be differentiated from an acute infection.

Paracoccidioides and AIDS

An association between paracoccidioidomycosis and AIDS has been reported. The clinical manifestations are variable, with predominance of an acute or subacute infection, cutaneous and bone lesions, generalized adenopathy, hepatosplenomegaly, and eventually association with tuberculosis.

Laboratory diagnosis

Direct examinations

The fungus can be easily identified in unstained preparations from smears of cutaneous lesions, pus of liquefying lymph nodes, and eventually in sputum. They are very typical spherical cells with a refringent wall, with single or multiple buds. The presence of multiple buds is characteristic of *P. brasiliensis*.

Cultures

Cultures are indicated for investigations. The culture medium used is Sabouraud dextrose agar with cycloheximide and chloramphenicol. Growth is slow, around 30 days, with cottony colonies (mycelial phase) at room temperature. In cultures at 37°C or in BHIA creamy colonies (yeast-like phase) develop.

Inoculations

Inoculations are also indicated for investigations, and are carried out in guinea pig testis, hamster, albino rat, camondongo (mouse), and the chorioallantoic membrane of embryonate eggs.

Histopathology

Histopathology is very useful for the diagnosis. It reveals a granulomatous infiltrate with epithelioid and giant cells and abscess formation. The fungus spores are within giant cells or free in the infiltrate. The spores show single or multiple buds. The presence of multiple buds, giving the appearance of a ship steering wheel, is characteristic of the species. The fungus spores are best seen with PAS or GMS stain. The molecular identification of *P. brasiliensis* by PCR in tissue could be useful for the diagnosis.[4]

Serology

Serology can be useful in the diagnosis but is indispensable during and after treatment.

A decrease in serological titer confirms the clinical improvement and a rise after treatment reveals a relapse. There are many techniques but immunodiffusion is most frequently used. With an antigenic preparation having about 90% gp43, immunodiffusion provides a specificity of 98.9% and a sensitivity of 84.3%. Crossed immunoelectrophoresis has similar sensitivity and specificity. The immunoenzymatic method, ELISA, using antigenic preparation with gp43, is also useful for diagnosis and follow-up. The immunoblotting technique is also promising.

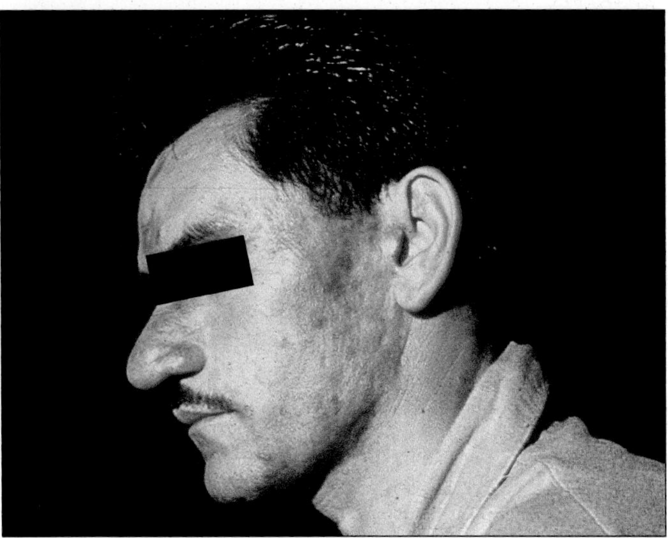

Figure 19.20 Regression of cutaneous and visceral lesions after treatment with amphotericin B.

Treatment

The azoles are the indicated drugs and itraconazole is the first choice. The dose is 200 mg/day for 12–24 months according to clinical and serological improvement. Radiologic evaluation of the pulmonary lesions is very important. Adverse reactions are rare, including hepatotoxicity, which was found with ketoconazole. This was the first azole introduced in the treatment of paracoccidioidomycosis: it is very effective but has some adverse reactions, including hepatotoxicity.[5]

Fluconazole is also effective at a dose of 200–400 mg/day with elective indications for involvement of the nervous system.[6]

Other triazole derivatives which have been successfully tested include saperconazole, voriconazole, and posaconazole.[7] There is a report of a case of paracoccidioidomycosis successfully treated with terbinafine.[8]

Amphotericin B intravenously is very effective and can be used as initial treatment in severe and extensive cases and in treatment-resistant cases (Figs 19.19 and 19.20).[9] The initial dose is 0.25 mg/kg, followed by 0.5 mg/kg and then 1.0 mg/kg per day or on alternate days. The total dosage in one series was 30–80 mg/kg. Amphotericin B is nephrotoxic.

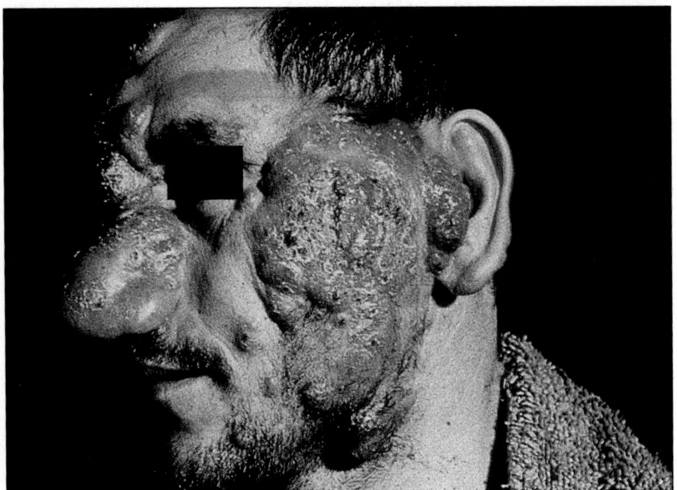

Figure 19.19 Extensive lesions of paracoccidiodomycosis before treatment.

The sulfonamides were the first effective drugs used in paracoccidioidomycosis. Currently the combination of sulfamethoxazole–trimethopim, at a daily dose of 800–1600 mg sulfamethoxazole and 160–320 mg trimethoprim, can be used as maintenance therapy as a substitute for triazole therapy.

References

1. Lutz A. Uma mycose pseudococcidica localizada na bocca e observada no Brasil. Contribuição ao conhecimento das hyphoblastomicoses americanas. Bras Med 1908; 22:121–124.
2. Almeida F. Estudos comparativos do granuloma coccidioidico nos Estados Unidos e no Brasil. Novo genero para o parasito brasileiro. An Fac Med Univ São Paulo 1930; 5:125–141.
3. Fava Netto C, Raphael A. Reação intradermica com polissacaride do *Paracoccidoides brasiliensis*. Rev Inst Med Trop São Paulo 1961; 13:161–165.
4. Gomes GM, Cisalpino PS, Taborda CP et al. PCR for diagnosis of paracoccidioidomycosis. J Clin Microbiol 2000; 38:3478–3480.
5. Cucê LC, Wroclawski EL, Sampaio SAP. Treatment of paracoccidioidomycosis with ketoconazole. Rev Inst Med Trop São Paulo 1981; 23:82-85.
6. Diaz M, Negroni R, Montero-Gei F et al. A pan American 5 year study of fluconazole therapy for deep mycoses in the immunocompetent host. Clin Infect Dis 1992; 14 (suppl.):S68–S76.
7. Carrilo-Munoz AJ, Brio S, Qundóz G. Una nueve generacion de farmacos antifungicos. Rev Iberoam Micol 2001; 18:2–5.
8. Ollague JM, Zurita AM, Calero G. Paracoccidioidomycosis (South American blastomycosis) successfully treated with terbinafine. Br Jr Dermatol 2000; 143:188–191.
9. Dillon NL, Sampaio SAP, Habermann MC et al. Delayed results of treatment of paracoccioidomycosis with amphotericin B plus sulfamides versus amphotericin B alone. Rev Inst Med Trop São Paulo 1986; 28:263–266.

Penicilliosis marneffei

Michael B. Smith, Seema Patel, Jeffery A. Meixner and Michael R. McGinnis

Synonyms: Penicilliosis

Key features:

- *Penicillium marneffei*
- Southeast Asia
- Respiratory infection with dissemination to skin
- Amphotericin B and itraconazole

Introduction

Penicilliosis marneffei is an opportunistic infection that occurs primarily in patients who have AIDS that reside in Southeast Asia. The disease has been described in patients living in other parts of the world who have a travel history to the endemic area. The sole etiologic agent of this disease is the thermally regulated dimorphic fungus *Penicillium marneffei*. Even though a sexual stage for this hyphomycete may exist, it has yet to be discovered.

Following inhalation of conidia, the fungus develops into an intracellular yeast that reproduces by fission. This reproductive process readily distinguishes *P. marneffei* from the intracellular yeast of *Histoplasma capsulatum*, which produces blastoconidia within phagocytic cells. The similarity of the yeast forms of these two dimorphic fungi has resulted in some instances of misidentification of the etiologic agent in some patients, especially in earlier case reports describing infection in patients living in Southeast Asia. Owing to the increased frequency of worldwide travel, penicilliosis marneffei should be considered in the differential diagnosis when intracellular yeasts are detected in tissue sections.

Therapy involves the use of amphotericin B, followed immediately by itraconazole. The relapse rate following successful therapy in AIDS is approximately 50%. For this reason, itraconazole suppressive therapy is required for life in these patients.[1] Primary prophylactic therapy is beneficial in high-risk patient populations to prevent infection. Individuals living in northern Thailand have a substantially higher instance of penicilliosis marneffei than individuals living in other parts of Southeast Asia.

Pathogenesis and etiology

It is believed that the infection is initiated following the inhalation of conidia with subsequent dissemination to lymph nodes, liver, spleen, lung, intestine, bone marrow, and skin. The fungus is probably a soil hyphomycete that grows on organic plant material. It has been isolated from soil as well as from captured bamboo rats that live in underground burrows. When isolation data are plotted on a topographic map of the endemic area, the fungus appears to be associated with higher elevations. This observation is supported by the 6.8% frequency of *P. marneffei* infection in AIDS patients living in northern Thailand compared to the frequency of 0.4–1% in those living in central, northeast, and south Thailand.[2] The infection has been reported among HIV-infected persons in Thailand, Myanmar (Burma), Vietnam, Cambodia, Malaysia, northeastern India, Hong Kong, Taiwan, and southern China, as well as persons living in the USA, the UK, France, Germany, Italy, the Netherlands, Sweden, Switzerland, Australia, and Japan after visiting the endemic region.[3] Penicilliosis marneffei is consistently found in AIDS patients who have low CD4 (+) T-cell lymphocyte counts. An average CD4 (+) T-cell lymphocyte count of 63.8 cells/μl was noted for a cohort of patients studied at Chiang Mai University, Thailand.[4] The presence of penicilliosis marneffei is one of the indicators of AIDS in Thailand.

The reticuloendothelial system is the primary target of *P. marneffei*. *P. marneffei* can cause two clinical types of the disease; focal and fatal progressive, disseminated infections. Symptoms of infection include fever (97–99% of patients), anemia (78–86% of patients), weight loss (76–100% of patients), generalized lymphadenopathy (58% of patients), hepatomegaly (51% of patients), diarrhea, chronic coughing, and typical skin lesions consisting of papules having central necrotic umbilication (71–81% of patients)[5–7] (Fig. 19.21). Oral lesions usually occur in patients with disseminated disease and manifest as shiny papules, erosions, shallow ulcers covered with whitish yellow, necrotic slough, or a combination of all of these. The lesions may occur on the palate, gingiva, labial mucosa, tongue, and oropharynx. In advanced cases of AIDS, the fungus often disseminates by hematogenous means to various organs, especially the skin. Skin disease appears as multiform rashes and as molluscum contagiosum-like papules in late stages of infection.

Patient evaluation, diagnosis, and differential diagnosis

Because the fungus disseminates by hematogenous means, bone marrow aspirates, blood smears, and biopsies of skin and superficial lymph nodes are excellent specimens for diagnosis.[8] ELISA and latex agglutination tests have been developed for the serologic

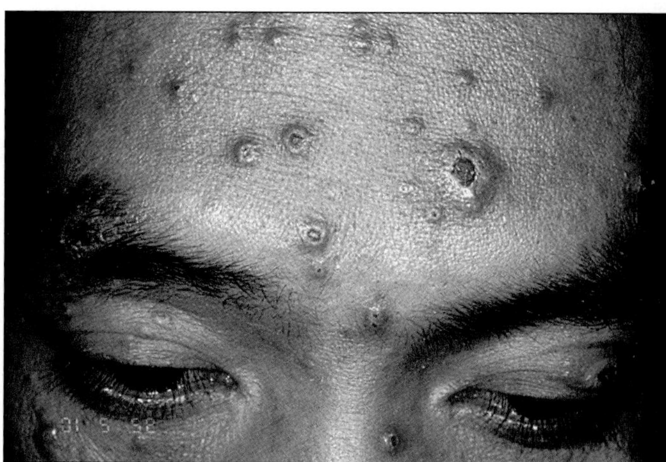

Figure 19.21 Cutaneous lesions following hematogenous dissemination of *Penicillium marneffei* in a patient with acquired immunodeficiency syndrome (AIDS).

diagnosis of penicilliosis marneffei.[9–11] The fungus is readily isolated from skin lesions, as well as blood and bone marrow. The signs and symptoms of penicilliosis marneffei have features in common with other infections seen in immunocompromised patients, including tuberculosis, molluscum contagiosum, cryptococcosis, and histoplasmosis.[12]

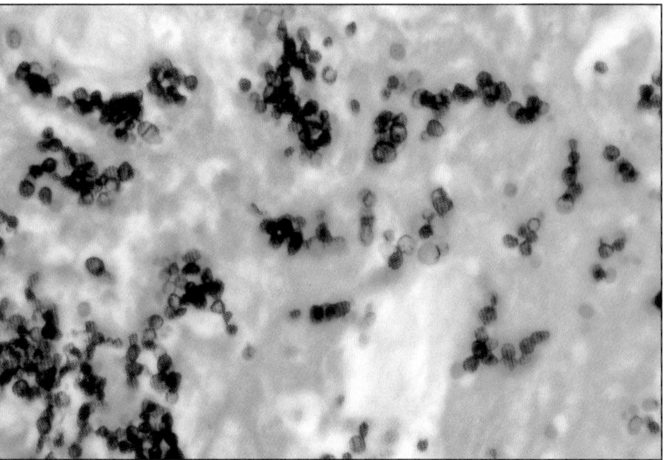

Figure 19.22 Lung tissue showing yeast cells of *Penicillium marneffei* reproducing by fission. Gomori methenamine silver, 1000x. (Courtsey of Dr. Chester Cooper Jr.)

Pathology

In tissue, the histologic manifestations of *P. marneffei* infection can be variable, ranging from distinct to poorly formed granulomas, to a mixed suppurative histiocytic reaction. Similarly, the fungus, which grows as a yeast at 37°C, also shows morphologic variability. The yeasts, which may be found intracellularly in histiocytes or extracellularly, can be oval, spherical, or elongate in shape, and can range from 3 to 12 μm along their longest axis (Fig. 19.22). When found in histiocytes they are more often at the smaller end of their range, oval, and show less variation in size and shape than when present extracellularly, where elongate, slightly curved "sausage-shaped" yeasts may be found. Because the size and some features of the morphology of *P. marneffei* overlap that of other pathogenic fungi, particularly *H. capsulatum*, careful observation by the histopathologist of the absence of blastoconidium development on the part of *P. marneffei* is important. *P. marneffei*, which reproduces in vivo by fission, will demonstrate the presence of cross-walls or transverse septa in yeasts rather than budding. Although the cross-walls can be seen on routine stains, they are especially well demonstrated using a silver impregnation stain such as GMS, Grocott's, or the PAS stain. Identification of these cross-walls is diagnostic of *P. marneffei*.

Treatment

Itraconazole and ketoconazole are the drugs of first choice for mild to moderately severe forms of the disease, whereas parenteral therapy with amphotericin B may be required for seriously ill patients. The current recommended treatment regimen is amphotericin B 0.6 mg/kg per day for 2 weeks, followed by itraconazole 400 mg/day orally in two divided doses for 10 weeks.[7] After the initial treatment, immunocompromised patients should be given 200 mg/day itraconazole for life[1] because recurrence of the disease is common. Itraconazole primary prophylaxis in patients having CD4 (+) T-cell lymphocyte counts of less than 100 cells/μl can prevent both penicilliosis marneffei and cryptococcosis.[2]

References

1. Supparatpinyo K, Perriens J, Nelson KE et al. A controlled trial of itraconazole to prevent relapse of *Penicillium marneffei* infection in patients infected with the human immunodeficiency virus. N Engl J Med 1998; 339:1739–1743.
2. Chariyalertsak S, Supparatpinyo K, Sirisanthana T et al. A controlled trial of itraconazole as primary prophylaxis for systemic fungal infections in patients with advanced human immunodeficiency virus infection in Thailand. Clin Infect Dis 2002; 34:277–284.
3. Sirisanthana T, Supparatpinyo K. Epidemiology and management of penicilliosis in human immunodeficiency virus-infected patients. Int J Infect Dis 1998; 3:48–53.
4. Vanittanokom N, Sirisanthana T. *Penicillium marneffei* infection in patients infected with human immunodeficiency virus. Curr Top Med Mycol 1997; 8:35–42.
5. Sirisanthana T. *Penicillium marneffei* infection in patients with AIDS. Emerg Infect Dis 2001; 7 (suppl. 3):561.
6. Ranjana KH, Priyokumar K, Singh TJ et al. Disseminated *Penicillium marneffei* infection among HIV-infected patients in Manipur state, India. J Infect 2002; 45:268–271.
7. Sirisanthana T, Supparatpinyo K, Perriens J et al. Amphotericin B and itraconazole for treatment of disseminated *Penicillium marneffei* infection in human immunodeficiency virus-infected patients. Clin Infect Dis 1998; 26:1107–1110.
8. Mo W, Deng Z, Li S. Clinical blood routine and bone marrow smear manifestations of disseminated penicilliosis marneffei. Chin Med J 2002; 115:1892–1894.
9. Desakorn V, Simpson AJ, Wuthiekanun V et al. Development and evaluation of rapid urinary antigen detection tests for diagnosis of penicilliosis marneffei. J Clin Microbiol 2002; 40:3179–3183.
10. Panichakul T, Chawengkirttikul R, Chaiyaroj SC et al. Development of a monoclonal antibody-based enzyme-linked immunosorbent assay for the diagnosis of *Penicillium marneffei* infection. Am J Trop Med Hyg 2002; 67:443–447.
11. Chaiyaroj SC, Chawengkirttikul R, Sirisinha S et al. Antigen detection assay for identification of *Penicillium marneffei* infection. J Clin Microbiol 2003; 41:432–434.
12. Cooper CR Jr, McGinnis MR. Pathology of *Penicillium marneffei*. An emerging acquired immunodeficiency syndrome-related pathogen. Arch Pathol Lab Med 1997; 121:798–804.

Chapter 20

Meningococcal disease

Charles Moon and Jeffrey Meffert

Synonyms: Meningococcemia, meningococcal sepsis, meningococcal meningitis, cerebrospinal fever, epidemic cerebrospinal meningitis

Key features:

- Infections with bacteria of the species *Neisseria meningitidis* are the most common cause of community-acquired bacterial meningitis
- The disease may occur in seasonal epidemics and targets the young
- Severe flu-like symptoms predominate initially with nausea, vomiting, headache, severe myalgias, rash, and possibly sepsis, with or without meningeal signs
- 50% develop a petechial or purpuric cutaneous eruption with predilection for the trunk and limbs
- Early recognition and treatment with penicillin or appropriate empiric cephalosporin therapy will decrease mortality

Introduction

Meningococcemia presents as a flu-like illness in an otherwise healthy child or young adult. Initial symptoms may include a petechial or purpuric rash, headache, nausea, vomiting, myalgia, and fever with or without meningeal signs. The gold standard for diagnosis is isolation of *N. meningitidis* from sterile body fluids, to include cerebrospinal fluid (CSF) or blood. Treatment with appropriate systemic antibiotic agents must be initiated without delay if the diagnosis of systemic meningococcal infection is suspected. Aggressive management of shock and disseminated intravascular coagulation in an intensive care unit setting may also be required. This condition carries an approximate mortality rate of 10–15% if treated promptly, but a 90% fatality rate if left untreated. Recognition of cutaneous findings by the health care provider may help expedite the diagnosis and prevent delay in treatment.

History

Meningococcal disease was first described in 1805 after a meningitis outbreak occurred in Geneva.[1] However, it was not until 1882 that Anton Weichselbaum isolated the responsible pathogen from the CSF of an infected patient.[2] In 1909, immunologically distinct serotypes of the bacteria were identified.[3] The advent of sulfonamides and penicillin and their use for chemoprophylaxis and treatment drastically reduced the incidence of disease and mortality rates during and after World War II.

Epidemiology

N. meningitidis exclusively infects humans and causes both endemic and epidemic infection. These attacks occur with seasonal variation, exhibiting the highest frequency in February and March, and the lowest in September. There is no sex predisposition. Large-scale epidemics still occur with devastating consequences in Africa, parts of Asia, countries of the former Soviet Union, and South America, but remain endemic in most western developed countries.[4]

There are at least 13 serogroups of *N. meningitidis*, determined by polysaccharide capsule composition, with the overwhelming majority of worldwide disease caused by serogroups A, B, C, Y, and W-135. The largest outbreaks, which originated in northern China and spread globally, were caused by strains of serogroup A. This serogroup still accounts for the majority of disease in Asia. In 1987 serogroup A strains spread from China to the Middle East, causing a massive epidemic among pilgrims during the Haj in Mecca. Today, major African epidemics are associated with serogroups A and C; however, the W-135 serogroup caused an epidemic in 2000 and 2001 among pilgrims returning from the Haj in Mecca, Saudi Arabia. In 2002, serogroup W-135 also emerged in Burkina Faso, killing approximately 1500. In most industrialized countries, serogroup B strains have been the predominant infectious strains.

In northwestern Europe, periodic hyperendemic infections have occurred in the last three decades. Similar group-B isolates have also emerged in Brazil, the USA, Israel, Australia, New Zealand, China, Thailand, Spain, North Africa, and northern Europe.[4]

An equatorial region of sub-Saharan Africa, referred to as the meningitis belt, displays a high burden of invasive meningococcal disease. The countries of Burkina Faso, Ghana, Togo, Benin, Niger, Nigeria, Chad, Cameroon, Central African Republic, The Sudan, Ethiopia, Mali, Guinea, Senegal, and Gambia comprise this region (Fig. 20.1). Outbreaks due to serogroup A and occasionally C occur annually in this hyperendemic region, causing predictable, devastating disease.[5]

Epidemic spread of meningococcal disease is not entirely understood but it appears that the occurrence of invasive meningococcal disease is determined by the virulence of certain bacterial strains, the susceptibility of the population, and certain risk factors (Box 20.1) that enhance transmission. The most important of these risk factors is nasooropharyngeal carriage.[6]

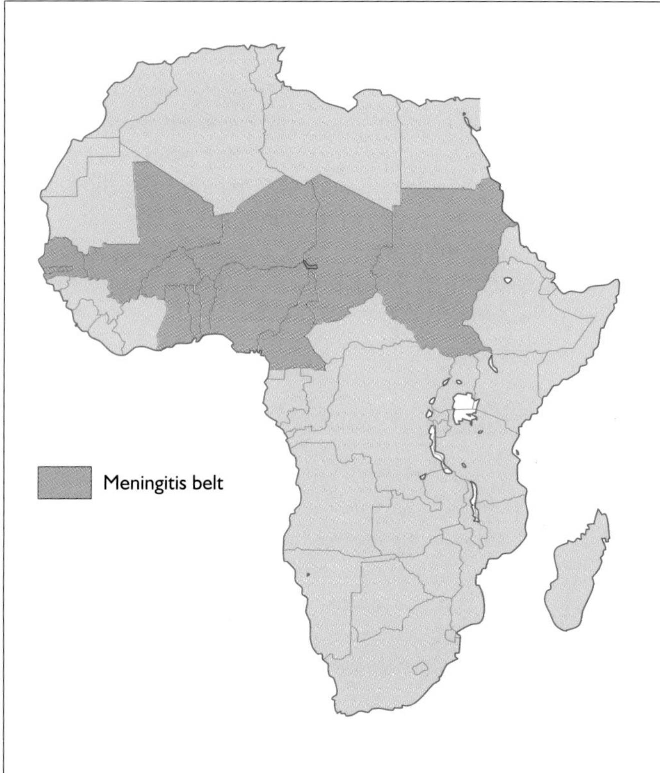

Figure 20.1 The countries of the meningitis belt.

Box 20.1 Risk factors for epidemics

Nasooropharyngeal carriage
Host risk factors
Smoking
Preceding respiratory tract infection

Box 20.2 *Neisseria meningitidis* virulence factors

Pili	**Lipoligosaccharide**
Opacity (adhesion) proteins	Polysaccharide capsule
Antigenic variation	Phase switching
Immunoglobulin A protease	

Pathogenesis

Neisseria meningitidis, a fastidious bacterium, is a Gram-negative kidney-bean-shaped diplococcal obligate aerobe. Of particular importance are virulence factors (Box 20.2 and Fig. 20.2), which allow the organism to invade tissue and evade immune responses. Phase switching and antigenic variation of these virulence factors further magnify the pathogenicity of these organisms.

Four conditions must exist before invasive meningococcal disease can occur. These include: (1) exposure to a pathogenic strain of bacteria; (2) colonization or nasopharyngeal carriage; (3) penetration of epithelial mucosa; and (4) survival of *N. meningitidis* in the host's blood stream.[7]

1. Meningococci are transferred from person to person by direct contact or via droplets. The carriage rate of meningococci is higher in lower socioeconomic classes, crowding, and in conditions where people from different regions congregate. Climatic conditions may play a role in bacterial survival after expulsion from the nasopharynx.[4]

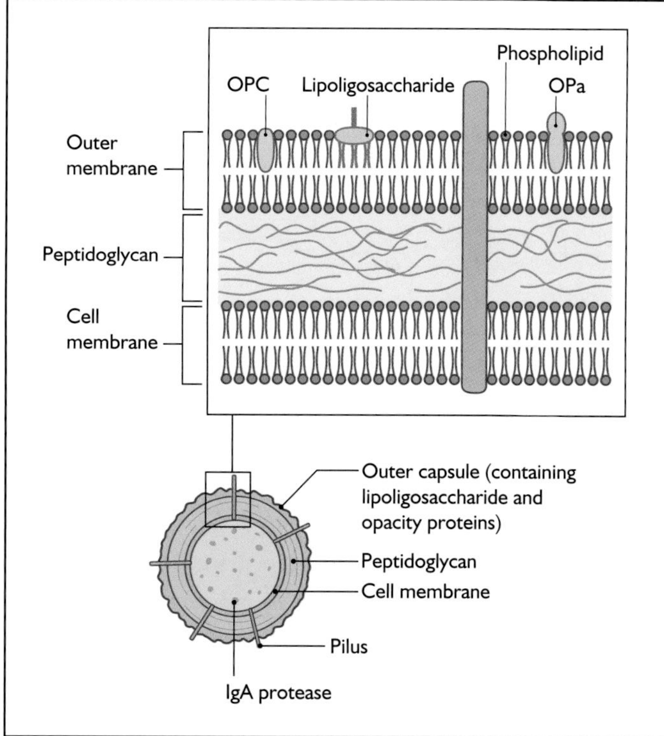

Figure 20.2 Schematic representation of *Neisseria meningitidis* structure and virulence factors.

2. The presence of a virulent strain colonizing the naso-oropharyngeal mucosa of a non-immune host precedes clinical disease. Colonization of mucosa most likely occurs if the ciliated epithelium is damaged by exposure to tobacco smoke, preceding viral or bacterial infections, and/or direct trauma. Pili, glycosylated protein appendages on the bacterial surface, are the major adhesins that facilitate attachment of meningococci to epithelial cells. Interaction with the host cell is also facilitated by adhesion proteins, dubbed opacity proteins (Opa proteins A, B, D and Opc), on the outer membrane of the bacteria.[4]
3. Penetration of the epithelial cell then follows. Upon contact, cytoskeletal changes mediated by adhesion molecules (pili, Opc, Opa) occur within the epithelial cell. This allows passage through the mucosal epithelium via phagocytic vacuoles for transport to the basolateral surface of the cell. It appears that a neisserial immunoglobulin A (IgA) protease cleaves lysosomal associated membrane protein, promoting bacterial survival inside epithelial cells during trafficking. This IgA protease can also be released by the cell and is responsible for cleaving host secretory IgA.[4]
4. Once in the blood stream, meningococci proliferate and survive by virtue of their polysaccharide capsule and lipooligosaccharide (LOS) coating in the setting of incomplete host defenses. Capsular polysaccharides provide a physical barrier, protecting against complement-mediated bacteriolysis and phagocytosis. LOS or endotoxin (similar in structure and effects to lipopolysaccharide (LPS), found in enteric Gram-negative pathogens) plays a role in infectivity. The release of endotoxin in the form of vesicular outer-membrane structures called blebs allows bacteria to evade host defenses (complement fixes on shed blebs instead of organism) and contributes to endotoxemia. High levels of endotoxin, in conjunction with massive cytokine release and unimpeded complement activation, promote septic shock, vessel wall damage, disseminated intravascular coagulation (DIC), and increased mortality.[4]

A naive or defective host immune system may further contribute to the pathogenicity of meningococci. Innate defenses such as complement-mediated bacteriolysis via the mannose-binding lectin or alternative complement pathway, and opsonization and phagocytosis, provide initial immune defenses since antibodies may take longer than a week to develop. Defects in these innate, early defenses (particularly deficiencies in the late-acting complement components C5–C8) may predispose individuals to rapid, invasive disease. Other factors, such as splenectomy, immunosuppressive drugs, cellular immune defects, or autoimmune diseases, may further contribute to host susceptibility.

Clinical features

Meningococcal disease may present with a variety of manifestations, ranging from a transient flu-like illness to fulminant disease with rapid clinical deterioration. Once the bacteria enter the blood stream and the host is unable to clear the infection rapidly, invasive disease, characterized classically into four presentations, will develop.[4,8]

1. Bacteremia without signs of shock. These patients may have a relatively low load of bacteria that is effectively cleared from the blood stream. In these cases, individuals present with a transient febrile, flu-like syndrome, and intense myalgias. These individuals do not develop meningeal signs or shock.
2. Acute meningococcemia with shock but no meningitis. These patients are septic, febrile, and often hypotensive at presentation. Patients will complain of headache, a rash, weakness, intense myalgias, and general malaise. Fever and vomiting are often the only presenting symptoms in young children, infants, and the elderly.
3. Acute meningitis without meningococcemia or signs of shock. These patients present with headache, fever, and meningeal signs but without evidence of bacteremia or shock. The spinal fluid parameters will suggest a bacterial process.
4. Acute meningoencephalitic manifestation (fulminant meningococcemia and meningitis). These patients may present obtunded with signs of advanced sepsis and meningeal signs. Abnormal behavior, nerve palsies, long tract signs, and seizures are variably present.

Since, headache, confusion, and stiff neck may be present in less than half of patients with invasive meningococcemia, cutaneous findings may be a helpful adjuvant in establishing the correct diagnosis. Cutaneous lesions are classically described as petechial, but may not always be present. They are small and have a smudged pale or gun-metal gray color, often with a vesicular center (Fig. 20.3).[9] Lesions are most commonly located on the extremities and trunk (Fig. 20.4), especially in areas where pressure is applied to the skin (i.e., belts, elastic straps), but may also be found on the head, palms, soles, and mucous membranes such as the soft palate and conjunctivae. These cutaneous lesions are the result of damage to small dermal blood vessels from the organisms, the immune system, and endotoxin. This damage leads to erythrocyte extravasation, thrombosis, and subsequent necrosis.[10] Typically, in

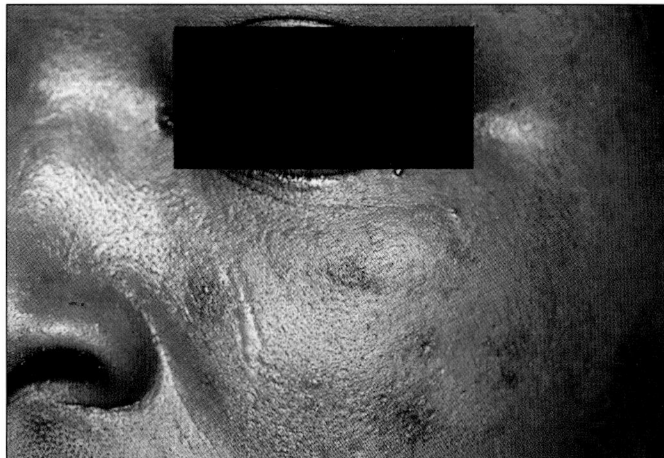

Figure 20.3 Early cutaneous lesions of meningococcemia. (Courtesy of Dr. Luc Van Kaer.)

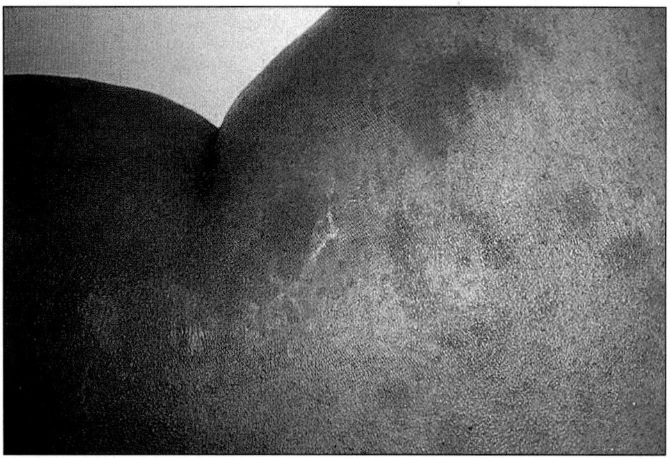

Figure 20.4 Cutaneous lesions of meningococcemia on the lower extremity. (Courtesy of Dr. Luc Van Kaer.)

fulminant meningococcal disease, skin lesions appear 6–18 h after onset of symptoms and may not be present in approximately 20% of patients. Extensive vesiculobullous, pustular lesions and hemorrhagic gangrenous areas resembling purpura fulminans can appear in patients with DIC (Fig. 20.5). These petechiae and hemorrhagic areas may be an important indicator not only of vessel wall damage, but also of thrombocytopenia related to DIC and impending hematologic complications. Aside from a variety of petechial or hemorrhagic lesions, a macular and papular rash suggestive of rubella may develop early in the course. This non-petechial eruption fades rapidly (hours to 2 days), and may be misdiagnosed as a viral xanthem.

Chronic meningococcemia is a unique entity associated with persistent meningococcal bacteremia. Clinically these patients present with fever, arthritis, and cutaneous lesions that may resemble those seen in chronic subacute gonococcemia. Initially fever is present, but this generally fades and the patient experiences arthralgias and joint edema, anorexia, weight loss, and myalgias. A rash usually accompanies the fever and fades as the fever recedes. The cutaneous lesions have a variety of manifestations, ranging

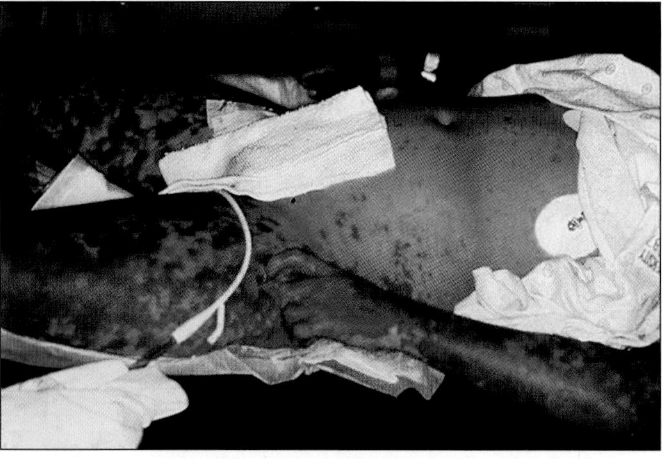

Figure 20.5 An example of purpura fulminans in this patient with fulminant meningococcal disease. (Courtesy of Dr. Luc Van Kaer.)

from pale or rose-colored macules (30% of cases), to erythema nodosum-like tender nodules, and petechiae or hemorrhagic lesions. The rash and fever recur weeks to months later with an average interval of 6–8 weeks. Untreated, this subacute illness may progress to acute meningococcemia, endocarditis, and meningitis.[11]

Rarely, meningococcemia may result in unusual septic complications, including arthritis, cranial nerve dysfunction, endocarditis, and pericarditis with tamponade. *N. meningitidis* may also cause a primary, acute bacterial conjunctivitis, more commonly seen in children. Progression to systemic disease may occur rapidly in approximately 20% of cases, so aggressive treatment is warranted. Meningococcal pneumonia is a well-recognized form of community-acquired disease. These patients have an excellent prognosis with a low incidence of sepsis and minimal cutaneous findings.

Patient evaluation, diagnosis, and differential diagnosis

Early diagnosis of meningococcemia may be difficult to establish. Typically, the patient will present non-specifically and may demonstrate transient clinical improvement, concealing impending deterioration. At this stage the neck is supple, overt signs of meningitis and shock are absent, and the initial skin manifestations appear more like a viral rash. Unfortunately, examination of body fluids at this stage is typically inconclusive. After the bacteria breach the blood stream and are not rapidly cleared, invasive disease, characterized by shock and meningitis, develops. At this stage, isolation of the organism is more easily performed, but the delay in instituting therapy may have grave consequences.

The gold standard for diagnosing invasive meningococcal disease is isolation of *N. meningitidis* from sterile fluids such as CSF, blood, skin, or synovial fluid. With meningitis, CSF examination reveals polymorphonuclear leukocytosis, increased protein, reduced glucose, and the presence of organisms on Gram-stained smears of fluid. In patients with meningitis alone, blood cultures may only be positive in one-third of patients. The organisms, however, are typically recovered from the CSF, even when overt signs of meningitis are lacking.[12] Cultures will be positive even when antibiotics are given within 1 h of CSF sampling. In cases of acute meningococcemia and shock, blood cultures will typically be positive in 100% of patients. At this stage, demonstration of organisms from skin lesions may provide another way of identifying the pathogen. Care must be exercised in demonstrating organisms from cutaneous lesions due to the presence of Gram-negative commensals commonly found on the skin. Some reports cite positive demonstration of organisms in 50–80% of skin aspirates, biopsies, or smears of lesions.[12] The positive demonstration of organisms from skin may confirm the diagnosis, but a negative finding does not exclude the possibility of meningococcemia.

Aside from Gram staining and culture, there are other available means of detecting *N. meningitidis* from body fluids. Kits utilizing latex beads coated with antibodies to capsular antigens are available for testing body fluids such as CSF and urine, but not blood.[13] These tests have low sensitivity for capsular serogroup B, however. PCR is yet another means of detecting organisms in body fluids. These tests have excellent sensitivity and may play a broader future

Box 20.3 Differential diagnosis for acute invasive meningococcal infection

Systemic bacteremias:
- *Neisseria gonorrhoeae*
- *Streptococcus pneumoniae* and group A streptococci
- *Staphylococcus aureus*

Staphylococcal toxic shock syndrome
Acute bacterial endocarditis
Rickettsial disease
Leukocytoclastic vasculitis
Leptospirosis
Viral infections
- Coxsackie
- Echoviridae
- Rubeola (measles)

role in rapidly identifying, typing strains in epidemics, and assessing antibiotic sensitivity.[14]

As mentioned previously, establishing the diagnosis of invasive meningococcal infection is challenging since many conditions present with fever and a petechial or hemorrhagic eruption, with or without signs of meningitis (Box. 20.3). The following conditions, if encountered, should prompt consideration of meningococcal disease.[15]

Acute bacteremias

Systemic bacteremias can cause a fulminant picture not unlike invasive meningococcal disease. This includes organisms such as *Streptococcus*, *Staphylococcus*, *Haemophilus*, and conditions such as endocarditis (especially if staphylococcal in origin). Often patients with these conditions will have petechial or hemorrhagic eruptions. DIC may be present, leading to areas of massive hemorrhage and gangrene, like those seen in fulminant meningococcal infections. Neurological symptoms may be present due to embolization and cerebral implantation of organisms (especially in cases in endocarditis). The presence of a heart murmur, splinter hemorrhages, Osler's nodes, and Janeway lesions may help distinguish endocarditis from meningococcemia. In many cases when the patient is profoundly ill, appropriate broad-coverage antibiotics are required while awaiting species identification.

Toxic shock syndrome

This multisystem disorder is also characterized by similar constitutional symptoms and fever, with various cutaneous manifestations and hematological disturbances. Although blood cultures may be positive in 15% of cases, most of the symptoms are caused by toxic shock syndrome toxin-1 produced by *Staphylococcus aureus* infection or colonization.

Viral infection

Viral infections can cause fever, a petechial eruption, and aseptic meningitis, often following a non-specific upper respiratory infection. This is particularly true of Echo- and Coxsackie viruses. Measles is another viral condition that may be considered, but the presence of cough, coryza, conjunctivitis, and Koplik spots may help distinguish this entity.

Leukocytoclastic vasculitis

This is a common cause of petechiae. The absence of fever or acute illness may help distinguish this entity, although they may be present in cases such as Henoch–Schönlein purpura or other systemic vasculitides.

Rickettsial disease

Rocky Mountain spotted fever often causes intense headache, a cutaneous eruption that may be petechial, and fever. The presence of a tick bite and travel or residence in an endemic area may be helpful clues to this diagnosis.

Leptospirosis

This condition is characterized initially by an acute febrile syndrome, which is followed by aseptic meningitis and rash. Hemorrhagic cutaneous and systemic manifestations may be seen with specific serotypes of leptospirosis (Weil's syndrome).

Acute gonococcemia

Acute gonococcemia, caused by *Neisseria gonorrhoeae*, is an entity that may bear a resemblance to meningococcal infection. Typically, disseminated gonococcal infection is characterized by fever, polyarthralgias with arthritis, tenosynovitis, and rarely meningitis (the arthritis–dermatitis syndrome). This may closely mimic the chronic form of invasive meningococcal infection (see Box. 20.4 for the differential diagnosis of chronic meningococcal infection). The cutaneous manifestations of these two entities, however, have different distinguishing features. The lesions of gonococcemia typically appear acrally, around joints, are few in number, and evolve from petechiae or papules into vesicles or pustules on a necrotic or hemorrhagic base (Fig. 20.6).

Pathology

A biopsy of the classic cutaneous lesion associated with invasive meningococcal disease reveals vasculitis, fibrin thrombi, and fibrin extravasation in the small blood vessels of the dermis. Infiltrates of neutrophils and lymphocytes are seen around vessels and there is some mild leukocytoclasia. Pustular lesions reveal epidermal and subepidermal collections of neutrophils. Gram-negative intracellular diplococci within neutrophils may be seen at high power using tissue Gram stains (Fig. 20.7).[16]

Box 20.4 Disease characterized by periodic fever, skin lesions, and joint involvement that resemble chronic meningococcemia

Subacute bacterial endocarditis
Acute rheumatic fever
Ratbite fever
Gonococcemia
Brucellosis

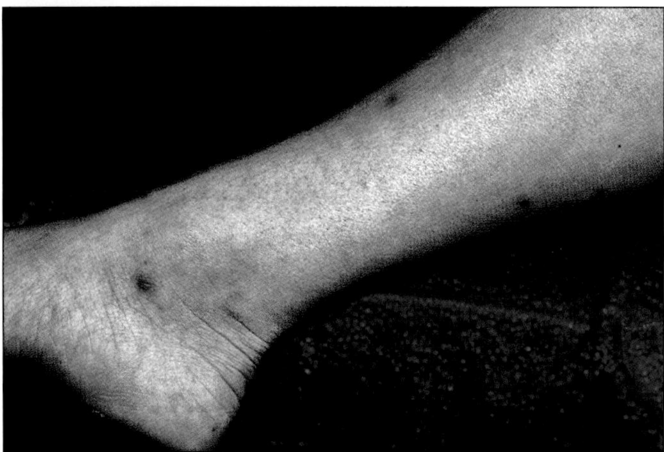

Figure 20.6 Classic cutaneous lesions associated with disseminated gonococcal infection.

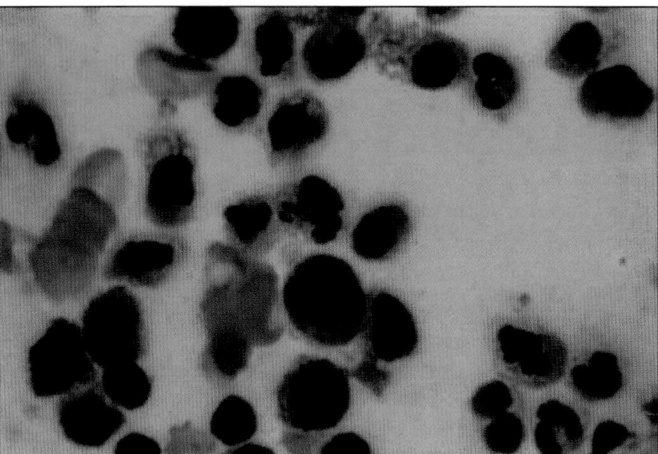

Figure 20.7 Note the neutrophil with intracellular Gram-negative diplococci in the center of this photomicrograph of a peripheral blood smear. (Courtesy of Dr. Luc Van Kaer.)

Treatment

The principles of treatment involve appropriate antibiotic selection, aggressive supportive care, and carriage eradication for patients and contacts. The mortality in developed countries with access to medical care and antibiotics is typically under 10%. A less favorable outcome can be expected with inadequate medical services or in non-epidemic random cases where the diagnosis may be overlooked. Once the diagnosis of invasive meningococcal disease is suspected, there should be no delay in instituting proper medical care.

The development of antibiotics in the last century has revolutionized the treatment of meningococcal infections and has decreased mortality and postinfectious sequelae. First-line antibiotic treatment is penicillin G with 4 million units IV/IM every 4 h for 5–14 days or 7 days after fever has resolved. Penicillin should not be introduced intrathecally due to the risk of severe neurotoxicity. Treatment of chronic meningococcemia does not typically require such high doses. Some cases of relative resistance have been reported secondary to reduced affinity of penicillin-binding proteins and rare reports of high-level resistance due to β-lactamase-producing strains have emerged in the UK, the USA, and Spain. In penicillin-allergic patients, chloramphenicol can be effectively substituted. This antibiotic should be administered IV at 50–100 mg/kg per day up to a maximum of 4 g/day or 1 g q.i.d. As with penicillin, rare reports of chloramphenicol-resistant strains have emerged.[17]

Third-generation cephalosporins may be used for the empiric treatment of meningitis in children. Specifically, ceftriaxone and cefotaxime achieve levels in the CSF several magnitudes higher than the susceptibility of meningococcus to these agents. A regimen of 10–14 days of therapy is generally sufficient for cases of invasive meningococcal infection.[18] Although penicillin is still the agent of choice for meningococcal infection, these cephalosporins may be beneficial for empiric treatment of bacterial meningitis, in cases of penicillin-resistant meningococci, drug hypersensitivity reactions that preclude the use of penicillin or chloramphenicol, and in situations where once-daily dosing is necessary.[4,17,18]

Eradication of nasal carriage in the patient and close contacts is an important aspect of therapy. Close contacts are generally defined as household contacts, college dormitories, long-term care hospitals, nursery schools, day-care centers, and military barracks. Medical hospital or office-based personnel are generally not at risk unless there is an intimate exposure where exchange of secretions could have occurred (mouth-to-mouth resuscitation). When penicillin is used for treatment, there may still be colonization with the infecting strain of *N. meningitides*. It is generally accepted that rifampin is an effective form of therapy and can eradicate carriage for 6–10 weeks after treatment, but rifampin-resistant meningococci have emerged in approximately 10–30% of treated patients. Minocycline has been used for carriage eradication and is efficacious, but the side-effect of vertigo may have limited its use. Ciprofloxacin, ofloxacin, and azithromycin single-dose oral therapy is also effective in eradicating nasopharyngeal carriage. Single-dose IM ceftriaxone has also been shown to eradicate nasal carriage for 14 days after therapy. See Box 20.5 for recommended antibiotic eradication strategies.[4,17,19]

Aside from rapid institution of appropriate antimicrobial therapy, aggressive supportive measures are often necessary to improve outcomes in cases of invasive meningococcal disease. Most importantly, it is important to recognize individuals with signs of fulminant meningococcal disease since these patients will have

Box 20.5 Suggested prophylaxis/eradication strategies

Rifampin
- Adults: 600 mg PO q 12 h × 4 doses
- Children > 1 month: 10 mg/kg q 12 h × 4 doses
- Children < 1 month: 5 mg/kg q 12 h × 4 doses

Ciprofloxacin
- Adults: 500 mg PO single dose

Ofloxacin
- Adults: 400 mg PO single dose

Ceftriaxone
- Adults 250 mg IM single dose
- Children <15 years 125 mg IM single dose

Azithromycin
- Adult 500 mg PO single dose

Box 20.6 Indicators of poor prognosis

Extremes of age
Rapid development of symptoms
Absence of meningitis
Progressive or widespread skin lesions
Shock demonstrated by slow capillary refill
Acral coolness
Moderately elevated or normal C-reactive protein serum concentration
Absence of leukocytosis
High concentrations of cytokines (interleukin-6, tumor necrosis factor, interleukin-1, interferon-gamma)

the highest mortality. Indicators of fulminant meningococcal disease and poor prognosis are shown in Box 20.6.[4]

Polysaccharide vaccines have been developed from groups A, C, Y, and W-135 of *N. meningitidis* and a quadrivalent vaccine is available that confers protection for these four subtypes. These vaccines have proven safe and effective in preventing meningococcal disease in individuals over 2 years of age.[20] Common side-effects include irritability in children and injection site reactions. The vaccines seem to be poorly immunogenic in children younger than 2 years of age and currently there is no effective group-B vaccine. In these situations, chemoprophylaxis, as described above, is indicated in lieu of vaccination for secondary cases of meningococcal disease. Immunization protection has a lag of 1–2 weeks, as would be expected for adequate antibody production, but may confer resistance, although variable, for up to 3 years.[17]

References

1. Vieussaeaux M. Mémoire sur le maladie qui a régné à Genève au printemps de 1805. J Med Chir Pharmacol 1805; 11:163.
2. Weichselbaum A. Ueber die Aetiologie der akuten Meningitis cerebrospinale. Fortschr Med. 1887; 5:573.
3. Dopter C. Etude de quelques germes isolés du rhino-pharynx, voisins du méningocoque (parameningocoques). CR Soc Biol (Paris) 1909; 67:74.
4. Van Deuren M, Brandtzaeg P, Van de Meer JWM. Update on meningococcal disease with emphasis on pathogenesis and clinical management. Clin Microbiol Rev 2000; 13:144–166.
5. Riedo FX, Plikaytis BD, Broome CV. Epidemiology and prevention of meningococcal disease. Pediatr Infect Dis 1995; 14:643–657.
6. Stephens DS. Unlocking the meningococcus: dynamics of carriage and disease. Lancet 1999; 353:941–942.
7. Schwartz B, Moore PS, Broome CV. Global epidemiology of meningococcal disease. Clin Microbiol Rev 1989; 2 (suppl.):S118–S124.
8. Wolfe RE, Birba CA. Meningococcal infections at an army training center. Am J Med 1968; 44:243–255.
9. Feldman HA. Meningococcal infections. Adv Intern Med 1972; 18:177.
10. Sotto MN, Langer B, Hoshino-Shimizu S et al. Pathogenesis of cutaneous lesions in acute meningococcemia in humans: light, immunoflourescent, and electron microscopic studies of skin specimens. J Infect Dis 1976; 133:506.
11. Ploysangam T, Sheth AP. Chronic meningococcemia in childhood: case report and review of the literature. Pediatr Dermatol 1996; 13:483.
12. Hoyne AL, Brown RH. 727 meningococcal cases, an analysis. Ann Intern Med 1948; 28:248–259.
13. Muller PD, Donald PR, Burger PJ et al. Detection of bacterial antigens in cerebrospinal fluid by latex agglutination test in 'septic unknown' meningitis and serogroup B meningococcal meningitis. S Afr Med J 1989; 76:214.
14. Ni H, Knight AI, Cartwright K et al. Polymerase chain reaction for diagnosis of meningococcal meningitis. Lancet 1992; 340:1432.
15. Weinberg AN, Morton NS. Gram-negative coccal and bacillary infections. In Freedburg IM, Eisen AZ, Wolff K et al, eds. Fitzpatrick's dermatology in general medicine, 5th edn. New York: McGraw-Hill; 1997:2232–2237.
16. Weedon D. Cutaneous infections and infestations-histological patterns. In: Weedon D, ed. Skin pathology, 2nd edn. Edinburgh: Churchhill Livingstone; 2002:527–528.
17. Apicella MA. *Neisseria meningitidis*. In Mandell ML, Bennett JE, Dolin R, eds. Principles and practices of infectious diseases, 5th edn. Philadelphia: Churchill Livingstone; 2000:2228–2242.
18. Neu HC. Cephalosporins in the treatment of meningitis. Drugs 1987; 34:S135–S153.
19. Centers for Disease Control and Prevention. Control and prevention of meningococcal disease and control and prevention of serogroup C meningococcal diseases. Evaluation and management of suspected outbreaks. Morb Mortal Wkly Rep 1997; 46(RR-5):1–22.
20. Ball R, Braun MM, Mootrey GT. Safety data on meningococcal polysaccharide vaccine from the vaccine adverse event reporting system. Clin Infect Dis 2001; 32:1273.

Chapter 21

Staphylococcal and streptococcal pyodermas

Paul M. Benson and Ulrich R. Hengge

Key features:

- Pyodermas caused by Gram-positive cocci are a significant cause of morbidity and comorbidity in developing countries
- Antibiotic resistance, empiric and inadequate therapy, and cost of new antibiotics impede efforts to reduce prevalence of cutaneous skin infections
- Toxin production is associated with increased severity and mortality of infections
- Poststreptococcal glomerulonephritis may occur
- Lack of resources (clean water, sanitation, public health surveillance) contributes to morbidity and persistence of pyodermas

For the future, the main challenge is to keep the wealthier parts of the world, where most medical research and development takes place, interested in the problems of their less affluent tropical neighbors. Many of these drug-resistant tropical infections do not respect international borders, and their ecology is likely to change with increasing international travel and global warming.

Introduction

Throughout the tropical world and developing countries, the Gram-positive cocci, *Staphylococcus aureus* and *Streptococcus pyogenes*, are a major health problem and a significant cause of morbidity among both children and adults. No large-scale epidemiological studies have been performed recently but numerous regional and local prevalence surveys of bacterial pyodermas attest to the widespread nature of these infections. In a 1993 survey of skin diseases in rural East Africa, the prevalence of dermatoses in children was 32%, with over a quarter of these dermatoses (27%) being bacterial infections.[1] The lack of skilled dermatological care, paucity of affordable antibiotics, and an alarming increase in the prevalence of antibiotic-resistant organisms are cited as reasons for the high levels of cutaneous infections in these regions. Equally important, however, is the need to address socioeconomic issues such as poverty; high household density (crowding); lack of clean water; chronic debilitating conditions such as malnutrition, intestinal parasites and malaria, and inadequate health education, which contribute to a persistence of cutaneous infections in the developing world. Bacterial pyodermas along with dermatophytoses and scabies represent the "dermatoses of poverty" which will not decrease until living standards improve.

The relationship between the human host and bacteria is a complex interplay of factors, including virulence of the pathogen, toxin production, size of the inoculum, intrinsic host defenses, integrity of the skin, and nutritional and immunological status of the host and environmental factors such as heat, humidity, and occlusion. In developing countries and the tropics certain factors, such as nutritional status, vitamin deficiencies, lack of sanitation and hygiene as well as heat and humidity play much larger roles in initiation and maintenance of skin diseases than in industrialized nations. An effective approach to reducing the burden of cutaneous infections requires not only an awareness of the pathogens and antibiotic susceptibilities, but also of the factors which lead to persistence of disease. This chapter will examine skin infections caused by the two groups of medically important Gram-positive cocci, *Staphylococcus aureus* and *Streptococcus pyogenes*.

Table 21.1 Differential diagnosis of impetigo

Tinea corporis	Annular, scaly, erythematous patches, intensely pruritic; vesicles may be present	Potassium hydroxide-positive, fungal culture
Herpes simplex	Grouped tense vesicles on an erythematous, edematous base; shallow, coalescing erosions	Tzanck prep, DNA, culture
Varicella	Febrile prodrome; tense vesicles on base ("dewdrop on rose petal"); crops of lesions in various stages	Tzanck prep, DNA, culture
Scabies	Punctate papulovesicles, burrows in web spaces of fingers, axillae, areolae, genitalia; intense pruritus	Scabies prep
Contact dermatitis	Sharply demarcated erythema with blisters and scaling	Epicutaneous testing

Classification of skin infections caused by Gram-positive cocci

Bacterial skin infections (pyodermas) may be primary (i.e., impetigo, ecthyma, cellulitis) when they arise on normal skin or secondary when they complicate existing conditions such as atopic dermatitis, dermatophytosis, and scabies. Infections caused by Gram-positive cocci (Table 21.1) are also classified as either superficial or deep.

Staphylococcal infections of the skin

The superficial staphylococcal pyodermas are classified as follows:

- Impetigo and bullous impetigo
- Folliculitis
- Furunculosis and carbunculosis
- Paronychia

Impetigo and bullous impetigo

Synonyms:

- Impetigo: impetigo contagiosa, impetigo vulgaris
- Bullous impetigo: tropical impetigo, impetigo bullosa

Key features:

- Worldwide, primarily caused by *Staphylococcus aureus*, greater frequency of *Streptococcus pyogenes* in the tropics; also mixed infections
- Two forms: impetigo contagiosa (non-bullous) and bullous impetigo (caused by toxin-secreting *Staphylococcus aureus*)
- Primary and secondary types exist
- Streptococci colonize normal skin; staphylococci may colonize the anterior nares
- Acute glomerulonephritis may complicate streptococcal skin infections

History

The word "impetigo" is a Middle-English (fourteenth-century) derivation of the Latin word "impetere," literally meaning "to attack." It has come to mean a pustular skin condition, usually involving the face, characterized by the formation of scabs and crusts.

Epidemiology

Impetigo (non-bullous impetigo) occurs most frequently in children, with an equal distribution of males and females. It is common in hot, humid climates which encourage the growth of staphylococci on the skin. Worldwide, the non-bullous form of the disease is now caused predominantly by *Staphylococcus aureus*, with a minority of cases caused by *Streptococcus pyogenes* (group A β-hemolytic streptococci), or both.

Bullous impetigo, caused exclusively by strains of *Staphylococcus aureus* which secrete a toxin (exfoliatin), occurs most often in children under the age of 2.[2]

Clinical findings

The early clinical presentation of impetigo is that of grouped, fragile, thin-roofed vesicles which rapidly become cloudy pustules and then rupture. The resulting secondary lesions consist of patches of honey-colored, erythematous and crusted erosions which are most often found on the face, neck, and extremities. In most cases, patients are otherwise well but regional lymphadenopathy may be present.[3]

In temperate climates bullous impetigo is more common in newborns, but in warm tropical environments it may present as an acute bullous eruption of the axillae, groin, and hands in adults. In the neonatal period, it develops within the first 2 weeks of life with lesions initially developing on the face and hands. Later, lesions may generalize to cover large parts of the body. Bullae are typically large, tense, and cloudy and rupture easily, leaving a shiny, varnish-like crust over the affected area.

Histopathology

A skin biopsy of an intact lesion shows an accumulation of neutrophils below the stratum corneum of the epidermis with a few rounded acantholytic cells. Numerous Gram-positive cocci are seen. In the bullous form, a thin layer of stratum corneum forms the roof of the blister which is filled with inflammatory cells and bacteria.

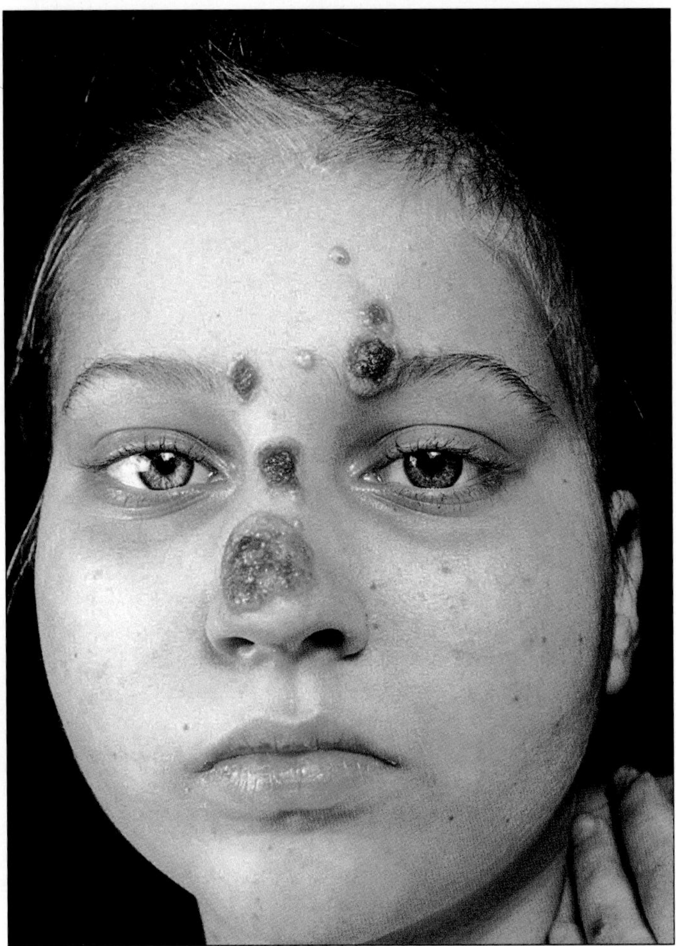

Figure 21.1 Impetigo contagiosa. Several plaques with yellowish crusts on the face.

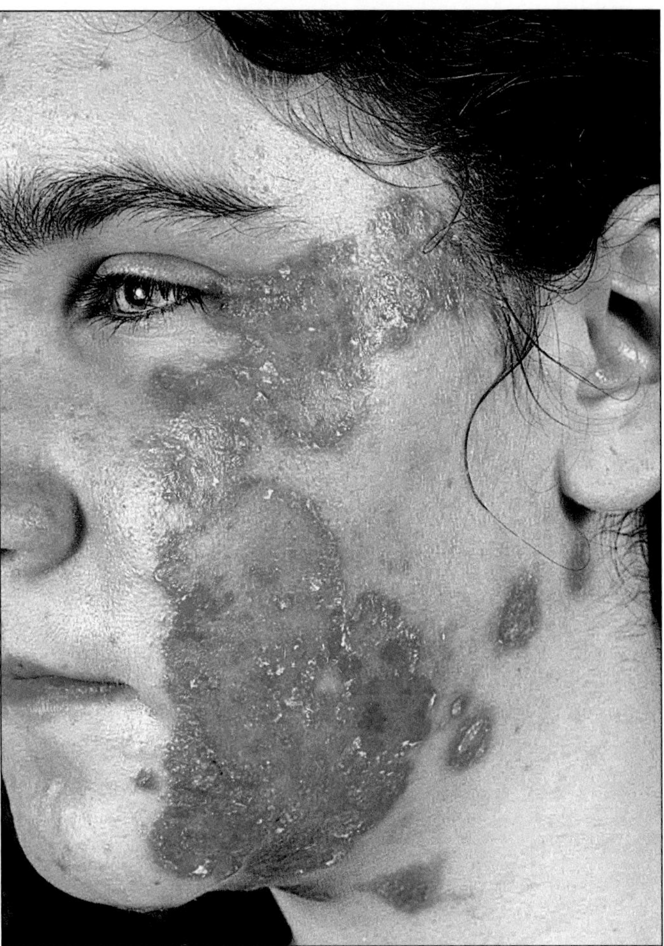

Figure 21.2 Tinea in the face complicated by impetigo. Sharply demarcated erythema with yellowish crusts on the left cheek.

Diagnosis and differential diagnosis

Primary non-bullous impetigo is generally diagnosed on clinical grounds, although laboratory support is occasionally necessary (Fig. 21.1). It is important to remember that impetigo frequently complicates several underlying dermatoses such as scabies, insect bites, atopic dermatitis, or dermatophytosis (Fig. 21.2). Therefore, it is important to accurately diagnose and treat any underlying disorder to reduce the risk of relapse (Table 21.1).

In situations where laboratory confirmation is important (epidemics, failure to respond to previous therapy, concern over nephrogenic streptococci), a Gram stain from an intact pustule or the base of the erosion will show Gram-positive cocci in chains (streptococci) or clusters (staphylococci). Culture on selective media with antibiotic sensitivities is necessary when methicillin resistance is suspected or when there is a failure to respond to appropriate therapy.

Table 21.2 Therapeutic options for non-bullous staphylococcal impetigo

Topical agents
Bacitracin ointment
Mupirocin cream, ointment
Erythromycin
Oral agents
Erythromycin
Dicloxacillin
Oxacillin
Cephalexin

Treatment

The decision to use topical or oral antibiotics must be made on the basis of extent of disease, age and health status of the patient, presence of constitutional symptoms, and response to previous therapy. Table 21.2 outlines therapeutic options for treating non-bullous impetigo. Limited disease can be treated with frequent washing with hot soapy water followed by twice- or three times-daily application of a topical antibiotic for a week. For more extensive disease systemic antibiotics are recommended.

Folliculitis

Synonyms: Impetigo of Bockhart, superficial pustular folliculitis

Key features:

- *Staphylococcus aureus* is the usual pathogen
- Other pathogens include *Candida, Pseudomonas, Pityrosporum*, herpes simplex virus as well as chemical irritants and human immunodeficiency virus (HIV)-associated eosinophilic folliculitis
- Tense yellowish pustules are pierced centrally by a hair; usual locations are the scalp, face, axillae, upper back, inguinal area, buttocks, and extremities
- Diagnosis is made on Gram stain, potassium hydroxide, Tzanck prep, or culture if needed
- Topical antibiotics are given for localized disease, while oral antibiotics are administered for widespread, resistant, or deeper folliculitis

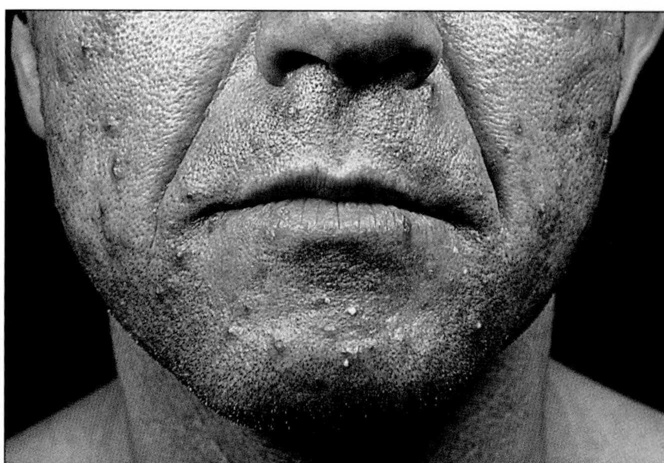

Figure 21. 4 Numerous small folliculitis lesions, some of which are crusted in the beard area: also called beard folliculitis.

History

The term "folliculitis" is a derivation of the Latin word "folliculus," literally meaning "follicle," therefore an inflammation or infection of a follicle.

Epidemiology

Folliculitis is more common in those who are obese or have diabetes mellitus. There are many causes, including bacteria (Gram-positive; occasionally Gram-negative, i.e., "hot tub folliculitis"), yeasts (*Candida albicans*, *Pityrosporum*), viruses (herpes simplex), sterile inflammation (eosinophilic folliculitis), and various chemicals.

Clinical findings

The hallmark lesion of staphylococcal folliculitis is an intact pustule pierced by a hair (Fig. 21.3). Lesions may occur over any area of hair-bearing skin but are particularly common on the scalp, face, axillae, upper back, inguinal folds, buttocks, and the extensor surfaces of the arms and legs. The pustules may be painless, painful, or pruritic and are often clustered in a hair-bearing area. Gram-negative folliculitis is frequently caused by *Enterobacter*, *Klebsiella*, *Escherichia coli*, *Pseudomonas aeruginosa*, and *Proteus mirabilis*. Antibiotic treatment selected depends on the infectious organism. Beard folliculitis is common and may develop into deeper abscesses (Fig. 21.4).

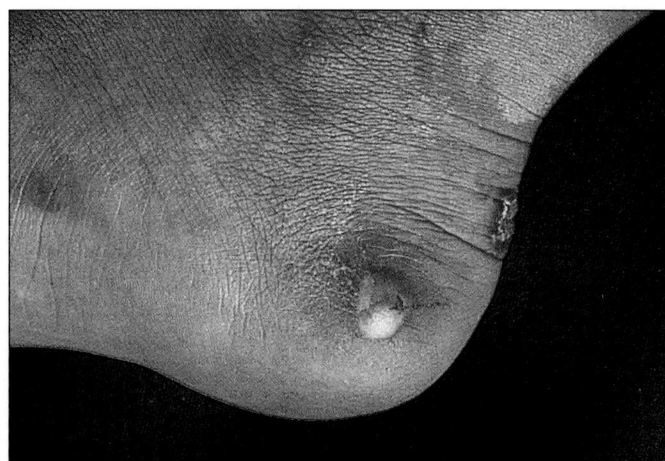

Figure 21.3 Folliculitis: a large pustule containing staphylococci on the heel.

Furuncles and carbuncles

Synonyms: Furuncle: abscess, boil

Key features:

- A deep suppurative extension of a primary abscess
- Emergency surgical and antibiotic treatment are required

Furuncles (abscesses) develop from infected hair follicles and expand by destruction of perifollicular tissue (Fig. 21.5). Several furuncules may coalesce and form carbuncles. Recurrent or multicentric furuncles may indicate immunodeficiency, diabetes, hypergammaglobulinemia, or chronic granulomatosis.

Antibiotic resistance

An alarming increase in staphylococcal resistance to affordable antibiotics has been reported worldwide and is due in part to the widespread, indiscriminate use of antibiotics for questionable indications, often in subtherapeutic doses.[4] For example, recent surveys have found that methicillin-resistant *Staphylococcus aureus* accounts for almost 50% of hospital-acquired staphylococcal infections in the USA. Two patterns of resistance are emerging: a hospital-acquired, highly drug-resistant organism and a community-acquired isolate with a more limited resistance pattern which is susceptible to penicillinase-resistant penicillins. These findings have important health implications for developing countries with limited resources and burgeoning health issues.

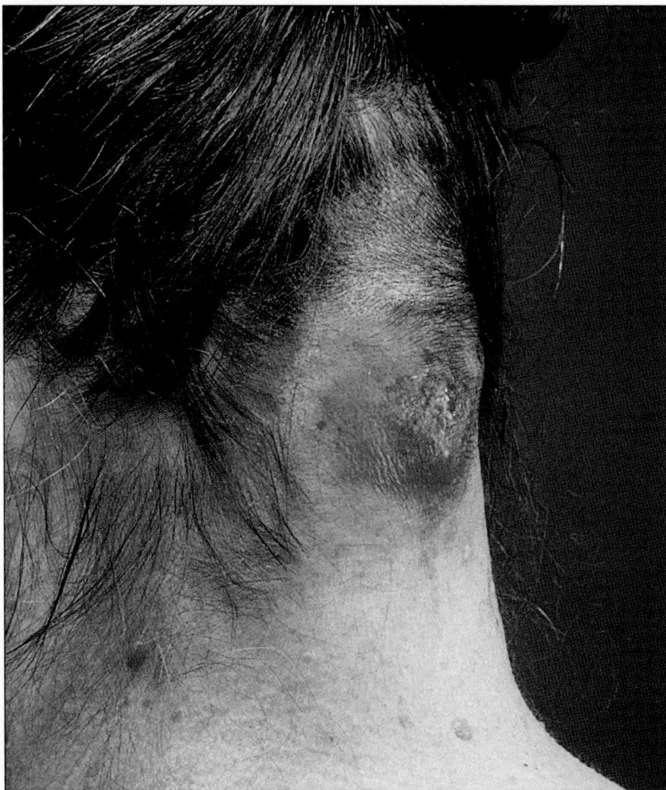

Figure 21.5 Highly inflammatory abscess in the neck with incipient purulation.

Streptococcal pyodermas

Streptococcal infections of the skin are classified as follows:

- Ecthyma infectiosum
- Perianal streptococcal dermatitis and vulvovaginitis
- Erysipelas and cellulitis
- Streptococcal necrosis.

Ecthyma infectiosum

Key features:

- Children, elderly, and malnourished individuals are at risk
- Lesions are present on the lower legs, ankles, and feet; they may be single or multiple
- A thick, gray-yellow adherent crust overlies a painful, punched-out ulcer
- Regional lymphadenopathy, lymphangitis, cellulitis, and sepsis may occur
- Lesions result in scarring
- Oral or parenteral semisynthetic penicillin or cephalosporin is the preferred treatment

Introduction

Ecthyma represents a deep, ulcerative form of impetigo occurring on the lower extremities that results in scarring. The disorder may rarely lead to complications such as lymphangitis, suppurative lymphadenitis, cellulitis, and bacteremia. There is debate over which Gram-positive coccus is primarily responsible for causing the disease. Both group A β-hemolytic streptococci (*Streptococcus pyogenes*) and *Staphylococcus aureus* have been isolated from primary lesions.[5,6]

Epidemiology

The incidence worldwide is unknown but it is less common than impetigo. There does not appear to be any racial or ethnic predilection. Predisposing factors include heat and humidity, poor hygiene, malnutrition, and crowding. The disease is more common in children, the elderly, diabetics, and immunosuppressed (HIV-infected) individuals. During the Vietnam war, streptococcal ecthyma of the legs and feet was the most common cutaneous bacterial infection reported.[7]

Clinical presentation

The primary lesion, which frequently develops after minor trauma, is a vesicle or small bulla. The blister enlarges and then ruptures, leaving a thick, adherent yellow-gray crust. Removal of the crust reveals a punched-out ulcer with an elevated and indurated border (Fig. 21.6). The ulcers may be solitary or multiple, 0.5–3.0 cm or more in diameter, and can be quite painful. Regional lymphadenopathy is common but lymphangitis, suppurative lymphadenitis, and cellulitis are rare. Extension beyond the dermis into the underlying subcutaneous fat, muscle, and tendon may occur and lead to gangrene and sepsis.

Untreated, the lesions heal slowly over several weeks. A shallow hyperpigmented or hypopigmented scar results. Acute poststreptococcal glomerulonephritis has been reported to occur in approximately 1% of cases.[6]

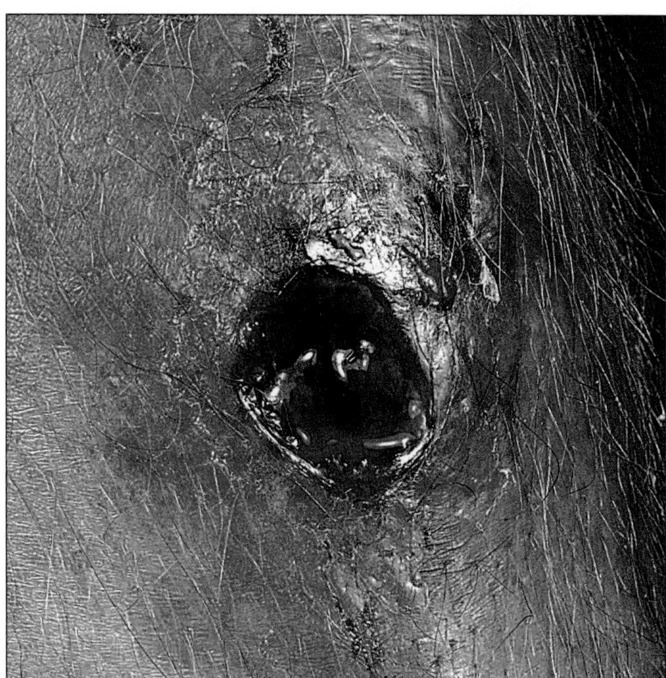

Figure 21.6 Ecthyma caused by *Streptococcus pyogenes:* a sharply demarcated ulcer on the shin with prominent perilesional inflammation.

Erysipelas

Synonyms: St. Antony's fire

Key features:

- The initial lesion expands rapidly through lymphatic vessels
- The presentation (blistering or hemorrhagic erysipelas) or course (recurrent erysipelas) may be atypical
- Appropriate treatment and management are key to resolution

Erysipelas is a superficial bacterial skin infection that characteristically extends into the cutaneous lymphatics (Fig. 21.7). While this infection is classically caused by *Streptococcus pyogenes* and occurs on the face, recent studies have indicated a shift in the distribution and etiology of this disease along with a dramatic increase in incidence and severity manifesting as streptococcal necrosis (Fig. 21.8).

Predisposing factors, such as minor trauma, venous insufficiency, stasis ulcerations, inflammatory dermatoses, dermatophyte infections, insect bites, and surgical incisions, have been implicated as portals of entry. Cases of erysipelas have been reported in all age groups, but it does appear that infants, young children, and elderly patients are the most commonly affected groups.

Clinical Presentation

Clinically, erysipelas presents as an acutely expanding overly warm fiery-red erythema, frequently on the face or chin. Symptoms may include fever, malaise, burning, tenderness, and chills. Lymphangitis and tender draining lymph nodes may be present.

Besides the typical presentation, leukocytosis, elevated erythrocyte sedimentation rate, and increased C-reactive protein are laboratory signs of erysipelas. Other useful tests include urinanalysis screening for hematuria/proteinuria, and antistreptolysin O and anti-DNAase B titers. Bacterial cultures are most often negative due to the intralymphatic spread of organisms. Biopsy and imaging studies are usually not necessary.

The histology of erysipelas includes marked dermal edema, vascular dilatation, and streptococcal invasion of lymphatics and tissues. This bacterial invasion results in a dermal inflammatory infiltrate consisting of neutrophils and mononuclear cells.

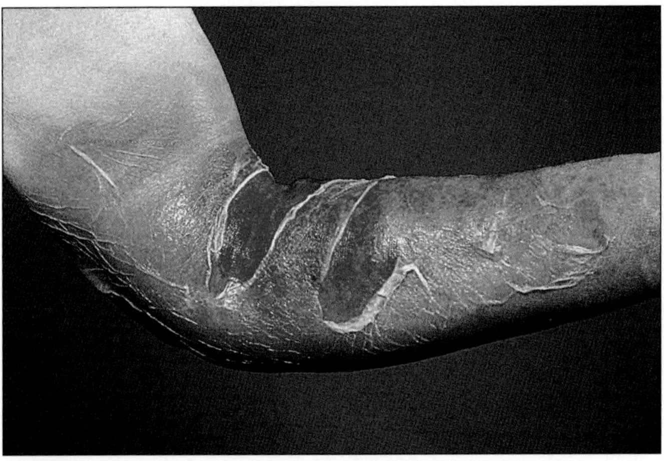

Figure 21.7 Rapidly expanding erythema with epidermolysis representing erysipelas.

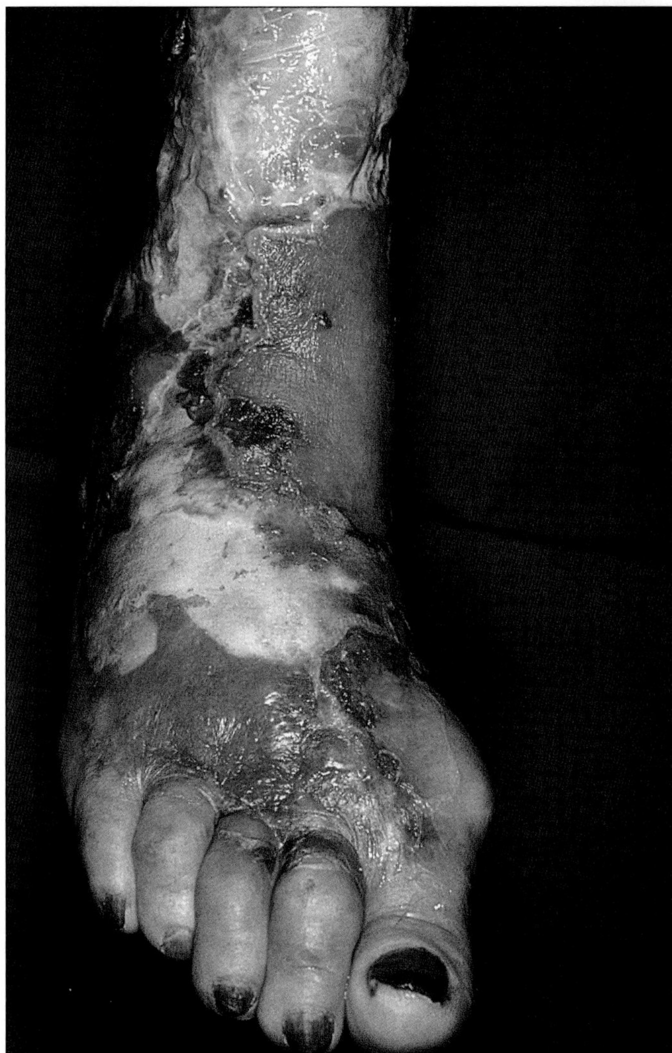

Figure 21.8 Necrotizing deep ulcerations and blisters caused by *Streptococcus pyogenes* as part of streptococcal necrosis.

Differentials include acute eczema, angioneurotic edema, cellulitis, allergic or irritant contact dermatitis, and drug eruptions.

Treatment

Elevation and rest of the affected limb and saline wet dressings should be applied to reduce local swelling and inflammation. Systemic penicillin has remained the first-line drug for therapy. Penicillin administered orally or intramuscularly is sufficient for many cases of erysipelas and should be given for 10–14 days. A cephalosporin or macrolide, such as erythromycin or azithromycin, may be used if the patient has an allergy to penicillin. Selection of an antibiotic with coverage for *Staphylococcus aureus* is not necessary for non-facial infections, but it should be considered in patients who do not improve with penicillin. Facial erysipelas should be treated empirically with a penicillinase-resistant antibiotic, such as dicloxacillin to cover for possible *S. aureus*. Roxithromycin has been reported to be extremely effective in the treatment of erysipelas.

Complications occur in 10–15% of patients with erysipelas. The most common complications include abscess, gangrene, and thrombophlebitis. Less common complications (<1%) are acute glomerulonephritis, endocarditis, septicemia, and streptococcal toxic shock syndrome. Predisposed patients may develop local recurrence, and this can lead to disfiguring and disabling healing reactions, such as elephantiasis nostras verrucosa. The prognosis for patients with erysipelas is excellent.

Cellulitis

Synonyms: Skin infection: group A streptococci, *Staphylococcus aureus*, *S aureus*, group B streptococci, fungal cellulitis, *Escherichia coli* cellulitis, *E coli* cellulitis, gas gangrene

Key features:

- Infection of the dermis and/or subcutaneous fat caused by bacteria (group A streptococci and *Staphylococcus aureus*)
- Warmth, erythema, edema, and tenderness as hallmarks
- Penicillinase-resistant synthetic penicillin (eg. dicloxacillin) or a first-generation cephalosporin are used for treatment in combination with cool packs

Introduction

The word cellulitis literally means inflammation of the cells. It generally indicates an acute spreading infection of the dermis and subcutaneous tissues resulting in pain, erythema, edema, and warmth.

Cellulitis may progress to serious illness by uncontrolled spread. No predilection exists for race, gender and age with the exception of facial cellulitis that is more common in adults older than 50 years and in children up to 3 years; and perianal cellulitis (children). Patients with peripheral vascular disease, diabetes, immunodeficiency, after lymphadenectomy or mastectomy are predisposed.

Bacterial (group A streptococci and *Staphylococcus aureus*) and rarely fungal infections cause cellulitis. Cellulitis in infants may present as sepsis, most commonly caused by group B streptococci. *Streptococcus pneumoniae* may cause a particularly malignant form of cellulitis, typically in an immunocompromised host characterized by violaceous color and bullae. This entity is frequently associated with tissue necrosis, suppuration, and blood stream invasion.

Clinical presentation

Clinical hallmarks of cellulitis include local warmth, erythema, edema, tenderness and lymphangitis. Fever may also be present. Complete blood count, blood cultures (culture and gram stain from lesion are of limited use) can be helpful in making the diagnosis. In severe clinical cases, particularly with crepitus, radiographs may show gas in the tissues (differential diagnoses: fasciitis and gangrene).

Treatment

The goals of therapy are to eradicate the infection and prevent complications. Empiric coverage for group A streptococci and *S aureus* should be provided. Acceptable outpatient regimens include penicillinase-resistant synthetic penicillin (eg. dicloxacillin) or a first-generation cephalosporin (e.g. cephalexin). Alternatively, long-acting parenteral cephalosporin (ceftriaxone) may be administered. Differential diagnoses include burns, severe contact dermatitis, erysipelas, gas gangrene, impetigo and toxic epidermal necrolysis.

Complications occur as bacteremia, sepsis, abscesses, lymphangitis and thrombophlebitis.

Gas gangrene

Synonyms: *Clostridium perfringens*, clostridial myonecrosis, emphysematous gangrene, gangrenous emphysema, progressive emphysematous necrosis

Key features:

- Rare infection by exotoxin-producing clostridial species
- Crepitance, edema, foul-smelling serosanguinous discharge, brownish skin discoloration and bullae represent typical clinical signs
- Wide debridement and surgical excision in combination with antibiotics are the mainstays of therapy

Introduction

Gas gangrene is caused by exotoxin-producing clostridial species. Traumatic gas gangrene (most common infection type) occurs through direct inoculation of a contaminated ischemic wound and occasionally after a surgical procedure. *Clostridium perfringens* causes 80-95% of cases of gas gangrene. Gas gangrene is an infectious disease emergency due to rapid onset of myonecrosis, gas production, and sepsis. About 900-1000 cases occur per year. Incubation period is usually fewer than 3 days, with rapid onset of symptoms. Infection can advance rapidly.

Clinical presentation

Local findings may be rather insignificant. Pain is usually out of proportion to physical findings. Crepitance, edema, foul-smelling serosanguinous discharge and brownish skin discoloration and bullae may occur. When muscle tissue has become ischemic, systemic findings (e.g. tachycardia, altered level of consciousness), will develop with progression to toxemia and shock occurring rapidly. Fever is often low grade early in the disease.

Lab studies should include Gram stain of bullae fluid or muscle tissue, complete blood count (hemolysis and anemia secondary to release of toxins), liver function tests, electrolytes, myoglobin, and a coagulation panel.

Plain radiographs and computed tomography may reveal soft tissue gas within the fascial planes.

Differential diagnoses include cellulitis, deep venous thrombosis and thrombophlebitis, myositis (e.g., streptococcal myositis, acute streptococcal hemolytic gangrene), phlegmasia coerulea dolens (deep venous thrombosis with venous obstruction) and other causes of gas in soft tissues (e.g., pneumomediastinum, pneumothorax, fractured larynx or trachea).

Treatment

Resuscitation, supplemental oxygen, and aggressive volume expansion may be indicated.

Use vasoconstrictors only if absolutely necessary; they can decrease perfusion to already ischemic tissue. Tetanus toxoid and immune globulin may be administered if indicated.

Wide debridement and excision (fasciotomy, debridement, or amputation) are the mainstays of therapy. Antibiotics (aminoglycosides, penicillinase-resistant penicillins, or vancomycin) may not penetrate the ischemic muscle but are important adjuncts to surgery. The use of hyperbaric oxygen is controversial. Tetanus immune globulin is used for passive immunization of patients with presumptive tetanus spore containing wounds.

Early diagnosis and aggressive treatment are the keys to decreasing mortality. Mortality from traumatic gas gangrene is greater than 25%. Mortality from nontraumatic gas gangrene caused by C *septicum* ranges from 67-100%.

Necrotizing fasciitis

Synonyms: Fournier's gangrene, Meleney's ulcer, flesh-eating bacteria, Cullen's ulcer.

Key features:

- Rare infection with high morbidity and mortality
- Early in the course of the disease, necrotizing fasciitis may appear quite benign. Pain may be out of proportion to physical findings
- Rapidly spreading erythema and tissue necrosis. As it progresses, the infection gives way to dusky or purplish skin discoloration and fascial necrosis
- Wide debridement and surgical excision in combination with antibiotics are the mainstays of therapy

Introduction

Necrotizing fasciitis can occur after trauma or around foreign bodies in surgical wounds, or it can be idiopathic, as in scrotal or penile necrotizing fasciitis. Typically, there is a sudden onset of pain and swelling at the site of trauma or recent surgery. Necrotizing fasciitis is a progressive, rapidly spreading, inflammatory infection located in the deep fascia, with secondary necrosis of the subcutaneous tissues. The majority of necrotizing soft tissue infections contain anaerobic bacteria, usually in combination with aerobic gram-negative organisms. Hydrogen, nitrogen, hydrogen sulfide, and methane accumulate in tissues because of reduced water solubility. Because of the presence of gas-forming organisms, subcutaneous air has classically been described but is only rarely detected in necrotizing fasciitis.

In necrotizing fasciitis, group A hemolytic streptococci and *Staphylococcus aureus*, alone or in synergism, are frequently the initiating infecting bacteria. However, other aerobic and anaerobic pathogens may be present, including *Bacteroides*, *Clostridium*, *Peptostreptococcus*, Enterobacteriaceae, *Proteus*, *Pseudomonas*, and *Klebsiella*. Anaerobic streptococci, occasionally seen in drug addicts, and *Vibrio vulnificus*, most often seen in persons with diabetes mellitus or cirrhosis of the liver, cause many forms of nonclostridial myonecrosis. The male-to-female ratio is 2-3:1 in persons from 40 to 60 years of age.

Clinical presentation

The patient usually appears moderately to severely toxic, but early on, the patient may look deceptively well. Typically, the erythema spreads over the course of hours to days (Fig. 21.9). As it progresses, the infection gives way to dusky or purplish skin discoloration near the site of insult. The initial necrosis appears as a massive undermining of the skin and subcutaneous layer. Fascial necrosis is typically more advanced than the appearance suggests. Without treatment, secondary involvement of deeper muscle layers may occur, resulting in myositis or myonecrosis. There may be accompanying general signs, such as fever and severe systemic reactions.

Work-up for suspected necrotizing fasciitis includes complete blood count, electrolytes, liver function tests and arterial blood gas. Local radiographs can reveal the presence of gas in subcutaneous fascial planes. Magnetic resonance imaging reliably detects fascial necrosis with absent gadolinium contrast enhancement in T1 images. Tissue biopsies from the periphery are the best method to use when diagnosing necrotizing fasciitis and for culturing.

Differential diagnoses may include cellulitis, epididymitis, gas gangrene, hernias, testicular torsion and toxic shock syndrome.

Treatment

Aggressive treatment may reduce morbidity and mortality. Immediate antibiotic treatment is mandatory. If streptococci are the identified major pathogens, the drug of choice is penicillin G,

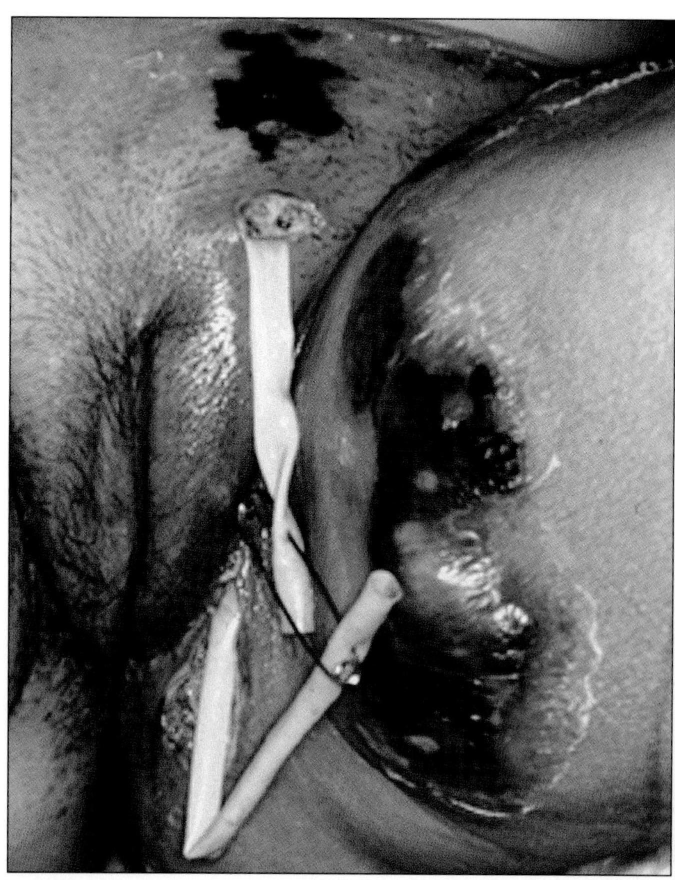

Figure 21.9 Purulent necrotizing fasciitis in a 63-year old woman with a 3 day history of onset.

with clindamycin as the alternative. To ensure adequate treatment, there must be coverage for aerobic and anaerobic bacteria. The anaerobic coverage can be provided by metronidazole or third-generation cephalosporins. Gentamicin, combined with clindamycin or chloramphenicol, has been proposed as a standard coverage. Ampicillin may be added to the basic regimen to treat enterococci if indicated by Gram stain. Early and aggressive debridement is important to improve the patient's outcome. Hyperbaric oxygen therapy has been propagated by special emergency centers.

Complications are not limited to, but frequently manifest as renal failure and septic shock. The overall morbidity and mortality is 70-80%.

References

1. Schmeller W. Community health workers reduce skin diseases in East African children. Int J Dermatol 1998; 37:370–377.
2. Park R. Impetigo. E-medicine 2002. Available online at: http://www.emedicine.com/emerg/topic283.htm (accessed August 31, 2004).
3. Ratz J, Ward DB. Impetigo. E-medicine 2004. Available online at: http://www.emedicine.com/med/topic1163.htm (accessed August 31, 2004).
4. Bär A, Hantschke D, Mirmohammadsadegh A et al. Spectrum of bacterial isolates in HIV-positive patients with skin and soft tissue infections (SSTI): emergence of methicillin-resistant staphylococci. AIDS 2003; 17:1253–1256.
5. Duve S, Voack C, Rakoski J et al. Extensive inguinal lymphadenitis: ecthyma with inguinal lymphadenitis. Arch Dermatol 1996; 132:823–826.
6. Davis L, Mays C. Ecthyma. E-medicine; November 5, 2001. Available online at: http://www.emedicine.com/derm/topic113.htm (accessed August 31, 2004).
7. Allen AM, Taplin D, Twigg L. Cutaneous streptococcal infections in Vietnam. Arch Dermatol 1971; 104:271–280.
8. Kaul R, McGreer A, Low DE et al. Population-based surveillance for group A streptococcal necrotizing fasciitis: clinical features, prognostic indicators, and microbiologic analysis of seventy-seven cases. Ontario Group A Streptococcal Study. Am J Med 1997; 103:18–24.
9. Fournier A. Grangrene foudroyante de la verge. Semaine Medicale 1883: 3; 345–347.

Chapter 22

Mycobacteria

- Tuberculosis ▪ *Leninha Valério do Nascimento*
- Leprosy ▪ *Anne E. Burdick, Virginia A. Capó and Stacy J. Frankel*
- Atypical mycobacteriosis ▪ *Rogerio Neves Motta and Andréa Neiva dos Reis*

Tuberculosis

Leninha Valério do Nascimento

Synonyms: Tisic, scrofula

Key features: Mycobacteria, tuberculosis, tuberculides

Introduction

Tuberculosis is an infectious disease that mainly affects the lungs, lymphatic ganglia, bones, joints, skin, intestines, and other organs.[1]

Cutaneous tuberculosis occurs when the bacillus reaches the skin by an exogenous or endogenous route from the infection foci within the organism itself.

History

Hippocrates (460–475 BC) called the disease phthisis (tisic), and this name particularly referred to the pulmonary form of the disease.

For many years, tuberculosis was suspected to be of infectious origin. This was only confirmed upon discovery of the bacillus by Robert Koch in 1882.

Epidemiology

For about a decade, we have been observing a recrudescence of pulmonary tuberculosis in all countries of the world, independent of human immunodeficiency virus (HIV) infection.

Tuberculosis in the USA had decreased to a 5–6% index by 1984. By contrast, from 1985 to 1991, there was an 18% increase in the number of tuberculosis cases.[2]

The increase of this "new tuberculosis" has a few peculiarities: HIV infection constitutes a new collective risk factor because HIV-positive patients may be carriers of, or be suffering from, tuberculosis; they also show a roughly 6% resistance rate. Oddly enough, in spite of this recrudescence of pulmonary tuberculosis, there has not yet been an apparent increase in cases of cutaneous tuberculosis. Nonetheless, this "new tuberculosis" has stimulated progress in diagnostic methods (genomic diagnosis). It has also been discussed in the context of the nosology and etiology of cutaneous tuberculides.[3]

Pathogenesis and etiology

Cutaneous tuberculosis occurs when *Mycobacterium tuberculosis* reaches the skin by an exogenous or endogenous route from infection foci within the organism itself. It may also be caused by *M. bovis* and *M. africanum* and, more rarely, by bacillus Calmette-Guérin (BCG).

Following *M. tuberculosis*[1,4] infection and phagocytosis by the antigen-presenting cells (APC), macrophages and T cells interact with mycobacterial antigens and release lymphokines (interleukin and interferon) on the surface of these APCs. Some of these lymphokines are responsible for activating and self-regulating class II antigen expression of the major histocompatibility complex (MHC) and interleukin 2 receptors (IL-2R) on T lymphocytes.[4]

After an organism's first contact with the bacillus and its products, there emerges an immunoallergic state which varies considerably from person to person. This reaction state is evaluated through a tuberculin test: Mantoux reaction or purified protein derivative (PPD). This is a more useful method by which to identify an infected individual.

Clinical features

Primary cutaneous tuberculosis complex, tuberculous chancre

The primary infection from tuberculosis usually occurs in the lungs. It may exceptionally present on the skin. When an individual who has a tuberculous past comes into contact with the Koch bacillus through a continuous skin solution, an initial lesion forms at the point of contact. The lesion is a nodule or papule. It is firm and consistent and measures roughly 2 cm in diameter. Its color is red or violet. The lesion is painful and after a few days it starts ulcerating and is covered over by a dark and adherent crust. The ulcer's inner area is granulous and exudes slightly. Three to 8 weeks after infection lymphangitis and satellite adenitis arise, and this constitutes the primary cutaneous tuberculosis complex.[1]

The ulcerous lesion is rich in bacilli, which are easily demonstrable in the exudate within the first few days of infection. The lesion is localized on the face and in the limb extremities. In 10% of cases, it may be accompanied by erythema nodosum. The lesion appears on the skin 2–4 weeks after inoculation. Within approximately 30–45 days spontaneous regression occurs, leaving a scar. Mantoux reaction is negative at the outset. It becomes positive with resolution of the process. At the outset, the histopathologic examination shows non-specific cellular infiltrate that is rich in bacilli, and at times small foci of necrosis. Three to 6 weeks later, the infiltrate suffers a transformation, showing a tuberculoid structure with rare bacilli.[1]

The main differential diagnosis is with sporotrichosis, syphilis, tularemia, and other mycobacterias.

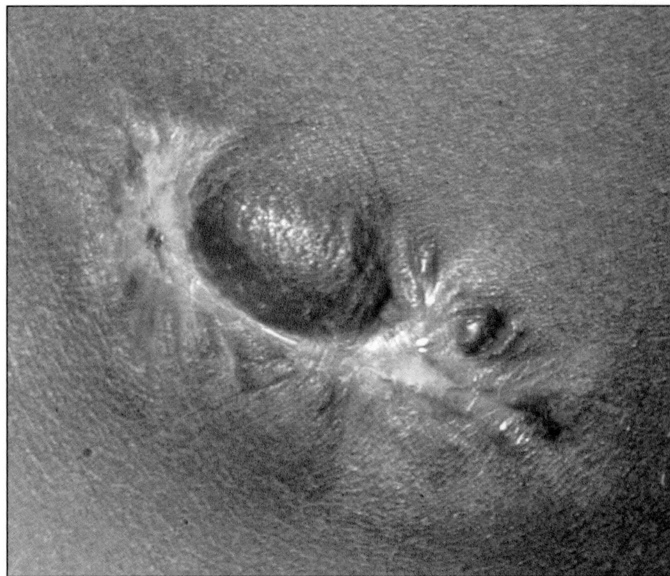

Figure 22.1 Tuberculous colliquativa cutis.

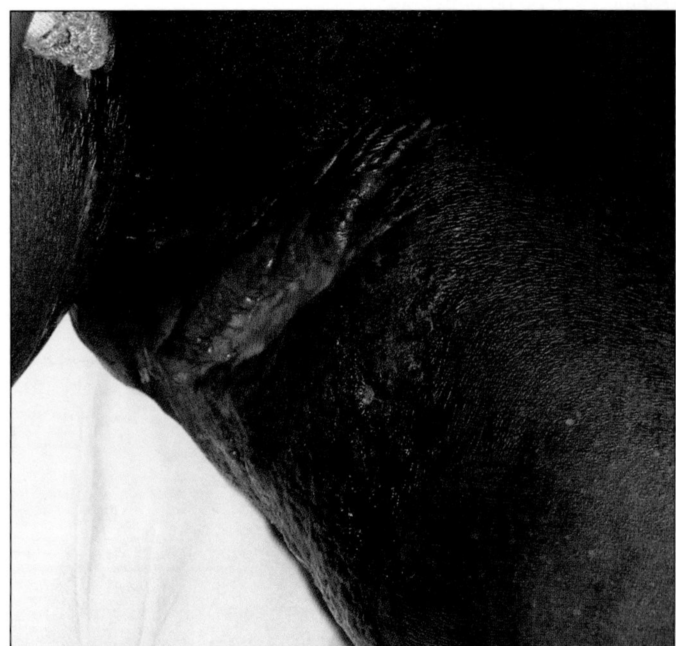

Figure 22.2 Ulcerated scrofuloderma.

Tuberculosis colliquativa cutis (scrofuloderma)

This form of tuberculosis is relatively frequent in the environment in Mexico and other tropical countries. It results from the contiguous involvement of the underlying skin of other tuberculous foci, and commonly of tuberculosis lymphadenitis, bone and joint tuberculosis, tuberculous epididymitis, or after BCG vaccination.[5] It affects all ages, with a higher prevalence in children, adolescents, and the elderly.

Onset is through a firm, consistent and deep nodule that adheres to the skin, and that is purple-red or erythematous violet in color. It progresses toward fluctuation, suppuration, and fistulization. The secretion is cloudy and viscous. At times, it is partially hemorrhagic, while at others the eliminated material is thick and purulent (Fig. 22.1). This aspect may persist for months. It may progress to elliptical and circular ulcers (Fig. 22.2). The lesion may be solitary or multiple, with a confluent tendency toward forming large infiltrated masses that intercommunicate via fistulous trajectories. The involution leaves these scars depressed, retractable, adherent, or hypertrophic (Fig. 22.3). The localizations are the parotid, submandibular, and supraclavicular regions, as well as the lateral surfaces of the throat.

This progressive description characterizes the tuberculous gummas of the skin, which may also be observed in the limbs and trunk, including the groin (Fig. 22.2). Coexistence with an active pulmonary process is relatively common.

It may be differentiated from atypical mycobacteriosis, sporotrichosis, actinomycosis, coccidioidomycosis, and lymphogranuloma venereum.

Acute miliary cutaneous tuberculosis

This is a clinical form specific to infancy. It is severe and rare, and often has a lethal outcome. It almost always afflicts allergic children with a progressive primary pulmonary lesion and subsequent dissemination in the blood.

In some cases, progression is fulminant with rapid aggravation of the process, resulting in death within a few days. The lesions are papules, tubercles, pustules, and purple spots disseminated over the entire body. Sensitivity to tuberculin is usually negative.[1]

The differential diagnosis proceeds as follows: atypical mycobacteriosis, syphilic gumma, deep mycosis, sporotrichosis, actinomycosis, severe forms of conglobate acne, and suppurative hydradenitis.

Tuberculosis verrucous cutis

Also known as anatomic tuberculosis or verruca necrogenica, this is a form of localized and progressive tuberculosis in which reinfection

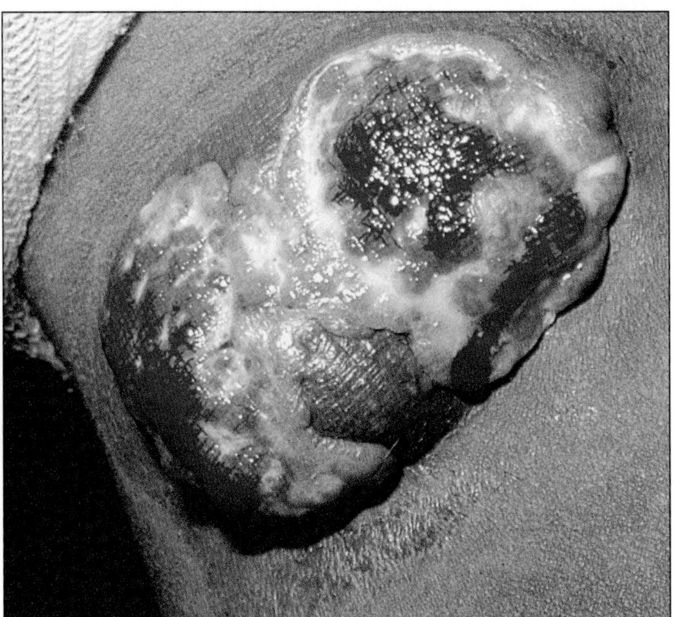

Figure 22.3 Hypertrophic scars of scrofuloderma.

occurs by a hematogenic route. It usually arises by propagation of the contiguous focus or by an external route (inoculation of the germ proceeding from tuberculous material), and commonly in persons working with tuberculous patients or animals. The preferential localization is in the limb extremities, mainly the hands and foot.[6] It is initiated by a tubercle slowly progressing to form plaque and verrucous lesions. The progression is centrifugal at the edges, with a tendency to central scarring that may persist for several years and be cured spontaneously.

PPD reveals a high degree of hypersensitivity. The differential diagnosis is made with atypical mycobacteriosis, North American blastomycosis, Majocchi granuloma, chromoblastomycosis, verrucous epidermal nevus, hypertrophic lichen planus, iododerma, bromoderma, and verruca vulgaris.

Tuberculosis lupus (lupus vulgaris)

In the early twentieth century, this condition was common in certain European countries. There is a high prevalence of the disease in regions where the climate is humid and cold.

The following clinical forms are considered: plane, hypertrophic, ulcerative, and cicatricial.

The mucosa (oral, nasal, pharyngeal, and conjunctival) may primarily be affected by extension of the cutaneous lesions.

Clinically, the lesions are tuberous, growing centrifugally, slowly and progressively. They are localized with high frequency in exposed areas: the face (nose, malar regions, and ears), hands and forearms and sometimes produce cervical adenitis. Vitropressure shows a characteristic "apple jelly" aspect. The central part of the lesion has an atrophic cicatricial aspect. It may destroy cartilage in the nasal septum and ears, and retract the natural orifices and eyelids, causing mutilations. The lesions regress and leave peculiar atrophic scars.

Microscopic examination shows typical tuberculosis, rare bacilli, and discrete caseation.

The following must be considered in the differential diagnosis: late-onset syphilis, paracoccidioidomycosis, leishmaniasis, sarcoidosis, discoid lupus erythematosus, lymphocytoma cutis, tuberculoid leprosy, and pyodermitis vegetans.

Tuberculosis cutis orificialis (ulcerous, cutaneous, and mucosa tuberculosis)

This disorder occurs in the mucosa and on skin close to natural orifices. It is due to self-inoculation of mycobacteria proceeding from an internal tuberculous focus. It is a rare form that may occur at any age. It is most common in middle-aged and older adults.

Small yellow or red nodules appear in the mucosa and later begin to ulcerate. The edges are poorly defined and consistency is soft. The lesion surface is covered by a pseudomembranous material that frequently exhibits multiple yellowed tubercles and eroded vessels. The lesions may be solitary or multiple, and are extremely painful.

Histopathology shows intense non-specific cellular infiltrate and areas of necrosis. In the depths of the dermis, tubercles may be found with caseation and the bacillus is easily identified.

The differential diagnosis is often made with the following: aphthous ulcers, carcinomas, and syphilis.

Erythema induratum (Bazin's disease)

This disorder is characterized by erythematous nodules that are not very precise, and are preferentially localized on the posterior part of the legs (calves) and, at times, on the anterior part of persons with tuberculin hypersensitivity (Fig. 22.4). The lesions are almost always symmetrical. They are localized in the subcutaneous tissue and progress until they provoke adherence of the overlying epidermis, and finally end up hardening. They may regress spontaneously, leaving depressed and atrophic areas with superficial scaling.

Histopathologic examination reveals lobular panniculitis, tuberculoid granuloma, caseous necrosis and, rarely, bacilli. The vascular

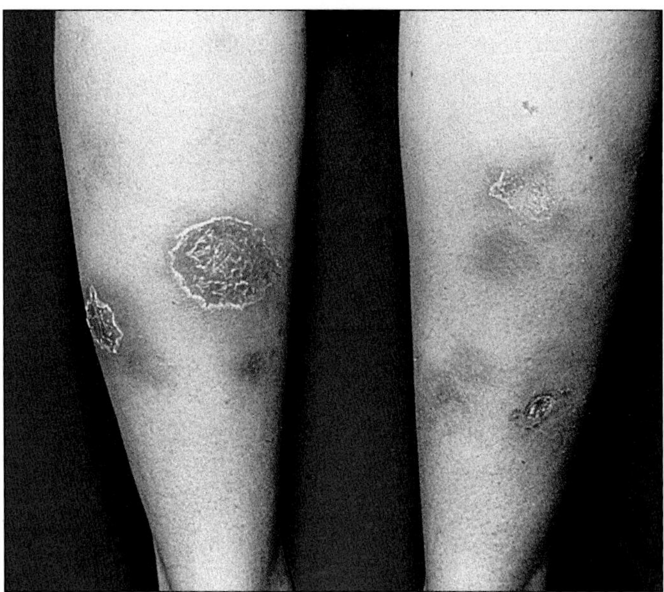

Figure 22.4 Erythema induratum.

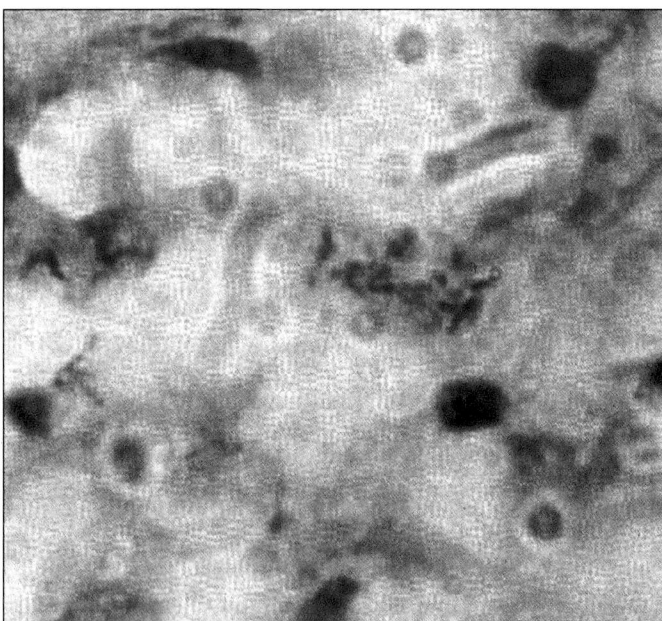

Figure 22.5 *Mycobacterium tuberculosis.*

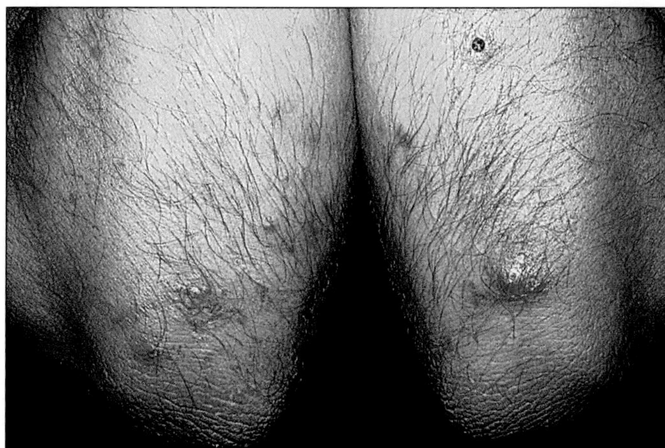

Figure 22.6 Papulonecrotic tuberculids.

alterations are vasculitis with thickening of the tunics, thrombosis, and consequent necrosis (Fig. 22.5).

Some authors include erythema induratum, i.e., Bazin's disease, among the tuberculids. We have adopted the criteria Rabello[7] proposed, which were convincing enough to include the disease as a form of tuberculosis.

Recently, polymerase chain reaction (PCR) techniques have helped confirm the diagnosis of erythema induratum, which differs from idiopathic nodular vasculitis.[2,8,9]

Papulonecrotic tuberculid

This disease affects youths, adolescents and even children. It results in cutaneous reinfection from the internal tuberculous focus by a hematogenic route.

It is manifested by dark-red or purple-colored papules that are firm and localized most commonly on the face and ears, elbows, knees, surface of the extensor forearms (Fig. 22.6), legs, dorsal aspect of the hands, and buttocks. The papules vary in size from 2 to 8 mm, become pustular or necrotic, and progress toward healing.

The localization and aspect of the scars are piecemeal, and at times allow for a retrospective diagnosis.

Mycobacteria DNA may be found on PCR in 50% of papulonecrotic tuberculid cases.

The differential diagnosis is as follows: secondary papulopustule syphilis, acute chickenpox-like lichenoid pityriasis, Churg–Strauss granuloma, lymphomatoid papulosis, perforating granuloma annulare, perforating collagenosis, and leukocytoclastic vasculitis.

Lichenoid cutaneous tuberculosis (lichen scrofulosorum)

This is a rare form, specific to childhood and adolescence. It may coexist with pulmonary, ganglionar, and bone tuberculosis.

It is characterized by small papular lesions which are yellow-red to brown-red in color. The lesions are shiny with a discoid form. They persist as unaltered and asymptomatic for several months.

It may be mistaken for lichen planus, lichenoid syphilis, eczema, lichen nitidus, and sarcoidosis.

Diagnosis

The main elements in the diagnosis of the diverse clinical forms of cutaneous tuberculosis are as follows:[3,10]

1. Clinical and epidemiologic history
2. Bacterioscopy – study of alcohol-acid-resistant bacilli in lesions
3. Culture – the culture medium used is Lowenstein–Jensen. The radiometric method uses the carbon dioxide principle of bacteria, which has C14 and leads to shortening the time needed to develop the *M. tuberculosis* colonies (Bactec)
4. Histopathology
5. Tuberculin test – PPD or Mantoux
6. PCR
7. Immunohistochemistry, mainly immunostaining with anti-BCG antibodies, is more effective

With the advent of acquired immunodeficiency syndrome (AIDS), it is recommended that all cases of cutaneous tuberculosis have a HIV serology test performed because these diseases require longer-term treatment.

Treatment

For all forms of cutaneous tuberculosis, the multidrug regimen is recommended.

The drugs and doses used are as follows: isoniazid (5 mg/kg), rifampicin (10 mg/kg), pyrazinamide (15–30 mg/kg) daily for 2 months. The isoniazid and rifampicin are continued for 4–10 months. If resistance to isoniazid is suspected, ethambutol (15 mg/kg per day) is added to the therapeutic regimen. In HIV-positive patients, three-drug regimen therapy is administered for 18–24 months.

References

1. Nascimento LV, Neves RG. Tuberculose cutânea. In: Talhari S, Neves RG, eds. Dermatologia tropical. Rio de Janeiro: MEDSI; 1995:267–281.
2. Odom RB, James WD, Berger TG. Mycobacterial diseases. In: Andrews' diseases of the skin. Clinical dermatology, 9th edn. Philadelphia, PA: WB Saunders; 2000:417–426.
3. Grosshans E. Tuberculosis. In: Bessis D, Guilhou YY, eds. La pathologie dermatologie en médecine interne. Rueil: Arnette; 1999:453–457.
4. Sehgal VN. Cutaneous tuberculosis. Dermatol Clin 1994; 12:645–653.
5. Tan H, Karakuzu A, Arik A. Scrofuloderma after BCG vaccination. Pediatr Dermatol 2002; 19:323–325.
6. Gruber PC, Whittan LR, Vivier A. Tuberculosis verrucosa cutis on the sole of the foot. Clin Exp Dermatol 2002; 27:188–191.
7. Rabello FE. Tuberculose cutânea indurativa de Bazin. Conference in Brazilian Academy. Rio de Janeiro: 1980.
8. Penneys NS, Leonardi CL. Look S et al. Identification of *Mycobacterium tuberculosis* DNA in five different types of cutaneous lesions by the polymerase chain reaction. Arch Dermatol 1999; 129:1594–1598.
9. Seckin D, Hizel N, Demirhan B et al. The diagnostic value of polymerase chain reaction in erythema induratum of Bazin (letter). Br J Dermatol 1997; 137:1011–1012.
10. Nascimento LV. Tuberculose cutânea indurativa (thesis). Rio de Janeiro: 1982.

Leprosy

Anne E. Burdick, Virginia A. Capó and Stacy Frankel

Synonyms: Hansen's disease

Key features:

- Anesthetic skin lesions
- Thickened peripheral nerves
- Acid-fast bacillus *Mycobacterium leprae* on skin smear and biopsy
- Extent of clinical disease varies with cell-mediated immunity to *M. leprae*
- Th1 cytokines are prevalent in tuberculoid type, Th2 in lepromatous type
- Reactional states can occur before, during, and after treatment
- Rifampin and dapsone for paucibacillary leprosy, plus clofazimine for multibacillary disease, can cure the infection but neuropathy and deformities may persist

Introduction

Leprosy is a mycobacterial infection caused by *Mycobacterium leprae* which affects primarily the skin, peripheral nerves, eyes, and mucous membranes of the upper respiratory tract. Most of the world's population is immune to this bacillus. The disease is transmitted via airborne droplets from, or direct prolonged skin contact with, an untreated person. The incubation period ranges from a few months to 20 years. The primary clinical manifestations are anesthetic skin lesions which, depending on the individual's immune status to *M. leprae*, may vary in number from one or few in limited tuberculoid leprosy to numerous in diffuse lepromatous leprosy. If left untreated, the disease may result in progressive damage to peripheral nerves, causing motor and sensory loss, hand and foot deformities, disability, and enacted or felt social stigma.

Global travel has become more common and there is significant immigration of individuals from endemic leprosy areas to other parts of the world. In non-endemic areas leprosy is often misdiagnosed or there is delay in the diagnosis. In a British study, 82% of the 28 patients had a mean lag time of 3 years from first symptom until time of diagnosis, with one patient as long as 15 years.[1] The misdiagnoses of these patients included cellulitis, vasculitis, ulnar nerve entrapment, soft-tissue infection, arthritis, gout, and filariasis. Early accurate diagnosis of leprosy with appropriate treatment prevents transmission of disease, nerve damage, and subsequent morbidity.

History

Humans have been infected with leprosy for centuries. Typical bone abnormalities have been identified in Egyptian mummies. Leprosy was described in the Bible, but it probably described a different condition, possibly psoriasis. In 1862, Rudolph Virchow described the presence of vacuolated macrophages and peripheral nerve damage in lepromatous leprosy. In 1873, Armauer G. Hansen identified the causative intracytoplasmic organism in macrophages and Schwann cells.

Individuals with leprosy have always been stigmatized. The fourteenth-century Parisian Ceremony of Separation involved a symbolic funeral and infected individuals were required to wear a "clapper" to warn others of their approach. In Japan, affected individuals were removed from their families and sent to remote leprosaria until the mid-twentieth century, for which the Prime Minister apologized in 2001 and gave financial remuneration.[2] In the USA, patients at the national leprosarium in Louisiana were not allowed to vote until 1946. In 1991, the member countries of the World Health Organization, by means of a resolution of the Health General Assembly, declared the intention of eliminating leprosy as a health problem by the year 2000. In that very same year the task force for leprosy established general guidelines for the elimination of leprosy.

Nowadays, the worldwide situation shows a drastic reduction of the number of countries where leprosy is still a health problem: from 122 countries in 1981, to only 24 in 1999. Calculations suggest that roughly 10 million people have been cured since the multidrug therapy was introduced.

Epidemiology

Statistics

At the end of 2002, the World Health Organization (WHO) estimated that the prevalence of leprosy worldwide was 524 311 individuals (Fig. 22.7). There were 620 672 new cases of leprosy detected in 2002, as reported by 110 countries (Fig. 22.8). Eighty-three percent of leprosy patients live in six countries (Brazil, India, Madagascar, Mozambique, Nepal, and Tanzania). India had the highest prevalence and incidence of new cases.[3] According to the WHO there are between 2 and 3 million people with permanently disabilities due to leprosy.[4] Other reports estimate that 7 million treated leprosy patients have permanent disabilities from the disease.[5]

The registered leprosy cases worldwide have decreased from 5.4 million in 1985 to below 1 million in 2001. In recent years, the WHO has worked to eliminate leprosy as a public health problem and its goal is to reduce the prevalence of leprosy to less than one case per 10 000 people nationally. As part of its elimination program, the WHO changed its definition of a leprosy case to an individual with clinical and/or pathological evidence of leprosy who has not completed a full course of treatment. Treated patients with late reactions or permanent disabilities were eliminated from this case definition. Although there has been a significant decline in the prevalence of leprosy, the annual incidence of new leprosy cases has remained stable at approximately 650 000–685 000 over the last decade. Some argue that the recent decline in worldwide prevalence of leprosy is due to the new case definition rather than an actual decrease in disease incidence.[6]

Among Latin-American countries Brazil contributes the largest number of patients followed by Paraguay. Nevertheless, many countries in this area of the world show prevalence below 1 per 10 000 at the national level, although at the subnational level they still have large numbers of patients. For example, the recent situation in Cuba has been that of a low endemic prevalence, with a national prevalence of 0.56 cases per 10 000 population in 1996 and 0.4 cases in 2001. However, the national rate varies between areas – as low as 0.1 cases per 10 000 population in the provinces of Holguín and Villa Clara and with hotspots as high as 1.1 in Camagüey and 0.9 in Guantánamo. In Havana City, the 2001 prevalence was 0.2 cases per 10 000 population.

In the USA, the number of leprosy patients is low. In 2002, there were 133 newly registered cases in the National Hansen's Disease Program (NHDP). Over two-thirds were multibacillary cases and approximately one-third of cases were from California. Other areas considered endemic for leprosy are Hawaii, Louisiana, New York, Puerto Rico, and Texas. Eighty-one percent of these new cases were immigrants, mostly from Mexico and the Philippines.[7]

Demographics

Leprosy has a bimodal age distribution, with one peak between 10 and 15 years of age and a second peak between 30 and 60 years of age. Children represent about 15% of leprosy cases[5] and tend to have limited disease, often having self-healing lesions of leprosy. However, in a non-endemic area of northern India, of 132 children with leprosy, 59% had borderline tuberculoid disease and 20.4%

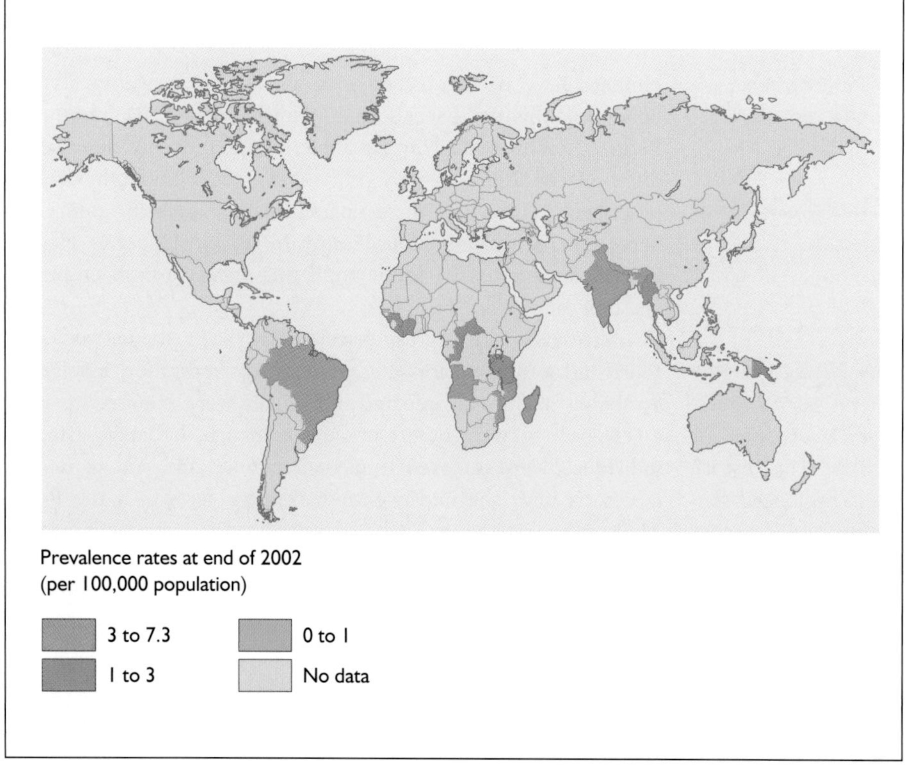

Figure 22.7 The prevalence rates of leprosy worldwide at the end of 2002. (Courtesy of the World Health Organization.[3])

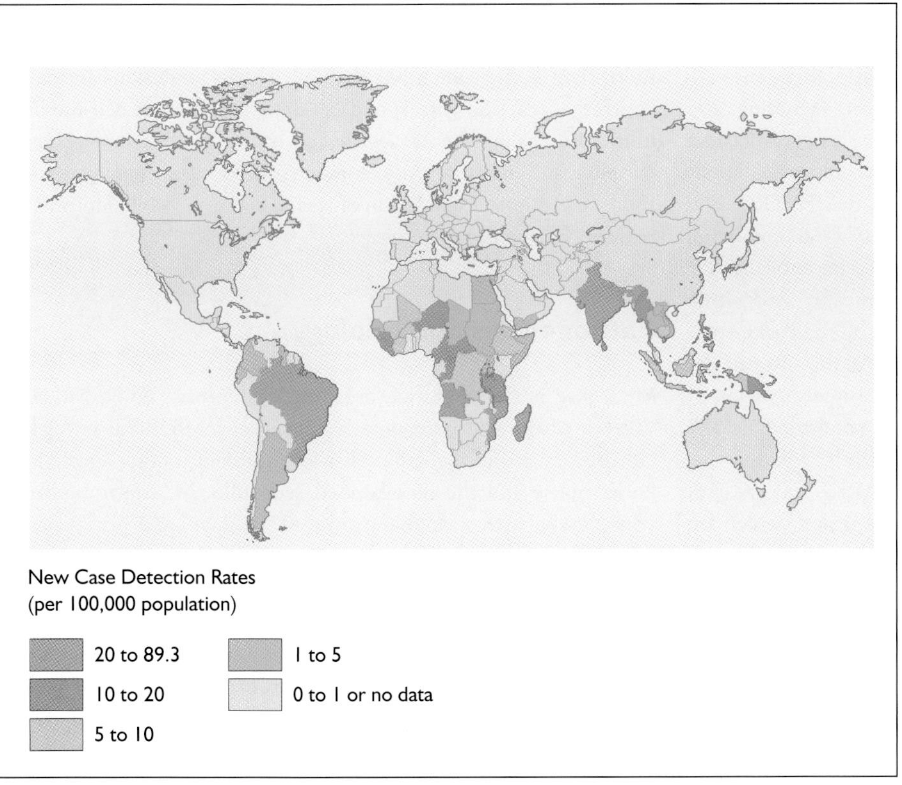

Figure 22.8 New case detection rates of various countries in 2002. (Courtesy of the World Health Organization.[3])

had borderline lepromatous disease.[8] The proportion of affected males and females is equal in children. In adults, however, significantly more males are affected than females.

Transmission of the organism is thought to be via nasorespiratory spread of airborne droplets from the nasal mucosa by sneezing or from the upper respiratory mucosa by coughing. Prolonged direct contact with open untreated skin lesions is another means of transmission. The infection then spreads hematogenously to the skin, nerves, and other organs.

While the major natural reservoir for leprosy is untreated multibacillary patients, paucibacillary patients may represent a weak source of infection.[5] Non-infected nasal carriers of *M. leprae*, as demonstrated by PCR, range from 5 to 10% in endemic populations and may serve as another reservoir for infection.[9,10] Nine-banded armadillos in south-central USA are also natural hosts for *M. leprae* (Fig. 22.9). Anecdotal reports suggest that occupational handling of these animals may result in infection.[11] Other animal reservoirs include the chimpanzee in Sierra Leone and the sooty mangabey monkey in Nigeria.[12,13] The incubation period for leprosy is very long and ranges from a few months to 5 years – an incubation period of 20 years has been reported.[14]

Susceptibility

The US NHDP estimates that more than 95% of individuals are not susceptible to leprosy, even after significant exposure.[14] Others have estimated that 0.5% of individuals infected with *M. leprae* will develop clinical disease.[15] Individuals who develop leprosy demonstrate an impaired cell-mediated immune response to the *M. leprae* bacillus. Multiple studies in various populations have shown that HIV type 1 infection does not affect susceptibility to leprosy, nor does it affect the clinical or histological spectrum of the disease. However, one case report described the presentation of leprosy as an immune reconstitution phenomenon after highly active antiretroviral therapy.[16]

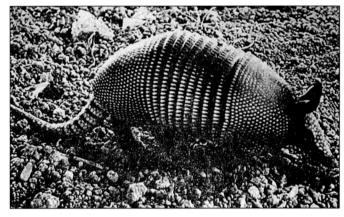

Figure 22.9 The nine-banded armadillo, a natural reservoir for *Mycobacterium leprae*.

Genetic studies

Recent studies have demonstrated a significant role of genetics in the susceptibility to leprosy. There are high concordance rates of leprosy among identical twins. Early studies showed an association of human leukocyte antigen (HLA) DR2 with tuberculoid disease. An Indian study did not find an association between susceptibility to leprosy and HLA types, but identified a region on chromosome 10p13 as the susceptibility locus for leprosy.[17] In a Southeast

Asian population with multibacillary disease, it was concluded that the NRAMP1 gene, which controls susceptibility to mycobacterial infections in mice, is one of several leprosy susceptibility genes.[18]

A genomic study of 86 Vietnamese families, including 205 siblings with leprosy, revealed a susceptibility gene on chromosome 6q25.[19] A subsequent study of two different ethnic populations defined specific variants of the 5′ region of the PACRG and PARK2 genes as worldwide risk factors for leprosy. One population included 197 Vietnamese families, each with two parents and one leprosy-affected child, and reported a significant association between leprosy and 17 markers that are shared by the Parkinson's disease gene PARK2 and the coregulated gene PACRG. Two of the most significant markers were clustered in the promoter region of these two Parkinson's genes. This finding was confirmed in 587 Brazilian leprosy cases and 388 non-infected controls.[20] Supporting this genetic susceptibility is the fact that the PARK2 and PACRG genes are expressed by Schwann cells and macrophages, which are the primary host cells of *M. leprae*.

In a microarray analysis of approximately 12 000 genes of six tuberculoid lesions and six lepromatous lesions, a distinct gene expression profile correlated with each clinical form of the disease. In addition, increased gene expression of the leukocyte immunoglobulin-like receptor family was reported in lepromatous lesions.[21]

The lepromin test

The lepromin test is a prognostic test of an individual's cell-mediated immunity to *M. leprae* but has limited practical use. It involves the intradermal injection of 40 million bacilli/ml heat-killed *M. leprae* derived from infected armadillos. The injection site is evaluated at 1–2 days and 3 weeks. The Fernández reaction occurs within the first 2 days and represents a delayed-type hypersensitivity reaction. At 3 weeks, the Mitsuda reaction is measured. A positive Mitsuda reaction is described as an indurated lesion of more than 4 mm which histologically shows granuloma formation. A positive reaction corresponds to the acquisition of cell-mediated immunity against the *M. leprae* and occurs in tuberculoid leprosy patients and most leprosy contacts. Borderline leprosy patients show an indurated skin lesion of less than 3 mm, while lepromatous patients have a negative reaction.[13]

Pathogenesis and etiology

M. leprae is the causative organism of leprosy. While *M. leprae* was one of the first human pathogens discovered, it has never been cultured in artificial media. However, animal models exist in the nude mouse and the nine-banded armadillo. *M. leprae* multiplies very slowly, with a doubling time of 12 days, and grows best at 27–33°C.[13]

M. leprae is an obligate intracellular rod with a multilayered cell wall. While all mycobacteria have lipid-rich cell walls, *M. leprae* is distinct in that its outermost layer contains phenolic glycolipid-1 (PGL-1) (Fig. 22.10). PGL-1 was the first antigen discovered to be specific to the *M. leprae* bacillus. Antibody titers to PGL-1 have been shown to be higher in multibacillary patients compared with paucibacillary patients.[22] PGL-1 has been shown to mediate the interaction with laminin 2 on the basal lamina of the Schwann cell axon of peripheral nerves, thereby determining the neural predilection of *M. leprae*.[23]

The role of PGL-1 in the demyelination of Schwann cells was demonstrated by in vitro studies of cocultures of dorsal root ganglia and Schwann cells. *M. leprae* bound to myelinating and non-myelinating Schwann cells. The bacteria and also purified PGL-1

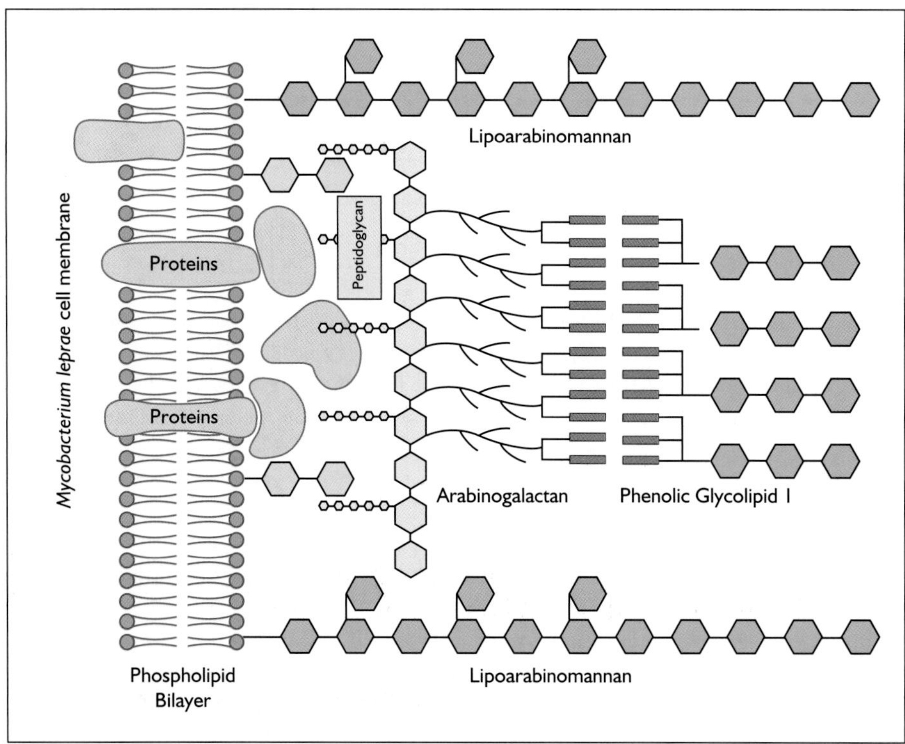

Figure 22.10 *Mycobacterium leprae* multilayered cell wall with phenolic glycolipid-1 (PGL-1) in the outer layer. (Reproduced with permission from the *Annual Review of Microbiology* vol. 41 ©1987 by Annual Reviews www.annualreviews.org.)

caused rapid demyelination of the myelinating Schwann cells and directly invaded the non-myelinating Schwann cells. *M. leprae* was shown to be able to demyelinate these cells without immunologic involvement, using mice that lacked functional B and T cells and that received *M. leprae* into their nerves, where the same attachment and demyelination phenomenon occurred.[24]

While the pathogenesis of leprosy has not been fully elucidated, it is well accepted that the host's cell-mediated immunity to *M. leprae* correlates with the clinical manifestations of the disease. The Ridley–Jopling classification of leprosy, introduced in 1962, delineates the spectrum of disease. This classification includes five types of leprosy ranging from the limited tuberculoid (TT) and borderline tuberculoid (BT) cases to the more extensive borderline borderline (BB), borderline lepromatous (BL), and lepromatous (LL) cases.

Tuberculoid leprosy is characterized by strong cell-mediated immunity to *M. leprae* which controls bacterial growth. Clinically, tuberculoid patients present with localized nerve involvement and few skin lesions. At the other end of the Ridley–Jopling spectrum, lepromatous patients lack cell-mediated immunity to *M. leprae* and present with extensive nerve involvement and numerous skin lesions with uncontrolled bacterial replication (Fig. 22.11). In these two polar forms of leprosy, skin lesions contain different T-lymphocyte subsets and express different cytokine patterns. Histologically, tuberculoid lesions are composed of well-formed granulomas. CD4+ T lymphocytes comprise the central core of the granuloma and CD8+ cells line the periphery in the proportion 2:1.[25] At the lepromatous pole, the lesions are composed of diffuse granulomatous inflammation without well-formed granulomas and contain mostly CD8+ cells.

Distinct cytokine patterns are expressed in tuberculoid and lepromatous lesions. Tuberculoid lesions express Th1 cytokines, including interleukin (IL)-2, IL-12, and interferon-γ, which activate macrophages and circulating monocytes, fostering the granulomatous response against intracellular pathogens. Lepromatous lesions demonstrate primarily Th2 cytokines, including IL-4 and IL-10. This results in impaired cell-mediated immune responses to *M. leprae*, a strong humoral response to the mycobacteria, and significant antibody production.[26]

The role of interferon-γ in the pathogenesis of leprosy has been studied. A signaling lymphocyte activation molecule (SLAM) is expressed on lymphocytes and increases interferon-γ production. Tuberculoid lesions were found to have a higher expression of SLAM, compared with lepromatous lesions.[27] Another study investigated for interferon-γ knockout mice infected with *M. leprae*. While these animals had bacterial growth, histologically they formed granulomas that were not well organized. Therefore, the infected knockout mice demonstrated an immune response to *M. leprae* which the investigators related to a borderline leprosy lesion.[28]

Granulysin, an antimicrobial protein that is released by CD4+ T cells, plays a role in the host's defense against leprosy. Granulysin has been shown to gain access to intracellular pathogens by a pore-forming molecule called performin. A study of eight lepromatous and eight tuberculoid patients revealed a sixfold greater frequency of granulysin-expressing CD4+ T cells in tuberculoid lesions compared to lepromatous lesions. However, the levels of performin were similar.[29]

Toll-like receptors (TLRs) are part of the innate immune defense system against infectious pathogens. It has been shown that TLR2 and TLR1 were more strongly expressed in tuberculoid lesions compared with lepromatous lesions.[30] Schwann cells in skin lesions from leprosy patients were found to express TLR2. The activation of TLR2 with *M. leprae* lipopeptides triggered the apoptosis of Schwann cells. This provides a mechanism for the activation of immune responses, contributing to the nerve damage in leprosy.[31]

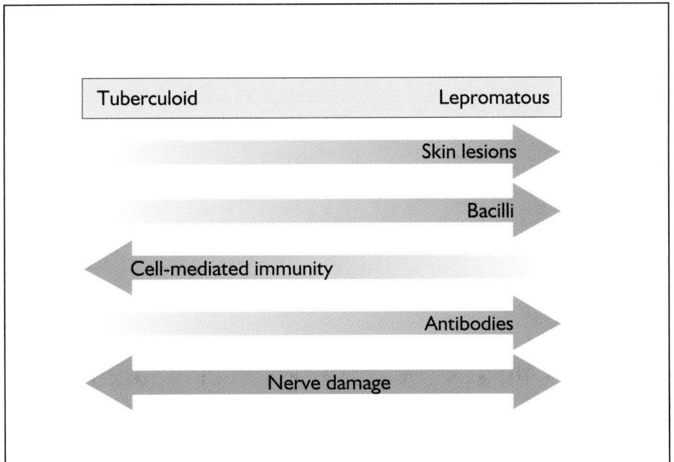

Figure 22.11 The spectrum of leprosy. At the tuberculoid end, patients have high cell-mediated immunity to *Mycobacterium leprae*, fewer bacteria with fewer antibodies, and skin lesions. Lepromatous patients have low cell-mediated immunity to *M. leprae*, extensive skin lesions, and numerous bacteria and antibodies. Nerve damage can occur throughout the spectrum. (Courtesy of Dr. Robert L Modlin.)

Clinical features

Clinical manifestations of leprosy are found in the skin, peripheral nerves, mucous membranes of the upper respiratory tract, the anterior chamber of the eye, and the testes. Skin lesions are the main clinical presentation and are most commonly seen on the buttocks, thighs, face, trunk, and the lateral aspects of the extremities. Warmer areas, such as the axilla and scalp, are usually spared. Since *M. leprae* has a predilection for cooler areas of the body, peripheral nerves in the face, neck, and limbs are particularly affected. Nerve damage develops before diagnosis, during treatment, or after completion of adequate antibiotic therapy.

Upon exposure to *M. leprae*, most individuals are resistant to the bacillus and do not develop infection. However, of the small percentage of people who develop leprosy, the disease begins with the indeterminate form. The majority of indeterminate cases resolve spontaneously. However, if the lesions do not resolve, the individual will develop one of the types of leprosy depending on his or her cell-mediated immunity to *M. leprae*. At one end of the spectrum, individuals develop limited disease, and at the other end of the spectrum, patients develop extensive skin disease with numerous systemic manifestations. The extent of the disease correlates with the type of leprosy, as classified by the Ridley–Jopling scale.

The Ridley–Jopling classification system is based on clinical features, bacterial index, histopathology findings, and the individual's cell-mediated immunity to *M. leprae*. Patients with tuberculoid disease (TT) and lepromatous disease (LL) represent the polar ends of the spectrum and are immunologically stable. These patients do not change their cell-mediated immunity to *M. leprae* during the course of their disease and therefore never change their Ridley–Jopling classification. Patients with borderline disease (BT, BB, BL) comprise the middle portion of the spectrum and can experience shifts in their cell-mediated immunity to *M. leprae*. The immunity of borderline patients is unstable. If their immunity against the bacillus improves, the borderline patient moves towards the tuberculoid end of the disease spectrum and experiences a type-1 reaction. If their specific immunity weakens, they shift towards the lepromatous type, with a downgrading reaction (Fig. 22.12).

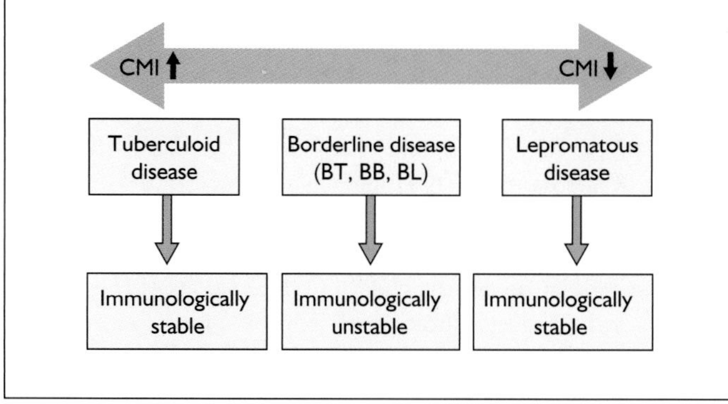

Figure 22.12 The immunologic spectrum of leprosy. Tuberculoid and lepromatous disease are at the polar ends and are immunologically stable. Borderline disease is immunologically unstable, and patients may move toward the tuberculoid or lepromatous pole. BT, borderline tuberculoid; BB, borderline borderline; BL, borderline lepromatous; CMI, cell-mediated immunity.

Slit skin smears have a high specificity (nearly 100%) for leprosy; however, the sensitivity of this tool is generally low because not all leprosy patients will be smear-positive.[32] Skin smears are used to assess the bacterial load of a leprosy patient and to follow the response to therapy. In the USA, slit smears are generally performed initially to aid the diagnosis and then annually to monitor response to treatment. A bloodless sample of tissue pulp is obtained from three to six sites: the earlobes, elbows, knees, and/or active skin lesions. The skin is pinched to render it bloodless and a scalpel is used to make a small incision (3–5 mm long and 2–3 mm deep). The inner area of the slit is scraped, the material is transferred to three areas on a glass slide and Fite Faraco acid-fast staining is performed to demonstrate the bacilli. The bacterial index is reported at each site using a semilogarithmic scale. The range is from none found to 6+, representing over 1000 acid-fast bacilli per one oil immersion field (Table 22.1). The bacterial index for a patient is obtained by averaging the values obtained at the sites tested. It has been estimated that the bacterial index declines between 0.6 and 1.0 per year in a patient on treatment[13] (Table 22.2). Studies have demonstrated that the combination of typical anesthetic skin lesions, enlarged peripheral nerves, and skin smear positivity increases the sensitivity of diagnosis of leprosy. The US NHDP considers that the presence of anesthetic skin lesions with acid-fast bacilli in skin smears or biopsies is diagnostic for leprosy.[14]

Table 22.1 Skin smear bacterial index

Very numerous	+6	Over 1000 bacilli per oil immersion field
Numerous	+5	100–1000 bacilli per oil immersion field
Moderate	+4	10–100 bacilli per oil immersion field
Few	+3	1–10 bacilli per oil immersion field
Very few	+2	1–10 bacilli per 10 fields
Rare	+1	1–10 bacilli per 100 fields
None found	NF	No AFB seen on entire site

Semilogarithmic scale NF (none found) to 6+ indicates total bacterial load of patient. AFB, acid-fast bacteria.

In 1980, the WHO created a two-group classification into which the Ridley–Jopling five-group classification is incorporated. Paucibacillary (PB) disease includes indeterminate, tuberculoid, and borderline tuberculoid leprosy, and multibacillary (MB) disease incorporates borderline (BB), borderline lepromatous patients (BL), and lepromatous (LL) leprosy (Fig. 22.13). In countries where histological evaluation of biopsy specimens is not available or too costly, the WHO recommends using skin smear results and number of skin lesions to diagnose a patient as paucibacillary or multibacillary.

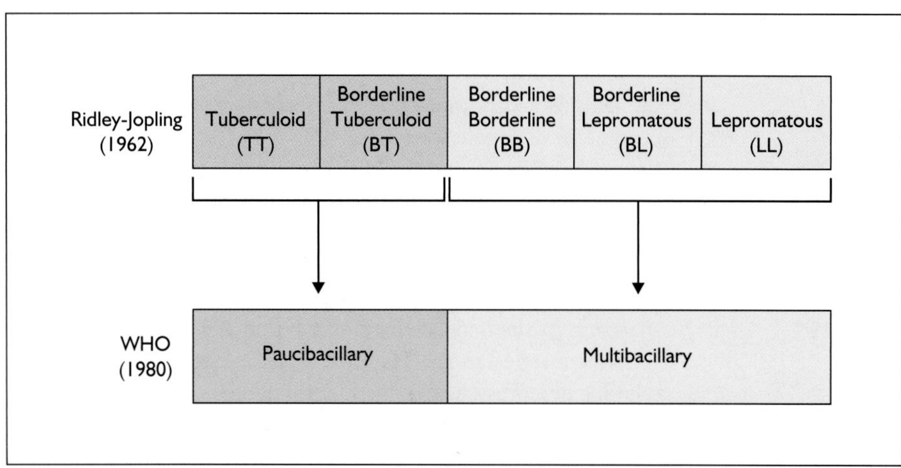

Figure 22.13 The Ridley–Jopling classification and the World Health Organization (WHO) classification for treatment. Note: Indeterminate disease is also paucibacillary.

Table 22.2 Bacterial indices of one patient from 1996 to 1999, demonstrating how the indices decreased with therapy

Skin site	04/18/1996	05/13/1998	08/25/1999
Right knee	+5*	+3	+2
Right elbow	+3*	+2	+1
Right ear	+2	+2	NF
Left knee	+5*	+3	+2
Left elbow	+2	+2	NF
Left ear	+4*	+2	NF

*Presence of globi; NF, none found.

Indeterminate leprosy

Indeterminate leprosy presents with one or a few ill-defined macules that are hypopigmented in dark-skinned individuals or erythematous in pale-skinned individuals (Fig. 22.14). While the lesion is usually anhidrotic, sensation is often intact and there is usually no nerve involvement. More than half of indeterminate cases resolve spontaneously. If not, they may progress to any disease type on the Ridley–Jopling spectrum.[14] At this stage classification depends on a good selection of the biopsy site and the study of serial histological sections. Histologically, minimal inflammation around skin adnexae with selective infiltration of nerve bundles by inflammatory cells is characteristic of indeterminate disease (Fig. 22.15). Slit smears are typically negative and the bacterial index is 0.

Tuberculoid leprosy

In tuberculoid leprosy, cell-mediated immunity against *M. leprae* is high. There is localized infection with fewer than five skin lesions asymmetrically distributed on the face, trunk, and buttocks. The typical lesion is a solitary, hypopigmented, sharply defined plaque with a raised border (Fig. 22.16). The central portion of the plaque may be erythematous or hypopigmented and the plaque may be scaly. Tuberculoid leprosy lesions are hypoesthesic or anesthetic and often have an absence of hair (Fig. 22.17). Due to disturbances in the autonomic innervation, tuberculoid lesions demonstrate early loss of sweating. Peripheral nerve enlargement may occur and, if it does, it is usually localized to one peripheral nerve early in the course of disease. Histologically there are well-formed epithelioid cell granulomas with Langhans' giant cells surrounded by a dense infiltrate of lymphocytes around nerve bundles, neurovascular bundles, and sweat glands. Epithelioid cell granulomas in the upper dermis may erode the basal layer of the epidermis. Nerve bundles may be replaced by epithelioid cell

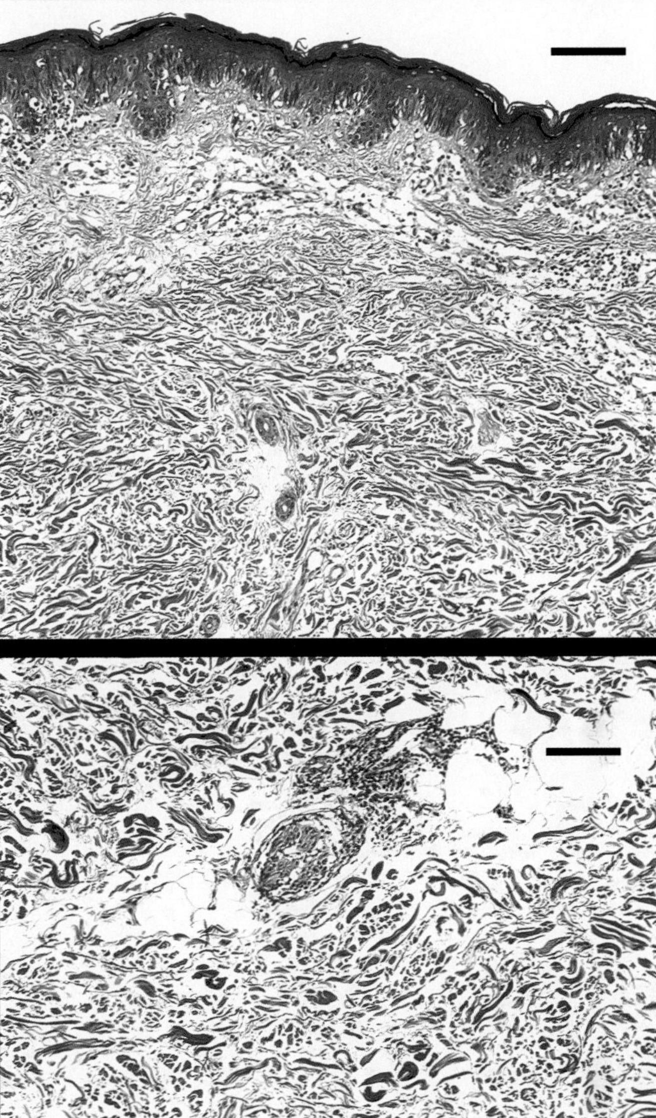

Figure 22.15 Histology of indeterminate leprosy. This classification should only be used to designate a definite diagnosis of leprosy in an early minimal lesion in which the extent of the infiltrate is insufficient to distinguish lepromatous from tuberculoid types. Top: The upper dermis contains mild, non-specific, chronic inflammatory infiltrates. Bottom: Perineural or endoneural inflammation, shown here in the lower dermis, is a distinguishing feature, as is the demonstration of acid-fast organisms which are rare (not shown), and require the examination of several Fite-stained sections. Original magnification, 10x; bar, 100 μm. (Courtesy of Dr. David M. Scollard.)

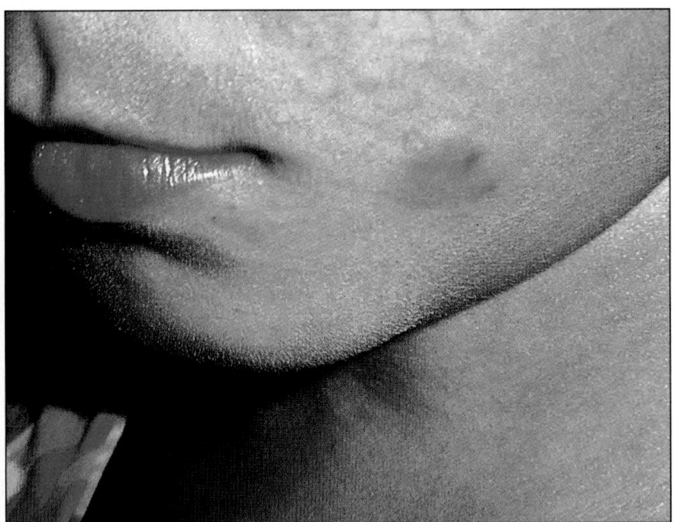

Figure 22.14 Indeterminate leprosy. Ill-defined macule that is slightly elevated and hypopigmented in a 9-year-old girl. (Courtesy of Dr. Omar Lupi.)

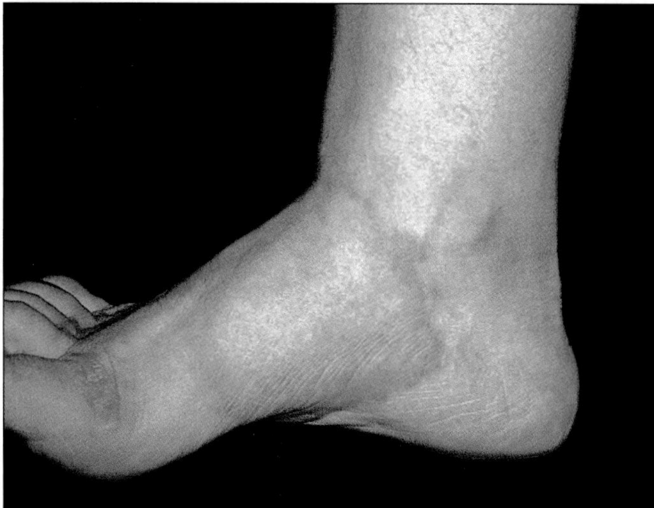

Figure 22.16 Tuberculoid leprosy. Solitary, hypopigmented, sharply defined plaque with a raised border. (Courtesy of Dr. Omar Lupi.)

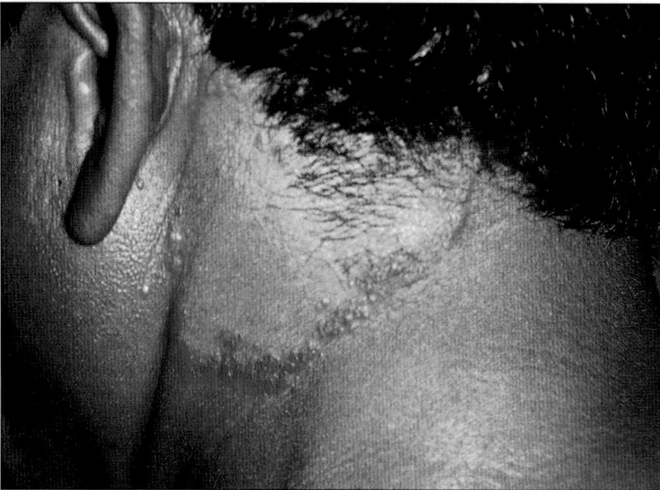

Figure 22.17 Tuberculoid leprosy. Sharply defined plaque with a raised border and an absence of hair. (Courtesy of Dr. Omar Lupi.)

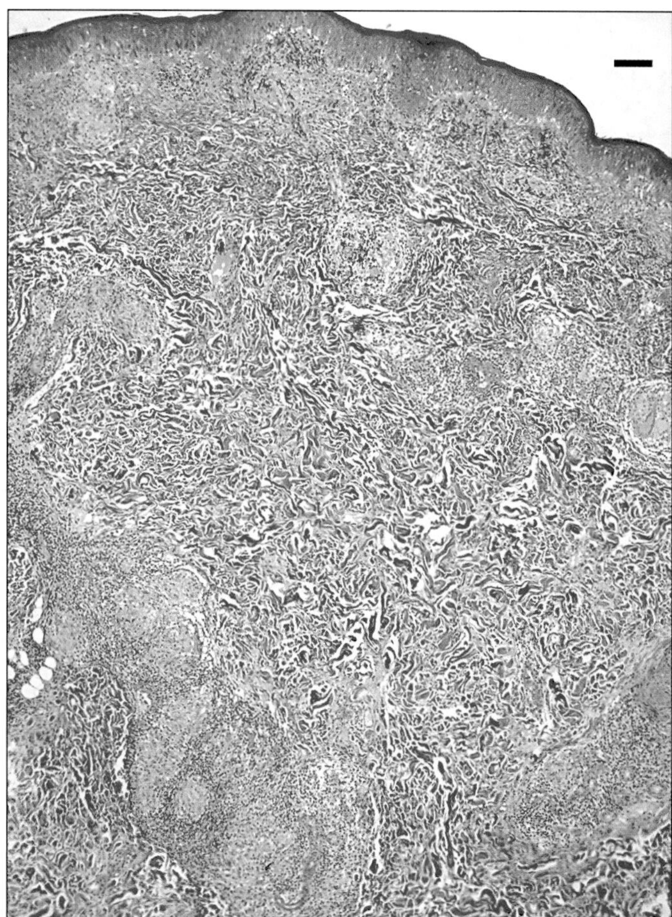

Figure 22.18 Histology of tuberculoid leprosy (TT). Well-formed granulomatous inflammatory infiltrates are observed in the dermis, with central epitheloid macrophages, a peripheral mantle of lymphocytes, and occasional multinucleated giant cells. The granulomas are often associated with nerves. *Mycobacterium leprae* are rare and detection requires examination of several Fite-stained sections. Differentiation of these granulomas from those of cutaneous tuberculosis and sarcoidosis may be very difficult. Original magnification, 5×; bar, 100 μm. (Courtesy of Dr. David M. Scollard.)

granulomas with central caseation. Characteristically, nerve bundles will massively enlarge in the deep dermis. Therefore, biopsy skin samples should be deep enough to get adipose tissue. Tuberculoid leprosy is the histological variant with the strongest presence of lymphocytes around granulomas. There are rare or few bacilli on biopsy although quite often bacilli can be found at a site where no inflammation or granuloma formation occur (Fig. 22.18). The bacterial index on slit smears is either 0 or 1.

Borderline leprosy (BT, BB, BL)

Borderline leprosy includes borderline tuberculoid (BT), borderline borderline (BB), and borderline lepromatous (BL) leprosy. Borderline tuberculoid leprosy patients have anesthetic discrete plaques similar to those in tuberculoid leprosy. However, there are multiple lesions, usually more than five and fewer than 10. Lesions are larger, less well-defined, and often contain satellite papules. Several peripheral nerve trunks are asymmetrically enlarged and neuropathy often results. Bacterial indices range from 0 to 2.

In borderline borderline leprosy, patients present with numerous asymmetrical annular plaques (Fig. 22.19). The classic lesion of borderline borderline disease is the dimorphic lesion which has features of both tuberculoid and lepromatous lesions. Dimorphic lesions are typically annular with poorly demarcated outer borders and sharply defined, "punched-out" centers (Fig. 22.20). Patients may experience symmetrical or asymmetrical nerve hypertrophy and/or neuritis. The bacterial index ranges from 3 to 4.

Borderline lepromatous patients may also have dimorphic lesions. They typically have symmetric bilaterally distributed lesions with widespread small macules, papules, and nodules of various sizes and shapes. These patients' lesions are mostly lepromatous in nature but also contain aspects of tuberculoid lesions. There is widespread asymmetric peripheral nerve involvement. The bacterial index is 4 or 5.

In the histologic presentation, as in the clinical presentation, borderline leprosy shows aspects of both tuberculoid and lepromatous disease. Ill-defined granulomatous inflammation and nerve infiltration are present. Acid-fast staining reveals bacilli (Figs 22.21

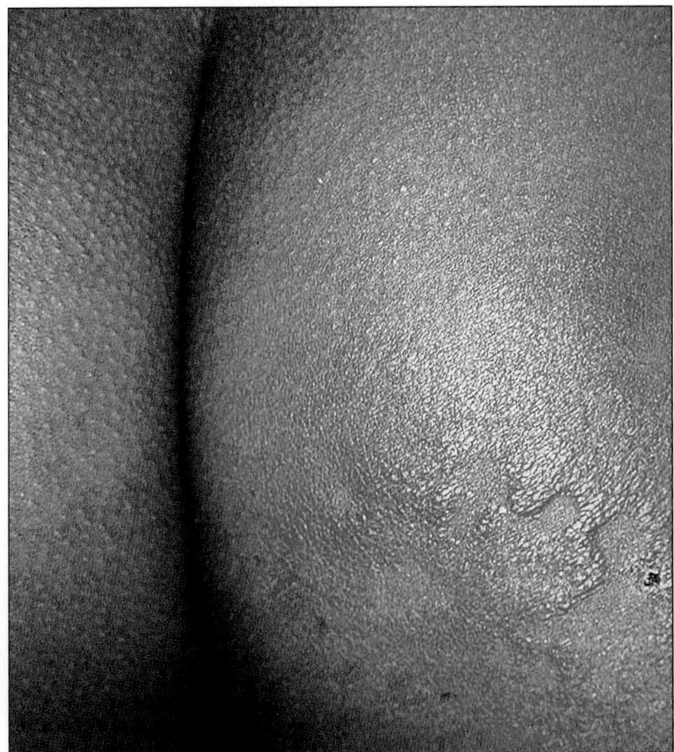

Figure 22.19 Borderline leprosy. Typical annular lesion with poorly demarcated outer borders and sharply defined "punched-out" centers. (Courtesy of Dr. Omar Lupi.)

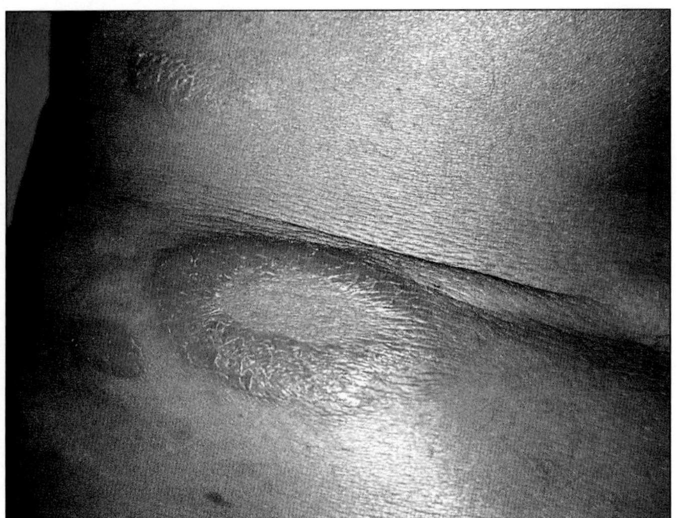

Figure 22.20 Borderline leprosy. Numerous asymmetrical annular plaques with "punched-out" centers. (Courtesy of Dr. Omar Lupi.)

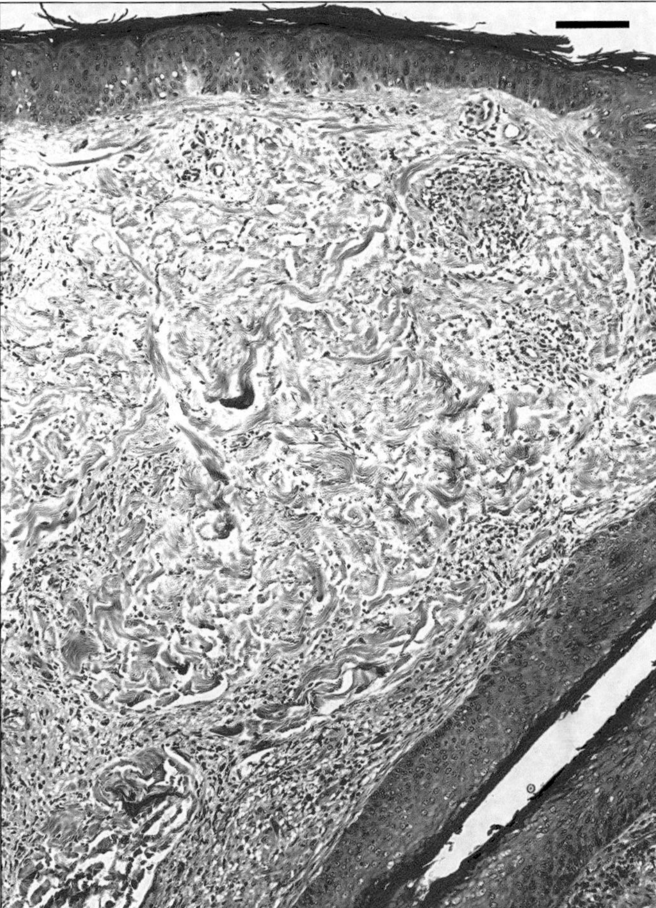

Figure 22.21 Histology of borderline tuberculoid (BT) leprosy. A linear or irregular granulomatous inflammatory infiltrate is observed at any or all levels of the dermis. In the upper dermis, it may extend to the basal layer of the epidermis. The granulomas contain epitheloid macrophages and variable numbers of lymphocytes, but are not as tightly organized as those of tuberculoid (TT) lesions. Acid-fast organisms are uncommon or rare (not shown) and their detection may also require examination of several Fite-stained sections; bacilli are often more easily found within or near cutaneous nerves. Original magnification, 10×; bar, 100 μm. (Courtesy of Dr. David M. Scollard.)

and 22.22). There are hallmarks that help in the histology classification of the lesions. For example, Langhans' cells are only present in tuberculoid disease and borderline tuberculoid lesions. Vacuolated giant cells can be found in borderline leprosy and lepromatous leprosy lesions. Epithelioid cells are present in tuberculoid disease, borderline tuberculoid and borderline borderline lesions. Moreover, some epithelioid cells can also be seen in borderline leprosy. Histiocytes and foamy macrophages are present in borderline lepromatous and Lepromatous leprosy lesions. Dense non-specific inflammatory infiltrates are found in tuberculoid disease and in borderline lepromatous although more remarkable in the first. Clear subepidermal zoning is preserved from borderline borderline to Lepromatous leprosy lesions. Lamination of the perineurium is more characteristic of borderline lepromatous and lepromatous leprosy.

Lepromatous leprosy (LL)

Due to an absence of cell-mediated immunity in lepromatous leprosy, *M. leprae* proliferates freely and this results in widespread systemic disease. The initial skin lesions are erythematous or hypopigmented disseminated, small macules that have poorly defined borders. Peripheral nerve damage occurs late in this type of leprosy and therefore sensation remains intact in early lepromatous lesions compared to the characteristic anesthetic tuberculoid lesion. As the disease progresses, many lesions become infiltrated and widely distributed in a bilateral pattern. In advanced lepromatous disease, ear helices may become infiltrated and earlobes may become pendulous. There is usually a loss of the lateral eyebrows and

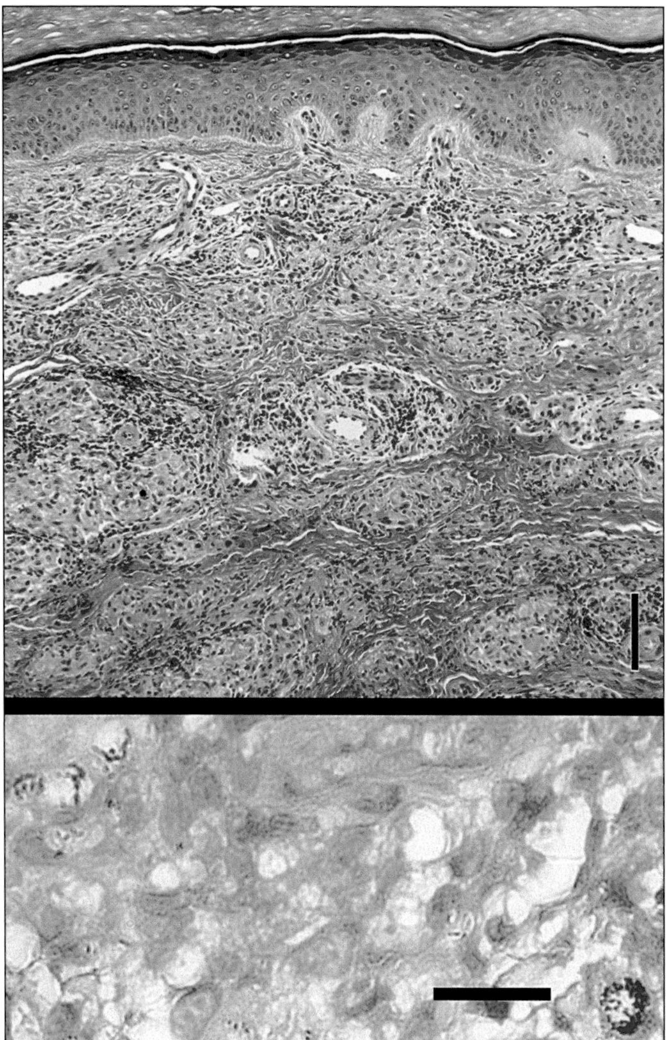

Figure 22.22 Histology of borderline lepromatous (BL) leprosy. Top: Poorly organized, linear, or irregular aggregates of lymphocytes and foamy histiocytes are observed at all levels of the dermis. In the upper dermis, the inflammation is separated from the basal layer by a Grenz zone. Bottom: Fite stains easily reveal moderate to large numbers of acid-fast organisms within foamy histiocytes and cutaneous nerves. Perineural reaction often leads to "onion-skin" thickening of the perineurium in BL lesions. Original magnification: hematoxylin & eosin, 10×; bar, 100 μm; Fite stain, original 40×, bar, 20 μm. (Courtesy of Dr. David M. Scollard.)

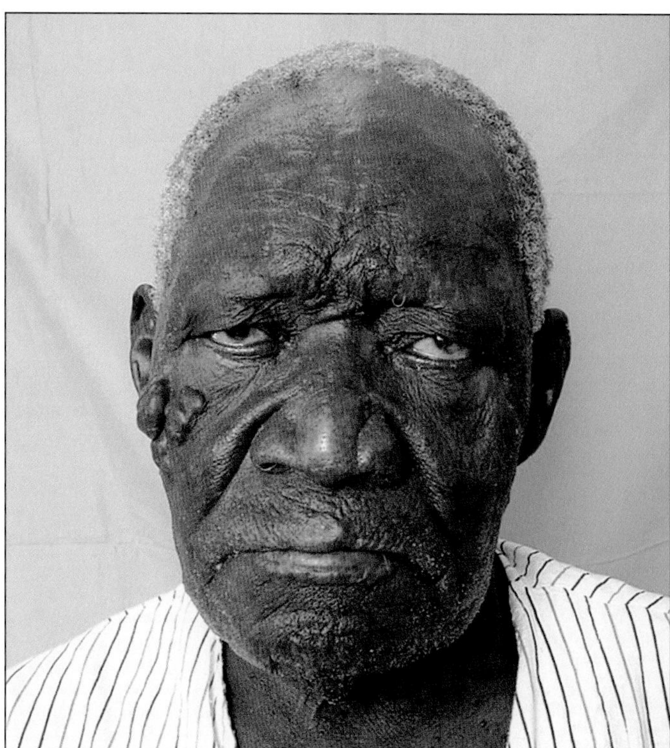

Figure 22.23 Leontine facies after longstanding lepromatous leprosy.

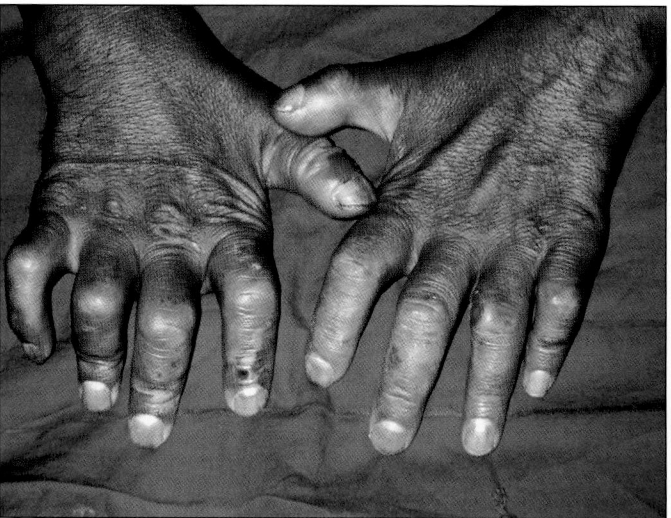

Figure 22.24 Permanent nerve damage of the ulnar and median nerves causing a claw-hand deformity. (Courtesy of Dr. Omar Lupi.)

sometimes eyelashes (madarosis). Bacterial infiltration of facial skin causes the classic leonine facies appearance of untreated lepromatous patients (Fig. 22.23). Most advanced untreated lepromatous patients have a glove-and-stocking neuropathy with claw-finger and toe deformities (Fig. 22.24).

M. leprae invades the nasal mucosa of most lepromatous patients, leading to local edema which manifests itself as nasal stuffiness, increased nasal secretions, and epistaxis. These symptoms may precede the diagnosis of leprosy.[5] Destruction of the nasal cartilage and intrinsic nose bone may result in perforation of the nasal septum and the pathognomic "saddle-nose deformity" of untreated advanced lepromatous leprosy (Fig. 22.25).

In lepromatous patients, multiorgan invasion by bacilli occurs. Lesions on the oral mucosa may develop on the palate and tongue.[15] Destruction of the uvula may also occur. Patients may present with hoarseness due to vocal cord edema. *M. leprae* has been identified in the liver, spleen, testes, bone marrow, and lymph nodes. It rarely causes local destruction of bones: X-rays can show changes in the cancellous part of the bones with patchy rarefication and loss of trabeculae. In the feet, there may be bony collapse, particularly at the metatarsal head and neck and the tarsal area.[33] In addition, peripheral neuropathy can result in ulcers of the hands and feet which may become secondarily infected. Osteomyelitis may also develop. In men, testicular invasion may produce atrophy,

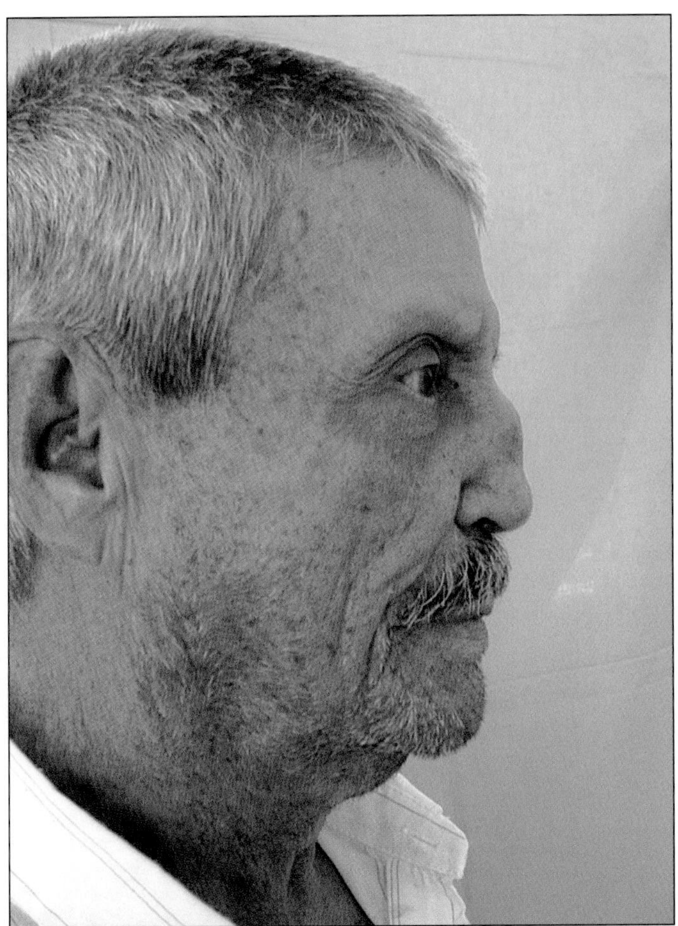

Figure 22.25 Saddle-nose deformity. Longstanding unattended lepromatous leprosy may produce the destruction and collapse of the nasal cartilage. If the disease progresses the proper bones of the nose may also collapse and the nose will look like a saddle horse. Note the absence of the eyebrow and eyelashes.

sterility, and gynecomastia. Although *M. leprae* has rarely been demonstrated by histology in the kidneys of leprosy patients, immune complex glomerulonephritis has been documented on many occasions and renal insufficiency as well as renal failure has developed in untreated patients.[15]

A silent neuropathy may also develop insidiously in leprosy patients. These patients manifest a functional deficit of a major nerve trunk without clinical evidence of neuritis.[34] An Ethiopian report of 158 multibacillary patients described 33 of their 56 patients with neuritis as being of the silent neuropathy type.[35] Sensation loss occurs gradually with an initial loss of thermal discrimination, followed by a loss of tactile perception, and finally pain. However, proprioception remains intact (Fig. 22.26).

Histologically, lepromatous leprosy (LL) reveals a clear Grenz zone between the epidermis and the granulomas in the dermis. The inflammatory infiltrate is composed of confluent aggregates or sheets of foamy macrophages, usually with a sparse lymphocytic component. The foamy macrophages are called Virchow or leprae cells which are loaded with *M. lepra* bacilli. Acid-fast staining reveals innumerable bacilli seen dispersed and also in clusters called globi (Fig. 22.27) The bacterial index is 5–6.

Histoid leprosy is a unique presentation of lepromatous disease in which the skin lesions consist of firm, non-tender, dermatofibroma-like papules and nodules (Fig. 22.28). Histologically, the macrophages have a spindle-cell appearance like fibroblasts.

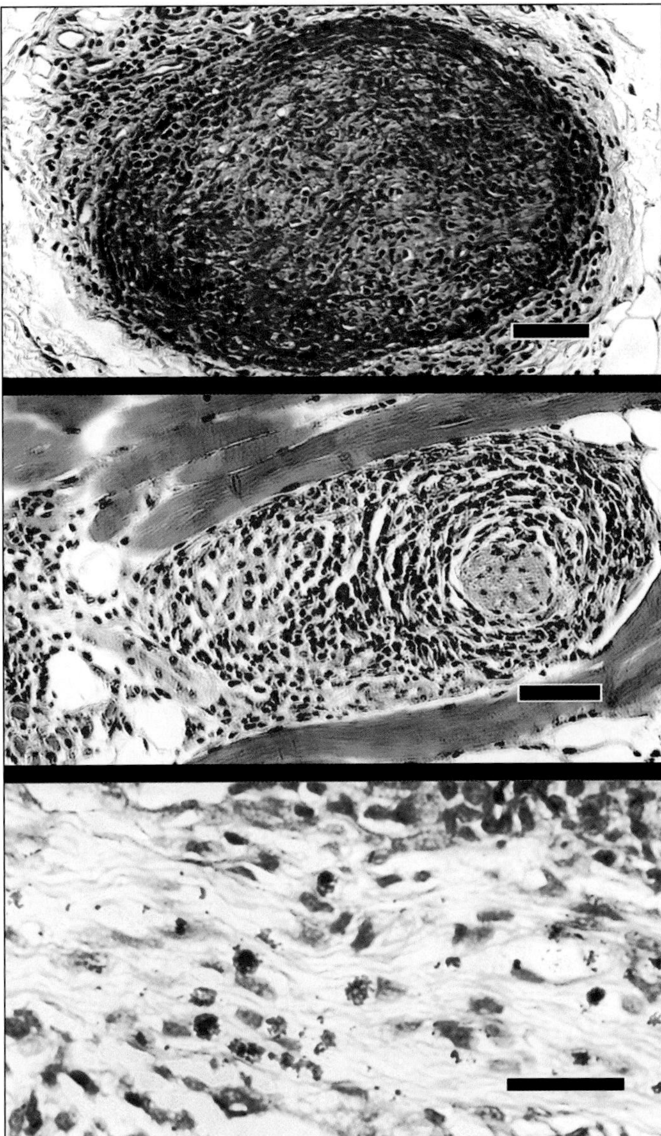

Figure 22.26 Infection and inflammation of cutaneous nerves: histology. Perineural and endoneural involvement are characteristics of *Mycobacterium leprae* infection, with differing degrees of host response. Top: Granulomatous replacement of a deep dermal nerve is seen in a borderline tuberculoid lesion. This results in conspicuous enlargement of the nerve. Original magnification 100×; bar, 100 μm. Middle: In borderline lepromatous lesions, strong perineural proliferation may result in the "onion-skin" thickening shown here in a nerve in the deep dermis. Bacilli (not shown) are numerous. Original magnification 100×, bar, 100 μm. Bottom right: In lepromatous lesions, nerves may be heavily infected, as shown in this Fite-stained section, with minimal perineural inflammation. Nerve function may be surprisingly well preserved for a prolonged period of time, even in such heavily infected nerves, but without treatment they will ultimately become fibrotic and non-functional. Original magnification 400×, bar, 20 μm. (Courtesy of Dr. David M. Scollard.)

Eye disease

Ocular disease represents a major cause of morbidity in all types of leprosy patients.[36] In tuberculoid disease, the ocular manifestations are due to invasion of nearby nerves. Involvement of the trigeminal

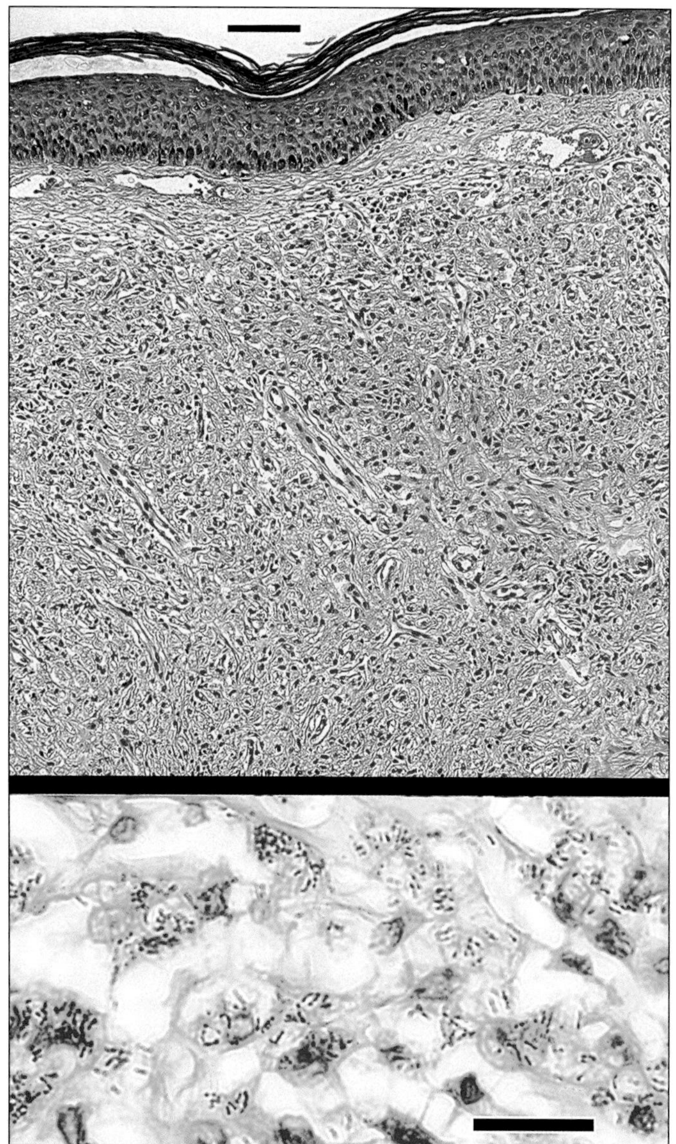

Figure 22.27 Lepromatous leprosy (LL): histology. Top: A Grenz zone is present. The inflammatory infiltrate is composed of confluent aggregates or sheets of foamy macrophages with a sparse lymphocytic component. Cutaneous nerves are inflamed and infected but display little or no perineural reactions. Bottom: Fite stains easily reveal very large numbers of *Mycobacterium leprae* within histiocytes and cutaneous nerves. Original magnification: top, hematoxylin & eosin 10×; bar, 100 μm. Bottom, Fite stain, original magnification 40×, bar, 20 μm. (Courtesy of Dr. David M. Scollard.)

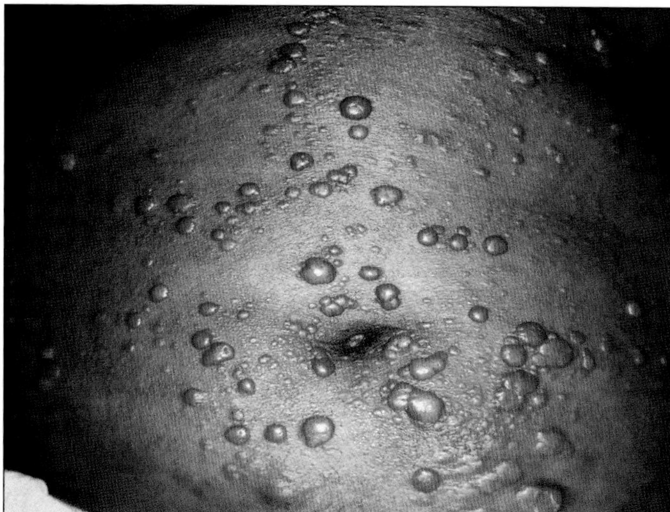

Figure 22.28 Histoid leprosy. Firm, non-tender, dermatofibroma-like papules and nodules with a diffuse distribution. (Courtesy of Dr. Omar Lupi.)

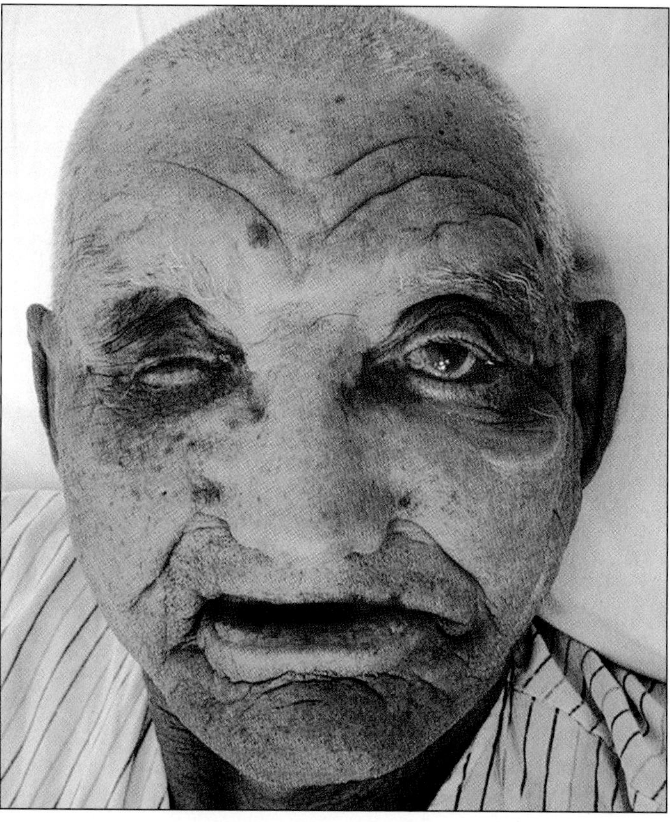

Figure 22.29 Lagophthalmos. Eye disease may be severe in leprosy patients. Facial nerve involvement may result in the inability to blink and to close the eyes (lagophthalmus) favoring eye dryness and corneal injury or infection that will need enucleation.

nerve causes sensory damage to the cornea and conjunctiva, resulting in decreased spontaneous blinking, unawareness of dryness, foreign bodies, and injuries. Involvement of the facial nerve causes motor weakness or paralysis of the orbicularis oculi muscle, which results in the inability to blink forcefully, and lagophthalmos (inability to close the eye) (Fig. 22.29). There is also loss of protective blinking, which leads to dry eyes, and keratitis caused by injury and/or infection. In lepromatous disease, bloodborne *M. leprae* invades the cooler anterior chamber of the eye, including the cornea, episclera, sclera, conjunctiva, ciliary body, and iris. This is usually asymptomatic and visible after more than 4 years of leprosy onset. Invasion of the cornea may lead to opacities and decreased vision. Painful episcleritis, scleritis, and iridocyclitis may occur during inflammatory reactional states. Iridocyclitis can cause cataracts, glaucoma, and blindness (Fig. 22.30). Prolonged corticosteroid use (either by mouth or in the form of eye drops) is a cause of subcapsular posterior cataracts in leprosy patients. In lepromatous disease, *M. leprae* invades the nasolacrimal duct and

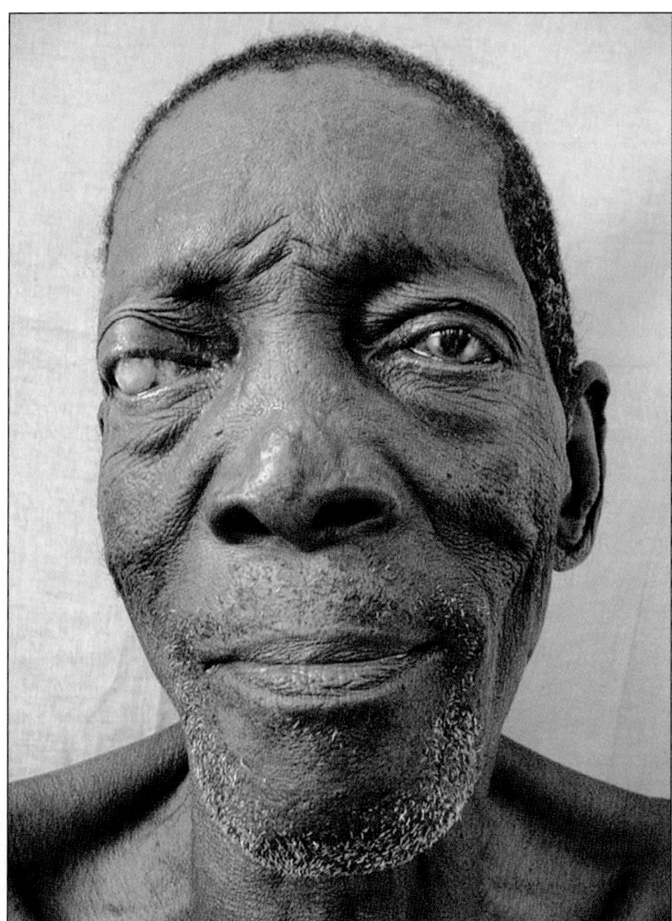

Figure 22.30 Opacity and blindness. Painful scleritis, iridocyclitis and invasion of the cornea may lead to the opacity of the cornea and blindness.

may cause either an increase or decrease in tearing. Blockage of the duct may result from dacrocystitis.[15]

Hand and foot injury

Damage to the feet may occur in all forms of leprosy due to peripheral motor and sensory neuropathy. In lepromatous disease, *M. leprae* rarely directly invades the bone. Loss of sensation predisposes patients to injury, ulceration, and chronic infections, including osteomyelitis. Patients are unaware of the injury or infection due to the absence of pain and continue to use the infected foot, which prevents healing. The dry skin that results from damage to the autonomic nervous system is easily injured and small fissures can provide entry for bacterial or fungal pathogens.[33] Similar to foot injury, injuries to the hands of leprosy patients are the result of sensory, motor, and autonomic nerve damage predisposing patients to repetitive injuries and deformities.

Pregnancy in leprosy

The US NHDP advises females of childbearing potential to avoid pregnancy until treatment is completed since pregnancy may precipitate the first symptoms of leprosy, neuritis, and the erythema nodosum leprosum.[14] Reversal reactions are more common during the postpartum period since a woman's cell-mediated immunity is recovering during this time. The possible risk of in utero transmission in an untreated pregnant women is reported to be very small.

Reactions in leprosy

Four reactions may complicate leprosy.[37] They occur in 25–50% of patients.[14] There are no known factors to predict reactions; however, tuberculoid patients do not have reactional states. The type 1 reversal reaction occurs only in borderline patients (BT, BB, and BL). It represents an acute increase in cell-mediated immunity against *M. leprae* and has also been referred to as an upgrading reaction. The type 2 reaction is erythema nodosum leprosum (ENL). This only occurs in BL and LL patients and represents an antigen–antibody immune complex reaction. A third and less well-recognized reaction is a downgrading reaction that arises in untreated or non-compliant patients when they experience a shift in their immunity toward the lepromatous pole of the leprosy spectrum. Clinically, these patients present with new lesions, fever, and malaise. They are difficult to distinguish from a patient with a type 1 reaction. Finally, Lucio's reaction is a rare vasculitic reaction in patients who have untreated Lucio's leprosy (diffuse lepromatous skin infiltration). Lucio's leprosy is seen primarily in Mexico and Central America but has also been reported in the USA and other countries.

The type 1 reversal reaction is a delayed-type hypersensitivity reaction. It usually occurs within the first 6–12 months after beginning therapy and is characterized by acute inflammation due to the upgrading of cell-mediated immunity against *M. leprae*. The immunologic basis of this reaction is thought to be due to a shift from a Th2 to a Th1 T-cell response.[38] Although this is favorable in terms of decreasing the bacterial load, clinically the patients develop erythema, warmth, and edema of preexisting or seemingly resolved leprosy lesions (Fig. 22.31). Patients may also present with hand and foot edema. Nerve involvement presents with pain or swelling in one or more peripheral nerves, or as new onset of sensory or motor loss. A reversal reaction with nerve involvement constitutes a medical emergency. Delay in treatment may result in permanent nerve damage with claw-hand deformity or facial paralysis.

In an ENL reaction, *M. leprae* antigens and antibodies form immune complexes that deposit in skin, blood vessel walls,

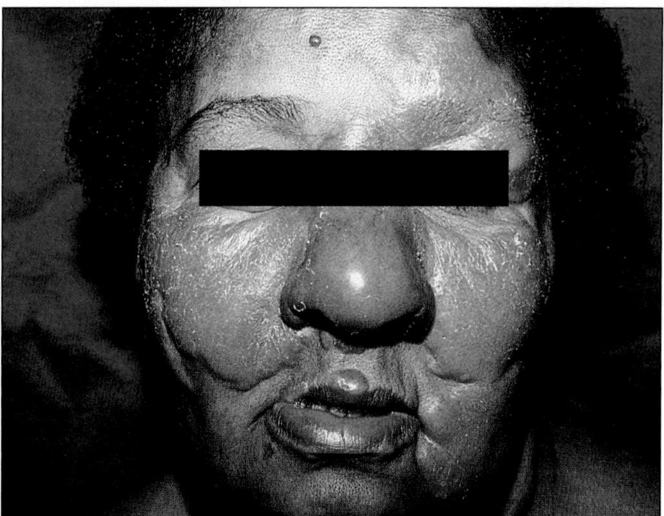

Figure 22.31 Type I reversal reaction, in a borderline patient. Massive infiltration of the face; edematous lesions affecting the nose and lips. (Courtesy of Instituto de Dermatologia Rubem David Azulay, Rio de Janeiro, Brazil.)

nerves, and other organs. ENL is characterized by new crops of tender, erythematous papules, plaques, nodules and bullae (Figs 22.32–22.33). The reaction is often associated with fever, polyarthralgia, myalgia, malaise, and neuritis. Other systemic findings include rhinitis, epistaxis, and orchitis. Rarely, proteinuria or hematuria occurs. In the kidney an immune complex glomerulonephritis rarely develops. If untreated, serious nerve damage can occur. Similar to reversal reactions, ENL may present with hand and foot edema. Both type 1 and type 2 reactions can develop after appropriate antibiotic therapy since the *M. leprae* antigens persist. Histologically, ENL shows an acute inflammatory infiltrate superimposed on the chronic granulomatous inflammation of borderline lepromatous and lepromatous leprosy (Fig. 22.34).

The fourth reaction is known as Lucio's phenomenon and is restricted to patients with Lucio leprosy, which is a diffuse nodular form of lepromatous leprosy. Lucio leprosy, also known as "la lepra bonita," was first described in 1948 by Latapí and Chevez. Although most reports of Lucio leprosy come from Mexico and Costa Rica, case reports have originated from numerous other countries, including Argentina, Brazil, Cuba, Paraguay, the USA, Spain, South Africa, India, Polynesia, and Southeast Asia.[39] Lucio's phenomenon is a vasculitic reaction that only occurs in untreated patients. It is characterized by tender purpuric lesions, which become necrotic and ulcerated. Although generally restricted to the extremities, lesions may progress to involve the trunk. The ineffective cell-mediated immunity to *M. leprae* allows for massive bacillary multiplication in these patients. However, their humoral immune system is intact and responds to the overwhelming amounts of *M. leprae* antigens with the production of vast quantities of antibodies. A severe immune complex reaction ensues, causing a destructive vasculitis and skin necrosis.

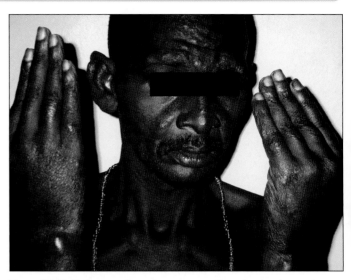

Figure 22.33 Erythema nodosum leprosum, type II reaction, in a lepromatous patient. Marked bilateral edema of the hands and infiltrated lesions on the earlobes, nose, and eyebrows. (Courtesy of Serviço de Dermatologia da Policlinica Geral de Rio de Janeiro, Rio de Janeiro, Brazil.)

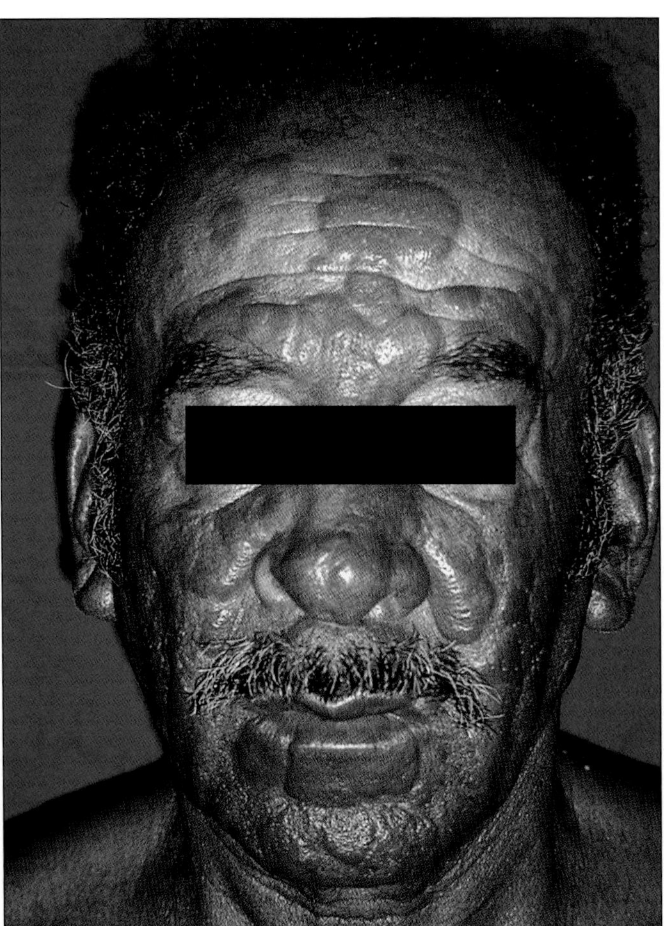

Figure 22.32 Erythema nodosum leprosum, type 2 reaction, in a lepromatous patient with new crops of tender, erythematous papules, plaques, and nodules. (Courtesy of Dr. Omar Lupi.)

Patient evaluation and diagnosis

Accurate and timely diagnosis of leprosy is important to prevent neuropathy, subsequent morbidity, and transmission to contacts. The length of time between the onset of symptoms to the diagnosis is shorter in endemic areas for leprosy compared to non-endemic areas.

The WHO defines a leprosy case as an individual who has at least one of the following: anesthetic skin lesion, thickened peripheral nerve, and positive skin smears. However, some leprologists recommend that a leprosy case should be a person with one thickened nerve and either a solitary hypopigmented skin lesion or a functional neurologic impairment typical of leprosy.[32]

During the clinical evaluation of a suspected leprosy patient, a personal and family history of leprosy should be elicited. A positive history of nosebleeds, persistent nasal congestion, painful elbows, changes in sensation or motor function or areas of numbness, burning in the hands or feet, and recurrent ulcers or "cellulitis" of the hands and feet may be helpful diagnostic clues. A thorough physical examination focusing on skin and peripheral nerves should be performed. The skin should be examined for hypopigmented or erythematous anesthetic patches or plaques and also for areas of decreased sweating. Neurosensory testing can be done using a cotton wisp or Semmes–Weinstein nylon monofilament. The eyes should be closely examined for pupil size, conjunctival erythema, and the ability to close the eye completely. Patients with borderline or lepromatous disease should be referred to an ophthalmologist

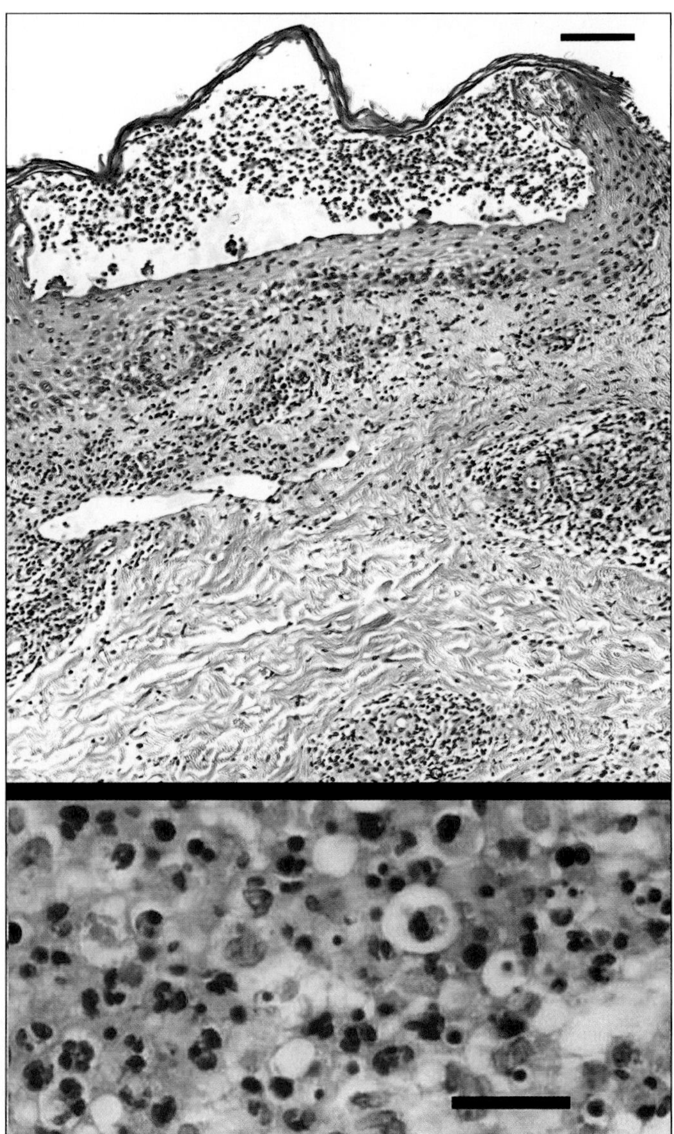

Figure 22.34 Erythema nodosum leprosum (ENL), type 2 reaction. Top: An acute inflammatory infiltrate is superimposed upon the chronic inflammation of lepromatous or borderline lepromatous leprosy, that may produce blistering lesions, as shown here. Bottom: If the cutaneous nodules are biopsied within 24 h of their development, collections of polymorphonuclear leukocytes can be found, with or without a clear association with cutaneous blood vessels. These acute inflammatory foci may also be observed in the subcutis. Original magnification: top, hematoxylin & eosin, 10×; bar, 100 μm; bottom, hematoxylin & eosin, original magnification 40×; bar, 20 μm. (Courtesy of Dr. David M. Scollard.)

to determine whether any ocular involvement exists. Peripheral nerves should be palpated for enlargement and tenderness, particularly the greater auricular, ulnar, radial, posterior tibial, and common peroneal nerves (Fig. 22.35). In addition, motor function related to these nerves should be assessed. The hands and feet should be examined for muscle atrophy, ulcerations, claw-hand deformities, footdrop, and secondary infections. Male patients should be examined to identify edema or nodules of the testicles. When possible, 4-mm-diameter punch biopses should be performed at the active border of suspected skin lesions. Skin smears should be done to quantify the patient's bacterial load, which will help to classify the patient's disease.

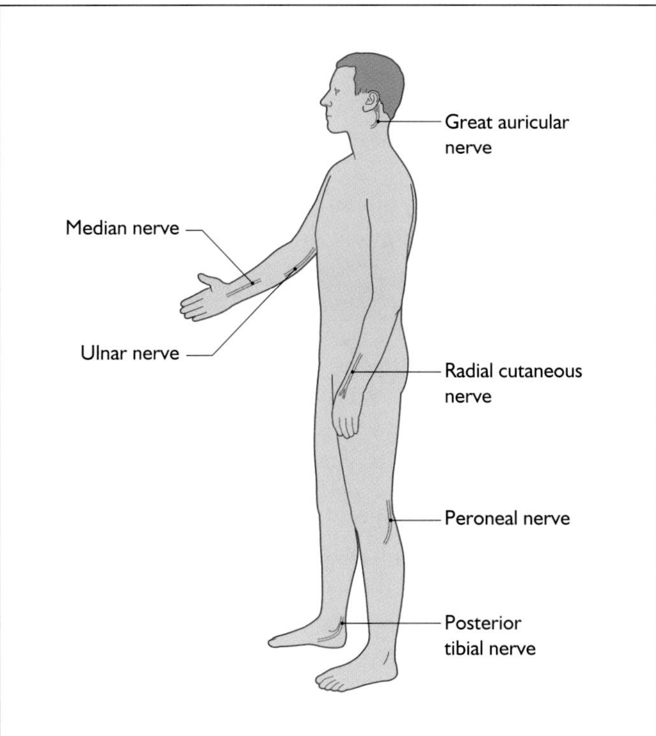

Figure 22.35 The sites at which peripheral nerves are most commonly palpable in leprosy.

Differential diagnosis

Leprosy can present with a variety of lesions and symptoms. The primary diseases to be included in a differential diagnosis of indeterminate leprosy are vitiligo, pityriasis alba, postinflammatory hypopigmentation, and pinta. A Wood's light examination is helpful to demonstrate the depigmented patches of vitiligo. A history of atopy, prior eruption, and country of origin or travel will aid in distinguishing these other conditions. Tuberculoid lesions and borderline tuberculoid lesions are typically anesthetic and can be distinguished from similar lesions of tinea corporis, tinea faciale, and tinea versicolor. A potassium hydroxide preparation aids in discriminating between these diseases. Other papulosquamous diseases, including psoriasis vulgaris, pityriasis rosea, T-cell lymphoma, parapsoriasis, lupus erythematosus, syphilis and sarcoidosis should be considered. Granuloma annulare may appear similar to a BT lesion.

Determining whether a patient has leprosy or sarcoidosis can present a diagnostic challenge since sarcoidosis can present clinically with indurated skin lesions, although histologically the granulomas are non-caseating. In leprosy-endemic areas dermatologists tend to make a diagnosis of leprosy for a patient with sarcoidosis.[40] Rarely, a patient may present with concomitant leprosy and sarcoidosis.[41] Reticulum staining of type III collagen fibers can be helpful, since in infectious processes this network appears to be disrupted and in sarcoidosis the reticulum network is preserved.

PCR has been used in the detection of *M. leprae* in biopsy specimens of patients suspected of having leprosy. In endemic regions, high sensitivity and specificity have been reported in detecting *M. leprae*.[42] However, PCR is highly unlikely to be positive, even in established leprosy cases when bacilli are rare or not detectable with careful histologic search of Fite-stained sections. In non-endemic populations it is recommended to use PCR in patients with acid-fast bacilli present on microscopy who have atypical histopathologic and clinical features which may obscure the diagnosis.[43,44]

Other systemic diseases must also be considered. Madarosis of the lateral third of the eyebrows can also be seen in thyroid disease. The peripheral neuropathy of multibacillary patients needs to be distinguished from diabetic neuropathy and other peripheral neural disorders. Electromyelogram (EMG) testing in leprous neuropathy demonstrates segmental slowing of nerve conduction velocity of clinically involved nerves.[45] A clinical pathologic case presentation of a borderline leprosy patient details the neurological differential diagnosis. The EMG results show small sensory fiber loss with intact deep tendon reflexes and the sural nerve biopsy is often diagnostic.[46] While leprosy is the most common cause of peripheral nerve thickening, the rare conditions of Charcot–Marie–Tooth disease and Dejerine–Sottas disease can be ruled out by inquiring about family history.[5] Since amyloid can rarely manifest as peripheral nerve thickening, other signs of this disease should be pursued.

Treatment

Treatment with dapsone, a weakly bactericidal sulfone, began in the 1940s. Before then, chaulmoogra oil from the fruit of the Cambodian *Hydnocarpus* tree fruit was used in parts of Asia without effect. In 1982 the WHO recommended multidrug therapy (MDT), which was modified in 1997. Rifampin is a bactericidal drug and clofazimine is weakly bactericidal but works synergistically with dapsone. After 1 week of treatment patients are no longer infectious.[14]

The WHO treatment regimen for paucibacillary leprosy is 6 months of daily dapsone 100 mg and monthly supervised rifampin 600 mg for 6 months.[47] For paucibacillary patients who have a single leprosy lesion, WHO recommends a single dose of rifampin 600 mg, ofloxacin 400 mg, and minocycline 100 mg. The WHO treatment regimen for multibacillary leprosy is monthly rifampin 600 mg and monthly clofazimine 300 mg given under supervision and daily dapsone 100 mg in combination with clofazimine 50 mg for 12 months.

In the USA, the NHDP treatment regimen for paucibacillary leprosy is 1 year of daily rifampin 600 mg and daily dapsone 100 mg. If active neuritis develops, the NHDP recommends that a third drug (usually clofazimine) should be added. For multibacillary leprosy, the NHDP recommendation is 24 months of daily rifampin 600 mg, daily dapsone 100 mg, and daily clofazimine 50 mg. If clofazimine is refused due to its hyperpigmentation, daily minocycline may be included. The NHDP recommends monthly rifampin dosing only if a patient is on concomitant prednisone. The NHDP has advised that alternative drugs can be used if there is drug intolerance or resistance. These drugs are ofloxacin 400 mg daily, levofloxacin 500 mg daily, and clarithromycin 500 mg twice daily.[47]

The WHO reported relapse risks after 9 years of completing treatment of 1.07% for paucibacillary and 0.77% for multibacillary leprosy, respectively. However, a few studies of multibacillary patients with high bacterial indices (+4 to +6) on slit smears reported higher relapse rates after WHO therapy – as high as 20% in one study.[36]

Clofazimine may have poor patient acceptance due to its skin pigmentation, but should be encouraged since it has strong anti-leprosy activity when combined with dapsone and it decreases the possibility of ENL. Rifampin decreases the effectiveness of prednisone, oral anticoagulants, oral contraceptives, and other drugs. Therefore, if a patient is on prednisone, rifampin is given once a month or discontinued and an appropriate alternative drug is started.

The US NHDP recommends that if a patient is on dapsone alone, according to earlier treatment guidelines, a clinical evaluation and a biopsy of the skin at the site of an old lesion should be done. If there is no evidence of active disease, dapsone should be stopped.

Baseline laboratory monitoring should include glucose-6-dehydrogenase, complete blood count (CBC), liver function tests, and urinalysis.[14] A CBC and liver function tests should be repeated every 6 months for patients on dapsone and/or rifampin.

Reversal reactions

For mild reversal reactions or ENL reactions, antipyretics and analgesics such as Aspirin and ibuprofen 400 mg three times daily are helpful. For a severe reversal reaction, prednisone 0.5–1 mg/kg daily should be started immediately to prevent further motor and sensory damage and given for 4–6 months, followed by a slow taper. Calcium with vitamin D and alendronate is advised. Gabapentin 300 mg nightly or 600 mg three times daily and amitriptyline 50–150 mg nightly have been used to ameliorate neuropathic pain in leprosy. Splinting the affected limb in a functional position has been advocated; however, this is controversial due to the concern of further muscle atrophy. Warmth to the affected nerve may alleviate some discomfort.

For chronic reversal and ENL reactions, the NHDP recommends increasing the clofazimine.[47] The clofazimine dose for such reactions is 100 mg three times daily for 4–6 weeks followed by a reduction in dose to 100 mg twice daily for several months. It can be given in combination with prednisone in order to reduce the corticosteroid dose. However, it takes 6 weeks for clofazimine to be effective and it will cause more hyperpigmentation and gastrointestinal side-effects. Thalidomide is of no benefit in reversal reactions. In patients with chronic ENL, precipitating factors, such as intestinal parasitic or other immune-compromising infections, and pregnancy, should be considered.

For severe ENL in men and postmenopausal or surgically sterilized women, thalidomide 100 mg every night or twice daily up to four times daily is the treatment of choice. Due to the sedative effect of thalidomide, some leprologists recommend the drug to be taken at night. Since thalidomide is teratogenic contraceptive measures and strict monitoring of female patients of childbearing potential with pregnancy tests must be performed.

Lesions and symptoms resolve within 48–72 h and the dose can be tapered gradually over a period of weeks to months to a maintenance dose of 50–100 mg daily. For patients who can take thalidomide, prednisone at a dose of 0.5–1 mg/kg daily to twice a day for several months is also effective, followed by a slow taper. Calcium with vitamin D supplements and alendronate should also be given. Prednisone is effective in combination with thalidomide during acute severe ENL reactions. Prednisolone is preferable for patients with hepatic disease. For patients who have completed MDT and are being treated with corticosteroids for reactional states, the US NHDP recommends restarting dapsone.[47]

The duration of therapy for pediatric patients is the same as adults for both paucibacillary and multibacillary disease. However, pediatric dose is adjusted according to body weight: dapsone 1 mg/kg daily, rifampin 10 mg/kg daily, and clofazimine 1 mg/kg daily. Minocycline and fluoroquinolones are avoided in children and during pregnancy. Rifampin is also avoided during pregnancy. Pregnant patients can be treated with clofazimine, dapsone, and, if necessary, prednisone. During lactation, standard MDT is used with a minimal risk to the infant.

For persons with HIV disease the potential interactions of rifampin with antiretroviral medications, especially the protease inhibitors, must be considered. It is important to determine whether an HIV-infected person has active tuberculosis before starting standard MDT since rifampin would mean monotherapy for the patient's tuberculosis.[47]

Downgrading reactions are treated with leprosy drugs, as is Lucio's phenomenon. The latter is also treated with supportive care. Patients with neuropathy often require periodic neurosensory evaluation, special orthopedic shoes, orthotics, or electromyelograms of affected nerves, as well as podiatry, physical or occupational therapy, and frequent ophthalmology and neurology consultations. Patients with neuropathic ulcers require aggressive wound care, callus debridement, periodic skin biopsies of chronic ulcers to rule out Marjolin's ulcer, bacterial cultures of infected ulcers, and radiographs and/or bone scans to rule out osteomyelitis underlying chronic ulcers and calluses. Mouse foot pad inoculation is rarely performed to rule out drug resistance. An immediate ophthalmology consultation is required if a patient develops iridocyclitis, for which atropine and corticosteriod drops are prescribed. Artificial tears are often recommended for lagophthalmos or decreased lacrimation. Orchitis may accompany an ENL reaction or occur independently and responds well to prednisone.

Close follow-up of patients who have completed leprosy treatment is important. WHO recommends follow-up for 2 years for paucibacillary leprosy and 5 years for multibacillary leprosy. The NHDP recommends annual evaluations for 5 years for paucibacillary patients and 8 years for multibacillary patients. All contacts who have lived in a patient's household during the 3 years prior to treatment should be examined once if their contact had paucibacillary disease and annually for 5 years for multibacillary contacts.

It is sometimes difficult to determine whether a patient is having a reversal reaction rather than a relapse. A patient can be determined to have a reversal reaction if the new lesions appear within 1 year of completing treatment (lesions of a relapse occur later), the lesions are edematous and/or painful (lesions of a relapse are asymptomatic), the lesions resolve with prednisone (lesions of a relapse do not), and the lesions develop rapidly within a few days to weeks (lesions of a relapse develop over months).

Personal treatment

Prior to slit smear testing, a eutectic mixture of local anesthesia, lidocaine, and prilocaine, is applied to the selected sites since this is a painful procedure in all but advanced lepromatous patients.[48] Patients with preexisting or subsequent anemia are prescribed 75 mg of dapsone daily or 50 mg dapsone daily, which is the minimal effective dose. If a patient develops a reversal reaction rifampin is discontinued and changed to daily ofloxacin 400 mg. After 2 years on an NHDP treatment regimen, if a patient still has positive slit smears, rifampin is discontinued and dapsone 100 mg daily is continued until there is bacillary negativity. Experience in three patients adding mycophenolate mofetil (1 g twice daily) to high doses of prednisone for severe reversal reactions did not permit the reduction of prednisone.

Chemoprophylaxis

It has been reported that a single BCG vaccination reduces the risk of developing leprosy by 50% and a subsequent randomized controlled study in Malawi found that a second BCG vaccination offered an additional 50% protection against leprosy. A South Indian study reported enhanced protection with BCG vaccination and the addition of killed *M. leprae*,[49] an observation that was not described in the Malawian study.[50]

Dapsone chemoprophylaxis has been shown to be effective in reducing the incidence of leprosy among household contacts and is given in some countries.[51] The NHDP does not generally recommend preventive treatment for pediatric contacts.[14]

To prevent injury to insensitive hands and feet, patients should be instructed to monitor their skin daily, check their footwear, and use gloves when cooking. Patients should be educated about the disease and its possible sequelae.

References

1. Lockwood DN, Reid AJC. The diagnosis of leprosy is delayed in the United Kingdom. Q J Med 2001; 94:207–212.
2. Sims C. Japan apologizes to lepers and declines to fight isolation ruling. NY Times 2001; May 24:A3.
3. World Health Organization Leprosy Elimination Project. Status report 2003. Draft. Geneva: World Health Organization; 2004.
4. Smith CM, Smith WC. Leprosy at the cutting edge: 2000 to 2005, and beyond. Trop Doctor 2002; 32:46–48.
5. Lockwood DNJ. Leprosy. Medicine 2001; 29:17–20.
6. Lockwood DN. Leprosy elimination – a virtual phenomenon or a reality? Br Med J 2002; 324:1516–1518.
7. Pfeifer LA. A summary of Hansen's disease in the United States – 2002. Epidemiology and Statistical Services 14 Mar 2003. Available online at: http://www.bphc.hrsa.gov/nhdp/Epidemiology_REHABILITATION.htm (accessed August 5, 2004).
8. Kaur I, Kaur S, Sharma VK et al. Childhood leprosy in northern India. Pediatr Dermatol 1991; 8:21–24.
9. Klaster PR, van Beers S, Madjid B et al. Detection of *Mycobacterium leprae* nasal carriers in populations for which leprosy is endemic. J Clin Microbiol 1993; 31:2947–2951.
10. Harman KE, Lockwood DN, Black M. Never take things at face value. Lancet 1998; 352:1190.
11. Bruce S, Schroeder TL, Ellner K et al. Armadillo exposure and Hansen's disease: an epidemiologic survey in southern Texas. J Am Acad Dermatol 2000; 43:223–228. Availabale online at: http://www.eble.org/scripts/om.dll/serve (accessed August 5, 2004).
12. Jacobson RR, Krahenbuhl JL. Leprosy. Lancet 1999; 353:655–660.

13. Steger JW, Barrett TL. Leprosy. In: Zajtchuk R, ed. Textbook of military medicine: military dermatology. Falls Church, VA Office of the Surgeon General, Dept of Army, USA; 1994:319–354.
14. National Hansen's disease programs. Standards of care for Hansen's disease in the United States. Louisiana, USA: 2003.
15. Hastings RC, Gillis TP, Krahenbuhl JL et al. Leprosy. Clin Microbiol Rev 1988; 1:330–348.
16. Lawn SD, Wood C, Lockwood DN. Borderline tuberculoid leprosy: an immune reconstitution phenomenon in a human immunodeficiency virus-infected person. Clin Infect Dis 2002; 35:1–3.
17. Buschman E, Skamene E. Leprosy susceptibility revealed. Int J Lepr 2003; 71:115–118.
18. Abel L, Sanchez FO, Oberti J et al. Susceptibility to leprosy is linked to the human NRAMP1 gene. J Infect Dis 1998; 177:133–145.
19. Mira MT, Alcais A, Van Thuc N et al. Chromosome 6q25 is linked to susceptibility to leprosy in a Vietnamese population. Nat Genet 2003; 33:412–415.
20. Bleharski JR, Li H, Meinken C et al. Use of genetic profiling in leprosy to discriminate clinical forms of the disease. Science 2003; 301:1527–1530.
21. Mira MT, Alcais A, Van Thuc N et al. Susceptibility to leprosy is associated with PARK2 and PACRG. Nature 2004; 427:636–640.
22. Maeda SM, Rotta O, Michalany NS et al. Comparison between anti-PGL-1 serology and Mitsuda reaction: clinical readings, microscopic findings and immunohistochemical analysis. Lepr Rev 2003; 74:263–274.
23. Ng V, Zannazzi G, Timplt R et al. Role of the cell wall phenolic glycolipid-1 in the peripheral nerve predilection of *Mycobacterium leprae*. Cell 2002; 103:511–524.
24. Rambukkana A, Zanazzi G, Tapinos N et al. Contact-dependant demyelination by *Mycobacterium leprae* in the absence of immune cells. Science 2002; 296:27–31.
25. Modlin RL, Hofman FM, Taylor CR et al. T lymphocyte subsets in the skin lesions of patients with leprosy. J Am Acad Dermatol 1983; 8:182–189.
26. Stafani MM, Martelli CL, Gillis TP et al. In situ type 1 cytokine gene expression and mechanisms associated with early leprosy progression. J Infect Dis 2003; 188:1024–1031.
27. Garcia VE, Quiroga MF, Ochoa MT et al. Signaling lymphocytic activation molecule expression and regulation in human intracellular infection correlate with Th1 cytokine patterns. J Immunol 2001; 167:5719–5724.
28. Adams LB, Scollard DM, Ray NA et al. The study of *Mycobacterium leprae* infection in interferon-γ gene-disrupted mice as a model to explore the immunopathologic spectrum of leprosy. J Infect Dis 2002; 185 (suppl. 1):S1–S8.
29. Ochoa MT, Stenger S, Sieling PA et al. T-cell release of granulysin contributes to host defense in leprosy. Nature Med 2001; 7:174–179.
30. Krutzik SR, Ochoa MT, Sieling PA et al. Activation and regulation of Toll-like receptors 2 and 1 in human leprosy. Nature 2003; 9:525–532.
31. Oliveira RB, Ochoa MT, Sieling P et al. Expression of Toll-like receptor 2 on human schwann cells: a mechanism of nerve damage in leprosy. Infect Immun 2003; 71:1427–1433.
32. International Leprosy Association Technical Forum. Diagnosis and classification of leprosy. Lepr Rev 2002; 73:S17–S26.
33. Brand PW. The insensitive foot (including leprosy). In: Jahss MH, ed. Disorders of the foot, vol. 2. Philadelphia, PA: WB Saunders; 1982:1266–1267.
34. Lockwood DN. Kellersberger memorial lecture 1998: nerve damage in leprosy: a problem for patients, doctors and scientists. Ethiop Med J 1999; 37:133–139.
35. van Brakel WH, Khawas IB. Silent neuropathy in leprosy: an epidemiologic description, Lepr Rev 1994; 65:350–360.
36. Joffrion VC, Brand ME. Hansen's disease of the eye, a general outline. Lepr Rev 1984; 55:105–114.
37. Burdick AE. Leprosy including reactions. In: Berth-Jones J, Coulson I, Heyman WR et al, eds. Treatment of skin disease: advanced therapeutic strategies. London: Mosby; 2002:336–339.
38. Yamamaur M, Uyemura K, Deans RJ et al. Defining protective responses to pathogens: cytokine profiles in leprosy lesions. Science 1991; 254:277–279.
39. Ang P, Tay YK, Ng SK et al. Fatal Lucio's phenomenon in two patients with previously undiagnosed leprosy. J Am Acad Dermatol 2003; 48:958–961.
40. Levy E, Lantis S. Sarcoidosis? Leprosy? Arch Dermatol 1971; 103:349–350.
41. Burdick AE, Hendi A, Elgart GW et al. Hansen's disease in a patient with a history of sarcoidosis. Int J Lepr 2000; 68:307–311.
42. Job CK, Jayakumar J, Williams DL et al. Role of polymerase chain reaction in the diagnosis of early leprosy. Int J Lepr 1997; 65:461–464.
43. Scollard DM, Gillis TP, Williams DL. Polymerase chain reaction assay for the detection and identification of *Mycobacterium leprae* in patients in the United States. Am J Clin Pathol 1998; 109:642–646.
44. Williams DL, Scollard DM, Gillis TP. PCR based diagnosis of leprosy in the United States. Clin Microbiol Newslett 2003; 25:57–61.
45. Said G. Leprous neuropathy. In: Mendell JR, Kissel JT, Cornblath DR, eds. Diagnosis and management of peripheral nerve disorders. New York: Oxford; 2001:551–564.
46. Chad DA, Hedley-Whyte ET. Case 1 – 2004: a 49-year-old woman with asymmetric painful neuropathy. N Engl J Med 2004; 350:166–176.
47. Joyce MP, Scollard DM. Method of leprosy. In: Rakel RE, Bope ET, eds. Conn's current therapy 2004. Philadelphia, PA: WB Saunders; 2004:100–105.
48. Burdick AE, Lehrer, KA, Barquin L. Use of eutectic mixture of local anesthetics: an effective topical anesthetic for slit-smear testing of patients with Hansen's disease. J Am Acad Dermatol 1997; 37:800–802.
49. Gupte MD, Vallishayee RS, Anantharaman DS et al. Comparative leprosy vaccine trial in South India. Ind J Lepr 1998; 70:369–388.
50. Karonga Prevention Trial Group. Randomised controlled trial of single BCG, repeated BCG, or combined BCG and killed *Mycobacterium leprae* vaccine for prevention of leprosy and tuberculosis in Malawi. Lancet 1996; 348:17–24.
51. International Leprosy Association. Summary of the report of ILA technical forum. Int J Lepr 2002; 70:S3–S5.

Atypical mycobacteriosis

Rogerio Neves Motta and Andréa Neiva dos Reis

Synonyms: Atypical mycobacteria (ATM), non-tuberculous mycobacteria, mycobacteria other than tubercle bacilli, potentially pathogenic environmental mycobacteria

Key features:

- Atypical mycobacteria (ATM) often cause systemic disease and mycobacterial infection may present solely as cutaneous lesions
- Skin and soft-tissue infections can result from direct inoculation or dissemination or may occur as a complication of surgery
- Clinically, the lesions consist of an erythematous surface studded with discharging pustules and fistulous openings, mixed with tender verrucous prominences
- There are no subcutaneous and bone alterations
- The ulcerated skin lesion is not painful and measures 2–4 cm in diameter
- Most cases occur in the extremities and initially present as nodules. Ulceration with abscess formation often follows
- Lesions usually last 8–12 months

Introduction

ATM are important human pathogens and differ from tuberculus mycobacteria because most are ubiquitous and saprophytic in the environment, especially in water. About 10% of mycobacterial infections seen in clinical practice are caused by ATM or non-tuberculous bacteria. These pathogens are among the most common opportunistic infections in advanced HIV disease. It is not easy to detect ATM by traditional methods such as Ziehl–Neelsen stain or by culture on specific media. At present, about 50 species of ATM have been identified but a few are considered potential human pathogens: *M. avium*, *M. intracellulare*, *M. chelonae*, *M. kansasii*, *M. marinum*, *M. fortuitum*, *M. gordonae*, and *M. ulcerans*. The third most common mycobacterial infection after tuberculosis and leprosy is *M. ulcerans*, the cause of Buruli ulcer. *M. avium–M. intracellulare complex* (MAC) are predominant species in HIV-infected persons. The immunological status of a person determines the prognosis of the disease: disseminated or localized. These organisms are not communicable person-to-person and are often strikingly resistant to antituberculous drugs.[1]

History

In the 1950s Timple and Runyon established that mycobacteria other than *M. tuberculosis* and *M. leprae* could cause disease in humans and classified these organisms based on pigment production, growth rate, and colonial characteristics: photochromogens (group I) grow slowly on culture media (>7 days). Their colonies change from a buff shade to bright yellow or orange after exposure to light. Scotochromogens (group II) also grow slowly but demonstrate pigmented colonies when incubated in the dark or the light. Non-photochromogens (group III) mycobacteria grow slowly and lack pigment in the dark or light. Rapid growers (group IV) also lack pigment, but they grow in culture within 3–5 days. Collectively, these four groups have been called the "atypical mycobacteria" (group I), "non-tuberculous mycobacteria" (group II), "mycobacteria other than tubercle bacilli" (group III) or "potentially pathogenic environmental mycobacteria" (group IV). Group I includes *M. kansasii*, *M. marinum*, and *M. simiae*; group II includes *M. xenopi*, *M. scrofulaceum*, *M. szulgai*, *M. gordonae* and *M. flavescens*; group III includes *M. avium* complex, *M. haemophilum*, *M. malmoense*, *M. terrae*, and *M. ulcerans*; and group IV includes *M. abscessus*, *M. fortuitum*, *M. chelonae*, and *M. smegmatis*.

ATM cause four clinical syndromes: (1) pulmonary disease; (2) lymphadenitis; (3) skin or soft-tissue disease; and (4) disseminated disease in AIDS. *M. avium* and *M. intracellulare* (known together as MAC) are the most common causes of pulmonary disease, lymphadenitis, and disseminated disease. All four clinical syndromes appear to be increasing in frequency, particularly in immunosuppressed hosts. Disease in patients who are immunocompetent usually consists of localized skin and soft-tissue infections.[2]

Epidemiology

Since 1982, the frequency of diseases attributed to non-tuberculous mycobacteria has increased, especially in AIDS patients and those who are immunocompromised secondary to cancer, organ transplantation, or administration of immunosuppressive drugs. Nosocomial infections may occur following hospitalization or surgery.

In contrast to *M. tuberculosis*, interpersonal transmission does not occur with non-tuberculous mycobacteria; these bacteria are ubiquitous and may be found everywhere in the environment. Their natural habitats are water, soil, and animals.

One such survey, published in 1982 by the Centers for Disease Control and Prevention (CDC), suggests that 65.2% of the total mycobacteria pathogens isolated were *M. tuberculosis* and 34.8% were ATM. Of the atypical mycobacterial isolates, about 60% were MAC; 20% *M. fortuitum–chelonae* complex; 10% *M. kansasii*; with *M. scrofulaceum*, *M. marinum*, *M. xenopi*, *M. szulgai*, and *M. malmoense* comprising the remaining 10%. *M. ulcerans* is not included because the survey was not in an *M. ulcerans*-endemic area. *M. leprae* is not included in this survey because it has not been cultured in vitro.

In 1990, the overall prevalence of atypical mycobacterial infections was estimated at about 2/100 000 population in the USA, with over one-half the cases due to MAC, and the largest population of patients being white males who are not infected with AIDS.[1] If MAC infections in AIDS patients were included, the percentage of infection in white males would be even higher.

Cutaneous infections with ATM are relatively rare in the USA; they are much more common in immunocompromised hosts, in particular those with HIV or leukemia or those undergoing immunosuppressive therapy. These infections cause little mortality but can cause morbidity, especially when they are not diagnosed and treated effectively; cutaneous atypical mycobacterial infections can often resolve on their own without intervention.

ATM infection is more common in men than women, especially in older patients; this probably relates to the decline in health in such patients.

Distribution of ATM appears to be worldwide; however, some organisms are only found in limited areas (e.g., *M. ulcerans* in Central Africa, Australia, New Guinea, Mexico, Central America, and South America). Some species are common in relatively similar geographical areas. For example, although MAC and *M. fortuitum–chelonae* complex are found almost worldwide, in the USA they are more common in the southeastern and Gulf-coast states, while *M. kansasii* is more prevalent in the Midwestern and central parts of the country.[3]

M. marinum, the fish tuberculosis agent, can be isolated in fresh water, seawater, and swimming pools, where the bacteria accumulate on the walls of the pool.

Pathogenesis and etiology

Because its first pathogenic representative was not identified until 1938, the recorded history of atypical mycobacterial infections is relatively short. With little or no human-to-human carriers among the more than 30 species, infection is usually the result of opportunistic encounters between patient and pathogen. These soil-and-water saprophytes will infect only humans under certain conditions.[3]

For the establishment of mycobacteriosis, compromise of host defenses is generally required. First, local tissue defects can be observed; thus the destruction of the integrity of skin or mucous membranes by wounds and injuries facilitates the development of cutaneous mycobacteriosis.

Second, it has been clearly demonstrated that reduction of the cell-mediated immune reactions increases the intracellular multiplication of mycobacteria. So mycobacteriosis is often associated with underlying diseases such as cancer, leukemia, viral infection, and organ transplant or with immunosuppressive therapies including steroids, chemotherapy, or radiation therapy.[4]

In patients with AIDS, disseminated infection with positive blood cultures is the most common clinical presentation. Occurrence depends on the degree of immunodeficiency; they are usually only seen in persons with a CD4 count <100 cells/mm^3. In 95% of cases, the isolated strains belong to MAC.

Clinical features

Mycobacterium marinum disease

Humans acquire the infection through traumatized skin lesions exposed to contaminated water or wounds in contact with marine animals or their products. Patients present with an isolated nodule, typically on the upper extremity.

A slightly tender, red, indurated area develops in the skin within a 1–6-week incubation period and then progresses to single or grouped multiple, brownish-red papulonodules that slowly become violaceous; the skin lesions may eventually ulcerate to drain pus or they may form slightly verrucous papules or plaques resembling psoriasis. They are usually located on the elbows (most common), knees, hands, and feet. In about 25% of cases, secondary nodules can be seen along the course of the lymphatics of the involved extremity in a sporotrichoid pattern.[4]

Mycobacterium kansasii disease

Cutaneous involvement may occur in normal or previously traumatized skin, and is commonly seen in patients with immunodeficiency. Clinical manifestations include red-to-violaceous indurated papules or plaques; pustular, ulcerated, crusted, or verrucous papules or nodules; cellulitis; abscesses; joint pain including arthritis, synovitis and bursitis; and a sporotrichoid adenopathy of an involved extremity.

Mycobacterium szulgai disease

This organism is distributed worldwide with no known natural reservoirs.

Red, tender nodules on the extremities, trunk, or neck may become fluctuant and drain spontaneously.

Mycobacterium scrofulaceum disease

The infection usually occurs in healthy-appearing children and, rarely, in adults as unilateral cervical adenopathy high in the neck, with minimal pain or tenderness. Occasionally the involved nodes may remain stationary and then regress, leaving residual fibrosis and calcification; more commonly the nodes progress and soften, with eventual rupture and drainage.

This organism also occasionally appears as scattered, multiple, subcutaneous abscesses and in a sporotrichoid pattern.[5]

Mycobacterium xenopi disease

Immunocompromised patients may have cutaneous involvement when they have underlying bone or soft-tissue involvement such as epididymitis, osteomyelitis, lymphadenitis, arthritis, or sinus tract development.

Mycobacterium gordonae disease

Cutaneous infection occurs as small, tender, red-blue papulonodules 0.5–1.5 cm in diameter with mamillated or ulcerated surfaces and with or without proximal lymphangitic spread in a sporotrichoid pattern.

After inoculation from a penetrating wound, infection may produce spreading, diffuse inflammation, with the wound discharging serosanguineous material accompanied by systemic signs of toxicity, such as fever, chills, nausea, and vomiting.

Mycobacterium avium–intracellulare complex

Primary skin lesions are very rare and their presence strongly suggests immunocompromise in any patient.

Skin involvement includes red-bordered plaques or crusted ulcerations which range from limited numbers of lesions to spreading, extensive lesions. With dissemination of disease, multiple granulomas, pustules, ulcerations, and generalized adenopathy have been reported.

Other manifestations include cervical adenitis in children or adults, subcutaneous nodules, sporotrichoid spread, panniculitis, fasciitis, and synovitis.[2]

Mycobacterium ulcerans disease

Almost all lesions occur on extremities; they begin as injuries or insect bites that do not heal but instead become indurated, with eventual necrosis and spreading ulceration.

Otherwise, the lesion appears as a single, firm, sometimes pruritic papule that becomes more indurated and fluctuant over several weeks and then breaks down into a spreading, punched-out ulceration with classically undermined edges. There is little pain or tenderness associated with the ulceration and the skin beyond the involved border. The ulceration usually extends only down to muscle, with rare bony involvement.

This disease should be considered in any patient with a relatively painless, chronic, progressive ulcer on an extremity in an endemic area.

Mycobacterium haemophilum disease

The skin lesions usually occur in multiple locations on the extremities and occasionally on the trunk, with red-to-violaceous papules that gradually enlarge to become tender, crusted, ulcerated nodules or abscesses and fistulas draining purulent material.

Mycobacterium malmoense disease

The patients develop tender, red, dermal nodules scattered on the extremities and trunk.

Mycobacterium fortuitum–chelonae complex

Most infections follow trauma or surgery and manifest themselves about 3–4 weeks after the initiating event as tender, red, indurated areas or as an inflamed or cold abscess, any of which may break down and drain. Occasionally, firm, red-brown, non-tender, subcutaneous nodules arise at scattered sites in the skin as a result of dissemination from prior surgery or trauma sites (Fig. 22.36).[5]

These organisms may cause solitary draining cervical lymphadenopathy. A sporotrichoid pattern of lymphangitic spread has also been seen.

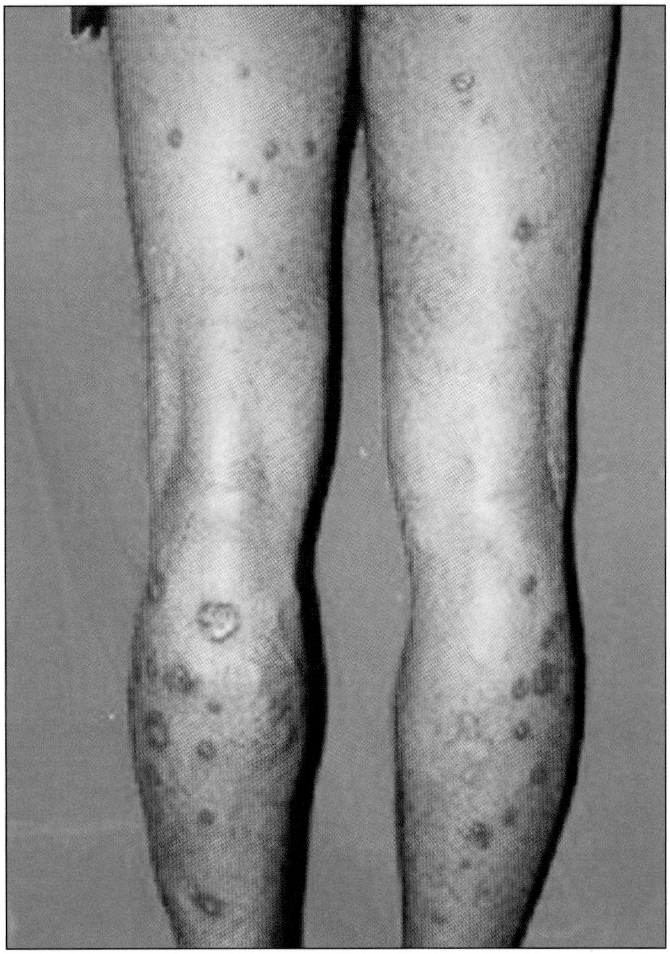

Figure 22.36 *Mycobacterium fortuitum-chelonae* complex. (Courtesy of Dr. Fernando Ferry, Dr. Cassio Ferreira, Dr. Carlos Mantins and Dr. Alvimar Ferreira.)

Patient evaluation, diagnosis, and differential diagnosis

The optimal way to diagnose ATM is by performing a culture of the tissue. This should be performed at multiple temperatures – 25, 37, and 42°C – to ensure that the cultures grow out all possible pathogens (Table 22.3 and Box 22.1).[2]

The development of DNA fingerprinting technology, especially pulsed-field gel electrophoresis, has been suggested as a diagnostic tool.

Pathology

The varying histopathologic findings of *M. kansasii*, for example, show acute suppuration, non-necrotic tubercles, or caseation. In general, the findings are similar to tuberculosis.

Skin lesions may show granulomas with areas of necrosis or foci of acute and chronic inflammation without well-formed granulomas. Other tissues may show caseating or non-caseating granulomas.

Box 22.1 Differential diagnosis of atypical mycobacteria

Actinomycosis
Pyoderma gangrenosum
Sarcoidosis
Wegener's granulomatosis
Yaws
Cellulitis
Coccidioidomycosis
Cutaneous manifestations of human immunodeficiency virus (HIV) disease
Erythema induratum (nodular vasculitis)
Nocardiosis
Atypical mycobacteria
Mycobacterium marinum
M. kansasii
M. scrofulaceum
M. chelonae
M. avium–intracellulare
M. gordonae
Papulonecrotic tuberculosis

Table 22.3 Colony growth as a function of temperature

	Temperature range (in °C)			
Atypical mycobacteria	24–25	30–32	35–37	42–43
Group I				
M. marinum	+	+ (7–14)*	N	N
M. kansasii	S	S	+ (10–20)*	N
Group II				
M. szulgai	S	S	+ (12–25)*	N
M. scrofulaceum	S	S	+ (>10)*	N
M. xenopi	N	N	+	+ (14–28)*
M. gordonae	S	S	+ (20–50)*	N
Group III				
M. avium–intracellulare	+	±	+ (10–21)*	±
M. haemophilum	S	+ (15–30)*	N	N
M. ulcerans	N	+ (28–60)*	S	N
M. malmoense	S	S	+ (15–60)*	N
Group IV				
M. fortuitum–chelonae complex	+	+	+ (3–5)*	N
M. smegmatis	+	+	+	+ (3–5)*

*Number of days necessary for growth at optimum temperature.
+, good growth; ±, growth may or may not occur; S, slow growth; N, no growth.

In patients with AIDS and in other immunocompromised hosts, many of the histologic characteristics of chronic diseases are absent.[2]

Treatment

The drug of choice depends on the sensitivity of an organism. *M. kansasii* is most susceptible to antituberculosis medications and can be treated with minocycline. *M. scrofulaceum* is not sensitive to medications, and surgical removal is often required. Combinations of medications based on sensitivities should also be used. *M. szulgai* is sensitive to medications. *M. haemophilum* may be sensitive to *p*-aminosalicylic acid and rifampin or rifabutin. For *M. fortuitum* and *M. abscessus*, combinations of medications that include ciprofloxacin, clarithromycin, amikacin, cefoxitin, and tobramycin, among others, have been used.[5]

Mycobacterium ulcerans infection

After tuberculosis and leprosy, Buruli ulcer disease (caused by infec-tion with *M. ulcerans*) is the third most common mycobacterial disease in immunocompetent people (Figs 22.37 and 22.38). Buruli ulcer is endemic in at least 32 countries, predominantly in areas of tropical rainforests; most patients are children and women who live in rural areas near rivers or wetlands. The emergence of Buruli ulcer disease in West African countries over the past decade has been dramatic. Current evidence suggests that the infection is transmitted through abraded skin or mild traumatic injuries after contact with contaminated water, soil, or vegetation;

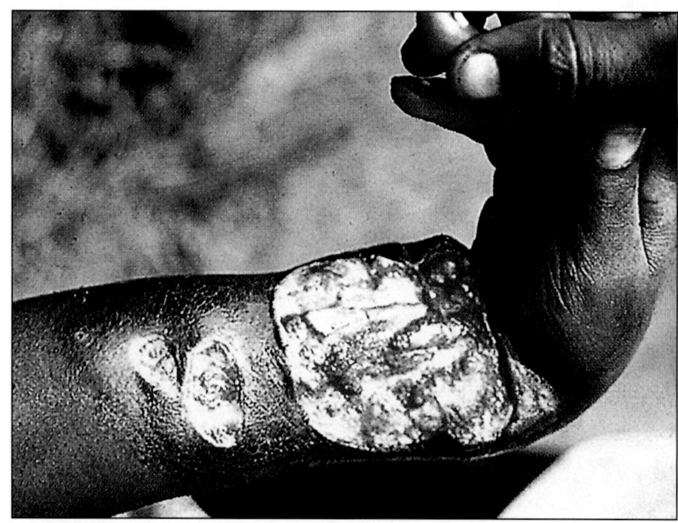

Figure 22.37 Typical Buruli ulcer in a Nigerian child. (Reproduced from Peters W and Pasvol G (eds). Tropical Medicine and Parasitology, 5th edition, Mosby, London 2002.)

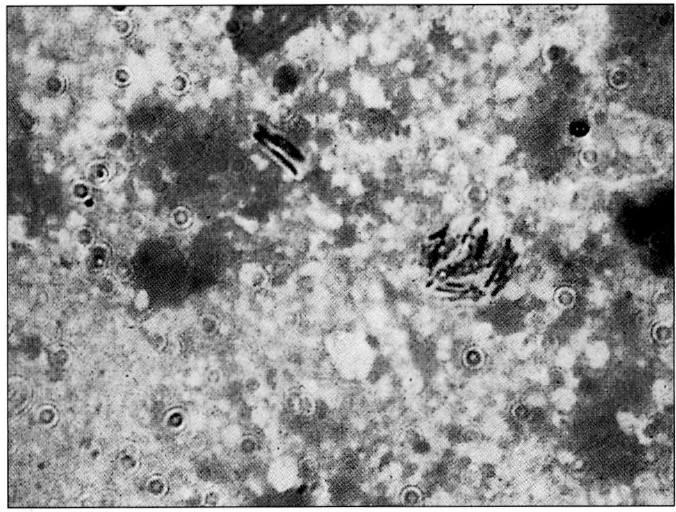

Figure 22.38 *Mycobacterium ulcerans* in a section of an ulcer. (Reproduced from Peters W and Pasvol G (eds). Tropical Medicine and Parasitology, 5th edition, Mosby, London 2002.)

there is one unconfirmed preliminary report of possible transmission by insects. The clinical picture ranges from a painless nodule to large, undermined ulcerative lesions that heal spontaneously but slowly. Most patients are children. The disease is accompanied by remarkably few systemic symptoms, but occasionally secondary infections resulting in sepsis or tetanus cause severe systemic disease and death. Extensive scarring can lead to contractures of the limbs, blindness, and other adverse sequelae, which impose a substantial health and economic burden. Treatment is still primarily surgical, and includes excision, skin grafting, or both. Although BCG has a mild but significant protective effect, new vaccine developments directed at the toxins produced by *M. ulcerans* are warranted. In West Africa, affected populations are underprivileged, and the economic burden imposed by Buruli ulcer disease is daunting. Combined efforts to improve treatment, prevention, control, and research strategies are urgently needed.[6]

Bacteriology

M. ulcerans belongs to the large group of environmental mycobacteria. It is a slowly growing acid-fast and alcohol-fast microorganism that is best cultured in egg-yolk-enriched Löwenstein–Jensen medium at 32°C. Attempts to culture the microorganism from clinical specimens fail in over half of all cases. Standard techiniques require much time for isolation and identification. If carbon-14 is added to the culture medium, a radiometric assay (BACTEC system) may detect growth much more quickly. DNA sequences specific for *M. ulcerans* have been amplified by means of PCR.[7]

Clinical features

In most African patients with Buruli ulcer disease, the subcutaneous tissue is the primary focus of infection. A firm, non-tender nodule indicates the first stage of disease, but preulcerative lesions also include plaques, which consist of larger areas of indurated skin, and edema. In the second stage, ulceration takes place. Coalescent necrosis of the subcutaneous fat with vascular occlusion results in sloughing and secondary ulceration of overlying skin, with typically undermined edges. Many acid-fast bacilli are present in the slough, but necrosis extends well beyond the site where *M. ulcerans* can be isolated (Fig. 22.38). Initially, a negative tuberculin (or burulin) skin response is seen. Several investigators have found that, when spontaneous healing occurs, the skin-test result becomes positive. The healing process may result in scarification, ankylosis, and contractures. Another presentation of *M. ulcerans*, although rare, is osteomyelitis.[8]

Treatment

Medical care

Rifampin may promote healing of preulcerative and small lesions, but it is ineffective in treatment of large ulcers. Some advocate postexcision treatment with rifampin alone or in combination with clofazimine. Hyperthermia with a 40°C water bath, such as a circulation water jacket, has shown significant effects in anecdotal reports. The use of hyperbaric oxygen has also been reported as effective in a small number of patients.

Surgical care

Excision is the treatment of choice for most lesions. Subcutaneous nodules or small ulcerations may be excised. After excision, the skin can be closed. Large lesions are often excised with skin graft closure.[9]

References

1. Collina G, Morandi L, Lanzoni A et al. Atypical cutaneous mycobacteriosis diagnosed by PCR. Br J Dermatol, 2002; 147:781–784.
2. Scheinfeld NS. Atypical mycobacterial diseases. Emedicine 2003; September: 1–15. Available online at: http://www.emedicine.com (accessed August 5, 2004).
3. Dailloux M, Laurain C, Weber M. Water and nontuberculous mycobacteria. Wat Res 1999; 33:2219–2228.
4. Johnston JM, Izumi AK. Cutaneous *Mycobacterium marinum* infection ("swimming pool granuloma"). Clin Dermatol 1987; 5:68–75.
5. Woods GL, Washington JA II. Mycobacteria other than *Mycobacterium tuberculosis*: review of microbiologic and clinical aspects. Rev Infect Dis 1987; 9:275–294.
6. Hayman J. Postulated epidemiology of *Mycobacterium ulcerans* infection. Int J Epidemiol 1991; 20:1093–1098.
7. Palomino JC, Portaels F. Effects of decontamination methods and culture condition on viability of *Mycobacterium ulcerans* in the BACTEC system. J Clin Microbiol 1998; 35:1097–1100.
8. Van der Werf T, Van der Graaf T, Tappero JW et al. *Mycobacterium ulcerans* infection. Lancet 1999; 354:1013–1018.
9. Mather MK, Flowers F et al. Buruli ulcer. E medicine 2003; August: 1–6. Available online at: http://www.emedicine.com (accessed August 5, 2004).

Chapter 23

Rickettsial infections

Katie R. Pang, Jashin J. Wu, David B. Huang, Rita de Sousa, Fátima Bacellar and Stephen K. Tyring

Introduction

The rickettsiae were named after Howard Taylor Ricketts, a University of Chicago investigator who lost his life during research in epidemic typhus. The rickettsial diseases have existed since antiquity and have influenced human evolution and history. Through famines and wars, these diseases have shaped the outcomes of many human events. Even now, when wars are less likely to be won or lost by the personal spread of a rickettsial disease such as epidemic typhus, the new threat of their use in bioterrorism hangs over the twenty-first century. In this chapter, we review these diverse diseases by examining the pathogenesis, epidemiology, clinical manifestations, and treatment of the tropical rickettsiae.

Pathogenesis

The maintenance of any *Rickettsia* in its natural cycle does not require transmission to humans.[1] However, investigation of the mechanisms occurring in rickettsial diseases has a valid purpose in advancing medical therapies and in fighting bioterrorism. All of the rickettsiae share many of the same general mechanisms of pathogenesis, which we will review below.

Rickettsia–host cell interaction

Rickettsiae attach to a protein-dependent receptor on the host cell membrane and induce focal host cell cytoskeletal rearrangements at the site of attachment, which results in their entry into the host cell by a mechanism requiring rickettsial metabolic activity.[2] Rickettsial outer membrane protein A (Omp A) and Omp B are adhesins of *R. japonica*, and OmpA is an adhesin of *R. rickettsii*.[3] The bacteria lyse the phagosomal membrane and enter the cytosol prior to phagolysosomal fusion, thus avoiding exposure to the lysosomal enzymes.[4] In the cytosol, they acquire their nutrients (such as glutamate and amino acids) and a part of their energy requirements through an adenosine diphosphate (ADP)/adenosine triphosphate (ATP) transporter. The spotted fever group (SFG) rickettsiae use cell-to-cell spread, whereas the typhus group rickettsiae burst open the massively infected host cell.[5]

Rickettsiae have a relatively long generation time (8–10 h), and the reasons for this are not clear.[1] Slow growth might be a good survival strategy to avoid harming the human host or the arthropod vector, but it would seem a poor approach to horizontal transmission from their rodent host to the uninfected feeding arthropod hosts.

Mechanisms of cell injury

Endothelial cells infected by *R. rickettsii* produce reactive oxygen species (ROS) that damage the infected cells via lipid peroxidation of host cell membranes.[6] The oxidative stress-mediated injury of cultured endothelial cells results in depletion of host components such as glutathione and increased levels of catalase, which increase the concentration of hydrogen peroxide. This reduces enzymes such as catalase, glutathione peroxidase, and glucose-6-phosphate dehydrogenase (G6PD) that are host defenses against ROS-induced damage.[7] The antioxidant molecules, α-lipoic acid and desferroxamine, in the infected endothelial cell culture system decrease ROS-induced damage.

There is less strong evidence that a rickettsial protease or phospholipase A_2 plays a role in the pathogenesis.[4,8] It is believed that phospholipase A_2 and ROS may act together synergistically in damaging the host cell.

In the absence of immune effectors, rickettsiae can kill infected cells.[9] However, some immune effector mechanisms such as CD8 cytotoxic T lymphocytes can eliminate infected cells by inducing apoptosis.[10] An immunopathologic effect can occur if the infected target of these cytotoxic T lymphocytes is extensive at the time of their clonal expansion and activation.[1] The death of *Rickettsia*-infected cells typically appears to be necrosis. Activation of NF-κB by a direct *R. rickettsii*-mediated, proteosome-independent mechanism halts apoptosis.[11] This would allow prolonged intracellular rickettsial survival and growth, but does not always prevent apoptosis.[10]

Pathophysiology

Increased vascular permeability results from copious foci of adjacent networks of endothelial cells of the organ's microcirculation. Fluid leaks from the blood stream, causing edema and hypovolemia. Edema in the lungs and the brain, which lacks lymphatics to remove interstitial fluid, can create a dangerous situation. Fluid in the air spaces of the lung limits gas exchange, leading to hypoxemia. Edema of the brain eventually prevents the blood from entering or exiting. Hypovolemia leads to poor perfusion of organs such as the kidney, leading to renal failure. The general and localized effects of multiple lesions in the central nervous system may cause loss of neurologic function corresponding to the area of the brain involved. However, focal lesions in other vital organs are not sufficiently extensive to result in organ failure. Hepatic infection may result in focal death of a small number of the liver cells sufficient to cause elevated serum transaminase concentrations, but not hepatic failure.

Mechanisms of tissue and organ damage

It is believed that thrombus-mediated vascular occlusion also plays a role in severe rickettsioses.[12] However, disseminated intravascular coagulation (DIC) rarely occurs, and postmortem studies of fatal cases reveal that thrombi are few and are a physiological response to endothelial denudation.[1] Animal models given lethal or sublethal doses of rickettsiae demonstrated that DIC does not occur and that fatal rickettsiosis is not a thrombotic disease.[13]

The pathogenic mechanisms regarding the vascular permeability changes associated with rickettsial infections have not been described. Multiple mechanisms may explain the increased vascular permeability seen in patients with rickettsial diseases. Extensive endothelial denudation may explain some of the changes in the most heavily affected segments of the vasculature, but probably could not explain the systemic manifestations of moderately to severely ill patients.[1]

Another hypothesized mechanism suggests an active role of the endothelium. Its ability to express an activated phenotype on rickettsial infection and to kill rickettsiae intracellularly implies an active role. *Rickettsia*-infected endothelial cells can interact with leukocytes, which in turn migrate and secrete cytokines. It is also possible that rickettsiae stimulate the production of a unique profile of chemokines and cytokines and this may explain the significant changes in permeability.

A third hypothesized mechanism is direct triggering of increased vascular permeability by intraendothelial rickettsiae through changes in the proteins and the cytoskeleton of the interendothelial junctional complexes, such as the adherens and tight junctions.[1] Circulating endothelial cells during rickettsial infection suggest that changes in the adhesiveness of these cells may play a role. These viable, circulating endothelial cells may establish new foci of infection in the capillaries.

Host defenses

Host defense is based on cytokine activation of intraendothelial killing of rickettsiae and the clearance of rickettsial infection by CD8 cytotoxic T-lymphocyte activity.[14] In the mouse model, tumor necrosis factor-α (TNF-α) and interferon-γ (IFN-γ) act together to activate nitric oxide synthase 2-dependent intraendothelial elimination. However, in humans, TNF-α, IFN-γ, interleukin-1β (IL-1β), and RANTES activate intracellular killing of rickettsiae by three different mechanisms in different host cell types when investigated in vitro.[14] The antirickettsial mechanisms include ROS, nitric oxide, and limitation of availability of tryptophan via its degradation by indoleamine-2, 3-dioxygenase.

Early in the course of infection, natural killer cells are effectors of antirickettsial innate immunity by secretion of IFN-γ.[15] Antibodies to epitopes of OmpA and OmpB (but not lipopolysaccharides) also add to immune protection against SFG rickettsiae.

Gaps in scientific knowledge

No rickettsial virulence factors, except for adhesins, have been found despite the availability of rickettsial genomes. Important unidentified essentials of the *Rickettsia*–host cell interaction include the host cell membrane receptor for the rickettsial adhesin(s) and the rickettsial method of escape from the phagosome.[1] The gene encoding the rickettsial phospholipase A_2 has not been found yet, and there are no data to support the hypothesis that it plays a role in phagosomal escape.

There is a need for more in vivo data in rickettsial research.[1] The in vivo effect of cytotoxic T-lymphocyte activity on cytokines has not been determined yet. In animal models, the role of ROS-mediated endothelial injury has not been ascertained. The exact mechanism of increased vascular permeability has not been elucidated. The roles of host-derived immune and inflammatory mediators have not been examined fully.

The lack of experimental models also hinders the advancement of rickettsial research.[1] The development of an SFG rickettsial disease model incorporating tick-bite transmission could help reveal the importance of tick saliva in modulating the early events in the skin and lymphatic vessels. An animal model of aerosol transmission would be essential for studies related to the use of rickettsiae as agents of bioterrorism.

There is also a lack of translational research in human subjects. Intracellular rickettsial elimination has been studied in human endothelial cells in vitro, but what actually occurs in the human body remains unknown.

The spotted fever group

Mediterranean spotted fever (MSF)

Synonyms: Boutonneuse fever, Marseilles fever, Kenya tick typhus, Indian tick typhus, Israel tick typhus

History

MSF was described by Conor and Bruch in Tunisia in 1910.[16] These researchers, working in Tunis at the Pasteur Institute, published a dispatch for the Society of Exotic Pathology, describing a new

Table 23.1 Etiology and epidemiology of spotted (SFG) fever group rickettsial disease

Geographic distribution	Disease	Organism	Principal tick vectors
Africa	Boutonneuse fever	*Rickettsia conorii*	*Rhipicephalus, Haemaphysalis*
Asia	North Asian tick typhus	*Rickettsia sibirica*	*Dermacentor, Haemaphysalis, Hyalomma*
	Oriental (Japanese) spotted fever	*Rickettsia japonica*	Not yet identified
Australia	Queensland tick typhus	*Rickettsia australis*	*Ixodes holocyclus*
Americas	Rocky mountain spotted fever Rickettsialpox	*Rickettsia ricketsii* *Rickettsia akari*	*Rhipicephalus sanguineus, Amblyomma cajennense, Dermacentor variabilis* and *D. andersoni* *Liponyssoides sanguineus*

disease characterized by an abrupt and high fever, headache, chills, and eruptive elements. This new nosological entity was referred to as fièvre boutonneuse de Tunisie.

The first descriptions of the disease in Europe were reported in Italy by Carducci (1920) and Olmer in France (1925).[17] Subsequently, other clinical and epidemiological aspects of the disease were defined. Pièri and Brugeas of Marseille in 1925 reported the presence of a "tache noire" at the site of rickettsial inoculation by tick bite.[18] In 1930, Durand and Conseil implicated the tick species *Rhipicephalus sanguineus* as the vector and reservoir of the disease in Northern Africa.[19] Brumpt, in his publication *Longévité du virus de la fièvre boutonneuse* (*Rickettsia conorii*) *che-tique, Rhipicephalus sanguineus*, named the etiological agent *Rickettsia conorii* in honor of Conor.[20]

The different places where the disease was described led to different designations, including: Boutonneuse fever, Marseille fever, MSF, febre escaro-nodular, Kenya tick typhus, Indian tick typhus, Astrakhan fever, and Israel tick typhus. During the First International Congress of Mediterranean Hygiene in 1932, the name "Boutonneuse fever" was adopted as the correct term for the disease.

Etiologic agent

MSF is a tick-borne infectious disease caused by *R. conorii*-complex strains. *R. conorii* is a small (0.3–0.5 × 1–2 μm), coccobacillary Gram-negative obligatory intracellular bacterium that belongs to the SFG of rickettsiae. The SFG includes most rickettsial species, including pathogenic and non-pathogenic bacteria. Non-pathogenic bacteria should be understood to be rickettsiae that have not been detected by polymerase chain reaction (PCR) or isolated from human samples.

R. conorii is the most frequently isolated and has the widest geographical distribution of the SFG *Rickettsia* species. The *R. conorii* complex includes different isolated strains from humans and ticks, and although they have some genotypic and phenotypic differences, they are considered the same species.[21] This complex includes the prototype strains such as Moroccan (Casablanca) and 7RC (Malish), and other strains such as Kenya tick typhus, M-1, Simko, Indian tick typhus, Manuel, Astrakhan fever *Rickettsia* and Israeli tick typhus *Rickettsia* strains.

There are countries like Portugal where MSF cases are caused by two strains of *R. conorii* complex. The Portuguese patients' isolates reveal the presence of *R. conorii* 7RC and Israeli tick typhus *Rickettsia* (Itt) strains. The latter strain was isolated in 1997 for the first time in Portugal from a patient's blood.[22] This strain was previously only known to be present in Israel.[23]

Rhipicephalus sanguineus (the brown dog tick) is the main vector and reservoir of *Rickettsia conorii* in the Mediterranean basin, Northern Africa, and India. Rickettsiae are maintained in nature by transovarial and transstadial transmission in ticks and are transmitted by saliva while the tick feeds.[24] It is important to note that humans are only incidental hosts and do not play a role in propagating the organism in nature.[25]

Epidemiology

R. conorii has been identified in India, Pakistan, Morocco, Israel, Russia, Ukraine, Ethiopia, Africa, and southern Europe. In the last few decades there has been an increase in reported MSF cases from France, Italy, Portugal, Spain, and Israel. It has been suggested that this increase is related to favorable climatic factors that influence tick activity.[26–29] During 1972–1981, Israel reported the highest MSF incidence rate ($6.2/10^5$ inhabitants), but this rate decreased over the years to $0.9/10^5$ inhabitants in 1994 and subsequent years.[30] Based on available data from other MSF endemic countries, Portugal currently has the highest reported incidence rate at $9.8/10^5$ inhabitants.[31]

Another important point regarding the prevalence of infection in endemic regions is that a relatively high proportion of the population has antibodies to SFG rickettsiae, despite the absence of a prior clinical history of MSF. Different studies conducted in these endemic regions show a seroprevalence of 7.6–13.7% in southern Portugal, 18.3% in Israel, 11.5% in Barcelona (Spain), 10.6% in Sicily (Italy), 4.2% in coastal Croatia, 12% in Corsica, 18% in southern France, and 6.7–12.4% in the Marseilles region of France.[32–34] It is difficult to determine if this high prevalence of antibodies is due to undiagnosed MSF or asymptomatic infection with *R. conorii* or another *Rickettsia* species.

The disease is characterized by a seasonality, which is related to the activity and seasonal dynamics of the ticks. The majority of the cases in the Mediterranean area occur during June to September

(81–88%), peaking in July and August when immature stages of the tick predominate. Nevertheless, some countries such as Portugal have reported cases throughout the whole year, since climatic conditions are suitable for *Rhipicephalus sanguineus* activity.[35]

The highest incidence of MSF is typically reported among children, especially in the 1–4-year group, and shows no statistical differences between genders. Although there have been some reported deaths in children, most severe and fatal cases are associated with people above 55 years old, a risk factor for severity of the disease. *R. conorii* has always been considered to produce a less severe disease than *R. rickettsii*. However, severe forms of MSF have been reported in 6% of patients, and, a case fatality rate of 1.4–10% has been reported for hospitalized patients in France, Israel, Portugal, and Spain.[36] Moreover, in southern Portugal where the incidence rate of disease is around 60/10^5 inhabitants, the fatality rate in 1997 reached 32.3% in hospitalized patients. Further investigations indicated that therapeutic delay was not implicated in this mortality, but host factors might have been implicated.[31]

R. conorii has been shown to have high genetic homology but more genetic diversity than *R. rickettsii*. There are cross-reactive proteins and lipopolysaccharide antigens, and cross-protection between these species.

Clinical manifestations

MSF is characterized by generalized endothelial infection of the microvasculature, and the main clinical features are due to the injury of blood vessels caused by rickettsial infection. The histopathological phenomenon of vasculitis can involve all the organs, not only the skin, and it can also have serious manifestations when the lungs and brain are affected.[37]

The incubation period ranges from 3 to 7 days after the tick bite, but it can be longer and this fact may be related to the bacterial inoculum size. During the onset of disease for 2–3 days, the observed symptoms are non-specific and difficult to distinguish from more common illnesses. Patients complain of severe headache, fever, and myalgia, but other symptoms early in the course can include malaise, anorexia, chills, nausea and/or vomiting, abdominal pain, diarrhea, and photophobia. After this period, the disease is characterized by fever (90–100%) greater than 39°C. The fever will usually decrease, and apyrexia occurs after 4–6 days. Severe myalgias, mainly in the lower limbs, arthralgias, sweating, chills, hepatomegaly, splenomegaly, conjunctivitis, and photophobia have been reported. Between the third and fifth febrile day, 50–90% of patients develop a rash, which initially consists of pink macules and then evolves to 2–5-mm macules and papules that are hardly ever pruritic. The lesions then spread centripetally from the extremities, within 24–48 h involving the entire body, including palms and soles. Spotless MSF cases have also been reported.[38–40] The rash usually persists for about 10–20 days after the remission of clinical symptoms.

In severe cases, vascular damage can result in a purpuric (15% of patients) or petechial (2%) rash, which is generally indicative of a bad prognosis. Patients may suffer other hemorrhagic manifestations such as epistaxis, hemoptysis, hematemesis, and upper gastrointestinal hemorrhage. Other reported complications include mental status changes, meningoencephalitis, jaundice, seizures, renal and hepatic failure, respiratory symptoms, myocarditis, and uveitis. Most severe MSF cases can result in septic shock, non-cardiogenic pulmonary edema, adult respiratory distress syndrome, multiorgan failure, and fulminant death within 24 h of admission.[31,39,40] Although injury to vascular endothelium stimulates activation of the coagulation system, platelets, and fibrinolysis with frequent thrombocytopenia, true DIC rarely occurs. Peripheral gangrene of the fingers and toes occasionally necessitates amputation (Fig. 23.1).

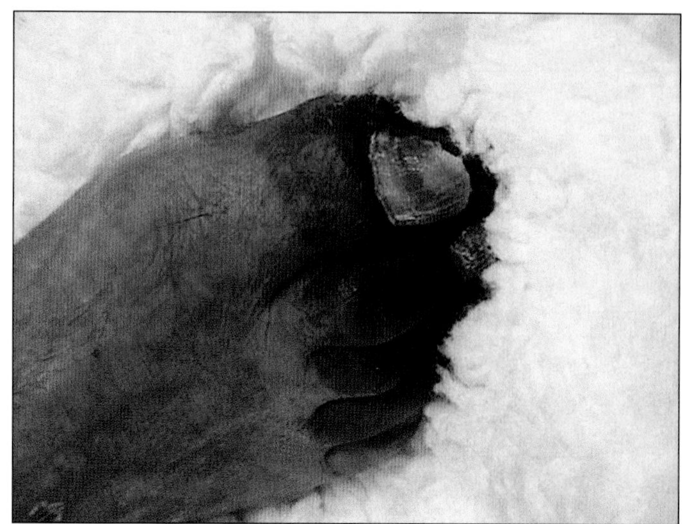

Figure 23.1 Gangrene of the toes associated with Mediterranean spotted fever.

Most patients with MSF also develop focal epidermal and dermal necrosis, an eschar or "tache noire" resulting from proliferation of rickettsiae at the site of the tick bite.[41] This sign shows a black crust approximately 1 cm in diameter but it may be variable and surrounded by an erythematous areola (Fig. 23. 2).

The presence of eschar in patients with MSF varies in different series from 30% to 90% of cases. Often, the detection of the eschar is difficult because it is hidden in some parts of the body such as the axilla, palpebra related to oculoglandular syndrome, groin, or submammary fold. Human infection with the Israeli tick typhus *Rickettsia* strain in Israeli patients has been reported to be similar

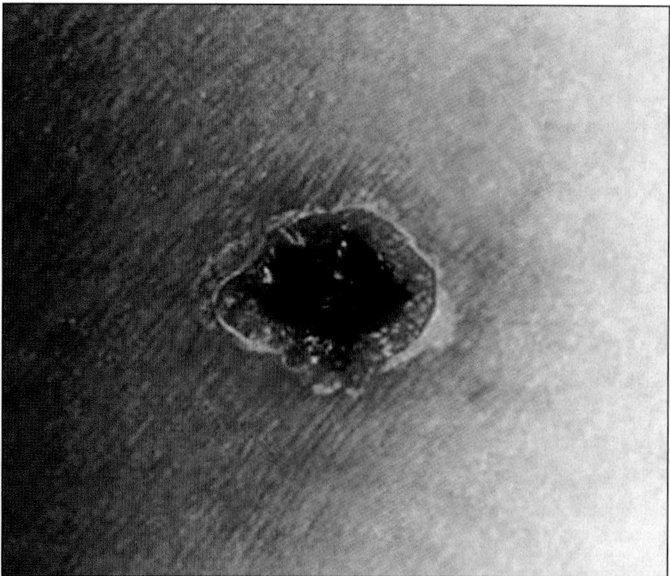

Figure 23.2 Eschar at the site of a tick bite in Mediterranean spotted fever.

to *R. conorii* 7RC infection, but the typical eschar at the inoculation site is usually lacking.[39] Nevertheless, a prospective study of Portuguese MSF patients infected with the Israeli tick typhus *Rickettsia* strain showed that some patients had an eschar and that there are no statistically significant differences between the presence or absence of the eschar between patients infected with *R. conorii* strain 7RC or the Israeli tick typhus strain (R. Sousa, unpublished work, 2004).

Laboratory findings are usually not very contributory for the diagnosis in the acutely ill patient, although the presence of thrombocytopenia caused by comsumption of platelets in hemostatic plugs (in foci of endothelium severely injured by rickettsiae) is usually a criterion for patient hospitalization instead of ambulatory treatment. The detection of thrombocytopenia in hospitalized patients can reach 80%. Other characteristic abnormalities include elevated erythrocyte sedimentation rates ranging between 15 and 40 mm/h, and alterations in coagulation factors (e.g., decreased prothrombin activity). Leukocytosis or leukopenia has been observed in 20–30% of patients. Elevated liver enzymes, muscular enzymes such as creatine phosphokinase (CPK), aldolases, and less specific enzymes such as lactate dehydrogenase (LDH) are usually present. Impaired renal function occurs with increased levels of creatinine in 17–77% of patients. Hyponatremia of less than 130 mmol/l occurs in 23–63.2% of patients.

Risk factors predisposing to severity of cases include old age, G6PD deficiency, diabetes, chronic alcoholism, and cardiac problems. Delay in treatment is sometimes associated with severity of illness and death.[42–45]

Patient evaluation, diagnosis, and differential diagnosis

The diagnosis of rickettsial illness is mainly clinical and epidemiological, since serologic evidence of infection occurs no earlier than 7–10 days after the onset of illness. Therefore, the clinician has to rely on a high index of suspicion, especially if the patient is a resident of an endemic area, and therapy must be instituted on clinical grounds, because severe illness and complications may develop and the disease may unexpectedly take a rapid, fatal course. For the differential diagnosis, the epidemiological context should be considered in relation to the season, contact with animals, outdoor activities, and travel. Detection and identification of the tick species can also assist in epidemiological diagnosis of the disease.

The differential diagnosis of the early clinical manifestations includes influenza, viral hepatitis, infectious mononucleosis, leptospirosis, typhoid fever, Gram-negative or Gram-positive bacterial sepsis, rubeola, meningococcemia, disseminated gonococcal infection, secondary syphilis, toxic shock syndrome, drug hypersensitivity, idiopathic thrombocytopenic purpura, thrombotic thrombocytopenic purpura, Kawasaki syndrome, and immune complex vasculitis. The triad of fever, rash, and headache should alert the physician to consider a rickettsial cause.

Physicians should also be aware of the atypical signs and symptoms of rickettsioses. In the USA, it has been reported that up to 11% of patients with Rocky Mountain spotted fever (RMSF) never develop a rash, similar to what occurs in MSF.[38,46] It has also been reported that MSF caused by the Israeli tick typhus strain can have an insidious course of a flu-like illness with a mild rash, and the typical eschar may not be readily identified; it is rarely, if ever, seen in patients from Israel.[47]

The gold standard for confirming the diagnosis for infectious diseases is the isolation and identification of the etiologic agent from patients' blood or tissues. However, other tests, such as immunohistochemistry, PCR on skin biopsy specimens, and immunologic detection of rickettsiae in circulating endothelial cells can be useful during the acute phase of illness, where no antibodies can be detected.[48]

Nevertheless, the diagnosis of rickettsial disease is most often confirmed by serological tests, because isolation and other procedures require specialized laboratories; usually serum is the only available sample.

Indirect immunofluorescent assay remains the most widely used serological technique for diagnosis of rickettsial diseases. Demonstration of a fourfold or greater rise in antibody titer (cut off: immunoglobulin M (IgM) with titers ≥ 64 or/and IgG titers ≥128) should be achieved between acute and convalescent sera (normal ranges depend on the laboratory). Other serological techniques, such as enzyme-linked immunosorbent assay (ELISA), complement fixation, or latex agglutination, have been applied to the detection of antibodies in patients with MSF, but these tests do not allow differentiation of the infecting strain among the SFG rickettsiae. Western blot and cross-adsorption immunoassays can assist in differentiating between SFG.[49] Serologic differention between infections with various *R. conorii* complex strains is still difficult, and the best method is isolation or PCR amplification from blood or skin. Isolation of rickettsiae is performed by shell-vial assay from heparinized blood (leukocytic cell buffy coat), or skin biopsy samples before antibiotic therapy. PCR-based methods for the detection of rickettsiae are attractive and can give sensitive and specific alternatives to culture. Although heparinized blood can be used for PCR amplification, blood collected in ethylenediaminetetraacetic acid (EDTA) or sodium citrate is preferred because heparin can inhibit the PCR reaction. Detection strategies based on recognition of sequences that encode the 17-kDa protein, citrate synthase, OmpA, and OmpB outer membrane proteins have been described.[48]

Treatment

First-line therapy for *R. conorii* infection is similar to that of other *Rickettsia* infections: doxycycline (200 mg/day) or tetracycline (25 mg/kg per day). Other effective regimens are chloramphenicol (2 g/day for 7–10 days) or ciprofloxacin (1.5 g/day for 5–7 days). The prompt administration of appropriate antibiotic therapy is the most effective measure for minimizing disease and preventing fatalities. Early antibiotic therapy is especially important in some rickettsioses, in which severe disease can develop and which resists attempts at intervention. Some authors state that most fatal cases, e.g., RMSF, are a result of difficulties in establishing the diagnosis and delay in beginning treatment.[50] Nevertheless, other studies of severe MSF did not associate therapeutic delay with fatal outcome and conclude that host factors might be strongly associated with mortality.[51]

Prevention

Since MSF is a zoonotic disease, the main vectors and reservoirs are found in nature and their eradication is impossible. Nevertheless, preventive measures can reduce disease transmission:

- Keep domestic areas free of animal ectoparasites
- Perform a regular control of domestic animals' hygiene

- Avoid exposure to ticks, especially if there are outside activities
- Use of tick repellents, wearing protective clothing
- Doing a routine examination of the entire body
- Prompt removal of ticks prevent inoculation of rickettsiae.

DNA fragments of two genes encoding major outer membrane proteins of spotted fever group rickettsiae (rOmpA and rOmpB) from *R. conorii* and *R. rickettsii* were tested as DNA vaccines.[52] Mice given DNA immunizations were conferred with partial protection against virulent *R. conorii* challenge, but only when DNA immunizations were followed by booster immunizations with the homologous recombinant proteins.[52] Immunization with plasmid DNA in an animal model resulted in cell-mediated production of IFN-γ.[52]

North Asian tick typhus (Siberian tick typhus)

North Asian tick typhus is caused by *R. sibirica*, which is rod-shaped, 0.3 × 10 μm in size, with a capsule-like coat thicker than that of other spotted fever group rickettsiae. *R. sibirica* is transmitted by *Dermacentor, Haemaphysalis*, and *Hyalomma* ticks and *Microtus fortis* mammals and hedgehogs. It is found in China (Fujian, Heilongjiang, Inner Mongolia, and Xinjiang province), the Czech Republic, Pakistan, Siberia, and Slovakia.[53] The *Dermacentor nuttallii* tick in Siberia is a vital reservoir of *R. sibirica*.[54] Only recently, since China has become more open to the west, have rickettsial diseases been studied in the country. Early serologic data from China did not distinguish infection of one spotted fever group from that of another. Healthy volunteers ($n = 154$) in Inner Mongolia showed antibodies in 11% to *R. sibirica* and 26.6% to *R. akari*. A study in Jinghe, Xinjiang Province, demonstrated an overall seropositivity of 62.5%.[55]

Restriction fragment length polymorphism (RFLP) analysis of PCR-amplified gene fragments was used to characterize 24 isolates of *R. sibirica* obtained in Russia. Only a single *R. sibirica* genotype was found. However, another study, also using RFLP and PCR, showed that two new strains, BJ-93 and 053, were genotypically identical with *R. sibirica*.[56] Three new isolates of *R. sibirica* were obtained in China and designated NH-95, BJ-95, and BHJ-95.[57]

The signs and symptoms of North Asian tick typhus are similar to those in Boutonneuse fever. Starting after a short incubation period, a generalized, erythematous, maculopapular rash appears distally. Fever, headache, and myalgia may occur, and the patient may develop regional lymphadenopathy. The symptoms typically resolve in 7–14 days. The risk of acquiring North Asian tick typhus during travel to endemic regions of Asia is unknown. A prospective study examined 13 paleontologists on expedition to Mongolia.[58] Four had acute illness, characterized by rash, fever, headache, and lymphadenopathy, and all had IgM and IgG antibodies to *R. sibirica*. Only two of the four infected patients were aware of tick bites. The other nine paleontologists with no illness and people who went on expeditions to other areas of the world did not have antibodies to *R. sibirica*. Even in the absence of recognized tick bites, travelers to regions endemic for *R. sibirica* are at risk of contracting North Asian tick typhus.

As with the other rickettsial spotted fevers, optimal therapy relies on a member of the tetracycline family or chloramphenicol. A study showed that therapy with galavit reduced manifestations and mortality in experimental animals infected with North Asian tick typhus.[59] There is no available vaccine yet, and prevention of this disease is tick control.

Oriental spotted fever

Oriental spotted fever, or Japanese spotted fever, is caused by *R. japonica*, which was first isolated in 1986 in Japan.[60] The vector has not been identified but is thought to be a tick species. Oriental spotted fever resembles the other spotted fever diseases, especially MSF and Siberian tick typhus, in that patients present with rash (100%), fever (100%), malaise (90%), eschar (48%), and headache (22%). The rash begins on the extremities, generalizes in a few hours, becomes petechial after about 4 days, peaks in about 10 days and then resolve after 14 days. The eschars seen on the hands, feet, neck, trunk, or shoulders, resolves after 7–14 days, and is not associated with tender regional or generalized lymphadenopathy. There have been reports of Japanese spotted fever with central nervous system involvement, including meningitis, back stiffness, and psychosis with stupor. Oriental spotted fever can be diagnosed by indirect immunoperoxidase or immunofluorescence assays, with antigens from *R. japonica* or other spotted fever group rickettsioses. Patients should be started empirically on doxycycline or minocycline therapy before the diagnosis is confirmed serologically.

Queensland tick typhus

Epidemiology

Queensland tick typhus is caused by *R. australis*, which is limited to eastern Australia. This rickettsial organism was first described in 1946 among Australian soldiers in northern Queensland and was subsequently designated Queensland tick typhus. *R. australis* and *R. rickettsii* share 53% DNA relatedness as determined by DNA–DNA hybridization studies. *R. australis* appears to have species-specific and group-reactive protein epitopes as monoclonal antibodies specific for protein antigens of *R. akari* and *R. rickettsii* do not cross-react with *R. australis*. It is believed that there is transovarial or transstadial transmission in ticks. *Ixodes holocyclus*, the principal human biting tick in Queensland and New South Wales, is the vector of Queensland tick typhus. This tick is an indiscriminate feeder, attacking both domestic and wild animals, and is mostly located near the coast. Spring and summer are the peak seasons of *R. australis* infection.

Clinical manifestations

Clinical symptoms are typically abrupt in onset. Early symptoms include fever, malaise, headaches, a local skin lesion, and/or tender localized lymphadenopathy (71%). In the initial reports, fever was shown to last an average of 7.5 days. The skin lesions occurred an average 4–5 days after the onset of symptoms. The rash is often macular or maculopapular, evolving to petechial lesions. The skin rash may progress to an eschar at the site of a tick bite in 50% of infected persons, or present as papules, pimples, "bruised areas," or "bite marks." The distribution of the skin rash is often blotchy, sparse, and generalized, and it may involve the palms and soles.

One-half of infected patients requires hospitalization and an average hospitalization duration of 6 days.[61] In one case series, 1 of 50 hospitalized patients died.[61]

Diagnosis

The diagnosis of *R. australis* is determined by clinical suspicion. Persons from an endemic region or who travel to eastern Australia with typical skin lesions and serological evidence of rickettsial infection should increase the clinician's suspicion of infection with this species. Biopsied skin lesions are non-specific but may show vasculitis with a mononuclear cell infiltrate.[61] Laboratory abnormalities are similar to the other rickettsial species such as leukopenia, thrombocytopenia, and minor abnormalities in hepatic and renal function. Also, similar to the other rickettsial species, serological tests are useful for diagnosis of *R. australis* based on its specific antigen. The available tests include the indirect florescent antibody, latex agglutination, and solid-phase immunoassay. These tests are sensitive and specific within 1–2 weeks of onset of illness.

Treatment

The recommended therapy for *R. australis* is doxycycline (200 mg/day) or tetracycline (25 mg/kg per day). Alternative regimens are chloramphenicol (2 g/day for 7–10 days), ciprofloxacin (1.5 g/day for 5–7 days), and ofloxacin (400 mg/day for 5–7 days).

Rocky mountain spotted fever (RMSF)

Epidemiology

RMSF, also known as Brazilian spotted fever when diagnosed in Brazil, is caused by the tick-borne obligate intracellular coccobacillus *Rickettsia ricketsii* (Fig. 23.3). The name RMSF is a misnomer, since the disease is found throughout the USA, Central and South America, most commonly in the southeastern and south-central parts (mid-Atlantic states) of the USA, and patients with the disease may have "spotless" skin. These factors may make the diagnosis of RMSF difficult early in the course of the disease.

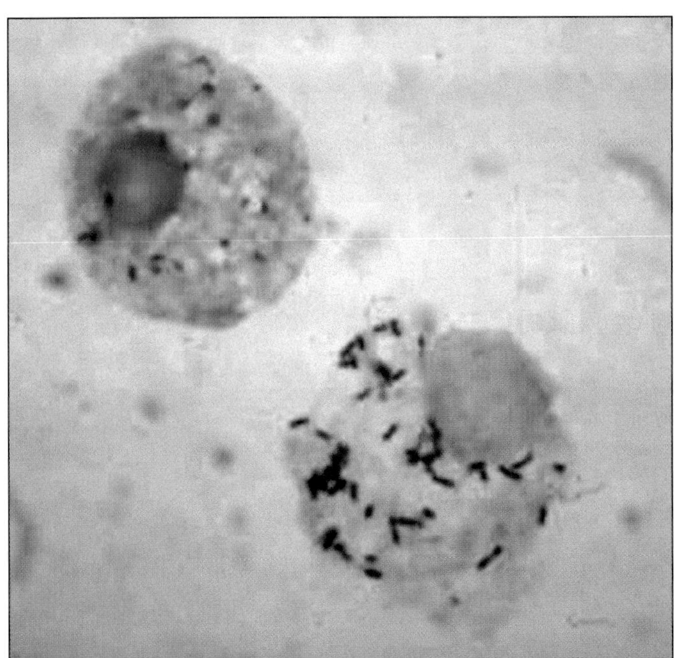

Figure 23.3 Intracellular *Rickettsia rickettsii* in Rocky Mountain spotted fever (RMSF). (Courtesy of Centers for Disease Control and Prevention.)

The primary reservoirs for *R. rickettsii* are ticks, and the most common tick vectors in Central and South America are the species *Rhipicephalus sanguineus* and *Amblyomma cajennense*. The most common tick vector in the eastern USA is the American dog tick, *Dermacentor variabilis*, and in the west, the Rocky Mountain wood tick, *D. andersoni*. The most common seasonality of RMSF is spring and summer, but cases have occurred at every month of the year. Humans are incidental hosts and acquire the infection from zoonotic reservoirs, usually dogs and wild rodents. Only adult ticks feed on humans, while the larval and nymph ticks feed on animals. The tick bite is painless, and, as the tick feeds on blood, *Rickettsia* are activated from a dormant state to a virulent state and are transmitted with the tick's salivary secretions to the host's dermal blood vessels. Transmission of the infection requires the tick to be feeding on and attached to the host for at least 6 h. There is also the possibility of person-to-person transmission of infection, as 4.4% of RMSF cases occur in a family member of a patient with RMSF, and there have been cases of familial clusters of RMSF. It is more likely, however, that there was a common (but unrecognized) environmental source of infection.

Pathogenesis

R. rickettsii causes systemic disease in humans by infecting endothelial cells of the small vessels of all major organs, thereby effecting irreversible damage in the dermis, lungs, heart, kidneys, gastrointestinal tract, brain, skeletal muscle, and other sites. Edema and damage of endothelial cells result in local thrombosis, infarction, and increased vascular permeability with extravasation from the systemic and pulmonary circulations. Infection in vascular smooth-muscle cells and contiguous endothelial cells leads to the classic skin lesions. Similarly, glial nodules develop in the central nervous system. These lesions then result in intravascular volume depletion, edema, oliguria, hypoproteinemia, hypotension, and non-cardiogenic pulmonary edema. Due to changes in microvascular permeability by *R. rickettsii*, infected sites may bleed, and these vascular lesions result in the organ damage seen in RMSF. This microvascular involvement results in the rash, headache, myalgias, and gastrointestinal symptoms commonly associated with RMSF, and can lead to gangrene, pulmonary hemorrhage and edema, acute respiratory distress syndrome, myocarditis, acute renal failure, meningoencephalitis, and cerebral edema.

Clinical manifestations

The severity of clinical disease is variable, but RMSF is the most lethal tick-borne infection in the USA, with a case fatality rate of 3–5% but ranges from 13–25% in untreated individuals. The mean incubation time of RMSF is 7 days after the bite, with a range of 2–14 days. Diagnosis can be difficult, especially early in the disease since the classic triad of rash, fever, and headache is only present in 3% of patients in the first few days. The initial presentation is commonly a flu-like syndrome, with fever, often greater than 39°C, headache, myalgias, nausea, vomiting, and malaise. Gastrointestinal symptoms, commonly nausea and vomiting, may be the only symptoms of the disease early in the course. Patients

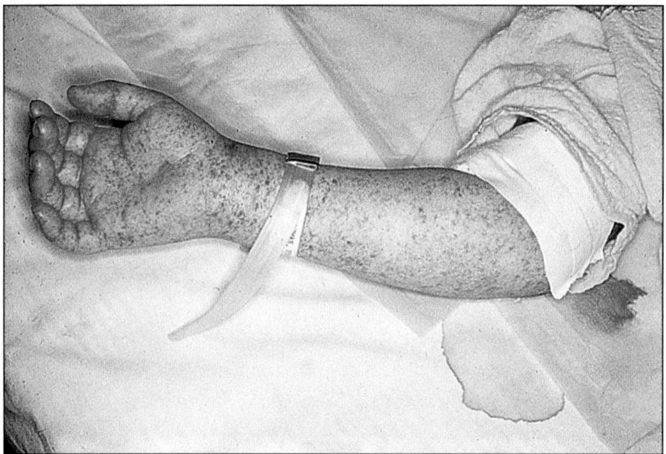

Figure 23.4 Macules, papules, and petechiae of Rocky Mountain spotted fever in a 4-year-old child on day 8 of the illness. The lesions are more hemorrhagic distal to the site of the tourniquet (Hess test) (Reproduced from Peters W and Pasvol G (eds). Tropical Medicine and Parasitology, 5th edition, Mosby, London 2002, image 44.)

can have lymphadenopathy, splenomegaly, and periorbital edema, which is a sign of severe disease.

RMSF is a multisystemic disease, but skin manifestations may be the only signs suggestive of rickettsial infection. The rash of RMSF usually appears about 3–5 days after onset of fever as 1–5-mm blanching erythematous macules at the wrists and ankles (Fig. 23.4), which in half of cases then develop into maculopapular lesions with central petechiae (Fig. 23.5). The lesions classically spread centripetally and spare the face. There may be scar formation in areas of focal skin necrosis, and gangrene can develop as a result of direct vascular injury from *R. rickettsii*. In patients with fulminant RMSF, the skin lesions may be different from classic lesions and may be thrombotic without the usual perivascular inflammatory response, making the diagnosis elusive. About 10% of patients with RMSF have no rash; this "spotless" variant is more often seen in older patients, males, and African–Americans (due to pigmentation). It may be due to the biologic properties of the organism, unknown host factors, or early initiation of antibiotics, and has no correlation with severity of disease.

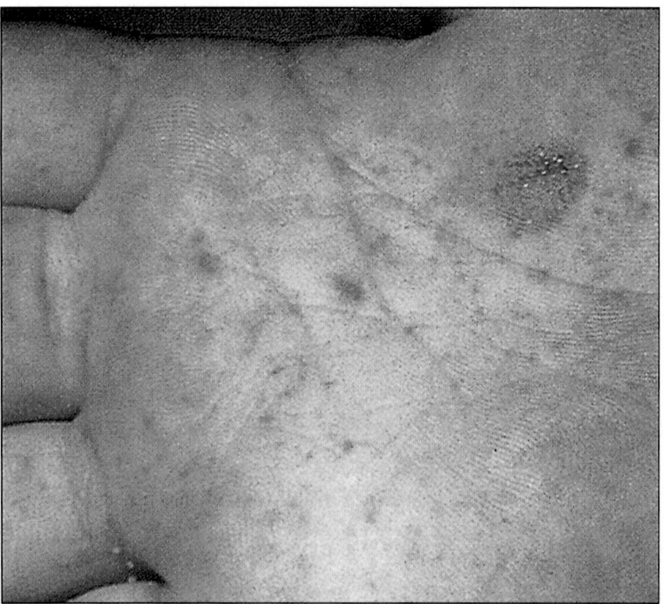

Figure 23.5 Macules and papules of the palm in Rocky Mountain spotted fever (Reproduced from Peters W and Pasvol G (eds). Tropical Medicine and Parasitology, 5th edition, Mosby, London 2002, image 45.)

The pulmonary manifestations are secondary to vascular permeability in the pulmonary microcirculation, correlate with the overall severity of the infection, and can include interstitial pneumonitis, pleural effusion, or acute respiratory distress syndrome. Especially at the beginning of the clinical disease, patients may predominantly have gastrointestinal symptoms, with nausea and vomiting, abdominal pain, and diarrhea, which may obscure the diagnosis of RMSF. Hepatomegaly has been noted in nearly all fatal cases. In severe cases, patients may develop acute renal failure, acute tubular necrosis or acute glomerulonephritis. Cardiac manifestations are rare, with myocarditis seen in a minority of cases. Neurologic manifestations include severe headache, which is a common early symptom, lethargy, photophobia, meningismus, amnesia, psychosis, and deafness. Patients can also have ataxia, sensory neuropathy, cranial nerve palsies, and seizures, all of which can confuse the diagnosis with enteroviral aseptic meningitis and arboviral encephalitis, diseases which have the same seasonality and age distribution as RMSF. The cerebrospinal fluid is often either normal or may contain white blood cells or elevated protein levels. Ocular manifestations are also common, with possible conjunctivitis, flame-shaped hemorrhages, and papillar edema. In severe cases of RMSF, patients often have acute renal failure, and even in milder cases, there may be significant increases in blood urea nitrogen. While myalgias are common, few cases with high elevations of creatine kinase have been reported.

The list of diseases in the differential diagnosis for Rocky Mountain spotted fever is long because of the non-specific complaints, frequent absence of rash at initial presentation, and lack of a history of tick bite. Patients frequently present on the second or third day of the illness, while the rash presents on the third or fourth day. Many patients are initially diagnosed with viral infection of the respiratory or gastrointestinal tract, or fever of unknown origin. Other tick-borne illnesses, including ehrlichioses, Lyme disease, babesioses, and other rickettsial diseases, are also in the differential diagnosis because they present with fever and non-specific symptoms. With the development of rash, misdiagnosis is still common because the lesions may have a non-specific appearance. At this stage, diseases that may be confused with RMSF include meningococcemia and atypical measles. Meningococcemia may be distinguished by the earlier appearance of rash that does not evolve like that of RMSF, leukocytosis, and Gram's stain, while atypical measles, associated with patients who were vaccinated with the killed measles vaccine between 1963 and 1976, may be more difficult to distinguish due to the similarity of its rash to that of RMSF. Because of this broad differential diagnosis, initial appropriate antibiotic therapy is begun in only 28–42% of cases.[62]

Diagnosis

The diagnosis of RMSF is made mostly on a clinical basis. Laboratory tests may support the diagnosis but are non-specific. It is difficult to be certain of the diagnosis unless skin biopsy with appropriate staining is done. The complete blood count is usually unremarkable, and the most common electrolyte abnormality is hyponatremia, which is present in 50% of patients. Serologic confirmation of RMSF, with complement fixation, indirect immunofluorescence assay (IFA), and latex agglutination, detect antibodies to *R. rickettsi* and depend on an acute titer above a specific threshold value or a fourfold increase in titer between acute and convalescent values. IFA is thought of as the gold standard even though there may be cross-reaction with other rickettsiae of the spotted fever group. Direct immunofluorescence or immunoperoxidase staining of fresh or fixed skin biopsy specimens can show evidence of RMSF at the time of appearance of the rash, around the first week of the illness. The immunoflurorescent staining method has a sensitivity of about 70% and specificity of almost 100%, while immunoperoxidase staining has a sensitivity of about 90% and specificity of nearly 100%.[63] Ideally, skin biopsies should be obtained before starting antibiotic therapy.

Treatment

Treatment should be started empirically because diagnostic tools are not available early in the course of the illness. The preferred treatment is at least 7 days of doxycycline, for adults, 200 mg/day or 3 mg/kg, whichever is higher, and for children less than 45 kg, 4.4 mg/kg, because doxycycline has a broad spectrum of coverage for other tick-borne illnesses that are in the differential diagnosis. Chloramphenicol is also effective in RMSF, but its use is limited to cases where doxycycline is contraindicated due to its association with a higher rate of fatalities than treatment with tetracyclines, the possibility of idiosyncratic reactions, and its uncertain efficacy in the treatment of other tick-borne illnesses that are in the differential diagnosis. Doxycycline is not contraindicated for children with suspected RMSF because the risk of tooth damage is not significant in short-term therapy and is outweighed by the benefit of the therapy for a disease that may be severe. *R. rickettsii* is commonly resistant to penicillins, cephalosporins, aminoglycosides, trimethoprim–sulfamethoxazole, and erythromycin. In fact, sulfa drugs can worsen the disease.

The prognosis is most affected by prompt diagnosis and early initiation of antibiotic therapy. Mortality is associated with absent or delayed onset of rash and delayed start of antibiotics, and more common if coma, seizures, renal failure, jaundice, or hepatomegaly are present. Fulminant cases can be fatal in the first 5 days and are seen primarily in African–Americans with G6PD deficiency who present with hemolysis. The best method of preventing RMSF is the use of insect repellents like diethyltoluamide (DEET) and permethrin, checking the skin for and removing ticks after outdoor exposure, and educating the public and health care professionals about the disease. Currently there is no effective vaccine to prevent RMSF, but efforts have been made to develop killed and live attenuated vaccines.

Rickettsialpox

Epidemiology

Rickettsialpox is caused by the organism *Rickettsia akari*, a small obligate intracellular bacterium with a cell wall similar to that of Gram-negative bacteria, and has the same lipopolysaccharide antigens as the other members of the spotted fever rickettsial group.[64] *Liponyssoides sanguineus*, a blood-sucking mite that feeds on rodents, is the arthropod vector for rickettsialpox.[65] The reservoir for rickettsialpox is the house mouse, *Mus musculus*, and humans are only infected if mice or other preferred hosts are not available. *R. akari* is maintained by transovarial transmission in mites, so human transmission is not essential.

Clinical manifestations

The disease begins with a primary cutaneous lesion at the site of inoculation by the mite and, after a usual incubation period of 9–14 days, rickettsialpox progresses into a febrile illness, followed by a secondary papulovesicular eruption.[66] The systemic symptoms are self-limited, typically resolving in 1–2 weeks, and may be severe, but no fatalities have been reported.[67]

The primary lesion is usually a solitary papule, may be seen on any part of the body, and can appear as soon as 24–48 h after the bite.[66] It can present with tenderness,[67] pruritus,[66] erythema, and induration of 1.0–2.5 cm in diameter, or be asymptomatic.[68] The papule soon transforms into a vesicle with cloudy or opaque fluid, which then ruptures and leaves a large area of induration that surrounds the eschar. Regional tender lymphadenopathy is frequently seen in the area draining the eschar, which resolves after about 4 weeks and can leave a small scar.[66]

Systemic symptoms, always with fever and malaise, appear suddenly about 1 week after the primary lesion. The temperature can reach up to 41°C but usually peaks between 38°C and 40°C[66] and gradually defervesces after 1 week.[69] Patients can also have chills that precede the fever and are followed by drenching sweats and myalgias. Other possible symptoms include conjunctival injection, photophobia, rhinorrhea, sore throat, cough, generalized lymphadenopathy, anorexia, nausea, or vomiting.[65]

The onset of the generalized cutaneous eruption usually occurs about 48–72 h after the systemic symptoms begin, but can follow several hours to 9 days after the generalized symptoms. There may be 20–40 non-pruritic lesions measuring 0.2–1.0 cm, consisting of erythematous macules, papules, and papulovesicles,[65] and the rash may affect the face, trunk, and extremities, including the palms and soles.[66] Characteristic lesions are round, with a small vesicle or pustule in the center; and some vesiculate and form a crust while others do not. Scarring from these secondary lesions does not occur.[66] Some patients may also have an enanthem, usually on the palate, which resembles the cutaneous lesions but lasts less than 48 h.[68]

Diagnosis

There are no specific laboratory findings in rickettsialpox. A common finding is mild leukopenia ranging from 2400 to 4000 white blood cells/mm^3, with a relative lymphocytosis. There may be a slight elevation of the erythrocyte sedimentation rate, and proteinuria, which is secondary to fever. Although blood cultures are negative, *R. akari* from patients' blood can be found after intraperitoneal inoculation into susceptible mice.[70] Except for one reported case of the serum of a 33-year-old man with rickettsialpox that showed a greater than fourfold increase in the titers of Proteus OX-2 and OX-19, the Weil–Felix test usually does not detect antibodies to *R. akari*.[71] However, serum antibodies can be detected by complement fixation studies within 10 days of the start of generalized symptoms, with titers peaking after 3–4 weeks in untreated patients, and after 6–8 weeks in patients treated with antibiotics.[66]

The histopathology of the primary lesions, or eschars, shows extensive necrosis and inflammation of the dermis and subcutaneous tissue, while papulovesicles show superficial edema and frank separation of the epidermal–dermal junction, which forms a subepidermal vesicle. The perivascular infiltrate may be lymphohistiocytic or vasculitic, with fibrin in the lumen and walls.[65] Direct immunofluorescence, using an anti-*R. rickettsii* globulin conjugated with fluorescein isothiocyanate, was found by Kass et al. to be positive in the eschars of five out of seven patients but in only one papulovesicular lesion out of nine patients, likely because there is a higher number of organisms at the site of inoculation.[65]

The differential diagnosis includes varicella, infectious mononucleosis, gonococcemia, echovirus (types 9 and 16), coxsackievirus A (types 9 and 16), and coxsackievirus B (type 5).[72] Rickettsialpox most resembles varicella but can be distinguished based on several factors. Vesicles of varicella are on an erythematous base, while those of rickettsialpox develop from papules. Varicella does not present with eschars and will show multinucleate giant cells in a Tzanck smear while lesions of rickettsialpox will not.

Treatment

Doxycycline 100 mg PO q 12 h for 2–5 days is the treatment of choice.[64] Rickettsialpox also responds to chloramphenicol but its use is limited due to the idiosyncratic reactions to chloramphenicol and the self-limited nature of the disease. Treatment should be withheld in children unless the symptoms are severe, when a 2-day course of doxycycline, which is brief and unlikely to cause tooth and bone deposition, may be used.[66] Rodent control helps reduce outbreaks of rickettsialpox.

The typhus group

Epidemic typhus

Synonyms: Louse-borne typhus, classic typhus, sylvatic typhus

Epidemiology

Epidemic typhus is caused by *Rickettsia prowazekii*, which is transmitted by the body louse (*Pediculus humanus corporis*). The life cycle is initiated when the body louse (Fig. 23.6) feeds on patients infected with primary epidemic typhus or by Brill–Zinsser disease, the recrudescent form of epidemic typhus. The organism reproduces in the alimentary tract of the louse, begetting numerous progeny that wait for defecation of the louse. When the louse takes a blood meal, it defecates, and when the host scratches the wound, it contaminates the wound with *R. prowazekii*-infected feces. Close personal contact or sharing of clothes is required to spread the lice from person to person. Epidemic typhus is usually spread in the cold winter months since migration of populations and crowding allow proliferation of lice. Infected lice typically die within 1–3 weeks from obstruction of the alimentary tract, and they do not pass the *Rickettsia* to their offspring.

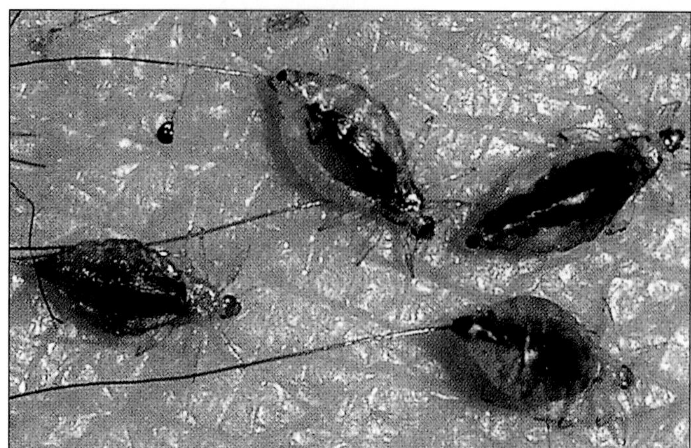

Figure 23.6 The body louse, *Pediculus humanus corporis*, transmits *Rickettsia prowazekii*, the cause of epidemic typhus (Reproduced from Peters W and Pasvol G (eds). Tropical Medicine and Parasitology, 5th edition, Mosby, London 2002, image 33.)

The first epidemics caused by epidemic typhus occurred in the late fifteenth century. Between 1918 and 1922 in Eastern Europe, it is estimated that 30 million cases occurred, resulting in 3 million deaths.[73] During World War II, cases occurred in North Africa and in the concentration camps of Eastern Europe. The most recent epidemics have been reported in Central and South America and Africa.

In 1922, the last outbreak of epidemic typhus in the USA occurred. Since then, most of the cases were due to Brill–Zinsser disease in immigrants or concentration camp survivors from Eastern Europe.[74] In 1975, *R. prowazekii* was isolated from the southern flying squirrel (*Glaucomys volans*).[75] Most cases of epidemic typhus reported from the southeastern USA have been associated with contact with flying squirrels.[75] Cases have been reported in Georgia, Massachusetts, North Carolina, Pennsylvania, Tennessee, Virginia, and West Virginia.[76]

Clinical manifestations

The typical course of epidemic typhus is 1–3 days of malaise before severe headeache, myalgia, rash, fevers, and chills develop.[77] In a study of 60 Ethiopian patients with epidemic typhus, all patients had fever and headache, 33% had a petechial rash, and 5% had a macular erythematous rash.[77] Around the fifth day, the rash begins in the axillary folds and upper trunk and spreads centrifugally to the extremities and occasionally to the soft palate

Table 23.2 Etiology and epidemiology of typhus group rickettsial disease

Geographic distribution	Disease	Organism	Principal tick vectors
Africa, Americas, Asia	Epidemic typhus	*Rickettsia prowazekii*	*Pediculus humanus corporis*
Worldwide	Murine (endemic) typhus	*Rickettsia typhi*	*Xenopsylla cheopis, Ctenocephalides felis*
Asia, Australia	Scrub typhus	*Rickettsia (Orientia) tsutsugamushi*	*Leptotrombidium*

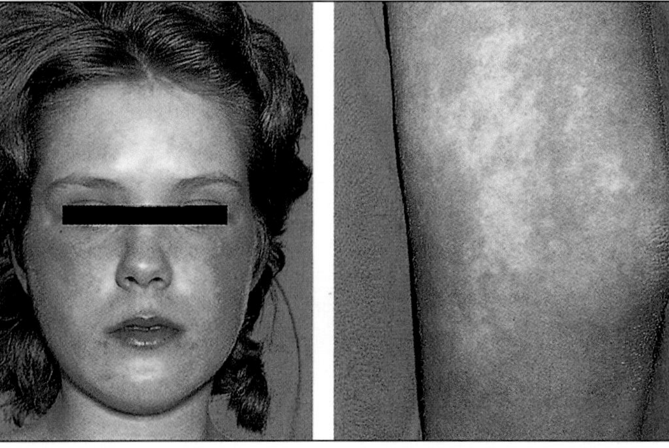

Figure 23.7 Erythematous macules of the face and extremities early in the course of epidemic typhus (Reproduced from Peters W and Pasvol G (eds). Tropical Medicine and Parasitology, 5th edition, Mosby, London 2002, image 35.)

and conjunctiva, but spares the palms and soles (Fig. 23.7). This is in contrast to the rash of RMSF, which begins in the extremities and spreads centripetally. The epidemic typhus rash appears initially as non-confluent erythematous macules that blanch on pressure, but after several days the rash becomes maculopapular and petechial.

In uncomplicated epidemic typhus, fever usually resolves after 2 weeks of illness if untreated, but recovery of strength typically takes 2–3 months. With appropriate antibiotics, fever resolves within 72 h of the start of therapy. Headache resolves after 7 days of therapy. Other neurological symptoms aside from headache range from nuchal rigidity to coma.

The complications include gangrene and vasculitis-induced cerebral thrombosis. Gangrene affects symmetric fingers and toes (Fig. 23.8). Treatment is medical in most cases, but severe gangrene may require amputation. Neurological deficits from cerebral thrombosis may take 2–4 weeks to resolve, but residual deficits are not common. The mortality from epidemic typhus is variable, with the highest rates in those over 60 years of age.

Diagnosis

For many years, the Weil–Felix agglutination reaction was the standard for serologic diagnosis, but there is a significant cross-reactivity between the ricksettsiae and a lack of specificity.[78] More sensitive tests include the microimmunofluorescent and plate microagglutination tests.[77] Acute and convalescent serum can be used to determine a fourfold rise in specific antibody titers. Also, in the past, it was difficult to differentiate between *R. prowazekii* and *R. typhi* due to antigenic similarity; antibody absorption tests were needed. Using monoclonal and polyclonal antibodies, typhus can be diagnosed on skin biopsies. However, now PCR can accurately detect *R. prowazekii* and differentiate between the rickettsiae.[79] A real-time PCR duplex assay has recently been developed that can differentiate *R. prowazekii* from eight of the spotted group rickettsiae, *R. typhi*, and *R. canada*.[79]

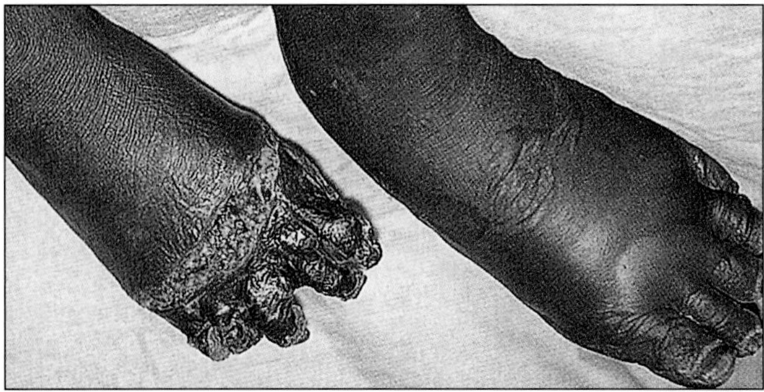

Figure 23.8 Gangrene of the feet in an Ethiopian patient with epidemic typhus (Reproduced from Peters W and Pasvol G (eds). Tropical Medicine and Parasitology, 5th edition, Mosby, London 2002, image 36.)

Laboratory abnormalities include elevations of aspartate aminotransferase and lactate dehydrogenase in most patients and mild thrombocytopenia in about 40% of patients. These abnormalities resolve with 14 days of treatment. The white blood cell count is typically normal, but may be high in a few patients.

Treatment

The most highly effective therapies are the tetracyclines and chloramphenicol. Doxycycline has been shown to be effective in a single oral dose, but the standard recommended treatment is 200 mg once a day for 5 days.[80] If the patient is too ill to take oral medication, the tetracyclines and chloramphenicol can be administered intravenously. Delousing the patient is also essential to prevent the cycle of reinfection.

Prevention of epidemic typhus is performed by decreasing the population of the body louse, which can be achieved by regular bathing, washing of infested clothes, and use of insecticides. Clothes treated with permethrin can eliminate lice even after several washings. Doxycycline prophylaxis can provide some protection if taken in endemic areas and may also interrupt a typhus outbreak.[77]

Vaccine for *R. prowazekii*

The first typhus vaccines were developed in the 1970s using crude antigen or formalin-killed *R. prowazekii*.[50] Although they provided some level of protection, they were only indicated for those at the highest risk of acquiring epidemic typhus, and they had undesirable toxic reactions and difficulties in standardization.[50]

Because of the obligate intracellular existence of the rickettsial agents, a vaccine capable of eliciting a strong cell-mediated immunity is essential. DNA vaccination provides prolonged antigen expression, and immunization with recombinant plasmid DNA, consisting of a bacterial plasmid that includes the gene of interest, represents a promising method in DNA vaccine research. Further, inducing an immune response to a single bacterial protein using a genetic vaccine allows the opportunity to develop diagnostic tests that could differentiate immune individuals from infected individuals and would aid in determining if *R. prowazekii* was intentionally spread within the population. A search for an effective vaccine against *R. prowazekii* is currently underway, and one laboratory has amplified 24 target genes using PCR to be transferred into DNA vaccine vectors, which is being tested in a rat model.[81]

Brill–Zinsser disease

Until the start of the nineteenth century, no clear distinction could be made between typhus and typhoid. In 1896, Nathan Brill noted sporadic cases of a typhoid-like illness with negative blood cultures during an epidemic of typhoid fever in New York City.[82] His clinical summary of 221 cases differentiated the disease clearly from typhoid.[83] Since it was non-communicable and did not have a deadly course, he also felt it was not typhus.

In the early 1930s, Hans Zinsser used bacteriological and epidemiological methods to show that Brill-Zinsser disease was an imported form of classical typhus representing recrudescence of infections originally acquired in Europe.[84] He believed that such a recurrence could produce a nidus for epidemic spread if the mouse–louse–human cycle could occur. Subsequently, *R. prowazekii* was isolated from ill patients with Brill–Zinsser disease, and these patients could infect lice feeding on them.[85] Brill–Zinsser disease was isolated from the lymph nodes of two Russian immigrants who had come to the USA more than 20 years earlier.[86]

It is thought that a weakening immune system or stress may reactivate the infection.[73] The clinical symptoms are typically milder than primary epidemic typhus and more closely resemble the symptoms of murine typhus.[76] Brill–Zinsser patients do not have specific IgM antibody and have elevated IgG antibody to *R. prowazekii*. Treatment is the same as with primary epidemic typhus.

With the continuing epidemics of epidemic typhus in Russia and the immigration of eastern Europeans into North America over the last few decades, cases of Brill–Zinsser continue to be reported in the USA[87] and Canada.[88]

Murine typhus (endemic typhus)

Epidemiology

R. typhi, an obligate intracellular bacterium, has been found worldwide. In the USA; most cases are in south Texas and southern California. These infected areas typically have inadequate vector and reservoir control. *R. typhi* is the cause of murine typhus, also known as endemic typhus. The peak prevalence of murine typhus occurs during the summer and early fall. In Texas, the peak prevalence is April through June.[89]

R. typhi was discovered in 1926 by Maxcy.[86] It is a zoonosis, found most commonly in temperate and subtropical seaboard regions, and is responsible for epidemics. *R. typhi* causes a mild illness but occasionally disease is severe, leading to death. *R. typhi* has been identified in cat fleas and infected individuals with exposure to fleas.[90] Murine typhus is transmitted by the feces of infected fleas into the bite wounds of the flea. *R. typhi* and *R. felis* share some antigenic and genetic components present on the major protein antigen, the rickettsial outer membrane protein B.[91] However, genotypic characterization of the gene for a 17-kDa lipoprotein (citrate synthase) and 16S ribosomal RNA distinguishes between these species.[91]

Clinical manifestations

The clinical symptoms of *R. typhi* are non-specific and typically occur 1–2 weeks after exposure to infected fleas. Symptoms may include fever (96%), headache (45%), chills (44%), myalgia (33%), nausea (33%), rash (18–50%), and neurological signs and symptoms (1–45%).[89] When a rash is identified, the appearance is described as macular or maculopapular (78%), most often distributed on the trunk (88%), with involvement of the extremities (>45%) and occasional involvement of the palms and soles.[89] The neurological signs and symptoms may include confusion, stupor, seizures, or ataxia. Ten percent of infected patients require hospitalization, and up to 4% of these patients die.[89]

Diagnosis

The diagnosis of murine typhus is based on clinical suspicion and supporting serological laboratory confirmation. As with the other *Rickettsia* species, serological tests used for diagnosis of *R. typhi* based on its specific antigen include the indirect fluorescent antibody, latex agglutination, and solid-phase immunoassay.[92] These tests are sensitive and specific within 1–2 weeks of onset of illness.[89] A shell-vial assay can be used to confirm infection during the acute phase of illness. This assay is not widely available and is considered dangerous and difficult. Other tests available for laboratory confirmation of rickettsial infection include PCR amplification of rickettsial nucleic acids in peripheral blood and immunomagnetic retrieval of circulating endothelial cells coupled with immunocytological demonstration of intraendothelial cell involvement.[93,94]

Laboratory features may suggest involvement with *R. typhi* infection. Mild leukopenia and thrombocytopenia are seen in 25–50% of patients in the first 7 days of illness. The most common laboratory abnormality is an elevated serum aspartate aminotransferase level (90–92%).[89] Other hepatocellular enzymes – alanine aminotransferase, alkaline phosphatase, and lactate dehydrogenase – may be elevated. Endothelial damage caused by *Rickettsia* infections can lead to hypoalbuminemia and serum electrolyte abnormalities such as hyponatremia (60%) and hypocalcemia (79%).

Treatment

The first-line therapy of mild to moderate *R. typhi* infection is doxycycline (200 mg/day) or tetracycline (25 mg/kg per day).[80] Other effective regimens are chloramphenicol (2 g/day for 7–10 days) or quinolones such as ciprofloxacin (1.5 g/day for 5–7 days) and ofloxacin (400 mg/day for 5–7 days).[95,96] In severe infections, intravenous doxycycline or chloramphenicol (50–75 mg/kg per day in four divided doses) is the preferred agent of treatment. These regimens should be continued at least 48–72 h after defervescence before switching to oral therapy. Most patients become afebrile after 72 h of therapy.

Scrub typhus

Epidemiology

Scrub typhus, a febrile disease caused by *Orientia tsutsugamushi*, is endemic to the area bounded to the north by northern Japan and southeastern Siberia, to the south by Queensland, Australia, and to the west by Pakistan.[97] The disease was first described in 1899, and was responsible for much morbidity in US troops in World War II and the Vietnam war. The main reservoir of the organism and the vector for transmission of the infection to humans are chiggers of the species *Leptotrombidium (Trombicula) akamushi* and *L. deliense*, or larval tromiculid mites (Fig. 23.9), which inhabit rural habitats like scrub forests, tall grasslands, or plantations.

Clinical manifestations

O. tsutsugamushi, an obligate intracellular organism, is different from *Rickettsia* species because of its lack of peptidoglycan and

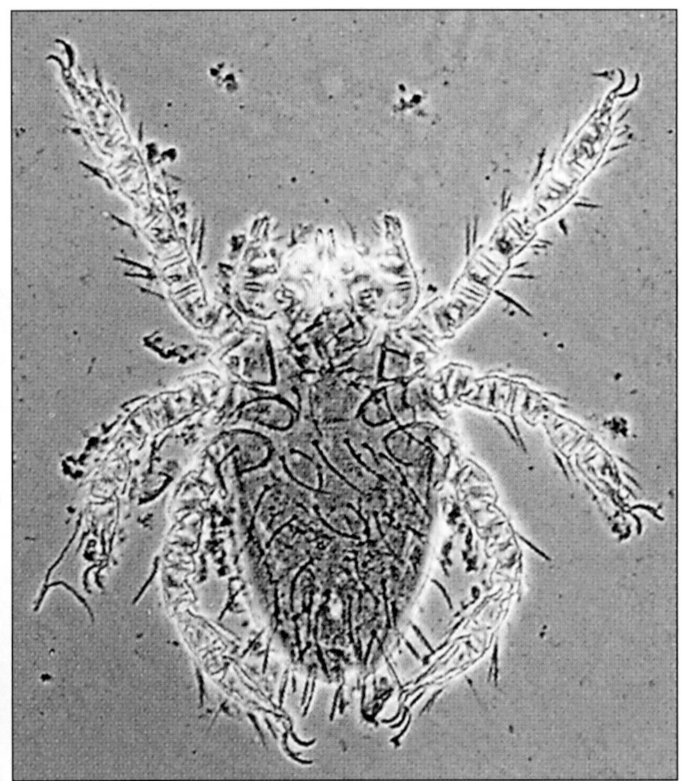

Figure 23.9 A larval trombiculid mite, the vector of *Orientia tsutsugamushi*, the cause of scrub typhus (Reproduced from Peters W and Pasvol G (eds). Tropical Medicine and Parasitology, 5th edition, Mosby, London 2002, image 39.)

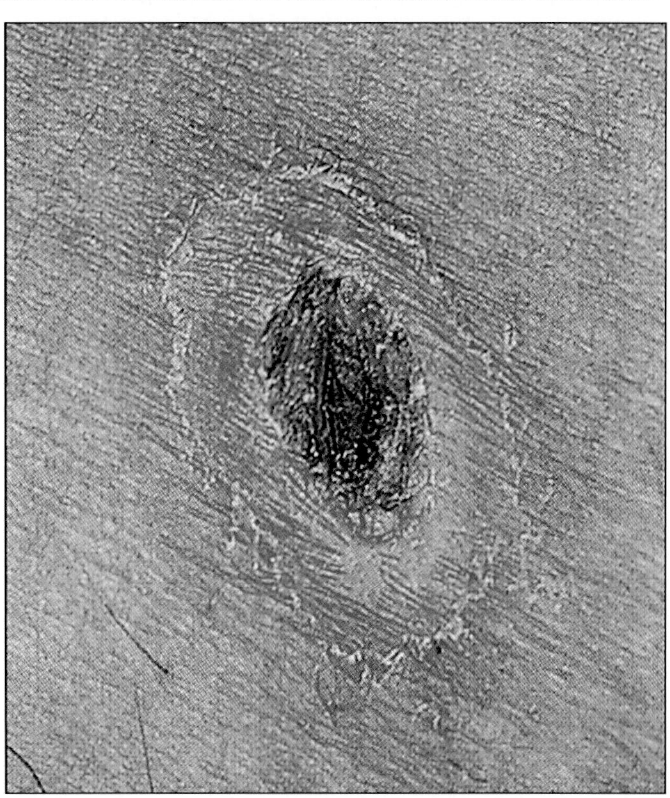

Figure 23.10 Eschar on the abdomen of a Thai patient with scrub typhus at the site of the mite bite (Reproduced from Peters W and Pasvol G (eds). Tropical Medicine and Parasitology, 5th edition, Mosby, London 2002, image 40.)

lipopolysaccharide and its distinct antigenic variants,[98] but there is enough cross-reactivity with antigens from *Rickettsia* such that serologic diagnosis can be made with the indirect fluorescent antibody test.[98] The disease is more common after periods of heavy rainfall, when mites proliferate. As the infected chigger feeds on a human host, *O. tsutsugamushi* is inoculated and then multiplies at the wound, forming a painless small papule after about 2 days. The papule enlarges, then vesiculates and necroses in the center, forming a black crust, or eschar[97] (Fig. 23.10). These lesions are associated with tender or suppurative regional lymphadenopathy. The organisms disseminate and cause vasculitis and perivasculitis of small blood vessels in multiple organs, particularly affecting the central nervous system and causing meningitis, encephalitis, and deafness;[99] the kidneys, liver, and lungs may also be damaged. Because there are different infecting strains of *O. tsutsugamushi*, the severity of disease can vary with the strain's virulence,[100] and the mortality rate of untreated patients can range from 1 to 60%.

The incubation period for the disease is 6–18 days, and the presenting symptoms commonly include fever up to 40°C, chills, and headache. Patients can also have anorexia, cough, myalgia, and nausea.[101] The less common physical findings are generalized lymphadenopathy (85%), eschar (46%), most often in the calf area but also found in the groin, axilla, and inguinal area, splenomegaly (43%), and maculopapular rash (34%) that appears at days 3–8 of the febrile illness and persists for an average of 4.2 days. Some patients can also have deafness, tinnitus, and conjunctival injection.[97]

The rash usually begins with macular lesions on the trunk that spread centripetally and can then become papular (Fig. 23.11). Neuropsychiatric symptoms are common, including confusion, delirium, slurred speech, and nuchal rigidity. Nine out of 72 patients presented with meningitis or encephalitis in one report.[99] Cerebrospinal fluid studies show results that resemble a viral or tuberculous meningitis picture.[99] In up to one-third of patients, deafness and tinnitus result.

Treatment with appropriate antibiotics decreases the duration of illness and the risk of death.[100] Fever resolves after 48 h in treated patients. Without antibiotics, fever usually persisted an average of 14 days, and up to 50% of patients died.[97] Patients who are untreated also can suffer complications such as acute respiratory

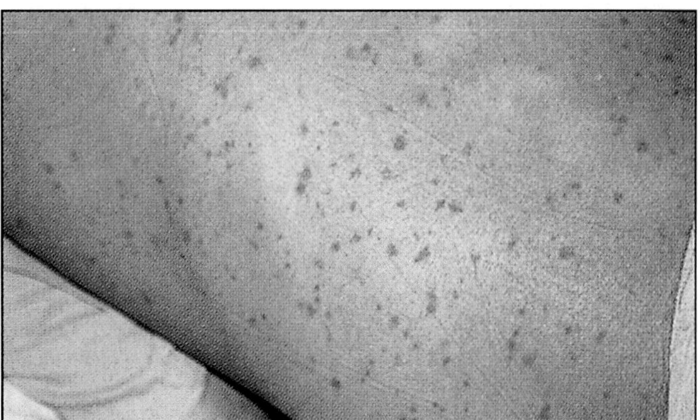

Figure 23.11 Macules and papules of scrub typhus usually appear on the sixth or seventh day of illness and are mainly distributed on the trunk, thighs, and upper arms (Reproduced from Peters W and Pasvol G (eds). Tropical Medicine and Parasitology, 5th edition, Mosby, London 2002, image 41.)

distress syndrome, renal failure, coma, hyperbilirubinemia, blindness, deafness, cognitive defects, and ataxia.[97]

Diagnosis

A high index of suspicion for scrub typhus must be maintained with febrile patients who have a history of travel in endemic areas. Some patients may not have the classic rash and eschar but have generalized lymphadenopathy and lymphocytosis that may confuse the diagnosis with infectious mononucleosis.[101] While serologic confirmation of the diagnosis is pending, treatment should be started empirically.

The diagnosis of scrub typhus can be made through several serological methods. The indirect fluorescent antibody test is more sensitive and specific than the more widely available Weil–Felix agglutination test,[99] and a peak in antibody titer after the second week of illness is seen. With the immunoperoxidase assay, which is easier to perform than the indirect fluorescent antibody test and just as sensitive and specific,[99] a fourfold increase in convalescent titers confirms the diagnosis of scrub typhus. PCR can also be used to detect the DNA of *O. tsutsugamushi* from peripheral blood and skin biopsy specimens.[102] Although the gold standard for diagnosing scrub typhus is the IFA assay, it requires specialized training and equipment and is done in only a few reference laboratories. Because of this, a sensitive, rapid lateral flow assay that detects *Orientia tsutsugamushi*-specific IgG/IgM antibodies is being developed.[103]

Patients usually have a normal white blood cell count, with lymphocytosis in the majority of cases. About 50% of patients have elevated aspartate aminotransferase, and 20% have proteinuria.[101]

Other diagnoses that must be considered include other rickettsial diseases, typhoid fever, brucellosis, leptospirosis, infectious mononucleosis, toxoplasmosis, and Dengue fever.[100]

Treatment

Appropriate antibiotic therapy includes either tetracyclines or chloramphenicol, but in one comparative study tetracyclines were found to reduce fever and other symptoms more quickly.[104] Some strains of *O. tsutsugamushi*, however are resistant to chloramphenicol. Fourteen days of tetracycline 2 g/day or doxycycline 200 mg/day, the recommended course of therapy,[105] is also effective at reducing relapses of scrub typhus, which are more common if patients are started on shorter courses of therapy during the first 5 days of the illness.[104] Ciprofloxacin was found in an animal model to be as effective as chloramphenicol,[106] and in one case report, it successfully treated a patient.[105]

Infection with a particular strain of *O. tsutsugamushi* provides immunity to that strain only, and patients can have subsequent episodes of scrub typhus if exposed to a heterologous serotype.[100] Because of the multiple antigenic strains of *O. tsutsugamushi*, a prophylactic vaccine for scrub typhus has not been created. Individuals who travel in endemic areas can prevent scrub typhus by taking doxycycline 200 mg/week,[107] using insect and mite repellent, and refraining from lying or sitting on the ground.

Rickettsial infections and bioterrorism

In 1996, a US law was enacted to prevent terrorists from gaining access to dangerous infectious agents.[108] Along with 10 other bacteria, *R. prowazekii* and *R. rickettsii* were listed as hazardous agents with severe restrictions on their study. A committee with expertise in public health, infectious diseases, and microbiology gathered to categorize infectious diseases into levels of potential threats of bioterrorism.[109] Centers for Disease Control category A was considered the most severe group; *R. prowazekii* was placed in category B, and *R. rickettsii* was placed in category C.[110] However, it has been argued that *R. prowazekii* belongs in category A, and that *R. rickettsii* and *R. typhi* also belong in category A, or at least in category B.[110]

There is a real threat of the rickettsial diseases being used as bioweapons. In the 1930s, the USSR developed *R. prowazekii* as a biologic weapon, and in the late 1930s to 1940s, Japan conducted field and human testing of typhus as a biologic weapon in northeastern China.[111] Further, *R. prowazekii* was an active area of bioweapon research in the USSR during the 1970s and thereafter.[111]

There are several characteristics of the biologic agents used for terrorism: high and stable infectivity, especially by small-particle aerosol; high level of virulence; low minimum infectious dose; clinical similarity of the bioterrorism agent to more common diseases; difficulty in distinguishing between bioterrorism and natural transmission; low level of immunity in the target population; easy person-to-person communicability; the diagnosis strikes terror in the population; and difficulty of therapy.[110]

R. typhi in dried flea feces and *R. prowazekii* in dried louse feces are highly infectious and stable for long periods of time.[112,113] Further, aerosols containing *R. conorii*, *R. prowazekii*, *R. rickettsii*, and *R. typhi* have caused many laboratory infections.[114,115] In a lyophilized state, *Rickettsia* can also be preserved stably, milled to 1–5 μm particles, and treated to prevent electrostatic clumping for aerosol dispersal. The minimum infectious dose (ID_{50}) for some rickettsial pathogens is one or two organisms.[116]

Manifesting similarly to the severe viral hemorrhagic fevers, RMSF (23–25% mortality) and epidemic typhus (10–60% mortality) are among the most severe infectious diseases in humans. *R. typhi* and *R. conorii* cause life-threatening illness in special populations (e.g., the elderly, persons with G6PD deficiency).[117]

The clinical manifestations of the rickettsioses may resemble other more common diseases, leading to delayed accurate diagnosis and therapy. Further, with the exception of *R. prowazekii*, the enzootic nature of many rickettsial diseases complicates the distinction between an act of bioterrorism and natural transmission. Since rickettsial diseases are endemic in many areas of the world, identification of the infectious source would be difficult. However, the sudden occurrence of a few human cases of typhus in non-endemic areas or an epidemic should set off the alarm for a possible bioterrorism attack.

In developed countries, there is a low level of immunity to typhus and spotted fever group diseases. High levels of susceptibility exist in these nations, and a high attack rate would be expected in populations exposed to an infectious aerosol. However, these diseases are not transmissible from person to person. The introduction of *R. prowazekii* to an indigent population infested with human body lice (*Pediculus humanus corporis*) could result in a devastating spread.

The degree of fear generated by a particular infectious disease diagnosis depends more upon media presentation and public perception rather than scientific basis. It is likely that an epidemic of any of the rickettsial diseases would not cause mass panic, even though they have the potential for high morbidity and mortality.

Successful treatment of the rickettsial diseases is dependent upon a rapid and accurate diagnosis and use of an antimicrobial agent to which *Rickettsia* is susceptible. Even now, patients with epidemic typhus and RMSF are misdiagnosed and treated with an empiric antibiotic that is not rickettsiostatic or rickettsiocidal.[118] Popular empiric first-line drugs against febrile illnesses (e.g., β-lactams and aminoglycosides) have no effect on rickettsiae.

In theory, it would be relatively simple for any bioterrorism lab to transform any *Rickettsia* to a chloramphenicol- and tetracycline- resistant strain by electroporation of resistance genes and selection of transformants under antimicrobial pressure. It is believed that a tetracycline-resistant strain of *R. prowazekii* has already been developed in the USSR.[110] This leads to the possibility that a *R. prowazekii* bioweapon has already been developed that is resistant to all antibiotics.

The most dangerous species is *R. prowazekii*, followed by *R. rickettsii* and *R. typhi*. *R. prowazekii* engineered to antimicrobial resistance meets all of the criteria of the most dangerous infectious diseases except for person-to-person communicability. However, the needs for biodefense against rickettsiae are the same as the needs for public health measures against these diseases throughout the world. The most urgently required innovations would be effective acute diagnostics and therapies for typhus group and spotted fever group rickettsioses, and a cross-protective typhus group vaccine.

Conclusion

The Rickettsiaceae family of microbes is widespread and maintained in nature through reservoirs of mammals and arthropod vectors. This family of microbes is a significant cause of morbidity and mortality and is likely underrecognized and underdiagnosed. The worldwide public health impact as a result of the Rickettsiaceae family is large. Numerous rickettsial strains have been isolated from ticks, fleas, and other vectors from many countries, and it is likely that many additional strains will be identified in the future. Prevention methods are crucial in controlling the tick and flea vectors and potential flea hosts, especially in persons who spend extended periods of time outdoors or work with animals (e.g., farmers, hunters, veterinarians, forestry workers, military training). All cases should be promptly reported to local public health authorities. Current effective treatments include tetracycline, chloramphenicol, and quinolones. Unfortunately, no vaccine of proven effectiveness currently exists, but recovery from natural infection will confer a solid, long-lasting immunity to reinfection.

References

1. Walker DH, Valbuena GA, Olano JP. Pathogenic mechanisms of diseases caused by *Rickettsia*. Ann NY Acad Sci 2003; 990:1–11.
2. Li H, Walker DH. Characterization of rickettsial attachment to host cells by flow cytometry. Infect Immun 1992; 60:2030–2035.
3. Uchiyama T. Role of major surface antigens of *Rickettsia japonica* in the attachment to host cells. In Kazar J, Raoult D, eds. Rickettsiae and rickettsial diseases. Bratislava: Publishing House of the Slovak Academy of Sciences; 1999:182–188.
4. Walker DH, Feng HM, Popov VL. Rickettsial phospholipase A_2 as a pathogenic mechanism in a model of cell injury by typhus and spotted fever group rickettsiae. Am J Trop Med Hyg 2002; 65:936–942.
5. VanKirk LS, Hayes SF, Heinzen RA. Ultrastructure of *Rickettsia rickettsii* actin tails and localization of cytoskeletal proteins. Infect Immun 2000; 68:4706–4713.
6. Eremeeva ME, Dasch GA, Silverman DJ. Quantitative analyses of variations in the injury of endothelial cells elicited by 11 isolates of *Rickettsia rickettsii*. Clin Diagn Lab Immunol 2001; 8:788–795.
7. Hong JE, Santucci LA, Tian X et al. Superoxide dismutase-dependent, catalase-sensitive peroxides in human endothelial cells infected by *Rickettsia rickettsii*. Infect Immun 1998; 66:1293–1298.
8. Temenak JJ, Anderson BE, McDonald GA. Molecular cloning, sequence and characterization of cjsT, a putative protease from *Rickettsia rickettsii*. Microb Pathog 2001; 30:221–228.
9. Feng H, Popov VL, Yuoh G et al. Role of T lymphocyte subsets in immunity to spotted fever group rickettsiae. J Immunol 1997; 158:5314–5320.
10. Walker DH, Olano JP, Feng HM. Critical role of cytotoxic T lymphocytes in immune clearance of rickettsial infection. Infect Immun 2001; 69:1841–1846.
11. Sahni SK, VanAntwerp DJ, Eremeeva ME et al. Proteasome-independent activation of nuclear factor kappaB in cytoplasmic extracts from human endothelial cells by *Rickettsia rickettsii*. Infect Immun 1998; 66:1827–1833.
12. Shi RJ, Simpson-Haidaris PJ, Marder VJ et al. Post-transcriptional regulation of endothelial cell plasminogen activator inhibitor-1 expression during *R. rickettsii* infection. Microb Pathog 2000; 28:127–133.
13. Schmaier AH, Srikanth S, Elghetany MT et al. Hemostatic/fibrinolytic protein changes in C3H/HeN mice infected with *Rickettsia conorii* – a model for Rocky Mountain spotted fever. Thromb Haemost 2001; 86:871–879.
14. Feng HM, Walker DH. Mechanisms of intracellular killing of *Rickettsia conorii* in infected human endothelial cells, hepatocytes, and macrophages. Infect Immun 2000; 68:6729–6736.
15. Billings AN, Feng HM, Olano JP et al. Rickettsial infection in murine models activates an early anti-rickettsial effect mediated by NK cells and associated with production of gamma interferon. Am J Trop Med Hyg 2001; 65:52–56.
16. Conor A, Bruch A. Une fièvre éruptive observée en Tunisie. Bull Soc Pathol Exot Fil 1910; 8:492–496.
17. Olmer D. Sur une infection épidermique, avec exantheme, de nature indeterminée. Marseille Méd 1925; 2:1291–1293.
18. Pièri A, Brugeas C. Un nouveau cas d'exanthème infectieux épidémique de nature méditerranée. Marseille Méd 1925; novembre.
19. Durand P, Conseil E. Transmission expérimentale de la fièvre boutonneuse par *Rhipicephalus sanguineus*. CR Acad Sci 1930; 190:1244.

20. Brumpt E. Longévité du virus de la fièvre boutonneuse (*Rickettsia conorii*, n. sp) chez la tique, *Rhipicephalus sanguineus*. CR Hebd Sci Mém Soc Biol 1932; 110:1199–1202.
21. Walker DH, Feng HM, Saada JI et al. Comparative antigenic analysis of spotted fever group rickettsiae from Israel and other closely related organisms. Am J Trop Med Hyg 1995; 52:569–576.
22. Bacellar FC, Beati L, França A et al. Israeli spotted fever *Rickettsia* (*Rickettsia conorii* complex) associated with human diseases in Portugal. Emerg Infect Dis 1999; 5:835–836.
23. Goldwasser RA, Klingberg W, Steiman Y et al. The isolation of strains of rickettsiae of the spotted fever group in Israel and their differentiation from another members of the group by immunofluorescence methods. Scand J Infect Dis 1974; 6:53–62.
24. Burgdorferi W, Varma MGR. Trans-stadial and transovarial development of diseases agents in arthropods. Annu Rev Entomol 1967; 12:347–376.
25. Rehacek J, Tarasevich IV. Acari-borne rickettsiae and rickettsioses in Euroasia. Bratislava: Veda Publishing House; 1988:1–343.
26. Walker DH. Rickettsial diseases in travelers. Travel Med Infect Dis 2003;1:35–40.
27. Mansueto S, Tringali G, Walker DH. Widespred, simultaneous increase in the incidence of spotted fever group rickettsioses. J Infect Dis 1986; 154:539–540.
28. Segura-Porta F, Font-Creus B, Espejo-Arenas E et al. New trends in Mediterranean spotted fever. Eur J Epidemiol 1989; 5:438–443.
29. Raoult D, Tissot DH, Caraco P et al. Mediterranean spotted fever in Marseille: descriptive epidemiology and the influence of climatic factors. Eur J Epidemiol 1992; 8:192–197.
30. Aharonowitz G, Koton S, Segal S et al. Epidemiological characteristics of spotted fever in Israel over 26 years. Clin Infect Dis 1999; 29:1321–1322.
31. Sousa R, Nobrega SD, Bacellar F et al. Mediterranean spotted fever in Portugal: risk factors for fatal outcome in 105 hospitalized patients. Ann NY Acad Sci 2003; 990:285–294.
32. Espejo-Arenas E, Font-Creus B, Alegre-Segura MD et al. Seroepidemiological survey of Mediterranean spotted fever in an endemic area (Valles Occidental, Barcelona, Spain). Trop Gregr Med 1990; 42:212–216.
33. Raoult D, Dupont HT, Chicheportiche C et al. Mediterranean spotted fever in Marseille, France: correlation between prevalence of hospitalized patients, seroepidemiology, and prevalence of infected ticks in three different areas. Am J Trop Med Hyg 1993; 48:249–256.
34. Bacellar F, Nuncio MS, Rehacek J et al. Rickettsiae and rickettsioses in Portugal. Eur J Epidemiol 1991; 7:291–293.
35. Bacellar F, Sousa R, Santos A et al. Boutonneuse fever in Portugal: 1995–2000. Data of a state laboratory. Eur J Epidemiol 2003; 18:275–277.
36. Walker DH, Herrero-Herrero JI, Ruiz-Beltran R et al. The pathology of fatal Mediterranean spotted fever. Am J Clin Pathol 1987; 87:669–672.
37. Walker DH, Mattern WD. Rickettsial vasculitis. Am Heart J 1980; 100:896–906.
38. Brouqui P, Dupont HT, Drancourt M et al. Spotless boutonneuse fever. Clin Infect Dis 1992; 14:114–116.
39. Yagupsky P, Wolach B. Fatal Israeli spotted fever in children. Clin Infect Dis 1993; 17:850–853.
40. Amaro M, Bacellar F, Franca A. Report of eight cases of fatal and severe Mediterranean spotted fever in Portugal. Ann NY Acad Sci 2003; 990:331–343.
41. Walker DH, Occhino C, Tringali GR et al. Pathogenesis of rickettsial eschars: the tache noir of boutonneuse fever. Hum Pathol 1988; 19:1449–1454.
42. Grillo-Reina A, Perez-Jimenez F, Escauriaza J et al. Fiebre botonosa. Estudio de los factores pronósticos. Rev Clin Esp 1982; 164:387–390.
43. Raoult D, Perrimont H, Lena D et al. Hemolysis with Mediterranean spotted fever and glucose-6-phosphate-dehydrogenase deficiency. Trans R Soc Trop Med Hyg 1986; 80:961–962.
44. Lucero M, Moya M, López L et al. Fiebre botonosa mediterránea en pacientes de edad avanzada. Med Geriatr 1988; 1:24–28.
45. Mártin-Farfán A, Fernández CJ, Torrecillas FC et al. Estudio clínico-epidemilógico de 164 casos de fiebre botonosa. Rev Clin Esp 1985; 176:333–339.
46. Sexton J, Corey GR. Rocky mountain "spotless" and "almost spotless" fever: a wolf in sheep's clothing. Clin Infect Dis 1992; 15:439–448.
47. Gross EM, Yagupsky P. Israeli rickettsial spotted fever in children. A review of 54 cases. Acta Trop 1987; 44:91–96.
48. Raoult D, Roux V. Rickettsiosis as paradigms of new or emerging infectious diseases. Clin Microbiol Rev 1997; 10:694–719.
49. Raoult D, Dash G. Line blot and Western blot immunoassays for diagnosis of Mediterranean spotted fever. J Clin Microbiol 1989; 27:2073–2079.
50. Walker DH. Biology of rickettsial diseases. Early vaccines. Boca Raton, FL: CRC Press; 1988.
51. Sousa R, Nobrega SD, Bacellar F et al. Mediterranean spotted fever in Portugal: risk factors for fatal outcome in 105 hospitalized patients. Ann NY Acad Sci 2003; 990:285–294.
52. Crocquet-Valdes PA, Diaz-Montero CM, Feng HM et al. Immunization with a portion of rickettsial outer membrane protein A stimulates protective immunity against spotted fever rickettsiosis. Vaccine 2001; 20:979–988.
53. Chen Z, Chen M, Zhong J et al. Using PCR/RFLP to detect spotted fever group *Rickettsia* in ticks and rodents collected in Ninghua, Fujian province. Zhonghua Yu Fang Yi Xue Za Zhi 2002; 36:106–108.
54. Rydkina E, Roux V, Rudakov N et al. New rickettsiae in ticks collected in territories of the former Soviet Union. Emerg Infect Dis 1999; 5:811–814.
55. Kaplan LI. Other spotted fevers. Clin Dermatol 1996; 14:259–267.
56. Zhang JZ, Fan MY, Bi DZ et al. Genotypic identification of three new strains of spotted fever group rickettsiae isolated in China. Acta Virol 1996; 40:215–219.
57. Chen M, Fan MY, Bi DZ et al. Detection of *Rickettsia sibirica* in ticks and small mammals collected in three different regions of China. Acta Virol 1998; 42:61–64.

58. Lewin MR, Bouyer DH, Walker DH et al. *Rickettsia sibirica* infection in members of scientific expeditions to northern Asia. Lancet 2003; 362:1201–1202.
59. Nelyubov MV. Cytokines in the pathogenesis of Astrakhan spotted fever and North Asian scrub typhus: problems of immunocorrection. Bull Exp Biol Med 2002; 134:165–167.
60. Oikawa Y, Takada N, Fujita H et al. Identity of pathogenic strains of spotted fever rickettsiae isolated in Shikoku district based on reactivities to monoclonal antibodies. Jpn J Med Sci Biol 1993; 46:45–49.
61. Sexton DJ, Dwyer B, Kemp R et al. Spotted fever group rickettsial infections in Australia. Rev Infect Dis 1991; 13:876–886.
62. Kirkland K, Wilkinson W, Sexton D. Therapeutic delay and mortality in cases of Rocky Mountain spotted fever. Clin Infect Dis 1995; 20:1118–1121.
63. Dumler S, Gage W, Pettis G et al. Rapid immunoperoxidase demonstration of *Rickettsia rickettsii* in fixed cutaneous specimens from patients with Rocky Mountain spotted fever. Am J Clin Pathol 1990; 93:410–414.
64. Walker D, Dumler J, Radulvis S. Spotted fevers and rickettsialpox. In Ronald A, ed. Infectious disease: a treatise on infectious processes. Philadelphia, PA: JB Lippincott; 1994:969–978.
65. Kass EM, Szaniawski WK, Levy H et al. Rickettsialpox in a New York City hospital, 1980 to 1989. N Engl J Med 1994; 331:1612–1617.
66. Brettman LR, Lewin S, Hozman RS et al. Rickettsialpox: report of an outbreak and a contemporary review. Medicine 1981; 60:363–372.
67. Rose H. The clinical manifestations and laboratory diagnosis of rickettsialpox. Ann Intern Med 1949; 31:871–883.
68. Sussman L. Kew Gardens' spotted fever. NY Med 1946; 2:27–28.
69. Greenberg M, Pellitteri O. Rickettsialpox. Bull NY Acad Med 1947; 23:338–351.
70. Huebner R, Stamps P, Armstrong C. Rickettsialpox – a newly recognized rickettsial disease: I. Isolation of the etiological agent. Public Health Rep 1946; 61:1605–1614.
71. Jacobson J, Desmond E, Kornblee L et al. Positive Weil–Felix reactions in a case of rickettsialpox. Int J Dermatol 1989; 28:271–272.
72. Feigin R, Snider R, Edwards M. Rickettsial disease. In Cherry J, ed. Textbook of pediatric infectious diseases. Philadelphia: WB Saunders; 1992:1847–1865.
73. Saah AJ. *Rickettsia prowazekii*. In Mandell GL, Bennett JE, Dolin R, eds. Principles and practice of infectious diseases, 4th edn. New York: Churchill Livingstone; 1995:1735–1737.
74. McDade JE, Shepard CC, Redus MA et al. Evidence of *Rickettsia prowazekii* infections in the United States. Am J Trop Med Hyg 1980; 29:277–284.
75. Duma RJ, Sonenshine DE, Bozeman FM et al. Epidemic typhus in the United States associated with flying squirrels. JAMA 1981; 245:2318–2323.
76. Baxter JD. The typhus group. Clin Dermatol 1996; 14:271–278.
77. Perine PL, Chandler BP, Krause DK et al. A clinico-epidemiological study of epidemic typhus in Africa. Clin Infect Dis 1992; 14:1149–1158.
78. Kaplan JE, Schonberger LB. The sensitivity of various serologic tests in the diagnosis of Rocky Mountain spotted fever. Am J Trop Med Hyg 1986; 35:840–844.
79. Jiang J, Temenak JJ, Richards AL. Real-time PCR duplex assay for *Rickettsia prowazekii* and *Borrelia recurrentis*. Ann NY Acad Sci 2003; 990:302–310.
80. Raoult D, Drancourt M. Antimicrobial therapy of rickettsial diseases. Antimicrob Agents Chemother 1991; 35:2457–2462.
81. Coker C, Majid M, Radulovic S. Development of *Rickettsia prowazekii* DNA vaccine: cloning strategies. Ann NY Acad Sci 2003; 990:757–764.
82. Lutwick LI. Brill–Zinsser disease. Lancet 2001; 357:1198–1200.
83. Brill NE. An acute infectious disease of unknown origin: a clinical study based on 221 cases. Am J Med Sci 1910; 139:484–502.
84. Zinsser H. Varieties of typhus virus and the epidemiology of the American form of European typhus fever (Brill's disease). Am J Hyg 1934; 20:513–532.
85. Murray ES, Snyder JC. Brill's disease: II, etiology. Am J Hyg 1951; 53:22–32.
86. Price WH. Studies on the interepidemic survival of louse borne epidemic typhus fever. J Bacteriol 1955; 69:106–107.
87. Green CR, Fishbein D, Gleiberman I. Brill–Zinsser: still with us. JAMA 1990; 264:1811–1812.
88. Portnoy J, Mendelson J, Clecner B. Brill–Zinsser disease: report of a case in Canada. Can Med Assoc J 1974; 111:166.
89. Dumler JS, Taylor JP, Walker DH. Clinical and laboratory features of murine typhus in south Texas, 1980 through 1987. JAMA 1991; 266:1365–1370.
90. Azad AF, Sacci Jr JB, Nelson WM et al. Genetic characterization and transovarial transmission of a typhus-like *Rickettsia* found in cat fleas. Proc Natl Acad Sci USA 1992; 89:43–46.
91. Radulovic S, Higgins JA, Jaworski DC et al. Isolation, cultivation, and partial characterization of the ELB agent associated with cat fleas. Infect Immun 1995; 63:4826–4829.
92. Kelly DJ, Chan CT, Paxton H et al. Comparative evaluation of a commercial enzyme immunoassay for the detection of human antibody to *Rickettsia typhi*. Clin Diagn Lab Immunol 1995; 2:356–360.
93. Carl M, Tibbs CW, Dobson ME et al. Diagnosis of acute typhus infection using the polymerase chain reaction. J Infect Dis 1990; 161:791–793.
94. Drancourt M, George F, Brouqui P et al. Diagnosis of Mediterranean spotted fever by indirect immunofluorescence of *Rickettsia conorii* in circulating endothelial cells isolated with monoclonal antibody-coated immunomagnetic beads. J Infect Dis 1992; 166:660–663.
95. Raoult D, Gallais H, DeMicco P et al. Ciprofloxacin therapy for Mediterranean spotted fever. Antimicrob Agents Chemother 1986; 30:606–607.
96. RuizBeltran R, Herrero JIH. Evaluation of ciprofloxacin and doxycycline in the treatment of Mediterranean spotted fever. Eur J Clin Microbiol Infect Dis 1992; 11:427–431.
97. Watt G, Strickman D. Life-threatening scrub typhus in a traveler returning from Thailand. Clin Infect Dis 1994; 18:624–626.

98. Ohashi N, Tamura A, Sakurai H et al. Characterization of a new antigenic type, Kuroki, of *Rickettsia tsutsugamushi* isolated from a patient in Japan. J Clin Microbiol 1990; 28:2111–2113.
99. Silpapojakul K, Ukkachoke C, Krisanapan S et al. Rickettsial meningitis and encephalitis. Arch Intern Med 1991; 151:1753–1757.
100. Saah A. *Rickettsia tsutsugamushi*. In Dolin R, ed. Principles and practice of infectious diseases, 4th edn. New York: Churchill Livingstone; 1995:1740–1741.
101. Berman S, Kundin W. Scrub typhus in South Vietnam, a study of 87 cases. Ann Intern Med 1973; 79:26–30.
102. Sugita Y, Nagatani T, Okuda K et al. Diagnosis of typhus infection with *Rickettsia tsutsugamushi* by polymerase chain reaction. J Med Microbiol 1992; 37:357–360.
103. Wilkinson RRD, Ching WM. Development of an improved rapid lateral flow assay for the detection of *Orientia tsutsugamushi*-specific IgG/IgM antibodies. Ann NY Acad Sci 2003; 990:386–390.
104. Sheehy T, Hazlett D, Turk R. Scrub typhus, a comparison of chloramphenicol and tetracycline in its treatment. Arch Intern Med 1973; 132:77–80.
105. Raoult D, Drancourt M. Antimicrobial therapy of rickettsial diseases. Antimicrob Agents Chemother 1991; 35:2457–2462.
106. McClain J, Joshi B, Rice R. Chloramphenicol, gentamicin, and ciprofloxacin against murine scrub typhus. Antimicrob Agents Chemother 1988; 32:285–286.
107. Twartz JC, Shirai A, Selvaraju G et al. Doxycycline prophylaxis for human scrub typhus. J Infect Dis 1982; 146:811–818.
108. Atlas RM. Biological weapons pose challenge for microbiology community. ASM News 1998; 64:383–389.
109. Rotz LD, Khan AS, Lillibridge SR et al. Public health assessment of potential biological terrorism agents. Emerg Infect Dis 2002; 8:225–230.
110. Walker DH. Principles of the malicious use of infectious agents to create terror: reasons for concern for organisms of the genus *Rickettsia*. Ann NY Acad Sci 2003; 990:739–742.
111. Alibek K. Biohazard. New York: Random House; 1999.
112. Silverman DJ, Boese JL, Wisseman CL. Ultrastructural studies of *Rickettsia prowazekii* from louse midgut cells to feces: search for "dormant" forms. Infect Immun 1974; 10:257–263.
113. Traub R, Wisseman CL, Farhang-Azad A. The ecology of murine typhus – a critical review. Trop Dis Bull 1978; 75:237–317.
114. Johnson JE, Kadull PJ. Rocky Mountain spotted fever acquired in a laboratory. N Engl J Med 1967; 277:842–847.
115. Pike RM. Laboratory-associated infection: summary and analysis of 3921 cases. Health Lab Sci 1976; 13:105–114.
116. Azad AF, Traub R. Experimental transmission of murine typhus by *Xenopsylla cheopis* flea bites. Med Vet Entomol 1989; 3:429–433.
117. Raoult D, Zuchelli P, Weiller PJ et al. Incidence, clinical observations and risk factors in the severe form of Mediterranean spotted fever among patients admitted to hospital in Marseilles 1983–1984. J Infect 1986; 12:111–116.
118. Raoult D, Maurin M. *Rickettsia* species. In Yu VL, Merigan TC, Barriere SL, eds. Antimicrobial therapy and vaccines. Baltimore, MD: Williams and Wilkins; 2001:568–574.

Chapter 24

Ehrlichioses

Juan P. Olano

Synonyms: Human monocytotropic ehrlichiosis (HME, caused by *Ehrlichia chaffeensis*), human granulocytotropic anaplasmosis (HGA, formerly known as human granulocytotropic ehrlichiosis, caused by *Anaplasma phagocytophilum*), ehrlichiosis ewingii (caused by *E. ewingii*).

Key features:

- Fever, history of tick bite/tick exposure. Signs and symptoms are non-specific
- Macular or maculopapular rash in approximately 30% of patients with HME. 2–5% in cases of HGA. In HME cases, rash is more frequent in the pediatric population (67%)
- Leukopenia and thrombocytopenia are frequent in the first week of illness
- Detection of serum antibodies by indirect immunofluorescent assay (IFA) is the gold standard for diagnosis. Detection of *Ehrlichia/Anaplasma* DNA in blood during the acute phase of the disease by polymerase chain reaction (PCR) is useful for diagnosis
- Treatment of choice is doxycycline hyclate

Introduction

Bacteria of the genera *Ehrlichia* and *Anaplasma* are obligate intracellular bacteria with ultrastructural characteristics of Gram-negative bacteria. They reside in cytoplasmic vacuoles of their target cells, called morulae, and have evolved in close association with arthropods and a eukaryotic host.

Human ehrlichioses comprise three different diseases: (1) HME, caused by *E. chaffeensis*; (2) HGA, caused by *A. phagocytophilum*; and (3) ehrlichiosis ewingii, caused by *E. ewingii* (Table 24.1). *Ehrlichia* and *Anaplasma* have been known for almost a century as veterinary pathogens. The target cells for these three pathogens are monocytes/tissue macrophages for *E. chaffeensis* and polymorphonuclear neutrophils (PMN) for *A. phagocytophilum* and *E. ewingii*. All three pathogens cause systemic disease and can produce dermatologic manifestations such as macular or maculopapular rashes that most commonly involve the trunk and the extremities (Fig. 24.1).

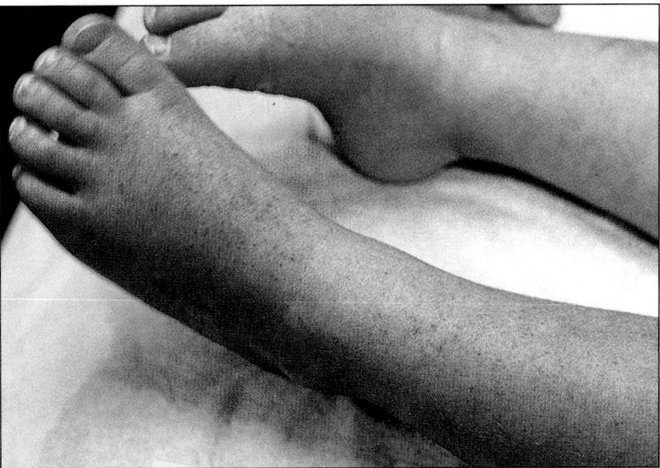

Figure 24. 1 Macular rash in a patient with human monocytotropic ehrlichiosis. (Courtesy of Dr. Edwin Masters.)

Table 24.1 Human ehrlichioses

Disease	Agent	Geographic distribution	Treatment
Human monocytotropic ehrlichiosis	*Ehrlichia chaffeensis*	USA	Doxycycline
Human granulocytotropic anaplasmosis	*Anaplasma phagocytophilum*	USA, Europe	Doxycycline
Ehrlichiosis ewingii	*Ehrlichia ewingii*	USA	Doxycycline

History

Ehrlichial pathogens have been known for almost a century as causes of disease in animals. In 1987, the first case of HME was described in the USA and its pathogen cultivated, sequenced, and characterized as a new *Ehrlichia* (*E. chaffeensis*) in 1991. In 1994, a second ehrlichiosis was described based on 16S rRNA sequencing. Its pathogen was cultivated later and named human granulocytotropic ehrlichiosis (HGE) agent. A new classification of all ehrlichial organisms based on genetic sequencing was recently published and the HGE agent was reclassified as *A. phagocytophilum*.[1] In 1999, a third uncultivable agent named *E. ewingii* was associated with a second form of granulocytotropic ehrlichiosis in humans (ehrlichiosis ewingii). The history of human ehrlichioses continues to evolve as new information becomes available in both North America and around the world.

Epidemiology

E. chaffeensis, *A. phagocytophilum*, and *E. ewingii* are part of zoonotic cycles in which they are transmitted transstadially through all maturation cycles of the tick vectors (larvae, nymphs, and adults). The larval and nymphal forms of tick vectors acquire a blood meal for molting during which they can acquire ehrlichiae from an ehrlichiemic mammal. There is no evidence of transovarial transmission of ehrlichiae in which larval progeny would be infected by an adult female tick.

Human granulocytotropic anaplasmosis

HGA has been well described in the USA and Europe. Endemic areas in the USA include the northeastern states and the upper Midwest, where the tick vector is most abundant. In Europe HGA has been described in several countries, including the Netherlands, Norway, Slovenia, Spain, Sweden, Switzerland, and the UK.[2] The main vectors in the USA and Europe are *Ixodes scapularis* and *I. ricinus*, respectively. Well-described mammal reservoirs in Europe include sheep, goats, deer, and mice. In the USA, the main reservoirs are mice, cotton-tail rabbits, white-tail deer, and rats. The presence of *A. phagocytophilum* in nymphal and larval forms is as high as 25% in areas of high endemicity. As of 1997, a total of 449 cases had been reported to the Centers for Disease Control (CDC).[3] However, this number is probably an underestimate of the true prevalence. The male-to-female ratio is approximately 4:1 and HGA has a definite seasonal distribution with most cases being diagnosed during the spring and summer, when tick vectors are most actively looking for blood meals.

Human monocytotropic ehrlichiosis

HME is most prevalent in the south-central, southeastern, and mid-Atlantic states, where the vector *Amblyomma americanum* (lone star tick) is most abundant and the population of white-tail deer, its main mammal reservoir, is increasing. Other less important reservoirs include coyotes and goats. Serologic evidence of HME has also been described in other continents, including South America, Africa, and Asia, although isolation of *E. chaffeensis* or demonstration of its DNA by PCR in humans has not been described outside the USA. As of 1997, 742 cases had been reported to the CDC.[3] The prevalence of HME is most likely underestimated. In fact, a prospective study conducted in southeast Missouri between 1997 and 1999 revealed a high incidence of HME.[4] The male-to-female ratio is also 4:1 and the distribution is seasonal, with the highest number of cases being diagnosed in the spring and summer. Because of the latitude of the endemic area, tick vectors for HME are active for longer periods of time as opposed to HGA vectors.

Ehrlichiosis ewingii

E. ewingii has not been isolated in culture in the laboratory. Its association with humans was demonstrated by detection of its DNA in the blood of ill patients. The main vector is also the lone star tick and therefore the distribution of the disease is similar to that of HME. White-tail deer are also reservoirs for this bacterium. *E. ewingii* seems to affect mostly immunosuppressed patients, including patients with human immunodeficiency virus (HIV). In dogs, it is responsible for canine granulocytotropic ehrlichiosis.

Pathogenesis and etiology

Human granulocytotropic anaplasmosis

The port of entry is through a skin bite by an infected tick. Attachment of the tick vector for 24–48 h is required for transmission to occur. The early events after inoculation by the tick bite are largely unknown but it is likely that *Anaplasma phagocytophilum* is internalized by circulating PMN. Internalization is mediated by adhesion of the bacterium to P-selectin, a membrane protein present in PMN.[5] Intracellular survival of *A. phagocytophilum* in a cell which is specialized in killing foreign invaders is based on several factors, including inhibition of phagolysosomal fusion and inhibition of critical enzymes needed for production of reactive oxygen species (ROS). Several cytokines also play a role in the pathogenesis of HGA. In animal models, interferon-γ (IFN-γ) induces production of nitric oxide which in turn helps control the infection. Interleukin-8 (IL-8) recruits PMN to the site of infection, therefore favoring infection of other PMN. Other cytokines which are found elevated in animal models of infection include tumor necrosis factor-α (TNF-α), IL-1β, and IL-6 but their role in pathogenesis in not well understood. In humans, high levels of IFN-γ and low levels of IL-10 and IL-4 were seen during the acute phase of the disease. In animal models immune evasion by *A. phagocytophilum* is mediated by antigenic variation of a 44-kDa protein gene that belongs to a multigene family. This process of antigenic variation under immune pressure has not been convincingly demonstrated in humans. Antigenic variation probably allows *A. phagocytophilum* to persist in the natural host for long periods of time.

Human monocytotropic ehrlichiosis

Inoculation occurs via a tick bite after 24–48 h of tick attachment to the host's skin. *E. chaffeensis* then gains access to the target cells (tissue macrophages and monocytes). Both the adhesin and the receptor have not been identified but plausible candidates include a 120-kDa glycoprotein and a protein of the selectin family, respectively. Once inside the cell, *E. chaffeensis* inhibits phagolysosomal fusion and upregulates transferrin receptors on the cytoplasmic vacuole to increase intravacuolar iron, necessary for *E. chaffeensis* survival. The immune response also involves several cytokines, including IL-1β, IL-6, IL-8, IFN-γ, and TNF-α. In a murine animal model developed recently, fatal outcome was associated with high levels of TNF-α. Immune evasion is probably mediated by a multigen family of 28-kDa proteins. Based on results in animal models, both cellular and humoral immune responses are important in clearing infections caused by *A. phagocytophilum* and *E. chaffeensis* from infected hosts.

The pathogenesis of infections caused by *E. ewingii* is virtually unknown. *E. ewingii* seems to be a less virulent pathogen than its counterparts discussed in this review, as shown by its prevalence in immunosuppressed patients.[6]

Clinical features

Human granulocytotropic anaplasmosis

A. phagocytophilum shares its vector with two other human pathogens, *Borrelia burgdorferi* and *Babesia* spp. Therefore, both synchronous and sequential infections with these two pathogens have been described. The clinical spectrum of HGA is variable and ranges from mildly symptomatic to more severe infections. Infections caused by *A. phagocytophilum* are less severe than infections caused by *E. chaffeensis*. In fact, neurologic manifestations in HGA are rare, but rather common in HME. Clinical signs and symptoms are non-specific and the onset is rather abrupt, with high fever, chills, headache, and malaise for 24–48 h followed by other non-specific manifestations such as anorexia, nausea, vomiting, abdominal pain, myalgias, arthralgias, and skin rash in only 2–5% of cases. The skin rash is macular or maculopapular and is rarely present from the beginning of the illness. Cases of HGA presenting as atypical pneumonitis have been described. In some series hospitalization was necessary in up to 50% of cases and its case-fatality rate ranges from 0.5 to 1%.[7,8] Rare reported complications include diffuse alveolar damage, rhabdomyolysis, myocarditis, plexopathy, and demyelinating polyneuropathies.[8]

Human monocytotropic ehrlichiosis

Signs and symptoms usually appear 7–10 days after the tick bite. They are non-specific and include high fever, malaise, headache, chills, nausea, vomiting, myalgias, arthralgias, abdominal pain, lymph-adenopathy, and skin rash that is more common than in HGA. The rash is macular or maculopapular or less commonly petechial and is present in up to 33% of cases of HME. Only 6% of cases have a skin rash at the time of initial presentation. The incidence in the pediatric population can be as high as 67% of cases.[8–11] The rash mostly affects the trunk and the extremities. Manifestations related to the central nervous system include delirium, confusion, stupor, ataxia, vertigo, neck stiffness, and coma. Complications are varied and include acute respiratory insufficiency due to diffuse alveolar damage, acute renal insufficiency due to acute tubular necrosis, cardiomyopathy, and hemorrhagic complications secondary to severe thrombocytopenia. Both HGA and HME are usually followed by months of asthenia and the appearance of opportunistic infections such as mucosal candidiasis and oral herpes infections due to an ill-defined immunosuppression after the acute phase resolves. HME tends to be more severe in HIV patients, in whom case-fatality rates are higher.

Patient evaluation and diagnosis

The diagnosis of ehrlichiosis/anaplasmosis should be suspected in every patient who presents with fever and a history of tick bite or potential tick exposure. As mentioned before, signs and symptoms associated with human ehrlichioses are non-specific. Suggestive laboratory data include leukopenia and thrombocytopenia that can occur in up to two-thirds of patients at the time of presentation, either alone or in combination. During the second week of illness, patients usually develop a reactive lymphocytosis with the presence of atypical lymphocytes in some cases. These lymphocytes are of the γ-δ T-cell type and their significance is unknown. The absence of either leukopenia or thrombocytopenia does not rule out the diagnosis. Other laboratory data include elevation of C-reactive protein and increased erythrocytesedimentation rate, both of which are non-specific. Mild elevation of hepatic transaminases can also be found at the time of presentation.

Human granulocytotropic anaplasmosis

The diagnosis of HGA is first suspected in the laboratory by the presence of the characteristic intracellular morulae present in PMN examined in blood smears. Intracellular morulae have been demonstrated in up to 50% of patients in the upper Midwest. Visualization of morulae requires training and a high index of suspicion, and must be differentiated from other cytoplasmic abnormalities, such as toxic granulations and Döhle bodies.

The gold standard for diagnosis of HGA is demonstration of anti-*Anaplasma* serum antibodies by IFA.[2,12] Standardization, accuracy, and reproducibility studies are underway across the nation. Normal ranges and diagnostic titers are developed by each laboratory based on their standardization procedures. In general, titers of 1:80 or greater are considered positive. Demonstration of seroconversion or quadruplication of serum titers in two samples taken 2–3 weeks apart or single titers of 1:320 or greater are considered diagnostic of acute HGA. Other serologic methods available in a few research laboratories around the country are based on the demonstration of antibodies by enzyme-linked immunosorbent assay (ELISA) or Western immunoblotting against specific *Anaplasma* proteins derived from *A. phagocytophilum* grown in cell monolayers or recombinant proteins. The most promising proteins are in the 42–49-kDa range and appear both sensitive and specific. In many cases serologic diagnosis is retrospective, since it is based on the demonstration of seroconversion in a period of 2–3 weeks. Therefore, diagnosis in the acute phase is difficult. Detection of *Anaplasma* DNA from peripheral blood by PCR represents an excellent alternative for this purpose, although reproducibility and standardization are far from ideal. Gene targets for PCR that have been used include the 16S rRNA subunit gene, *groesl*, *epank*-1, *msp*-2, *ftsZ*, and the 100–130-kDa protein genes. Sensitivity of PCR varies from 50 to 87% and specificity is close to 100% provided DNA amplicon contamination is not present in the laboratory. PCR testing is available in a few research laboratories around the country. Isolation of *A. phagocytophilum* is done in highly specialized laboratories, is cumbersome, and has been more successful than isolation of its counterpart, *E. chaffeensis*. This procedure is done using monolayers derived from a human leukemia cell line of myeloblastic differentiation (HL60). Postmortem diagnosis is possible by immunohistochemical demonstration of morulae in PMN in different organs using either polyclonal or monoclonal antibodies in postmortem formalin-fixed tissues.

Human monocytotropic ehrlichiosis

Clinical diagnosis is suspected when a patient consults for fever of 2–3 days' duration, associated with a history of tick-bite exposure and other non-specific signs and symptoms mentioned previously. Visualization of intracytoplasmic morulae in peripheral blood monocytes is rare (7–17% of cases). The preferred method of diagnosis for HME is also IFA.[2,12] Dilutions of 1:64 or greater are considered positive. Either seroconversion or quadruplication of serum antibody titers is considered diagnostic of HME. Single serum titers of 1:256 or greater is also highly suggestive of acute HME. Detection of *E. chaffeensis* DNA from peripheral blood by PCR has also been used for diagnosis during the acute phase of the disease. Target genes include the 16S rRNA subunit, 120-kDa protein gene, *nadA* gene, *ftsZ* gene, and the variable-length polymerase chain reaction target (VLPT) gene. Sensitivity and specificity are similar to the ones described for HGA. In general the sensitivity is higher in patients who consult early during the disease process in whom circulating ehrlichiae are higher than in cases evaluated late in the disease process in whom the immune response is better developed and therefore the levels of circulating ehrlichiae are lower. Monolayers derived from canine (DH82) and human monoblastic leukemia cell lines (THP-1) are used for this purpose. Rapid inoculation of the blood samples into the cell monolayers after drawing the blood from the patient seems to be a critical factor in isolating ehrlichiae in the laboratory. Postmortem diagnosis in paraffin-embedded tissues is also possible in cases of *E. chaffeensis* infection using either monoclonal or polyclonal antibodies.

A pitfall for the serologic diagnosis of HME and HGA is the presence of cross-reacting antibodies between *A. phagocytophilum* and *E. chaffeensis*. In these cases, PCR demonstration of DNA is helpful. In addition, titers against one of the infectious agents are usually higher (fourfold) than against the other agent.

The diagnosis of *E. ewingii* is based exclusively on PCR amplification of *E. ewingii* DNA from peripheral blood. Serologic diagnosis is very difficult due to the presence of abundant cross-reacting antibodies to *E. chaffeensis* because of their close genetic relationship.

Pathology

Organs affected in cases of HGA and HME include the bone marrow, spleen, liver, skin, lungs, and, in cases of HME, the central nervous system. In cases of HGA the intracytoplasmic morulae are present in PMN and in cases of HME they are present in tissue macrophages. Both *A. phagocytophilum* and *E. chaffeensis* have also been observed in secondary target cells to a much lesser degree such as endothelium. All affected organs reveal parenchymal and perivascular lymphohistiocytic infiltrates (Figs 24.2 and 24.3). In the central nervous system, there is evidence of meningoencephalitis with lymphohistiocytic infiltrates in meningeal and parenchymal vessels in cases of HME.

Treatment

Recommendations for treatment are mostly based on empiric data. Double-blind randomized clinical trials are not available. Few publications have addressed the issue of in vitro antibiotic susceptibility testing for both *A. phagocytophilum* and *E. chaffeensis*. These studies, although valuable, are far from being standardized and therefore interpretation is difficult.

The treatment of choice is doxycycline hyclate. The recommended dosage for adults is 100 mg b.i.d. for 2 weeks. In children,

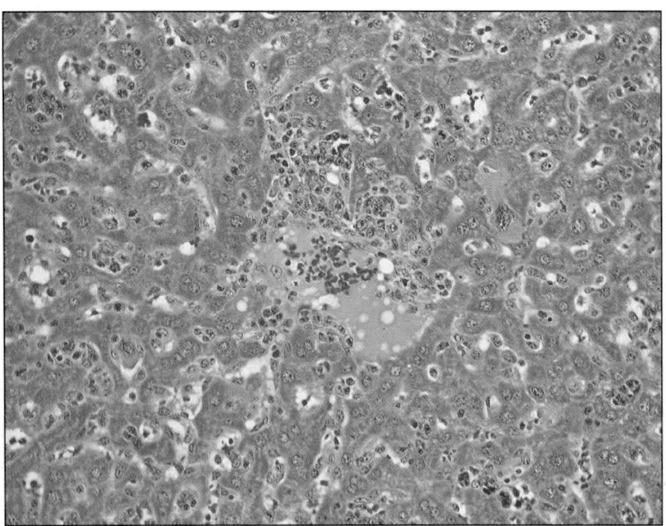

Figures 24.2 Perivascular and parenchymal lymphohistiocytic infiltrates in the liver of a murine animal model of HME. Hematoxylin and eosin stain (200×).

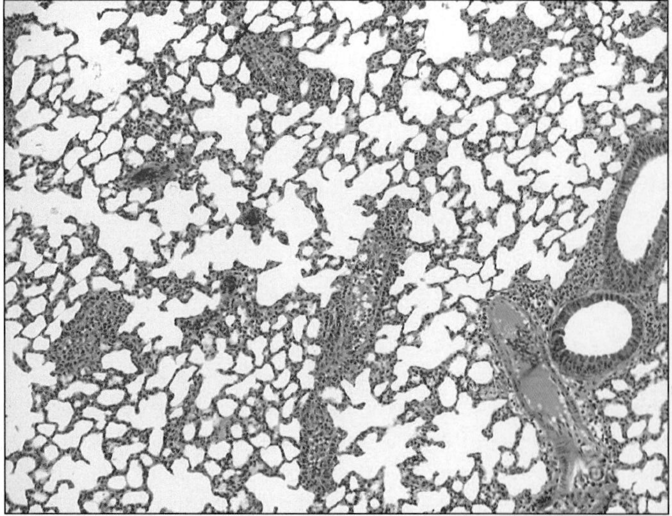

Figure 24.3 Perivascular and parenchymal lymphohistiocytic infiltrates in the lungs of a murine animal model of HME. Hematoxylin and eosin stain (100×).

the recommended dosage is 2.2 mg/kg b.i.d. in patients with body weight less than 40–45 kg. An excellent alternative is tetracyclines, although side-effects are more common. For patients in whom tetracyclines or doxycycline hyclate are absolutely contraindicated, rifampin represents a good alternative. During pregnancy, rifampin seems to be a good alternative to doxycycline/tetracyclines. However, no randomized double-blind studies exist to back up this statement. The evidence so far is anecdotal. Chloramphenicol is currently not recommended as an alternative treatment for ehrlichioses. Fluoroquinolones show some promise in vitro and anecdotal reports in vivo. However, resistance to fluoroquinolones has already been demonstrated in vitro for *E. chaffeensis*.

The best prophylaxis for ehrlichioses is to avoid tick bites during the time at which ticks are most active, looking for blood meals. Close inspection of the skin is advised in endemic areas and manual detachment of the tick is recommended. Antibiotic prophylaxis after the tick bite is controversial.

References

1. Dumler JS, Barbet AF, Bekker CP et al. Reorganization of genera in the families Rickettsiaceae and Anaplasmataceae in the order Rickettsiales: unification of some species of *Ehrlichia* with *Anaplasma*, *Cowdria* with *Ehrlichia* and *Ehrlichia* with *Neorickettsia*, descriptions of six new species combinations and designation of *Ehrlichia equi* and 'HGE agent' as subjective synonyms of *Ehrlichia phagocytophila*. Int J Syst Evol Microbiol 2001; 51:2145–2165.
2. Paddock CD, Childs JE. *Ehrlichia chaffeensis*: a prototypical emerging pathogen. Clin Microbiol Rev 2003; 16:37–64.
3. McQuiston JH, Paddock CD, Holman RC et al. The human ehrlichioses in the United States. Emerg Infect Dis 1999; 5:635–642.
4. Olano JP Masters E, Hogrefe et al. Human monocytotropic ehrlichiosis, Emerg Infect Dis 2003; 9:1579–1586.
5. Herron MJ, Nelson CM, Larson J et al. Intracellular parasitism by the human granulocytic ehrlichiosis bacterium through the P-selectin ligand, PSGL-1. Science 2000; 288:1653–1656.
6. Paddock CD, Folk SM, Shore GM et al. Infections with *Ehrlichia chaffeensis* and *Ehrlichia ewingii* in persons coinfected with human immunodeficiency virus. Clin Infect Dis 2001; 33:1586–1594.
7. Bakken JS, Krueth J, Wilson-Nordskog C et al. Clinical and laboratory characteristics of human granulocytic ehrlichiosis. JAMA 1996; 275:199–205.
8. Olano JP, Walker DH. Human ehrlichioses. Med Clin North Am 2002; 86:375–392.
9. Fishbein DB, Dawson JE, Robinson LE. Human ehrlichiosis in the United States, 1985 to 1990. Ann Intern Med 1994; 120:736–743.
10. Fishbein DB, Kemp A, Dawson JE et al. Human ehrlichiosis: prospective active surveillance in febrile hospitalized patients. J Infect Dis 1989; 160:803–809.
11. Schutze GE, Jacobs RF. Human monocytic ehrlichiosis in children. Pediatrics 1997; 100:E10.
12. Walker DH. Diagnosing human ehrlichioses. Am Soc Microbiol News 2000; 66:287–291.

Chapter 25

Bartonellosis

Francisco G. Bravo

- History
- Microbiology

Clinical syndromes

- Carrión disease
- Bacillary angiomatosis
- Cat-scratch disease
- Trench fever

Bartonella bacilliformis was described almost 100 years ago as the cause of Carrión disease but remained a medical curiosity until the description of bacillary angiomatosis (BA) in the late 1980s. *Bartonella* has received great attention since, and research on the matter has flourished. This is a group of bacteria that are selective mammalian pathogens requiring specific vectors to be transmitted. Some bacteria in this group are capable of stimulating endothelial cells in vitro and inducing angiogenesis in vivo, producing substances that are analogous to endothelial growth factor.[1] The mechanism of action for such a phenomenon seems to be phosphorylation of mitogen-activated protein kinase (MAPK) which is significantly expressed by the endothelial cells of verruga peruana (VP).[2] *B. bacilliformis* is known to induce immunosuppression in cases of Oroya fever (OF), by lowering the number of T-helper lymphocytes.[3] Both *B. bacilliformis* and *B. henselae* are capable of entering red blood cells by the action of specific proteins called deformins, causing hemolytic disease in human and cats.[4] Different species of *Bartonella* have different mammalian reservoirs: *B. bacilliformis* and *B. quintana* have a predilection for humans, whereas *B. henselae* and *B. clarridgeae* seems to prefer felines. The preferences of *B. bacilliformis* for humans and *B. henselae* for cats may be explained on the basis of red-blood-cell receptor differences as well as the characteristic motility of *B. bacilliformis*.

History

The first condition linked to this bacterium was Carrión disease. Caused by *B. bacilliformis*, it has two remarkable different clinical phases: systemic involvement characterized by fever, septicemia, and anemia (OF), and later, an eruptive phase of angiomatous papular and nodular skin lesions (VP). Although the reported cases were restricted to small endemic areas of Peru and Ecuador, the condition was briefly mentioned in major textbooks of medicine.

The history of VP goes back hundreds of years. Pottery from pre-Inca cultures such as the Huaylas shows human faces with papular lesions that could be interpreted as those of the eruptive phase of VP.[5]

In colonial times (sixteenth and seventeenth centuries) a chronicle described an epidemic outbreak of bleeding, oozing, exophytic lesions, affecting the face and body of Spanish troops belonging to Francisco Pizarro (the conqueror of Peru), in the area of Coaque, Ecuador.

By the 1870s, nothing was known about the relation between the eruptive angiomatous lesions known as VP and a systemic disease, of extremely high mortality, affecting a group of workers on the trans-Andean railroad in the central Sierra. The disease was named Oroya fever, after the location where most cases were detected.

By 1872 the possibility that VP and OF were parts of the same unique process was raised. That current of opinion led to the experiments conducted by Daniel Alcides Carrión.[5]

Carrión was a medical student, born in 1857, who developed a great interest in VP and OF. On August 17, 1885, in a self-promoted experiment that took his scientific curiosity to an extreme, and lacking complete awareness of the risk involved, he was inoculated with material from verruga. He was expecting to develop just the anemia, not the febrile illness. Unfortunately, the disease went on to its most severe state: first, fever, then, severe anemia, and, finally it provoked his death on October 5, 1885, at the age of 28. Carrión's experiment, at the expense of his own life, proved that the diseases were truly part of a unity as well as establishing that the disease was transmissible.

In 1909 Alberto Barton, a Peruvian doctor working at the Guadalupe Hospital of Callao, discovered the presence of what he called "X bodies" inside the red blood cells of patients affected by OF; this is considered the first description of the etiological agent and hereafter the bacteria was called *Bartonella*.

Bartonella became a medical curiosity, although interesting research continued to be done on a minor scale in Peru, the USA, UK, and France.

Before the 1980s the etiology of cat-scratch disease (CSD) was unknown. After an original publication implicating a new bacterial agent, *Afipia felis*, in the etiology of CSD, later reports failed to confirmed that observation; however, there was agreement on the bacterial origin of the disease, and also its capability of being stained with silver techniques. Those were the arguments used by LeBoit et al. to establish the link between CSD and a disease described by Stoler in New York, in 1984, affecting AIDS patients.[6,7] Once the microorganism causing the disease (by then named bacillary angiomatosis) was isolated, it was described as part of a different genus named *Rochalima*; retrospective genetic analysis allowed scientists to classify it as a member of the *Bartonella* group.

The *Bartonella* group can be used as a model for the mechanism of endothelial cell growth. As such, they may have an impact not only on the treatment of vascular proliferating tumors but on the treatment of malignant tumors in general that are dependent on blood supply for continuous growth.

Microbiology

The *Bartonella* family is best classified as belonging to the α_2 subgroup of bacteria, in the Protobacteriae class, that also includes closely related microorganisms such as *Brucella*, *Agrobacterium*, *Afipia*, and *Rickettsia*.

These bacteria are mammalian intracellular pathogens that require a vector for their transmission. The family had only one element, *Bartonella bacilliformis*, up until 1993. By then, DNA-DNA hybridization data and comparisons of existing 16S rRNA gene sequences gave sufficient evidence for merging the *Rochalimae* genus with *Bartonella*. Similar studies have led to the incorporation of *Grahamella* species in the same genus in 1995.

The prototype bacterium is *B. bacilliformis*, and currently the family includes 15 species, five of which are known to cause disease in humans: *B. bacilliformis*, *B. quintana*, *B. henselae*, *B. elizabethae*, and *B. clarridgeiae* (Table 25.1). The 16S rRNA gene sequence homology puts *B. elizabethae* as the closest relation to *B. bacilliformis*, followed by *B. henselae* and *B quintana*. *Afipia felis*, a putative agent causing CSD, is in fact closer to *Rickettsia* than to *Bartonella*. The close relation with other bacteria such as *Agrobacterium tumefaciens* becomes more intriguing if one takes into consideration that this last organism is capable of inducing tissue proliferation in infected plants, similar to what is seen in VP and BA.[8]

The members of this family can be described as Gram-negative, oxidase-negative, fastidious, aerobic rods. Although they are intracellular microorganisms in vivo, they are not obligate intracellular pathogens, which is another difference from the *Rickettsia* family. *B. bacilliformis* has a unique polar flagellum adapted for motility.

The organisms are difficult to grow. They require blood agar media, and temperature and CO_2 requirements vary depending on the species. Growth is optimal at 37°C, with the exception of *B. bacilliformis*, which requires lower temperatures of 25–28°C. *B. bacilliformis* is also unique because it grows better with no CO_2 supplements. The primary isolates are obtained after a period of 12–14 days, but this may extend up to 45 days. First subcultures are also difficult, with colony formation taking 10–15 days. Repeated subcultures may take only 3–5 days but with subsequent variations in morphology.

Clinical syndromes

Carrión disease

Synonyms: Carrión disease, Oroya fever (hematic phase), Verruga peruana (eruptive phase)

Key features:

- *Bartonella bacilliformis*
- Living or traveling to endemic areas
- Oroya fever: febrile state, anemia, hemolysis
- Verruga peruana: eruptive angiomatous papules and nodules

Carrión disease is the best current denomination for those clinical features associated with *B. bacilliformis*. The systemic, febrile disease is named OF, and represents the hematogenous phase. The cutaneous disease of eruptive angiomatous lesions is denominated VP and is considered a self-resolving condition. Both can be seen as a sequence, affecting the same patient, although most cases will develop either OF or VP. It is frequently said that OF is most common and more severe in patients who are foreigners to endemic areas; some recent reports tell us that this is not always the case.[5] VP seems to be more common in locals, especially in children.

Table 25.1 Diseases caused by members of the Bartonella family

Agent	Natural host	Vector	Disease in the immunocompetent	Disease in the immunosuppressed
B. bacilliformis	Human	Lutzomya	Carrion disease (OF, VP)	
B. quintana	Human	Louse	Trench fever	Bacillary angiomatosis
B. henselae	Cat	Flea	Cat-scratch disease	Bacillary angiomatosis–peliosis
B. clarridgeiae	Cat	Flea	Cat-scratch disease	
B. elizabethae	Human	Louse	Bacteremia–septicemia	

Epidemiology

The disease has been confined for a long time to specific regions of Peru and Ecuador, with only a single epidemic occurring in Colombia in 1939. The endemic areas in Peru are located in the northern Andes, and it was always said to follow a very specific range of altitudes, 500–3200 m above sea level. Over the last 5 years the descriptions of outbreaks in lower regions, in the limit between the Sierra and the Amazon forest, seem to indicate a change in the distribution of vectors, the incorporation of new vectors in the transmission of the disease, and the possibility of migratory workers acting as potential mobile human reservoirs. The main vector is a sand fly, *Lutzomya verrucarum*, which is also a vector for cutaneous leishmaniasis. The insect is always close to human dwellings and most infections are produced by female biting habits at sunrise and sunset.

Pathogenesis and etiology

B. bacilliformis is transmitted by the *Lutzomya* bite. Once inoculated, the bacteria reach the blood stream and rapidly invade the red cells (it is the only bacterium known to do so). Through the action of specific proteins called deformins, invagination of the cell membrane is induced and this is incorporated into the cell. It reaches 100% parasitism, induces hemolysis and is then captured by the reticuloendothelial system. From then on the microorganism enters a dormant state, to reappear later in the interstice of eruptive verrugas.

Clinical findings

Once an individual has been infected by *Bartonella*, the infection may follow a subclinical course or evolve into a febrile illness known as OF. The incubation period is 61 days, with a range of 10–210 days. The patient will experience a gradual appearance of fever, malaise, headache and mild chills; generalized weakness as well as back and extremity pain follow. Then, the development of severe anemia will dominate the clinical picture. The anemia is hemolytic in nature. This is a remarkable distinct bacterium, where the infectious agent can actually be seen in peripheral smears inside erythrocytes. Profound paleness, jaundice, and dyspnea are signs of the ongoing hemolytic process. Hepatosplenomegaly and generalized lymphadenopathy may develop. Changes in mental status, from mild somnolence to coma and seizures, represent progressive central nervous system involvement. Complications seen during this period include severe edema, non-cardiogenic pulmonary edema, myocarditis, and hemorrhagic pericarditis.

The OF state may last 2–4 weeks. Up to 30% of patients may develop opportunistic infections such as *Salmonella*, *Toxoplasma*, *Plasmodium*, *Histoplasma*, as well as *Staphylococcus* septicemia. Untreated OF may have high mortality rates, from 30 to 80%. With appropriate antibiotic treatment this rate can be reduced to less than 9%.

A recent outbreak outside the endemic area has shown some special features that are worth mentioning. The estimated mortality rates were lower than expected, compared to the classical endemic areas; also many patients with fever, malaise, and serological evidence of disease did not develop anemia at all. Such a finding raises the possibility of variable degrees of virulence, in relation to different strains of *B. bacilliformis*. Small surveys in well-known endemic areas have shown serological evidence of infection in up to 60% of the local population, indicating a larger than expected number of patients developing a subclinical infection and becoming human reservoirs.[9]

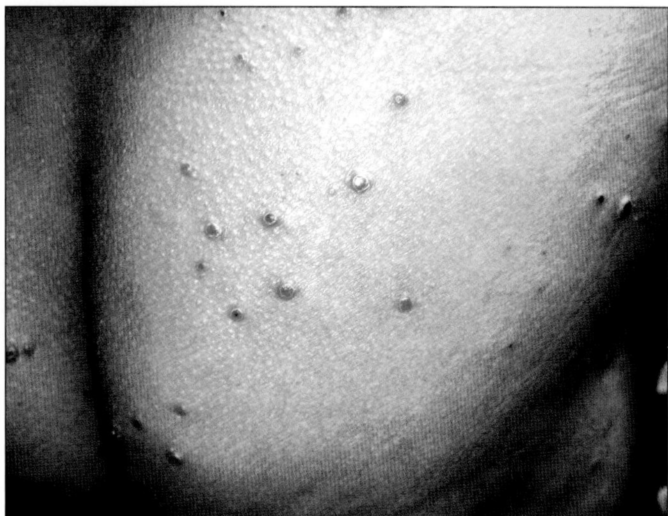

Figure 25.1 Miliary type of verruga peruana.

The most relevant form of Carrión disease for the dermatologist is the eruptive phase known as VP. This phase is characterized by the progressive appearance of one to several angiomatous lesions. The disease is most commonly seen in children, and can be located anywhere in the body, with a special predilection for the extremities. Mucous membrane involvement has been rarely described, as far as the larynx and the rectum. There are three classical types of lesions: the miliar type (Fig. 25.1), a more superficial, reddish papule with a collaret; the nodular type, which is larger, located deeper, and covered by intact epidermis, and the mular type (Figs 25.2 and 25.3), which is identical to the nodular type but with an angiomatous, eroded surface. Interestingly, some patients in the VP stage will have systemic symptoms, and a few may even have fever, anemia, and positive peripheral blood smears. VP is very

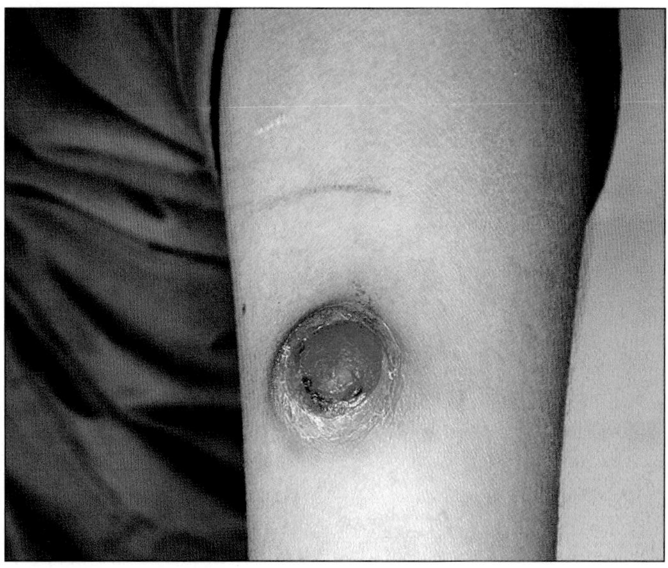

Figure 25.2 Mular type of verruga peruana.

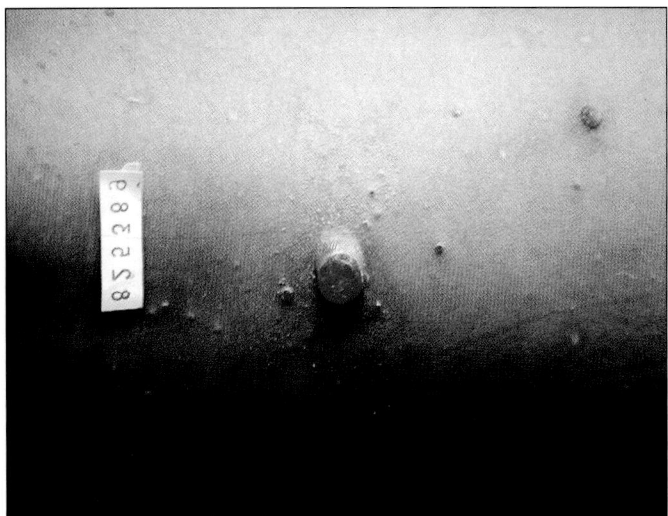

Figure 25.3 Another verruga peruana, mular type. Similarities to pyogenic granuloma and bacillary angiomatosis are evident.

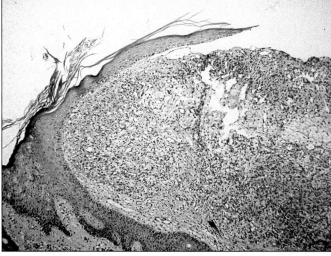

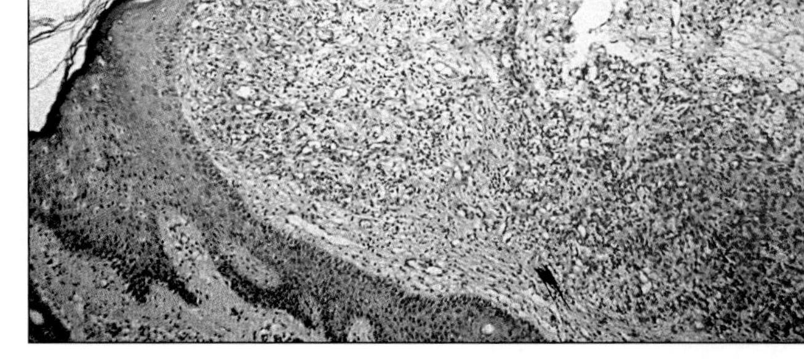

Figure 25.4 Verruga peruana showing the confluent vascular proliferation, collaret, and no septa. Hematoxylin and eosin 40×.

similar to what is seen in BA, reinforcing the idea of similar bacteria producing similar clinical pictures. For those who have had the opportunity to see cases of both diseases, no clinical difference can be established between cutaneous lesions of VP and those of BA.

Diagnosis and differential diagnosis

Diagnosis of OF is based on clinical findings: fever, headache, arthralgia, and evidence of hemolytic anemia. The most useful laboratory test is a peripheral blood smear, looking for the presence of bacteria parasitizing red blood cells. Additional methods include blood culture (quite difficult in the case of *B. bacilliformis*) and Western blot, which has demonstrated high sensitivity and specificity.

At this point the differential diagnosis will include any febrile processes, such as malaria, typhoid fever, yellow fever, typhus, and brucellosis.

Diagnosis of VP is made on the basis of clinical and histological findings. Warthin–Starry staining will show bacilli in the stroma of the vascular lesion. The differential diagnosis includes pyogenic granuloma, hemangioma, adnexal tumors, Kaposi sarcoma, angiolymphoid hyperplasia with eosinophilia, and even Spitz nevus.

Pathology

The histological findings of VP are remarkable for the presence of a proliferating vascular reaction, in a way similar to a granulation tissue. As opposed to pyogenic granuloma, no septa will be seen separating the tissue in lobules (Fig. 25.4). Sheets of cells, a mixture of endothelial cells (Figs 25.5 and 25.6) and round cells (dermal dendrocytes) will account for most of the cellular component. The blood vessels will be small, better formed than in Kaposi sarcoma, and the fascicular arrangement that is so common in KS will be seen in only a minority of cases. An interesting clue to the diagnosis of VP will be the focal presence of neutrophils, sometimes even forming abscesses in the middle of the perivascular stroma. The purple bodies of BA will not be seen in VP. The same collaret described in pyogenic granuloma will also be seen in VP, accounting for its clinical presence.

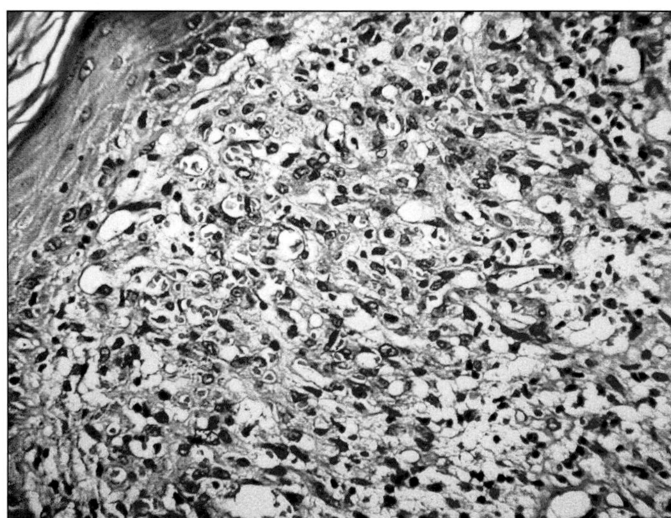

Figure 25.5 Higher power showing the vascular proliferation. Hematoxylin and eosin 100×.

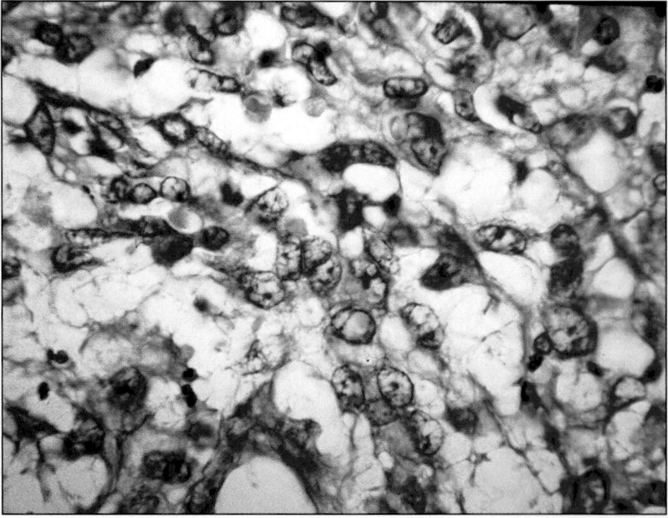

Figure 25.6 Verruga peruana: vascular proliferation and large endothelial cells. Hematoxylin and eosin 400×.

One remarkable finding is the capability of VP for mimicking malignant neoplasm, such as carcinomas, sarcomas (Figs 25.7 and 25.8), and lymphomas (Fig. 25.9), as stated by Arias-Stella and coworkers.[10] Also the clinical self-involution so characteristic of VP lesions in a 3–4-month period may manifest itself as a progressive conversion from the classical histology to a pattern very similar to pyogenic granuloma and cherry angiomas.

Warthin–Starry staining will allow visualization of the *Bartonella* in the interstice, although never in the amount seen in BA. Even though most pathologists working in endemic areas will easily make a histological diagnosis of VP, a clear distinction between VP and BA under the microscope will not be possible, unless one takes into consideration the clinical data. Specific immunostaining for *B. bacilliformis* has recently been developed.

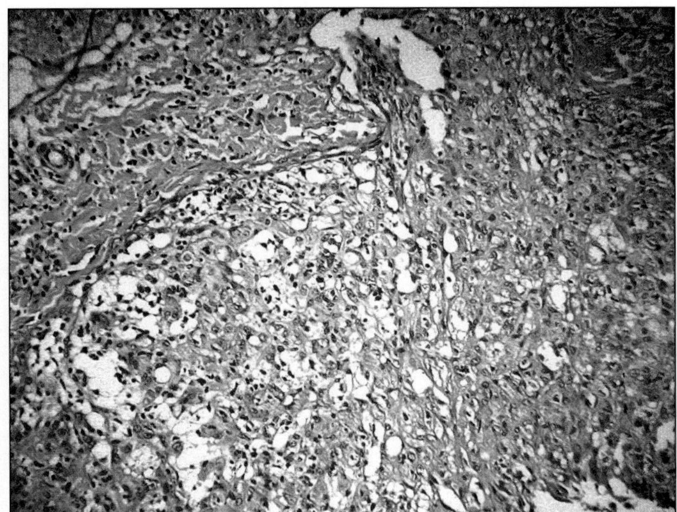

Figure 25.7 A more sarcomatous , spindle-cell pattern of verruga peruana. It may be confused with Kaposi sarcoma . Hematoxylin and eosin 100x.

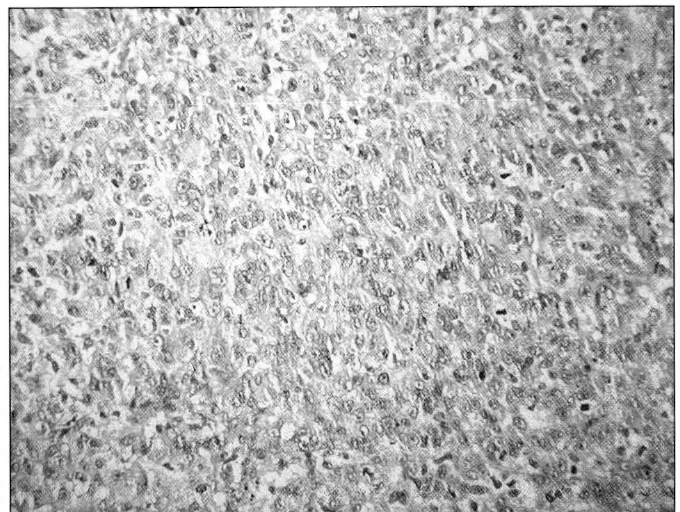

Figure 25.8 Solid, spindle-cell pattern of verruga peruana. Hematoxylin and eosin 100x.

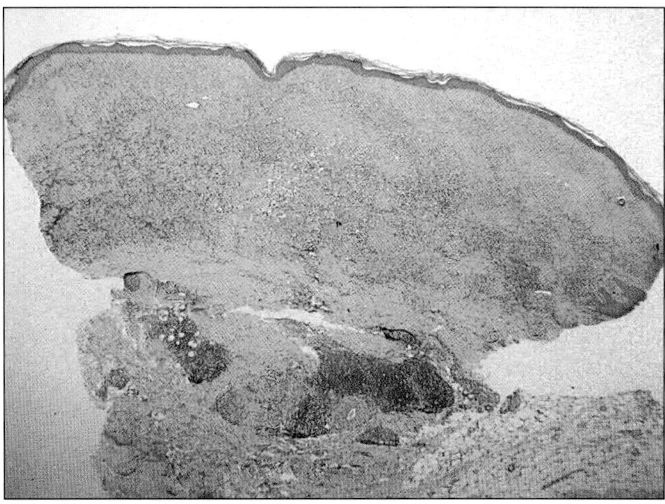

Figure 25.9 Verruga peruana mimicking lymphoma. Hematoxylin and eosin 20x.

Treatment

Treatment of choice of OF should include an antibiotic that will also show activity against bacteria such as *Salmonella*; the drug of choice is chloramphenicol, although in recent years ciprofloxacin has been demonstrated to be a valid alternative.

The drug of choice for the treatment of VP is oral rifampicin, with ciprofloxacin as a valid alternative.

Bacillary angiomatosis

Key features:

- *Bartonella henselae* and *B. quintana*
- Most cases are seen in immunosuppressed patients
- Angiomatous eruptive lesions are seen
- There is peliosis
- For *B. henselae*, contact with cats and fleas is important
- For *B. quintana*, poor living conditions and contact with lice are significant

The report of Stoler et al.[6] of a new condition in HIV patients triggered a new line of clinical and basic research in a field that, until then, went almost ignored. BA, as a new syndrome of reactive vascular proliferation induced by bacteria, even more in the context of acquired immunodeficiency syndrome (AIDS), aroused great interest in dermatologists, infectious disease specialists, pathologists, and microbiologists. The bacterial origin was suspected from the beginning, but LeBoit et al.[7] were the first to link the organism to the causative agent of CSD. First described in human immunodeficiency virus (HIV) patients, it was later reported in patients suffering from other kinds of immunosuppression, such as renal transplant patients, those in chemotherapy, and even in immunocompetent patients.[11]

Epidemiology

Despite all the excitement provoked by BA, it was never a common condition. The reported incidence in Germany and Brazil was 1.2–1.4 cases per 1000 HIV-infected patients.[12] It is actually even more rare nowadays, probably because of the effective treatment of the HIV condition and subsequent less immunosuppression, as well as the frequent administration of macrolide antibiotic therapy for *Mycobacterium avium* prophylaxis.

Pathogenesis and etiology

The two bacteria capable of inducing BA are *B. henselae* and *B. quintana*. *B. henselae* has been well studied in cats, in which it is capable of inducing prolonged bacteremia and systemic disease. *B. henselae* has been consistently isolated from cat fleas. The history of previous traumatic contact with cats has frequently been reported in patients with BA due to *B. henselae*, but not to *B. quintana*. This latter organism has been linked to small outbreaks of septicemia in homeless people suffering from lice infestation. In fact, there was a temporary association of such an outbreak in Seattle, Washington, and a simultaneous occurrence of *B. quintana*-associated BA cases seen in San Francisco, California, from January to June, 1993.[13] Risk factors for *B. quintana*-associated BA in the context of HIV infection include low socioeconomic status, homeless conditions, and lice infestations. BA associated with *B. henselae* does not seem to occur in outbreaks, but in a rather constant fashion throughout the year.

BA occurs frequently in HIV patients with a past or present history of opportunistic infection. Most will have low counts of CD4+ T cells, in the range of 100 cells/mm^3 or less.

Clinical features

The common clinical manifestations of BA include cutaneous and subcutaneous lesions of a vascular nature, asymmetric lymphadenopathy, and abdominal symptoms associated with fever (anorexia, nausea, vomiting, and abdominal pain).

Cutaneous lesions have been described under different morphologies such as red, angiomatous, polypoid papules (similar to the miliary lesions of VP) (Fig. 25.10) or subcutaneous nodules and deep-seated tumors (similar to nodular and mular types of VP) (Figs 25.11 and 25.12). The number of lesions may vary from just one to hundreds. They may erode, bleed, and become crusty. Dry, hyperkeratotic plaques have been reported in dark-skinned individuals.[14] The distribution of lesions is widespread and involvement of oral, anal, conjunctival, and gastrointestinal mucosa is not uncommon. Laryngeal lesions leading to airway obstruction as well as lung involvement have been reported. Central nervous system involvement with isolation of *Bartonella* from the cerebrospinal fluid has also been described.

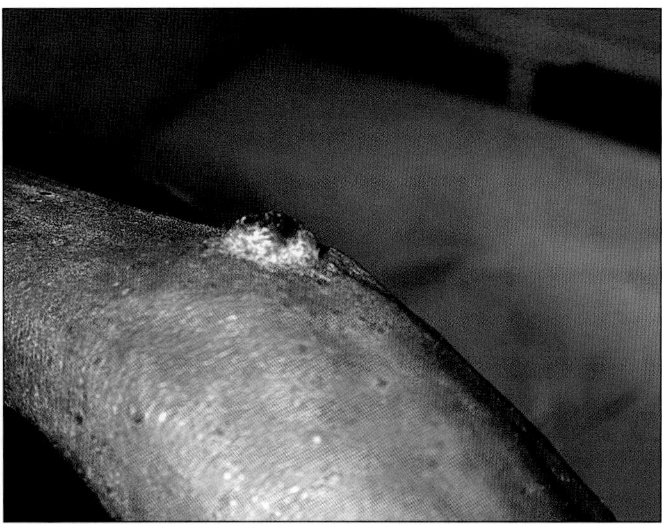

Figure 25.10 Bacillary angiomatosis, angiomatous type. Similarity with verruga peruana is remarkable.

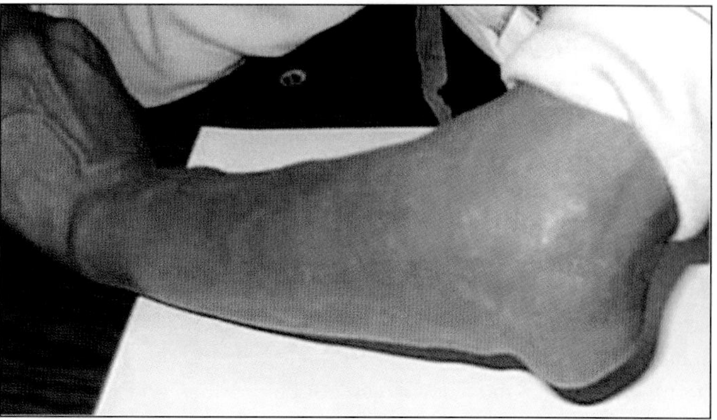

Figure 25.11 Bacillary angiomatosis on elbow.

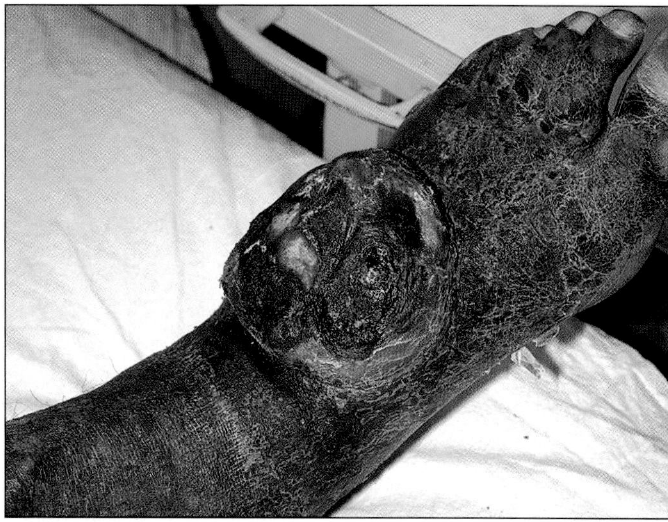

Figure 25.12 Bacillary angiomatosis, verrucous type.

Subcutaneous lesions may be mobile or fixed to deeper tissues; they are sometimes tender and may feel firm or rubbery on palpation. Underlying bone involvement may occur, ranging from simple cortical erosions to extensive geodes. It is usually very painful, most commonly affecting the radius, fibula, or tibia. Subcutaneous and bone lesions are strongly associated with infection by *B. quintana*.

Asymmetric lymphadenopathy is also a common presentation, and a marker for *B. henselae* infection. There is no suppuration or draining from affected lymph nodes but it is common to see coexistent skin lesions. Changes in the lymph node are identical to the histological changes described in the skin and soft tissue.

Peliosis, which consists of the presence of cystic, blood-filled spaces in the liver parenchyma, was reported as early as 1952 in the context of chronic disease such as tuberculosis, advanced cancer, or associated with the use of certain drugs such as anabolic steroids. By 1990 peliosis hepatitis was described in HIV patients who also presented with signs of BA. The presence of bacilli adjacent to the stromal changes and blood-filled spaces and the characteristic staining of the microorganism with the Warthin–Starry technique made evident its causative role in the development of the syndrome. Parenchymal peliosis, a term that includes liver and spleen involvement, is seen exclusively in BA caused by *B. henselae*.[15] It is reported in up to one-third of patients with BA, and is clearly associated with increased alkaline phosphatase levels.[13]

The diagnosis is usually made based on the classical histology of the cutaneous and parenchyma lesions, culture, serology, or polymerase chain reaction (PCR) testing. *Bartonella* can be isolated from the blood of patients with BA more commonly than from biopsy material. Serology testing, by either immunofluorescent antibody or enzyme-linked immunosorbent assay (ELISA), was initially developed for diagnosis of BA and later applied to the study of CSD and other bartonelloses. These tests are considered very sensitive, although sometimes they are lacking in species specificity. Species can be identified by PCR analysis of biopsy samples and blood isolates.

The main differential diagnosis from a clinical point of view will be Kaposi's sarcoma and VP. Histology in the first case, and epidemiological data in the second, will allow the clinician to rule out such entities. The possibility of BA should be considered when dealing with angiomatous lesions of an uncertain nature, from recurrent pyogenic granulomas to disseminated eruptive angioma, even in the absence of immunosuppression.[16,17]

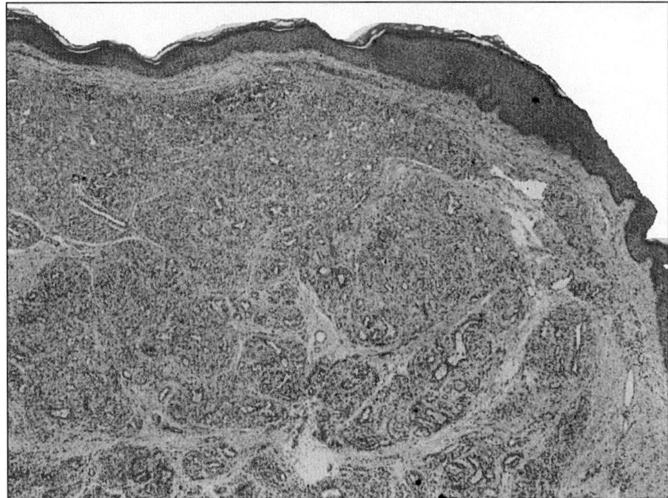

Figure 25.14 Bacillary angiomatosis: vascular pattern with septa. Hematoxylin and eosin 20×.

Pathology

The histopathological changes of skin and subcutaneous lesions consist of a proliferation of small blood vessels, either organized in a lobular pattern (Figs 25.13 and 25.14), separated by fibrous septa, or as confluent aggregates, with a solid interstitial component of round, epithelioid cells. The endothelial cells may project into the lumina. Focal necrosis of the interstitial component as well as focal, randomly distributed aggregates of neutrophils and nuclear dust will be seen through out the lesions (Fig. 25.15). The location of the process may vary, from very superficial, with collaret formation, to mid-dermis, subcutaneous tissue, or into the fascia and muscular tissue. The general appearance will be quite similar to VP; the spindle pattern, so common in Kaposi's sarcoma, will be absent in BA. The presence in the interstitium of purple, granular material, readily seen on hematoxylin and eosin (H&E) staining (Fig. 25.16), will represent aggregates of bacilli that stained with Warthin–Starry (Fig. 25.17). Several authors have raised the possibility that *B. henselae* induces the formation of isolated angiomatous lesions indistinguishable from pyogenic granulomas, in immunocompetent individuals. A recent study has shown a higher incidence of *B. henselae*-positive serology in patients with pyogenic granulomas, compared with matched controls with classical cherry angiomas.[18]

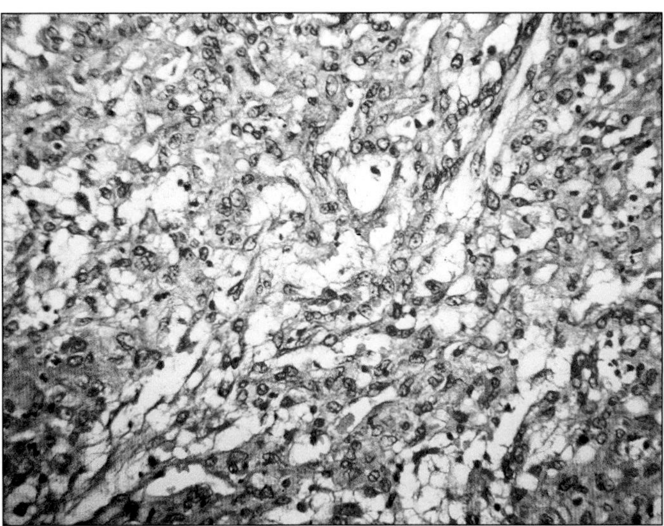

Figure 25.15 Bacillary angiomatosis: the pattern of vascular proliferation and the presence of nuclear dust. Hematoxylin and eosin 100×.

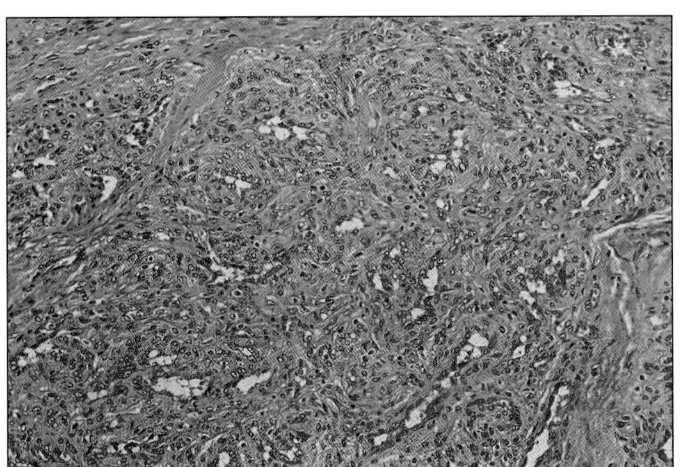

Figure 25.13 Bacillary angiomatosis: lobular pattern, well-defined blood vessel. Hematoxylin and eosin 40×.

Treatment

Therapy of BA and peliosis is based on the use of erythromycin or doxycycline for prolonged periods; recurrence is commonly seen

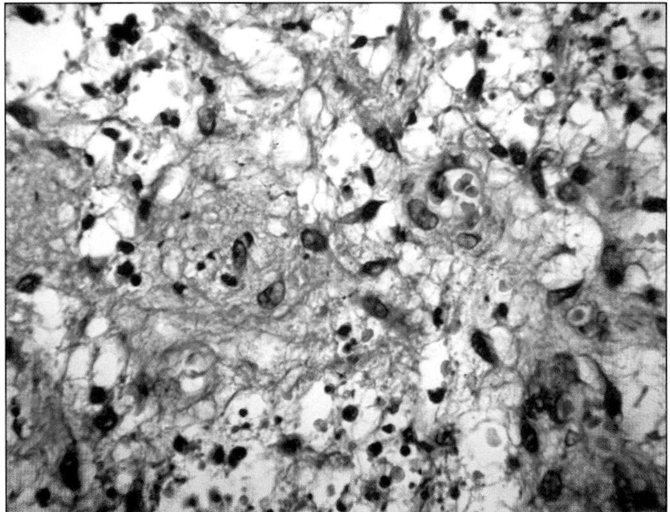

Figure 25.16 Bacillary angiomatosis: nuclear dust and interstitial purple material. Hematoxylin and eosin 400x.

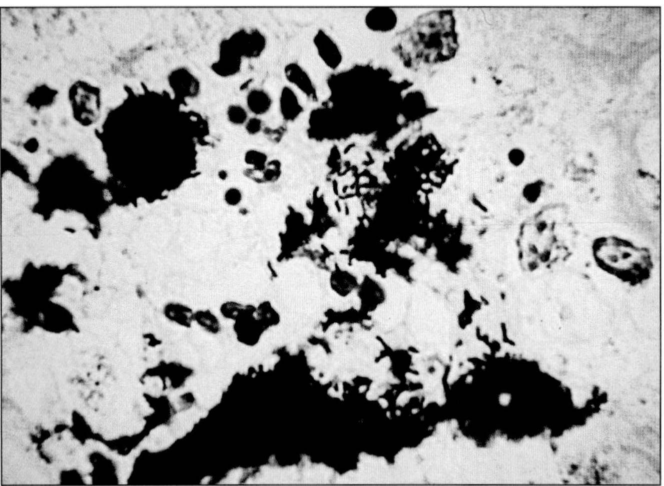

Figure 25.17 Aggregates of bacilli, the equivalent of the purple material seen on hematoxylin and eosin. Warthin–Starry staining 1000x.

unless there is an improvement of the immunological status. In such cases, lifelong treatment is recommended.

Cat-scratch disease

Key features:

- *Bartonella henselae*
- *Bartonella clarridgeiae*
- Traumatic contact with cats
- Lymphocutaneous syndrome, most common in the axilla and neck
- Spontaneous resolution

Whereas Carrión disease and BA are expressions of overwhelming infection with large bacterial load, with subsequent bacteremia and angiogenesis induced by the microorganism, CSD is the expression of an overwhelming inflammatory reaction of an immunocompetent host against a small bacillary load, with a rather effective control of the infection at the level of the lymph node.

Epidemiology

Since the original description of Debre of "le maladie de griffes de chat," in 1950, great advances have taken place regarding the etiology, clinical course, and prognosis of CSD.[8,19,20] This is the most common of all bartonelloses, affecting immunocompetent patients. There are an estimated 24 000 cases of CSD in the USA, giving rise to 2000 admissions per year. The estimated incidence in ambulatory patients is 9.3 per 10 000 population per year. There is a seasonal distribution: CSD is more common in the fall and winter. CSD has a worldwide distribution, with cases described in North and South America, Europe, Africa, and Asia. The main population affected is children, with 80% of patients 21 years old or younger.

Pathogenesis and etiology

Regarding etiology, the most significant advances began with the establishment of its bacterial origin in 1983, when researchers detected the presence of bacilli, using Warthin–Starry stain, in the lymph node tissue of a patient with CSD. In the late 1980s, while developing serological techniques for the diagnosis of BA, blood samples from CSD patients were found to be reactive for *B. henselae*, leading investigators to assess *Bartonella* as the causative agent. Dolan, in 1993, was able to isolate *B. henselae* from lymph nodes of patients with CSD.[8] In 1994, similar studies using PCR assays detected the presence of *B. henselae* in 21 of 25 lymph nodes of similar patients. It is now accepted that the cause of CSD in most cases is *B. henselae*, and, to a lesser extent, *B. clarridgeiae*. Cats are considered to be the main mammalian reservoir, and the flea is a potential vector. About 28% of cats in the USA have positive serology for *B. henselae*; 8% are positive in Switzerland and 50% in the Netherlands. The cat flea (*Ctenocephalides felis*) carries *B. henselae* in its feces.

Clinical features

The clinical manifestations are those of a lymphocutaneous syndrome. Contact with cats, especially with kittens, is considered one of the diagnostic criteria. This contact may vary from just licking to traumatic contact, including scratching or biting. Cats with fleas are more likely to transmit the disease.

The inoculation lesion develops in more than 90% of patients, and is usually associated with the trauma site. It evolves through erythematous, vesicular, and papular stages, persisting from 1 to 3 weeks. Two weeks after the inoculation a regional lymphadenopathy will develop, most commonly on the axillae, neck, and submandibular region. The nodes are tender, enlarged, 1–5 cm, with overlying erythema. More than 80% will have only one enlarged node, a few will have local satellites, but generalized lymphadenopathy is considered rare. Most patients will have a gradual resolution, but up to 20% will have persistent lesions lasting for several months. Suppuration may be present in up to one-third of patients. One-third will have fever greater than 38°C, that may last for 1–2 weeks. Up to 20% of patients with CSD will have a positive PCR test in their blood, suggesting that bacteremia does occur in those patients.

The Parinaud syndrome will be seen in 2–3% of patients. This is an oculoglandular syndrome, with unilateral conjunctivitis and preauricular lymphadenopathy. An ocular granuloma may be present. It is said that, in such cases, the conjunctival mucosa was the port of entrance, either by direct trauma from the animal or by the patient's own contaminated hand. Occasionally, an angiomatous histology has been seen in primary lesions located in the conjunctiva.

Neurological involvement occurs in 2% of cases, including encephalitis, seizures, myelitis, peripheral neuropathy, and retinitis. The encephalopathy will manifest itself as headaches and mental status changes 2–3 weeks after the lymphocutaneous syndrome. Transient Bell's palsy and peripheral neuropathy may also be seen.

Systemic involvement will be expressed as abdominal pain, with hepatosplenomegaly. A mononucleosis-like syndrome has also been reported.

The occurrence of erythema nodosum is important for the dermatologist, with skin eruption and fever taking place 1–6 weeks after the regional lymphadenopathy.

Diagnosis and differential diagnosis

Diagnosis of CSD is based on three of the four following criteria: (1) contact with a cat with a primary lesion; (2) regional lymphadenopathy; (3) characteristic histological findings on the node; and (4) a positive intradermal testing. This last criterion has been now changed to a positive serology testing, by immunofluorescent antibody, with a reported 50–95% sensitivity.

Pathology

The histology of CSD adenitis is different from what is seen in BA. The findings will evolve from lymphoid hyperplasia to subsequent formation of granulomas, developing central necrosis and stellate microabscesses, with neutrophils (Fig. 25.18). Multiple giant cells may be seen. Clumps of bacteria will not be detected on regular H&E staining but will stain with Warthin–Starry. PCR may be used in negative cases.

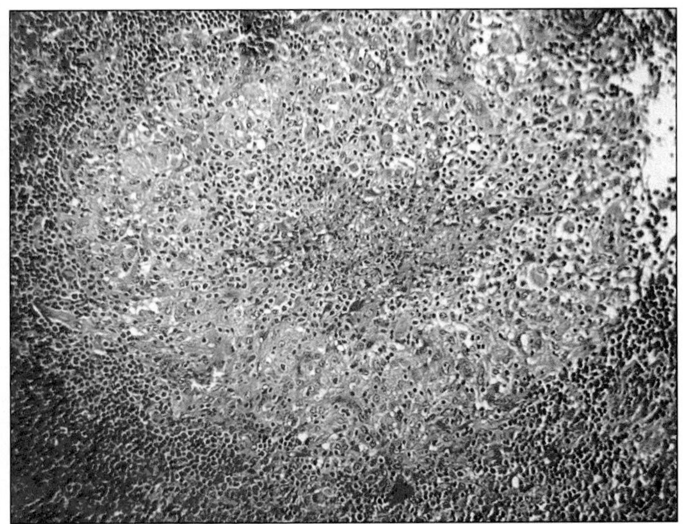

Figure 25.18 Cat-scratch disease: granuloma with central necrosis and neutrophils in the lymph node. Hematoxylin and eosin 20x.

Treatment

For the most part, CSD will have a benign course. The little influence of antibiotic therapy on the clinical course may be a reflection of the small bacterial load and the intense inflammatory reaction. Most clinical findings are an expression of the intensity of the inflammatory response. In cases where antibiotic therapy is indicated, several drugs can be used, including rifampin, ciprofloxacin, gentamicin, trimethoprim and sulfamethoxazole, clarithromycin, and azithromycin. One placebo-controlled study using azithromycin therapy resulted in a more rapid diminution in size of infected lymph nodes.[21] Most cases of CSD occurring in normal hosts do not require antiinfective therapy for resolution of infection.

Trench fever

Synonyms: Quintana fever, shinbone fever, shank fever, His–Werner disease, Wolhynian fever

Key features:

- *Bartonella quintana*
- Fever
- Chills
- Recurrent pattern every fifth day
- Retroorbital pain

Trench fever is the second oldest bartonellosis known to humans, although its current bacterial classification is just a decade old. Initially described in World War I, it was an important cause of mortality for both sides in the conflict. Cases have been described in Poland and other countries of Eastern Europe, Russia, North Africa, and China. Some serological surveys have suggested the presence of the bacteria in the Americas, but there is no report of trench fever as such in the western hemisphere.

The etiological agent is *B. quintana*, and its vector of choice is the body louse. The presence of the bacteria in the louse has been confirmed by PCR testing, particularly in homeless people.[22]

Clinical features

This is a febrile process, with an incubation period that extends from 5 to 20 days. The spectrum goes from mild to severe, recurrent disease. Febrile episodes last for 5–7 days and recur every 3–5 days, hence the name quintana (i.e., fifth).

Characteristically, the patient develops fever, malaise, chills, profuse sweating, anorexia, headache associated with retroorbital pain, conjunctiva redness, myalgia, arthralgia, and osteomuscular pain, especially in the neck, back, and leg (shinbone fever). A maculopapular rash is seen in over 80%, located on the trunk.

Diagnosis

Diagnosis of trench fever should be considered when dealing with any febrile patient, especially in the context of epidemiological data. Isolation from the blood of patients using chocolate and sheep blood agar will be essential for the specific diagnosis. Serology using immunofluorescent antibody techniques is also helpful in making a definitive diagnosis. The differential diagnosis should include typhus, typhoid fever, *Borrelia* infections, and malaria.

Treatment

The natural course is towards spontaneous resolution. Effective drugs against *B. quintana* include chloramphenicol and tetracycline, with quick remission of symptoms in a couple of days.

References

1. García FU, Wojta J, Broadley KN et al. *Bartonella bacilliformis* stimulates endothelial cells in vitro and is angiogenic in vivo. Am J Pathol 1990; 136:1125–1135.
2. Arbiser JL, Weiss SW, Arbiser ZK et al. Differential expression of active mitogen-activated protein kinase in cutaneous endotelial neoplasms: implications for biologic behavior and response to therapy. J Am Acad Dermatol 2001 ; 44:193–197.
3. Patrucco R. Estudio de los parametros inmunológicos en pacientes portadores de la enfermedad de carrión (bartonelosis humana). Diagnostico 1983; 12:138–144.
4. Iwaki-Egawa S, Ihler GM. Comparison of the abilities of proteins from *Bartonella bacilliformis* and *Bartonella henselae* to deform red cell membranes and to bind to red cell ghost proteins. FEMS Microbiol Lett 1997; 157:207–217.
5. Maguiña C. Bartonellosis o enfermedad de carrión: nuevos aspectos de una vieja enfermedad. Lima: AFA Editores; 1998.
6. Stoler M, Bonifiglio T, Steigbigel R et al. An atypical subcutaneous infection associated with acquired immune deficiency syndrome. Am J Clin Pathol 1983; 80:714–718.
7. LeBoit P, Berger T, Egbert B et al. Epithelioid hemangioma-like vascular proliferation in AIDS: manifestation of cat scratch bacillus infection. Lancet 1988; 1:960–963.
8. Anderson BE, Neuman MA. *Bartonella* spp. as emerging human pathogens. Clin Microbiol Rev 1997; 10:203–219.
9. Chamberlin J, Laughlin LW, Romero S et al. Epidemiology of endemic *Bartonella bacilliformis*: a prospective cohort study in a Peruvian mountain valley community. J Infect Dis 2002; 186:983–990.
10. Arias-Stella J, Lieberman PH, García-Caceres U et al. Verruga peruana mimicking malignant neoplasm. Am J Dermatopathol 1987; 9:279–291.
11. Cockerell CJ, Bergstresser PR, Myrie-Williams C et al. Bacillary epithelioid angiomatosis occurring in an immunocompetent individual. Arch Dermatol 1990; 126:787–790.
12. Gazineo JLD, Trope BM, Maceira JP et al. Bacillary angiomatosis: description of 13 cases reported in five reference centers for AIDS treatment in Rio de Janeiro, Brazil. Rev Inst Med Trop Sao Paulo 2001; 43:1–6.
13. Koehler JE, Sanchez MA, Garrido CS et al. Molecular epidemiology of *Bartonella* infections in patients with bacillary angiomatosis-peliosis. N Engl J Med 1997; 337:1876–1883.
14. Cockerell CJ, LeBoit PE. Bacilllary angiomatosis: a newly characterized, pseudoneoplastic, infectious, cutaneous vascular disorder. J Am Acad Dermatol 1999; 22:501–512.
15. Mohle-Boetani JC, Koehler JE, Berger TG et al. Bacillary angiomatosis and bacillary peliosis in patients infected with human immunodeficiency virus: clinical characteristics in a case–control study. Clin Infect Dis 1996; 22:794–800.
16. Schwartz RA, Nychay SG, Janniger CK et al. Bacillary angiomatosis: presentation of six patients, some with unusual features. Br J Dermatol 1997; 136:60–65.
17. Smith KJ, Skelton HG, Tuur S et al. Bacillary angiomatosis in an immunocompetent child. Am J Dermathopatol 1996; 18:597–600.
18. Lee J, Lynde C. Pyogenic granuloma: pyogenic again? Association between pyogenic granuloma and *Bartonella*. J Cutan Med Surg 2001; 5:467–470.
19. Maguiña C, Gotuzzo E. Bartonellosis, new and old. Infect Dis Clin North Am 2000; 14:1–22.
20. Spach DH, Koehler JE. Bartonella-associated infections. Infect Dis Clin North Am 1998; 12:137–155.
21. Conrad DA. Treatment of cat-scratch disease. Curr Opin Pediatr 2001; 13:56–59.
22. Maurin M, Raoult D. *Bartonella (Rochalimaea) quintana* infections. Clin Microbiol Rev 1996; 9:273–292.

Chapter 26

Bacterial sexually transmitted disease

Introduction

Bacterial sexually transmitted diseases (STDs) have become an important medical challenge worldwide, especially among the tropical countries. The ubiquitousness of STDs affects all nations and races, but is particularly evident in developing countries. Insufficient health care centers, inadequate laboratory capabilities, and the unavailability of appropriate drug regimens of treatment perpetuate the prevalence of these STDs. However, it is important to appreciate that underservicing of areas and regions is not found exclusively in developing countries, but is evident in developed regions as well.

Syphilis is still a public health problem in many countries and some ethnic manifestations of the disease, especially among black populations, make it one of the most interesting dermatological diseases nowadays. Pinta, bejel, and yaws are uncommon and non-venereal treponematoses have been almost eradicated from most countries but are still observed in some areas of South America (Amazon rain forest), Middle East, and North Africa. These diseases were identified as human pathogens in early hominids, millions of years ago, because of the bone patterns associated with these infections.

Chlamydial and gonococcal infections are common worldwide but the high endemicity in some tropical countries will allow the identification of some uncommon signs and symptoms associated with these diseases, such as the esthiomenic syndrome of lymphogranuloma venereum (LGV) and gonococcal ophthalmia in newborns.

The huge impact of human immunodeficiency virus (HIV) infection is especially clear among the STDs. It is well recognized that any previous STD is associated with an increased risk for HIV infection, particularly those characterized by genital ulcers such as syphilis, granuloma inguinale, and chancroid. Bacterial STDs are still a major threat to human health worldwide and should be considered as important infections.

Chlamydia

Omar Lupi, Renata A. Joffe and René Garrido Neves

Introduction

Members of the order Chlamydiales are obligate intracellular Gram-negative bacteria. The order Chlamydiales has one family, the Chlamydiaceae, containing one genus, *Chlamydia*, and three species pathogenic to humans: C. *trachomatis*, C. *psittaci*, and C. *pneumoniae*.[1]

C. *trachomatis* is a strictly human pathogen, with a tropism for the genital and conjunctival epithelia. C. *trachomatis* consists of 19 different serovars.[1] Types A, B, Ba, and C infect mainly the conjunctiva and are associated with endemic trachoma; serovars D, Da, E, F, G, Ga, H, I, Ia, J, and K are predominantly isolated from the urogenital tract and are associated with STDs, Reiter's syndrome, inclusion conjunctivitis, or neonatal pneumonitis in infants born to infected mothers. Serovars L1, L2, L2a, and L3 can be found in the inguinal lymph nodes and are associated with LGV.

Chlamydial infections

C. *trachomatis* is present in about 80% of patients with the venereal form of Reiter's syndrome – a disorder recognized by the clinical triad of arthritis, urethritis, and conjunctivitis. It is implicated as a possible agent of the disease and considered to have a trigger function. Circinate balanitis is the most common cutaneous finding, being reported in about 36% of patients (Fig. 26.1). Another common manifestation is keratoderma blennorrhagicum (15%), a scaling plaque-like process that resembles pustular psoriasis with a combination of crusting, exudation, and erosion associated with erythema (Fig. 26.2).

Epidemiology

C. *trachomatis* has the highest prevalence amongst young men and women. It is the most common STD in western countries.[2]

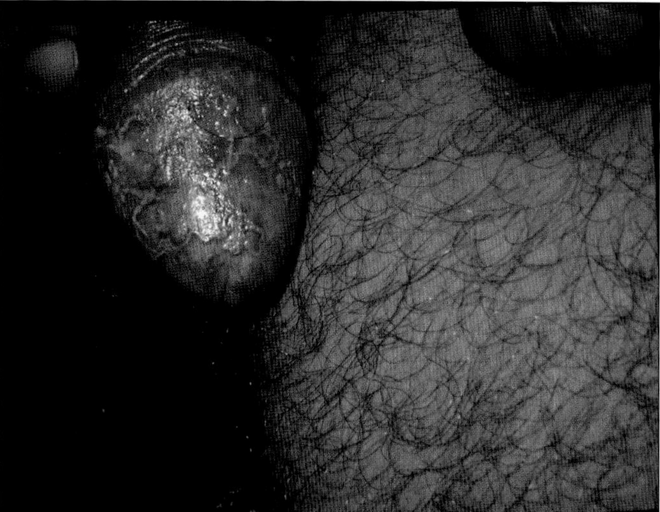

Figure 26.1 Circinate balanitis in a case of Reiter's syndrome.

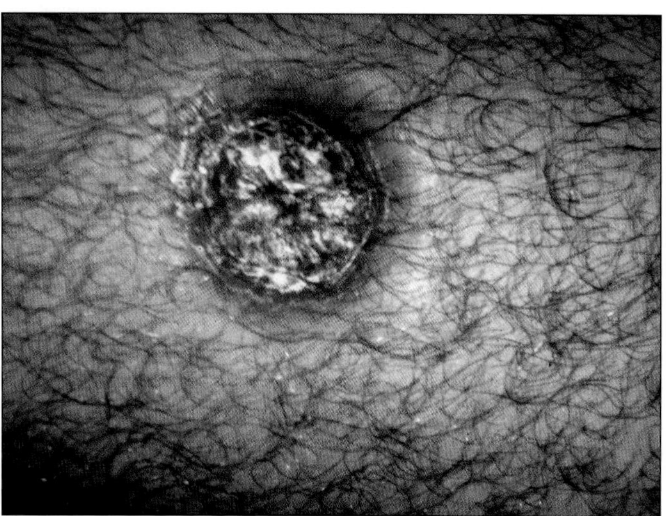

Figure 26.2 Keratoderma blennorrhagicum (Reiter's syndrome).

Worldwide, 89 million cases are estimated to occur each year.[3] Infection with this agent can be asymptomatic in up to 80% of women. Left undetected and untreated, *Chlamydia* can ascend the upper genital tract, causing inflammation and scarring in both the female and male reproductive tract. In women it is responsible for urethritis, cervicitis, pelvic inflammatory disease, and sequelae such as infertility and ectopic pregnancy. In men it can cause arthritis and epididymitis, which can result in urethral obstructions and decreased fertility in some cases. Neonates may present with conjunctivitis and pneumonia.

Lymphogranuloma venereum

Synonyms: Nicolas–Favre–Durand, tropical bubo, climatic bubo, d'emblé bubo, scrofulous bubo, subacute inguinal lymphogranulomatosis, inguinal lymphogranuloma[4]

Introduction

LGV is an uncommon STD with transient genital lesions followed by significant regional lymphadenopathy and systemic manifestations. LGV may progress to late fibrosis and tissue destruction in untreated cases.[5]

Epidemiology

The disease is almost always transmitted by sexual contact. Transmission has been attributed largely to asymptomatic female carriers. The main age of onset is 25 years, but the disease can be seen in any age group. Highest prevalence is found in young single male patients of low socioeconomic and educational status. Prostitutes and male homosexuals have a major role in the transmission of the disease.

Clinical manifestations

The clinical course of LGV is classically divided into three stages.[4]

Primary lesion The incubation period is extremely variable but has been estimated to be between 1 and 2 weeks. This transient primary lesion usually appears as a vesicle, small erosion, or an ulcerated area that lasts for 2–3 days.[6] The site of the primary lesion is usually around the genitals but may be anal, rectal, or oral, mainly in male homosexuals.

Secondary lesions, lymphadenitis, or bubo LGV is primarily a disease of the lymphatic system that progresses to lymphangitis. Adenopathy represents the most important objective element of the clinical exam and is unilateral in 60% of these cases. It usually occurs 2–4 weeks after onset of the primary lesion. In its earlier stages the adenopathy syndrome consists of painful inflammation and infection of the inguinal and/or femoral lymph nodes. In women, the deep pelvic nodes may also be involved. After several days they become matted, with a firm lobulated swelling not attached to the deep tissues. The overlying skin is often slightly reddened and edematous (Fig. 26.3), but later it may become thickened and develop a purple hue. In a short time the lymph nodes become

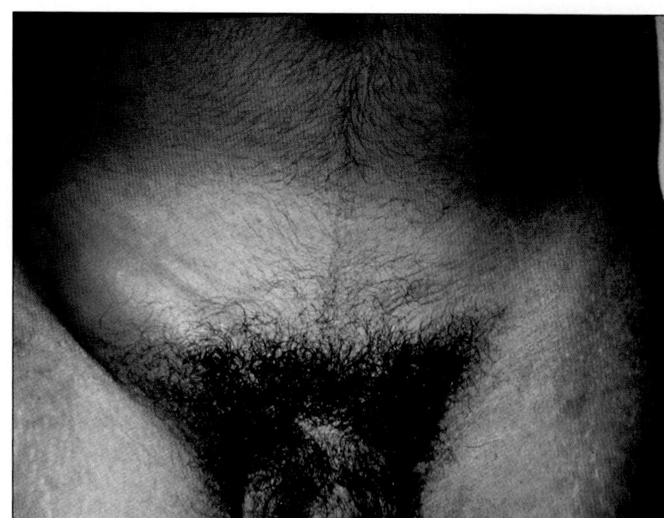

Figure 26.3 Lymphogranuloma venereum with massive inguinal lymphadenopathy.

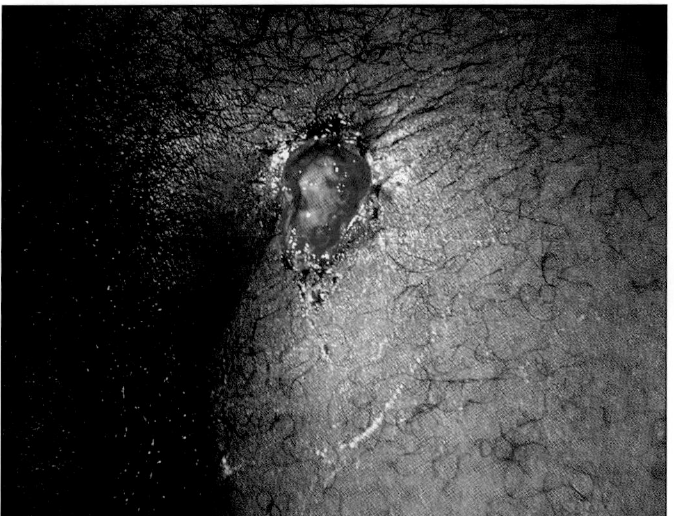

Figure 26.4 Bubo with spontaneous fistulization.

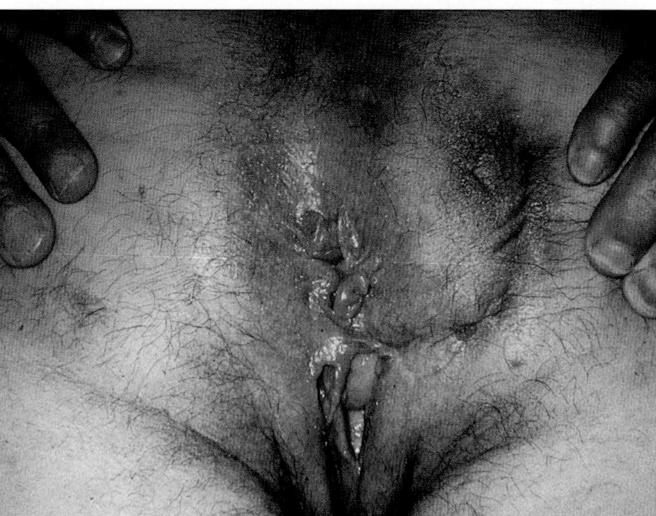

Figure 26.5 Later stage of lymphogranuloma venereum with perianal fistulas.

tender and fluctuant and are referred to as buboes. In the natural evolution of LGV, the nodes may undergo necrosis and spontaneous fistula tracts may develop (Fig. 26.4). These nodes may also become fluctuant and rupture in 30% of patients. Although most buboes eventually heal without complications, some may progress to develop chronic sinus formation. The emergence of many fistulous orifices explains the comparison made with a "watering can." There may be fever and chills during this stage of LGV, associated with other non-specific systemic symptoms such as headache, nausea, anorexia, and myalgia.[5]

Tertiary stage or the genitoanorectal syndrome This stage does not necessarily follow the lymphadenopathy. It involves a series of conditions, resulting from progressive spread of the disease with destruction of tissue in the involved areas, including proctitis, acute proctocolitis mimicking Crohn's disease, fistulae, strictures, and a chronic granulomatous disfiguring condition of the vulva (esthiomene). The lymph nodes rupture, causing hemorrhage and friability of the anorectal mucosa, with rectitis, tenesmus, mucosanguineous rectal discharge, and constipation. Later, as healing occurs, there is formation of strictures, fistulas, and abscesses with destruction of anal and rectal structures (Fig. 26.5).

Long-term complications

The destruction of lymph nodes may result in elephantiasis of the vulva or penis and scrotum. It represents late manifestations, which are rare today.[4] An association with rectal cancer has been reported. The esthiomenic syndrome, composed of vulvar ulceration followed by sclerosis and tegumentar hypertrophy, can occur in patients with LGV.

No studies have been performed on patients with concomitant HIV infection and LGV, and remarkably little anecdotal evidence regarding clinical features and treatment has been published. HIV appears to have no effect on the clinical presentation of the disease.

Diagnosis

LGV can be suspected on positive *Chlamydia* serology and isolation of *C. trachomatis* from the infected site. Samples must contain cellular material which is obtained for direct bacteriological exam and culture from affected lymph nodes by aspiration from fluctuant lymph nodes/buboes, from the ulcer base exudates, or from rectal tissue. Staining of the smear (Giemsa or fuchsin) reveals the intracellular corpuscles of Gamna–Miyagawa, which occur in some chlamydial infections (Fig. 26.6).

The culture on cycloheximide-treated McCoy cells of material from suspected LGV lesions is labor-intensive, expensive, and of restricted availability. Its sensitivity is 75–85% at best, and often closer to 50% in the case of the bubo aspirate.

A complement fixation test, using group-specific antigens, is typically positive within 2 weeks of the onset of disease. A titer of ≥1:16, in the presence of a compatible clinical syndrome, is suggestive of LGV. Titers >1:64 are considered diagnostic of LGV.[6] Serial samples with a 15-day interval frequently show a fourfold increment in titer in the acute stage of the disease. Indirect immunofluorescence represents a sensitive method but is not widely

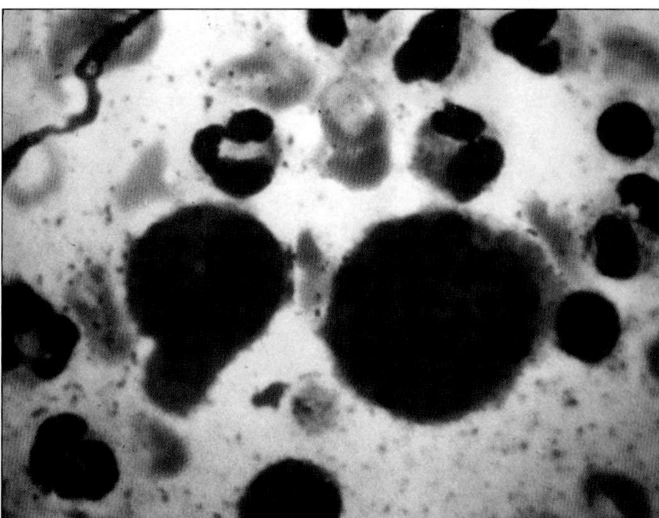

Figure 26.6 Staining of the smear (Giemsa, 400×) reveals the intracellular corpuscles of Gamna–Miyagawa.

available. Antibody titers do not necessarily correspond with disease activity and may not decline after treatment.[7] The microimmunofluorescence test is the only serological means of distinguishing between different serotypes of C. *trachomatis* and is the diagnostic test of choice.

Enzyme-linked immunosorbent assay (ELISA) is considered a convenient and objective method, suitable for ulcer scrapes or bubo aspirates. Sensitivity is lower than other methods (75–80%) and should be confirmed by another method. Monoclonal antibodies are an extremely sensitive method and have high specification in the diagnosis of the LGV, capable of preventing serological cross-reactivity among the causative, and other serotypes of, C. *trachomatis*.

Detection of nucleic acid is by DNA amplification techniques such as the ligase chain reaction (LCR) or polymerase chain reaction (PCR); these methods are becoming established for routine testing.

Differential diagnosis

The differential diagnosis includes chancroid, syphilis, ganglionar tuberculosis, cat-scratch disease, and Hodgkin's disease. Late manifestations must be distinguished from neoplastic skin disease, filariasis, rectal cancer, inflammatory bowel disease, and hidradenitis suppurativa.[5]

Treatment

No controlled double-blind treatment trials have been published on LGV.[4] The low incidence of the disease, its complex presentation, and its natural history have precluded any rigorous evaluation of management. Early treatment is important to reduce the chronic phase. Prolonged treatment (at least 3 weeks) is the norm.

Antibiotics

- First choice: doxycycline: 100 mg PO every 12 h, for 3 weeks
- Second choice: erythromycin: 500 mg every 6 h, for 3 weeks[7]

Other treatments include:

- Tetracyclines: 500 mg PO every 6 h, for 2–4 weeks
- Tianfenicol: 500 mg (2 capsules) PO every 8 h, for 2–3 weeks
- Sulfadiazine: 500 mg PO every 6 h, for 2–3 weeks
- Sulfisoxazole: beginning dose of 4 g PO and then 2 g for 2–3 weeks.

The activity of azithromycin against C. *trachomatis* suggests that it may be effective, but clinical data on its use are lacking.

After an initial course of treatment, patients should be seen at least every 3 months for 1 year. Retreatment should be given if there is clinical evidence of relapse. Sexual contacts should be treated similarly.

Pregnant and lactating women should be treated with the erythromycin regimen.

People who have had sexual contacts with a patient who has LGV within the 30 days before onset of the patient's symptoms should be examined, tested for urethral or cervical chlamydial infection, and treated.

The Centers for Disease Control recommend the same treatments for LGV in HIV-negative and HIV-positive patients, with the note that these patients may not respond as well to therapy and prolonged treatment may be required.[8,9]

Tense and fluctuant nodules should be aspirated, rather than incised and drained. Dilation and partial amputation of the rectum are measures occasionally indicated to correct rectal stricture. Vulvectomy and colostomy are seldom necessary.

Follow-up and prognosis

Patients should be followed clinically until signs and symptoms have resolved. This may occur within 3–6 weeks. However, there is also evidence of spontaneous remission in 8 weeks.

The prognosis is excellent for acute infections treated with appropriate antibiotics. The late disease becomes rarer each day, but severe lymphatic involvement is frequently irreversible. Malignant transformation of the genital lesions of elephantiasis and anorectal syndrome, more common in females, is considered exceptional.

References

1. Cevenini R, Donati M, Sambri V. *Chlamydia trachomatis* – the agent. Best Pract Res Clin Obstet Gynaecol 2002; 16:761–773.
2. Guaschino S, de Seta F. Update on *Chlamydia trachomatis*. Ann NY Acad Sci 2000; 900:293–300.
3. Stamm WE. *Chlamydia trachomatis* infections: progress and problems. J Infect Dis 1999; 179 (suppl. 2):S380–S383.
4. Mayaud P. National guideline for the management of lymphogranuloma venereum. Clinical Effectiveness Group (Association of Genitourinary Medicine and the Medical Society for the Study of Venereal Diseases) Sex Transm Inf 1999; 75 (suppl. 1):S40–S42.
5. Neves RG, Lupi O. Lymphogranuloma venereum. In: Borchardt KA, Noble MA, eds. Sexually transmitted diseases. New York: CRC Press LLC; 1997:217–225.
6. Brown TJ, Yen-Moore A, Tyring SK. An overview of sexually transmitted diseases. Part I. J Am Acad Dermatol 1999; 41:511–529.
7. Workowski KA. The 1998 CDC sexually transmitted diseases treatment guidelines. Curr Infect Dis Rep 2000; 2:44–50.
8. Rosen T, Brown TJ. Cutaneous manifestations of STDs. Med Clin North Am 1998; 82:1081–1104.
9. Czelusta A, Yen-Moore A, Van der Straten M et al. An overview of sexually transmitted diseases. Part III. Sexually transmitted diseases in HIV-infected patients. J Am Acad Dermatol 2000; 43:409–432.

Gonococcal infection

Mauro Romero Leal Passos and Renata de Queiroz Varella

Synonyms: Blennorrhagia, blennorrhea, "flow of seed"

Key features:

- Pandemic STD, only rarely spread by accidental contamination, mainly affects genital, rectal, oropharyngeal, and conjunctival mucosa.

Introduction

Gonorrhea is one of the most commonly reported diseases in the world. A few decades ago it was described as the second most common infectious disease, after flu. Gonorrhea in women, when not treated, can provoke infection of the upper genital tract, which can lead to ectopic pregnancy and infertility. In many developed countries, such as the USA, the rates of gonorrhea declined from 1970 to the mid-1990s. Nevertheless, these rates have gone up 7% since then. Dissemination to other parts of the body varies from 0.5 to 3%, mainly affecting the skin (dermatitis); gonococcus drug resistance is increasingly common, and as a consequence this disease still merits considerable attention.[1,2]

History

The first reports of urethral secretions date from the time of the Chinese emperor Huang Ti, in 2637 BC. It was known to the Egyptians, and Moses, father of the Hebrews, in 1500 BC, mentioned it in the Old Testament in Leviticus, indicating sanitary methods for its control. In 1838, Ricord defined gonorrhea as inflammation of the urethra due to various causes. Neisser, in 1879, identified the etiological agent, and called it gonococcus. In 1881, Credé demonstrated that silver nitrate could prevent ophthalmologic gonorrhea in newborns (Fig. 26.7). Leistikow made the first culture of this microorganism in 1882. After long years of using potassium permanganate solution in intraurethral irrigations and instillations, sulfa drugs appeared in the 1930s. In the following decade penicillin was able to cure nearly all cases. In the early 1960s, the selective Thayer–Martin culture medium facilitated research and etiological diagnosis.[3]

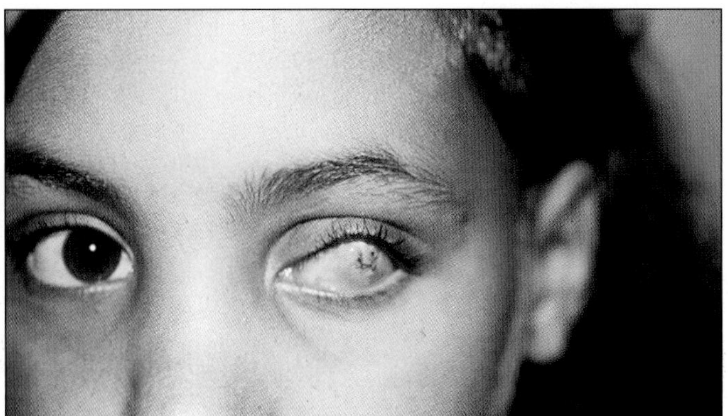

Figure 26.7 Severe sequel of neonatal ophthalmia. The mother reported that during pregnancy, her husband had a "little infection" in the penis, treated at the pharmacy. The woman was not treated during her pregnancy.

Epidemiology

The global map of the World Health Organization, with estimates of the number of annual new cases of the four main STDs, shows their importance for public health. Gonorrhea alone accounts for 62 million new infections per year. Obviously, the developing countries are the most affected. Nevertheless, this is still a serious public health problem all over the world, including the developed countries.

Adolescents and young adults (15–25 years old) are the most affected. However, gonococcus has been increasingly found in individuals over 50 years old. New medications for men (sildenafil: Viagra) and for women (hormonal replacement therapy), along with greater acceptance of and increased sexual activity in older people could be among the reasons for increasing STDs in this age group. On the other hand, sexual abuse of children with transmission of STDs has become increasingly common. Under these circumstances, gonorrhea, as a purulent bacterium, has a high degree of infectiousness.

The risk of sexual transmission by men infected with urethral gonorrhea is more than 90%, while in infected women the risk of transmission to sexual partners is 50–60%.[4]

Pathogenesis and etiology

In adults, gonococcus species are mainly pathogens of the columnar and non-cornified squamous epithelia. After contagion, the gonococcus initially avoids the reaction of immunological systems, thanks to fimbriae and external cytoplasmic membrane proteins. Through the protease, immunoglobulin A (IgA), mediated by the fimbriae and protein II, attaches to the host cell. The lipopolysaccharides impede ciliary activity and protein I promotes a closer contact between the gonococcus and the cell, followed by phagocytosis, and the gonococci are transported unharmed, in phagosomes, to the base of the cell, where they reproduce. From there, at some variable time afterwards, they are ejected to the subepithelial layers, initiating the local inflammatory process, exteriorization to the surface, and a possible invasion of the blood stream, provoking remote infections.[3]

It appears that the gonococcus prepares the way for subsequent infections by less aggressive microorganisms.

Neisseria gonorrhoeae is a Gram-negative intracellular polymorphonuclear bacterium, about 0.6–1 μm in diameter, reniform, grouped two by two, and joined at the concave side. It only grows in enriched media (Thayer–Martin) with vitamin supplements, using inhibitors such as vancomycin, colistin, and nystatin, at an optimal temperature between 35 and 36.5°C in 5% CO_2.

Clinical features

The incubation period varies from 2 to 10 days. However it can range from 24 h to 20 days.

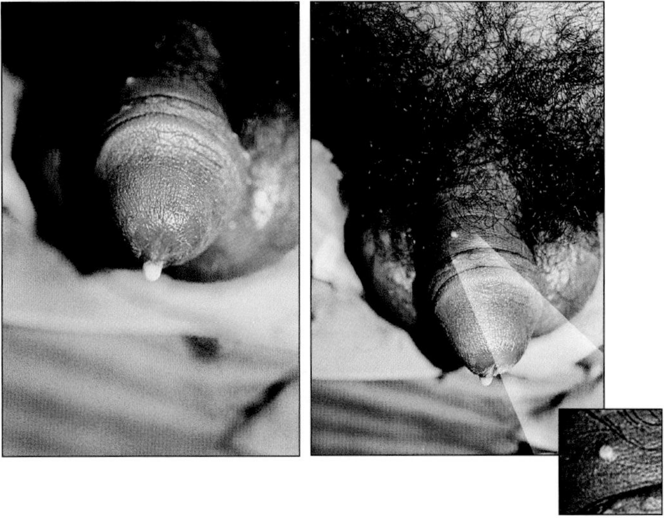

Figure 26.8 Typical clinical picture of purulent urethritis by gonococci. During the exam we noted a pustule on the penis (in the detail), which on bacterioscopy showed Gram-negative intracellular diplococci and the culture gave *Nesseria gonorrhoeae*. The patient had fever, cephalalgia, and myalgias, which indicate the beginning of a septicemic episode.

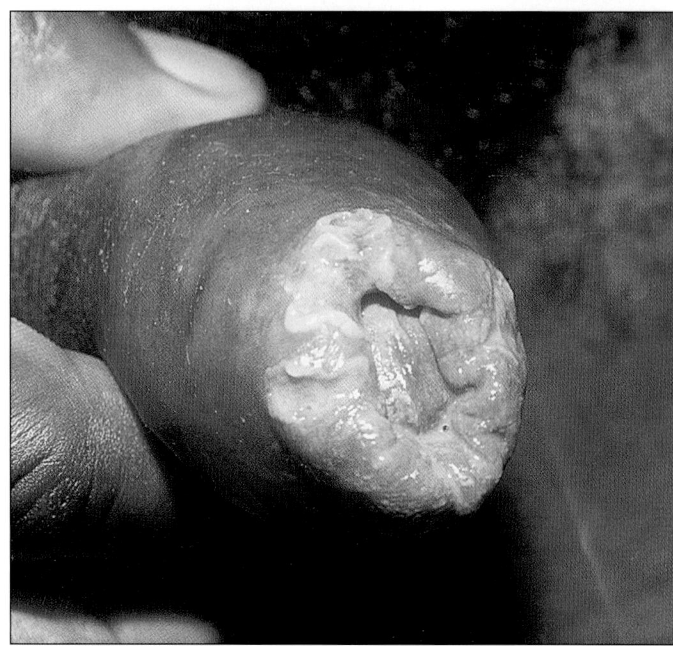

Figure 26.10 Patient with ulcerated balanoposthitis from an intense secretion of gonococcal urethritis. The preputium was long, the patient did not practice adequate hygiene, the skin became edematous, and fissures appeared and evolved to ulcers.

The clinical manifestations differ between sexes. In men, the symptoms begin with a sensation of stinging or intraurethral itching, with dysuria. Soon after, a urethral mucosal flow starts, that rapidly becomes mucopurulent, spontaneously flowing abundantly, or with very light pressure (Figs 26.8 and 26.9). The edges of the urethral meatus become edematous, with erythematosus (Figs 26.10 and 26.11). In women, gonococcal urethritis does not have such an exuberance of signs and symptoms as it does in men; the clinical manifestations are dysuria, a need to urinate, and, less frequently, a yellowish secretion (Fig. 26.12). Generally, cases of gonorrhea in women are explained by endocervicitis, which, associated with clinical history data, make it possible to suspect gonococcal infection.[2]

The most frequent complications in men are: balanoposthitis, littritis, cowperitis, prostatitis, epididymitis (Fig. 26.13), and urethral stenosis. In women the complications are: bartholinitis, infection of the upper genital tract (endometritis, salpingitis/inflammatory pelvic disease, pelviperitonitis) and peripatitis.

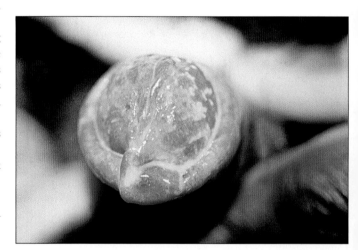

Figure 26.11 Gonococcal urethritis and fungal balanitis.

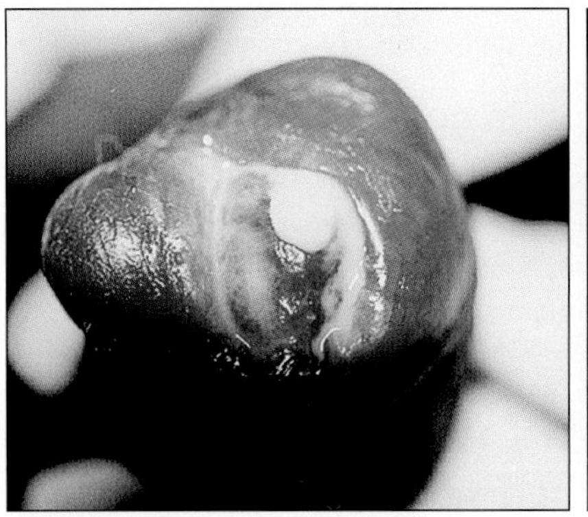

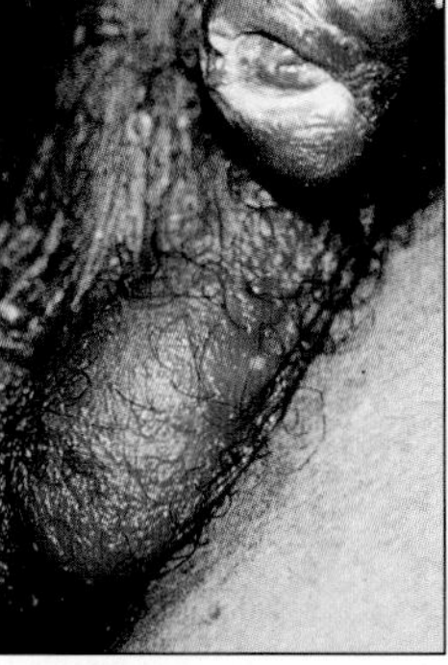

Figure 26.9 Urethritis together with gonococcal balanoposthitis with considerable edema and scabbing in the scrotum. The pus accumulated between the glans and the preputium, causing the deformity. Serology for human immunodeficiency virus was negative. The Venereal Disease Research Laboratory test was reactive 1:64.

In men, as well as in women, gonorrhea spreads to other parts of the body in 0.5–3% of affected patients and mainly affects the skin (dermatitis), articulations (arthritis) and, with less frequency, the heart valves (endocarditis) and the brain (meningitis).

Dermatitis

Approximately 50–75% of patients with disseminated gonococcal infection have cutaneous lesions, mainly in the nearby articular regions.

This clinical picture is composed of up to 10 small and painful lesions, which appear on the distal surfaces of extremities (Fig. 26.14). The lesion begins with a hemorrhagic macule, with

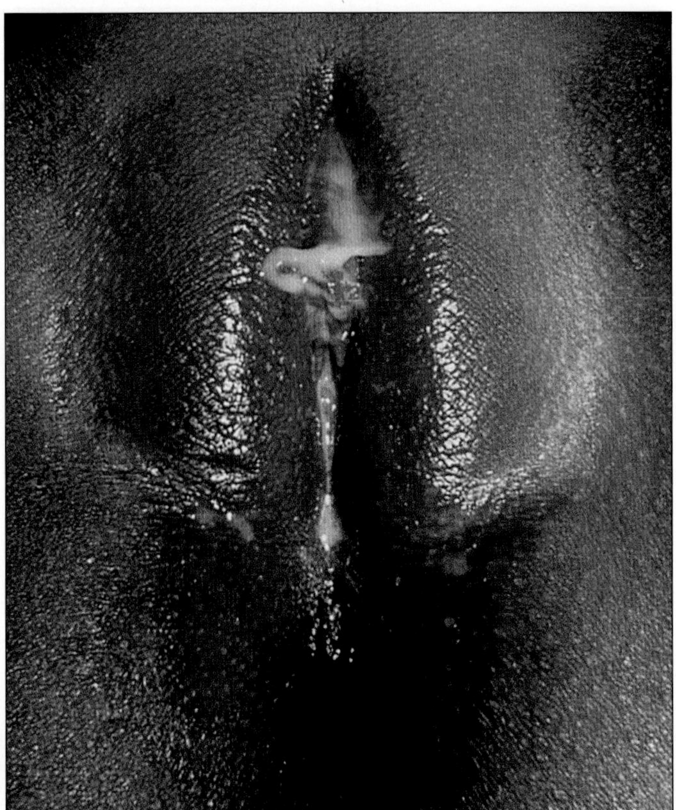

Figure 26.12 Gonococcal vulvitis in a child victim of sexual abuse.

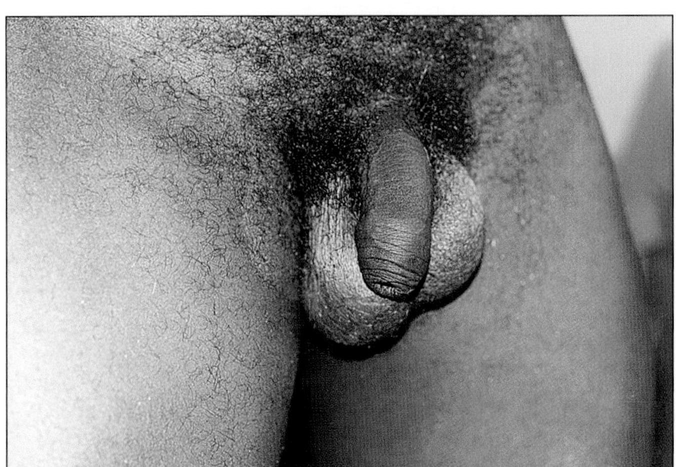

Figure 26.13 Patient with orchiepididymitis as a complication of gonococcal urethritis. Dermatomycosis on the inner surface of the thigh was associated with the testicular problems.

posterior pustulization, with a gray necrotic center, surrounded by a violet halo, which can evolve to form a crust (Fig. 26.15).

Buccopharyngeal gonorrhea is another tegumentar manifestation, usually with massive oral edema and erythematous aspect of the uvula, pustular areas in the pharynx, and irregular erosions on the upper surface of the tongue (Fig. 26.16).

The diagnosis can be made by demonstrating the microorganism in cutaneous lesions. Whenever one suspects gonococcemia, it would be prudent to obtain culture samples of all of the probably infected

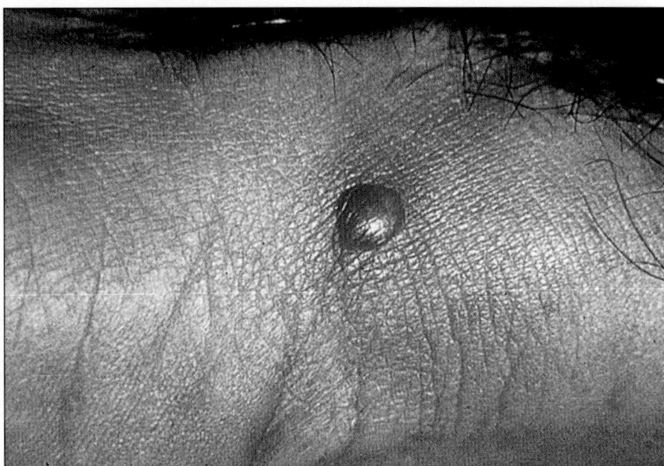

Figure 26.14 Gonococcal dermatitis, where it is possible to observe a pustule.

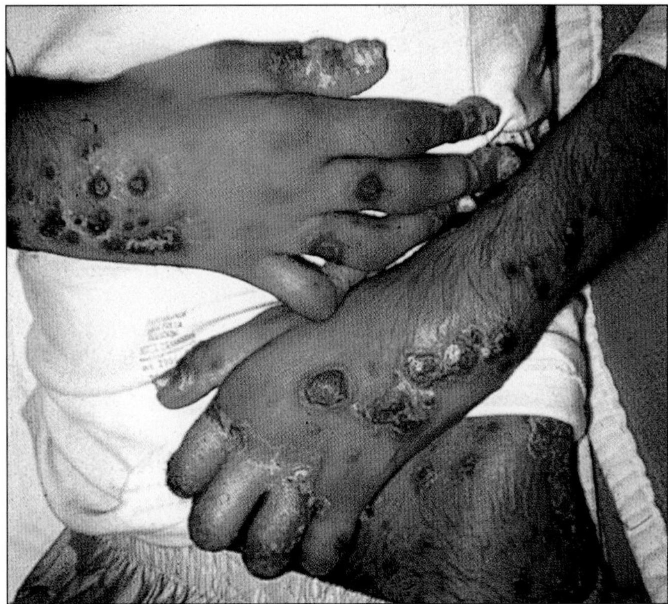

Figure 26.15 Rare case of gonococcemia, which signifies massive hematogenic dissemination of gonococci; it is normally more common in meningococcal disease. Diagnosis should include hemoculture. (Courtesy of Dr. J. C. Flichmann.)

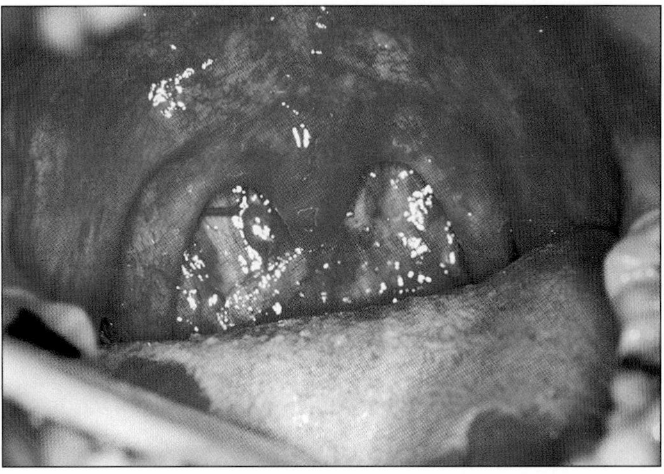

Figure 26.16 Buccopharyngeal gonorrhea. Observe edema and erythematous aspect of the uvula, pustular areas in the pharynx, and irregular erosions on the upper surface of the tongue. (Courtesy of Prof. L. C. Moreira.)

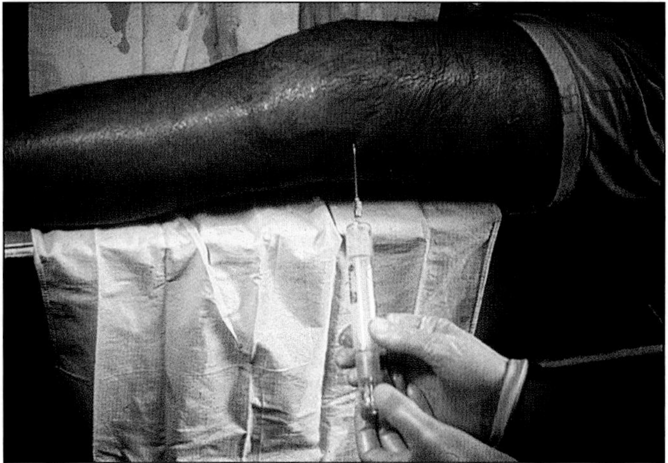

Figure 26.17 Patient with gonococcal arthritis; this is a bisexual man who also had gonococcal urethritis.

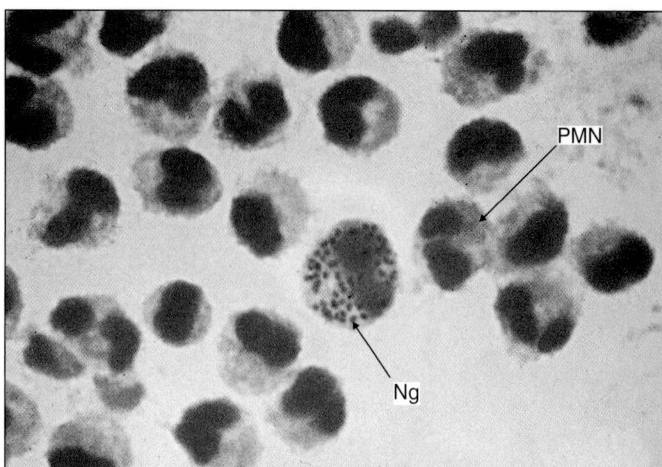

Figure 26.18 Presence of various Gram-negative intracellular reniform diplococci in some polymorphonuclear leukocytes (1000×).

areas, and also from the blood, as the latter tests positive in more than 50% of patients in the initial phase of the infection.[5,6] Differential diagnosis of gonococcemia lesions should be made, principally with meningococcemia lesions.

Arthritis

In young and sexually active people, gonococcal arthritis is the most frequent. It is present in more than 90% of cases of gonococcal septicemia, often being polyarticular. The symptomatology varies from arthralgia to acute arthritis, affecting mainly the wrist and knee. Synovial liquid can be removed by puncture; it will be serous or purulent, with high concentrations of proteins and low concentrations of glucose (Fig. 26.17). If it is not immediately treated, the infection can evolve to erosion of the cartilage, atrophy of the adjacent bone structures, and incapacitating arthritis.

It is only possible to demonstrate the gonococcus, by bacterial culture or by direct exam, in 50% of the cases. The investigation includes centrifugation of the liquid and examination of the sediment.

The differential diagnosis should be made in comparison with other types of septic arthritis, including rheumatoid arthritis, rheumatic fever, and Reiter syndrome.

Normally, the signs only show up on radiologic examination 20 days after the initial appearance of arthritis, frequently revealing a decrease in the articular space with subchondral cysts and articular osteoporosis.[5,6]

Patient evaluation, diagnosis, and differential diagnosis

Bacterioscopy of the urethral secretion with Gram staining can show bacteria in the interior of polymorphonuclear leukocytes (Fig. 26.18).

Culture

Thayer–Martin selective medium

In cases of acute urethritis in men, bacterioscopy is a good method of culture. In women, culture of material from the cervical canal is the best option. Nevertheless, if molecular biological techniques, PCR, and hybrid capture (HC), are available, they are extremely useful. They have a great practical advantage, as the same sample can also be used to test for *Chlamydia trachomatis* (Table 26.1).

Differential diagnosis

Men

The differential diagnosis in men is mainly non-gonococcal urethritis (*C. trachomatis, Mycoplasma hominis, Ureaplasma urealyticum,* or *Trichomonas vaginalis*), chemical urethritis (introduction of irritating substances into the urethra for prophylactic or curative purposes), and traumatic urethritis (due to the habit of expressing the gland to demonstrate secretion (milking). Men with painful and/or swollen testicles may have tumors or a twisted testicle.

Women

In women the differential diagnosis is endocervicitis, bartholinitis, and salpingitis (infection of the upper genital tract in women) by *Chlamydia*.

Table 26.1 Evaluation of laboratory methods[7]

Exam	Sensitivity (%)	Specificity (%)
Bacterioscopy by Gram:		
Urethra	90–95	95–99
Endocervix	45–65	90–99
Vagina, anus	Not recommended	
Culture		
Urethral section	94–98	>99
Endocervicitis	85–95	>99
Molecular biology: PCR, CH	95–98	>99

Treatment

Urethritis and acute endocervicitis

- Ciprofloxacin 500 mg PO single dose
- Ofloxacin 400 mg PO single dose
- Levofloxacin 250 mg PO single dose
- Gatifloxacin 400 mg PO single dose
- Cefixin 400 mg PO single dose
- Ceftriaxom 250 mg IM single dose
- Tianfenicol 2.5 g PO single dose
- Spectinomycin 2 g in a single IM dose

In chronic, extragenital and/or complicated infections, treatment regimens should not use single doses; rather classical doses and intervals should be implemented, for not less than 10 days.[8,9]

Note: Due to reports of resistance of gonococci to quinolones, these should be avoided for the treatment of gonococcal infections in the Asian Pacific area, including Hawaii and California in the USA.[10]

In men, the criterion for cure is basically clinical. In women it is necessary to make a culture of endocervical material, 7–10 days after the end of the treatment period.

Since infection with gonococci associated with C. *trachomatis* can exceed 30%, especially in young women, simultaneous treatment for this agent should also be started. In these situations the most commonly used treatment regimens are:

- Uncomplicated disease or infection of the lower genital tract by *Chlamydia* (urethritis, endocervicitis):
  - Azithromycin 1 g PO in a single dose
  - Doxycycline 100 mg PO every 12 h for 7 days
  - Doxycycline 200 mg PO once a day for 7 days
  - Erythromycin (stearate) 500 mg every 6 h PO for 7 days
- Complicated disease, or affecting the upper genital tract (endometritis, salpingitis/pelvic inflammatory disease), epididymitis, arthritis):
  - Doxycycline 100 mg, oral, 12/12 h or 200 mg oral once a day for 14 days.

Important

Treatment of a case of gonorrhea or other STD/genital infections requires immediate action. The syndrome approach permits immediate action, including a detailed investigation, whenever possible and indicated. Consequently the following should not be postponed:[8,9,11]

- Carry out an excellent clinical history.
- Perform a satisfactory physical exam.
- Advise counseling (health education).
- Offer Venereal Disease Research Laboratory (VDRL), HIV, and hepatitis testing.
- Emphasize adherence to treatment (therapy supervised at the doctor's exam).
- Emphasize the importance of consulting/treating sexual partners.
- Emphasize the importance of family planning.
- Emphasize the importance of periodic exams (gynecological, prostate).
- Make condoms available (male/female).
- Notify the official public health organizations of the case.
- Schedule a return visit by the patient.

Patients with immunodeficiency (acquired immunodeficiency syndrome (AIDS), neoplasias, malignancies, use of immunosuppressors) can have atypical and/or exaggerated responses to many infections. In these people the treatment may require a higher dose, more time, and even changes in the route of administration of the drugs. It is not uncommon to have to repeat the treatment regimen or hospital stay with intravenous medication.

If there is recurrence or persistence of the urethritis, administration of 2 g metronidazole in an oral single dose may be a satisfactory solution.

References

1. Dicker LW, Mosure DJ, Berman SM et al. Gonorrhea prevalence and coinfection with *Chlamydia* in women in the United States, 2000. Sex Transm Dis 2003; 30:472–476.
2. Hook III EW, Handsfield HH. Gonococcal infections in the adult. In: Holmes KK et al., eds. Sexually transmitted diseases, 2nd edn. New York: McGraw-Hill; 1994.
3. Sparling PF. Biology of *Neisseria gonorrhoeae*. In: Holmes KK et al., eds. Sexually transmitted diseases, 2nd edn. New York: McGraw-Hill; 1994.
4. Holmes KK, Johnson DW, Trostle HJ et al. An estimate of risk of men acquiring gonorrhea by sexual contact with infected females. Am J Epidemiol 1970; 91:170.
5. O'Brien JA, Stewart PJ, Mancini K et al. Disseminated gonococcal infection: a prospective analysis of 49 patients and a review of pathophysiology and immune mechanisms. Medicine 1983; 2:395.
6. Masi AT, Eisenstein BI. Disseminated gonococcal infection (DGI) and gonococcal arthritis (GCA): II. Clinical manifestations, diagnosis, complications, treatment and prevention. Semin Arthr Rheum 1981; 10:173.
7. Lewis JS. Seleção e avaliação de testes de controle de qualidade. In: Morse SA, Moreland AA, Holmes KK, eds. Atlas de doenças sexualmente transmissíveis e Aids, 2nd edn. Porto Alegre : Artes Médicas; 1997: 56–62.
8. Passos MRL, Almeida GL. Atlas de doenças sexualmente transmissíveis. Rio de Janeiro: Revinter; 2002.
9. Passos MRL. Doenças sexualmente transmissíveis, 4th edn. Rio de Janeiro: Cultura Médica; 1995.
10. Centers for Disease Control and Prevention. Sexually transmitted diseases treatment guidelines 2002. MMWR 2002; 51 (no. RR-6):37.
11. Brasil Ministério da Saúde. SPS. Coordenação nacional de doenças sexualmente transmissíveis e AIDS. Manual de controle das doenças sexualmente transmissíveis, 3rd edn. Brasília: Brasil Ministério da Sáude SPS; 1999.

Chancroid

Omar Lupi, Dominique Fausto Perez and Michelle Gralle Botelho

Synonyms: Chancroid, soft chancre, ulcus molle, soft ulcer, dwarf chancre, transient chancroid, phagedenic chancroid, follicular chancroid, papular chancroid, giant chancroid

Key features:

- Genital ulcer: small, dirty, necrotic, rounded or oval, painful, tender and has a tendency to bleed on touch
- Inguinal adenitis
- Caused by *Haemophilus ducreyi*, a Gram-negative coccobacillus
- STDs endemic in Asia, Africa, and the Caribbean
- In HIV-positive patients, the duration of the ulceration is longer, and the number of ulcers at initial presentation is greater than that in HIV-negative patients

Introduction

Chancroid is one of the classical genital ulcerative diseases. It is caused by the Gram-negative coccobacillus *Haemophilus ducreyi* and its principal mode of transmission is sexual intercourse. Chancroid is a public health problem because *H. ducreyi* and HIV facilitate each other's transmission.[1] Therefore, it is assumed that chancroid is one of the factors responsible for the rapid spread of HIV in endemic countries, such as in Africa.

History

Bassereau and Ricord, in France, first distinguished soft from indurated (syphilitic) chancres in 1852. Ducreyi, a bacteriologist at the University of Naples, identified the causative organism of chancroid in 1889.[2]

Epidemiology

The World Health Organization estimates that the annual global incidence of chancroid is approximately 6 million cases.[1] However, it is difficult to obtain an exact number of affected individuals because most patients do not seek medical attention and the available diagnostic methods have low sensitivity and specificity.

In endemic areas in Asia, Africa, and the Caribbean, the prevalence of chancroid ranges between 23% and 56%.[3]

There is a close geographical association between chancroid and HIV infection. In countries where chancroid is endemic, the HIV infection rates are the highest in the world.[2]

Although rare in the USA and Europe, sporadic outbreaks can occur. More recently, chancroid prevalence has declined markedly in countries such as China, the Philippines, Senegal, and Thailand.[2,4]

The disease affects mainly males. The mean male-to-female ratio is 20:1, so women may represent asymptomatic carriers of the organism. This high male-to-female ratio was studied in human models of infection. Women experimentally inoculated with *H. ducreyi* resolved their initial lesions more frequently than males without progressing to the pustular stage of the disease.[2] The mechanism underlying this gender difference is not currently known; female hormones may have suppressing effects on the parasite growth. Prostitutes and subjects with poor hygiene are most affected. The 18–45-year-old age group is the most vulnerable.[5]

Pathogenesis and etiology

Chancroid is an infectious disease caused by the Gram-negative, facultative anaerobic bacillus *H. ducreyi*.

H. ducreyi is a strict human pathogen and naturally infects genital and non-genital skin, mucosal surfaces, and regional lymph nodes. The disease is largely disseminated through sexual intercourse with an infected individual. The organism enters the skin and/or mucous membrane of the new host through microabrasions received during sexual intercourse.[5] The estimated transmission rate is 70%.[4] Lack of circumcision is associated with infection in men.[1]

By 48 h after inoculation, *H. ducreyi* is surrounded by neutrophils and macrophages and associated with collagen and fibrin.[6] Yet the parasite is not phagocytosed and it is resistant to the oxidative burst products of neutrophils, which represent its mechanism of virulence.

Clinical features

The incubation period for chancroid is short and varies between 3 and 7 days, rarely more than 10 days. The atypical variants of chancroid may have a long mean incubation period of 8–11 days. Patients with associated HIV may also have longer incubation periods.[2]

The disease typically begins as a small inflammatory papule at the site of inoculation: this papule rapidly becomes pustular and then ulcerates. The ulcer is small, dirty, necrotic, rounded or oval, painful, tender, and has a tendency to bleed on touch. Satellite ulcers, two to five in a cluster, are quite often present, and are more common in women than men (Fig. 26.19).

In males, lesions are most commonly found on the prepuce, on the frenulum, and on the glans (Fig. 26.20). In females, lesions are most commonly found on the vulva, cervix, and perianal area. Extragenital infection on hands, eyelids, lips, breasts, and oral mucosa have been reported (Figs 26.21 and 26.22).

Painful inguinal adenitis occurs in 50% of patients and is more common in men. The adenitis, usually unilateral, develops about a week after the appearance of the ulcer and may progress to a suppurative bubo (Fig. 26.23).

In HIV-positive patients, the duration of the ulceration is longer, and the number of ulcers at initial presentation is greater than that in HIV-seronegative patients.[3]

Systemic infection by *H. ducreyi* has never been observed.

Several clinical variants have been identified:[5,6]

1. Dwarf chancroid: a small, superficial, relatively painless ulcer.
2. Giant chancroid: a large granulomatous ulcer at the site of a ruptured inguinal bubo, extending beyond its margins.

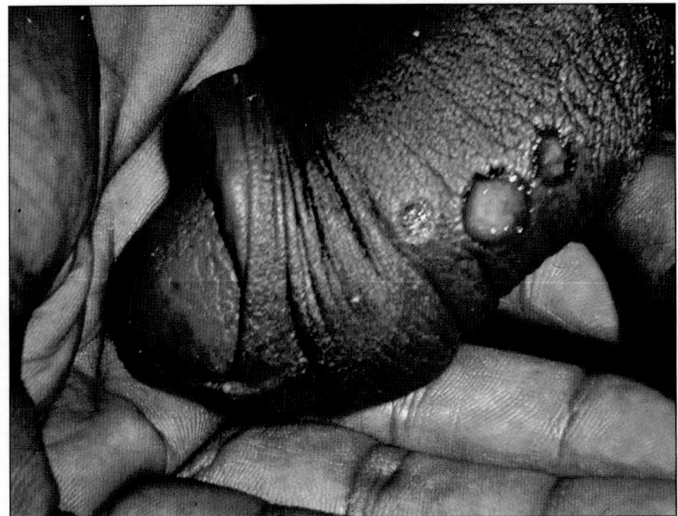

Figure 26.19 Chancroid. Small rounded and very tender ulcer with two satellite ulcers.

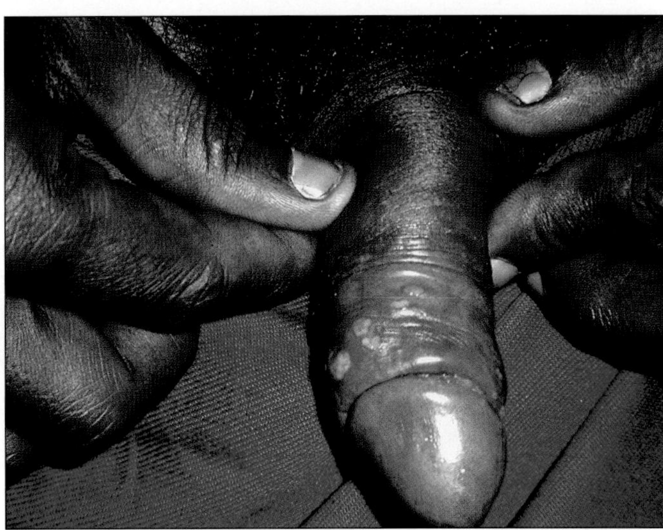

Figure 26.20 Chancroid. Cluster of ulcers on the prepuce, on the frenulum, and on the glans.

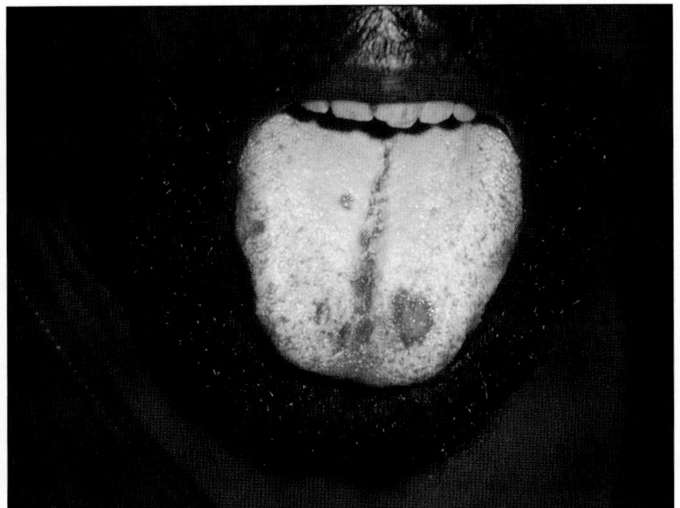

Figure 26.21 Extragenital chancroid affecting the tongue and palatum. (Courtesy of Dr. C. Maia).

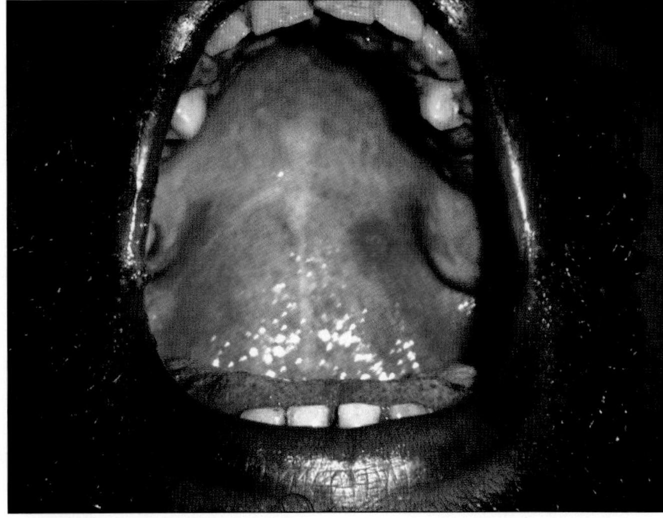

Figure 26.22 Extragenital chancroid affecting the tongue and palatum. (Courtesy of Dr. C. Maia).

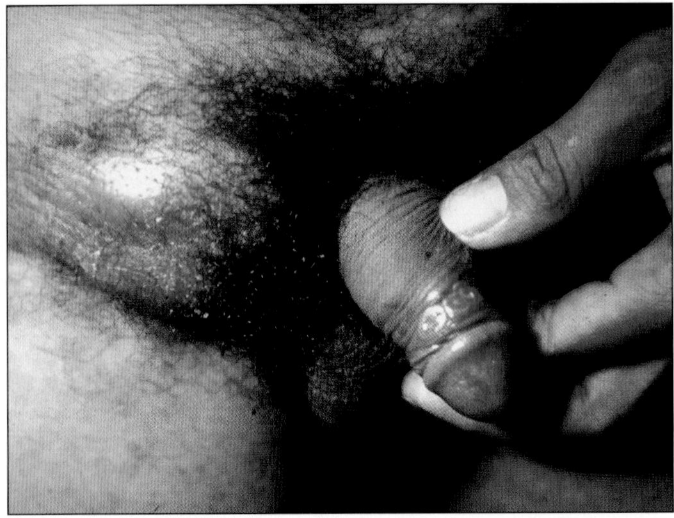

Figure 26.23 Chancroid. Painful unilateral adenitis and a cluster of ulcerative lesions on the prepuce.

3. Follicular chancroid: essentially seen in women in association with hair follicles of the labia majora and pubis: initial appearance is as a follicular pustule, later resulting in a classic ulcer at the site.
4. Transient chancroid (French: chancre mou volant): very superficial ulcers, which may soon heal, followed by a typical inguinal bubo.
5. Serpiginous chancroid: multiple ulcers coalesce, spreading by extension and autoinoculation.
6. Phagedenic chancroid (ulcus molle gangrenosum): caused by superinfection with fusospirochetes. The ulceration causes extensive destruction of the genitalia.
7. Papular chancroid (ulcus molle elevatum): a granulomatous ulcerated papule that might resemble donovanosis or condyloma lata.
8. Mixed chancroid: non-indurated, tender ulcers of chancroid together with an indurated, non-tender ulcer of syphilis with an incubation period of 10–90 days.

Diagnosis

The diagnosis of chancroid is based on a history of sexual intercourse and development of painful genital ulcers following the incubation period. Chancroid is also associated with tender inguinal lymphadenopathy or suppurative adenopathy. The following tests are diagnostic:[7]

- Gram stain of the ulcer exudates may demonstrate short, plump, Gram-negative rods in the classic "school-of-fish" appearance; however, *H. ducreyi* is difficult to demonstrate in Gram smears and frequently the material has polymicrobial contamination.
- Culture is the best widely available diagnostic method, although it is difficult to grow *H. ducreyi* in vitro (Fig. 26.24).
- PCR testing is the diagnostic test that has greatest sensibility and specificity. PCR testing is considered the gold-standard test for diagnosis, but it is expensive and not commercially available.
- A serologic evaluation for syphilis should also be performed.

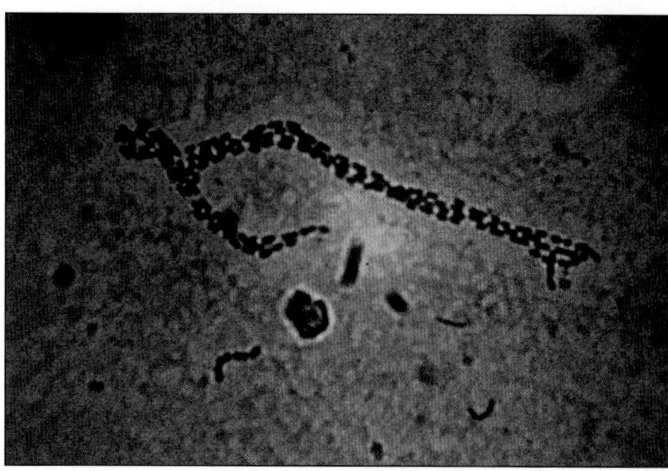

Figure 26.24 *Haemophylus ducreyi*. Culture showing Gram-negative rods in the classic "school of fish" disposition. (Courtesy Dr. M Passos.)

Differential diagnosis is shown in Table 26.2.

Superinfected traumatic lesions and non-infectious causes of genital ulceration, such as Crohn's disease or Behçet's syndrome, must be considered in the differential diagnosis.

Pathology

The histopathology is a useful complement to the diagnosis. The tissue below the floor of the ulcer can be arbitrarily divided into three zones. The more superficial zone consists of necrotic tissues and an inflammatory infiltrate. The broad mid-zone contains the new blood vessels with patchy proliferative changes on the one hand and degenerative changes on the other. The deeper zone shows a chronic inflammatory infiltrate of plasma cells and lymphocytes.

Treatment

Specific and prompt treatment of chancroid is imperative to reduce transmission rates and to prevent outbreaks. Patients should be told to avoid unprotected sexual intercourse during the treatment. The goal of the therapy is the eradication of the organism; for this purpose many antibiotics can be prescribed (Table 26.3).

Table 26.2 Differential diagnosis for chancroid

Disease	Incubation	Genital ulceration	Adenopathy	Etiology	Diagnosis
Syphilis	30–90 days	Round or oval, sharply defined, regular, indurated borders, non-tender, with smooth, brownish-red base, painless	Rubbery, movable, non-tender, non-suppurative, painless, uni- or bilateral	*Treponema pallidum*	Dark-field examination, serologic testing for antibodies
Herpes simplex	2–7 days	Small but grouped vesicular lesions that ulcerate Very painful	Tender, painful, bilateral	Herpes simplex virus (HSV)-2 and, less commonly, HSV-1	Tzanck smear, Papanicolaou staining method, culture, HSV antigen detection, HSV DNA detection by polymerase chain reaction
Donovanosis	2 weeks to 3 months	Large spreading, exuberant ulcers, with bright-red granulating surface (ulcerovegetative)	True adenopathy is rare Subcutaneous nodule may be mistaken for lymph nodes (pseudobubo)	*Calymmatobacterium granulomatus*	Wright's or Giemsa's stain from a fresh biopsy permits the demonstration of Donovan bodies
Lymphogranuloma venereum	3–30 days	Soft, erythematous, painless erosion that heals spontaneously	Nodes that coalesce to form a firm, elongated, unilateral, immovable mass. The fistulization may form multiple openings	*Chlamydia trachomatis*, serologic varieties L1, L2, L3	Culture, complement fixation test (titer 1:64, or greater), polymerase chain reaction DNA

Table 26.3 Prescribed treatment for chancroid

Antibiotic	Dose	Route	Evidence-based medicine
Azithromycin	1 g single dose	PO	3[a] (8)
Ceftriaxone	250 mg single dose	IM	3[a] (8)
Ciprofloxacin	500 mg twice daily for 3 days	PO	3[a] (9)
Erythromycin	2 g four equally divided doses	PO	3[a] (9)

[a]Clinical trial >20 subjects.

Amoxicillin/clavulanate is no longer recommended because of *H. ducreyi* resistance to this antibiotic. In patients with concomitant *H. ducreyi* and HIV infection, a longer course of therapy and close monitoring are mandatory.

Drainage of fluctuant lymph nodes larger than 5 cm in diameter by needle aspiration can be done. If not treated, the chancroid can become complicated, with rupture of buboes and subsequent scarring and/or chronic sinus tract drainage. Phimosis and balanoposthitis may also occur. It is important to emphasize to patients that they should avoid high-risk sexual activities, such as unprotected sexual intercourse or sexual intercourse with high-risk partners.

References

1. Spinola SM, Bauer ME, Munson RS Jr. Immunopathogenesis of *Haemophilus ducreyi* infection. Infect Immun 2002; 70:1667–1676.
2. Steen B. Eradicating chancroid. Bull WHO 2001; 79:818–826.
3. Al-Tawfiq JA, Spinola SM. *Haemophilus ducreyi*: clinical disease and pathogenesis. Curr Opin Infect Dis 2002; 15:43–47.
4. Bong CT, Harezlak J, Katz BP et al. Men are more susceptible than women to pustule formation in the experimental model of *Haemophilus ducreyi* infection. Sex Transm Dis 2002; 29:114–118.
5. Sehgal VN, Srivastava G. Chancroid: contemporary appraisal. Int J Dermatol 2003; 42:182–190.
6. Bauer ME, Goheen MP, Townsend CA et al. *Haemophilus ducreyi* associates with phagocytes, collagen, and fibrin and remains extracellular throughout infection of human volunteers. Infect Immun 2001; 69:2549–2557.
7. Lewis DA. Diagnostic tests for chancroid. Sex Transm Inf 2000; 76:137–141.
8. Martin DH, Sargent SJ, Wendel GD Jr et al. Comparison of azithromycin and ceftriaxone for the treatment of chancroid. Clin Infect Dis 1995; 21:409–414.
9. Malonza IM, Tyndall MW, Ndinya-Achola JO et al. A randomized, double-blind, placebo-controlled trial of single-dose ciprofloxacin versus erythromycin for the treatment of chancroid in Nairobi, Kenya. J Infect Dis 1999; 180:1886–1893.

Donovanosis (granuloma inguinale)

Márcio Lobo Jardim, Letícia P. Spinelli and Omar Lupi

Synonyms: Granuloma inguinale, granuloma venereum, chronic venereum ulcer, granuloma donovani, ulcerating granuloma of the pudenda

Introduction

Donovanosis is an indolent, progressive, ulcerative, granulomatous skin disease caused by *Calymmatobacterium granulomatis*, formerly known as *Donovania granulomatis*. It mainly affects the skin and subcutaneous cell tissue of the genital and perianal areas and inguinal region; less frequently it affects other regions of the skin, mucosa, and even the internal organs.

It is probably spread by both homosexual and heterosexual sexual contact, as well as by non-sexual means. Untreated, it shows no tendency to go into spontaneous remission and in later stages it may be severely debilitating.

Many terms have been proposed for this disease: inguinal granuloma, venereum granuloma, tropicum granuloma, pudendi tropicum granuloma, contagious granuloma, ulcerating granuloma, sclerosing granuloma, chronic venereum ulcer, and granuloma donovani.[1,2]

History

Donovanosis was first described in 1882 by McLeod, in Madras, India: McLeod named it serpiginous ulcer.[3] Many other names have been suggested, but, aside from granuloma inguinale, only the term donovanosis persists.

In 1905, Donovan demonstrated the causative agent of the disease, and classified it in the protozoa group.[4] He described the bipolar-staining, intracellular inclusions in macrophages from lesion exudate (termed Donovan bodies).

In 1912, in a very well-established work, Aragão and Viana[5] published their conclusions about the etiological agent, proposing the name *Calymmatobacterium granulomatis*.

In the twentieth century, other names were given to this microorganism, such as *Donovania granulomatis* and *Klebsiella granulomatis*, despite the research of Brazilians Aragão and Vianna. After detailed bacteriological, clinical, and therapeutic studies, the bacteria was called *Calymmatobacterium granulomatis*.

Anderson, in 1943, established the bacterial nature of Donovan bodies, when he cultivated the microorganism in the vitelline embryonic yolk sac. Requirements for growth on artificial media were established in 1959.

In 1950, Marmell and Santora introduced the term donovanosis, as a homage to Donovan.

Epidemiology

Sporadic cases of donovanosis occur worldwide, with recent reports from developed countries such as Canada, France, Italy, Sweden, and Japan. Endemic foci are usually only seen in tropical and subtropical areas, such as New Guinea, Brazil, central Australia, the Caribbean, and parts of India.

The sexually transmitted nature of donovanosis is controversial: it appears, from clinical and epidemiological observations, that it is not only transmitted by sexual intercourse. Strong arguments indicate the importance of sexual contact: the lesions are more frequent in the genital or anal region; the disease is more frequent in the sexually active group, and it is localized anally in male homosexuals. The possibility of non-venereal transmission is suggested by the occurrence of disease in sexually inactive children, and the infrequency of infection in partners repeatedly exposed to open lesions, and in sexually active people (e.g., prostitutes) in some endemic areas.

Sehgal and Prasad[6] published a donovanosis case which they considered an example of non-venereal transmission in adults, since the lesions were restricted to the arms, face, and neck, with no evidence of lesions on the genital, inguinal, or oral regions.

Some authors, such as Jardim,[7] affirm that contact with carriers of donovanosis does not always result in infection in a normal individual, and that whether the skin is healthy or broken does not seem to enhance the transmission of the disease. It has also been pointed out that infection only occurred when fragments of affected tissue or pus aspirated from pseudobuboes were implanted in or inoculated on subcutaneous tissue of human volunteers.

It seems clear, however, that donovanosis is one of a class of diseases causing genital ulceration that may predispose individuals to the transmission of HIV.

Although many authors affirm that the disease attacks men more than women, the tendency today is to consider that it affects both men and women. Some authors, such as Kuberski,[8] Lal and Nicholas,[9] and Lynch,[10] observed more cases among men, while Bhagwandeen[11] and Ribeiro[12] reported that most of their cases were female. Other authors report that the disease is more frequent among male homosexuals.

As regards age, the consensus is that most cases involved young adults (20–40 years old) – the age range that is likely to be experiencing greater sexual activity.

Although reports of the disease in children and the elderly are rare, Banerjee[13] observed the disease in a 6-month-old child, while Ribeiro[12] published a case of a 94-year-old patient with donovanosis.

Pathogenesis and etiology

The causative agent is termed *Donovania granulomatis*. It is a Gram-negative rod, sometimes cocobacilli, measuring 0.5–1.5 μm wide by 1.0–2.0 μm long, presenting round extremities. These microorganisms are steadfast and have a polysaccharide and fibrous capsule.

They appear isolated or form bunches inside large mononuclear macrophages (corpuscles of Donovan), and are also found in extracellular spaces. The cellular wall is Gram-negative, similar to the wall of *Klebsiella*, although *Klebsiella* has not yet demonstrated any correlation with this bacteria.

It has been demonstrated in fecal flora, and there is evidence from electron microscopy that it may share a bacteriophage with Enterobacteriaceae.

The microorganisms stain with greater intensity in the extremities than in the center, varying from deep blue to black, while the capsule is red. They can be stained by Giemsa, Leishman, or Wright.

Antibodies against the organism may be detected by the complement-fixation test, although it is of little diagnostic value. Circulating antibody, which does not affect the relentless course of untreated disease, has raised the possibility that a defect in cell-mediated immunity may predispose the patient to clinical illness, as is the case in the other diseases caused by intracellular organisms (e.g., leprosy and tuberculosis).[1,2]

Clinical features

The incubation period is poorly defined and may range from 2 weeks to 3 months. According to Rajam[14] it is 2 weeks to 1 month; Greenblatt and Torpin[15] assert it is 42–50 days, while Lal and Nicholas[9] claim it is 3 days to 6 months. Experimental human inoculation has produced lesions after a latency period of 21 days.

The disease begins as single or multiple subcutaneous nodules, which erode through the skin, producing a very well-defined ulceration that grows slowly and bleeds readily on contact (Fig. 26.25). From this point, the manifestations are directly linked to the tissue responses of the host, the originating localized or extensive forms, and may even be visceral lesions through hematogenous dissemination. The subcutaneous nodule, if large enough, may be mistaken for a lymph node, giving rise to the term pseudobubo. True adenopathy and general symptoms are rare.

The bottom of the lesion is soft and beefy-red (Fig. 26.26). The edges are irregular, elevated, well-defined, and indurated. In recently formed lesions, the bottom is filled with serosanguineous secretion, while in old lesions, the surface becomes granulated and the secretion is seropurulent and has a fetid odor.

In men, the penis, scrotum, and glans are the most common sites of primary lesions; in women, the commonest sites are the labia minora, vulva, vagina, cervix, and pubis.

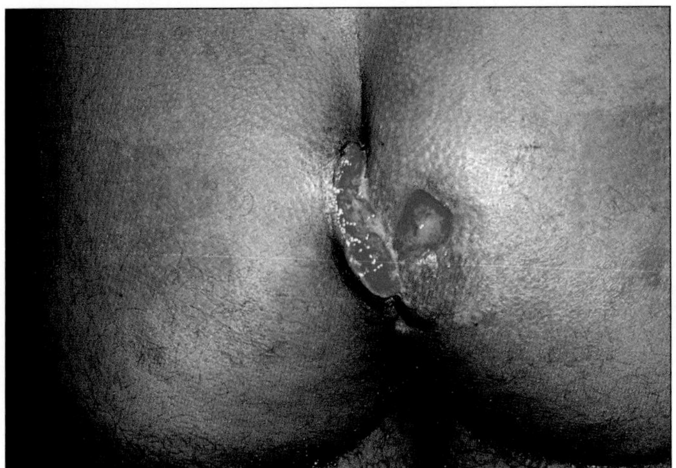

Figure 26.25 Donovanosis. Very well-defined ulceration that grows slowly and bleeds readily on contact. (Courtesy of Dr. Omar Lupi.)

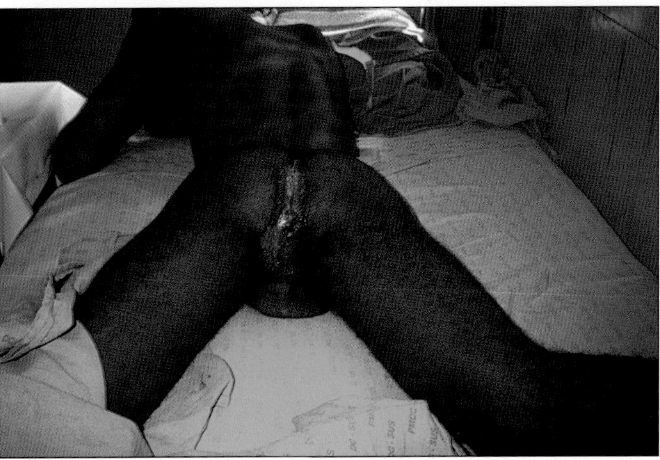

Figure 26.27 Donovanosis. Perianal lesions. (Courtesy of Dr. Andreia Mateus.)

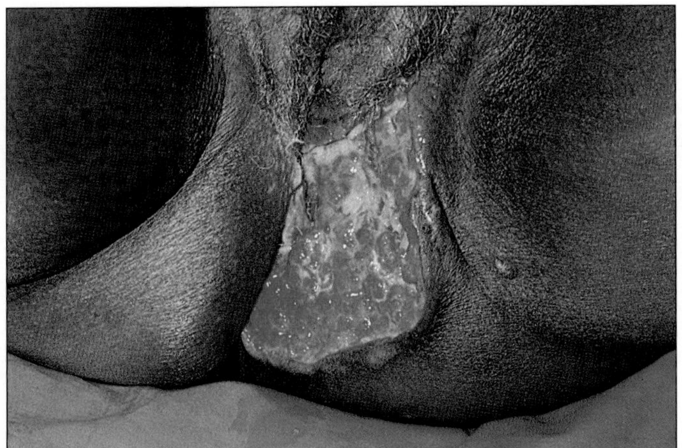

Figure 26.26 Donovanosis. The bottom of the lesion is soft and beefy-red. (Courtesy of Dr. Omar Lupi.)

In most cases of donovanosis described in the literature, localization is restricted to cutaneous areas and mucosa of the genitalia and anal, perianal, and inguinal regions, where the lesion generally initiates as a small papule or painless nodule that ulcerates and grows as it develops (Figs 26.27 and 26.28). Through autoinoculation, satellite lesions merge and join, covering extensive areas.

The lesion may present as a vegetating mass or tends to form fibrous or keloid tissues, sometimes leading to deformity of the genitalia, paraphimosis, or elephantiasis.

Superinfection with fusospirochetal organisms may give rise to necrotic lesions with massive tissue destruction, similar to so-called phagedenic chancroid.

Extragenital donovanosis occurs in 3–6% of cases, with occasional systemic involvement, notably in the gastrointestinal tract and bone, including the bony orbit and orbital skin. Almost all cases of extragenital donovanosis are from endemic areas.

The localization of the disease away from the anogenital site can be explained by the following: hematogenous dissemination to organs, such as the liver, lungs, bones, and spleen; continuity or contiguity to adjacent pelvic organs; lymphatic dissemination; and autoinoculation.

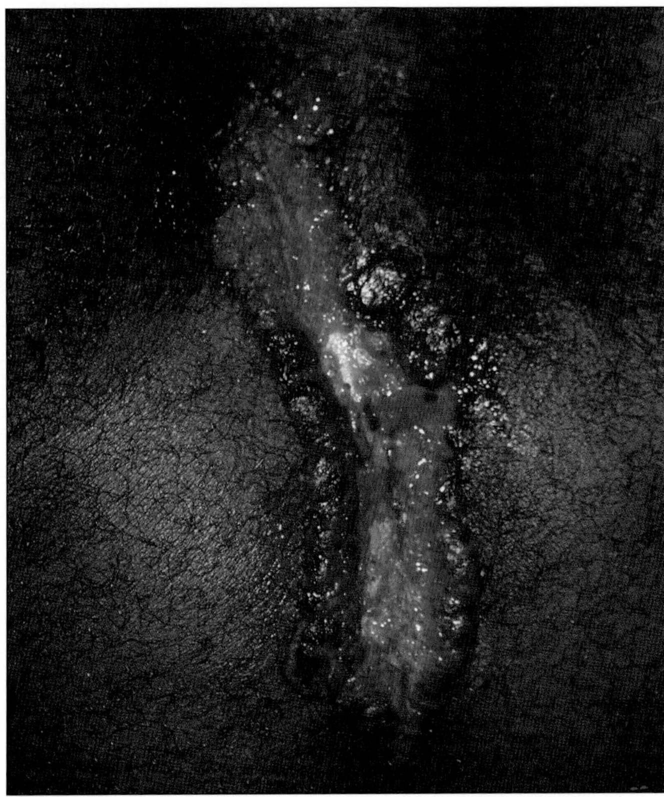

Figure 26.28 Donovanosis. Closer view of perianal lesions. (Courtesy of Dr. Andreia Mateus.)

Jardim[7] proposed a clinical classification:

Genitals and perigenitals
1. ulcerous
2. with hypertrophic edges
3. with plane edges
4. ulcerovegetating
5. vegetating
6. elephantiasic

Extragenital
Systemic.

In HIV-positive patients and predominantly in patients with AIDS, donovanosis may assume a completely abnormal clinical development. This situation can complicate both the diagnosis and treatment.

Patient evaluation, diagnosis, and differential diagnosis

The clinical diagnosis of donovanosis, based on history and appearance, may be fairly accurate in endemic areas. The correct diagnosis can be made if appropriately selected laboratory techniques are used to confirm the presumed clinical aspects.

The organism is difficult to cultivate and demands special growth nutrients and factors for its development. It can be cultivated in vivo in the chick embryonic yolk sac and in vitro in culture means enriched with egg yolk. It is always an arduous and expensive procedure, and of low reproducibility.

Laboratory diagnosis requires a crush or touch preparation stained with Wright or Giemsa stain from a punch biopsy specimen.

The most suitable clinical material are fragments of subsuperficial tissue of an active granulation area. A collection should be made of five to six tissue samples of different areas, radially, just below the edges of the lesions. The biopsy should be obtained before cleaning the lesion and removing necrotic tissue with saline solution and sterilized gauze, to prevent contamination. Scrapings from the base of the lesion or exudate aspirated from pseudobuboes can also be used. The diagnostic Donovan bodies are seen as deeply staining, bipolar, safety-pin-shaped rods in the cytoplasm of macrophages.

Many pathologies are clinically similar to donovanosis: primary syphilis, chancroid, LGV, neoplasia, condyloma acuminatum, leishmaniasis, deep mycosis, cutaneous tuberculosis, atypical mycobacteriosis, and cutaneous amebiasis. They can be differentiated by demonstrating the specific causal agent or on histopathological examination.[1,2]

Pathology

Preferably the biopsy should be done on the edge of the lesion, where the pathological modifications are more substantial.

The coloration usually made by hematoxylin and eosin is not ideal to demonstrate Donovan bodies in the interior of histiocytes or macrophages.

Histologically, the skin exhibits a massive cellular reaction, predominantly polymorphonuclear, with occasional plasma cells and, rarely, lymphocytes. The marginal epithelium demonstrates acanthosis, elongation of rete pegs, and pseudoepitheliomatous hyperplasia. These latter changes are highly suggestive of early malignancy and squamous cell carcinoma. Hypertrophic and cicatricial forms demonstrate the appropriate increase in fibrous tissue. Typically, large mononuclear cells containing numerous cytoplasmic inclusions (Donovan bodies) are scattered throughout the lesions. These are considered to be diagnostic of donovanosis and are often best demonstrated with special stains, such as Giemsa stain, Delafield hematoxylin, Dieterle silver stain, and the Warthin–Starry stain.

The differential histological diagnosis includes rhinoscleroma, histoplasmosis, leishmaniasis, and squamous cell carcinoma.[1,2]

Treatment

There is a varied therapeutic arsenal for the treatment of donovanosis. The medications can be used alone or in combination:

- Streptomycin 1 g/day IM for 20–30 days
- Sulfamethoxazole 800 mg + trimethoprim 160 mg 12/12 h PO, for 20–30 days
- Tetracycline 500 mg 6/6 h PO for 30–60 days
- Doxycycline 100 mg 12/12 h PO for 30–60 days
- Erythromycin 500 mg 6/6 h PO for 30–60 days
- Chloramphenicol 500 mg 6/6 h PO for 15 days
- Tianfenicol 500 mg 8/8 h PO for 15–20 days
- Gentamicin 30 mg 12/12 h IM for 15 days
- Ampicillin 500 mg 6/6 h PO for 20–30 days
- Amoxicillin 500 mg 8/8 h PO for 20–30 days
- Lincomycin 500 mg 6/6 h PO for 20–30 days.

With the recent emergence of new macrolides, drugs of low toxicity which are very well tolerated, mainly azithromycin which has excellent permanency in the tissues, are being tested. The therapeutic results have been encouraging.

The response may be monitored by clinical appearance and serial biopsy specimens examined for persistent presence of Donovan bodies. In early cases, the prognosis for complete healing is good. In late cases, irreparable tissue destruction may have supervened and radical surgery may be required.[1,2]

References

1. Passos MRL. Donovanosis. In: Kenneth AB, Noble MA, eds. Sexually transmitted diseases – epidemiology, pathology, diagnosis and treatment. Los Angeles: 1997:103–116.
2. Rothenberg RB. Granuloma inguinale. In: Freedberg IM, Eisen AZ, Wolff K et al. Fitzpatrick´s dermatology in general medicine, 5th edn. New York: McGraw Hill; 1999:2595–2598.
3. Hammar L. The dark side to donovanosis: color, climate, race and racism in South American venereology. J Med Humanit 1997; 18:29–57.
4. Donovan RF. Ulcerating granuloma of the pudenda. Int Med Gaz 1905; 40:414.
5. Aragão HD, Viana G. Pesquisas sobre o granuloma venéreo. Mem Inst Oswaldo Cruz 1912; 13:45.
6. Sehgal VN, Prasad AL. Donovanosis current concepts. Int J Dermatol 1986; 25:8–16.
7. Jardim ML. Donovanose em pacientes portadores de AIDS. An Bras Dermatol 1990 ; 65:175–177.
8. Kuberski T. Granuloma inguinale (donovanosis). Sex Dis 1980; 7:29–36.
9. Lal S, Nicholas C. Epidemiological and clinical features in 165 cases of granuloma inguinale. Br J Vener Dis 1970; 46:461.
10. Lynch GPJ. Sexually transmitted disease: granuloma inguinale,

lymphogranuloma venerium, chancroid and infectious syphilis. Clin Obst Gynecol 1978; 21:2.
11. Bhagwandeen BS. Granuloma venereum (granuloma inguinale) in Zambia. East Afr Med J 1977; 54:637–642.
12. Ribeiro J. Granuloma inguinale. Practitioner 1972; 209:628–630.
13. Banerjee K. Donovanosis in a child of six months. J Ind Med Assoc 1972; 59:293.
14. Rajam RV. Donovanosis. WHO monograph 24. Geneva: WHO; 1954.
15. Greenblat RB, Torpin R. Experimental and clinical granuloma inguinale. JAMA 1939; 113:1109–1116.

Syphilis

Sinésio Talhari and Carolina Talhari

Synonym: Lues

Key features:

- Syphilis is an infectious, chronic, systemic, venereal, and congenital disease with a myriad of clinical presentations
- It can mimic many other diseases and immune-mediated processes in advanced stages, and is known as "the great imitator"
- The disease comprises four stages: primary, secondary, latent, and late
- Patients in the late stage may manifest cutaneous, cardiovascular, and central nervous system disease[1]

Introduction

Syphilis is a genital ulcerative disease, which facilitates the transmission of HIV, contributing to the increase of its spread. It has been reported that the disease may accelerate the development of immunodeficiency in HIV-infected persons, even increasing the risk of rapid progression to neurosyphilis and its complications. Untreated maternal syphilis may result in preterm delivery, stillbirth, neonatal death, and infant disorders such as deafness, neurologic impairment, and bone deformities.[1–3]

History

According to recent studies, the disease may be a New World mutation of yaws. Syphilis received its present name from the poem by Fracastoro in 1530 about a wealthy and handsome shepherd, "Syphilus," who contracted a repulsive disease as a punishment for blasphemy to the Sun God. In 1905, *Treponema pallidum* was identified by Fritz Schaudinn and Erich Hoffman as the causative agent of syphilis. Lues is the name for plague[1,4].

Epidemiology

Syphilis is most common in sexually active young adults, especially in the group of 20–29 years, followed by adolescents and middle-aged persons. Men have a higher incidence than women.[2,3] The disease has no racial preference; it has been directly correlated to socioeconomic factors, such as poverty, lack of hygiene, crowded urban communities, and also to risk-taking behaviors such as sexual promiscuity and drug abuse.[5]

According to the *Sexually Transmitted Disease Surveillance 2001*,[6] the number of primary and secondary syphilis cases increased by 2.1% in 2001 compared to 2000, the first increase since 1990. This increase was only observed among men and was due to several reports of syphilis outbreaks in men who have sex with men.[5] A high rate of HIV coinfection and high-risk sexual behavior among these men was also reported. On the other hand, the total number of syphilis cases among women has decreased every year since 1990. Between 2000 and 2001 this decrease was 19.5%.[6] These numbers have contributed to the elevation of the male-to-female case ratio of syphilis from 1.4:1 to 2.1:1 during the same period. The male-to-female case ratio of syphilis has increased constantly since 1996, when it was 1.1:1.[6]

The decrease in syphilis rates reported in women may explain the decline of congenital syphilis rates in the USA. In the last decade, the average annual percentage decrease of the congenital syphilis rate was 19.8%. In 2000 the overall rate of congenital syphilis was 14.0 per 100 000 live births and in 2001 this rate had decreased to 11.1/100 000.[6]

Congenital syphilis is still an important health problem in many developing countries. For example, in 1998, the congenital syphilis rate in Brazil was 1.2 per 1000 live births.[1,5]

From 1990 to 1996, cases of syphilis have decreased in all ethnic and racial groups in the USA.[6] From 1997 to 2000 the rates were stable in these groups, except in African–Americans, among whom the rates declined. Between 2000 and 2001, the cases among this same group showed a decline of 9.8%, but the rates have increased 40% among whites, 31% among Hispanics, 67% among Asian/Pacific Islanders, and 75% among American Indians/Alaska natives.[6]

According to the World Health Organization, the estimated worldwide number of new cases of syphilis in 1999 was 12 million, being 140 000 in western Europe and 100 000 in North America. Syphilis is still highly prevalent in many developing countries and in some areas of North America, Asia, and Europe, especially Eastern Europe.[6]

Pathogenesis and etiology

The causative agent of venereal syphilis is the spirochete *T. pallidum*, a motile, Gram-negative, bacterium.[1,2]

The infection is virtually always transmitted by direct contact with infectious lesions, generally through sexual contact. It can also be transmitted transplacentally from mother to unborn child and less frequently through blood transfusion. Humans are the only known reservoir.[3]

The treponeme penetrates the skin through intact mucosal membranes and abrasion on epithelial surfaces. It disseminates rapidly through blood vessels and lymphatics, provoking obliterative endarteritis, periarteritis, and plasma cell-rich mononuclear infiltrates as primary histologic features. After an incubation period of 10–90 days (average of 3 weeks), a primary lesion or chancre develops at the site of inoculation. It heals spontaneously after an average of 30 days.[7]

The secondary lesions develop about 4–10 weeks after the appearance of the chancre. Patients may experience malaise, myalgias, fever, arthralgias, generalized body rash, and lymphadenopathy. During this stage, more than 30% of patients have abnormal findings in the cerebrospinal fluid, showing early involvement of the central nervous system. Symptomatic secondary syphilis resolves without treatment in the majority of patients. These patients become non-infectious.[7]

About 6 months after the secondary stage, patients will develop an asymptomatic latent stage. This latent stage may persist with positive serology without clinical manifestations for life in two-thirds of the patients. The other patients develop tertiary syphilis which may involve gummatous, cardiovascular, and/or neurologic manifestations.[1,2,5]

Syphilis is classified into two stages: early- and late-stage. The early stage, with an average duration of 1 year, comprises primary and secondary syphilis and the beginning of the latent stage; the late stage is characterized by the manifestations of tertiary syphilis and latent syphilis.[1]

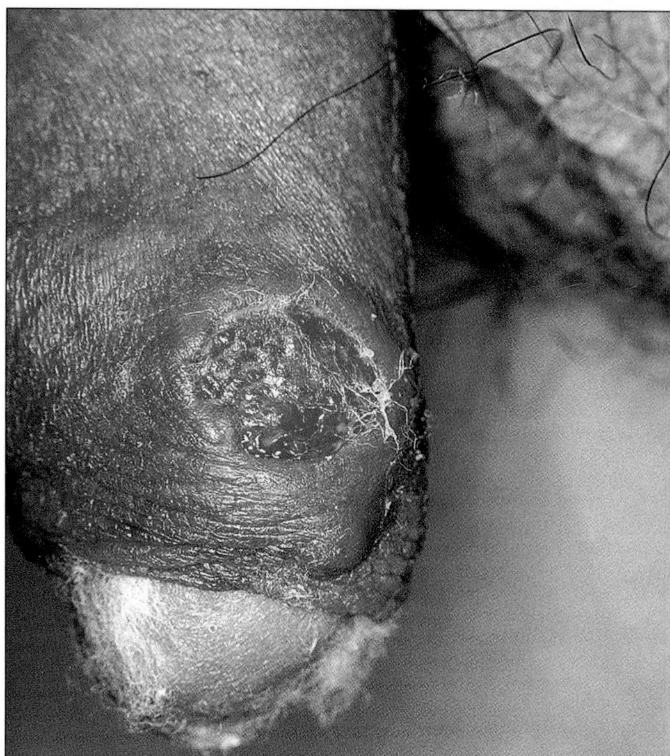

Figure 26.29 Primary syphilis or chancre.

Clinical features

Early syphilis

After an incubation period of 10–90 days (an average of 3 weeks) the first clinical manifestation of syphilis appears; that is the primary syphilis or chancre. Characterized by a shallow, smooth, and clean base, it is a painless ulcer. The borders of the ulcer are raised and indurated. In men the chancre is localized more frequently on the glans, the coronal sulcus, and the foreskin (Fig. 26.29); in women, the labia, fourchette, urethra, and perineum are the most frequent locations of the chancre. The lip is the most frequent location of the extragenital chancre.[2,3,8]

The chancre may be located in any part of the body and in 15–30% the chancre goes unnoticed. Quite frequently the primary lesion is an atypical ulcer, simulating herpes simplex, pyoderma, chancroid, traumatic ulcers, and others. Enlarged and painless lymph nodes located unilaterally in the inguinal area are frequent.

Untreated, the chancre persists from 1 to 6 weeks and disappears spontaneously.[1]

Lesions of secondary syphilis appear after or even in the presence of the chancre, after 3–12 weeks or later. Clinically it is characterized by macular eruption of pink color (roseola syphilitica) that resembles allergies and viruses like measles or rubella (Fig. 26.30). Slowly, there is an evolution of these lesions to papules, papulosquamous eruptions, nodules, and plaques (Figs 26.31–26.33). Annular, serpiginous, concentric, or arcinate configurations may be

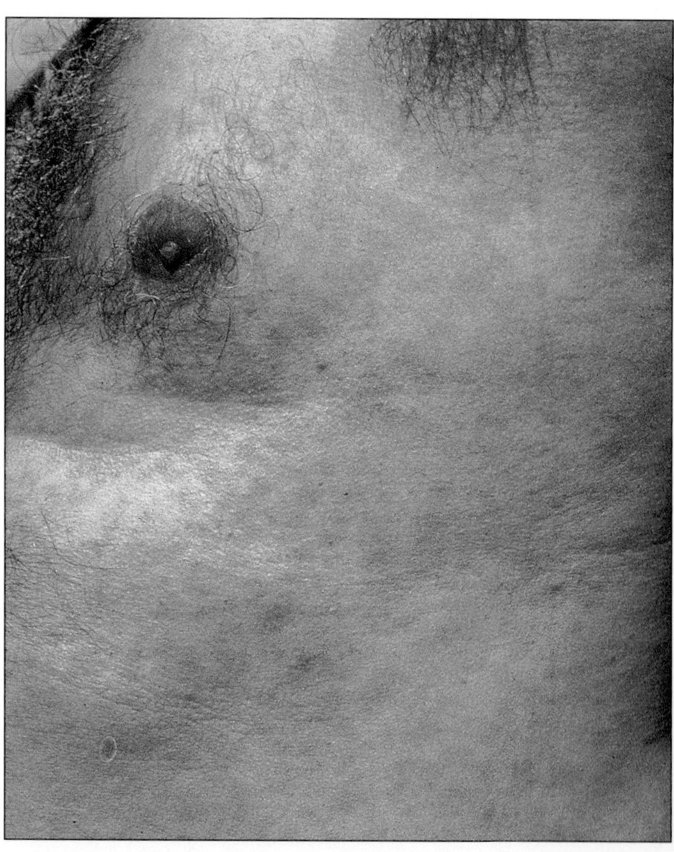

Figure 26.30 Secondary syphilis: roseola syphilitica.

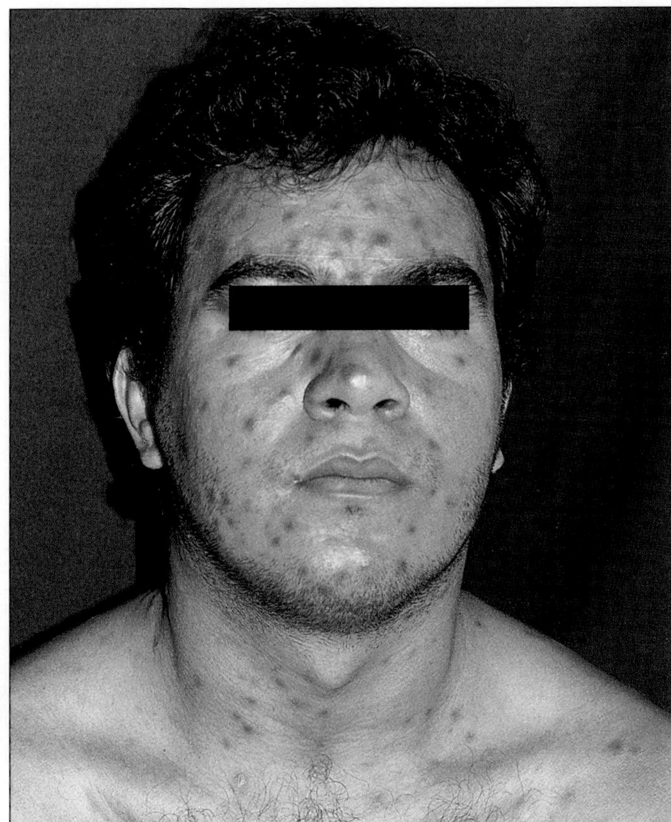

Figure 26.31 Secondary syphilis: disseminated papular lesions.

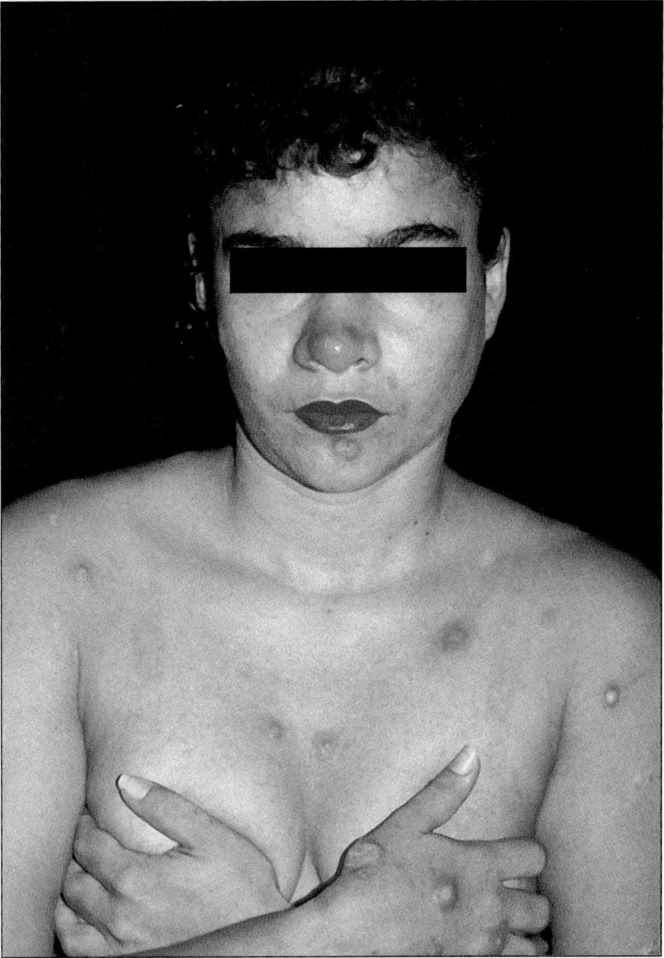

Figure 26.32 Secondary syphilis: papular and nodular lesions.

seen (Fig. 26.34). These lesions may resemble leprosy, psoriasis, and lichen planus.[8]

The palms and soles are frequently involved and the lesions may become hyperkeratotic (Figs 26.35 and 26.36). The lesions on palms and soles are quite typical of secondary syphilis (Fig. 26.37).

Secondary syphilis is often observed on the mucous membranes. These lesions are extremely infectious. The three clinical manifestations are condylomata lata, mucous patches, and pharyngitis. Condylomata lata are located mainly in the anogenital areas and are characterized by moist, oozing papules, which become flattened and macerated; these lesions are frequently confused with venereal warts (Fig. 26.38).[5,9]

Alopecia is another manifestation observed in patients with secondary syphilis (Fig. 26.39). Hair loss is more common on the scalp and occasionally affects the eyebrows and beard; it may be in patches, generalized, or combined. It is observed in 3–7% of patients and may be the only sign of secondary syphilis.[10]

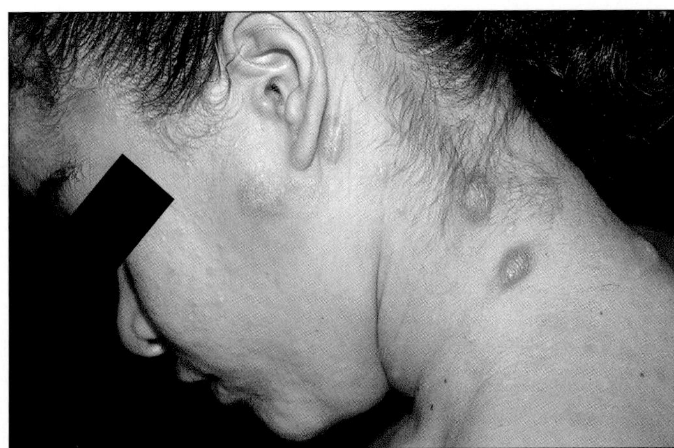

Figure 26.33 Close-up of figure 26.32.

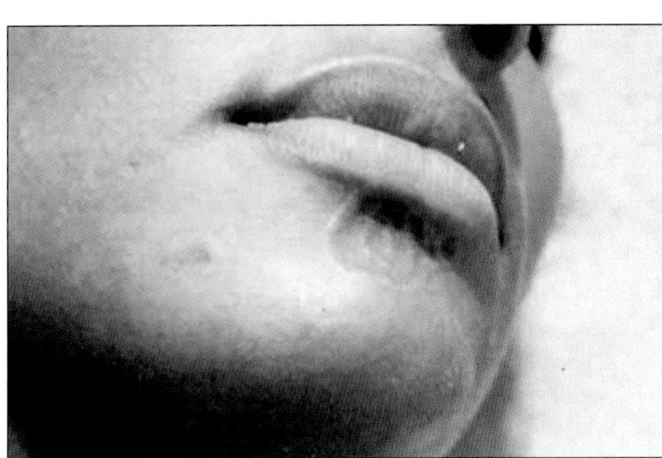

Figure 26.34 Secondary syphilis : annular lesions.

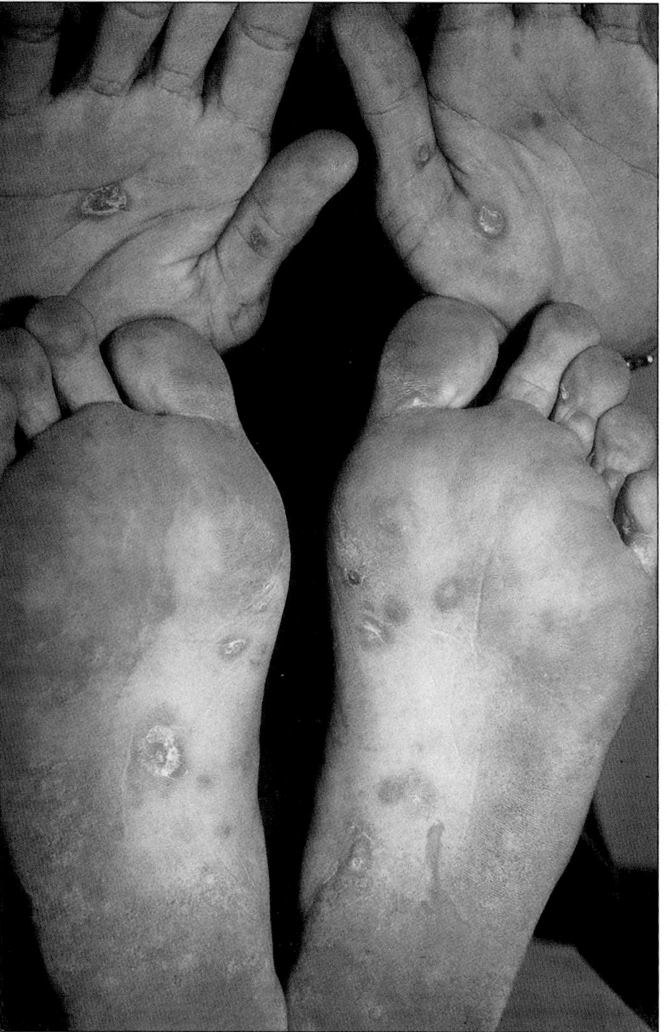

Figure 26.35 Secondary syphilis: hyperkeratotic lesions on palms and soles.

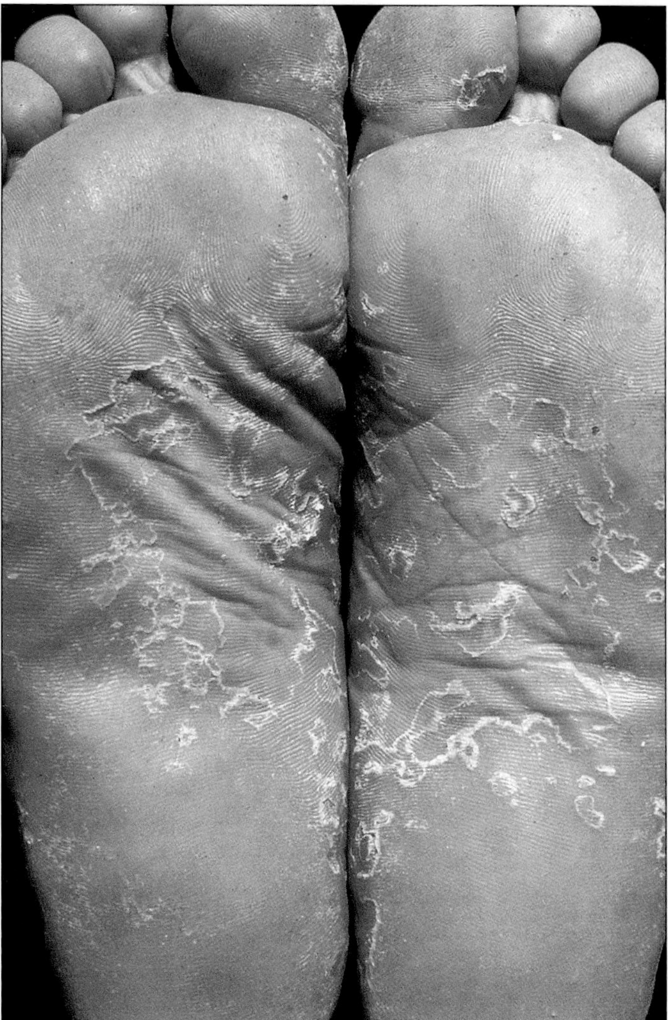

Figure 26.36 Secondary syphilis: hyperkeratotic and squamous lesions, resembling tinea.

Nail plate abnormalities such as onycholysis, splitting, fissuring, and dystrophy are observed. Paronychia and ulceration of the nail bed are also described.

Ophthalmologic, auditory, musculoskeletal, hematologic, renal, hepatic, gastric, cardiopulmonary, and neurologic manifestations may be observed in secondary syphilis.[10]

Enlarged lymphnodes are present in 50–80% of patients with secondary syphilis. The inguinal, axillary, cervical, epitrochlear, femoral, and supraclavicular chains are the most frequently involved.[1,2,5,10]

Even without treatment, all the cutaneous and/or systemic manifestations will disappear spontaneously and the patient enters into the latent stage.

Late or tertiary syphilis

Approximately one-third of patients with untreated latent syphilis develop tertiary syphilis; the other two-thirds remain in latency for life. The three main presentations during late syphilis are late benign (tertiary) syphilis, cardiovascular disease, and neurosyphilis.[10]

The most important cutaneous manifestations related to late benign syphilis are infiltrated grouped papules that tend to ulcerate, nodular, noduloulcerative lesions, and gummas. These lesions may be mistaken for cutaneous tuberculosis, leishmaniasis, chromomycosis, sarcoidosis, sporotrichosis, psoriasis, and other cutaneous diseases.

Diffuse gummatous infiltration may involve mucous membranes, especially the palate, nasal mucosa, tongue, tonsils, and pharynx. Deep mycosis, tuberculosis, leishmaniasis, and malignant tumors must be differentiated from this clinical presentation of syphilis.[5,10]

The most important cardiovascular lesions are aortitis, aortic aneurysm, coronary ostial stenosis, aortic valvular incompetence, and myocardial disease.[5]

Before the introduction of penicillin, between 23 and 87% of cases progressed to clinical neurological disease. Among the most important neurological manifestations are:

- Acute syphilitic meningitis: occurring during the first year of infection
- Parenchymatous neurosyphilis: characterized by tabes dorsalis, general paresis, and optic atrophy

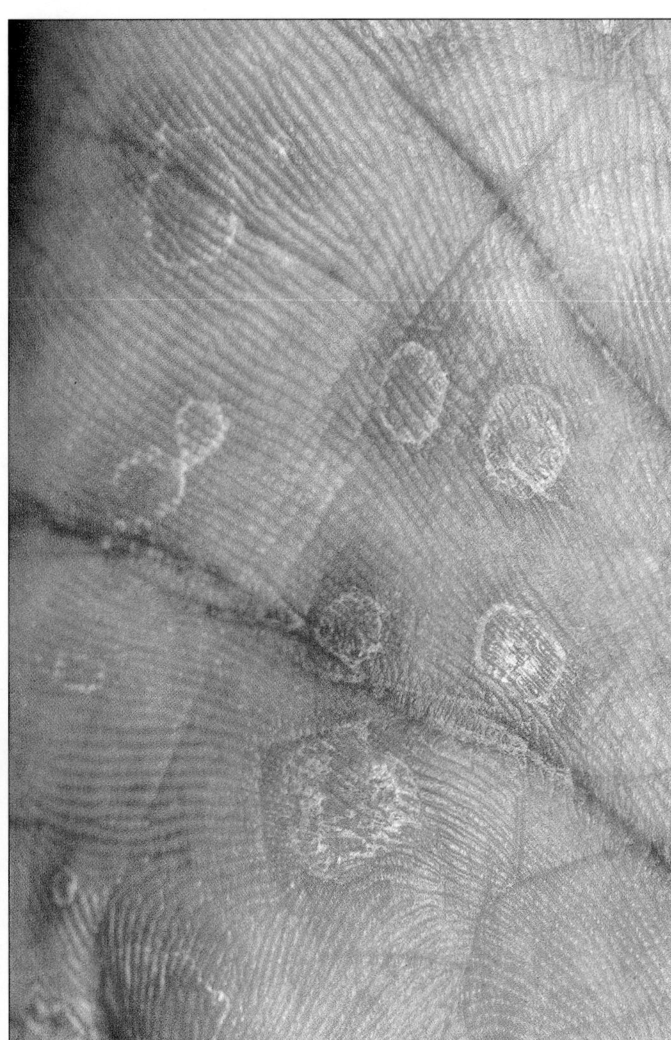

Figure 26.37 Secondary syphilis: Biet's collaret on palms.

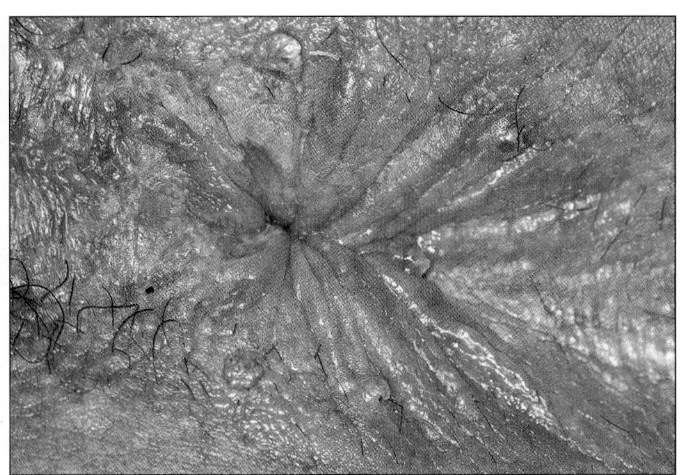

Figure 26.38 Secondary syphilis: condylomata lata on the perianal area.

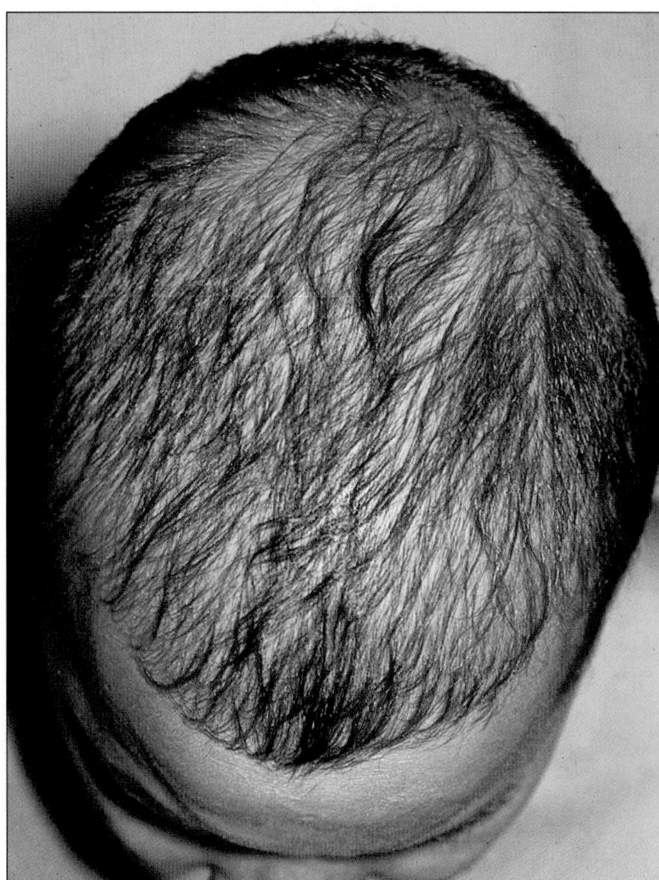

Figure 26.39 Secondary syphilis: patches of alopecia.

- General paresis: characterized by psychiatric, neurologic, or both symptoms.

Congenital syphilis

Without treatment, infected mothers usually transmit the disease to the fetus transplacentally or during delivery.

Syphilis may cause preterm delivery, stillbirth, congenital infection, or neonatal death. In general, the longer the duration of syphilis in the mother, the lower the possibility of the disease transmission to the unborn infant.[10]

Clinically, congenital syphilis is divided into early congenital syphilis and late congenital syphilis.

The manifestations related to early congenital syphilis occur within the first 2 years of life. The cutaneous lesions are similar to those observed in adults with secondary syphilis, except they are more infiltrated, with or without scale, and mainly located on the palms and soles; sometimes bullous lesions (syphilitic pemphigus) are observed (Figs 26.40–26.41). Ulcerations around the mouth, nose, or anus may heal with rhagades (depressed linear scars, or Parrot's lines).[2,5]

Low birth weight, lymphadenopathy, osteochondritis, hepatosplenomegaly, anemia, jaundice, thrombocytopenia, respiratory distress, rhinitis, and pseudoparalysis (Parrot) may also occur.[5]

Neurosyphilis occurs in 40–60% of all syphilitic infants.

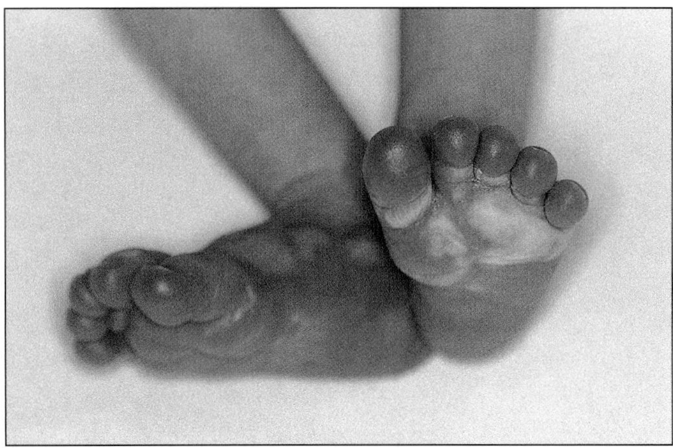

Figure 26.40 Congenital syphilis: syphilitic pemphigus.

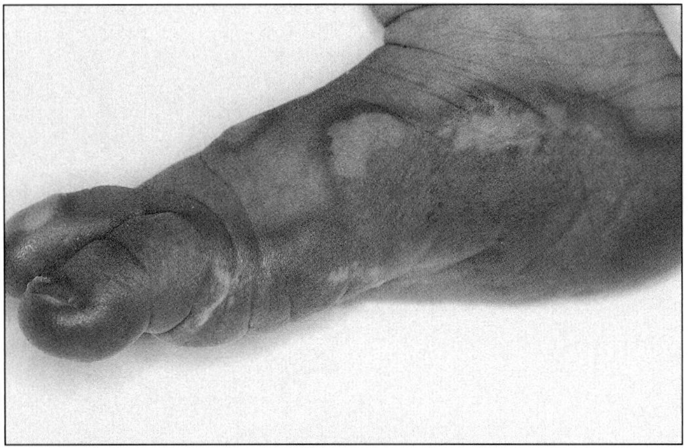

Figure 26.41 Congenital syphilis: same patient as in figure 26.40.

Manifestations of late congenital syphilis occur after the age of 2 years. This can be divided into two groups: active pathologic processes and stigmata, or malformations like frontal bossing, saber shins, dental malformations (Hutchinson's teeth), saddle nose, high arched palate, interstitial keratitis, retinitis, and scaphoid scapula.[10]

Asymptomatic neurosyphilis, bilateral eighth-nerve deafness, skin manifestations (similar to tertiary syphilis), bone manifestations, and paroxysmal cold hemoglobinuria are among the many manifestations that can occur in this type of syphilis.[5]

Syphilis and HIV infection

It is possible that syphilis may accelerate the development of immunodeficiency in HIV-infected patients, and HIV infection may cause reactivation of dormant syphilis.

Most of the HIV-positive patients, coinfected with syphilis, present the classical clinical manifestations of syphilis, the same serological pattern, and a good response to treatment. Some syphilitic patients with AIDS may present nodular, noduloulcerative, and necrotic cutaneous lesions (malignant syphilis).[1]

The prevalence of neurosyphilis is higher in AIDS patients. Neurosyphilis may be the first clinical manifestation of HIV infection, and a fulminant form (necrotizing neurosyphilis) has been reported more frequently in AIDS patients.

Treatment failures have been observed more commonly in patients with low CD4 counts.

All patients with AIDS must be tested for syphilis (and vice versa) and the cerebrospinal fluid of patients with the coinfection AIDS/syphilis must be tested for syphilis.

High VDRL titers may be observed in patients with the coinfection.[1]

Patient evaluation, diagnosis, and differential diagnosis

Chancre

The dark-field examination and histopathology are the most important tests for the confirmation of the diagnosis. These tests are not available in most health services in developing countries and, mainly for this reason, most patients are treated based on the clinical diagnosis. The Veneral Disease Research Laboratory (VDRL) becomes positive 4–5 weeks after infection, and the fluorescent treponemal antibody-absorption test (FTA-ABS) becomes positive at the third week of infection.[5,10]

Secondary, latent, and tertiary syphilis

The diagnosis is screened using the VDRL and rapid plasma reagin (RPR) test. FTA-ABS, *Treponema pallidum* hemagglutination assay (TPHA), microhemagglutination *Treponema pallidum* (MHA-TP) which is becoming the most widely performed treponemal test, and ELISA are specific confirmatory tests. The ELISA test is very sensitive (100%) in congenital syphilis.[5]

The VDRL and RPR are very useful and cheap but non-specific tests and cross-reactions may occur with lepromatous leprosy, Lyme disease, HIV-1, malaria, tuberculosis, and other diseases. In doubtful cases a specific test like FTA-ABS, TPHA, MHA, or ELISA is very important in a patient with strong clinical aspects of syphilis. If a specific test is unavailable, a course of treatment with penicillin is advisable.[5,6]

As a general rule, the later the syphilis, the lower the titer of the serologic tests.

Treatment

The drug of choice is penicillin.[5]

Early syphilis

Treatment for early syphilis is 2.4 million units of benzathine penicillin G i.m. 1 week apart for two doses.

If the patient is allergic to penicillin, tetracycline or erythromycin (500 mg p.o. four times daily for 15 days) is the drug of choice. Ceftriaxone, 250 mg daily or 1 g every other day IV for 10 days, is an alternative.

Late syphilis (except neurosyphilis)

Treatment for late syphilis is 2.4 million units i.m. 1 week apart for three doses.

Tetracycline or erythromycin for 30 days is recommended for patients who are allergic to penicillin. The dosage is the same as that recommended for early syphilis.

Neurosyphilis

Aqueous crystalline penicillin, 18–24 million units administered daily as 3.5–4 million units IV six times daily for 10–14 days, is the treatment of choice.

Pregnant women

The treatment is the same.

Children (acquired syphilis): early syphilis

Treatment for children is benzathine penicillin G 50 000 units/kg i.m. at a single dose; the treatment for late syphilis is the same dosage 3 weeks apart for two doses.

Congenital syphilis

For newborns the treatment is 50 000 units/kg IV of aqueous penicillin G every 12 h for the first 7 days of life. For the next 3 days the recommended treatment is aqueous penicillin in the same dosage every 8 h or 50 000 units/kg of procaine penicillin G IM daily for 10–14 days.

For postneonatal syphilis, benzathine penicillin G is used in a dose of 50 000 units/kg IM if the cerebrospinal fluid examination is negative. Intravenous aqueous crystalline penicillin must be used in cases of neurosyphilis. The standard dose is 50 000 units/kg IV every 4–6 h for 10–14 days.

References

1. Azulay DR, Azulay MM. Doenças sexualmente transmissíveis. In: Schecther M, Marangoni DV, eds. Doenças infecciosas: conduta diagnóstica e terapêutica, 2nd edn. Rio de Janeiro: Guanabara Koogan; 1998:210–219.
2. Azulay RD, Azulay DR. Treponematoses. In: Azulay RD, Azulay DR, eds. Dermatologia, 3rd edn. Rio de Janeiro: Guanabara Koogan; 2004:197–199.
3. Hay RJ, Adrians BM. Bacterial infections. In: Champion RH, Burton JL, Burns DA et al. Text of dermatology, 6th edn. London: Blackwell Science; 1998:95.
4. Ministério da Saúde. Manual de controle das doenças sexualmente transmissíveis, 3rd edn. Brasilia: Coordenação Nacional de DST/AIDS; 1999.
5. Sampaio SAP, Rivitti EA. Sífilis e treponematoses. In: Sampaio SAP, Rivitti EA, eds. Dermatologia, 1st edn. São Paulo: Editora Artes Médicas; 1998:122–129.
6. Division of STD Prevention. Sexually transmitted disease surveillance 2001. Atlanta, GA: Department of Health and Human Services; 2003.
7. Sanchez MR. Syphilis. In: Freedberg IW, Fitzpatrick TB, eds. Fitzpatrick's dermatology in general dermatology, 5th edn. New York: McGraw-Hill; 1999.
8. Tramont EC. *Treponema pallidum* (syphilis). In: Mandell GL, Bennett JE, Dolin R, eds. Principles and practice of infectious disease, 4th edn. New York: Churchill Livingstone; 1995:2117–2132.
9. Morton RS. The treponematoses. In: Champion RH, Burton JL, Ebling FJG, eds. Rook, Wilkinson and Ebling textbook of dermatology. London: Blackwell Scientific; 1992:1085–1126.
10. Talhari S, Neves RG. Sífilis. In: Talhari S, Neves RG, eds. Doenças sexualmente transmissíveis e manifestações cutâneas relacionadas à AIDS. Rio de Janeiro: Manaus, 2002:11–24.

Endemic treponematoses

Sinésio Talhari and Carolina Talhari

Introduction

The endemic and non-venereal treponematoses comprise pinta, endemic syphilis, and yaws. They are not sexually transmitted diseases at all but were included in this chapter because their etiologic agent is almost identical, both morphologically and antigenically, to *Treponema pallidum*, the agent of syphilis. These distinct and chronic diseases have predominantly affected economically disadvantaged, isolated rural areas of tropical and subtropical countries, and were once a major health concern in many Third-World countries. Speciation among these agents has to be based on clinical and epidemiological aspects since they are so related to each other and with *Trepomema pallidum*. The causative agents of endemic treponematoses are morphologically and serologically indistinguishable. Therefore speciation has to be based on clinical and epidemiological aspects.

Pinta

Synonyms: Pinta is also known as azula (blue), and mal de pinto (pinto sickness)

Key features:

- Pinta is a chronic infectious/contagious disease
- It is not sexually transmitted or congenitally acquired
- It is the most benign and unusual treponematosis and its only manifestation is on the skin
- It affects people of all ages[1,2]

History

The word pinta comes from the Spanish and means painted, spot, or mark. Pinta is considered the first treponematosis to occur in humans. It was described in Aztec and Caribbean Amerindians in the early years of the sixteenth century.[2,3] In 1938, *Treponema carateum* was recognized as the causative agent of pinta by Armenteros and Triana (Cuba).[2] Leon and Blanco in Mexico reproduced the disease by inoculating exudates into normal volunteers in 1942. Padilha Gonçalves established that pinta was a different treponematosis from syphilis or yaws.[2,4]

Epidemiology

Most patients acquire the infection during childhood. There is no difference between the two sexes. The indigenous population is the most affected.[1]

These treponematoses existed as an endemic disease in Brazil, Colombia, Ecuador, Peru, and Venezuela. The number of cases was less in Bolivia, Dominican Republic, El Salvador, Guatemala, Haiti, Honduras, and Nicaragua; it was occasionally seen in Cuba, Guadeloupe, Panama, Puerto Rico, and the Virgin Islands.[5] In Brazil this disease was supposed to be extinct until 1975, when 265 new cases of pinta were diagnosed among Baniwas, Canamari, Paumari, and Ticuna Indians.[2,4] These Indians lived in small communities on the banks of the Amazon, Içana, Juruá, Purus, and upper Negro rivers and some tributaries of the western Amazon river. Since 1979, no further cases of pinta have been reported to the World Health Organization from previously endemic areas.[2,4] The last report of cases from Colombia was in 1977. Cuba reported its last case in 1975; however, in 1998 a patient who had lived in Cuba for 7 years was diagnosed with pinta in Austria.[5] Today it is believed that the disease still exists in very isolated communities in remote rural areas of Mexico and South America, especially in a few scattered areas in the Brazilian Amazon rain forest.[4]

There is no proof of a spontaneous cure for the disease and because cell-mediated immunity is not completely effective, the infection persists indefinitely. Patients may harbor subclinical disease and be contagious for a long time. It has been said that pinta was man's best friend: it follows him to the grave![4]

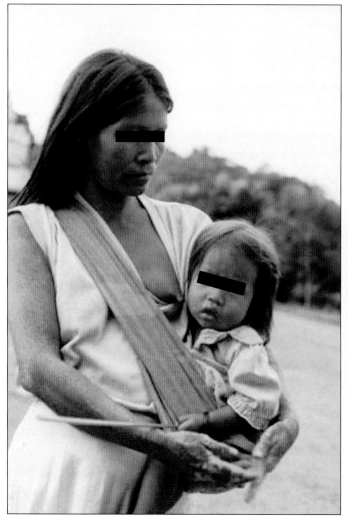

Figure 26.42 Pinta: transmission of pinta via direct contact with an infected person.

Pathogenesis and etiology

The disease is caused by *T. carateum*, an organism that is morphologically and antigenically identical to the etiologic agent of syphilis and yaws.[4]

The disease is usually acquired during early childhood and spreads through direct contact with an infected person or fomites (Fig. 26.42). The only known reservoir is humans. The treponeme enters the skin through small cuts, scratches, or other skin damage.[2]

Clinical features

Pinta is classified into two different clinical stages: primary- and late-stage.[4]

Primary stage

The primary stage is divided into two phases, an early phase or initial period, and a secondary phase or period of cutaneous dissemination. According to Padilha-Gonçalves,[6,7] the initial period appears 7–20 days after the treponeme inoculation. The primary lesions are characterized by erythematous papules, affecting most commonly the face, upper and lower extremities, or other exposed areas.[2,4] These lesions tend to grow in extension, producing erythematosquamous or erythematous, hyperpigmented plaques (Fig. 26.43), varying in size and shape (arciform, circinate, polycyclic, and serpinginous). Generally, the lesions are asymptomatic and eventually patients may complain of pruritus. Within 6 months to 2–3 years of the first lesions' appearance, hypochromic, erythematous, or erythematohypochromic patches appear, initiating the period of cutaneous dissemination. Those lesions present variable degrees of hyperkeratosis.[5,8] The lesions are small and sometimes nummular. They gradually enlarge and coalesce, affecting large areas of the body with normal skin in the center of the lesions (Fig. 26.44). These lesions are referred to as pintides, and are initially red to violaceous and later become slate-blue, brown, gray, or black. Lesions from different periods may be present in a single patient, forming polymorphic clinical features.[8,9]

Late stage

The hallmark of this stage, which appears 2–5 years after the first lesion, is the appearance of achromic patches, especially over body prominences, such as the dorsum of the hands, wrist, elbows, anterior part of the tibia, ankles, and dorsal and plantar areas of the foot. In this period, large hypochromic areas commonly appear on the upper extremities, trunk, and thighs.[4,9] One may observe cutaneous atrophy, achromic puntiform lesions, and multiple hyperchromic lesions, producing a mottled pattern (Fig. 26.45). The appearance of hypochromic patches with irregular borders and hypochromic macules is quite frequent on buttocks. Curiously, the

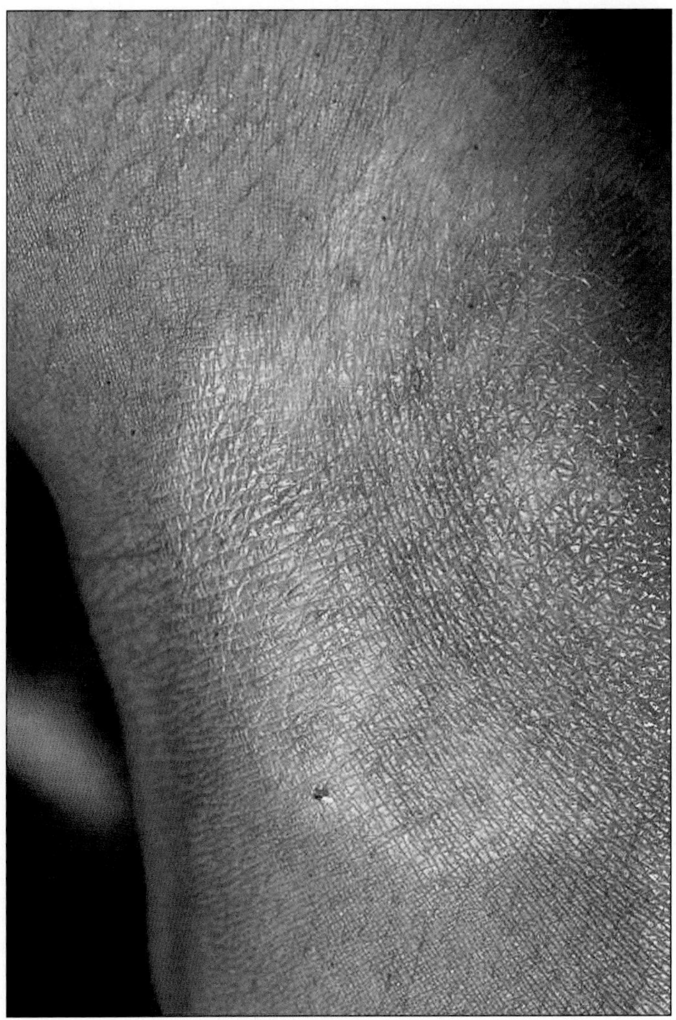

Figure 26.43 Pinta: primary stage; erythematous and erythematosquamous hyperpigmented plaques.

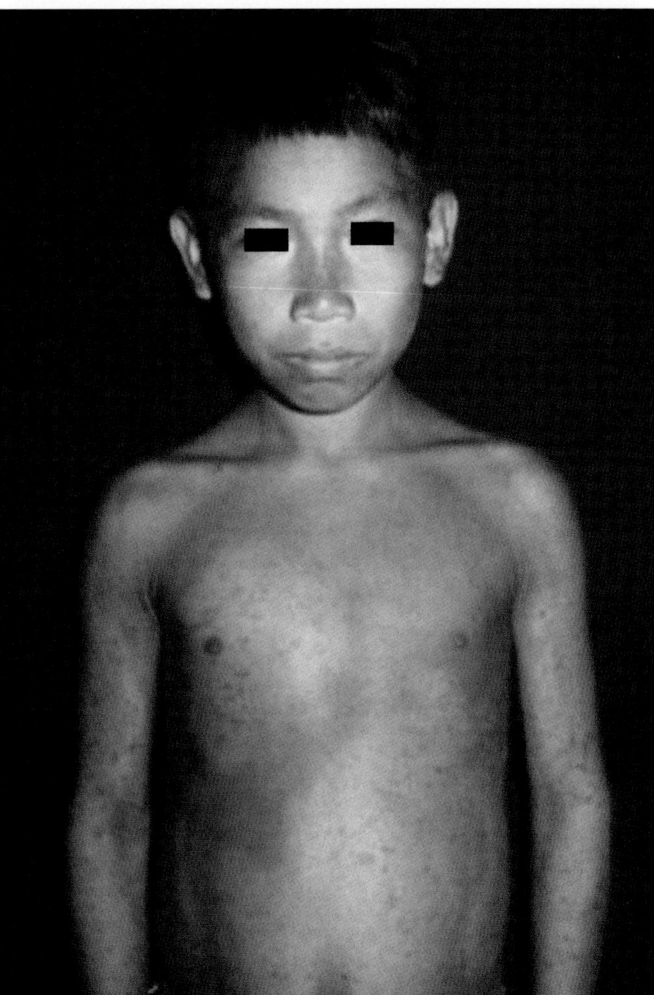

Figure 26.44 Pinta: period of cutaneous dissemination characterized by hypochromic patches.

groin, genital area, and the inner and upper parts of the thighs are often spared. Another very important aspect of the late phase of pinta is the appearance of hyperchromic and hyperkeratotic patches most commonly on exposed areas of the upper and lower extremities (Fig. 26.46). On the palmar surfaces hyperpigmented and achromic patches associated with hyperkeratosis are usually observed (Fig. 26.47(A)). Plantar hyperkeratosis is quite frequent (Fig. 26.47(B)). In some patients, even with a history of the disease, the cutaneous lesions may be confined to a limited area of the body. There is no evidence of involvement of other organs, even after many years of evolution.[5,10]

Patient evaluation, diagnosis, and differential diagnosis

The diagnosis may be made by:

- Dark-field microscopic examination from lymph obtained from the skin lesions.
- The most common serologic tests used are TPHA, FTA-ABS, MHA-TP, and non-treponemal serology tests such as the VDRL and RPR.[2,4,11]
- Animal inoculation: *T. carateum* cannot be cultured in vitro, but can be transmitted to chimpanzees. This method is not used for diagnosis.[4]

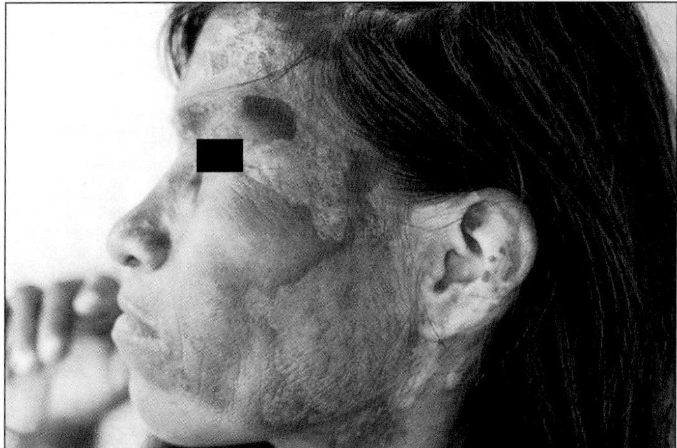

Figure 26.45 Pinta: hyperchromic, hypochromic, and achromic patches. Late stage.

- Histopathology is important for the diagnosis. The primary lesions are characterized by mild acanthosis, epidermal edema with lymphocyte migration, and liquefaction degeneration of the basal cell layer. In the dermis the changes consist of a slight lymphohistiocytic and plasmocytic infiltrate and a mild vascular reaction.[4] In the secondary stage the

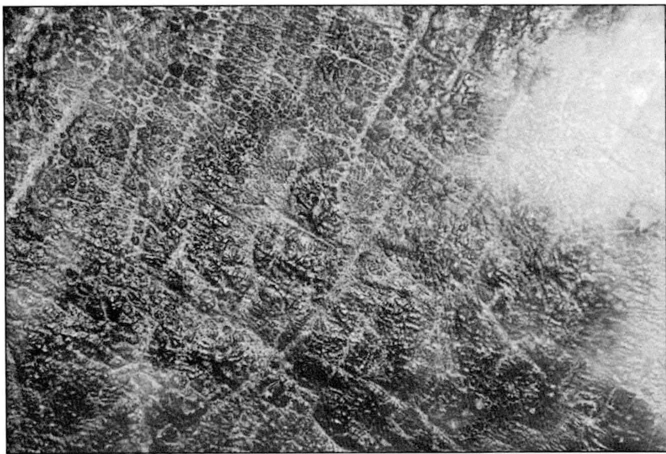

Figure 26.46 Pinta: hyperkeratosis, and achromic lesions. Late stage.

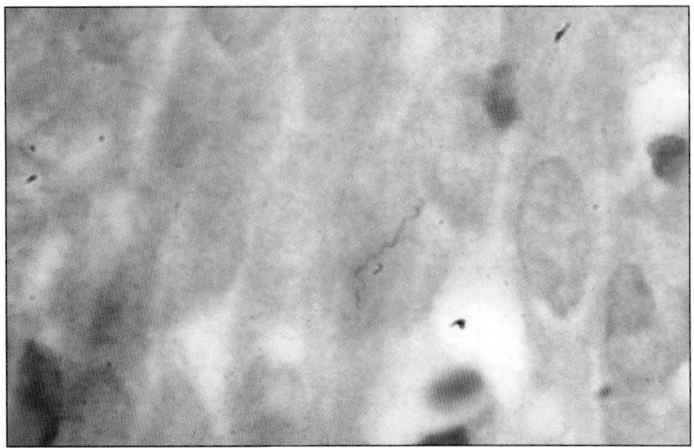

Figure 26.48 Pinta: presence of treponeme on the epidermis, shown on Warthin–Starry stain.

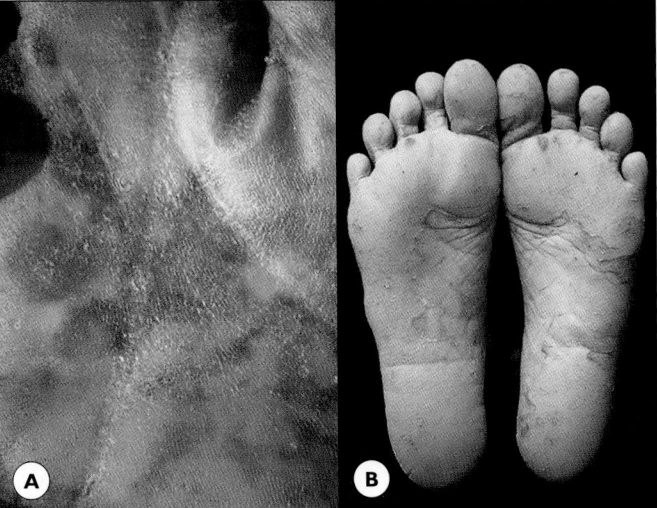

Figure 26.47 Pinta: (A) Hyperchromic and hyperkeratotic patches on the palmar surface. (B) Hyperkeratotic areas on the plantar surface.

hypochromic lesions are present with moderate hyperkeratosis, acanthosis, and spongiosis. There is a superficial infiltrate around the thickened vessels. In the erythematous and squamous lesions, the Malpighian layer is enlarged with hyperkeratosis and spongiosis. There is a lymphohistiocytic infiltrate in the dermis plus edema and vascular neoproliferation in the papillary dermis. In the achromic lesions there are hyperkeratosis, atrophy of the epidermis, complete absence of melanin in the papillary dermis and an inflammatory infiltrate. It is possible to demonstrate the presence of the treponeme in the epidermis through special stains like Warthin–Starry (Fig. 26.48) in all lesions, with the exception of achromic lesions.[2,5,12]

Initially pinta must be differentiated from tinea, psoriasis, erythema dyschromicum perstans, tinea versicolor, eczema, leprosy, cutaneous tuberculosis, and some clinical aspects of yaws and endemic syphilis.

After treatment, late pinta may be difficult to distinguish from vitiligo. In this case, the previous existence of pigmentation, hyperkeratosis, and other features of pinta are important.

Treatment

The recommended treatment for pinta, irrespective of the stage of the disease, is a single or divided dose of benzathine penicillin G (600 000–4 800 000 U). Within a few days, the hypochromic and erythematosquamous lesions disappear. Later, the hyperpigmented and recent achromic lesions disappear. The old achromic patches do not usually respond to the treatment, and persist for life.[2,4]

Endemic syphilis

Synonyms: Endemic syphilis is known by many local names: bejel (in Iraq, Mongolia, Russia, and Syria), skerljevo (in the Balkans), sibbins (in Scotland), radesyge (in the Scandinavian countries), njovera or dichuchwa (in southern Africa), and belesh or bishel (Bedouins of Saudi Arabia)[13]

Key features:

- The disease is a non-venereal chronic childhood treponematosis
- It occurs in isolated closed communities with poor hygienic conditions
- It affects the skin, mucous membranes, muscles, bone, and cartilage
- It is less invasive than venereal syphilis

History

Endemic syphilis is assumed to have existed before 8000 BC, most probably as a result of a mutation of *T. pallidum* as an adaptation to differing epidemiologic influences.

Epidemiology

The main reservoir of endemic syphilis is in children 2–15 years of age. Adults may also become infected. There is no clear sex preponderance.[13,14]

The disease was highly prevalent in dry, arid, hot, and temperate climates in the eastern hemisphere, especially in isolated and primitive rural and semiurban communities living under unhygienic conditions crowded together in small places such as huts or tents.

It used to be endemic in North Africa, Southwest Asia, Northern Europe, and the Eastern Mediterranean basin. Today it occurs primarily among nomadic and seminomadic tribes in Saudi Arabia, in the Turaiba area and sub-Saharan Africa.[13–15]

During the second decade of the nineteenth century the disease was eradicated in the regions of Inner Carniola and Carst (Slovenia) as a result of social and health changes. Compulsory medical examination of inhabitants in the affected area, treatment of patients, and preventive measures were initiated. Bulgaria has also eradicated the disease in treatment campaigns between 1958 and 1960.[15]

In 1987 the Programme for the Control of the Endemic Treponematoses (World Health Organization) reported a dramatic increase in cases of bejel in sub-Saharan Africa. A survey carried out in this region showed that 15–40% of children had serologic evidence of treponemal infection and 2–20% had initial lesions of endemic syphilis. In 1988, a survey among Bedouin tribes in the Middle East reported that bejel was prevalent in up to 27% of those born and bred in the desert.[13,14]

Pathogenesis and etiology

The organism responsible for endemic syphilis is *T. pallidum* subsp. *endemicum*, which is indistinguishable microscopically from the organisms of syphilis, yaws, or pinta.[13]

Endemic syphilis is a familial treponematosis that spreads usually among children and, less commonly, to adults. Adults who were not infected during childhood are at risk of contracting the disease later, especially from their own children. The disease is most probably transmitted directly via infected lesions on the skin and mucous membranes (frequently by kissing) and by contaminated fingers. Infections can also occur indirectly through infected drinking vessels or pipes. There is little, if any, evidence of congenital transmission. The infection is facilitated by promiscuity, lack of cleanness, little or no clothing, and by lesions with abundant secretions rich in treponemes.[13,16]

There is no evidence of direct transmission of treponemes by fomites, flies, or other insects.

Clinical features

Endemic syphilis is divided into an early and a late stage. The early stage includes a primary and secondary period and the late stage comprises the latent stage and tertiary disease.

Early stage

The primary lesion is rare in endemic syphilis when compared to yaws and pinta. An initial chancre is present in only about 1% of cases. It is believed, however, that the lesion is more common than reported, possibly being unnoticed because of its minimal size or its location due to the small inoculum involved. The primary stage is characterized by a small papule or ulcer, usually occurring on the nipples of breast-feeding women, on the mouth or the labial commissures rather than true chancre.[13,14,16]

Secondary lesions appear after an incubation period of 2–3 months. At this stage the typical lesions are shallow and relatively painless patches on mucous membranes, accompanied by hoarseness caused by syphilitic laryngitis. Angular stomatitis, non-itchy skin eruptions, and generalized lymphadenopathy with discrete, mobile, non-tender, firm nodes are also important secondary manifestations. Axillary and anogenital condylomata lata are other manifestations of this period. On a rare occasion, one may observe a macular, papular, or annular papulosquamous eruption. Alopecia can be present in small scattered irregular patches, producing a "moth-eaten" appearance. As in yaws, a painful osteoperiostitis may occur.[13,16]

Late stage

The late stage comprises the latent stage and the tertiary period.

In the latent stage there are no clinical signs or symptoms and the spinal fluid is normal. This stage occurs after early lesions have subsided and may last from 5 to 15 years. The treponemes can only be detected by reactive serologic tests.

The tertiary stage develops from 6 months to several years after the period of latency. It affects the skin, bones, and cartilage. Cardiologic and neurologic involvement is extremely rare, or even absent. According to Tabbara et al.,[17] the most frequently encountered ophthalmologic manifestations in 17 patients with clinical and serological evidence of endemic syphilis were uveitis, choroiditis, chorioretinitis, and optic atrophy.

The cutaneous manifestations of the tertiary stage are superficial nodular or tuberous lesions and deep gummatous lesions. The gummas are masses of granulomatous syphilitic tissue, which undergo necrosis. They tend to disappear after time, leaving characteristic atrophic, depigmented scars surrounded by hyperpigmentation. Gummata of the nasopharyx, larynx, skin, and bone (gangosa) are common in this stage and may progress to destructive chronic ulcers. The most frequently described long bone lesions are exostosis and periostitis, affecting especially the tibia (saber tibia) and fibula. The bones of the central part of the face are also affected, causing severe destructive lesions of the palate and nasal septum associated with difficulties with articulation and swallowing.[13,16]

Attenuated endemic syphilis

In 1985, Csonka and Pace[14] described a clinically attenuated form of endemic syphilis in Saudi Arabia. This survey showed a reduced number, severity, and duration of both early and late lesions. In attenuated endemic syphilis the majority of patients have latent disease and are asymptomatic. The main complaint was persistent pain in the legs, often associated with radiologic evidence of osteoperiostitis of the tibia and fibula. The authors hypothesized that persistent lesions are sustained by superinfection and that improvements in hygiene have resulted in a decrease in the incidence of reexposure.

Patient evaluation, diagnosis, and differential diagnosis

The diagnosis is based on epidemiologic, clinical, and laboratory findings. Positive serologic tests, the presence of treponemes in dark-field examination of exudates of skin lesions, and examination of skin biopsies usually confirm the diagnosis.[13,17]

The serologic tests are the same as those described for pinta.

Histopathological changes are identical to venereal syphilis, consisting of a perivascular infiltrate of plasmacytes and lymphocytes, intimal proliferation of veins and arteries, and a granulomatous infiltrate progressing to caseation in the late stage of the disease. The most characteristic finding which differentiates endemic and venereal syphilis from yaws and pinta is the intimal proliferation of the vessels.[14]

The differential diagnosis includes other treponematoses, especially venereal syphilis and yaws. Other dermatoses resembling early endemic syphilis are psoriasis, eczema, pityriasis rosea, lichen planus, leprosy, mycoses, herpes simplex, condyloma acuminatum, and many diseases presenting with a generalized rash.

Oral lesions of endemic syphilis must be differentiated from aphthosis, perlèche, vitamin deficiency, and herpes. The differential diagnosis of late-stage manifestations includes mycosis fungoides, leukemias, infiltrated types of rosacea, and facial granuloma. Mutilating nasopharyngeal lesions may resemble tuberculosis, leprosy, rhinoscleroma, rhinosporidiosis, mucocutaneous leishmaniasis, and South American blastomycosis.

Treatment

Treatment consists of long-acting penicillin preparations. Patients with active lesions, family members, all other contacts of patients and patients with latent infections must receive 1 200 000 units of benzathine penicillin G. The dosage for patients under 10 years old is 600 000 units. The dosage is the same for yaws and is administered as a single intramuscular injection. In cases of penicillin allergy, erythromycin or tetracycline is recommended. After treatment, early lesions heal within 2 weeks.[13,15]

The major parameters used to measure the response to treatment are changes in titers determined by quantitative non-treponemal tests. Treponemal tests may remain positive for life, despite therapy.

Yaws

Synonyms: Yaws is known by many names: pian in French, framböise (raspberry), bouba in Spanish, and parangi and paru in Malay[18]

Key features:

- Yaws is a chronic infectious, relapsing treponematosis caused by the spirochete *Treponema pallidum* subsp. *pertenue*
- It is not sexually or congenitally acquired
- The disease is characterized by three stages: an initial ulcer or cutaneous granuloma called the "mother yaws"; early non-destructive and late destructive lesions of the skin, bones, and periosteum
- The late manifestation may produce disabling deformities.[18]

History

Bone lesions found in skeletal remains of *Homo erectus* in Nairobi suggest that yaws had its origin in Africa during the middle Pleistocene period (1.5 million years ago).[19] The disease was brought to the New World by black slaves. The etiological agent was identified by Aldo Castellani in 1906 in Sri Lanka.

Epidemiology

Yaws is a disease particularly of childhood. Both sexes are equally affected.

This treponematoses affects especially rural populations in the rain forest areas of the world where high levels of humidity and rainfall prevail. Yaws, like endemic syphilis, is a disease of poverty.[18]

There were an estimated 50–150 million cases of active yaws in the early 1950s. The disease was distributed in regions between the tropics of Cancer and Capricorn, including areas of Africa, Asia, South and Central America, and the Pacific Islands.[20–22] More than 40 million people had the disease, varying from disseminated skin lesions to gross destruction of tissues, joints, and bones. A dramatic decline in the prevalence of yaws was brought about by the implementation of mass treatment campaigns with penicillin under the technical guidance of World Health Organization and with material support from the United Nations Children's Fund (UNICEF) in the 1950s and 1960s.[18] However, the persistence of poverty as well as the lack of public health surveillance and prophylactic control measures resulted in the resurgence of yaws in some tropical countries.

In the Central African Republic a survey conducted in 1987 in itinerant pygmies detected 15% of children with serologically confirmed yaws.[22] Outbreaks of yaws have been reported in the Solomon Islands; the last one was in 1988, despite mass population treatment campaigns conducted in 1984 and 1987. In 1990, an outbreak of yaws was also reported from a rural village in southern Thailand.[20]

A survey in 1988 in the northern region of Ecuador documented a prevalence of 16.5% of clinical cases and 96.3% of serological cases. In 1993, a second survey showed a reduction in the prevalence of clinical cases to 1.4% and of serological cases to 4.7%. Between 1993 and 1998, no other clinical case was detected and the serological prevalence in 1998 was 3.5%. In Indonesia, the site of the largest treatment campaign in the 1950s, widely dispersed foci of endemic infection continue to exist.[23]

As in many other countries, yaws was supposed to be eradicated in Nigeria. In 1994, 64 cases of yaws were encountered during an epidemiological survey for filariasis in the mid-Hawal river valley.[21]

Yaws seems to be endemic in rural Guyana. In 2000 a control program was implemented in this country. This program screened and treated 1020 children (14 years old or younger) with active lesions. These children were treated with oral penicillin V for 7–10 days. In 2001, 516 children were reexamined and active lesions retreated. The prevalence of yaws skin lesions fell from 5.1% to 1.6%, a 71% drop.[18]

In some African, South American, and Southwest Asian countries, the prevalence levels now approach the precampaign levels. It is estimated that, at present, at least 100 million children are at risk of acquiring yaws.[20–23]

Pathogenesis and etiology

Yaws is caused by *T. pallidum* subsp. *pertenue*.

These treponematoses are transmitted by direct skin contact with the exudates or serum from an open primary or secondary lesion. Spirochetes cannot enter intact skin: it must be facilitated by breaks in the skin from wounds, abrasions, scratches, or bites. Mechanical transmission by a fly, *Hippelates pallipes*, has been established but does not seem to be important.[18]

Clinical features

There are three clinical stages in yaws: primary, secondary, and tertiary.

Primary stage

The initial lesion of yaws is called "mother yaws." It arises at the site of entry of the organism anywhere on the skin, but most commonly on legs, feet, and buttocks. The lesion appears 9–90 days (average of 21) after inoculation. Mother yaws is an erythematous infiltrated papule or a group of papules on an erythematous base. Those lesions may enlarge rapidly and form a papillomatous, vegetative, "frambesiform" ulcer with a shiny, yellowish-red base. This base shows serous fluid, which may sometimes be bloody and may dry up, forming an adherent brownish crust. The lesions are round to oval, varying in size from 1 to 5 cm (Fig. 26.49). They are painless and are considered highly infectious. Treponemes are easily detected by dark-field examination. The clinical picture is usually modified by secondary infection. After several weeks to months, mother yaws frequently heals spontaneously, leaving an atrophic and hypopigmented or pitted scar surrounded by a darker halo. In 10% of patients, there is no primary stage; the disease passes directly into its secondary period.[18,24]

Systemic symptoms such as fever and joint pain are sometimes present, appearing before or with the primary lesion. Regional lymphadenopathy is present in most cases with discrete, non-suppurative, large, firm nodes. Without secondary infection, lymphadenopathy is painless.

Secondary stage

This stage is characterized by disseminated cutaneous lesions that appear in untreated cases after the healing of the initial lesion. The clinical picture of this stage is a widespread, often bilateral and symmetrical eruption. This eruption may be present in two main clinical features: a large one that resembles the mother yaws and is called "daughter yaws," pianoma or frambesia (Fig. 26.50) and a micropapular type, called miniature yaws. Patients may show both varieties simultaneously. Daughter yaws are smaller than mother yaws, and are multiple. Miniature yaws consist of lichenoid, firm, and pink papules which appear in crops around the mother yaws, forming later a miliary follicular eruption. The most commonly affected locations are the face, particularly the nose and mouth, and intertriginous moist surfaces, such as axillae, buttocks, anus, and vulva. Later the lesions may affect the trunk, head, and arms.[18]

The lesions may also be condylomatous, circinate, and annular, resembling tinea, or may even be present as a morbilliform eruption. Rarely, patients may show a macular eruption (yaws roseola) or hypochromic and squamous macules on the trunk.

Usually the soles present thick hyperkeratotic plaques with fissures and pain, forcing the patients, especially children, to walk with a peculiar gait, known as "crab yaws." Plantar granulomas may break down and result in painful ulcerations. The toe or finger nails can also be involved. The appearance of papillomas in the nail fold causes a paronychia that is called frambesial onychia or pianic onychia. The palms are less involved.[18,24]

Cutaneous lesions usually heal, leaving a hypochromic area. More destructive lesions and those with secondary infections may leave an atrophic scar.

Painful osteoperiostitis and polydactylitis of the hand, forearm, leg, and foot are the most common secondary bone lesions. These may be the first manifestations of the disease, especially in

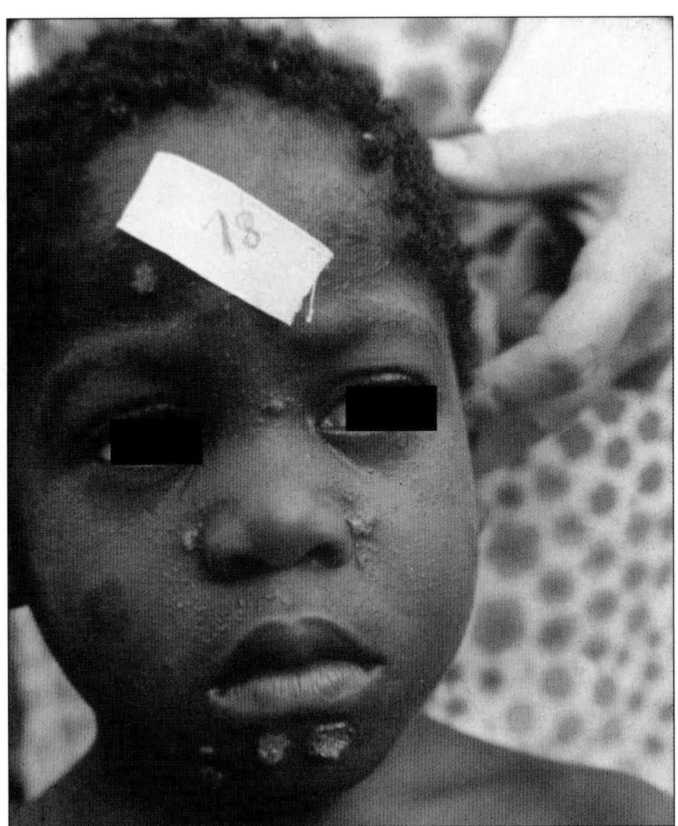

Figure 26.49 Primary stage of yaws: "mother yaws," erythematous infiltrated group of papules on an erythematous base. (Courtesy of Prof. A Basset and J. Malleville.)

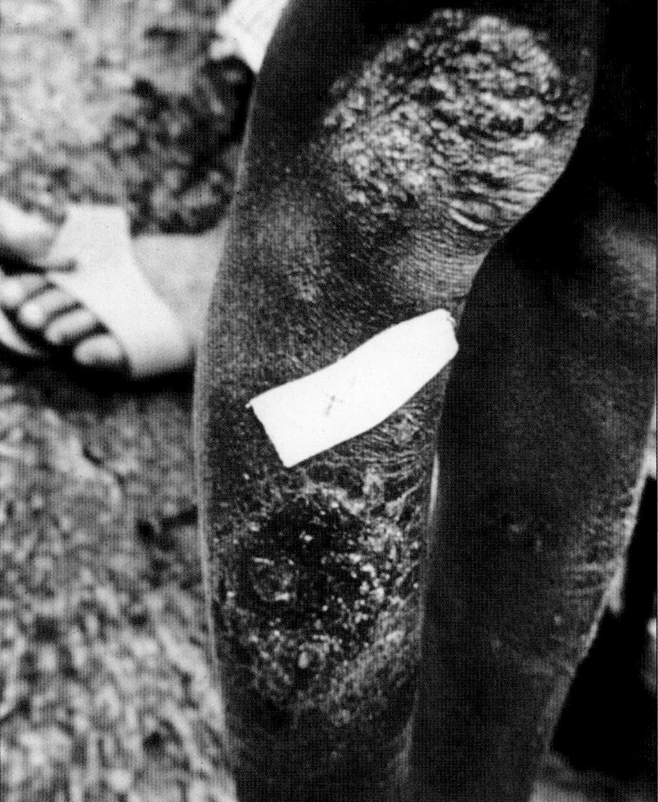

Figure 26.50 Secondary stage of yaws: "daughter yaws," pianoma or framboesia. The lesions on the lower limbs are circinated. (Courtesy of Prof. A Basset and J. Malleville).

children, with a rapid onset and spontaneous resolution after a few weeks or months. Periosteal thickening and reaction of underlying bone may also be seen in this stage of the disease.[24,25]

Lesions on the mucocutaneous junction may affect the mucosa, but true involvement of the mucous membranes is rare in yaws. There is no alopecia.

Systemic symptoms and signs, such as fever, headache, generalized adenopathy, and nocturnal bone pain, may be present in this stage.

Tertiary stage

Late yaws appears in untreated or undertreated patients several years after the initial lesion. It occurs in approximately 10% of cases. Lesions from earlier stages may be present in a single patient, overlapping with late yaws. There are asymptomatic cases for many years, where positive serological tests are the only evidence of the disease. This stage affects the skin, subcutaneous tissues, mucous membranes, bones, and joints. The presence of neurological, cardiovascular, and ophthalmological lesions is very controversial.[25,26] However, Román and Román have suggested that cardiovascular, neurological, and neuroophthalmologic complications can indeed occur in late yaws.[24]

The lesions of late yaws are characterized by nodular and tubercular pianides, gummatous lesions, palmar and plantar keratoderma, osteoarticular lesions, gangosa, goundou, and juxtaarticular nodes.[18]

- Nodular and tubercular pianides: groups of firm nodules or tubercles in a plaque with arciform borders. The lesion may ulcerate or heal, leaving an atrophic scar.
- Gummas: the lesion starts with a non-tender, mobile, single nodule that later ulcerates and discharges purulent material. Chronic ulcers may affect subcutaneous tissues, bones, and joints, leading to the formation of scar tissue with ankylosis and considerable deformity. Gummas may also be secondary to an underlying osteitis.
- Palmar and plantar keratoderma: this frequently occurs in late yaws and may also appear in earlier stages. The lesions consist of fissured, painful hyperkeratotic plaques with defined borders that usually cause disability.
- Osteoarticular lesions: hypertrophic periostitis, gummatous periostitis, osteitis, and osteomyelitis occur most commonly on the long bones, scalp, metatarsal, and metacarpal bones. Chronic osteitis can lead to anteroposterior curvature of tibia, resulting in the classic saber tibia.
- Gangosa: this is the palate and nasal septum destruction and perforation caused by the ulcerations. It starts with a nodule which ulcerates and progressively destroys the mucous, cartilaginous and osseous structure of septum, palate, and posterior pharynx. Gangosa means muffled voice in Spanish and reflects the peculiar nasal sound produced by the destruction described.
- Goundou: these are the exostoses of the nasal bridge and adjacent bones caused by subperiosteal deposition of new bone. The lesion may even obstruct the vision.
- Juxtaarticular nodes: these firm, round nodules vary in size and are located most commonly on the elbow, wrist, knee, and foot.[18]

Attenuated yaws

Since 1934, a clinically attenuated form of yaws has been described in areas of reduced transmission. The lesions tend to be solitary or consist of few lesions, which are small, flat, dry, gray, and often limited to the skin folds. This form is less contagious, and there is great potential for these cases to be missed during surveillance.

Patient evaluation, diagnosis, and differential diagnosis

Serological tests, such as RPR, VDRL, FTA-ABS, *T. pallidum* immobilization and *T. pallidum* hemagglutination assay can confirm the diagnosis. Dark-field microscopic examination, radiological and histopathological studies have also been used.[18,24]

Late yaws manifestations are usually clinically and serologically indistinguishable from late syphilis.

Initial yaws must be distinguished in particular from venereal syphilis. It can also resemble, eczema, ecthyma, scabies, tungiasis, sarcoid, warts, vegetating pyoderma, tropical phagedenic ulcer or mycobacterial ulcer, vegetating carcinoma, tuberculosis, sporotrichosis, leishmaniasis, pityriasis rosea, pityriasis versicolor, and psoriasis.

Late yaws skin manifestations can be identical to those of syphilis, leprosy, mucocutaneous leishmaniasis, rhinosporidiosis, rhinoscleroma, and South American blastomycosis. Keratoderma and hyperkeratosis of the palms and soles are indistinguishable from those of endemic syphilis and pinta. Bone lesions of yaws can mimic venereal syphilis, endemic syphilis, tuberculosis, osteomyelitis, and sickle-cell disease.

Treatment

Penicillin is still the drug of choice, being curative. The dosage recommended by a World Health Organization scientific group in 1980 is a single dose of 1.2 million units of benzathine penicillin G for early and late active cases. In children under 10 years of age, half of that dose is appropriate.[27]

References

1. Antal GM, Lukehart SA, Meheus AZ. The endemic treponematoses. Microb Infect 2002; 4:83–94.
2. Talhari S. Pinta. In: Talhari S, Neves RG, eds. Dermatologia Tropical. Rio de Janeiro: Medsi; 1995:291–300.
3. Engelkens HJ, Vuzevski VD, Stolz E. Nonvenereal treponematoses in tropical countries. Clin Dermatol 1999; 17:143–152.
4. Talhari S. Pinta: Aspectos clínicos, laboratoriais e situação epidemiológica no estado do Amazonas (Brasil). PhD thesis. São Paulo, Brazil: Escola Paulista de Medicina; 1988.
5. Medina R. Pinta: An endemic treponematoses in the Americas. Bol Oficina Sanit Panam 1979; 86:242–255.
6. Gonçalves AP. Pinta: presentation of 2 patients. An Bras Derm Sifilogr 1950; 25:185–186.
7. Gonçalves AP. Immunologic aspects of pinta. Dermatologica 1967; 135:199–204.
8. Woltsche-Kahr I, Schmidt B, Aberer W et al. Pinta in Austria (or Cuba?): import of an extinct disease? Arch Dermatol 1999; 135:685–688.
9. Kerdel Vegas F. Pinta. In: Rook A, Wilkinson DS, Ebling FJG et al., eds. Textbook of dermatology, vol. 1, 5th edn. Oxford: Blackwell Scientific; 1992:1121–1126.

10. Engelkens JH, Niemel PL, van der Sluis JJ et al. Endemic treponematoses. Part II. Pinta and endemic syphilis. Int J Dermatol 1991; 30:231–238.
11. Talhari S, Dourado HV, Alecrim WD et al. Pinta em população nativa do estado do Amazonas. Acta Amazônica 1975; 5:199–202.
12. Talhari S, Castro RM, Neves RG. Pinta among Indians in occidental Amazon. In: 17th World Congress of Dermatology volume of abstracts, part 2. Berlin: Internationl Society of Dermatology; 1987:26.
13. Sanchez MR. Endemic (nonvenereal) treponematoses. In: Freedberg IM, Eisen AZ, Wolff K et al., eds. Fitzpatrick's dermatology in general medicine, vol. 2, 5th edn. New York: McGraw-Hill; 1999:2581–2587.
14. Csonka G; Pace J. Endemic nonvenereal treponematoses (bejel) in Saudi Arabia. Rev Infect Dis 1985; 7 (suppl. 2):S260–S265.
15. Slavec ZZ. Skrljevo disease in Slovenia. Lijec Vjesn 2002; 124:150–155.
16. Koff AB, Rosen T. Nonvenereal treponematoses: yaws, endemic syphilis and pinta. J Am Acad Dermatol 1993; 29:519–535.
17. Tabbara KF, al Kaff AS, Fadel T. Ocular manifestations of endemic syphilis (bejel). Ophthalmology 1989; 96:1087–1091.
18. Kerdel Vegas F. Yaws. In: Canizares O, ed. Clinical tropical dermatology. London: Blackwell Scientific; 1975:79–86.
19. Rothschild BM, Rothschild C. Treponemal disease revisited: skeletal discrimination of yaws, bejel and venereal syphilis. Clin Infect Dis 1995; 20:1402–1408.
20. Tharmaphornpilas P, Srivanichakorn S, Phraesrisakul N. Recurrence of yaws outbreak in Thailand, 1990. Southeast Asian J Trop Med Public Health 1994; 25:152–156.
21. Akogun OB. Yaws and syphilis in the Garkida area of Nigeria. Zentralbl Bakteriol 1999; 289:101–107.
22. Herve V, Kassa Kelembho E, Normand P et al. Resurgence of yaws in Central African Republic. Bull Soc Pathol Exot 1992; 85:342–346.
23. Anselmi M, Moreira JM, Caicedo C et al. Community participation eliminates yaws in Ecuador. Trop Med Int Health 2003; 8:634–638.
24. Román GC; Román LN. Occurrence of congenital, cardiovascular, visceral, neurologic, and neuro-ophthalmologic complications in late yaws: a theme for future research. Rev Infect Dis 1986 ;8:760–770.
25. Mohamed KN. Late yaws and optic atrophy. Ann Trop Med Parasitol 1990; 84:637–639.
26. Smith JL, Israel CW. A neuro-ophthalmologic study of late yaws and pinta. Trans Am Ophthalmol Soc 1970; 68:292–300.
27. Scolnik D, Aronson L, Lovinsky R et al. Efficacy of a targeted, oral penicillin-based yaws control program among children living in rural South America. Clin Infect Dis 2003; 36:1232–1238.

Chapter 27

Other spirochetoses

- Borreliosis (Lyme disease) ▪ *Cláudia Pires do Amaral Maia and Ryssia Alvarez Florião*
- Leptospirosis ▪ *Mauricio Younes-Ibrahim and Omar da Rosa Santos*

Introduction

Spirochetoses other than syphilis are diseases with a restricted geographic distribution and are very common in tropical countries. Borreliosis and leptospirosis are zooanthroponoses with severe clinical manifestations and many dermatological findings.

It is interesting to point out that spirochetoses are common cause of infections among many mammals around the world. This ubiquitousness is related to the fact that spirochetes are ancient bacteria that infected eukaryotic cells from the very beginning of evolution. The theory of progressive sequential endosymbiosis proposed by some biologists, such as Lynn Margulis and Dorion Sagan, stated that the first eukaryotic cells originated from a fusion of other previous bacteria that originated the mitochondria (cyanobacteria), chloroplasts (ancient algae), and even the primitive nucleus (Archaea kingdom). According to this theory, spirochetes were presumably associated with the first cellular flagellum and mobility. In a certain way, spirochetes may represent our most ancient disease but also a great leap forward in evolution.

Borreliosis (Lyme disease)

Cláudia Pires do Amaral Maia and Ryssia Alvarez Florião

Synonyms: Lyme disease, cutaneous borreliosis, borreliosis, borrelial lymphocytoma, lymphadenosis cutis benigna, erythema chronicum migrans, erythema migrans, acrodermatitis chronica atrophicans (ACA)

Key features:

- This anthropozoonosis is endemic in North America and Europe
- It is caused by *Borrelia burgdorferi*, a spirochete
- The vector is the tick (*Ixodes ricinus* complex)
- Clinical manifestations:
  - Early stage: erythema migrans, borrelial lymphocytoma
  - Chronic stage: acrodermatitis chronica athrophicans
- Extracutaneous manifestations: nervous, cardiovascular, and musculoskeletal
- Diagnosis: clinical findings; epidemiologic history (endemic area, tick bite), serological tests (immunofluorescent antibody (IFA), enzyme-linked immunosorbent assay (ELISA), Western blot), histopathology, polymerase chain reaction (PCR)
- Treatment: antimicrobials (doxycycline, amoxicillin, ceftriaxone, cefotaxime, penicillin G)

Introduction

Lyme disease (LD) is an infectious syndrome caused by the spirochete *Borrelia burgdorferi* which is transmitted by ticks. It is an anthropozoonosis which can cause a spectrum of disease from the initial skin lesion, through widely varied symptoms and signs, to chronic neurologic and arthritic disability.[1–3] It has been widely reported throughout the USA, Europe, and many parts of the world. In recent years, there have been increasing gains in our knowledge of the disease, including studies of pathogenesis, and guidelines for diagnosis and treatment.[4]

History

The first erythema migrans (EM) cases were described in the early twentieth century by Afzelius and Lipschutz.[5] In 1977, Steere et al. studied in Lyme, Connecticut (USA) the association between EM and arthritis, and also nonspecific symptoms, cardiac and neurological manifestations, which were conclusively linked in 1982 with the recovery of a previously unrecognized spirochete from the tick vector and from infected patients.[4]

Epidemiology

LD is the most common vector-borne disease in North America and Europe. In 1999, over 16 000 cases of human LD were reported in the USA, where it occurs in the northeast, the Midwest and the west.[2] In Europe, LD is widely established in forested areas, with the highest reported frequencies in middle Europe and Scandinavia, particularly in Austria, Czech Republic, Germany, Slovenia, and

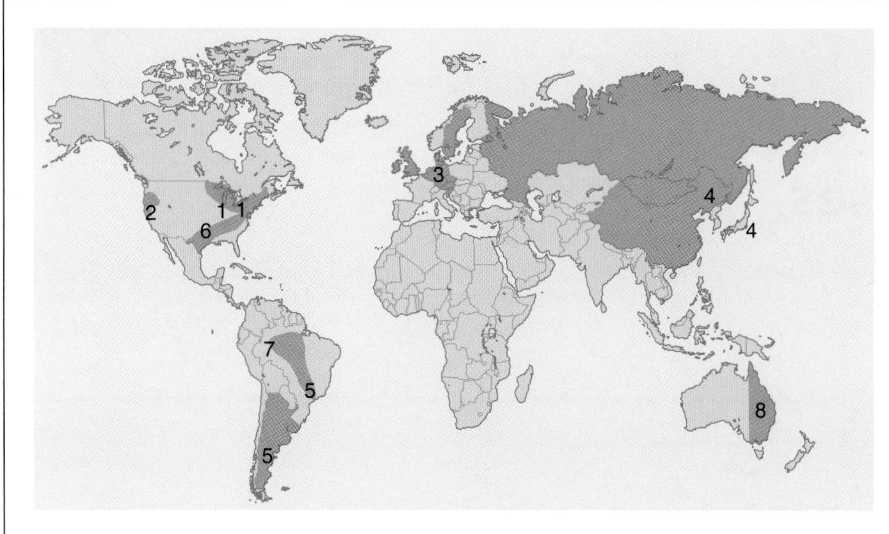

Figure 27.1 World distribution of the main Lyme disease tick vectors and identified spirochete genospecies: 1, *Ioxes scapularis (I. dammini)*: *Borrelia burgdorferi* sensu stricto; 2, *I. pacificus*: *B. burgdorferi* sensu stricto; 3, *I. ricinus*: *B. burgdorferi* sensu stricto, *B. garinii*, *B. afzelii*; 4, *I. persulcatus*: *B. japonica*; 5, *I. pararicinus*; 6, *Amblyomma americanum*: *B. lonestari* (Lyme disease-like illness); 7, *A. cajennense*, *A. aureolatum*, *I. didelphidis*, *I. loricatus* (Lyme disease-like illness); 8, *I. holocyclus* (Lyme disease-like illness).

Sweden. The infection is also found in Australia, Canada, China, Japan, northeast Africa, and Russia.[4] In South America, studies showed that antibodies to *B. burgdorferi* were present in the Argentinean population, and the disease was described in Bolivia.[6] In Brazil, human cases of LD have been reported and *B. burgdorferi* has been identified[7].

LD occurs in all age groups, in both sexes, and in all races. Who becomes infected is likely more to do with frequency and intensity of tick exposure than with any genetic predisposition. Children represent about 25% of cases, and men are infected more commonly than women. Most cases of EM develop in the late spring and early summer, when the nymphs are actively questing for their blood meal.[5]

Etiology

The etiologic agent, *B. burgdorferi sensu lato*, is a Gram-negative bacterium, and like other spirochetes, it is a helically shaped motile microorganism.[3] It has been subdivided into three genospecies causing the human disease: *B. burgdorferi sensu stricto*, *B. afzelii*, and *B. garinii*. Only the first species is found in the USA; however all three have been found in Europe, and *B. afzelii* is the dominant skin isolate. Antigenic differences between the three genospecies may explain the variability in the clinical manifestations in patients with LD.[1,3,8] *B. valaisiana* has been detected by PCR in the skin of a few patients with EM; another newly identified species, *B. lusitaniae*, has been found in Europe.[8]

LD is transmitted by ticks of the *Ixodes ricinus* complex. These ticks have larval, nymphal, and adult stages, in a 3-year life cycle.[9] All stages of ticks are capable of transmitting disease, but the nymphal stage is the most common. The risk of infection is largely dependent on the intensity of ticks, their feeding habits, and the animal hosts. Ticks are most commonly found attached to plants in grassy, wooded, bushy areas and are transferred by contact with animals or humans who are incidental hosts. Other possible vectors include mosquitoes, deer flies, and horse flies.[3]

In the northeastern and north central USA, *I. scapularis* (*I. dammini*) ticks are the most important vector, and *I pacificus* in the west.[4,9] In Europe, the principal vector is *I. ricinus*, and in Asia it is *I. persulcatus*.[4] In South America, *I. pararicinus* was observed in the bovine population of Argentina and Uruguay.[10] The identification of *Ambvlyomma americanum* as the vector in the USA of a distinct, uncultivable species of *Borrelia* known as *B. lonestari*, recognized as the etiological agent of an LD-like illness causing cutaneous lesions without systemic manifestations, has added the genus *Amblyomma* to the list of known vectors of this disease to humans.[4,11] In Brazil, an LD-like illness has also been observed, with clinical similarities to classical LD, although with some laboratory differences, which suggests that the causative agent is either a very different *Borrelia* or a microorganism of another genus transmitted by ticks other than those of the *I. ricinus* complex.[11] Recently, ticks of the species *A. cajennense*, *A. aureolatum*, *I. didelphidis*, and *I. loricatus* have been identified in that country in rodents and marsupials contaminated with spirochetes morphologically similar to those of the genus *Borrelia* (Fig. 27.1).[11]

Many mammals may serve as an intermediate host for *B. burgdorferi*, but the major reservoir hosts are deer and white-footed mice. Domestic animals, including dogs, cats, horses, and cattle from endemic areas, are also potential hosts.[3]

Pathogenesis

After a tick bite, the spirochete may be transmitted into the skin of the bitten host, and three outcomes are possible. First, the host defense mechanisms may overwhelm the spirochetal offense so that no disease develops. Second, the infection may become established but remain localized to the skin around the bite. Third, the infection may spread through the lymphatics or blood stream and become systemic.

After the tick bite, the *B. burgdorferi* migrate from the tick's midgut to the salivary glands, from where they find their way into the host. This fact probably explains the evidence from human and animal studies suggesting that tick bites of less than 24 h duration rarely result in infection. In many cases, no symptoms occur.[5]

Only a small percentage of tick bite leads to infection in untreated patients. The host defense mechanisms may limit the infection, but pathogen-related factors may also play a role. There is evidence that genes coding the outer-surface protein C (Osp C) may play a role in the invasiveness of a *B. burgdorferi* strain. It may explain why some patients develop more invasive disease.

Systemic invasion of the spirochete may occur early in the course of LD. The spirochetes can change their outer antigenic structure and migrate into the intracellular compartment – both strategies may help the organism to evade the host's immune defenses.[5]

In patients who develop EM, the incubation period ranges from 1 to 36 days, with a median of 7–10 days.[5]

The last factor regarding pathogenesis is the phenomenon of coinfection, which may occur in 10–15% of cases.[5] Other tick-borne pathogens, such as the agents of babesiosis, ehrlichiosis, and possibly others, can be transmitted by the same tick bite as the one that caused LD, and may modify the clinical manifestations and response to therapy.

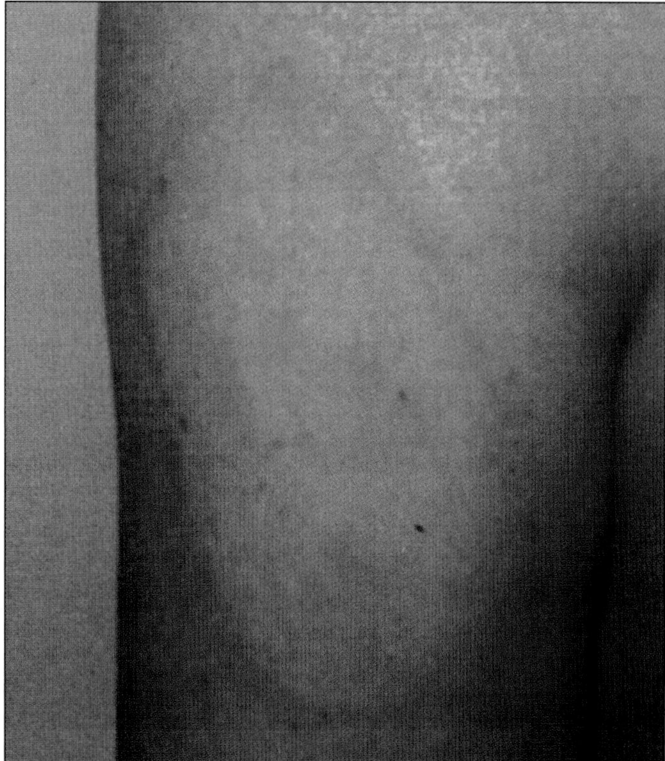

Figure 27.2 Erythema migrans. (Courtesy of Dr. Absalom Filgueira.)

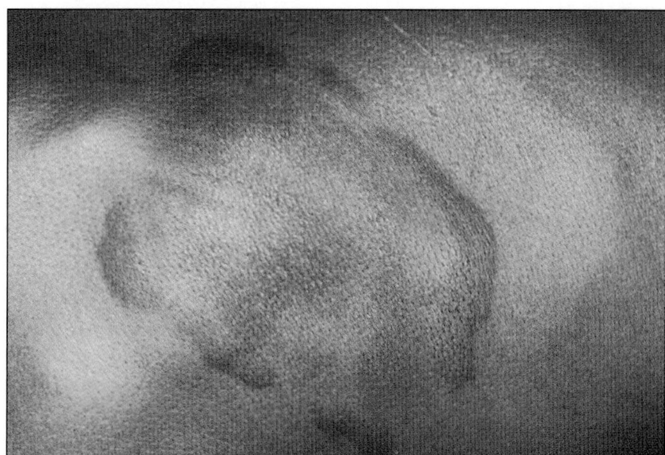

Figure 27.3 Erythema migrans. (Courtesy of Dr. Sinesio Talhari.)

Clinical features

The characteristic manifestations of cutaneous LD are an early eruption in EM and the chronic sequel – acrodermatitis chronica atrophicans (ACA).[1] The early lesion starts after a tick bite and is carried by the responsible spirochete for borreliosis which leaves a small macule or papule at the site, usually in the extremities, but it may be seen anywhere on the body.[1,3,10] A total of 70–80% of patients are unable to recall the bite. A week later (range 3–32 days) there is expansion of the red papule, changing to annular erythema where the site of the bite may clear or become vesicular or necrotic; the red peripheral ring grows up to 68 cm[10] (Figs 27.2 and 27.3). The central annular erythematous lesion shows elevation or the erythema fades away and the border may be slightly raised, warm, or bluish-red, sometimes accompanied by a burning sensation or, rarely, becoming painful or pruritic. Usually the ring formation enlarges at a rate of several centimeters per week. This typical EM happens in 85% of patients who are diagnosed with early LD. It is often accompanied by an acute flu-like illness.[1,3,10]

Multiple secondary annular lesions similar to the primary lesion, but smaller, and less migratory to the original lesion, can be found in 50% or less of patients (Fig. 27.4). There are cases which have 100 secondary lesions. These fade away at about a month but some eruptions may be present or recur over the following months. In Europe, during this early period a lymphocytoma or benign lymphocytic infiltrates may occur, and most commonly are found as bluish-red papular nodules in the earlobes of children or on the anterior chest of adults[1,3,4,10] (Fig. 27.5).

Hematogenous dissemination may cause frequent complications: arthritis (mono- or oligoarthritis, mostly found in the USA and involving large joints in early and late disease, migratory joint pains, 10% in the knees), neurologic (stiff neck, meningitis, Bell's palsy, Bannwarth's syndrome in Europe, and cranial and peripheral neuropathies) and cardiac manifestations (myocarditis, congestive heart failure, atrioventricular partial or complete block for a brief period). Non-specific findings are related: mild anemia, elevated erythrocyte sedimentation rate, elevated immunoglobulin M (IgM) level, and elevated liver function. Other signs and symptoms include fever, malaise, fatigue, headache, conjunctivitis, iritis, iridocyclitis, keratitis, retinal hemorrhage, nausea, vomiting, anorexia, hepatitis, splenomegaly, lymphadenopathy, myalgia, as well as cutaneous manifestations: urticaria, malar erythema, hemorrhagic blister, or erythema nodosum-like lesions. Transplacental transmission has been reported. In pregnancy LD was not associated with fetal malformations. In the late form of the disease, 10% of untreated patients may develop neurological problems, cardiac manifestations have been found in 5% and arthritis in up to 50%.[1,3,4,10]

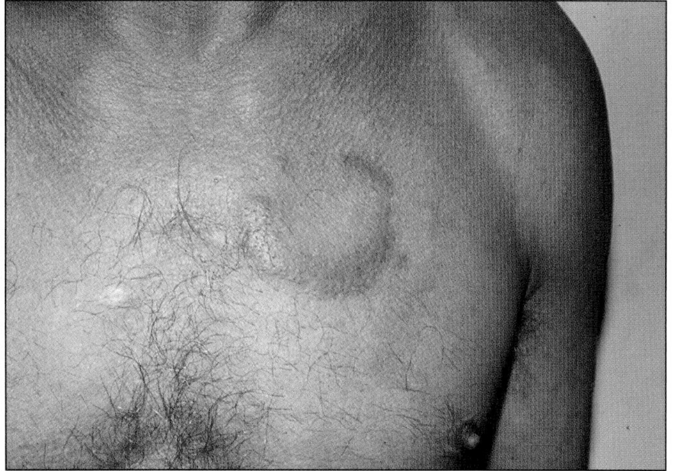

Figure 27.4 Erythema migrans: lesion with red outer rims and nearly complete clearing in the center. (Courtesy of Dr. Absalom Filgueira.)

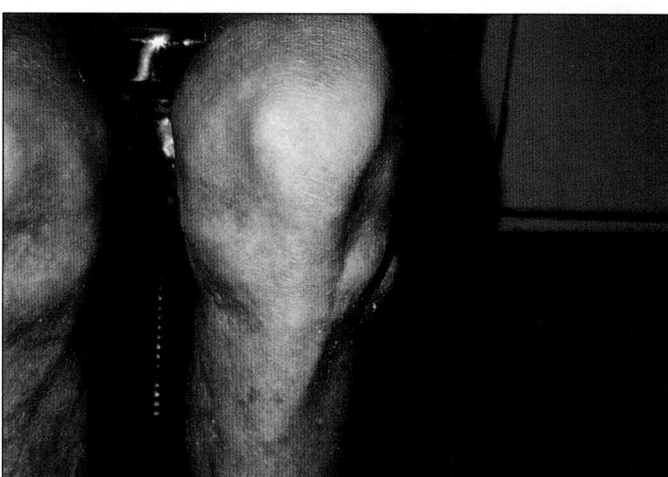

Figure 27.6 Acrodermatitis chronic atrophicans. Detail: thin skin with prominent vessels. (Courtesy of Dr. Absalom Filgueira.)

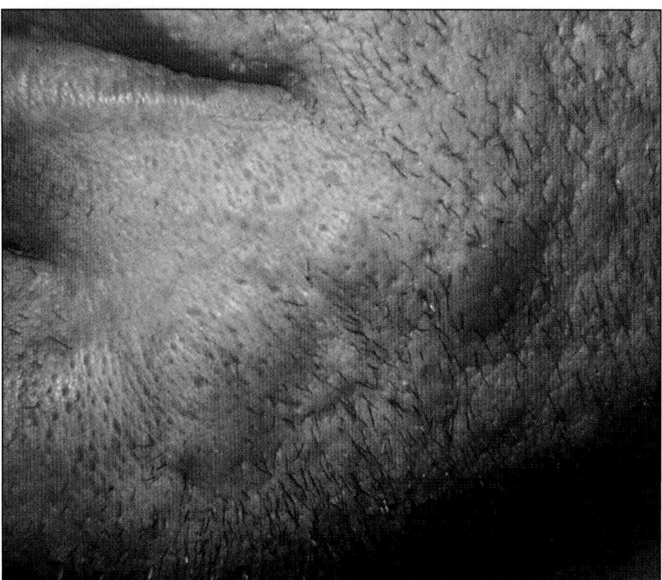

Figure 27.5 Borrelial lymphocytoma. Bluish-red papules and nodules. (Courtesy of Dr. Absalom Filgueira.)

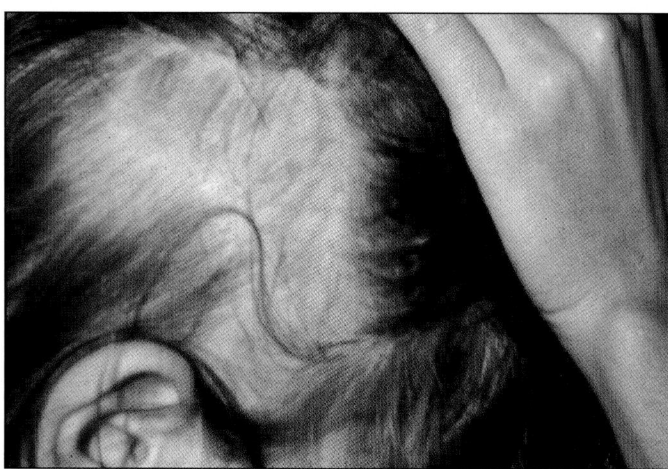

Figure 27.7 Morphea lesion in a girl who had erythema migrans. (Courtesy of Dr. Absalom Filgueira.)

In Europe ACA has been observed, involving most commonly cutaneous lower extremities, initially causing a bluish, erythematous swelling and edema that atrophies where the underlying blood vessels are easily seen (Fig. 27.6). Sclerodermoid-like features are related in some cases to fibrous thickness and indurated linear bands and nodules. Some patients may eventually present with late cutaneous sequelae: morphea (Fig. 27.7), atrophoderma of Pasini and Pierini, anetoderma, and lichen sclerosus.[1,10]

Some cases of LD begin with asymptomatic seroconversion, and remain asymptomatic, appearing to have been spontaneously cured, or they develop manifestations of disseminated or late LD as their initial clinical manifestation[12] (Fig. 27.8).

Disseminated and late LD are less responsive to antibiotic treatment than in early infection. Some individuals experience an ill-defined post-LD syndrome characterized by fatigue, headache, myalgias, arthralgias, and other constitutional symptoms after otherwise curative antibiotic therapy.[12]

Diagnosis

It is important to recognize that LD is a clinical diagnosis; any laboratory test used to supplement that evaluation should be interpreted in the context of careful investigation of the patient's history and physical examination, i.e., after thoughtful assessment of the probability that a patient actually has a borrelial infection.[2] In USA, the diagnosis is usually based on the recognition of the characteristic clinical findings, a history of exposure in an area where the disease is endemic, and, except in patients with EM, an antibody response to *B. burgdorferi*, interpreted according to the criteria of the Centers for Disease Control (CDC) (Table 27.1).[4]

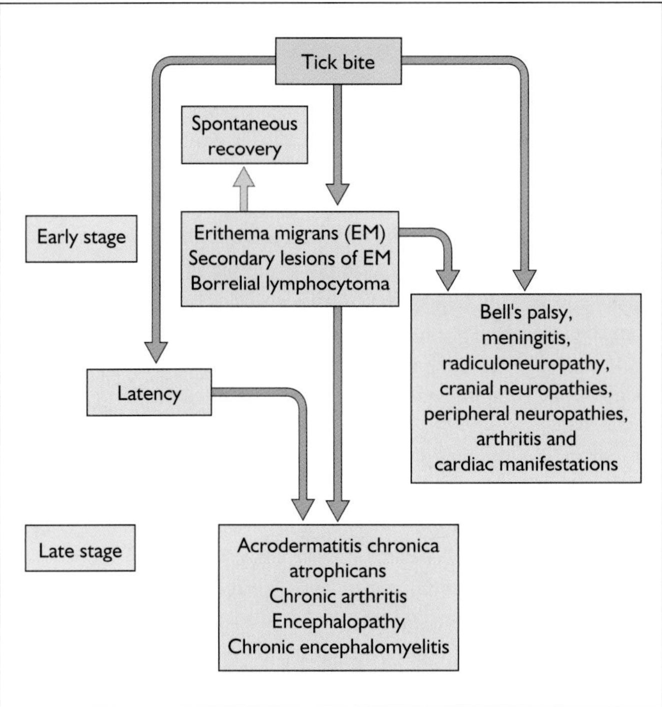

Figure 27.8 The evolution of Lyme disease.

Table 27.1 Case definition of Lyme disease for National Surveillance[a]

• Erythema migrans observed by a physician. The lesion expands slowly over days or weeks to form a large, round lesion, often with central clearing. For surveillance purposes, a solitary lesion must reach a size of at least 5 cm
• At least one subsequent manifestation and laboratory evidence: – Nervous system: lymphocytic meningitis, cranial neuritis, radiculoneuropathy, or, rarely, encephalomyelitis, alone or in combination. For encephalomyelitis, for surveillance purposes, there must be *Borrelia burgdorferi* antibody in the cerebrospinal fluid – Cardiovascular system: acute-onset , high-grade (second- or third-degree) atrioventricular conduction defects that resolve in days or weeks, sometimes associated with myocarditis – Musculoskeletal system: recurrent, brief attacks (lasting weeks to months) of objectively confirmed joint swelling in one or a few joints, sometimes followed by chronic arthritis in one or a few joints – Laboratory: isolation of *Borrelia burgdorferi* from tissue of body fluid or detection of diagnostic levels of *Borrelia burgdorferi* antibody by the two-test approach (enzyme-linked immunosorbent assay, Western blotting), interpreted according to the criteria of the Centers for Disease Control[b]

Modified from Steere AC. Lyme disease. N Engl J Med 2001;345:115–125.
[a]Adapted from recommendations made by the Centers for Disease Control.
[b]In an acute disease of less than 1 month's duration, immunoglobulin M (IgM) and IgG antibody responses should be measured in serum samples obtained during the acute and convalescent phases. Only the IgG response should be used to support the diagnosis after the first month of infection; after that time, an IgM response alone is likely to represent a false-positive result.

Immunoserologic tests for LD can only be used to assist a diagnosis process, and are most valuable when presentation is atypical or manifests with disseminated or late-stage infection.[12] The prevalence of seropositivity in high focal endemicity of LM may occur in 8–15%.[9,10]

Although the three genospecies of *B. burgdorferi* generally express similar antigens, significant differences do occur, which complicate the development of a single immunoserologic assay that is optimal for laboratory testing for LD.[2] There is little standardization among the numerous commercial kits for LD diagnosis.

The serologic tests for LD includes ELISA, immunoblotting (Western blot), and IFA. It is helpful to use a two-step process for testing. The first step employs a sensitive serologic test, such as ELISA or IFA. Specimens found to be negative are not tested further. All specimens with positive or equivocal results are tested by immunoblotting (high-specific). When immunoblotting is used in the first 4 weeks after the onset of disease, both IgM and IgG procedures should be performed.

The serological tests are insensitive during the first several weeks of infection. About 70–80% of LD patients will seroconvert within this 4-week period. In the event that a patient suspected to have early LD has a negative serology, evidence of infection is best obtained by testing paired acute- and convalescent-phase samples. Since specific IgG should be present in nearly all untreated patients after 1 month of infection, a positive IgM test result alone cannot be considered to support the diagnosis and may represent a false-positive result.[4]

After antibiotic treatment, antibody titers fall slowly but IgG and even IgM responses may persist for many years after treatment.[2,4,9]

In individuals vaccinated with recombinant OspA vaccine, ELISA and IFA assays utilizing the same strains of *B. burgdorferi* will not discriminate between vaccinated and naturally infected individuals.[2]

Many diseases have been reported to cause cross-reactivity in IgM and/or IgG assays, such as Epstein–Barr virus infection, bacterial endocarditis, syphilis, other spirochetal infections, and *Helicobacter pylori* infection.[2] The Venereal Disease Research Laboratory (VDRL) test is negative in LD.[10]

The culture of *B. burgdorferi* on artificial medium – Barbour–Stoenner–Kelly from a clinical sample (blood, skin and cerebrospinal fluid) – permits definitive diagnosis of infection, and is the most specific assay for detection of an early-phase infection. However, most laboratories are not capable of culturing organisms. In the late phase of LD, it is of limited value for detection of infection.[9]

The detection of *B. burgdorferi* is possible by PCR analysis from skin biopsy specimens, joint fluid, synovial biopsy specimens, or cerebrospinal fluid. It has a high sensitivity but PCR is not as specific as cultivation for an active infection confirmation. PCR should not be used as a screening assay, because it is expensive and is only performed in reference laboratories, so it is reserved for special situations.[9]

Other immunologic assays performed on a research basis have been developed to aid in clinical diagnosis of LD, such as the measurement of T-lymphocyte recognition of *B. burgdorferi* antigens, the detection of circulating immune complexes (IC), and a flow cytometry-based assay to detect borreliacidal antibodies.[2,9]

Pathology

Histopathologic findings of EM are not specific for the disease.[5] They show superficial and deep perivascular and interstitial infiltrates primarily composed of lymphocytes, histiocytes, and eosinophils, with some plasma cells, with angiocentric arrangement and in the interstitium or around the veins[3,7] (Fig. 27.9).

The numbers of *B. burgdorferi* in tissues during infection are low, so direct detection by microscopy is of limited application. Their detection in fixed-tissue sections is best achieved with silver stains (Warthin–Starry and Steiner) (Fig. 27.10), but artifacts may confuse results.[9]

Immunohistologic staining using polyclonal or monoclonal antibodies has been used to show spirochetes in patient tissues, but this is not a commonly performed procedure.[9]

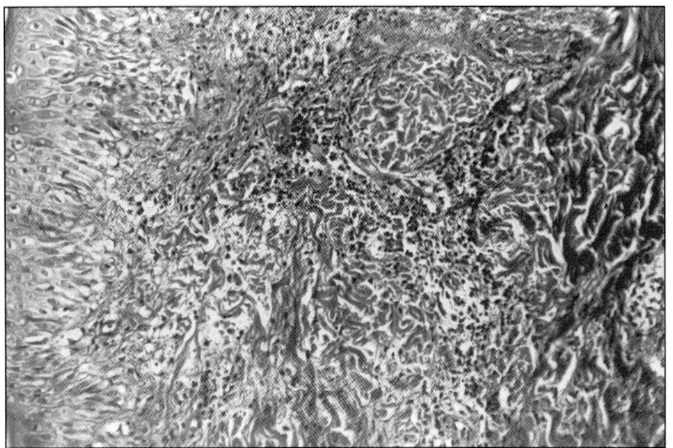

Figure 27.9 Inflammatory infiltrate in the dermis, interstitium, and around the veins, comprised of lymphocytes, histiocytes, and plasmocytes. Hematoxylin and eosin, ×200. (Courtesy of Dr. Itelvina S. de Melo, with permission from An Bras Dermatol 2003; 78:169–177.)

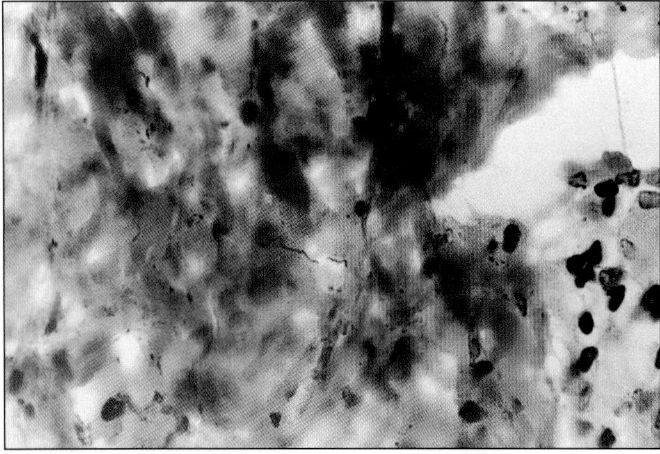

Figure 27.10 *Borrelia* spirochetes in the upper dermis: Warthin–Starry silver stain, ×1000. (Courtesy of Dr. Itelvina S. de Melo, with permission from An Bras Dermatol 2003; 78:169–177.)

Differential diagnosis

Many other cutaneous processes can mimic the early phase of EM: bacterial cellulitis, tinea corporis, hypersensitivity to tick or other insect bites, spider bites, contact dermatitis, pityriasis rosea, urticaria, granuloma annulare, erythema multiforme, erythema annular centrifugum, morphea, and fixed drug eruption. Borrelial lymphocytoma should be differentiated from histiocytoma, keloid, angioma, Kaposi's sarcoma, granuloma annulare, granuloma faciale, sarcoidosis, and lupus erythematosus.[5]

In the late phase, lesions on the lower legs can mimic circulatory insufficiency, perniosis, and dermatomyositis; fibrotic papules and nodules may be mistaken for rheumatic nodules or gouty tophi.[1]

Treatment

Prompt treatment of patients with early disease often leads to rapid resolution of symptoms and, perhaps more significantly, prevents late sequelae.[1,3] Cutaneous manifestations disappear after therapy; for lymphocytoma, resolution can take up to 6 months; the degenerative changes in acrodermatitis are not reversible.[1]

Some studies demonstrate that even an appropriate antimicrobial regimen may not always eradicate the spirochete. The treatment of disseminated LD, even for longer than 3 months, may not be sufficient (the spirochetes can remain in the serum, skin, and other tissues and clinical relapses can occur). It remains unresolved if the prognosis of patients with disseminated LD is improved with a longer initial treatment.[1] Extracutaneous manifestations of LD were described after an antimicrobial regimen in up to 10% of patients.[1]

The two first-line agents for oral treatment of LD are doxycycline and amoxicillin, for 14–21 days[1,4,5,13] (Table 27.2). Doxycycline is taken only twice daily; it is inexpensive, well tolerated, and has the advantage of treating any coinfecting ehrlichial or rickettsial organisms. Pregnant and lactating women and children younger than 9 years of age should be treated with amoxicillin, which can also be used for other patients. Tetracycline and penicillin are alternatives but are generally used less frequently. Other options are cefuroxime axetil administered twice daily. The first-generation cephalosporin (cephalexin), quinolones and trimethoprim–sulfamethoxazole are not adequate to treat *B. burgdorferi* infections. Erythromycin has underperformed the tetracyclines and β-lactam antibiotics.[5]

Lyme arthritis and other manifestations of lesser severity should be treated first with oral antibiotics. About 10% of patients with Lyme arthritis may persist with joint inflammation for months or even several years after 2 or more months of antibiotic therapy, despite either oral or intravenous treatment. The persistent arthritis should be treated with antiinflammatory agents or arthroscopic synovectomy if the results of PCR testing of joint fluid are negative.

For patients with severe extracutaneous manifestations, such as neurological and cardiac, parenteral antibiotics, such as ceftriaxone, cefotaxime, and penicillin G are recommended for 2–4 weeks. Ceftriaxone has excellent penetration into the cerebrospinal fluid.[3] For pregnant women, parenteral antimicrobials should be used in case the tick bite is suspected during the first trimester. If the patient is bitten later on during pregnancy and has no extracutaneous symptoms or signs, oral antimicrobials are sufficient.[1]

Table 27.2 Oral treatment of Lyme disease

Stage of disease	Drug	Dose
Early disease (local or disseminated) (14–21 days)		
Adults	Doxycycline	100 mg orally twice daily
	Amoxicillin	500 mg 3 times a day
Doxycycline or amoxicillin allergy	Cefuroxime axetil	500 mg orally twice daily
	Erythromycin	250 mg orally 4 times a day
Children	Amoxicillin	50 mg/kg per day orally in 3 divided doses
Penicillin allergy	Cefuroxime axetil	30 mg/kg per day orally in 2 divided doses
	Erythromycin	30 mg/kg per day orally in 3 divided doses
Neurologic abnormalities (early or late) (14–28 days)		
Adults	Ceftriaxone	2 g IV once a day
	Cefotaxime	2 g 3 times daily
	Penicillin G	3.3 million U IV every 4 h
Ceftriaxone or penicillin allergy	Doxycycline	100 mg orally 3 times a day[a]
Facial palsy alone	Oral regimens may be adequate	
Children	Ceftriaxone	75–100 mg/kg per day IV once a day
	Cefotaxime	150 mg/kg per day in 3 doses
	Penicillin G	200–400.000 U/kg per day in 6 divided doses
Arthritis	Oral regimens listed above for 30–60 days or IV regimens for 14–28 days	
Cardiac abnormalities		
First-degree atrioventricular block	Oral regimens listed above for 14–21 days	
High-degree atrioventricular block	IV regimens listed above	
Pregnant women	Standard therapy for manifestation of the ilness; avoid doxycycline	
Vaccination	L-OspA in adjuvant, 30 μg intramuscularly at 0, 1, and 12 months	

[a]This regimen may be ineffective for late neuroborreliosis.
Modified from Steere AC. Lyme disease. N Engl J Med 2001; 345:115–125.

The Jarisch–Herxheimer reaction may occur in about 15–20% of patients during the first 24 h of antimicrobial therapy.

Prevention

Protective measures may include avoiding tick-infested areas, wearing protective clothing, using repellents, skin inspection for early detection, and correct removal of ticks.[1,4]

Some authors believe that a single 200-mg dose of doxycycline effectively prevents LD when given within 72 h after the tick bite occurs.[4]

The development of an effective vaccine for LD represents a great advance in the control of the disease in the USA. Vaccination with recombinant OspA is safe and immunogenic in humans, effective in 76% of patients in preventing LD, after three injections, but it is no longer available.[1,4] A single antigen OspA vaccine is not effective in Europe and Asia, where more heterogeneous species of *B. burgdorferi* are present.[1,12] Protective immunity against *B. burgdorferi* b was demonstrated by other *B. burgdorferi* outer-surface proteins, for instance OspB and OspC.[1] Since antibody titers wane rather quickly, booster injections need to be given for 1–3 years to maintain protection.[4]

Vaccination is not recommended for individuals with minimal or no exposure to such ticks, or for children under 15 or for pregnant women.[4,12] The induction of inflammatory arthritis through an autoimmune mechanism is possible in genetically susceptible individuals.[12] As the vaccine is not uniformly effective, other protection measures should not be neglected.[12]

References

1. Hercogova J. Lyme borreliosis. Int J Dermatol 2001; 40:547–550.
2. Reed KD. Laboratory testing for suspected Lyme disease: possibilities and practicalities. Med Clin North Am 2002; 86:311–340.
3. Abele DC, Ander KH. The many faces and phases of borreliosis I. Lyme disease. J Am Acad Dermatol 1990; 23:167–186.
4. Steere AC. Lyme disease. N Engl J Med 2001; 345:115–125.
5. Edlow JA. Erythema migrans. Med Clin North Am 2002; 186:239–259.
6. Montoya FD, Moraga CH, Olavarría CL. Plaga de garrapatas en Santiago. Pediatr Dia 2000 ; 16 :365–366.
7. Melo IS, Gadelha AR, Ferreira LCL. Histopathological study of erythema chronicum migrans cases diagnosed in Manaus. An Bras Dermatol 2003; 78:169–177.
8. Weber K. Aspects of Lyme borreliosis in Europe. Eur J Clin Microbiol Infect Dis 2001; 20:6–13.
9. Bunikis J, Barbour A. Laboratory testing for Lyme disease: possibilities and practicalities. J Clin Microbiol 2002; 40:319–324.

10. Florião RA. Borrelyose de Lyme. Determinação de manifestações peculiares à BL entre os pacientes que frequentam o HUCFF. Thesis. Rio de Janeiro: Universidade Federal do Rio de Janeiro;1994.
11. Costa IP, Bonoldi VLN, Yoshinari NH. Search from *Borrelia* sp. in ticks collected from potential reservoirs in an urban forest reserve in the state of Mato Grosso do Sul, Brasil: a short report. Mem Inst Oswaldo Cruz 2002; 97:631–635.
12. Rahn DW. Lyme vaccine: issues and controversies. Infect Dis Clin North Am 2001; 15:171–187.
13. Verdon EM, Sigal LH. Lyme disease. Am Fam Phys 1997; 56:427–439.

Leptospirosis

Mauricio Younes-Ibrahim and Omar da Rosa Santos

Introduction

Leptospirosis is a worldwide zooanthroponosis caused by pathogenic spirochetes of the genus *Leptospira*. Rodents and a wide range of domestic and wild mammals are the main natural hosts for the 250-plus known serovars of the bacteria. Human leptospirosis is a potentially fatal but treatable infectious disease that, despite sanitation and scientific knowledge in the twenty-first century, still represents a veterinary and medical public health problem. Currently, human leptospirosis is rare in developed countries where anecdotal reports are usually related to circumscribed occupational or recreational activities. On the other hand, in tropical and developing countries where this infection is endemic in animals, it easily becomes an epidemic for humans as well, mainly during rainy–flooding seasons. Because recent changes in meteorological factors have altered global temperature and rainfall levels, the World Health Organization (WHO) now includes leptospirosis as one of the reemerging infectious diseases, since an increased epidemic risk for humans is associated with global climate changes.[1]

Human infections frequently occur by direct contact with the urine of an infected animal or indirectly through contaminated water, soil, or vegetation. In normal conditions, intact skin is an efficient barrier against *Leptospira* invasion. Usual portals of entry in humans are abraded skin and exposed conjunctival, nasal, and oral mucous membranes. Human infection may either be asymptomatic or present with a wide clinical spectrum, which is often a cause of misdiagnosis. Clinical manifestations may vary from mild, with non-specific influenza-like symptoms, to severe, with jaundice, hemorrhagic disorders, and dramatic multiorgan failure.[2]

History

Since 1886, when the German physician Adolf Weil described the classic form of infectious disease involving jaundice and nephritis, this condition became known as Weil's disease. After this first clinical observation, it was possible to separate leptospiral jaundice from the heterogeneous group of infections associated with icterus. Twenty years later, in Japan, Inada and coworkers succeeded in isolating the etiologic agent implicated in the clinical impairment and named it *Spirochaeta icterohaemorrhagiae*.

During the First World War many cases of leptospirosis were reported among troops, and several investigators in Europe, Asia, and the Americas confirmed the epidemiologic significance of *Leptospira* found in the urine of rats captured in areas where human leptospirosis had occurred. Soon, worldwide clinical and laboratory reports appeared and many different types of *Leptospira* were isolated and arranged into serogroups and serovars according to antigenic determinants. More recently, genotyping of leptospiral DNA has contributed to knowledge of leptospirosis by identifying important subserovar differences in virulence or host adaptation.[1,2]

Epidemiology

Leptospirosis requires close veterinary control because of its considerable medical and economical impact on human and agriculture activities. Microbiological surveillance data show pathogenic organisms found in every place of the world where they have been sought. Although human leptospirosis has been described in five continents, the disease is clearly most common in tropical and subtropical areas with high rainfall. The principal leptospiral reservoirs are species of the rodent family, followed by the widespread infection of domesticated mammals. There are various modes of horizontal and vertical transmission between species, but environment contamination by animal-infected urine is the most important source for human leptospirosis (Fig. 27.11). Of particular epidemiologic significance is the ability of these organisms to

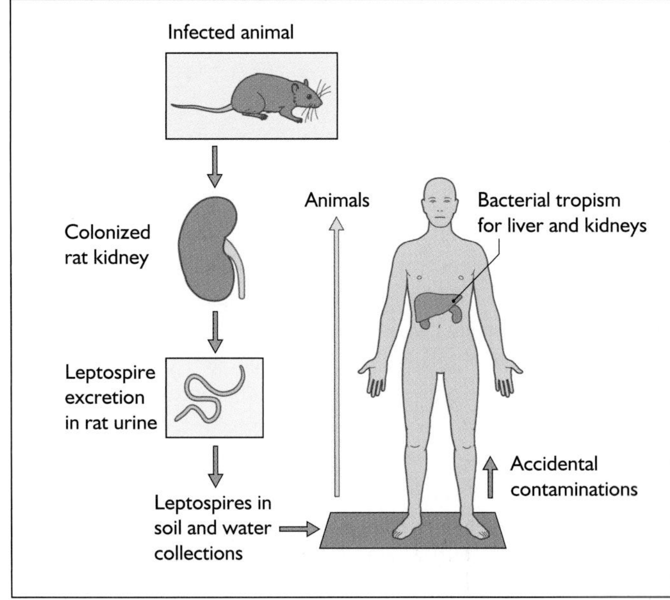

Figure 27.11 Usual cycle of *Leptospira*: rodents are the main reservoir and they excrete bacteria to the environment. Water and soil, in contact with humans, are sources of accidental contamination. (Courtesy of Dr. Ana Maria Miranda Pinto.)

grow and multiply within the host's tissues, especially in the lumen of the convoluted tubules of the renal cortex. They are excreted from renal tubules in the urine and the chronicity of leptospiruria may extend from months to years in various natural hosts. Usually, in different geographic regions, each *Leptospira* serovar is endemic in one or several animal species which, if they become adapted, may continue to shed spirochetes for their entire lifetime.

According to WHO, the incidence of human leptospirosis disease may range in different continents from 0.1 to over 100 cases per 100 000 habitants per year.[1] Seroprevalence studies indicate that subclinical infection is very common worldwide and the prevalence rates of human leptospirosis are underestimated. As urban rats are involved in human transmission, the rate of leptospirosis incidence is directly related to a combination of negative social, environmental, and hygiene conditions. Indeed, leptospirosis is an occupational hazard mainly to rice and sugar cane field workers, sewage workers, and miners. More recently, in developed countries human leptospirosis has been described in participants of ecotourism, triathlons, fishing, and other outdoor leisure activities where humans come into accidental contact with urine from infected wild rodents. The viability of bacteria outside their natural hosts is of fundamental importance to the human leptospirosis epidemiology and leptospires are able to retain their viability and pathogenicity for as long as 22 days in surface waters with pH 7.0–8.0.

Human leptospirosis can be correlated with the relative frequency of leptospirosis in the natural hosts of the regions studied. Men have higher incidence and prevalence of clinical disease than women. There is no agreement in the literature as to whether this is due to more frequent exposure since in some series individuals from both sexes presented with the same seroprevalence. On the other hand, despite their high environmental exposure and the similar seroprevalence to that found in adults, children have a lower incidence of clinical leptospirosis.

Pathogenesis and etiology

Leptospirosis is caused by motile spirochetes belonging to the family Leptospiraceae. This family comprises the genera *Leptospira* (pathogenic) and *Leptonema* (non-pathogenic). The taxonomy, based on antigenic relatedness, is currently being reviewed due to new tools for genetic classification. Both techniques subdivided the genus into two species: *L. biflexa* and *L. interrogans*, names derived from the microscopic shape of *Leptospira* (hook at both ends: *biflexa;* question-mark-shaped: *interrogans*). While *L. biflexa* is a free-living saprophyte not associated with disease, *L. interrogans* comprises 250 serovars, and is pathogenic for humans and many wild and domestic animals. Pathogenic leptospires are Gram-negative bacteria that have two periplasmic flagella and an outer envelope composed of a triple-layered structure containing proteins, polysaccharides, and lipids.[3]

Pathogenic *Leptospira* are aerobic microorganisms that divide by binary fission. Unlike most bacteria, instead of carbohydrates and amino acids, they use long-chain fatty acids and alcohols as sources of carbon and energy in their metabolism. Some serovars produce different lipases able to cause hemolysis that have been related to bacterial virulence. In the last 50 years, various studies were developed in order to understand the mechanism of interaction among hosts and *Leptospira*. In contrast to other Gram-negative bacteria, the lipopolysaccharide (LPS) extracted from *L. interrogans* differs from classical LPS of Enterobacteriaceae concerning structure and biological activities and was named lipopolysaccharide-like substance (LLS). Indeed, the leptospiral lipid A is neither toxic nor pyrogenic.

In 1986, Vinh et al.[3] claimed that a glycolipoprotein (GLP) fraction extracted from *Leptospira* was the active bacterial endotoxin. This concept remains current today, although the mechanisms involving the biologic effects of GLP are still not completely understood. Regarding the cellular pathophysiology of leptospirosis, our laboratory has shown that the GLP is a potent and specific Na^+, K^+-ATPase inhibitor, in all different species and tissues tested.[4] Also, we demonstrated that the non-esterified unsaturated fatty acid (NEUFA) components of GLP are the active inhibitors of the enzyme.[5] As Na^+, K^+-ATPase is ubiquitous on eukaryotic cells and is the main membrane transporter involved in epithelial polarity and cell transmembrane electric potential, it is currently accepted that the impairment in Na^+ and K^+ active transport could potentially be the origin of many cellular and organic dysfunctions observed in vivo during leptospirosis.[6]

Leptospirosis is a systemic and biphasic febrile illness that may involve different organs and systems. As an organ is colonized, it becomes more vulnerable to GLP action. Regardless of the site of leptospirae penetration into the body from the blood stream, the bacteria have preferential tropism to colonize the kidney and liver. As GLP is an endotoxin present on bacterial walls, it will establish interaction mainly with surrounding cells when it is released by bacterial lysis that results from an immune reaction and/or antibiotics. The relationship between the intensity of tissue colonization, organ dysfunction, and clinical manifestations is the current explanation for the hepatic and renal characteristic manifestations of the disease. Leptospirae have been found in different organs[7] but severe forms of leptospirosis resemble sepsis, and some systemic effects are not directly related to the presence of leptospirae. GLP extracted from pathogenic, but not from non-pathogenic, serovars induces mononuclear cells to produce cytokines.[8] According to classical Gram-negative bacterial sepsis, plasma cytokines are elevated in Weil's disease, although cytokine activation does not occur through the same LPS pathway.[8] Tumor necrosis factor-α (TNF-α) and interleukin-10 are increased but only TNF levels are associated with the severity of leptospirosis. More recently, it has been shown that *Leptospira* can activate T-cell subsets and produce Th1 cytokines as the patient develops disease or establishes host defenses.[9]

Clinical features

Leptospirosis is characteristically an acute infection with a biphasic course. After an incubation period between 4 and 21 days, a sudden onset of irregular fever (38–40° C) with chills, myalgia, headache, vomiting, ocular hyperemia, and skin lesions is usually present in this first phase, called septicemic or leptospiremic. This phase, in which microorganisms are found in the blood stream, aqueous humor, and liquor, lasts around 5–7 days and culminates with a host-specific immune response by IgM antibody. If antibodies are sufficient to combat, block, and eliminate bacterial proliferation, all symptoms disappear in a few hours. However, if bacterial colonization is maintained despite host immunologic responses, the patient progresses clinically to the immune phase. This new phase assists the disappearance of leptospires from the circulation as bacteria gain access and colonize tissues, especially in kidneys, liver, muscles, and brain, and from this moment *Leptospira* are present in the urine.

Clinical manifestations in the immune phase more often occur in infections by serovar *L. icterohaemorrhagiae* and may broadly vary from mild to moderate with up to 5–10% severe, often fatal, cases. The two chief presentations are as follows:

1. The anicteric form: fever, chills, headache, vomiting, lumbar and calf muscle pain, exanthema, and non-specific symptoms. Frontal migraine plus retroocular pain and photophobia are frequent; lung involvement with cough, chest pain and hemoptysis; conjunctival suffusions, generalized painful lymphadenitis mostly in the neck, pharyngeal injection, enlarged and painful liver (very frequent) and splenomegaly (around 20%) as well as questionable jaundice are seen. Several types of exanthema are possible: macular, maculopapular, erythematous, urticarial, and hemorrhagic. After a 7–10-day course, the disease abates; however, it may rarely recur after the third week, presenting with iritis, iridocyclitis, or chorioretinitis.
2. Weil's disease comprises pyrexia, severe icterus, oliguric or non-acute renal failure and hemorrhagic diathesis. Between the second and seventh days of jaundice, the appearance becomes ochre to bronze yellow, with pale stools and marked choluria, pruritus, and tender enlarged liver. Jaundice is due to hemolysis plus hepatic cholestasis. Cholestasis with normal or slightly elevated serum transaminases and high serum alkaline phosphatase and conjugated bilirubin are typical findings. Icterus itself does not mean high mortality in spite of the fact that most deaths occur among icteric patients.

Cutaneous involvement (Figs 27.12 and 27.13) is not usually emphasized, but is almost always distinct. Erythema of the chest, abdomen, and extremities is seen, but most extensor surfaces remain clear; the face and cheeks are usually spared. Morbilliform, maculopapular, erythematous, urticarial, or petechial and hemorrhagic exanthema, with or without furfuraceous desquamation, may resemble mumps, scarlet fever, or urticaria. Scleral and conjunctival injection or hemorrhages appear together with jaundice early in the course. Weil's disease includes all types of hemorrhagic skin lesions: petechiae, vibices, ecchymosis and others, concurrently with prominent jaundice. Children may suffer infarctions in parts of their hands and feet. Infection due to *L. interrogans* may cause erythema nodosum. *L. autummalis* serovar infection not infrequently exhibits pretibial 1–5-cm tender, slightly raised erythematous skin lesions (Fort Bragg pretibial fever). Herpetic mucous and cutaneous lesions can appear during leptospiral infection (Fig. 27.12E). Body sodium depletion states add to the signs and symptoms of cutaneous turgor loss. Rarely, the Jarisch–Herxheimer reaction can follow antibiotic treatment. Muscle pain from soft touch is typical and the biopsy shows sarcoplasmic degeneration, leptospiral organisms, areas of myolysis, and necrotic foci that may cause expressive rhabdomyolysis.

Capillary damage to endothelium produces extravasation of fluids, inflammatory and red cells, and spirochetes. Arterial hypotension is associated with a fast, weak, sometimes irregular pulse. A diffuse vasculitis elicits many clinical manifestations; it principally affects the capillaries, causing ubiquitous hemorrhage (epistaxis, hemoptysis, hematemesis, melena, rashes, conjunctival suffusions, bleeding in skeletal muscles as well as in the myocardium, pleural spaces, peritoneum, adrenals, kidneys, lungs, liver, and subarachnoid spaces) without intravascular coagulation but accompanied by thrombocytopenia and prolonged clotting time.

The myocardium may also be attacked and myocarditis, heart failure, arrhythmias, and electrocardiogram alterations are not rare: sudden death may ensue. Arterial hypotension is usual and several previously hypertensive subjects temporarily remain without need of their antihypertensive drugs. Cardiogenic shock sometimes takes place and may respond to prompt fluid administration. Gastrointestinal signs and complaints of melena, diarrhea and large hematemesis, cholecystitis without calculi, and overt pancreatitis may ensue; isolated hyperamylasemia is not rare. The central nervous system is harmed; headache, photophobia, blurred vision, nuchal rigidity, mental disturbances, seizures, frank encephalitis, and coma may occur. Ocular lesions, from conjunctivitis to uveal tract inflammation, are not uncommon. Lung involvement (20–70%) is manifested by cough, dyspnea, hemoptysis and respiratory failure. Acute respiratory distress syndrome (ARDS) seems to become more prevalent in Brazil and overwhelming pulmonary bleeding has been seen.[10]

Oliguria is frequent and slight proteinuria with hyaline and granular casts, leukocytes, and red cells is frequent. Acute renal failure (ARF) is due to tubular and interstitial lesions of both hypoxic and toxic nephropathy with interstitial edema, tubular cell necrosis, and frequent tubular basement membrane rupture. We have seen 181 cases of ARF in leptospirosis and 69% presented initially with oliguria. Typical paradoxical normal or hypokalemia (32%) was present (serum K level 3.7 ± 0.9 mmol/l) despite high creatinine levels (5.8 ± 2.4 mg%).[11]

Multiple organ failure has been reported and the emergency-room physicians must be aware of this possibility in order to start adequate treatment promptly, since early recognition makes the differ ence between recovery and death. Hypotension in the presence of vascular collapse associated with meningoencephalic changes, cerebrospinal fluid pleiocytosis, ARDS, oligoanuric ARF, hemorrhagic diathesis, and altered mental status heralds a poor prognosis.

Patient evaluation, diagnosis, and differential diagnosis

The evaluation of human leptospirosis infection depends on three factors: (1) virulence of the serovar; (2) the degree of bacterial infection; (3) the host immune response. Seroprevalence trials show the subclinical form of infection in most cases, which makes it easier to combat bacterial invasion. Humans react to *Leptospira* infection by producing specific anti-*Leptospira* antibodies. Seroconversion may occur as early as 5–7 days after the onset of disease but sometimes only after 10 days or longer. IgM antibodies usually appear earlier than IgG and generally remain detectable for months

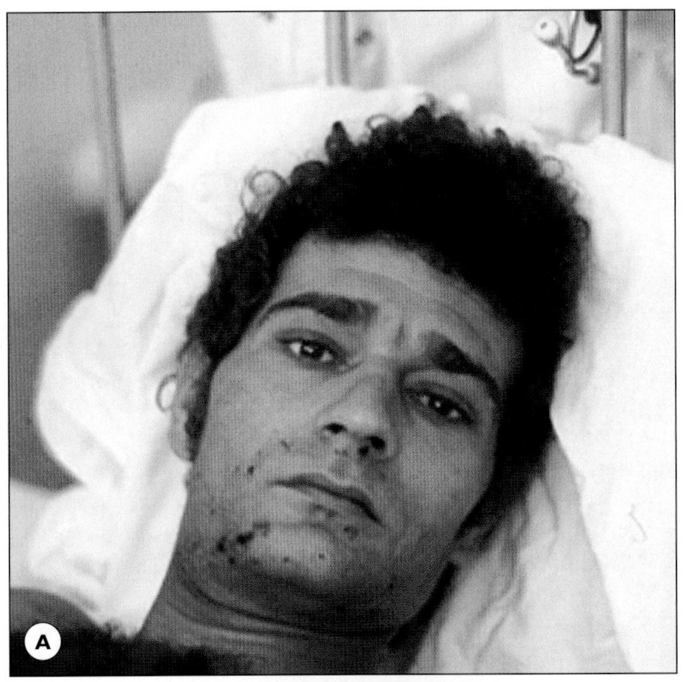

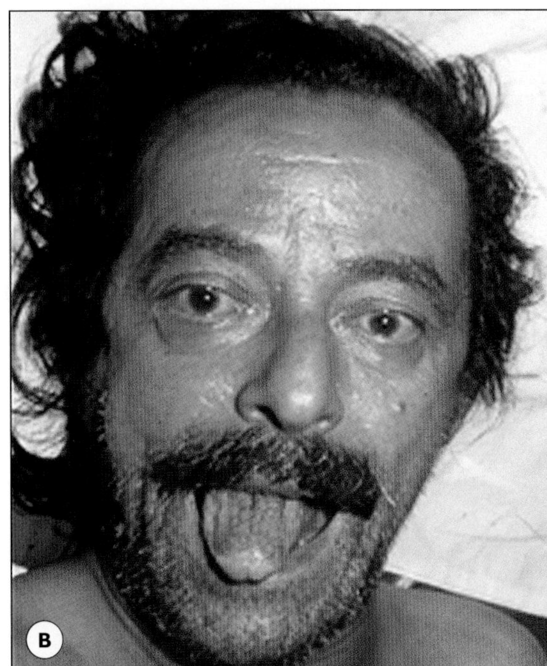

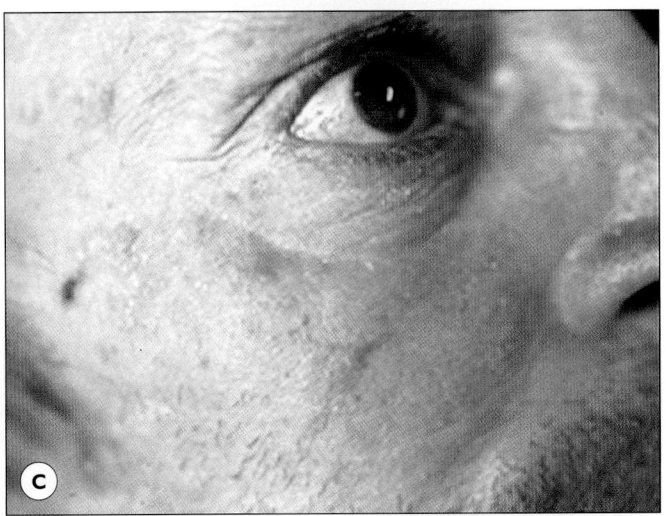

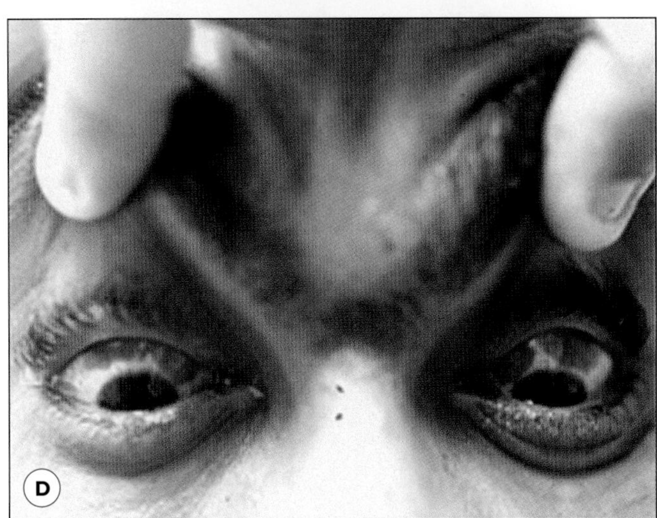

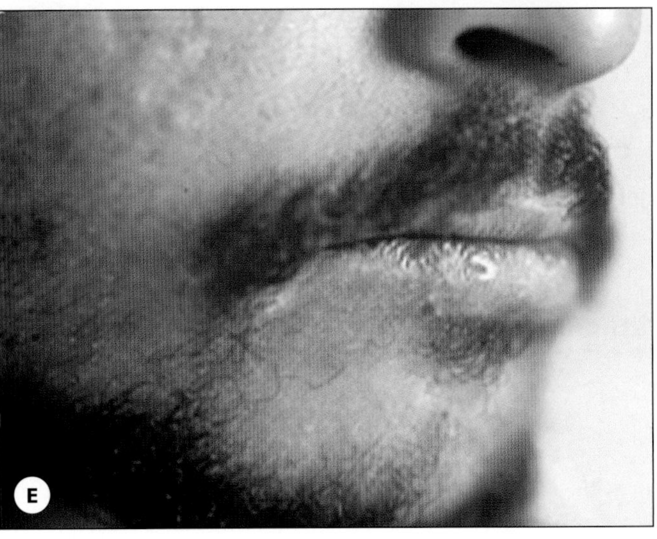

Figure 27.12 Skin manifestations in patients with leptospirosis: (A) Leptospirosis in convalescence. Icterus is still present with cutaneous vasodilatation and bleeding after shaving. (B) Icterus. Dehydration with saline repletion. Dry skin and mucosa with "parrot's tongue." Noticeable cutaneous vasodilatation. Bright eyes with conjunctival hyperemia and jaundice. (C) Jaundice and hyperemia plus cutaneous telangiectasia and petechia. Nasal redness. (D) Bilateral conjunctival jaundice and hemorrhage. (E) Cutaneous icterus with vasodilatation, petechiae, and labial herpetic lesions. (Courtesy of Dr. Ana Maria Miranda Pinto.)

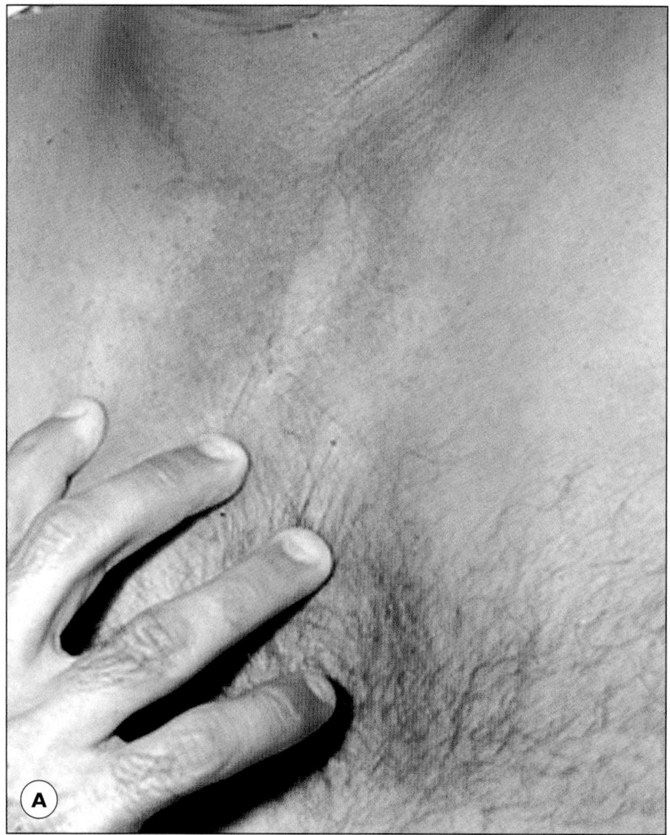

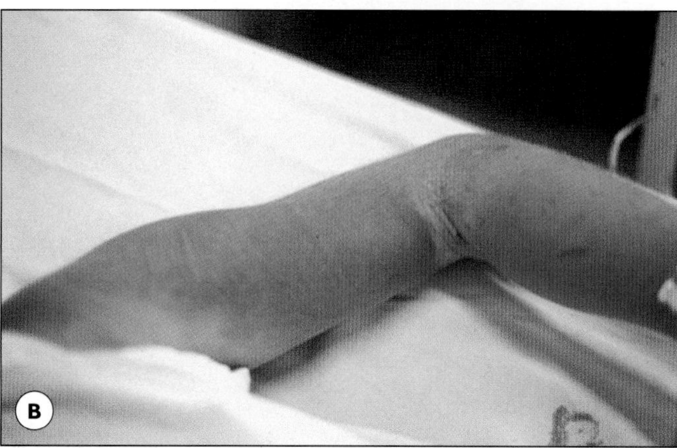

Figure 27.13 Skin manifestations in patients with leptospirosis. (A) Jaundice with marked vasodilatation; white dermographism on digital pressure; (B) extensive ecchymosis on deltoid and anterior brachial regions at sites of needle punctures. (Courtesy of Dr. Ana Maria Miranda Pinto.)

or even years, but at low titers. IgG antibodies may not be detected at all, or for only short periods, or may be detected for several years. The antibodies are usually directed against common antigens shared by other pathogenic *Leptospira* and are able to immunize the patient against infection by other serovars.

Due to improved treatment with antibiotics and dialysis, severe forms now have a better prognosis and mortality has considerably decreased. After acute disease, liver and renal recovery is usually complete. Mortality has been reported from 5% up to 50% or greater. In our series in Rio de Janeiro the 23-year cumulative mortality rate among leptospirotic hospitalized patients was around 10%.[12] However, during epidemic outbreaks, severe pulmonary involvement and multiorgan failure may result in higher mortality rates.

Diagnosis of leptospirosis is based on careful history and physical exam, assisted by cross-examination of epidemiological data and accurate suspicion.

The specific diagnosis is based on bacterial detection and may be performed by direct methods as culture of the bacteria (from blood, cerebrospinal fluid, urine, and tissues), dark-field microscopy, inoculation of infected patients' material on experimental animals, bacterial staining (with silver-Lavaditi stain, immunofluorescence, or immunoperoxidase) and by PCR. Indirect methods include the microscopic agglutination test (MAT) and ELISA. The MAT, by mixing infected serum with live or killed formalin-fixed *Leptospira*, detects both the agglutinating IgM and IgG responses; therefore, antibody responses elicited by recent or previous infection or vaccination cannot be distinguished with one single test. As a result, sequential serum sample analyses are required in order to establish the stage of the infection. Several commercial ELISA assays can detect agglutinating and non-agglutinating antibodies as early as 2 days after symptoms manifest. Since IgM and IgG responses can be identified separately, past infection or vaccination can be differentiated from acute infection, in contrast to MAT. Recently, the so-called LEPTO dipstick became commercially available; it is an IgM-specific dot-ELISA that contains broadly reactive leptospiral antigens capable of reacting with 22 different serovars and has been proven effective in diagnosing leptospirosis in endemic areas.[2]

Non-specific laboratory findings range from leukopenia to marked leukocytosis, thrombocytopenia, and high erythrocyte sedimentation rates. Cerebrospinal fluid may present with pleocytosis with a predominance of mononuclear cells, normal glucose concentration, and proteins exceeding 100 mg/dl. Serum biochemistry may show azotemia, hypokalemia, alkaline phosphatase elevated by 50% or more, serum transaminases (aspartate serum transaminase and serum glutamic oxaloacetic transaminase) at normal or slightly increased levels, and high bilirubin with predominance of the direct fraction, although gamma-glutamyl transpeptidase is rarely high. Low albumin and cholesterol levels may also be found. The prothrombin time is usually prolonged. Urinalysis frequently shows choluria, glycosuria, mild proteinuria, casts, cellular elements and, more rarely, hematuria and myoglobinuria.

The differential diagnosis demands a high index of precision and experience with diverse clinical presentations. Leptospirosis may be underdiagnosed among children, perhaps because the suspicion index is lower and the clinical manifestations are not infrequently mild. Several diseases must be considered in both endemic and non-endemic areas (Table 27.3).

Pathology

Necropsy studies from leptospirotic patients frequently show jaundice with a varied degree of discoloration. Scleras and serous membranes appear from slightly yellow to a deep greenish-yellow cast to the entire skin and mucosa. In the skin, hemorrhages, chiefly petechiae and extensive areas of ecchymosis, may be seen at sites of needle puncture (Fig. 27.13B). Petechiae are also observed in the serosal membranes, conjunctiva, renal pelvis, and mucosa of the gastrointestinal tract. The mouth and gums may be covered by partly

Table 27.3 Differential diagnosis of leptospirosis

Disease	Characteristics for differentiation
Dengue	Pyelonephritis
Q fever	Overwhelming adenovirus infection
Typhus	Gastroenteritis
Malaria	Meningoencephalitis
Viral hepatitis	Atypical pneumonia
Pulmonary tuberculosis	Viral hemorrhagic fevers
Influenza	Bacterial endocarditis
Brucellosis	Connective tissue disorders
Tularemia	Vasculitis
Erlichiosis	Hemolytic–uremic syndrome
Syphilis	Henoch–Schönlein purpura
Human immunodeficiency (HIV) infection	Thrombotic thrombocytopenic purpura
Sepsis	Snake bites
Yellow fever	Intoxications: carbon tetrachloride, chloroform, tetrachloroethylene
Hantaan virus	Hemorrhage, renal failure

clotted blood. Hemorrhage may be present in the retroperitoneal fat, omentum, subarachnoid space and pectorals, intercostals, psoas, and lumbar muscles.

In severe forms, interstitial and intraalveolar hemorrhages may also be present. The lungs are always congested, principally if there is associated myocarditis. Foci of acute interstitial inflammation, in the presence of lymphocytes and plasma cells, contribute to the development of respiratory failure.[10] Liver histopathology may vary from advanced degenerative changes to mild interstitial edema and vascular congestion. Liver biopsies done with no complications in 29 of 89 cases described by Correa-Lima[13] disclosed predominance of centrolobular cholestatic hepatitis. In the most exuberant cases, hepatocytes present with mitotic figures with bile pigment in their cytoplasm, and Kupffer cells may be hyperplastic. The sinusoids are congested with focal or diffuse hemorrhages and bile canaliculi may present with bile casts. Inflammatory phenomena are more marked in the periphery of the hepatic lobule and are associated with a moderate round-cell infiltrate in the periportal space. More rarely, advanced degeneration with necrotic foci may be distributed at random.[7] The mechanism of icterus in leptospirosis remains unknown. Light microscopy of liver biopsies discloses cholestasis and the ultrastructural study shows normal hepatocytes side by side with cells showing altered sinusoidal pole microvillus, suggesting the presence of a toxin effect over bile pigment excretion. In agreement, the presence of leptospiral antigen in portal tracts close to bile ducts was demonstrated by immunoperoxidase staining. A supposed GLP endotoxin-inhibitory effect on Na^+, K^+-ATPase from bile duct cells could impair sodium-dependent bile secretion and thus be a direct participant in the cholestatic mechanism during leptospirosis.

Renal alterations vary in intensity and nature depending on the duration of illness and usually include both interstitial nephritis and focal acute tubular damage. Injured nephrons are seen alternating with normal ones. A limited number of glomeruli may exhibit mild lesions with mild and focal swelling. Inflammatory foci are more prominent in the cortex and outer medulla with the presence of lymphocytes, macrophages, plasma cells and, occasionally neutrophils and eosinophils.

Treatment

The therapeutic approach must simultaneously consider infection control and preservation of metabolic balance. *Leptospira* are theoretically susceptible to a wide variety of antibiotics: penicillin G, tetracycline, doxycycline, ampicillin or amoxicillin are usually employed. Both prophylactic effect and early administration of antibiotics until the fourth day after beginning of symptoms are established. There are arguments about the value of antimicrobial therapy started late, after the onset of kidney and liver damage. A double-blind study concluded that penicillin G started even after the fifth day shortened the fever period and hospitalization time.[14] Another recent randomized trial including patients with severe forms showed that the group which started penicillin treatment after 4 days of symptomatic disease presented higher mortality than controls.[15] In some circumstances, presumptive administration of penicillin G may be life-saving, and the risk of a Jarisch–Herxheimer reaction following antibiotics in leptospirosis is too small to justify withholding them.

Metabolic balance in leptospirotic patients depends on the severity of disease manifestations. Hydroelectrolytic infusion is usually necessary for hemodynamic stability and renal perfusion. Oliguric patients usually start diuresis after 24–48 h treatment. In this way, normalizing plasma volume with intravenous fluid administration and/or dialysis together with plasma electrolyte correction is essential. Because paradoxical hypokalemia and low intracellular K^+ levels are frequent, careful potassium replacement must be considered despite the presence of acute renal failure.[16] Restoration of serum potassium to normal levels in leptospirotic patients correlates with recovery of renal function. Kaliuretic drugs such as loop diuretics as well as dopamine and digitalis must be avoided because their GLP synergic effects on Na^+, K^+-ATPase activity increase the risk of cardiac arrhythmias. Extrarenal purification may be necessary for the treatment of ARF and peritoneal or hemodialysis can be employed.

Vaccination

Since the 1960s animal vaccination has become the mainstay of leptospiral control in public health policies, thus one can expect a reduction of human leptospirosis. Animal vaccines are polyvalent and prepared from one to six serovars common to the species and to the specific geographical region. The duration of immune protection varies from a few weeks to over a year. Vaccination has been successful in controlling veterinary infection caused by serovars such as *L. pomoma* in swine and cattle, and *L. canicola* and *L. icterohaemorrhagiae* in dogs; however the ideal vaccine, which prevents all types of leptospirosis in all animal species, has not been found. Currently, human vaccination is indicated for people with occupational and special risk conditions. The variability of antigenic properties among the several serovars and the recommendation of annual revaccination are challenges for the development of a human vaccine against leptospirosis.

References

1. World Health Organization. Human leptospirosis: guidance for diagnosis, surveillance and control. Geneva: WHO; 2003.
2. Plank R, Dean D. Overview of the epidemiology, microbiology, and pathogenesis of *Leptospira* sp. in humans. Microb Infect 2000; 2:1265–1276.
3. Vinh T, Adler B, Faine S. Glycolipoprotein cytotoxin from *Leptospira interrogans* serovar *copenhageni*. J Gen Microbiol 1986; 132:111–123.
4. Younes-Ibrahim M, Burth P, Castro-Faria MV et al. Inhibition of Na, K-ATPase by an endotoxin extracted from *Leptospira interrogans*: a possible mechanism for the physiopathology of leptospirosis. CR Acad Sci Paris 1995; 318:619–625.
5. Burth P, Younes-Ibrahim M, Gonçalves FHFS et al. Purification and characterization of a Na^+, K^+ ATPase inhibitor found in an endotoxin of *Leptospira*. Infect Immun 1997; 65:2557–2560.
6. Younes-Ibrahim M, Buffin-Meyer B, Cheval L et al. Na, K-ATPase: a molecular target for *Leptospira interrogans* endotoxin. Braz J Med Biol Res 1997; 30:213–223.
7. Arean VM. Studies on the pathogenesis of leptospirosis. II. A clinicopathologic evaluation of hepatic and renal function in experimental leptospiral infections. Lab Invest 1962; 11:273–288.
8. Diament D, Brunialti MKC, Romero EC et al. Peripheral blood mononuclear cell activation induced by *Leptospira interrogans* glycolipoprotein. Infect Immun 2002; 70:1677–1683.
9. Klimpel GR, Matthias MA, Vinetz JM. *Leptospira interrogans* activation of human peripheral blood mononuclear cells: preferential expansion of TCR$\gamma\delta^+$ T cells vs TCR $\alpha\beta^+$ T cells. Immunology 2003; 71:1447–1455.
10. Carvalho CRR, Bethlem EP. Pulmonary complications of leptospirosis. Clin Chest Med 2002; 23:469–478.
11. Santos OR, Younes-Ibrahim M, Vieira LMSF et al. Insuficiência renal aguda na leptospirose humana. J Bras Nefrol 2000; XXII (suppl. 1):5.
12. Younes-Ibrahim M, Rosa Santos O. Hipótese para Insuficiência Renal Agunda Peculiar. An Acad Nac Med 1995; 155:26–35.
13. Correa-Lima MB. Contribuição ao estudo do fígado na leptospirose. Thesis. Rio de Janeiro, Brazil: Escola Medicina e Cirurgia; 1971.
14. Watt G, Padre LP, Tuazon ML et al. Placebo-controlled trial of intravenous penicillin for severe and late leptospirosis. Lancet 1988; 1:433–435.
15. Costa E, Lopes AA, Sacramento E et al. Penicillin at the late stage of leptospirosis: a randomized controlled trial. Rev Inst Med Trop S Paulo 2003; 45:141–145.
16. Seguro AC, Lomar AV, Rocha AS. Acute renal failure of leptospirosis: nonoliguric and hypokalemic forms. Nephron 1990; 55:146–151.

Acknowledgments

We are indebted to Dr. Ana Maria Miranda Pinto for the care of patients in Figures 27.12 and 27.13, and to Dr. Walter C. Franco for reviewing the manuscript.

Chapter 28

Anthrax, plague, diphtheria, trachoma and miscellaneous bacteria

- Anthrax ■ *Stephen K. Tyring*
- Plague ■ *Stephen K. Tyring*
- Diphtheria ■ *Mark Burnett and Martin Ottolini*
- Trachoma ■ *Frank Mwesigye*
- Miscellaneous bacteria ■ *Stephen K. Tyring*

Anthrax

Stephen K. Tyring

Synonyms: *Bacillus anthracis* toxins

Key features:

- Anthrax is a fatal disease in domestic livestock and in wild herbivores
- Humans are usually infected incidentally
- Most human disease is cutaneous, followed by oral–oropharyngeal, gastrointestinal, and inhalational
- Disease is mediated through toxins which cause edema, hemorrhage, and necrosis
- Mortality rate is high
- Diagnosis is clinical, biopsy, Gram stain, culture, or serology
- Treatment is with penicillin, ciprofloxacin, tetracycline, erythromycin, chloramphenicol, or streptomycin
- Prevention is via vaccination or quarantine of animals and avoidance/destruction of contaminated animal products

Introduction

Anthrax is found throughout tropical Africa, Asia, Central and South America as well as the Caribbean; it is due to the Gram-positive bacillus, *Bacillus anthracis*. Incidental infection of humans is usually due to contact with infected livestock or wild herbivores or animal products, e.g., meat, hides, wool. Dying and dead animals contaminate the soil with spores which subsequently infect other animals or humans. Recently the potential of the use of anthrax spores as weapons of bioterrorism has become a reality.

Over 95% of all clinical anthrax is cutaneous, resulting from spores entering abraded skin of persons skinning or butchering infected animals or persons subsequently handling the meat, hides, or wool. If untreated, 80% of the cutaneous infections become localized and 20% develop bacteremia and fatal septicemia.

Other presentations of anthrax include oral–oropharyngeal or gastrointestinal (from eating raw or undercooked meat) and inhalational (from contaminated wool or hides or from bioterrorism). The majority of these systemic presentations are fatal if not treated. Hematogenous spread can lead to meningoencephalitis. Death is from edema, hemorrhage, and necrosis secondary to anthrax toxins.

History and epidemiology

Anthrax spores can survive for years in dry soil and in other harsh environments. When these spores come into contact with wild animals or livestock, epidemics of anthrax can result, as was the case in Zimbabwe from 1978 to 1982.[1,2] Anthrax spreads to animals and humans from contaminated soil and from animal carcasses, but also from the bites of tabanid flies, e.g., horse flies and deer flies. Although most human cases of anthrax have been reported from Africa, southern Europe, and the Middle East, anthrax in livestock is reported regularly from west Texas to South Dakota. Although such cases in livestock can affect ranchers, butchers, and others who work with cattle, such reports are uncommon in the USA.

Persons who work with animal products such as hides in the textile industry and tanneries have been infected with anthrax, resulting in the majority of cases reported in the USA in the twentieth century being industry-related. In recent decades, however, such cases have become rare due to strict controls on animal products as well as the increasing use of synthetic fabrics.

In the twenty-first century anthrax has been used as a weapon in isolated cases of bioterrorism. The accidental release of anthrax in 1979 from a biological weapons facility in Sverdlovsk (now Ekaterinburg), Russia resulted in significant mortality in humans and in livestock.[3]

Pathogenesis

After entering the skin, anthrax spores germinate, resulting in a "malignant pustule," although pus is usually only seen if there is a secondary bacterial infection. Histology of the skin lesions reveals marked tissue destruction with extensive subepidermal edema, thrombosis of vessels, and hemorrhagic interstitium.[4] Toxin production results in generalized edema and non-pitting edema around the lesion. Although the draining lymph nodes respond to the infection, the bacterial capsule is antiphagocytic and bacteremia often results.

Inhalation anthrax results in phagocytosis of spores by alveolar macrophages, mediastinal widening, and bacteremia. As seen in the victims in Sverdlovsk, death is due to primary pneumonia.[3] Interestingly, anthrax is not found in the sputum in inhalation anthrax.[3]

Ingestion of meat contaminated with anthrax results in ulceration and hemorrhage at the points of entry in the submucosa, especially in the oropharynx and the ileocecal regions. Hemorrhagic ascites and diseased bowel segments are associated with bacteremia. Hemorrhagic meningitis can result from bacteremia in any clinical form of anthrax.

Although reinfection with anthrax has been reported, immunity can develop from subclinical infection and lasting protection usually results in survivors of clinical anthrax.[5,6] Measurable antibodies to the toxin and the capsule are found after infection. Anthraxin is a skin test for delayed-type hypersensitivity that has been reported to be useful.

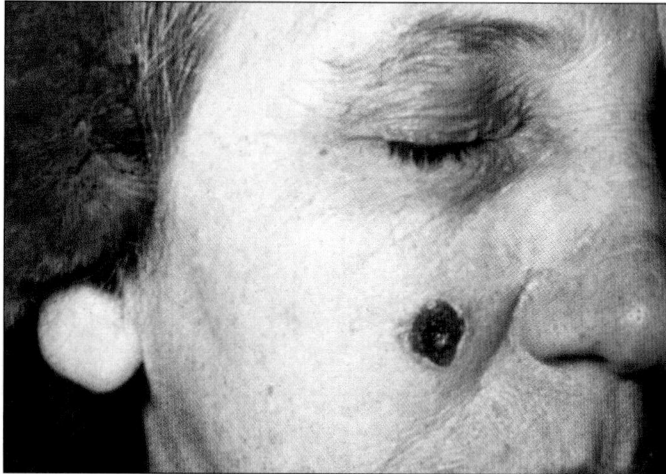

Figure 28.2 Anthrax ulcer on the face. (Courtesy of Centers for Disease Control and Prevention.)

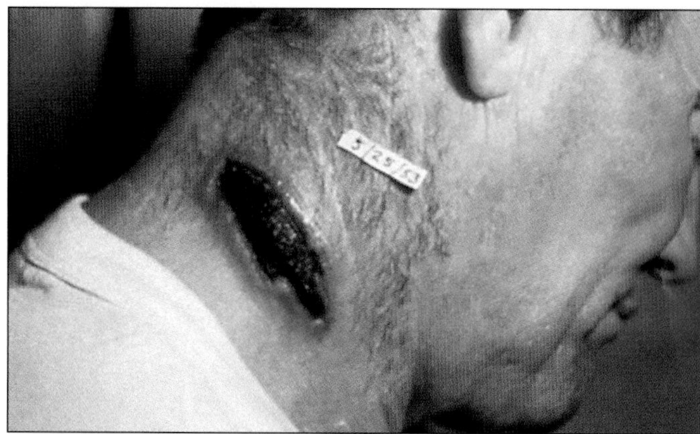

Figure 28.3 Anthrax eschar of the neck. (Courtesy of Centers for Disease Control and Prevention.)

Clinical manifestations of cutaneous anthrax

In humans clinical anthrax presents in one of three forms: cutaneous, inhalational, and oral–oropharyngeal/gastrointestinal. Over 95% of cases, however, are cutaneous.[7] In approximately 90% of cases, there is only one lesion, and it is usually on an exposed part of the body. The initial symptom is pruritus which follows infection by 3–10 days. The first sign, a papule a few millimeters in diameter, usually follows pruritus by only 1 day. During the next day, vesicles develop which surround the papule (Fig. 28.1). The vesicles coalesce and the papule ruptures, resulting in a 4–6-cm ulcer (Fig. 28.2). During the next few days the ulcer develops a thick, depressed, brown to black eschar which is adherent to the underlying tissue (Fig. 28.3). Non-pitting edema forms around the eschar and regional lymphadenopathy develops. If the lesion is on the neck, edema may become so extensive as to compromise respiration. The patients are usually afebrile and the skin lesions are usually painless. Some patients, however, do develop fever, headache, anorexia, nausea, and lethargy associated with the systemic effects of the toxin.

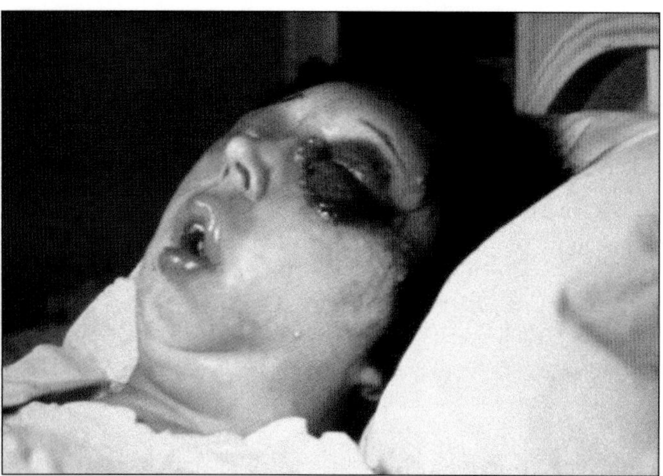

Figure 28.1 Anthrax of the eye on day 5. (Courtesy of Centers for Disease Control and Prevention.)

Over 80% of untreated cutaneous lesions remain localized and heal within 2–6 weeks, often resulting in scar formation. Almost 20% of untreated cutaneous lesions and the majority of systemic infections develop systemic bacteremia and are fatal.[8]

Diagnosis and differential diagnosis

In the setting of the signs and/or symptoms of anthrax and/or a history of (potential) exposure to the bacteria or spores, a Gram stain should be carried out on material from the vesicle fluid, ulcer base, or other appropriate clinical material for large, Gram-positive bacilli. Bacterial culture should be inoculated on the appropriate medium and serology performed using a specific inhibition enzyme immunoassay for antibodies directed against purified protective antigen. A biopsy should be taken from a characteristic cutaneous lesion and examined for the changes described above. Therapy must be initiated immediately to prevent the high rate of mortality and to reduce morbidity.

The differential diagnosis of cutaneous anthrax includes orf, staphylococcal skin lesions such as bullous impetigo, tularemia, plague, burns, cutaneous diphtheria, rickettsial eschar, and ecthyma gangrenosum.

Therapy

Considering the high mortality rate of anthrax, treatment must be started as soon as possible. Therapy of cutaneous anthrax is usually with oral potassium penicillin V or intramuscular procaine penicillin G. If the patient has a penicillin allergy, alternatives include tetracycline, ciprofloxacin, erythromycin, streptomycin, or chloramphenicol. Intravenous penicillin G along with intensive supportive care is the therapy of choice for systemic anthrax. Surgical excision or incision of the cutaneous lesions is not beneficial and can even exacerbate the injury.

Prevention

Use of control measures for animal anthrax will help prevent human anthrax. These measures include quarantine of animals suspected to have been exposed to anthrax, use of antibiotics, or destruction and incineration of infected animals and vaccination of livestock at risk for anthrax. Prevention of human anthrax also requires public awareness programs and vaccination for persons at high risk, i.e., the military.[9] Antibiotic prophylaxis can be protective if used properly.

References

1. Davies JCA. A major epidemic of anthrax in Zimbabwe, part I. Cent Afr J Med 1982; 28:291.
2. Sternbach G. The history of anthrax. J Emerg Med 2004; 26:354.
3. Meselson M, Guillemin J, Hugh-Jones M. The Sverdlovsk anthrax outbreak of 1979. Science 1994; 266:1202.
4. Lever WF, Schaumburg-Lever G. Bacterial diseases. In Lever WF, Schaumberg-Lever G, eds. Histopathology of the skin, 6th edn. Philadelphia: Lippincott; 1983:290–319.
5. Marcus H, Danieli R, Epstein E et al. Contribution of immunological memory to protective immunity conferred by a *Bacillus anthracis* protective antigen-based vaccine. Infect Immun 2004; 72:3471–3477.
6. Reissman DB, Whitney EA, Taylor TH Jr et al. One year health assessment of adult survivors of *Bacillus anthracis* infection. JAMA 2004; 291:1994–1998.
7. Godyn JJ, Siderits R, Dzaman J. Cutaneous anthrax. Arch Pathol Lab Med 2004; 128:709–710.
8. Sanderson WT, Stoddard RR, Echt AS et al. *Bacillus anthracis* contamination and inhalational anthrax in a mail processing distribution center. J Appl Microbiol 2004; 96:1048–1056.
9. Walker DH, Yampolska O, Grinberg LM. Death at Sverdlovsk: what have we learned? Am J. Pathol 1994; 144:1135.

Plague

Stephen K. Tyring

Synonyms: *Yersinia pestis*, bubonic plague, septicemic plague, pneumonic plague

Key features:

- Plague is a zoonotic infection in rodents and is transmitted by fleas
- Plague is due to a non-motile, non-sporulating, Gram-negative coccobacillus, *Yersinia pestis*
- Without therapy, most cases of bubonic plague and almost all cases of septicemic and pneumonic plague are rapidly fatal
- Plague is found in the western USA, in parts of South America, in southern Africa, and in eastern and southern Asia
- Therapy is with streptomycin, gentamicin, tetracycline, or chloramphenicol
- No vaccine is available, but control is by avoidance of areas with epizootic plague and control of fleas with insecticides

Introduction

For many centuries plague has appeared in epidemics, with significant mortality rates. Due to the understanding of the epidemiology of plague and the responsible organism, *Yersinia pestis*, control of the responsible rodents and fleas has markedly decreased the incidence of this infection. The availability of antibiotics in the second half of the twentieth century has allowed effective therapy of plague if the signs and symptoms are recognized in a timely manner.

History

Although there are biblical references to "plagues," it was not until 542 AD that a pandemic due to plague (i.e., *Y. pestis*) was described.[1] It lasted 100 years and devastated the populations of the Mediterranean and the Middle East. Following the increase in the rat population, the next recorded pandemic lasted from 1347 to 1350, resulting in 25 million deaths, approximately 25% of Europe. It was referred to as the "black death," possibly due to a hemorrhagic diathesis in some patients. Pandemics were subsequently recorded in London in 1665 and in the Far East in the late nineteenth century. By 1903 India was experiencing over one million deaths annually due to plague.[2] The infection made its appearance in the western hemisphere in Santos, Brazil, in 1899 and in the USA (in San Francisco) in 1909. The last epidemic of pneumonic plague was in Berkeley Hills, California, in 1919.[3] With the increased understanding of the epidemiology of plague in the late nineteenth century and the discovery of the responsible organism by Alexander Yersin in 1894, better control of the wild rodent population and rat-proofing of buildings and ships resulted in marked decreases in plague in the western hemisphere by the twentieth century.

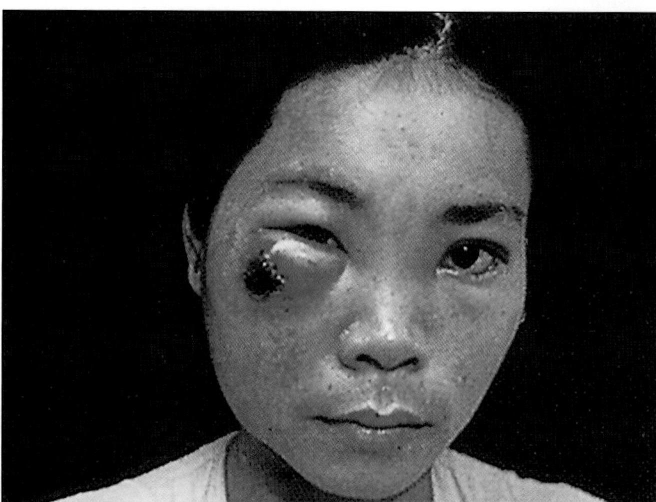

Figure 28.4 An eschar and local facial carbuncle resulting from the bite of a *Yersinia pestis*-infected flea. (Reproduced from Peters W and Pasvol G (eds). Tropical Medicine and Parasitology, 5th edition, Mosby, London 2002, image 63.)

Epidemiology

About 15 countries report plague to the World Health Organization each year. These cases are primarily from the western USA, Peru, East Africa, Southeast Asia, and India. *Y. pestis* exists in nature as a zoonotic infection in rodents and their fleas, and humans are incidentally infected, usually by flea bites and occasionally by handling infected animals or by inhalation.[4]

Pathogenesis

After gaining entrance into the body via a flea bite or inhalation, the organism causes bacteremia and septicemia, leading to death by disseminated intravascular coagulation (DIC), refractory hypotension, renal shutdown, and shock. Pneumonic plague results in acute respiratory distress syndrome (ARDS) and multilobar confluence.

Clinical

Bubonic plague

Approximately 2–6 days after infection, the patient with bubonic plague experiences fever to 38°C or greater, chills, headache, myalgias, arthralgias, and lethargy.[5] During the next day or two the patient suffers pain and tenderness in the regional lymph nodes draining the area of the flea bite. The bite often results in a papule, pustule, ulcer, or eschar (Fig. 28.4). The skin over the involved lymph nodes becomes erythematous, edematous, tense, and warm to the touch. The bubo of plague (Fig. 28.5) differs from the lymphadenopathy of most other etiologies by its rapid onset, marked tenderness, and systemic toxemia as well as the absence of cellulitis or ascending lymphangitis.

If appropriate antibiotic therapy is initiated in the acute state, bubonic plague usually responds rapidly, with decrease of fever and resolution of systemic symptoms in 2–5 days. The buboes, however, remain enlarged, tender, and sometimes fluctuant for 1 week or longer after successful therapy.

If therapy is not initiated acutely, bubonic plague progresses to systemic toxemia, tachycardia, prostration, agitation, confusion, convulsions, delirium, and death.

Septicemic plague

Patients with septicemic plague often present with endotoxemia and gastrointestinal symptoms, but without regional lymphadenitis.[6,7]

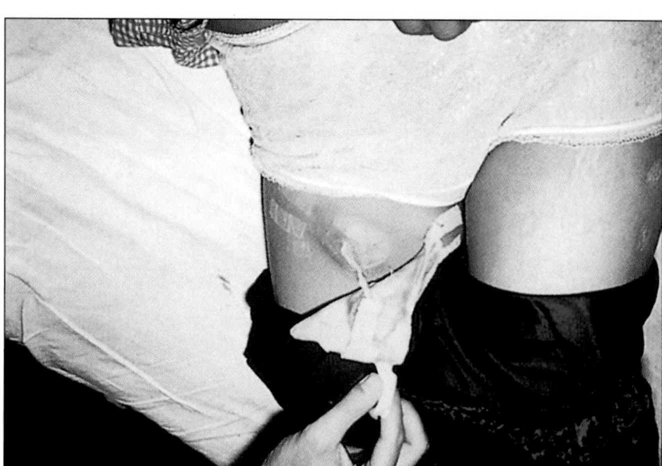

Figure 28.5 A bubo of the femoral lymph nodes in a patient with bubonic plague. (Reproduced from Peters W and Pasvol G (eds). Tropical Medicine and Parasitology, 5th edition, Mosby, London 2002, image 62.)

Plague is often not suspected initially until laboratory results indicate its presence. Without intensive supportive care and antibiotic therapy, septicemic plague can rapidly progress to DIC, manifested as petechiae, ecchymoses, and acral gangrene (Figs 28.6 and 28.7). In addition to DIC, refractory hypotension, renal shutdown, and ARDS usually result in shock and death, in the absence of therapy.

Pneumonic plague

The most rapidly developing and deadly form of plague is pneumonic plague. Within 2–4 days of infection, fever, chills, myalgias, arthralgias, dizziness, and lethargy develop. By the second day, the patient suffers from productive cough, tachypnea, dyspnea, hemoptysis, respiratory distress, chest pain, cardiopulmonary insufficiency, circulatory collapse, and sudden death.

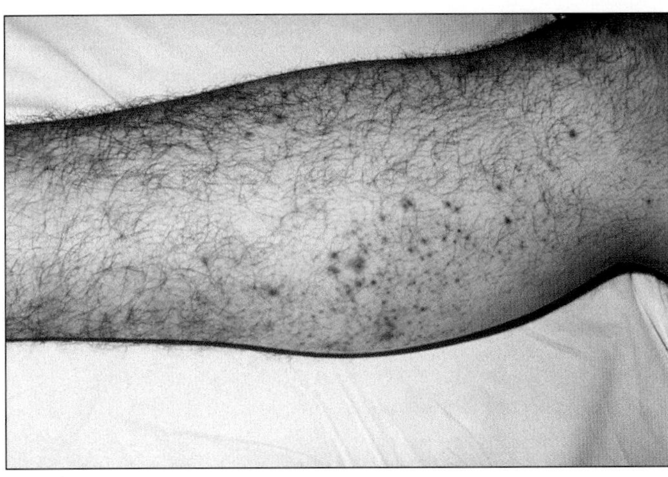

Figure 28.6 Petechiae on the leg of a patient with septicemic plague. (Courtesy of Centers for Disease Control and Prevention.)

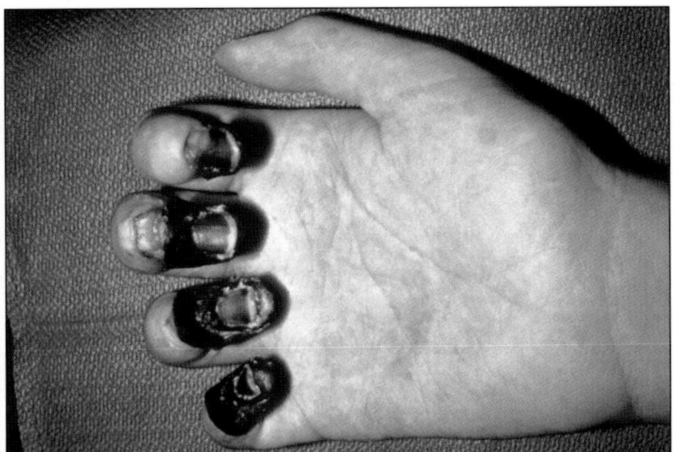

Figure 28.7 Acral gangrene from disseminated intravascular coagulation in a patient with septicemic plague (Courtesy of Centers for Disease Control and Prevention.)

Diagnosis and differential diagnosis

In order for the diagnosis to be made in time to initiate life-saving therapy, the physician must have a high index of suspicion from the patient's history of exposure to *Y. pestis*-carrying rodents and fleas as well as signs and symptoms suggestive of plague. Intensive supportive care and appropriate antibiotic therapy must be initiated immediately upon reasonable suspicion of plague. Gram, Wayson, and/or Giemsa stains and cultures must be taken of buboes, blood, lymph node aspirates, sputum, or tracheal samples and cerebrospinal fluid. The clinical specimens should also be examined using fluorescent antibody testing. Acute and convalescent serology should be taken[8] and a chest radiograph should be obtained. The peripheral leukocyte count is usually between 15 000 and 25 000/μl and sometimes exceeds 100 000/μl.

The differential diagnosis of bubonic plague includes lymphogranuloma venereum or localized lymphadenopathy due to other regional infections, but the symptoms of plague would not be expected in these conditions. The differential diagnosis of septicemic plague can include various gastrointestinal infections, and the differential diagnosis of pneumonic plague includes other causes of pneumonia.

Therapy

The drug of choice in treatment of plague is streptomycin, although gentamicin, tetracycline, and chloramphenicol can also be used. Buboes may require surgical drainage. Patients with plague also require intensive supportive care. Without antibiotic therapy, over 50% of patients with bubonic plaque will die, as will almost 100% of patients with septicemic or pneumonic plague.

Prevention

A safe and effective vaccine for *Y. pestis* is not available for humans,[9] but control of plague is best achieved by avoidance of areas with known epizootic plague, avoidance of diseased or dead animals, use of repellents, insecticides, protective clothing, and masks. Individuals with suspected pneumonic plague must be isolated and respiratory precautions taken. Antibiotic prophylaxis can be used for individuals who have to work in areas of plague outbreaks or care for plague patients.

References

1. Butler T. The black death past and present I. Plague in the 1980s. Trans R Soc Trop Med Hyg 1989; 83:458–460.
2. Update: human plague – India, 1994. MMWR Morbid Mortal Wkly Rep 1994; 43:722–723.
3. Kartman L. Historical and ecological observations on plague in the United States. Trop Geogr Med 1970; 22:257–275.
4. Cavanaugh DC. Specific effect of temperature upon transmission of the plague bacillus by the oriental rat flea *Xenopsylla cheopis*. Am J Trop Med Hyg 1971; 31:839–841.
5. Palmer DL, Kisch AL, Williams RL Jr et al. Clinical features of plague in the United States: the 1969–1970 epidemic. J Infect Dis 1971; 124:367–371.
6. Hull HF, Montes JM, Mann JM. Septicemic plague in New Mexico. J Infect Dis 1987; 155: 113–118.
7. Hull HF, Montes JM, Mann JM. Plague masquerading as gastrointestinal illness. West J Med 1986; 145:485–487.
8. Splettstoesser WD, Rahalison L, Grunow R et al. Evaluation of a standardized F1 capsular antigen capture ELISA test kit for the rapid diagnosis of plague. FEMS Immunol Med Microbiol 2004; 41:149–155.
9. Titball RW, Williamson ED. *Yersinia pestis* (plague) vaccines. Expert Opin Biol Ther 2004; 4:965–973.

Diphtheria

Mark Burnett and Martin Ottolini*

Synonyms: Diphtheria toxoid, diphtheria vaccine, pseudomembrane, *Corynebacterium diphtheriae* toxin

Key features:

- Diphtheria is a respiratory tract pathogen causing symptoms ranging from purulent nasal discharge to membrane formation with respiratory compromise
- The chronic non-healing skin lesions vary in appearance
- Toxin-induced cranial neuropathies causing demyelination typically result in dysphonia and regurgitation
- There may be toxin-induced myocarditis, with complications ranging from first-degree heart block to bundle-branch blocks and complete atrioventricular dissociation
- Toxin-induced tubular necrosis of the kidneys may also be a feature

Introduction

Although rarely seen in western Europe and the USA, diphtheria remains a significant pathogen in large areas of the developing world. Recent epidemics in Russia and the former Soviet Union in the early and mid-1990s illustrate how diphtheria can become a serious public health problem if significant percentages of the general population lack immunity. The dermatologic presentations of diphtheria vary and it is probably an often-overlooked diagnosis when patients from endemic regions present with chronic skin infections.

History

Descriptions of a disease likely to be diphtheria have been found as early as the fifth century BC in writings of Hippocrates. Sporadic epidemics ravaged sixteenth- and seventeenth-century Spain and eighteenth-century England. From 1735 to 1740 an outbreak of diphtheria in the New England colonies of America claimed the life of one in every 40 inhabitants.

It was not until the nineteenth century that this disease acquired its present name. Pierre Bretonneau, a French pathologist and clinician, first used the term "diphtherite" (from the Greek meaning skin or hide) to describe the throat membrane of those afflicted, as he thought that it resembled a piece of leather.[1] The organism was discovered by Klebs in 1883, and was definitively shown to be the causative agent by Loeffler in 1884. Antitoxin for therapy was developed prior to the turn of the century, and a toxoid was developed in the 1920s. Widespread vaccination was initiated in the USA in 1930s, and by 1935 diphtheria ceased being the most common infectious cause of mortality among American children.

*The views of the authors do not necessarily reflect the views of the U.S. Army and Air force.

Epidemiology

Humans are the only known reservoir for C. *diphtheriae*. Spread of infection is primarily through close contact via respiratory droplets or exudates from infected skin. Fomites and food-borne sources, especially contaminated milk, have also been reported. The incidence of diphtheria has declined dramatically since universal immunization began in western Europe and the USA in the 1930s and 1940s. In the USA of the 1920s the incidence of infection was 100–200 cases per 100 000 but since 1980 only 0.001 cases per 100 000 are reported annually. More than 150 000 cases were reported in Russia and the former Soviet Union during a recent epidemic and the disease remains endemic to large areas of the developing world. In the prevaccine era, children were most at risk of serious disease, but most cases now reported in western Europe and the USA are in adults with waning immunity. A recent survey of American children and adults found that the percentages of US residents with protective levels of diphtheria antibodies declined with age, from 91% at age 6–11 to approximately 30% in those aged 60–69 years.[2]

Pathogenesis and etiology

Corynebacterium diphtheriae is an irregularly staining, Gram-positive, non-motile, non-sporulating, pleomorphic bacillus that may appear slightly curved or club-shaped. Four morphologic variants described by colony type exist – *mitis, gravis, intermedius*, and *Bellanti* – all of which can be toxigenic or non-toxigenic. The toxigenicity of the C. *diphtheriae* organism depends upon the presence of a lysogenic β-phage (*tox* + phage) that induces the organism to produce an exotoxin. The exotoxin consists of a binding B domain and an enzymatically active A domain. The A domain inactivates elongation factor-2, inhibiting cellular protein synthesis. Initial infection most commonly involves the skin or the epithelium of the upper respiratory tract. Exotoxin release causes local tissue destruction and a coagulum of leukocytes, bacteria, fibrin, and necrotic tissue that forms the characteristic pseudomembrane of the upper respiratory tract. From the nidus of infection, exotoxin may then be carried to all tissues of the body, potentially causing myocarditis, neuritis, and tubular necrosis of the kidneys.

Clinical features

The most common clinical manifestation of C. *diphtheriae* infection is disease of the upper respiratory tract and/or cutaneous diphtheria.

Asymptomatic upper respiratory tract carriage of C. *diphtheriae* can last for weeks and is common in areas of the world where the disease is endemic. Symptomatic infections follow a brief incubation period of 2–7 days, and patients present with a low-grade fever, sore throat, and malaise. Anterior nasal infection, most commonly seen in infants, results in a purulent nasal discharge, which can cause a mild erosion of the external nares. Faucial infection, involving the posterior portions of the mouth and proximal oral pharynx, is the most common site of infection of the respiratory tract. An adherent white or dirty-gray membrane may develop on

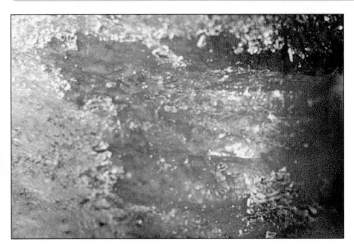

Figure 28.8 Eczematous form of cutaneous diphtheria. (Courtesy of the Centers for Disease Control and Prevention.)

one or both tonsillar pillars, extending to the uvula, soft palate, oropharynx, and nasopharynx. Cervical edema and adenopathy may cause the patient to develop a "bull-neck" appearance, which, coupled with pseudomembrane development, may lead to airway compromise. Infection of the larynx may uncommonly be a primary infection, or may spread from the proximal pharynx. Patients will typically be hoarse and may promptly develop respiratory compromise.

Cutaneous diphtheria is most commonly seen in tropical and subtropical areas, although it is also seen in homeless populations of the developed world.[3] More contagious than respiratory diphtheria, it can colonize any kind of lesion. Wounds, burns, pyoderma, eczema, and impetigo colonized with diphtheria can take on a highly varied appearance (Fig. 28.8). The classic appearance of cutaneous diphtheria is that of the ulcerative form of ecthyma diphthericum. It begins as a vesicle or pustule filled with straw-colored fluid which breaks to form single or multiple ulcerations measuring several millimeters to a few centimeters across (Fig. 28.9). The margins of the ulcerations may be slightly elevated or inverted. They may be painful and covered with a dark pseudomembrane or eschar. During the first several weeks of the illness the lesion becomes anesthetic, and after separation of the pseudomembrane a hemorrhagic base appears, sometimes with serosanguineous exudate drainage. Common areas involved are the lower legs, hands, and feet. Spontaneous healing may take weeks to months; with cases lasting up to a year being reported.[4] Coinfection may be common, with *Streptococcus pyogenes* or *Staphylococcus aureus* as frequent culprits.

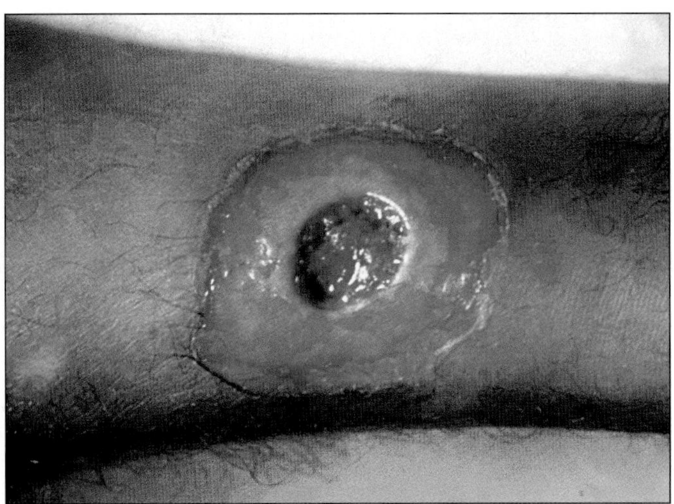

Figure 28.9 Ecthyma diphthericum. (Courtesy of the Centers for Disease Control and Prevention.)

Myocarditis as a result of exotoxin-mediated damage occurs in 10–20% of patients with oropharyngeal diphtheria and accounts for the most deaths relating to diphtheria today. Cardiac involvement is rarely seen in cases of cutaneous diphtheria. Initial presentations of cardiac involvement occur 1–2 weeks after the initial infection. Myocarditis can present as sinus bradycardia, first-degree atrioventricular block or ST-T wave changes. In more severe cases, there may be progression to bundle-branch blocks, atrioventricular dissociation, ventricular tachycardia, or congestive heart failure – all of which carry a poor prognosis. Cardiac pacing has been performed in patients with severe conduction defects, with some improvement in outcome.[5]

Exotoxin production of C. *diphtheriae* may also cause neurologic toxicity, more commonly in severe infections. Examination of the affected nerves under microscopy reveals degeneration of the myelin sheaths and axon cylinders.[6] Clinical manifestations, seen most typically after the first week of illness, include dysphonia and reflux as a result of paralysis of the soft palate and posterior pharyngeal wall. Peripheral neuropathies may develop and the motor nerves of the trunk, neck, and upper extremity may be affected. Resolution of symptoms may take months after severe infection.

Patient evaluation, diagnosis and differential diagnosis

The initial onset of symptoms of an upper respiratory tract diphtheria infection may be indistinguishable from a viral upper respiratory tract infection. Fevers are typically low-grade (<39.4 °C: 103.0 °F) and are accompanied by a sore throat and feelings of general malaise. Two physical findings that make this type of infection distinguishable from other similar infections are the presence of the characteristic pseudomembrane, and the development of a "bull-neck" appearance (Fig. 28.10). The pseudomembrane can be white-gray to brown in appearance and may initially involve one or both tonsils (Fig. 28.11). It then extends off the tonsils and can involve the nares, uvula, soft palate, pharynx, larynx, and tracheobronchial tree. Significant cervical soft-tissue edema and lymphadenopathy result in the "bull neck" which can contribute to airway compromise. Nasal diphtheria, seen typically in infants, results in a serosanguineous to mucopurulent nasal discharge (Fig. 28.12) and a croup-like illness in infants. Laryngeal diphtheria may present with hoarseness or stridor. Less clinically characteristic is cutaneous diphtheria, which can superinfect any type of skin lesion and may have a wide range of appearance. Ecthyma diphthericum, which may be covered by a dark pseudomembrane, is the classic ulcerative lesion and is pathognomonic for diphtheria.

Specimens for the diagnosis of respiratory diphtheria should be obtained with a cotton- or polyester-tipped swab, with samples obtained from the membrane or preferably beneath the edge of

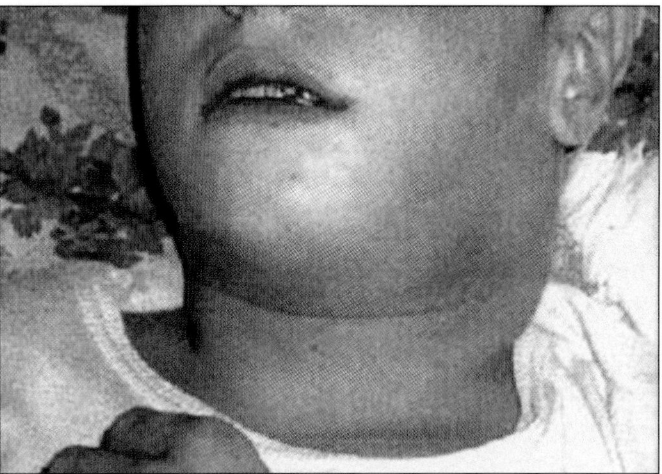

Figure 28.10 "Bull neck" of diphtheria. (Courtesy of the Centers for Disease Control and Prevention/Barbara Rice.)

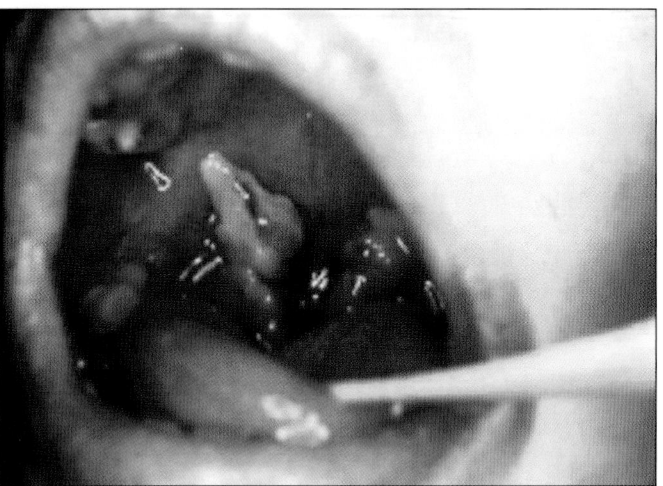

Figure 28.11 Pseudomembrane of diphtheria. (Courtesy of the James Bass Infectious Disease Photo Collection.)

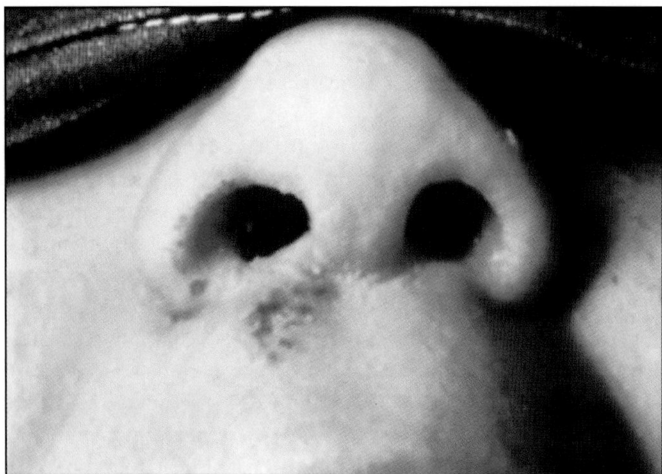

Figure 28.12 Nasal diphtheria. (Courtesy of the James Bass Infectious Disease Photo Collection.)

the membrane. Skin lesions should be cultured with swabs in any patient with respiratory diphtheria. Suspected cases of diphtheria should be plated on a sheep blood agar plate, as well as on selective medium such as cystine-tellurite blood agar or Tinsdale medium. The plates are read after 18–24 h at 37 °C, ideally in a 5% CO_2-enriched environment.[7] For further detection of the A and B subunits of the diphtheria (*tox*) gene, the Centers for Disease Control and Prevention have developed a real-time fluorescence polymerase chain reaction (PCR) assay sensitive enough to detect when two to three copies of the target gene are present. This is important as many clinical specimens only contain minute amounts of DNA.[8]

The differential diagnosis of diphtheria is somewhat limited. Faucial mononucleosis, bacterial and viral pharyngitis, and tonsillitis can all be suspected in an early diphtheria infection. The "bull-neck" appearance of diphtheria can resemble mumps or Vincent's angina. Acute epiglottis may be suspected after patients have begun to display airway compromise.

Treatment

For active disease, a combination of antitoxin and antimicrobial therapy is the current standard of care. As the condition of patients with diphtheria may deteriorate rapidly, a single dose of equine antitoxin should be administered on clinical grounds even before the diagnosis is culture-confirmed. Intravenous administration is preferred to neutralize toxin as rapidly as possible. A scratch test of a 1:1000 dilution of antitoxin in saline solution should be performed prior to antitoxin administration to evaluate for sensitivity to horse serum. If the patient is found to be sensitive to equine antitoxin, desensitization is necessary. In the USA, antitoxin can be obtained from the National Immunization Program of the Centers for Disease Control.

Antitoxin treatment dosages are based on pseudomembrane size and location, toxicity of patient, and duration of illness. Suggested dosages are as follows: pharyngeal or laryngeal disease of 48 h duration or less 20 000–40 000 U; nasopharyngeal lesions 40 000–60 000 U; extensive disease of 3 days or longer duration or diffuse swelling of the neck, 80 000–120 000 U. Antitoxin is not thought to be of value in cutaneous diphtheria, but some experts recommend 20 000–40 000 U of antitoxin if used, as toxic sequelae with higher doses have been reported. The use of intravenous immunoglobulin for the treatment of cutaneous or respiratory diphtheria has not been approved in the USA.[9]

Antibiotics should be used in conjunction with antitoxin in the treatment of active diphtheria infections. Erythromycin is the standard first-line treatment of choice, although a recent randomized trial of 44 Vietnamese children with diphtheria found four isolates resistant to erythromycin.[10] The recommended erythromycin dosage is 20–25 mg/kg every 12 h intravenously for 14 days, while benzylpenicillin G should be administered as 50 000 U/kg/day intramuscularly for 5 days, followed by penicillin VK by mouth at 50 mg/kg per day for 5 additional days for the treatment of respiratory diphtheria. Children can be treated with oral or intravenous erythromycin for 14 days, given penicillin G intramuscularly or intravenously for 14 days, or given penicillin

G intramuscularly for 14 days. Cutaneous diphtheria can be treated with either erythromycin or penicillin for a 10-day course following cleaning of the wound with soap and water.

Carriers may be treated with oral erythromycin or penicillin G for 7 days, or may be administered a single intramuscular dose of penicillin G benzathine (600 000 U for those weighing less than 30 kg and 1.2 million units for children weighing more than 30 kg and adults). Follow-up cultures are recommended at least 2 weeks after completion of therapy. If these cultures are positive, another 10-day course of erythromycin is indicated. Carriers should be actively immunized if this has not previously occurred, and can be reimmunized with a booster dose of diphtheria toxoid if a year has elapsed since their last booster dose.

Close contacts, regardless of their immunization status, are recommended to have cultures taken and should be observed for 7 days for disease development. Antibiotic prophylaxis is presumed to be beneficial and can be either with oral erythromycin (40–50 mg/kg per day for 7 days to a maximum of 2 g/day) or intramuscular penicillin G benzathine (600 000 U for those weighing <30 kg and 1.2 million U for children weighing >30 kg as well as adults).

Universal immunization is the most effective control measure. Infants and children receive a total of five doses of diphtheria toxoid between 2 months of age and their seventh birthday. Annual booster doses of diphtheria toxoid every 10 years after completion of the initial series result in persisting immunity. Immunization should be initiated or continued in those who are recovering from active disease, as disease does not always result in immunity.

References

1. English PC. Diphtheria and theories of infectious disease: centennial appreciation of the critical role of diphtheria in the history of medicine. Pediatrics 1985; 76:1–9.
2. McQuillan GM, Kruszon-Moran D, Deforest A et al. Serologic immunity to diphtheria and tetanus in the United States. Ann Intern Med 2002; 136:660–666.
3. Harnisch JP, Tronca E, Nolan CM et al. Diphtheria among alcoholic urban adults. Ann Intern Med 1989; 111:71–82.
4. Hofler W. Cutaneous diphtheria. Int J Dermatol 1991; 30:845–847.
5. Dung NM, Kneen R, Kiem N et al. Treatment of severe diphtheritic myocarditis by temporary insertion of a cardiac pacemaker. Clin Infect Dis 2002; 35:1425–1429.
6. Hadfield TL, McEvoy P, Polotsky Y et al. The pathology of diphtheria. J Infect Dis 2000; 181 (Suppl. 1):S116–S120.
7. Funke G, Bernard KA. Coryneform Gram positive rods. In Murray P, Barron EJ, eds. Manual of clinical microbiology, 8th edn. Washington, DC: ASM Press; 2003.
8. Mothershed EA, Cassiday PK, Pierson K et al. Development of a real-time fluorescence PCR assay for rapid detection of the diphtheria toxin gene. J Clin Microbiol 2002; 40:4713–4719.
9. Pickering LK, Baker CJ, Overturf GD et al. Diphtheria. In: American Academy of Pediatrics Red Book. Elk Grove: American Academy of Pediatrics; 2003:263–266.
10. Kneen R, Giao PN, Solomon T et al. Penicillin vs. erythromycin in the treatment of diphtheria. Clin Infect Dis 1998; 27:845–850.

Trachoma

Frank Mwesigye

Introduction

Trachoma is a contagious disease caused by the Gram-negative obligate intracellular bacteria of *Chlamydia trachomatis* subtypes. Humans are the natural host and transmission is strictly from human to human. *C. trachomatis* is associated with diseases ranging from blinding trachoma to sexually acquired genital infections and lymphogranuloma venereum (LGV).

Trachoma remains closely linked to poverty and is hidden in rural communities deprived of access to basic hygienic facilities. It is endemic in most developing countries in Africa, some parts of Latin America, Southeast Asia, India, China, the Middle East, and areas in Australia, as shown on the map (Fig. 28.13).

Individuals are affected independently of race and gender. Besides trachoma being a common eye disease of the conjunctiva and cornea through eye-to-eye transmission, genital-to-eye transmission remains another important route. Thus, there are two main ocular syndromes attributable to *C. trachomatis*: (1) classic trachoma and (2) sexually acquired inclusion conjunctivitis associated with urethritis, cervicitis, salpingitis, epididymitis, and neonatal pneumonia. It is therefore essential that patients with confirmed or suspected disease have their conjunctivae inspected. In addition, their sexual partners and, in case of neonatal ophthalmia, their parents are examined for possible concomitant genital infection.

History

The available medical reports are in conflict and it is difficult to be precise about the accurate history of trachoma. Its natural home is believed to have been Egypt[1] and trachoma was once known as "Egyptian ophthalmia." The name trachoma was used by a Sicilian physician, Pedanius Dioscorides (AD 40–91) in his *De Materia Medica*. Earlier it was believed to be a natural phenomenon due to noxious night vapor and sandiness of the soil. It was transported and spread to various countries by the Crusaders from Palestine, Muslim invaders, and the Spanish conquistadores. Trachoma was particularly noticed when the entire French and most of the British army fell victims to it during the Napoleonic campaign in Egypt, when the soldiers were sent home blind. Various views to

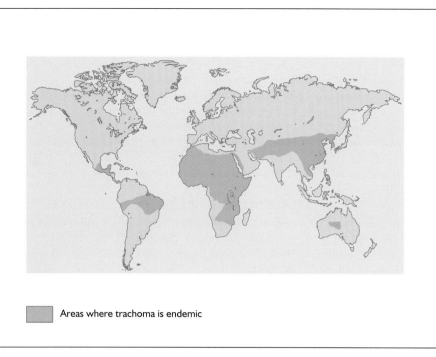

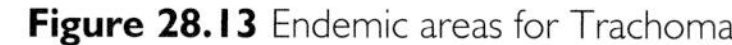
Figure 28.13 Endemic areas for Trachoma.

explain the disease remained controversial until 1907 when Halberstaedter and Prowazek discovered the causative organisms (Halberstaedter–Prowazek inclusion bodies). This work was completed in 1957 when T'ang et al. succeeded in identifying C. *trachomatis* as the cause of trachoma.[2] Trachoma remained a major public health concern in many countries, including western Europe and the USA, until it regressed and disappeared with the rising standards that accompanied industrialization and economic development.

Epidemiology

Ocular C. *trachomatis* infection occurs in two distinct epidemiological settings, which produce ocular syndromes that are often indistinguishable in early phases. There is the classic type that is potentially blinding and is spread by eye-to-eye transmission. It is sometimes described as endemic trachoma caused by C. *trachomatis* serotypes A, B, or C. The other type is the infection of the eye by sexually transmitted C. *trachomatis* serotypes D, E, F, G, H, I, J, or K, best known as paratrachoma. C. *trachomatis* serotypes A–K are sometimes referred to collectively as TRIC (**tr**achoma **i**nclusion **c**onjunctivitis) because they share many characteristics.

Trachoma affects all races, although there is often considerable ethnic difference in its incidence, probably because of similar social habits. In some areas trachoma is universal, affecting well over 90% of indigenous inhabitants, while in others it is rare or sporadic, being confined to individuals or smaller groups. Trachoma is a major public health problem worldwide. It is estimated that 6 million people are blind, 150 million are infected and need treatment, while 500 million are at risk of getting the disease. Trachoma is overwhelmingly associated with dirt, squalor, and intimate proximity of poverty. Its distribution is attributable to hot, dry, dusty climates with limited access to water. Other factors, such as low personal hygiene and increased eye-seeking flies attracted to purulent discharge around the eyes, play a big role.

The prevalence of active trachoma is greatest among children under 10 years and then decreases with age. This is probably because personal hygiene, which is a major factor in the transmission of trachoma, improves with age. The disease is spread either by direct contact of eye to eye during play or sharing a bed, conveyance on fingers, contaminated materials with infected secretions (towels, handkerchiefs, and others), eye-seeking flies, or coughing/sneezing.

Among children, the prevalence and severity of acute infection are equal between sexes. However, there is a general trend of chronic disease in the female. The female-to-male ratio of blinding disease is around 3 to 1, which may be explained by increased contact of females with a chronically actively infected child population.[3]

Seasonal epidemics of other bacterial causes of conjunctivitis that occur in areas where trachoma is endemic are complicating the epidemiology of trachoma. *Haemophilus influenzae*, *Streptococcus pneumoniae,* and *Moraxella* species are the major causes.

The sexually transmitted inclusion conjunctivitis is caused by C. *trachomatis* serotypes D–K, which also cause urethritis, cervicitis, and salpingitis, among others. In adults transmission is through direct contact of the eye with infected genital or urinary secretions. The modes of transmission include oral–genital sexual activities or genital–hand-to-eye spread of the infection. The disease may have remained relatively asymptomatic in the genital tract before ocular disease develops. Whereas trachoma is rare in economically developed countries, the reverse is true with ocular sexually transmitted chlamydial infection. In Europe, up to 18% of conjunctivitis is sexually related and caused by *Chlamydia*. There are 50 million new cases occurring each year. The disease is most prevalent among sexually active young adults between 20 and 35 years. In neonates, it is transmitted through contact with infected genital secretions during childbirth. Two-thirds of neonates from infected mothers have ocular infections.

Pathogenesis

Chlamydia infection spreads easily from person to person. The acute inflammation is generally localized to superficial epithelial or mucosal surfaces and may undergo spontaneous resolution without permanent complications. The host genetic factors appear to play a major role in susceptibility or resistance to C. *trachomatis* disease.[4] The development of trachoma requires repeated infections and subsequent reinfections cause more severe inflammation than the previous ones. Observation that multiple serial reinfections are responsible for the severity of the disease has led to the concept that the disease provokes and contributes an immunopathogenic response of the host to C. *trachomatis* infections. The initial infection presumably induces partial immune sensitization of the host. Later, the cell-mediated hypersensitivity responses to *Chlamydial* reinfection become responsible for exacerbated inflammation that causes severe disease with scarring sequelae. Experimentally induced trachoma in monkeys previously infected or immunized against C. *trachomatis* has caused more severe inflammation than in non-immunized ones. The sexually transmitted inclusion conjunctivitis does not inflict as much eye damage as trachoma. Even untreated disease rarely causes permanent ocular morbidity. This is probably because of lower innate pathogenicity. Also, frequent reinfection that may be necessary to provoke immune responses is rare in adults while the immune system in neonates is still immature.

Clinical features

Many studies have detected C. *trachomatis* in the absence of clinical disease. Also, active infection may remain asymptomatic and appears to cause little or no discomfort. On a different note, people believe that the disease is a fact of life because it is so common.

The onset of trachoma is between 5 and 14 days after exposure to the organisms transmitted directly from person to person through infected ocular secretions or indirectly through contact with infected materials from the eye or through eye-seeking flies. Infected children with active trachoma are the main reservoirs of the organisms in the community. Active trachoma is frequently a disease of young children, although blinding complications occur in adults in whom first infections have likely occurred many years before. Often, both eyes are affected, although initially the disease may first present asymmetrically. The disease is seen in its typical form on the upper tarsal conjunctiva, the limbus, and, to a lesser extent, the lower eyelid. Acute infection manifests as keratoconjunctivitis, varying from mild to severe in nature, which includes redness, irritation, photophobia, pain, swollen eyelids, and mucopurulent or purulent discharge. In early stages of the disease in children under 2 years of age, there is a papillary conjunctivitis without the typical well-developed lymphoid follicles. In later years, however, the disease progresses to a chronic follicular keratoconjunctivitis. The conjunctival lymphoid follicles that are flat or elevated, grayish, and measuring between 0.2 and 2 mm in diameter, represent a regular feature of trachoma. Scarring of the conjunctiva, from trachoma, appears as fine linear and small satellite scars in milder forms and as broader confluent scars in more severe cases. Quite often the follicles necrotize, leading to further scarring of the conjunctiva.

The major complications of trachoma are distortion of the lids, particularly the upper lid, with misdirection of individual lashes (trichiasis) and inward deformation of the lid margin (entropion). The abrasion of the cornea by sturdy lashes results in corneal ulceration, followed by opacity and permanent visual loss. Corneal lesions in trachoma include superficial punctate keratitis and extension of superficial blood vessels from the limbus into the edematous corneal epithelium (vascular pannus). The disease is more marked at the upper limbus, although the entire limbus is frequently involved. Systemic symptoms are rare, although associated rhinitis, upper respiratory tract infection, and preauricular lymphadenopathy have been reported.

The sexually transmitted ocular disease by C. *trachomatis* serotypes D–K is a milder disease than trachoma. Permanent visual damage rarely occurs. Although trachoma is almost exclusively a disease of developing poor countries, oculogenital infections are also prevalent in developed countries. The incubation period is 5–21 days. The symptoms may be acute or subacute keratoconjunctivitis, which initially may be indistinguishable from acute trachoma. A fine papillary reaction and follicles in the lower conjunctiva, as opposed to trachoma, where follicles are more frequent in the upper tarsal conjunctiva, are dominant findings. Conjunctival scarring and corneal pathology are rare. When the disease remains untreated, it may persist for years but generally only leads to limited sequelae.

The neonate is always infected through contact with infected genital secretions during passage through the birth canal and it is responsible for 40% of all ophthalmias of the newborn. Signs of infection begin 5–14 days postpartum, although they may be earlier if there is premature rupture of the membranes. The acute keratoconjunctivitis is often associated with a mucopurulent discharge. Follicles are absent, owing to immaturity of the immune system. It is important always to rule out bacterial infection, especially gonococcal and chemical conjunctivitis, and prophylactic silver nitrate is frequently administered in this age group. Classic teaching dictates that the signs of chemical and gonococcal ophthalmia in neonates appear within 72 h postpartum. In reality, the time of onset and severity of symptoms are never reliable clinical signs for determining the cause of neonatal ophthalmias. C. *trachomatis* must be included in the differential diagnosis of ophthalmias of the newborn, regardless of the time of presentation or the severity of symptoms.

Pathology

There is still considerable argument whether or not trachoma is an epitheliosis with strict localization of the causative organisms to the epithelial cells, yet the principal lesions are subepithelial. The characteristic cell inclusions are found and remain in the superficial epithelial cells of the mucous membrane. In the first few days of infection the epithelium thickens and becomes irregular, followed by degeneration and exfoliation of epithelial cells.

Two to four weeks later there is marked vascular dilatation and infiltration of the subepithelial tissue by lymphocytes, plasma cells, and other inflammatory cells. Frequently, these cells are organized in oval lymphoid aggregates known as follicles. It is interesting to note that, at this stage, the disease may remain self-limiting and can heal without significant permanent damage. However, probably arising because of frequent reinfections, chronic disease may cause severe inflammation with subepithelial hyperplasia, proliferation of connective tissue, fibrous membrane, squamous metaplasia, loss of goblet cells, degeneration of muscle fibers, especially Müller's muscle, and localized perivascular amyloidosis.[5] Consequently, there is subepithelial fibrosis and scarring of necrotic follicles, leading to conjunctival scars. The scar forms a network, leaving islands of relatively normal mucous membranes that protrude above the depressed scars. A cellular infiltration of the tarsus with subsequent degeneration leads to its deformity, which may also be worsened by mechanical contraction of the scarred conjunctiva.

Accessory lacrimal glands and ducts are compromised by subepithelial infiltration and scarring, which may lead to xerosis that worsens the overall pathological picture. In the cornea there is a diffuse superficial keratitis and dilatation of limbal capillaries which elongate and descend into the edematous epithelium causing micropannus formation. There is also subepithelial lymphoid infiltration with typical mature follicles, especially at the limbus, surrounded by a vascular network. When the limbal follicles eventually resolve, they leave behind ghost pits known as Herbert's pits.

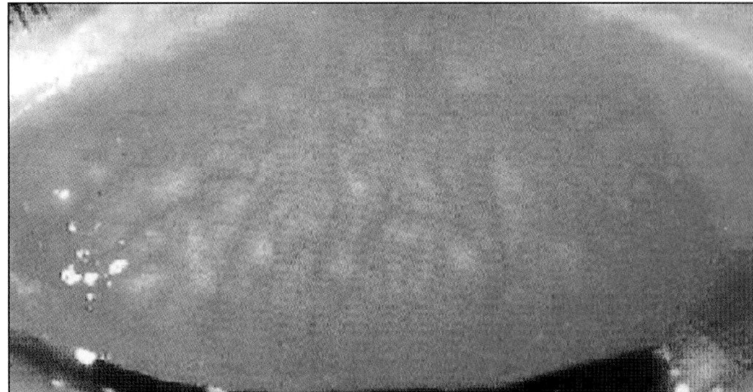

Figure 28.14 Follicular conjunctivitis (FT).

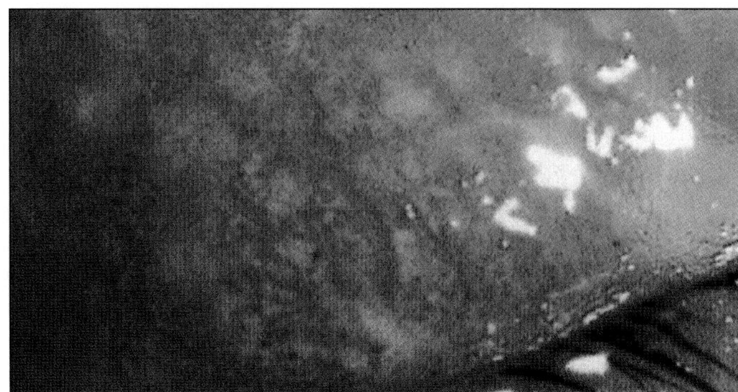

Figure 28.15 Intense, diffuse inflammation (TI) with papillary hypertrophy.

Diagnosis

Knowledge of the location and pattern of disease allows the accurate diagnosis and more expedient and successful management of trachoma. Quite often it is difficult to be certain about the diagnosis of trachoma in children whose examination under slit lamp is difficult. Also, because trachoma is rare in developed countries and the index of suspicion of the disease is extremely low or even absent, the sporadic cases of trachoma in these countries are frequently misdiagnosed.

The mere presence of C. *trachomatis* in the epithelial surface may not cause clinical disease as certain host factors (such as local immunity) may play an important role. Also, in the presence of classical signs, culture of organisms may be negative in up to half of all cases. This poses a huge diagnostic challenge to the clinician.

In practice, the clinical diagnosis has remained the most acceptable choice. Simplified World Health Organization grading schemes of follicular conjunctivitis (FT), intense inflammation (TI), scarring (TS), trichiasis (TT), and corneal opacity (CO) have been adapted (Figs 28.14–28.18). Each of these clinical signs may be present or absent; any two of them, however, are pathognomonic.

Vernal keratoconjunctivitis must be considered in the differential diagnosis of trachoma. Both vernal keratoconjunctivitis and trachoma affect young people, occur in hot, dry climates, and have a predilection for the limbus and the upper tarsal conjunctiva. When the two conditions occur simultaneously, they challenge the clinician with a diagnostic dilemma.[6]

However, in a typical case of vernal keratoconjunctivitis, the upper tarsal conjunctiva is covered with papillae that are hard,

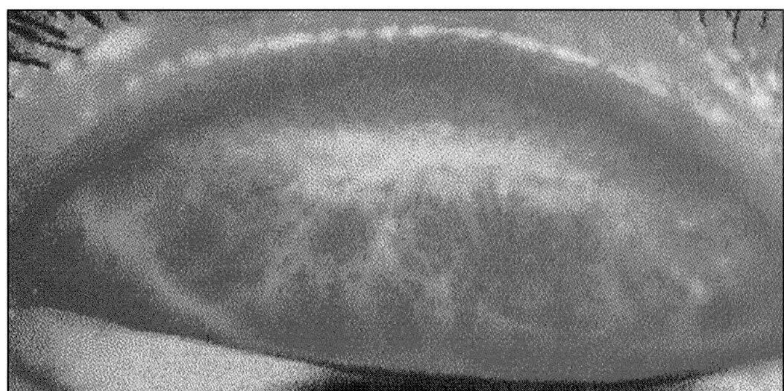

Figure 28.16 Linear and stellate scarring of upper eyelid tarsus (TS).

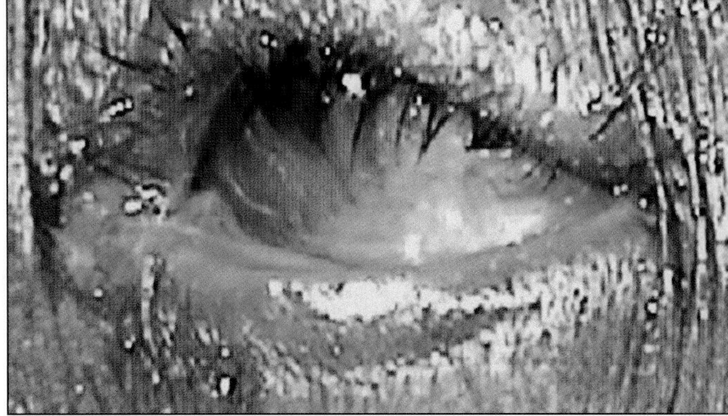

Figure 28.17 Trichiasis (TT) and cicatricial entropion of upper eyelid.

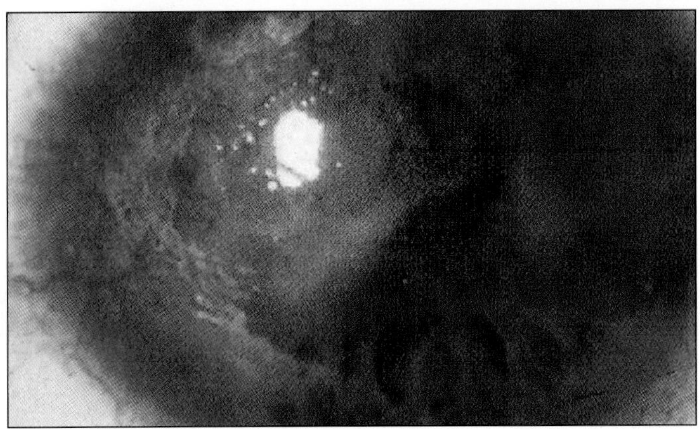

Figure 28.18 Corneal opacity (CO) from superficial fibrovascular pannus involving visual axis.

broad, and flattened so as to make the conjunctiva appear like an ancient pavement of cobblestones. These papillae are covered by copious delicate whitish films of mucus. In the limbus the papillae have a gelatinous appearance; they may coalesce and form a ridge along the limbus. Micropannus may be present. A history of seasonal exacerbation and/or associations with other allergic conditions is extremely important.

Trachoma is also included in the differential diagnosis of follicular conjunctivitis, toxic reactions, Parinaud's oculoglandular syndrome, Axenfeld's conjunctivitis, and viral infections. Follicular conjunctivitis may be clinically indistinguishable from trachoma and oculogenital conjunctivitis. The most common causes of follicular conjunctivitis include pharyngoconjunctival fever, epidemic keratoconjunctivitis, herpes simplex, molluscum contagiosum, and rubella. Among the points to be considered in the differential diagnosis of follicular conjunctivitis are accompanying skin lesions, upper respiratory infection, lymphadenopathy, and existing general systemic illnesses.

While much of the trachoma diagnosis is basically dependent on clinical signs, laboratory tests are still essential in supporting the diagnosis of clinically suspected disease in individual cases, monitoring individuals for effect of therapy and shifts in serotypes in a given population that might indicate the introduction of an agent from outside the community. Giemsa and fluorescent monoclonal antibody staining can offer a rapid diagnosis. Although the microscopic examination of Giemsa-stained smears has been the mainstay of diagnosis for a long time, fluorescent staining, which is about three times more sensitive in confirming the presence of *C. trachomatis* compared to Giemsa staining, is increasingly becoming more preferable.[7]

Culture of organisms is a very effective method in the diagnosis of chlamydial infection especially in sexually transmitted diseases. The high cost and delay before results are obtained render the method not suitable for mass screening. Nucleic acid (DNA) amplification techniques such as PCR and ligase chain reaction (LCR) are other methods that provide unique effective and sensitive means for detecting *Chlamydia* in clinical specimens from patients with trachoma, epididymitis, salpingitis, and reactive arthritis, and can be useful for mass screening as well.

Prevention

Trachoma remains a preventable disease. Both early treatment and economic empowerment may result in rapid reduction in the prevalence and severity of disease. International efforts to control the disease based on the SAFE strategy, which combines Surgery, Antibiotics, Facial cleanliness, and Environmental improvement, are encouraged. The Global Elimination of Trachoma as a disease of public health importance by 2020 (GET 2020) is currently the overall goal in trachoma control efforts.[8]

The current medical opinion for reducing or eliminating the *Chlamydia*-associated chronic syndromes that pose a serious public health threat through the development of an efficacious vaccine is not far-fetched. However, there are still major challenges towards this endeavor, although advances in chlamydial genomics and proteomics should enhance the identification of the likely chlamydial gene products that fulfill the antigenic requirements of a putative vaccine. Major inroads are needed into the construction and development of novel and effective delivery systems such as vectors and adjuvants.[9]

Many studies have found chlamydial infection in the absence of clinical disease. This carrier group constitutes a significant reservoir of infection. Ideally, treatment of all infected people without signs of disease should be carried out. Certainly, this is not attainable, thus treatment of individuals will be performed on the basis of clinical signs. In the developed western world, where trachoma is very rare and least suspected, the sporadic cases of trachoma are usually misdiagnosed and insufficiently treated. The increase in oculogenital sexually transmitted disease in these countries is a challenge that demands responsibility in the diagnosis and treatment of all chlamydial diseases, including trachoma.

Treatment

In uncomplicated active trachoma, tetracycline eye ointment has been the mainstay of treatment for the best part of half a century and still provides an affordable option with no evidence of clinically significant resistance in developing ocular strains of *C. trachomatis*. It can also be safely used in children and pregnant mothers. The ointment, used twice a day for 6 weeks, is effective and can prevent reinfection. Oral tetracycline given as a supplement to topical therapy is significantly better than ointment alone in reducing the intensity of the disease. Also systemic therapy clears the infection from non-ocular sites of carriage such as the nasopharynx and genitourinary tract. Systemic tetracycline should however not be given to children and pregnant mothers as it affects the teeth and bones of young children.

More recently, oral single azithromycin has proven to be more effective than tetracycline.[10] It shows excellent compliance, unlike the other drugs that have to be used frequently and for a long time. Moreover, there are sustained high levels of azithromycin in conjunctival and other tissues for up to 3 weeks after intake. In all cases of chlamydial infection, including trachoma, the response to chemotherapy is slow, occurring in some cases 9–18 weeks after starting treatment. Additionally, the response that may lead to clinical cure is short-lived before reinfection may take place again. The prolonged high levels of azithromycin in tissues make it even more suitable for the treatment of chlamydial diseases.[11] To sustain cure and minimize reinfection, biannual azithromycin therapy 20 mg/kg is recommended. The high cost suggests that, in the absence of donation programs, routine treatment with azithromycin is not a good use of resources in developing countries and the treatment of choice should remain topical tetracycline.

Treatment with sulfonamides has lost popularity because they have an unacceptably high rate of unwanted reactions, some of which can be serious. Rifampicin and erythromycin are other effective but expensive drugs. In order to prevent reinfection and complications in the genital tract, all sexual partners should be counseled and treated simultaneously.

References

1. Duke-Elder system of ophthalmology, vol. VIII. London: Henry Kimpton; 1965:260.
2. T'ang FF, Chang HL, Huang YT et al. Studies on the etiology of trachoma with special reference to isolation of the virus in chick embryo. Chin Med J 1957; 75:429–446.
3. Buchan JC, Zondervan M, Foster A. Trachoma: a review. Trop Doctor 2003; October: 33.
4. Mahdi-Olaimatu SM. Impact of host genetics on susceptibility to human *Chlamydia trachomatis* disease. Br J Biomed Sci 2002; 59:128–132.
5. Guzey M, Ozardali 1, Basar E et al. A survey of trachoma: the histopathology and mechanism of progressive cicatrization of eyelid tissues. Ophthalmologica 2000; 214:277–284.
6. Friedlaender NH. Vernal karatoconjunctivitis and trachoma. Int Ophthalmol 1998; 12:47–51.
7. Baveja UK, Hiranandani MK, Talwar P. Laboratory techniques for diagnosis of chlamydial infections of the eye. J Commun Dis 1997; 29:247–253.
8. Mabey DC, Solomon AW, Foster A. Trachoma. Lancet 2003; 362 :223–229.
9. Agietseme JU, Eko FO, Black M. Contemporary approaches to designing and evaluating vaccines against *Chlamydia*. Expert Rev Vaccines 2003; 2:129–146.
10. Bowmann RJ, Sillah A, Van-Dehn C et al. Operational comparison of single dose azithromycin and topical tetracycline for trachoma. Invest Ophthalmol Vis Sci 2000; 41:4074–4079.
11. Guzay M, Slan G, Ozardali I et al. Three day course of oral azithromycin vs. topical oxytetracycline.polymyxin in treatment of active endemic trachoma. Jpn Ophthalmol 2000; 44:387–391.

Miscellaneous bacteria

Stephen K. Tyring

A number of other tropical bacterial diseases with cutaneous manifestations occasionally present to physicians in temperate countries and are included in this chapter. These diseases include melioidosis, glanders, tularemia, *Vibrio vulnificus* infections, typhoid fever, psittacosis, and Q fever.

Melioidosis

Melioidosis is an opportunistic infection caused by the Gram-negative bacillus *Burkholderia (Pseudomonas) pseudomallei* and is most commonly reported from Southeast Asia in persons who have frequent contact with soil or surface water, such as rice paddies.[1] Because of this association, melioidosis is four times more common in males than females. It is also strongly associated with diabetes mellitus. The infection may be subclinical in otherwise healthy persons or fulminant and rapidly fatal in immunocompromised patients. In addition, melioidosis may be acute or chronic and localized or disseminated. It may be latent and reappear clinically at times of stress, as reported in American veterans of the Vietnam war.[2]

Clinical manifestations develop after an incubation period of 6 days (range of 1 day to 2 months) with high fever and rigors as well as occasional confusion, stupor, jaundice, and diarrhea. Common laboratory findings include anemia, neutrophil leukocytosis, coagulopathy, and renal and hepatic abnormalities.

Cutaneous manifestations are seen in 10–20% of patients and include cutaneous pustules (Fig. 28.19) or subcutaneous abscesses. The most common cutaneous manifestation in children is acute suppurative parotitis (Fig. 28.20). Pneumonia may result from inhalation of air borne bacteria (Fig. 28.21).

Treatment of melioidosis is intensive supportive care, draining of abscesses, and antibiotic therapy using β-lactam agents such as ceftazidime or amoxicillin and clavulanate, with or without

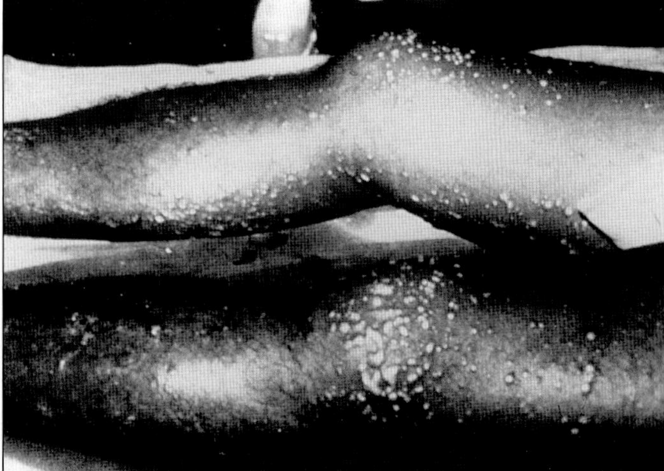

Figure 28.19 Multiple pustules of melioidosis on the legs of a rice farmer with nephrotic syndrome. (Reproduced with permission from Guerrant, Walker and Weller. Essentials of tropical diseases, 1st edn. Churchill Livingstone; 2001: Figure 31-3, p. 205.)

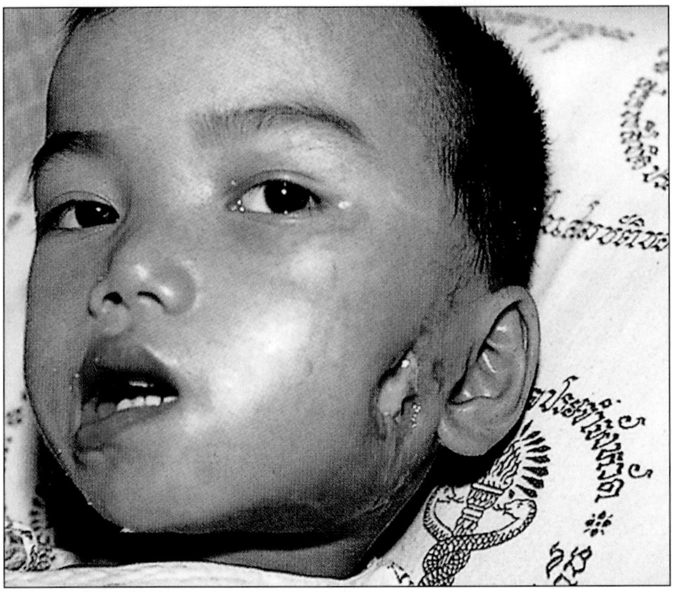

Figure 28.20 Parotid abscess of localized melioidosis. (Reproduced from Peters W and Pasvol G (eds). Tropical Medicine and Parasitology, 5th edition, Mosby, London 2002, image 594.)

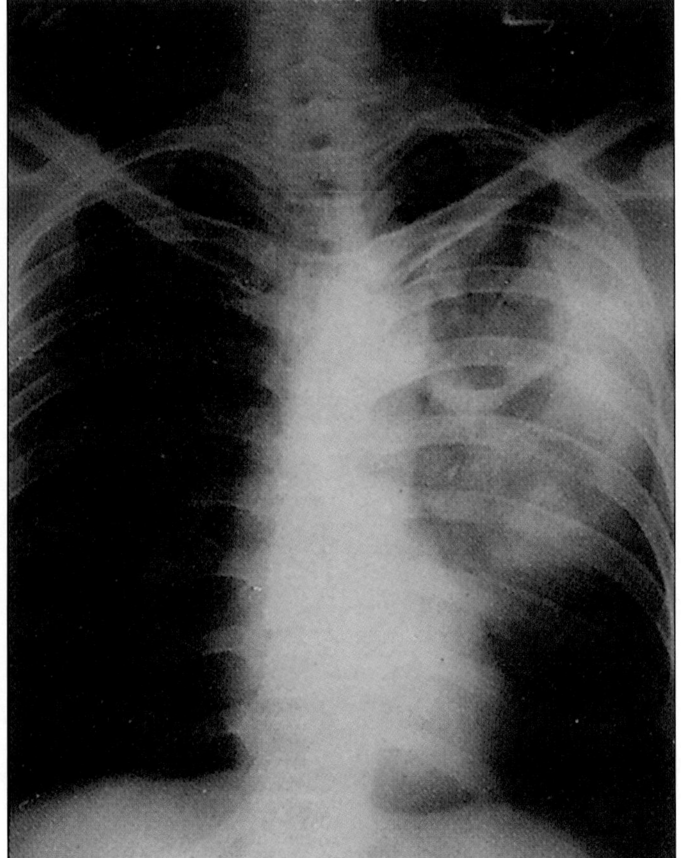

Figure 28.21 Left upper pneumonia due to melioidosis. (Reproduced with permission from Peters and Pasvol, Tropical Medicine and Parasitology, 5th edition. Mosby figure 593.)

co-trimoxazole. Antibiotics must be given for 20 weeks to avoid relapses.

Glanders

Glanders is caused by a Gram-negative bacterium, *Burkholderia (Pseudomonas) mallei*, and is usually acquired from horses, but may be transmitted from person to person. It is most common in Asia, Africa, and South America, but was reported in an American research microbiologist in 2001.[3] After an incubation period of 1 day to 2 weeks, glanders can present with fever and any of four clinical manifestations:

1. A nodule with lymphangitis at the site of inoculation; the nodule eventually breaks down and ulcerates.
2. Mucous membrane ulceration and granulomatous reaction.
3. Septicemia with cutaneous papules and pustules.
4. Pulmonary form with malaise, headache and pleurisy.

The treatment of glanders is with sulfadiazine.

Tularemia

Although not usually classified as a tropical disease, tularemia can be seen in Mexico and in the Far East. It is more likely to be acquired in the USA, Europe, or in the former Soviet Union. Tularemia is a zoonosis due to infection with a Gram-negative coccobacillus, *Francisella (Pasteurella) tularensis*; it is usually acquired from infected animals such as wild rodents, carnivores, and some species of birds. It can be seen in hunters who prepare animal carcasses, e.g., "rabbit fever," or can be acquired from the bites of mosquitoes, tabanid flies, or ixodid ticks. Clinical symptoms can be manifested as an ulceration at the site of primary infection (Fig. 28.22), followed by lymphadenopathy and fever (ulceroglandular disease). The majority of infections remain subclinical but septicemia as well as abdominal and pleuropulmonary forms can develop.[4] Streptomycin is the drug of choice, but other

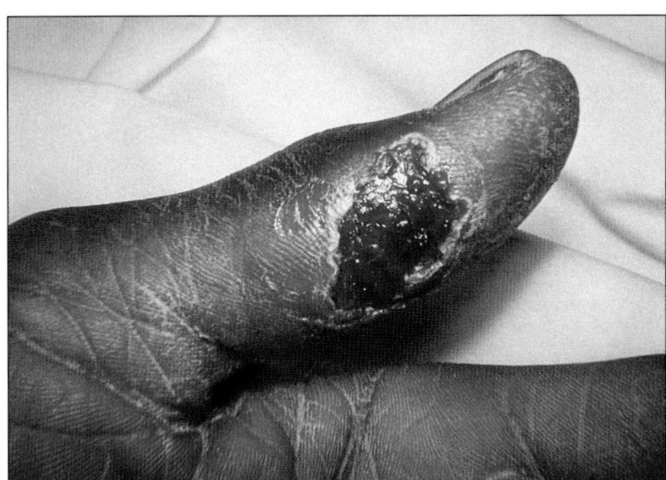

Figure 28.22 Cutaneous ulcer due to tularemia. (Reproduced from CDC, courtesy of Emory U./Dr. Sellers.)

aminoglycosides can be used successfully, as can tetracyclines, chloramphenicol, third-generation cephalosporins, rifampin and erythromycin. Prevention is by the use of gloves when handling wild animals, avoidance of ticks, and use of insect and tick repellents.

Vibrio vulnificus

Cutaneous manifestations can result from puncture wounds from shrimp, crabs, or various other sources of trauma (e.g., fishhooks) in salt water. Cellulitis, necrosis, and hemorrhagic bullae can develop, especially if the patient has alcoholic cirrhosis or diabetes mellitus (see Figure 35.23 in Chapter 35). Ingestion of seafood contaminated with *V. vulnificus*, especially raw oysters, in patients with such immunocompromising conditions can result in septicemia and widespread hemorrhagic bullae and can be fatal if not treated with intensive supportive care and systemic antibiotics.[5]

Other species of *Vibrio* can rarely have similar clinical manifestations.[6]

Other bacterial diseases

Cutaneous manifestations can be seen in a number of other tropical bacterial diseases, such as the erythematous macules known as "rose spots" of typhoid fever (see Figure 1.9 in Chapter 1) due to *Salmonella typhi*.[7] Extrapulmonary manifestations of psittacosis include Horder's spots (pink macules resembling "rose spots" of typhoid), acrocyanosis, superficial venous thrombosis, splinter hemorrhages, erythema multiforme, and erythema nodosum.[8] In addition, Q fever, due to *Coxiella burnetii*, can occasionally cause erythema nodosa and erythema annulare centrifugum.[9]

References

1. Chaowagul W, White NJ, Dance DAB. Melioidosis: a major cause of community-acquired septicemia in northeastern Thailand. J Infect Dis 1989; 159:890.
2. Leelarasamee A, Bovornkitti S. Melioidosis: review and update. Rev Infect Dis 1989; 11:413.
3. Srinivasan A, Kraus CN, DeShazer D et al. Glanders in a military research microbiologist. N Engl J Med 2001; 345:256–258.
4. Jacobs RF, Condrey YM, Yamauchi T. Tularemia in adults and children: a changing presentation. Pediatrics 1985; 76:818.
5. Tyring S, Lee P. Hemorrhagic bullae associated with *Vibrio vulnificus* septicemia. Arch Dermatol 1986; 122:818–820.
6. Newman C, Shepherd M, Woodward MD et al. Fatal septicemia and bullae caused by non-01 *Vibrio cholerae*. J Am Acad Dermatol 1993; 29:909–912.
7. Hoffner RJ, Slaven E, Perez J et al. Emergency department presentations of typhoid fever. J Emerg Med 2000; 19:317–321.
8. Semel JD. Cutaneous findings in a case of psittacosis. Arch Dermatol 1984; 120:1227.
9. Raoult D, Marrie T. Q fever. Clin Infect Dis 1995; 20:489.

Chapter 29

Scabies

Bart Currie and Ulrich R. Hengge

Synonyms: Scabies, *Sarcoptes scabiei*, itch mite

Key features:

- Ectoparasite spread from person to person
- Endemic disease and epidemics related to overcrowding and poverty
- Female mite burrows into epidermis and lays eggs
- Rash and itch are from papules/vesicles of individual mites in burrows plus secondary more generalized papular immune response
- Secondary bacterial pyoderma occurs
- More severe disease in the immunocompromised, including crusted (Norwegian) scabies
- Topical scabicides cure infection when correctly administered
- Treatment of contacts is essential to prevent reinfection

Introduction

Scabies has been recognized as a contagious disease for centuries. Although large epidemics have been related to poverty, overcrowding, and social upheaval such as in wars, endemic scabies persists in most tropical regions. In addition to the discomfort of the often intractable itch, secondary bacterial pyoderma is an important antecedent to systemic bacterial sepsis and post-streptococcal glomerulonephritis. Hyperinfestation (crusted or Norwegian scabies) is increasingly recognized in patients with acquired immunodeficiency syndrome (AIDS) and also in elderly individuals in nursing homes, who may be the focus for unexpected and initially unrecognized scabies outbreaks. Recent molecular epidemiological studies have shown scabies to be generally host-restricted, with human-to-human infection cycles not overlapping with those of animal scabies. Although definitive diagnosis of scabies requires microscopic visualization of a mite retrieved from a skin burrow, empirical treatment based on clinical suspicion remains far more common. The skin rash of scabies can be very variable and hard to distinguish from many other dermatological conditions. Furthermore, clinical care and availability of treatment are limited in many locations where scabies is endemic. Hence accurate global epidemiology is lacking and both overdiagnosis and underdiagnosis frequently occur.

History

Scabies has been known for millennia, and has been referred to in the Old Testament of the Bible as well as by Aristotle.[1] Scabies mites were described and drawn by the Italians Bonomo and Cestoni in 1689.[2] This has been described as the first definitive description of a parasitic organism being responsible for an infectious disease and preceded modern germ theory by almost two centuries.

Epidemiology

Classical accounts of the epidemiology of human scabies described large epidemics or pandemics that were said to occur in 30-year cycles, with intensity concomitant with major wars. Such pandemics have been documented for the periods 1919–1925, 1936–1949, and 1964–1979.[3] There has been much discussion whether this apparent cyclical pattern of scabies is a biological phenomenon or an oversimplification based on limited data of questionable accuracy. Even regional scabies data are limited, with diagnosis being mostly anecdotal: the disease is not notifiable to health authorities and published reports are usually based on interesting cases or small outbreaks. It has been noted that even during the "pandemic" periods, peak scabies years were different for different countries and the recent cycle peaking in the late 1970s reflected descriptions from North America and Europe. It has been shown that clearance of primary scabies infection correlates with development of immunity; on reinfection both humans and animals have a reduced parasitic burden and some previously infected individuals can eliminate a second infestation before clinical manifestations develop.[4,5] Therefore the concept of "herd immunity" as an explanation for cyclical pandemics has some biological plausibility. However this is countered by the documentation of ongoing scabies endemicity in many tropical and subtropical communities such as India, South Africa, Panama, and northern Australia.[6–9] Furthermore it is yet to be definitely established whether a history of infection with *Sarcoptes scabiei* will result in long-term immunity.

A unifying explanation for the classical pandemic descriptions and the current recognized endemicity is that scabies is indeed endemic in many regions because of overcrowding and the continuing new cohorts of susceptible young children who maintain the infection cycle, while exceptional crowding together of susceptible adult populations during war situations drove the epidemics. The documented high rates during war of other external arthropod parasites such as the lice *Pediculus humanus* and *Phthirus pubis* are consistent with this.[9]

Although data are lacking, it was estimated that there were around 300 million cases of scabies globally towards the end of the twentieth century. In recent surveys some remote Aboriginal communities in northern Australia had a prevalence of scabies based on clinical diagnosis as high as 50%, with scabies underlying up to 70% of group A streptococcal (*Streptococcus pyogenes*)-infected skin sores.[7]

Scabies is overall most common in young children, most likely reflecting both increased exposure and, in endemic situations, a lack of immunity. Scabies affects both sexes similarly, although mothers of young children appear more commonly infected than other adults in some studies.[8] An increase in the incidence of scabies is also observed in the elderly in nursing homes. This is likely to be multifactorial, including increased exposure, especially when related to index cases of crusted (Norwegian) scabies, possible immunodeficiency in the elderly, and decreased ability to kill mites by scratching in debilitated patients such as those with dementia and following strokes.

Although some studies have documented scabies rates to be higher or lower in certain ethnic groups, there is no evidence for biological susceptibility based on race. Ethnic differences in scabies are most likely to be related to differences in overcrowding, housing, socioeconomic and behavioral factors rather than racial origin.

The most consistent factor associated with scabies is overcrowding, presumably because this allows greatest opportunity for the close contact required for transmission of scabies mites from one infected individual to another person. Poverty and poor hygiene are often associated with overcrowding, but the evidence that they are independent risk factors for scabies is mostly lacking.[7] Indeed, scabies can occur in affluent circumstances if exposure occurs and scabies is endemic in many coastal tropical communities with plentiful access to water and with meticulous hygiene. It is possible that nutritional deficiencies associated with poverty may make individuals more susceptible to more severe scabies. In one study during a scabies epidemic in an Indian village there was a significant association between a high prevalence of scabies and poor nutritional status.

S. scabiei affects a wide range of animal species in addition to humans.[10] However, mite populations are generally host-species-restricted such that, for instance, *S. scabiei* var. *canis* and *S. scabiei* var. *suis* are rarely responsible for human cases, which result from infection with *S. scabiei* var. *hominis*. Recent molecular genotyping studies of scabies mites from humans and dogs support the concept of host-species-restricted cycles of transmission.[11] Occasional cases of human scabies have been described following exposure to dog scabies but these infections are considered to be self-limiting, with skin itch from reaction to the dog mites but usually no mite reproduction occurring in human skin and therefore no or very limited transmissibility to other humans. Scabies is common in some economically important livestock. For instance, it is estimated that scabies affects over half of pig herds worldwide, with control of scabies mange a serious productivity issue. Globally *S. scabiei* causes mange in many companion animals such as dogs and cats. Scabies is also responsible for epizootic disease in many wild animal populations.[7]

Pathogenesis and etiology

S. scabiei is a member of the family Sarcoptidae within the class Arachnida. The sarcoptid mites are obligate parasites of mammals and birds. Adult females are around 0.4 mm long and 0.3 mm wide, with males smaller, at up to 0.25 mm long and 0.2 mm wide. The body is opaque off-white in color and the legs and mouthparts are brown. Adults and nymphs have eight legs and larvae have six. On the dorsal and lateral surfaces are pairs of spine-like projections and some of the legs have stalked pulvilli (suckers) and/or spur-like claws (Fig. 29.1).

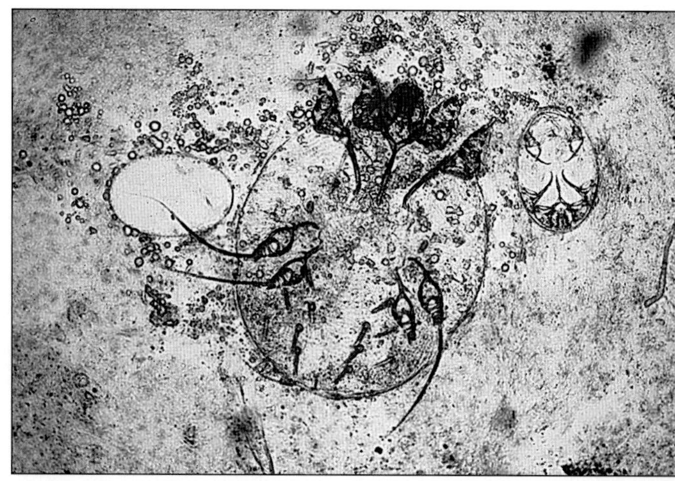

Figure 29.1 Female scabies mite with eggs – from skin scraping of crusted scabies.

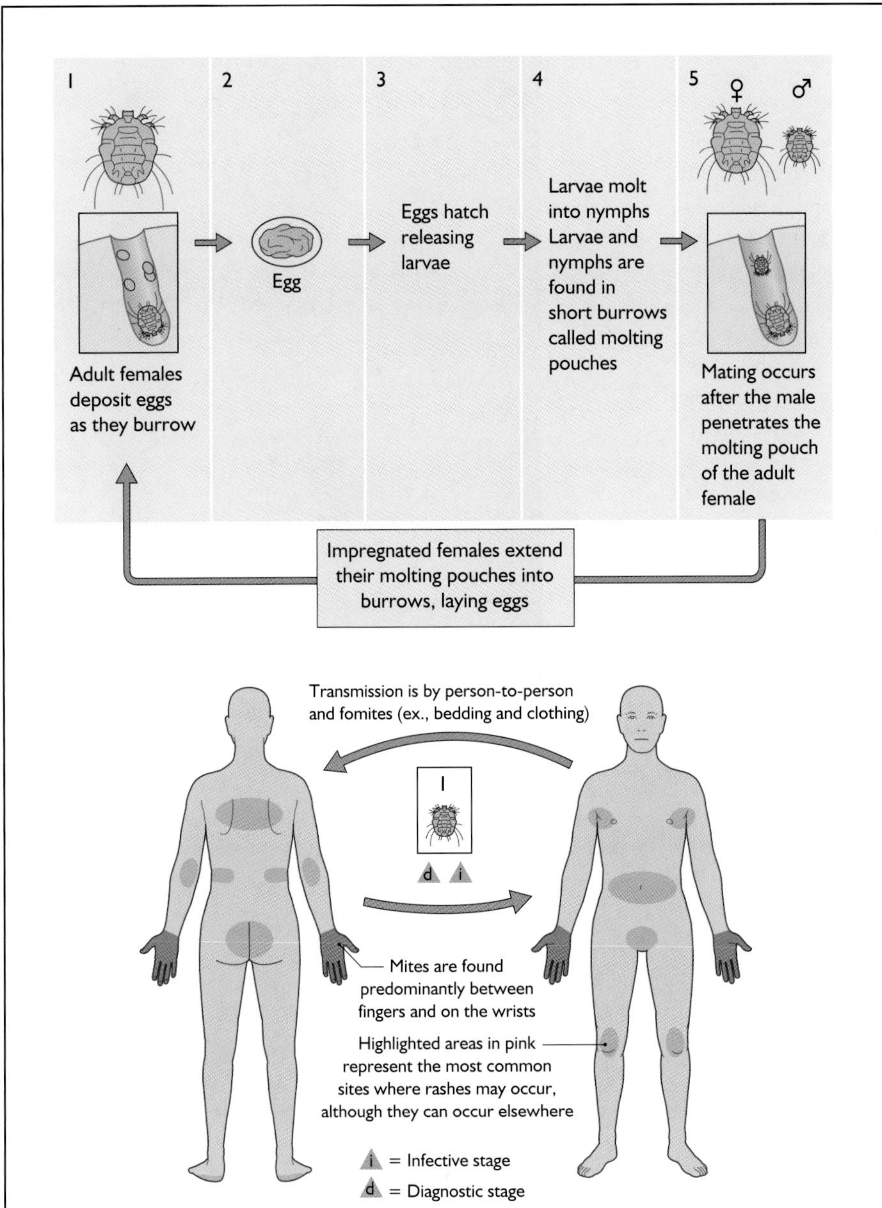
1
2
3
4
5
Adult females deposit eggs as they burrow
Egg
Eggs hatch releasing larvae
Larvae molt into nymphs
Larvae and nymphs are found in short burrows called molting pouches
Mating occurs after the male penetrates the molting pouch of the adult female
Impregnated females extend their molting pouches into burrows, laying eggs
Transmission is by person-to-person and fomites (ex., bedding and clothing)
Mites are found predominantly between fingers and on the wrists
Highlighted areas in pink represent the most common sites where rashes may occur, although they can occur elsewhere
= Infective stage
= Diagnostic stage

Figure 29.2 Life cycle of scabies.

After mating of adult male and female *S. scabiei* mites, the male dies and the female begins to lay eggs in the skin burrow within the stratum granulosum of the epidermis. The female lays 0–3 eggs/day for up to 6 weeks before dying. Larvae hatch 2–4 days after eggs are laid, cut through to the skin surface, and begin to dig burrows. Three to four days later the larvae molt into protonymphs which 2–3 days later molt into tritonymphs, from which an adult male or female emerges after a further 5–6 days (Fig. 29.2).

There have been differing opinions as to whether fertilization of female mites by male mites only occurs in burrows or also on the skin surface.[1–4] It therefore remains uncertain whether infection of new hosts is more commonly via the more numerous nymphal stages or by transmission of already fertilized adult female mites. However, skin entry can occur in less than 30 min and all life cycle stages can penetrate intact epidermis by secreting enzymes that dissolve skin, which is then ingested by the mite.

Classical studies by Mellanby showed that direct person-to-person body contact was generally necessary for transmission of scabies.[4] Only four new cases resulted from 272 attempts to infect volunteers who climbed into warm beds just vacated by heavily infected patients. This suggested that fomites such as clothing or exposure to mites shed on to floors or surfaces were unlikely means of infection. While probably generally true, the exception is the patient with hyperinfestation (crusted or Norwegian scabies), who can shed multiple skin flakes totaling thousands of mites daily. Mite survival in the environment requires moisture and increases with decreasing ambient temperature. However, mobility and host-seeking activity increase in warmer environments, with little movement possible below 20° C. Scabies mites can survive at least several days at moderate ambient temperatures in humid environments. Transmission via fomites as well as direct skin contact may therefore be occurring in nursing-home outbreaks and infections in hospital staff where a crusted scabies patient is the core transmitter. Similar transmission via shed mites is likely to occur in households in the tropics where a person with crusted scabies resides.

Intrafamilial transmission as the commonest means of infection is supported by epidemiological studies and more recently by molecular studies showing the genotypes of mites from household members to be more homogenous than those from separate households within a community.[7] Among adults sexual contact is an important means of transmission.

Although the cycle from egg to adult female is around 2 weeks, less than 1% of the laid eggs develop to adult mites and after experimental infection it may require 3–4 weeks for the presence of new adult females. On a normal host the average mite burden that develops is as few as 10–12 mites and after 3 months mite numbers usually decrease rapidly.[4] Both mechanical removal of the mites by scratching and development of the host immune response contribute to control of the mite population. Sensitization to mite antigens can be demonstrated a month following primary infestations, with both humoral and cellular responses against mite midgut cells resulting in inhibition of nutrient absorption.

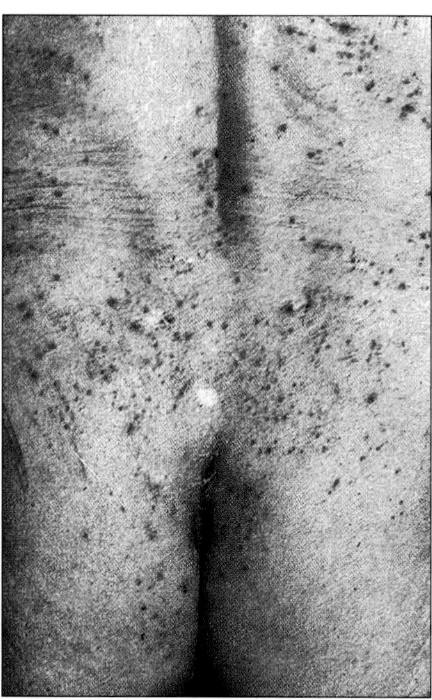

Figure 29.4 Papular lesions may occur as immunological reactions to mite excretions.

Clinical features

Scabies in adults and older children usually presents as an intensely pruritic rash, with the itch often worse at night. In primary infection the symptoms develop 3–4 weeks after infection. In those previously infected and therefore sensitized to mite antigens, rash and itch can occur within 24–48 h of a new infection. The rash of scabies is considered to result from varying combinations of two processes: (1) papular or vesicular lesions occurring at the site of burrows made by adult and larval mites; and (2) a more generalized pruritic and erythematous papular eruption which is unrelated to obvious individual mites and which is thought to be an immunological response (Figs 29.3 and 29.4).

Preferred sites for mites to burrow are where the stratum corneum is thin and soft and where there are few or no hair follicles (Box 29.1 and Fig. 29.5). In infants and small children and, more commonly, in both children and adults in tropical regions, the palms, soles, face, neck, and scalp may also be involved with mite-associated lesions. The more generalized skin rash is most commonly seen around the axillae, chest and abdomen, buttocks, and thighs.

Box 29.1 Sites of predilection for scabies mites to burrow

Web spaces between the fingers and adjacent sides of the fingers
Flexor surfaces of wrists
Extensor surfaces of elbows
Anterior axillary folds
Skin around the nipples (especially in women)
Periumbilical region
Pelvic girdle, including waist, lower buttocks, upper thighs
Penis (shaft and glans)
Extensor surfaces of knees
Lateral and posterior aspects of feet

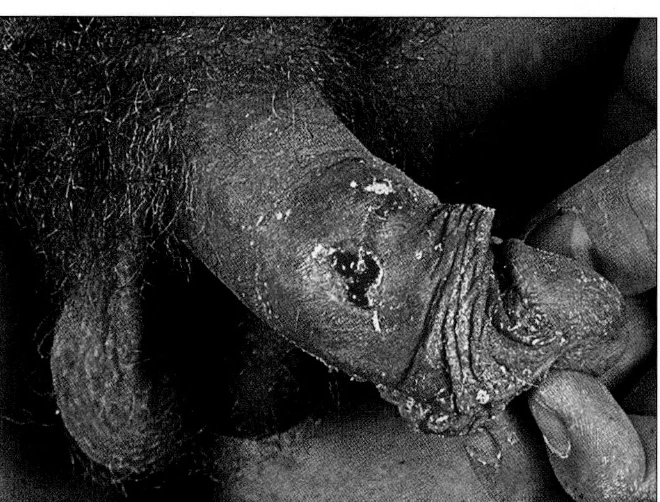

Figure 29.3 Papular vesicular and croded lesions occurring at the site of burrows made by adult and larval mites.

The classical diagnostic clinical sign of scabies is the burrow made by the adult female as it ingests and digests the horny layer of the epidermis. Burrows appear as serpiginous grayish, reddish, or brownish lines, 2–15 mm long. They are just visible to a trained unaided eye, but are difficult to see and classical burrows are often absent, even when the skin is inspected with magnification. Egg cases and mite fecal pellets are present inside the burrow. The papule at the burrow surface is usually small and erythematous, often excoriated or covered by a small blood clot. In infants and young children it can be vesicular or even bullous. Visible burrows appear to be less commonly seen in tropical regions, possibly

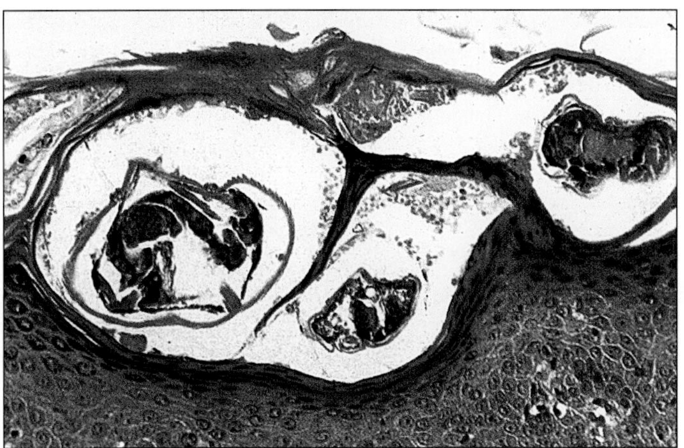
Figure 29.5 Section through a burrow showing mite parts below the stratum corneum.

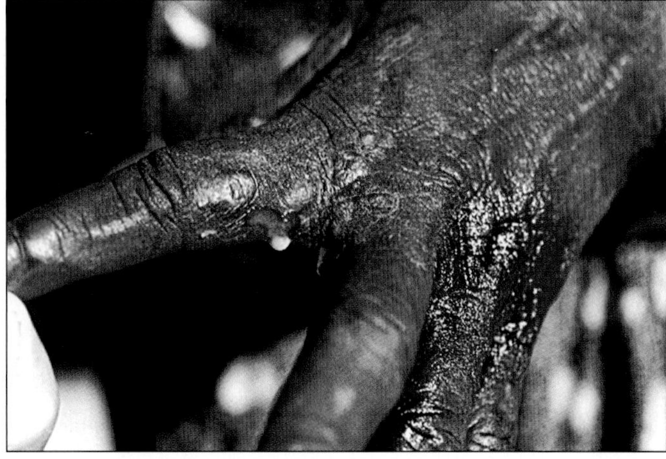
Figure 29.7 Scabies with secondary streptococcal infection.

because many presentations are not primary but repeat infections, where a more intense local inflammatory response may obscure the burrows and the more generalized immune response-related rash may be more prominent.

Other skin manifestations

While in suspected scabies the presence of visible burrows or papules in the web spaces between the fingers is adequate for diagnosis, there is a wide range of clinical appearances (Fig. 29.6). This often relates to the severity and extent of the inflammatory immune response, with any itchy generalized or local rash being possibly caused by scabies. Atypical appearances are more common in patients with longstanding scabies who may develop chronic excoriation and eczematization of limbs and trunk. However, young children can also have an extensive inflammatory response. Secondary bacterial infection of scabies lesions is frequent, with *Streptococcus pyogenes* and *Staphylococcus aureus* the common organisms (Figs 29.7 and 29.8). Scabies may therefore underly bacterial pyoderma, presenting as pustular or crusted sores, boils, cellulites, or lymphangitis/lymphadenitis.

Scabies may be hard to recognize in patients taking topical or oral steroids (scabies incognito) and in immunosuppression from

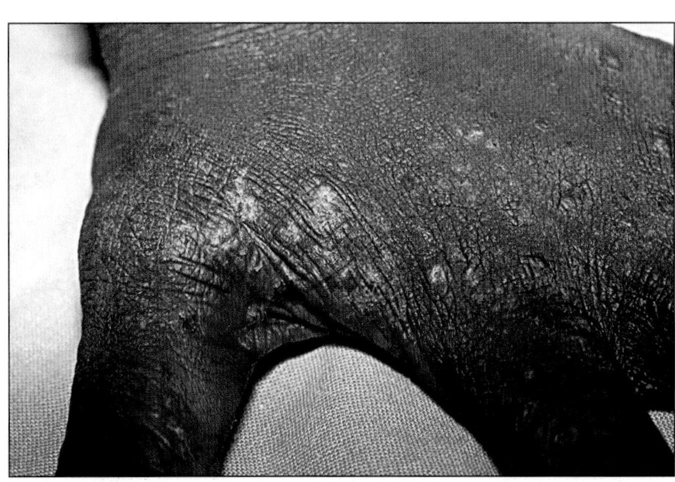
Figure 29.6 Scabies of the hand.

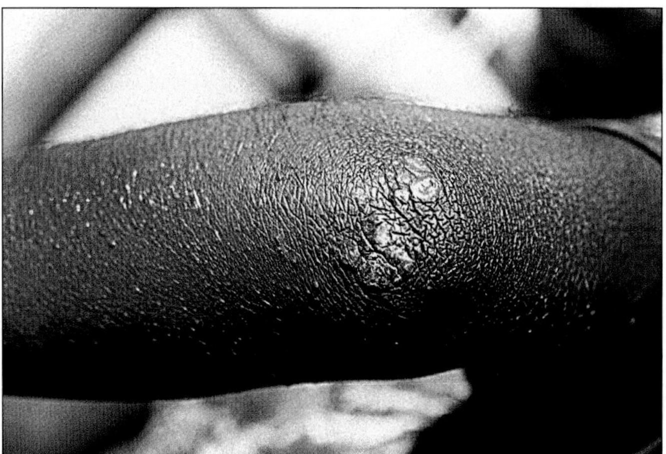
Figure 29.8 Scabies with secondary infection – elbow.

disease or of iatrogenic nature. After curative treatment of scabies the rash and itch may commonly persist for days to several weeks. However in a minority of cases a nodular reaction (nodular scabies) occurs and it may persist for months after mite-eradicating treatment. The firm, red-brown dome-shaped nodules are 5–8 mm in diameter, usually extremely itchy, and most common on the anterior axillary folds, groin, genitalia, buttocks, and periumbilical region.

Crusted scabies

While *Sarcoptes scabiei* infection and mite reproduction in humans are usually self-limiting, a small minority develop hyperinfestation, with estimated total mite numbers in the most severe cases up to over a million. This debilitating condition is crusted or Norwegian scabies, so called because it was first described among leprosy patients in Norway in 1848. Crusted scabies has also been noted in overtly immunosuppressed patients, such as with malignancies, chemotherapy, and transplant patients.[6] Most recently it has been increasingly recognized in advanced human immunodeficiency virus (HIV) infection.[12] Crusted scabies also occasionally occurs in malnutrition, in Down's syndrome, in the elderly and institutionalized, and in those with cognitive deficiency or physical debility who are unable to interpret properly, or respond to the itch by scratching.

Cases have been described in indigenous Australians who have no overt immunosuppression.[13] It has been hypothesized that such patients may have a specific immune deficit predisposing them to hyperinfestation. This is consistent with the association of crusted scabies with both leprosy and infection with human T-lymphotropic virus-1 (HTLV-1). There is no evidence of mite differences or increased virulence of mites in these cases, with normal scabies occurring in hospital staff infected from these "core transmitters."

The cardinal feature of crusted scabies is the development of hyperkeratotic skin crusts that may be loose, scaly, and flaky or thick and adherent. Skin flakes with thousands of mites can be shed daily on to bed linen or floors. While hands and feet are most commonly involved, the distribution is often extensive, including neck, scalp, and face as well as trunk and limbs, especially knees and elbows (Figs 29.9–29.13). Thick deposits of debris and mites accumulate beneath the nails, which are often dystrophic and thickened. Some cases may have crusting limited to one or several limbs, the back of the fingers and hands, or just the buttock region. Fissuring and secondary bacterial infection are common and regional lymphadenopathy is frequently present (Figs 29.14–29.16). The presence of itch is variable but can be intense, even in leprosy patients. A peripheral blood eosinophilia is common and serum levels of immunoglobulin E (IgE) are often extremely high. There is a high mortality in crusted scabies from secondary bacterial sepsis.

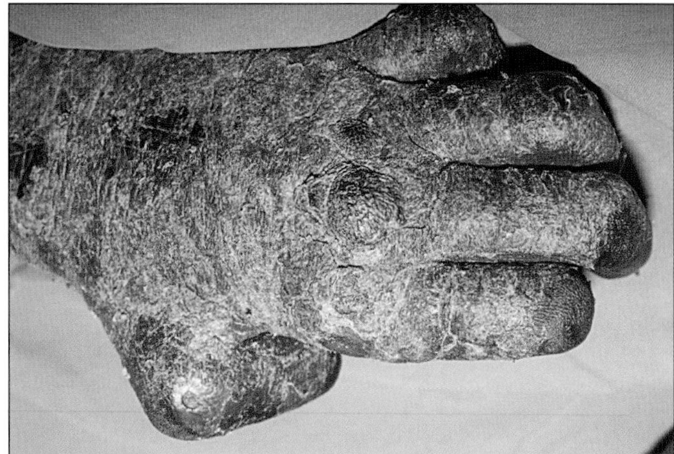

Figure 29.11 Crusted scabies in a patient with leprosy.

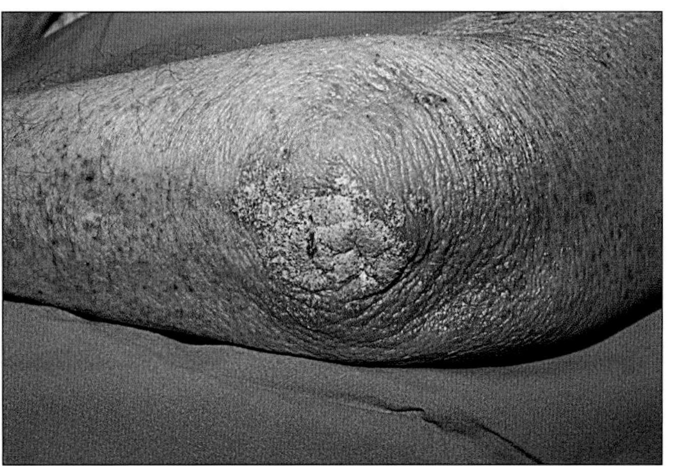

Figure 29.9 Crusted scabies of the elbow – immunosuppressed patient.

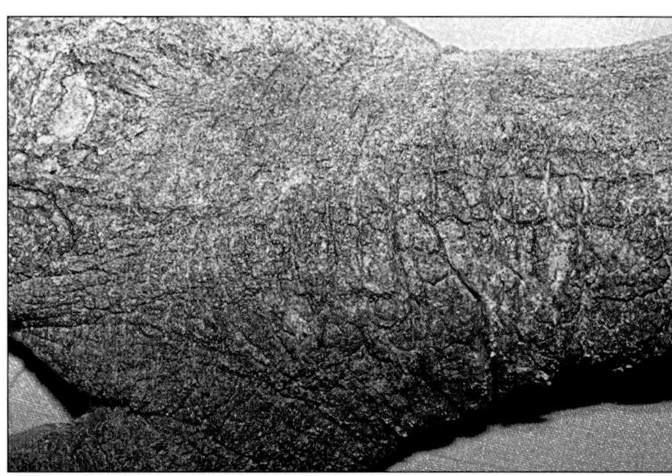

Figure 29.12 Crusted scabies of the hand and wrist.

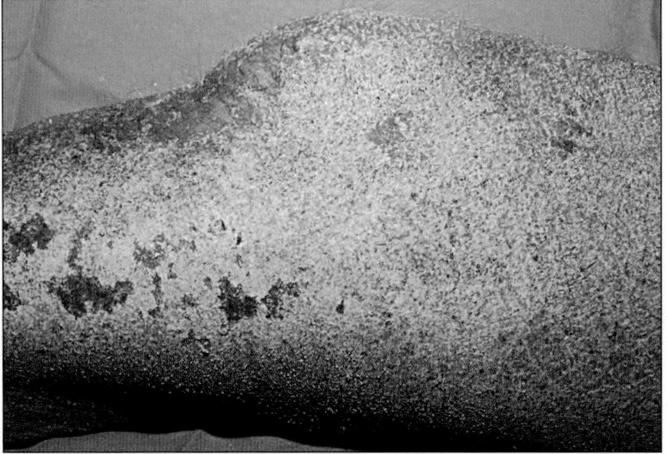

Figure 29.10 Same patient as in Figure 29.9.

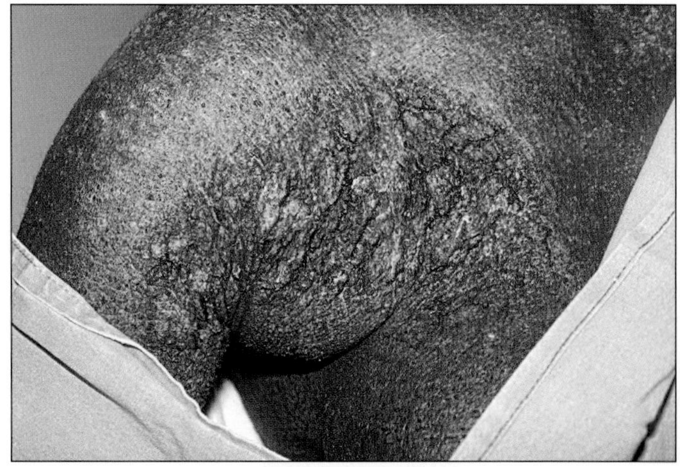

Figure 29.13 Crusted scabies of the shoulder.

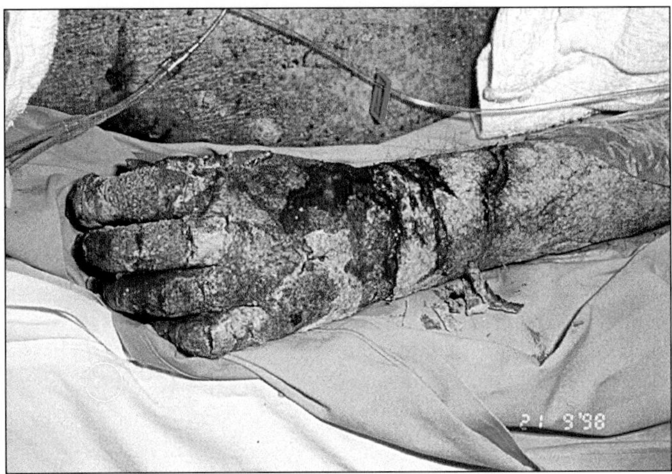

Figure 29.14 Fatal crusted scabies.

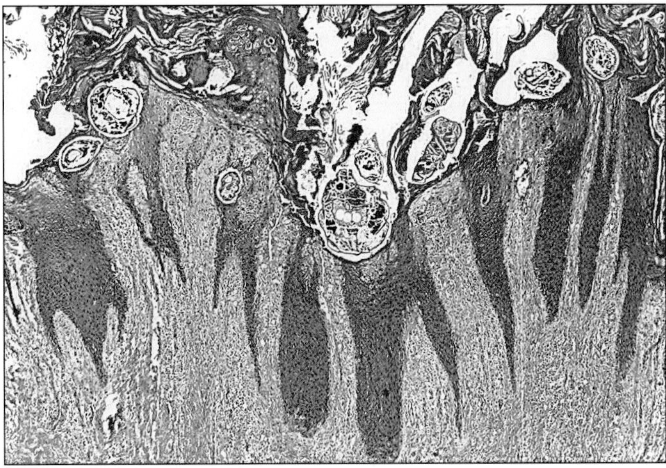

Figure 29.16 Skin biopsy of a fatal case of crusted scabies, showing mites in the epidermis, with hyperkeratosis and inflammatory response.

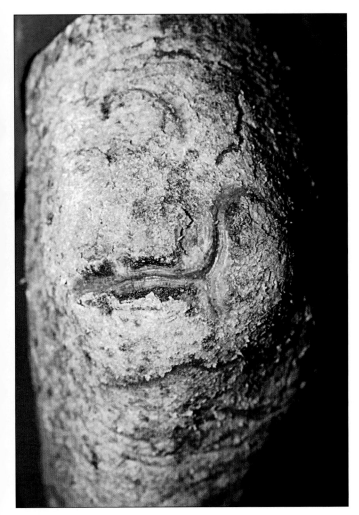

Figure 29.15 Severe crusted scabies with fissuring involving the leg.

Complications of scabies

As noted, secondary bacterial infection of scabies lesions is frequent, with *Streptococcus pyogenes* and *Staphylococcus aureus* as the most common organisms, although any bacteria colonizing skin can be involved. In crusted scabies sepsis from Gram-negative organisms such as *Pseudomonas aeruginosa* may occur alone or as polymicrobial sepsis in combination with *Streptococcus pyogenes* and/or *Staphylococcus aureus*. Streptococci and staphylococci have been isolated from mite fecal pellets and from skin burrows, with mites possibly facilitating bacterial spread. Sporadic and epidemic acute poststreptococcal glomerulonephritis are important complications of scabies with secondary bacterial infection. Acute poststreptococcal glomerulonephritis and systemic sepsis from skin bacteria are the two possible situations where complications of scabies may cause death. The metabolic burden of scabies can contribute to malnutrition, especially in severe scabies in infants and young children and in crusted scabies.

Patient evaluation, diagnosis, and differential diagnosis

Scabies should be considered in any patient presenting with a rash and itch. A recent history of scabies in contacts or household members should be sought and this increases the predictive value of a presumptive clinical diagnosis. Itch which is worse at night is also a useful predictor.

Although definitive diagnosis is by microscopic identification of the *Sarcoptes scabiei* mite, in suspected scabies the presence of visible burrows or papules/vesicles in the web spaces between the fingers is adequate for diagnosis. Magnifying glasses or dermatoscopes (5–10×) may help identify burrows. In any non-classical presentation it is recommended that skin samples be collected for microscopy if available (Boxes 29.2–29.4). However in scabies-endemic communities and primary care settings where microscopy is not available, presumptive treatment based on clinical suspicion is appropriate (Fig. 29.17).

Given the usually low number of mites present in scabies, the sensitivity of microscopy for confirming scabies is generally poor, although some dermatologists and trained health staff are expert at extracting mites from burrows. Difficulty in finding mites is especially common in atypical presentations and non-primary infections, where the inflammatory response may obscure the

Box 29.2 Sampling for mites

Identify a non-excoriated papule
Visualization of burrows can be facilitated by placing 2–3 drops of ink over the papule for 10 s then wiping clean with an alcohol swab
Place a drop of mineral oil over the burrow/papule
Gently scrape off the burrow/papule with a scalpel blade (e.g., #15), skin curette, or needle
Place the tissue on a glass slide, preferably with one drop of 10% potassium hydroxide, and apply coverslip
Examine under microscope at low power (10–100×) for mites, eggs, and eggshells
Presumptive treatment is recommended if scabies cannot reasonably be excluded or if it is a possible diagnosis and microscopy is unavailable

Box 29.3 Differential diagnosis of scabies

Impetigo and furunculosis
Eczema
Bites from mosquitoes, midges, fleas, lice, bedbugs, chiggers, or other mites
Tinea corporis
Paronychia
Papular urticaria and other allergic reactions
Dermatitis herpetiformis
Eczema herpeticum

Box 29.4 Differential diagnosis of crusted scabies

Psoriasis
Skin malignancy – lymphoma, Sézary syndrome
Tinea corporis and nail tinea
Syphilis

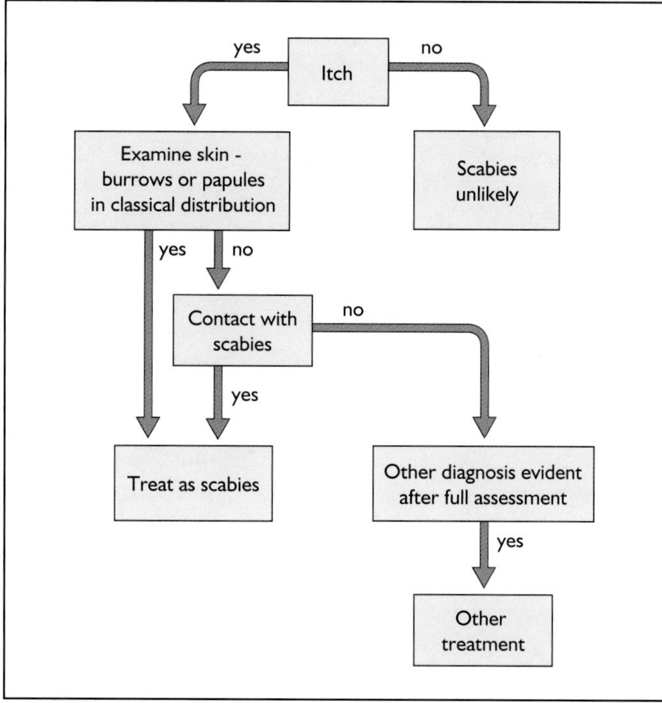

Figure 29.17 Presumptive treatment of scabies algorithm.

burrow location. Diagnosis in unsuspected scabies will sometimes be made by histological examination of formalin-fixed skin biopsies of undiagnosed rashes. In crusted scabies collection or scraping of the shedding skin flakes and hyperkeratotic areas will usually reveal multiple mites and eggs on microscopy, thus confirming the diagnosis (Fig. 29.1).

A number of commercial serology assays have been developed for the diagnosis of scabies in pigs and dogs, based on antibodies to whole-mite antigen preparations. These show cross-specificity between host *S. scabiei* varieties but have not been formally evaluated in human scabies. Furthermore, there is evidence that cross-specificity of scabies antigens with house dust mite allergens causes false-positive serology results in humans because of exposure to house dust mites, which is ubiquitous for people living in many locations. However, given the difficulties in obtaining a positive microscopic diagnosis, a serology assay of high specificity for active scabies infection would be of enormous benefit. Current studies of recombinant scabies antigens may lead to such an assay, although discriminating current infection from past exposure will be problematic, as for many serology assays. Efforts are also underway to find unique *S. scabiei* genetic fingerprints that may enable direct detection of mite DNA in skin samples. While blood eosinophilia and high IgE levels are common in scabies, they are also seen with many other endemic parasitic infections.

Pathology

Adult female mites reside in burrows within the stratum granulosum of the epidermis (Fig. 29.3). Eggs, egg cases, mite fecal pellets, and debris are also present in the burrow. The associated underlying inflammatory response includes varying intensity and combinations of lymphocytes, histiocytes, eosinophils, and polymorphs. In crusted scabies there is massive expansion of the keratin layer due to proliferation keratinocytes. Numerous adult mites, eggs, and larvae are also usually seen, some clearly associated with burrows but many just spread throughout the epidermis and on the skin surface. A more extensive underlying mixed inflammatory response is also usual in crusted scabies. In ordinary scabies CD4+ T lymphocytes predominate in the inflammatory response, whereas CD8+ T lymphocytes are more common in limited studies from crusted scabies patients.[7,14]

Treatment

The mainstay of scabies therapy is topical acaricides, although oral ivermectin is increasingly being used in certain circumstances, most notably crusted scabies (Box 29.5). Topical permethrin and oral ivermectin, where affordable, are currently considered the best treatment options.[15,16]

Permethrin, a synthetic pyrethroid, is more expensive than other agents but is now considered the treatment of choice for scabies in many countries, including the UK and the USA. The standard treatment for scabies is topical application of permethrin cream in a concentration of 5% and the 1% preparations used for treatment of head lice should not be used for scabies. It has been recommended for use in children over 6 months, but is widely used in younger infants. Permethrin is well tolerated, has low toxicity, is poorly absorbed by the skin, and is rapidly metabolized. A single overnight application was shown to be equally effective as lindane[17] (category 2 evidence in a randomized controlled trial (RCT)). However in vitro mite tolerance to permethrin has now been documented, with some reports of treatment failure in endemic indigenous communities in northern Australia.[7] The globally expanding resistance of head lice to permethrin suggests that continued surveillance for resistance in scabies is crucial (Table 29.1 and Box 29.6).

Benzyl benzoate, an ester of benzoic acid and benzyl alcohol, has been an effective scabies treatment for more than 60 years (category 4 evidence in a case series). Although in vitro studies show that it kills scabies mites faster than permethrin, it has been traditionally recommended to leave the lotion on the skin for 24 h. The main problem with benzyl benzoate is skin irritation in the first minutes after application. Although the discomfort usually rapidly decreases in severity after several minutes, the burning sensation is not uncommonly so painful that the lotion has to be washed off. It is generally recommended that the 25% emulsion be diluted in 3 parts water for children less than 2 years of age and in 1 part water for children 2–12 years old and in sensitive older children and adults, possibly reducing its efficacy. Central nervous system (CNS) toxicity has rarely been reported in children.

Table 29.1 Topical scabicides

Drug	Comments
Permethrin 5%	Very effective, little toxicity, expensive, drug of choice where affordable: category 2 evidence from randomized controlled trials
Benzyl benzoate 25%	Very effective, although a burning sensation is a problem for some people: category 4 evidence from case series
Gamma benzene hexachloride 1% (lindane)	Very effective, toxicity rare but serious – withdrawn in some countries: category 2 evidence from randomized controlled trials
Sulfur creams	Poor efficacy: category 3 evidence from comparative studies
Crotamiton 10%	Poor efficacy: category 3 evidence from comparative studies

Box 29.5 Summary of scabies treatment studies

In ordinary scabies

Topical permethrin and oral ivermectin are at least as effective as topical lindane (category 2 evidence from randomized controlled trials)

Topical permethrin may be superior to single-dose ivermectin but equivalent to two doses of ivermectin 2 weeks apart (category 2 evidence from a single unblinded randomized controlled trial)

In crusted scabies

Combined oral ivermectin and topical scabicide is superior to topical scabicide alone (category 4 evidence from case series)

Box 29.6 Use of topical scabicides

Apply to the whole body except eyes and mucous membranes
Supervised therapy is preferable
Leave on for 12–24 h before washing off
Treat all family members and close personal contacts, preferably at the same time
Wash clothing and bed linen in the normal fashion or store for 7 days in a bag
A repeat application of topical scabicide at 1–2 weeks is recommended in more severe scabies

Gammabenzene hexachloride 1% (lindane) is an organochlorine used for many years in scabies and with a demonstrated high cure rate[17,18] (category 2 evidence in RCTs). However, systemic absorption can occur, especially in young children and those with damaged skin: both CNS toxicity (mostly seizures)[19] and aplastic anemia are well documented. Although these serious complications are rare, they have resulted in lindane being withdrawn in some countries. There have also been reports suggesting occasional development of mite resistance to lindane.[20]

Crotamiton 10% cream has been widely used for scabies in children because of its low toxicity profile and the fact that it is well tolerated. However it has low and slow efficacy against *S. scabiei* and daily application for 3–5 days is recommended if it is to be used at all (category 3 evidence in comparative studies). It can be used for children less than 2 months of age if permethrin is not being used or is unavailable.

Sulfur compounds have been used to treat scabies for centuries. Although not active against scabies mites in vitro, when applied on the skin sulfur appears to elicit an active compound, possibly pentathionic acid, produced by skin microorganisms or epidermal cells. This may account for its apparent but limited efficacy (category 3 evidence in comparative studies). Sulfur creams are messy and smelly, can cause skin irritation, and require repeated application. Like crotamiton, they have a limited role, but 5% sulfur cream/lotion daily for 2–3 days is an alternative to permethrin in infants.

Although it is often recommended that topical therapy is only applied below the neck, scabies not infrequently involves the head and scalp in children and in the tropics also in adults, hence the general recommendation for whole-body application. Patient information sheets are useful educational aids, explaining the treatment and the importance of adequate acaricide application, warning against excessive use, and noting that the itch may take several days or even weeks to resolve, even though the mites are killed. The life cycle of *S. scabiei* supports repeat treatment at 1–2 weeks in more severe cases, to enable killing of nymphs hatched from eggs not killed by the initial treatment.

Oral ivermectin

Ivermectin is a chemically modified avermectin with a half-life of 36 h. It has a broad spectrum of activity against numerous nematodes and arthropod parasites. It has been widely used for treatment of sarcoptic mange in animals in topical, oral, and parenteral preparations. In humans it has been used since the mid-1980s, most commonly for the treatment of the filarial worm *Onchocerca volvulus* (causing river blindness), but also for *Wuchereria bancrofti* and *Brugia malayi* (causing filariasis). It is now the drug of choice for strongyloidiasis. Oral ivermectin for scabies is increasingly used worldwide, especially for crusted scabies.[15,16] Although CNS toxicity from ivermectin is well documented in certain dog varieties, the extensive use in filarial programs has shown excellent tolerance, with few adverse reactions. Limited reports of possible CNS toxicity in elderly nursing-home patients treated during scabies outbreaks have yet to be substantiated. Although no adverse outcomes have been reported with inadvertent use in pregnancy, ivermectin is currently not recommended for use in pregnancy or in children under 5 years of age.

An early study showed 100 μg/kg oral ivermectin to be as effective as topical benzyl benzoate in scabies, although methodology and follow up were problematic and apparent failures were common in both groups (category 3 evidence in an unblinded comparative study). Other studies using 200 μg/kg have shown up to 100% efficacy with oral ivermectin in ordinary scabies (category 4 evidence in a case series) and shown it to be at least as effective as lindane[18] (category 2 evidence in a double-blind "double-dummy" RCT). However one study comparing single-dose ivermectin (200 μg/kg) with topical 5% permethrin showed the permethrin regimen to be superior, with the authors suggesting that two doses of ivermectin at a 2-week interval were required to be as effective as single-application permethrin[21] (category 2 evidence in an unblinded RCT). It was suggested that ivermectin may not be effective against scabies eggs.

Initial case reports of successful treatment of refractory crusted scabies with oral ivermectin have been followed by several case series documenting treatment failure in more severe cases given 1–3 doses of ivermectin and proposing regimens using combined topical scabicide plus oral ivermectin, with dose numbers given dependent on the severity of the crusted scabies[12,13] (Box 29.7 and Table 29.2) (category 4 evidence in a case series).

Table 29.2 Ivermectin dosing regimens: 200 μg/kg dose (round dose/kg up, not down)

Ordinary scabies	Single dose
Crusted scabies	
Mild	Single dose or two doses: day 1 and 15
Moderate	Three doses: day 1, 15, and 29 or day 1, 2, and 8
Severe	Five doses: day 1, 2, 8, 9, 15
Extreme, recurrent	Seven doses: day 1, 2, 8, 9, 15, 22, and 29

Drug resistance and treatment failure

Many patients experience persistent symptoms for up to several weeks after curative treatment, often because of ongoing immune response to mite antigens (Box 29.8). However resistance of *S. scabiei* to lindane and benzyl benzoate has been reported, although rarely, and resistance to permethrin and ivermectin resistance may be emerging and is well documented for other parasites. Two confirmed cases of clinical and in vitro ivermectin resistance have now been documented.[22]

The "knockdown" insecticide action of permethrin and other synthetic pyrethroids results from slowing the gating kinetics of a neuronal, voltage-sensitive sodium channel. Potential resistance mechanisms include target sodium channel mutations in the

Box 29.7 Treatment of crusted scabies

Oral ivermectin: 200 μg/kg dose
Plus supervised topical scabicide such as permethrin or benzyl benzoate 2–3 times in the first week then weekly until cured
Plus keratolytic therapy with lactic acid/urea cream or salicylic acid cream initially daily (except when applying topical scabicide), until crusts are resolved
Isolate the patient to prevent scabies transmission to staff and family – use long-sleeved gowns, gloves, foot covers, and a single room where possible
Treat family members and close contacts with topical therapy
Use broad-spectrum antibiotics early for suspected secondary systemic bacterial sepsis

Box 29.8 Persistent symptoms despite scabies treatment

Incorrect initial diagnosis
Topical scabicide failure – incorrect or inadequate application
Topical scabicide failure – drug resistance
Ivermectin failure in crusted scabies – inadequate doses or drug resistance
Cured but continuing immune response to mite antigen (may be weeks)
Cured but secondary eczema
Cured but reaction to topical scabicide
Reinfection from untreated contacts or contaminated fomites

organism to make it less susceptible, removal of the drug by an efflux pump, such as P-glycoprotein, and enzymatic degradation of the drug. Of these, target alteration and enzymatic degradation are well-established causes of pyrethroid resistance in a range of insects and ectoparasites and surveillance for these in *S. scabiei* will be important given the expanding use of permethrin in humans for both head lice and scabies.

Ivermectin resistance in gastrointestinal nematodes has become a major problem in veterinary practice. Potential resistance mechanisms include mutations in the target glutamate-gated chloride channels in the organisms and alteration in P-glycoprotein expression, resulting in increased drug removal. Of interest, ivermectin is an inhibitor of P-glycoprotein as well as being potentially able to be removed by the efflux pump system. Surveillance for emerging ivermectin resistance in *S. scabiei* is important.

New topical acaricides

Concerns about toxicity and emerging resistance have resulted in a search for new topical scabicides. Promising agents include 5% tea tree oil, manufactured from the tree *Melaleuca alternifolia*.[7] Tea tree oil is a traditional medicine used by indigenous Australians and has been shown to have excellent activity against a range of bacteria, including methicillin-resistant *Staphylococcus aureus* (MRSA), yeasts and herpes simplex virus. It rapidly kills *Sarcoptes scabiei* in vitro and has been successfully used with oral ivermectin in refractory crusted scabies. Another essential oil recently successfully used for scabies is 20% lippia oil, extracted from the leaves of *Lippia multiflora Moldenke*, a shrub from the West African savannah. In both these essential oils terpenoids are the likely active components.

Community scabies programs

In small communities where scabies is endemic, whole-community treatment with topical permethrin has resulted in dramatic decreases in both scabies and streptococcal pyoderma[8,23] (category 4 evidence in a case series). The success and sustainability of such programs require considerable planning, resources, and follow-up. Oral ivermectin rather than topical therapy has been used in those aged over 5 years in one successful program.

References

1. Alexander JO. Scabies. In: Arthropods and human skin. New York: Springer-Verlag; 1984:227–292.
2. Montesu M, Cottoni F, Bonomo GC et al. Discoverers of the parasitic origin of scabies. Am J Dermatopathol 1991; 13:425–427.
3. Green MS. Epidemiology of scabies. Epidemiol Rev 1989; 11:126–150.
4. Mellanby K. The development of symptoms, parasitic infection and immunity in human scabies. Parasitology 1944; 35:197–206.
5. Arlian LG, Morgan MS, Rapp CM et al. The development of protective immunity in canine scabies. Vet Parasitol 1996; 62:133–142.
6. Chosidow O. Scabies and pediculosis. Lancet 2000; 355:819–826.
7. Walton SF, Holt DC, Currie BJ et al. Scabies: new future for a neglected disease. Adv Parasitol 2004; 57:309–376.
8. Taplin D, Porcelain SL, Meinking TL et al. Community control of scabies: a model based on use of permethrin cream. Lancet 1991; 337:1016–1018.
9. Fain A. Epidemiological problems of scabies. Int J Dermatol 1978; 17:20–30.
10. Arlian LG, Morgan MS, Arends JJ. Immunologic cross-reactivity among various strains of *Sarcoptes scabiei*. J Parasitol 1996; 82:66–72.
11. Walton SF, Choy JL, Bonson A et al. Genetically distinct dog-derived and human-derived *Sarcoptes scabiei* in scabies-endemic communities in northern Australia. Am J Trop Med Hyg 1999; 61:542–547.
12. Meinking TL, Taplin D, Hermida JL et al. The treatment of scabies with ivermectin. N Engl J Med 1995; 333:26–30.
13. Huffam SE, Currie BJ. Ivermectin for *Sarcoptes scabiei* hyperinfestation. Int J Infect Dis 1998; 2:152–154.
14. Cabrera R, Dahl MV. The immunology of scabies. Semin Dermatol 1993; 12:15–21.
15. Walker GJ, Johnstone PW. Interventions for treating scabies. Cochrane Database Syst Rev 2000:CD000320.
16. Roos TC, Alam M, Roos S et al. Pharmacotherapy of ectoparasitic infections. Drugs 2001; 61:1067–1088.
17. Schultz M, Gomez M, Hansen R et al. Comparative study of 5% permethrin cream and 1% lindane lotion for the treatment of scabies. Arch Dermatol 1990; 126:167–170.
18. Chouela EN, Abeldano AM, Pellerano G et al. Equivalent therapeutic efficacy and safety of ivermectin and lindane in the treatment of human scabies. Arch Dermatol 1999; 135:651–655.
19. Davies JE, Dedhia HV, Morgade C et al. Lindane poisonings. Arch Dermatol 1983; 119:142–144.
20. Roth W. Scabies resistant to lindane 1% lotion and crotamiton 10% cream. J Am Acad Dermatol 1991; 24:502–503.
21. Usha V, Gopalakrishnan Nair TV. A comparative study of oral ivermectin and topical permethrin cream in the treatment of scabies. J Am Acad Dermatol 2000; 42:236–240.
22. Currie BJ, Harumal P, McKinnon M et al. First documentation of *in vivo* and *in vitro* ivermectin resistance in *Sarcoptes scabiei*. Clin Infect Dis 2004; 39:E8–E12.
23. Wong L, Amega B, Barker R et al. Factors supporting sustainability of a community-based scabies control program. Australas J Dermatol 2002; 43:274–277.

Chapter 30

Pediculosis

Christine Ko and Dirk M. Elston

Synonyms:

- Infestation with *Pediculus humanus capitis* (synonym: head louse), pediculosis capitis
- Infestation with *Pediculus humanus humanus* (synonym: clothing louse, body louse), pediculosis corporis, vagabond's disease
- Infestation with *Pthirus pubis* (synonym: crab louse, pubic louse), pediculosis pubis

Key features:

- *Pediculus humanus capitis* infests the scalp
- *Pediculus humanus humanus* infests the clothing of humans and periodically bites the host
- *Pediculus humanus humanus* is the vector of epidemic typhus, relapsing fever, and trench fever
- *Pthirus pubis* infests pubic hair as well as hair on other parts of the body, including the scalp and eyelashes
- Pediculoses are transmitted either through contact (often sexual in the case of *Pthirus pubis*) or fomites
- Resistance to topical treatments is increasing worldwide; malathion, permethrin/pyrethrins, and lindane are mainstays that are still effective, especially if used on a rotational basis

Introduction

Infestation by sucking lice causes pediculosis. *Pediculus humanus capitis*, *P. humanus humanus*, and *Pthirus pubis* are the three types of lice that commonly parasitize humans. They are in the phylum Arthropoda, class Insecta, order Phthiraptera, suborder Anoplura, family Pediculidae or family Pthiridae. *Pediculus humanus humanus*, the body louse, and *P. humanus capitis*, the head louse, are variants of the same species.[1]

History

Lice have infested humans for thousands of years, and pediculosis remains a prevalent disease in affluent suburban schools as well as in inner-city populations. Despite the similarities between body lice and head lice, body lice (but not head lice) transmit typhus, trench fever, and relapsing fever. Interestingly, *Rickettsia prowazekii* and *Bartonella quintana* can be isolated from body lice and used not only in the epidemiological study of epidemic typhus and trench fever but also in the prediction of disease outbreaks in refugee populations. Human DNA, extracted from lice, can be used as forensic evidence.

Epidemiology

Pediculosis capitis

P. humanus capitis infests the scalp of humans and affects 6–12 million people per year in the USA alone. Infestation occurs in all seasons, but may be increased in warmer months. Head lice predominantly affect females, ages 3–12, in the pediatric population. Close head-to-head contact is thought be the most important mode of transmission,[2] but contact with infested fomites can spread lice as well. The anatomy of head lice adapts them better to grasp the more cylindrical hairs of Caucasians. This fact, in combination with factors such as the use of hair pomades, causes the incidence of pediculosis to be low in African–Americans.

Pediculosis corporis

P. humanus humanus is the cause of pediculosis corporis. Body lice transmit three diseases: louse-borne relapsing fever, epidemic typhus, and trench fever. *R. prowazekii*, the organism of epidemic typhus, has been isolated from body lice in Burundi, France, Peru, Russia, and Zimbabwe;[3] Russia[4] and Burundi[5] have both documented outbreaks. In the USA, a natural endemic reservoir of *R. prowazekii* is found in North American flying squirrels (*Glaucomys volans* and *sabrinus*). Following a natural disaster, typhus has the potential to spread from an endemic source and become a louse-borne epidemic. Body lice can carry and transmit both *R. prowazekii* and *B. quintana* simultaneously. In developed countries, pediculosis corporis most commonly affects the urban homeless,[6] and infestation correlates with blood serologies for *B. quintana*.[7]

Pediculosis pubis

Infestation with *Pthirus pubis* is commonly acquired sexually. Patients should be screened appropriately. Infestation is year-round but slightly increased in colder months.

Pathogenesis and etiology

Pediculosis capitis

The head louse is 1–2 mm in length, the size of a sesame seed. Head lice are wingless, dorsoventrally flattened, and elongated (Fig. 30.1). They have three pairs of legs tailored to clutch hairs and small anterior sucking mouth parts to obtain blood meals. Head lice can crawl rapidly, up to 23 cm/min. The egg cases, or nits, are difficult to remove as they are firmly cemented to the hair shaft (Fig. 30.2). Lice lay nits very close to the scalp in all climates except those that are very humid. Young lice hatch within 1 week and mature over 1 week. One female head louse lives about 16 days and can lay 50–150 nits.

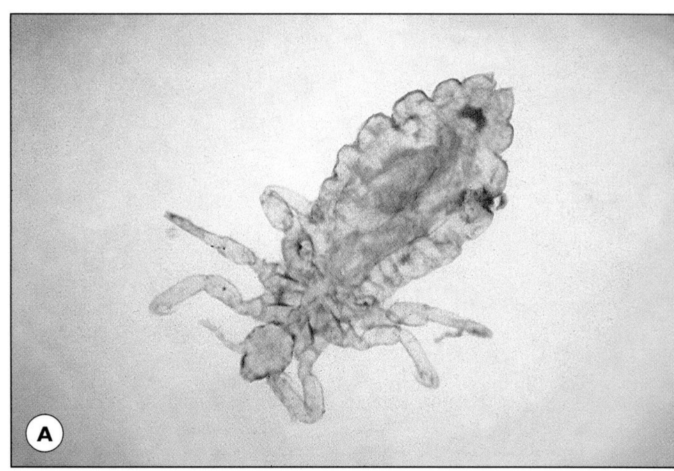

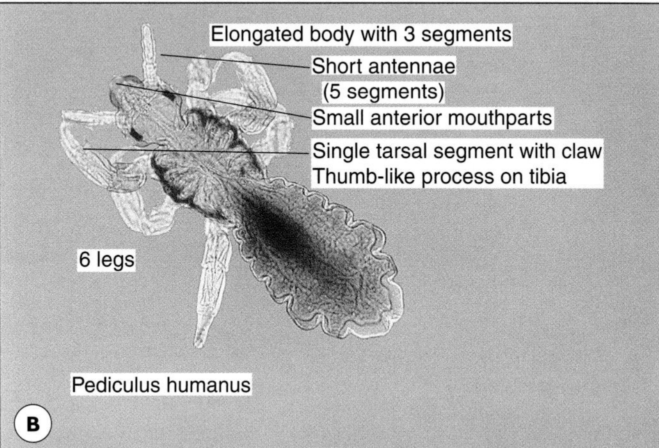

Figure 30.1 (A) Immersion oil mount of a head louse. (B) Identifying characteristics of a head louse. (Reprinted courtesy of *Cutis*.)

Pediculosis corporis

Larger than the head louse, the body louse is about 2–4 mm in length but is otherwise very similar in appearance to the head louse. The life span is on average 18 days, during which time females lay about 270–300 ova. Ova incubate 8–10 days and produce nymphs which need a 2-week period to mature to the adult form. Body lice are found in the seams of clothing and can take blood meals as infrequently as every 3 days.

Pediculosis pubis

Crab lice are about 0.8–1.2 mm in length. The first pair of legs are shortened with serrated edges and resemble crab claws. The length and width of crab lice are almost equal, which enables grasping of widely spaced pubic hairs (Fig. 30.3), although mobility is limited to about 10 cm/day. Females produce about 25 ova over an approximate 2-week life span. After a 1-week incubation, nymphs emerge and mature to adult forms over 2 weeks.

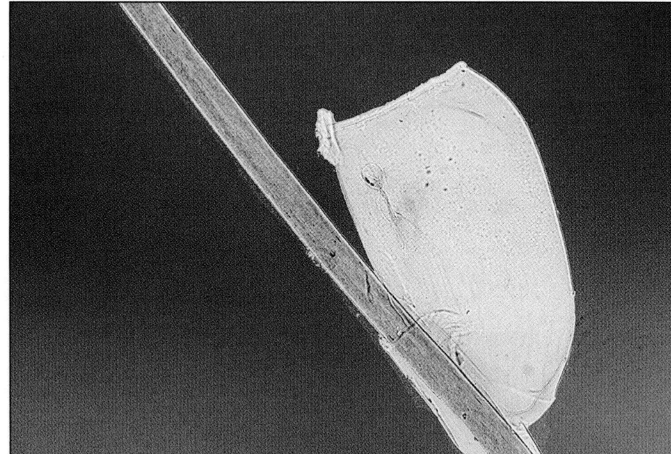

Figure 30.2 Head louse nit attached to a hair shaft.

Clinical features

Pediculosis capitis

Nits are often located in the retroauricular scalp and the occiput. As they are fixed to the hairs, they may be more easily visualized than the adult lice. Bite reactions result in pruritus. Excoriations, louse dung, and cervical lymphadenopathy may be noted. Secondary bacterial infection is common. A hypersensitivity rash, referred to as a pediculid, may mimic a viral exanthem. Bite reactions depend on the degree of host sensitivity to louse saliva or an injected anticoagulant.[8] Early bites produce little in the way of clinical symptoms. As the host develops immunity, papules with moderate pruritus are noted. Over time, there may be a shift to immediate

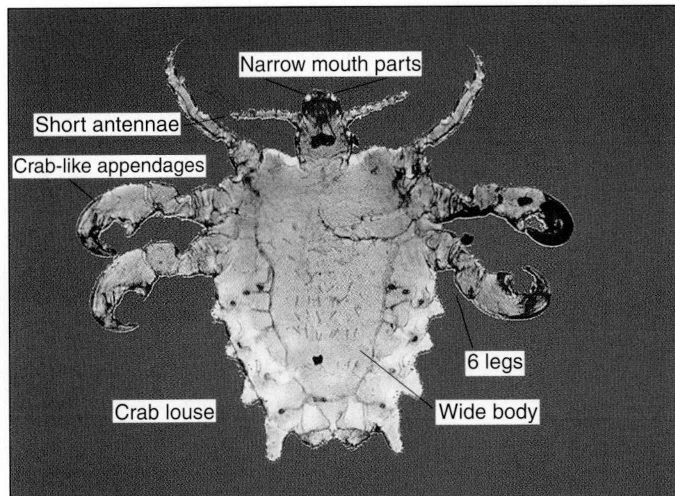

Figure 30.3 Identifying characteristics of a crab louse.

sensitivity with wheals and intense itching. Chronic infestation may produce smaller papules with mild pruritus. Interestingly, new bites may cause a recall phenomenon with reactivation of older bites.[9]

Pediculosis corporis

Body lice transfer to body hairs in order to feed and are otherwise located with their nits within clothing seams. Erythematous macules, papules, crusts, excoriations, and occasional lymphadenopathy are often secondary to extreme pruritus; serum, blood, and louse feces can stain clothing. Lesions are usually seen on the trunk, neckline, axillae, and waistline. Maculae caeruleae, bluish-gray macules secondary to lice bites, can be observed. Secondary infection is common. "Vagabond's disease" is the term for generalized lichenification and hyperpigmentation that result from chronic infestation and scratching.

Pediculosis pubis

The crab louse is found in the pubic region, as well as in adjacent and non-contiguous areas. Crab lice have been found on hairs of the chest, abdomen, legs, buttocks (Fig. 30.4), scalp, and even eyelashes. Pruritus leads to excoriation and secondary infection, and lymphadenopathy may be noted. Crab lice, like body lice, can cause maculae caeruleae, particularly over the lower abdomen and thighs.

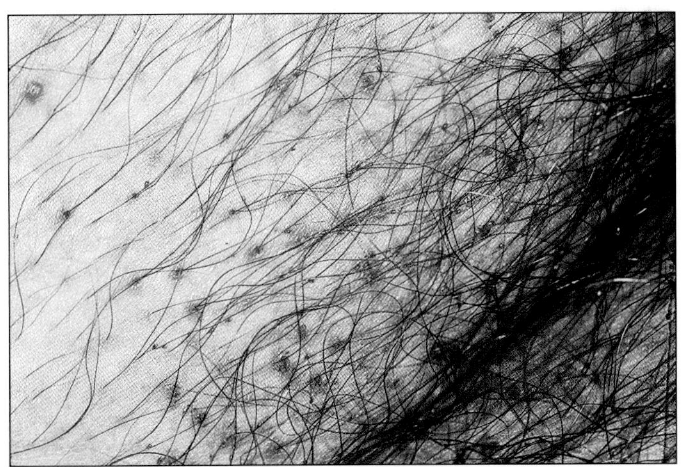

Figure 30.4 Crab louse nits.

Patient evaluation, diagnosis, and differential diagnosis

Pediculosis capitis

The observation of crawling head lice in scalp hair is diagnostic. Combing is a useful tool for screening, and visual inspection without combing will miss many cases of infestation. Nits alone only suggest active infestation when positioned no further than 5 mm from the scalp, although a caveat is in humid climates where viable nits may be located more than 20 cm from the scalp.

Inner-root sheath remnants (hair casts, pseudonits) may mimic nits. Hundreds of hair casts may be present (Fig. 30.5). Hair casts slide freely along the hair shaft, distinguishing them from nits, and the opaque amorphous hair cast is easily recognized microscopically (Fig. 30.6). White piedra, hair spray, dandruff, and trichodystrophies like monilethrix and trichorrhexis nodosa may mimic nits. Misdiagnosis can be circumvented by close examination of hair shafts.

Psocids are free-living louse-like insects in the class Insecta, order Psocoptera. Modern lice may have descended from psocids, so it is not surprising that psocids are capable of infesting the scalp. They are sometimes referred to as "booklice," despite the fact that they are not true lice. Psocids are 2–3 mm in size. A larger head,

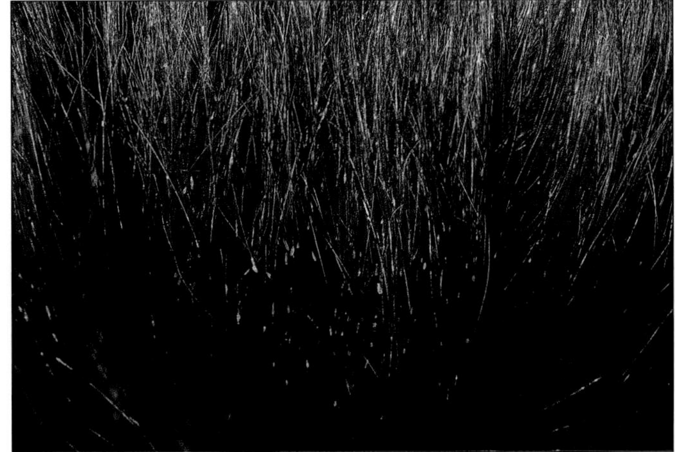

Figure 30.5 Hair casts.

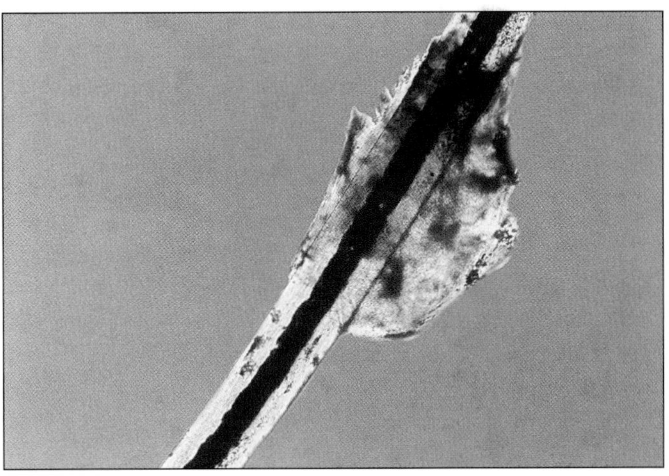

Figure 30.6 Microscopic mount of a pseudonit (hair cast).

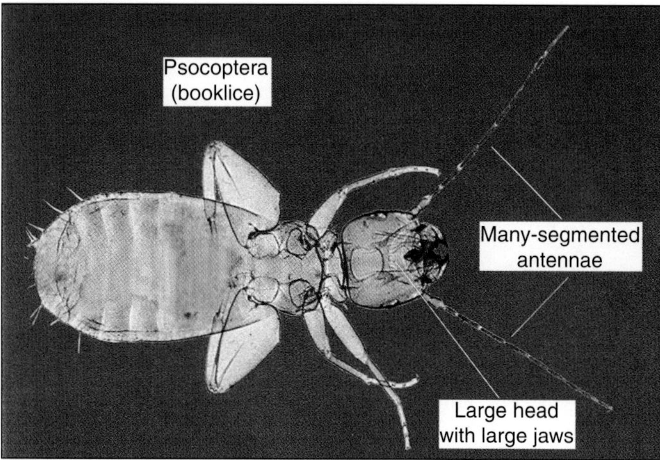

Figure 30.7 Identifying characteristics of a psocid. (Reprinted courtesy of *Cutis*.)

chewing mouth parts, bigger hind legs, and long antennae create a different morphology from that of the head louse (Fig. 30.7).

Pediculosis corporis

Clothing seams containing body lice or nits establish the diagnosis of pediculosis corporis. Lice are commonly found in warmer areas such as waistbands. Chronic infestation may be eczematous, suggesting atopy or contact dermatitis, or morbilliform, like a drug eruption or viral exanthem. Widespread excoriations may mimic scabies, and scabies mites and body lice can concurrently parasitize an individual. Certainly, refugee populations have been concomitantly infested with lice, scabies, mites, and fleas.

Pediculosis pubis

Crab lice (Fig. 30.8) are easily seen with the naked eye, and the diagnosis is seldom missed if suspected. White piedra or trichomycosis pubis can simulate nits. As in pediculosis corporis, the differential diagnosis includes contact dermatitis and scabies. Alternatively, irritant or allergic contact dermatitis resulting from home remedies or scabies infestation can certainly be superimposed on pediculosis pubis.

Pathology

Lice are ectoparasites, and take many small blood meals. Unlike ticks, they do not remain attached, and so are seldom represented in biopsy specimens. Biopsies of bite reactions may show crusting, evidence of excoriation, and a polymorphous dermal inflammatory infiltrate.

Treatment

Pediculosis capitis

Head lice are found on brushes, hats, combs, linens, stuffed animals, and upholstered furniture, although they prefer to remain in close proximity to the scalp. Eradication of lice can be accomplished without targeting fomites, but many patients prefer to vacuum, wash, dry-clean, or isolate items that have been in intimate contact with the scalp. Hats and scarves should be placed under each child's desk during school epidemics to minimize the risk of spread. Efforts to reduce transmission by fomites have not been proven necessary to achieve a cure, but may be worthwhile in cases of refractory infestation. The school nurse should perform louse-screening. Family members and playmates of infested children should be examined. Targeted therapy, treating only those with documented infestation, can be successful, and, unlike scabies, empiric treatment of contacts is generally not required. In larger-scale epidemics such as in refugee populations, pyrethroid-impregnated mosquito netting is a useful adjunct,[10] and louse repellents like piperonal may be constructive. However, the major determinant of effective treatment rests on eradication of scalp lice and ova.

Topical pediculicides remain the mainstay of treatment (Table 30.1). DDT was the first pediculicide and it was used extensively for pediculosis corporis during World War II. DDT is currently unavailable due to its environmental toxicity. Permethrin 1% (Nix), a synthetic pyrethroid, has an excellent safety profile and enjoys a healthy market share as an over-the-counter product in the USA. For 2–3 weeks after application, permethrin is retained on hair shafts, creating a residual effect. Permethrin disrupts sodium transport in lice, causing depolarization of neuromembranes and

Table 30.1 Pediculicidal treatments

Name	Pregnancy category	Instructions for use	Precautions
Permethrin 1% (5% also used)	B	Apply topically to body or dry scalp for 5–10 min, then rinse off; repeat in 1 week	Allergic/irritant dermatitis
Lindane	B	Apply topically to body or dry scalp for 5–10 min, then rinse off	Risk of seizures Allergic/irritant dermatitis
Pyrethrins	B	Apply topically to body or dry scalp for 5–10 min then rinse off. Repeat in 1 week	Allergic/irritant dermatitis
Malathion	B	Apply topically to body or dry scalp for 8–12 h then rinse off. Repeat in 1 week	Respiratory depression
Ivermectin	C	200 µg/kg PO × 1. Repeat in 1 week	Neurologic

respiratory paralysis. Knock-down resistance in lice commonly relates to sodium-gated channels, and appears to be a growing problem. Permethrin 5% (Elimite), an antiscabetic, has been used in an effort to overcome resistance to permethrin 1% but may be of limited value as resistance may be concentration-independent.

Lindane 1%, an organochloride, causes respiratory paralysis in arthropods. The actual neurotoxic potential in humans is quite low when used according to the manufacturer's instructions. However, as lindane is slowly metabolized, repeat applications result in escalating blood levels and are inadvisable, and such improper multiple applications were the likely cause of reported central nervous system neurotoxicity in children that caused California to prohibit sales of lindane. Lindane should be avoided if possible in young children and those with a history of seizure disorders.

Pyrethrins are a natural product of chrysanthemums, and individuals sensitive to Compositae plants can react adversely. Pyrethrins and permethrin have the same pediculicidal mechanism. Piperonyl butoxide potentiates the effect of pyrethrin.[11] There are several different brands of pyrethrin/piperonyl butoxide available in the USA (RID Mousse, RID Shampoo, A-200, R and C, Pronto, Clear Lice System), with different levels of treatment success, in part secondary to components of the vehicle. For example, A-200 shampoo contains benzyl alcohol, which is synergistic with pyrethrin.[11]

Malathion 0.5% (Ovide) causes respiratory paralysis in lice by being a weak organophosphate cholinesterase inhibitor. The active ingredient has an excellent margin of safety in humans, but killing of lice is unfortunately partially dependent on the flammable vehicle. Dipentene, terpineol, and 78% isopropanol are major constituents of the vehicle.[11] As malathion was not marketed in the USA for a significant period, little resistance is currently reported from North America. The product has been used more widely in the UK, and reports of resistance are correspondingly higher.

Resistance to pediculicides continues to emerge as an important issue. Patterns of resistance correspond to local patterns of drug use,[11] and cross-resistance to both pyrethrin and malathion has occurred in the UK. Furthermore, knock-down resistance to permethrin products commonly encompasses a broad range of related chemicals, regardless of whether or not they have been marketed in a given area. Therapeutic agents may be rotated, or used in combination, to decrease the development of resistance.

Lice have developed several different mechanisms to circumvent pediculicides. Knock-down resistance involves nerve insensitivity. DDT resistance is commonly related to glutathione-*S*-transferase. Enhanced drug metabolism is the basis of monooxygenase-based resistance, and synergistic agents such as piperonyl butoxide can override the resistance. Better topical agents are needed. Agents should be developed that occlude the respiratory apparatus of the lice and kill them consistently without any risk to the patient. Such an agent would have to be cosmetically elegant to enjoy a good market share.

It should be stressed that treatment failures can happen aside from drug resistance. Compliance and proper use of agents are important factors. Improper dilution or duration of application and differences in formulation may contribute to continued infestation. Application of products to wet hair dilutes pediculicides and decreases efficacy as lice temporarily close respiratory spiracles under wet conditions (Fig. 30.8). Hair conditioners may coat the hair, preventing therapies from binding. The ovicidal capability of all products are limited, with obligatory retreatment after 7–10 days. Some authorities choose a different agent for the second treatment. It should be noted that reinfestation from untreated contacts will mimic chemical resistance. Careful attention should be paid to close contacts. Simple field assays for resistance should be developed for use by practicing clinicians.

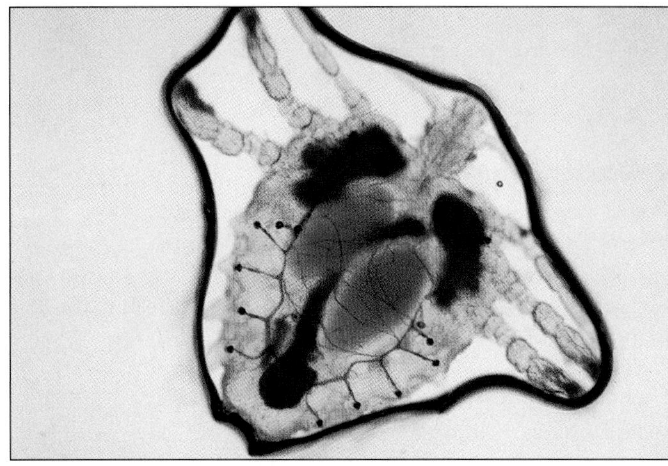

Figure 30.8 Immersion oil mount of a crab louse. The respiratory tract is seen as a black network.

Mechanical removal of lice and nits can be helpful, but generally should be regarded as an adjunct to chemical treatment rather than an alternative. Shaving of hair on the scalp or the body eradicates lice, but is seldom cosmetically acceptable. In the UK wet-combing is a popular modality that has had minor success in eliminating head lice.[12] Wet-combing is time-consuming and generally less effective than a chemical agent, although wet-combing is superior to combing dry hair due to water-induced temporary immobilization of lice. In place of water, diluted vinegar or commercial preparations of 8% formic acid can be applied to hair to allow easier combing.[13] In addition, a variety of enzymatic nit removal systems are available. Several brands of sturdy metal nit combs are accessible through the internet. Plastic combs are supplied with many chemical agents.

"Natural" topical treatments are numerous but of unproven effect. Sundry occlusive agents, including greasy ointments, petroleum jelly, pomades, oils, mayonnaise, and hair gels have been promoted as lethal to lice, but better agents that are cosmetically elegant, non-toxic, non-flammable, and easy to use are needed. Kerosene and *Lippia multiflora* essential oil are pediculocidal in vitro.[14] The safety of these agents has not been established. Combinations of coconut oil, anise oil, and ylang-ylang oil have shown some promise,[15] as have aliphatic alcohols, and these preparations may overcome permethrin resistance. Crotamiton (Eurax) is an antiscabetic with mild antipruritic properties that may poison lice.[16]

Trimethoprim–sulfamethoxazole (TMP/SMX) has also shown potential as a pediculicide. Permethrin in combination with TMP/SMX increases successful killing of lice.[17] The mechanism of action may involve killing the gut flora of the louse, with subsequent deficiency of B-vitamins. Levamisole, an antihelmintic and biologic immune response modifier that is approved by the US Food and Drug Administration as an anticancer agent, eradicated lice in a preliminary trial, but more study is needed.[18]

Ivermectin, both topical and oral, is a possible therapy for pediculosis, but the emergence of resistance is possible. Some evidence links ivermectin with neurotoxicity,[19] and definitive proof of safety and efficacy is absent.

Pediculosis corporis

Proper laundering of clothing or applying insecticide to clothing will destroy body lice. A pediculicidal application to the body will kill any lice adherent to body hairs and treat any concurrent infestation with other arthropods. A preventive measure is treating clothing with permethrin.

Pediculosis pubis

Pubic lice are commonly treated with malathion, permethrin, pyrethrins, and lindane. Crotamiton has in vitro pediculicidal activity against *Pthirus pubis*, but clinical data are lacking. Some authorities prefer to use a 5% permethrin cream, as the preparation has good patient acceptability and a low risk profile. Clothing and sheets should be laundered. Abstinence is advised until cured. Eyelash infestation has been treated with bland occlusive agents such as sterile petrolatum, but these will obscure vision. Fluorescein dye strips are an anecdotal treatment. Yellow oxide of mercury ointment should be avoided due to the potential for systemic mercury toxicity.

References

1. Leo NP, Campbell NJ, Yang X et al. Evidence from mitochondrial DNA that head lice and body lice of humans (Phthiraptera: Pediculidae) are conspecific. J Med Entomol 2002; 39:662–666.
2. Canyon DV, Speare R, Muller R. Spatial and kinetic factors for the transfer of head lice (*Pediculus capitis*) between hairs. J Invest Dermatol 2002; 119:629–631.
3. Roux V, Raoult D. Body lice as tools for diagnosis and surveillance of reemerging diseases. J Clin Microbiol 1999; 37:596–599.
4. Tarasevich I, Rydkina E, Raoult D. Outbreak of epidemic typhus in Russia. Lancet 1998; 352:1151.
5. Raoult D, Ndihokubwayo JB, Tissot-Dupont H et al. Outbreak of epidemic typhus associated with trench fever in Burundi. Lancet 1998; 352:353–358.
6. Sasaki T, Kobayashi M, Agui N. Detection of *Bartonella quintana* from body lice (Anoplura: Pediculidae) infesting homeless people in Tokyo by molecular technique. J Med Entomol 2002; 39:427–429.
7. Guibal F, de La Salmoniere P, Rybojad M et al. High sero-prevalence to *Bartonella quintana* in homeless patients with cutaneous parasitic infestations in downtown Paris. J Am Acad Dermatol 2001; 44:219–223.
8. Weir E. School's back, and so is the lowly louse. Can Med Assoc J 2001; 165:814.
9. Mumcuoglu KY, Klaus S, Kafka D et al. Clinical observations related to head lice infestation. J Am Acad Dermatol 1991; 25:248–251.
10. Rowland M, Bouma M, Ducornez D et al. Pyrethroid-impregnated bed nets for personal protection against malaria for Afghan refugees. Trans R Soc Trop Med Hyg 1996; 90:357–361.
11. Meinking TL, Serrano L, Hard B et al. Comparative in vitro pediculicidal efficacy of treatments in a resistant head lice population in the United States. Arch Dermatol 2002; 138:220–224.
12. Plastow L, Luthra M, Powell R et al. Head lice infestation: bug busting vs. traditional treatment. J Clin Nurs 2001; 10:775–783.
13. DeFelice J, Rumsfield J, Bernstein JE et al. Clinical evaluation of an after-pediculicide nit removal system. Int J Dermatol 1989; 28:468–470.
14. Oladimeji FA, Orafidiya OO, Ogunniyi TAB et al. Pediculocidal and scabicidal properties of *Lippia multiflora* essential oil. J Ethnopharmacol 2000; 72:305–311.
15. Mumcuoglu KY, Miller J, Zamir C et al. The in vivo pediculicidal efficacy of a natural remedy. Isr Med Assoc J 2002; 4:790–793.
16. Karacic I, Yawalker SJ. A single application of crotamiton lotion in the treatment of patients with pediculosis capitis. Int J Dermatol 1982; 21:611–613.
17. Hipolito RB, Mallorca FG, Zuniga-Macaraig ZO et al. Head lice infestation: single drug versus combination therapy with one percent permethrin and trimethoprim/sulfamethoxazole. Pediatrics 2001; 107:E30.
18. Namazi MR. Levamisole: a safe and economical weapon against pediculosis. Int J Dermatol 2001; 40:292–294.
19. Barkwell R, Shields S. Deaths associated with ivermectin for scabies. Lancet 1997; 349:1144–1145.

Chapter 31

Myiasis

Fábio Francescone and Omar Lupi

- Introduction
- Classification
- Pathophysiology
- Clinical manifestations
- Pathology
- Diagnosis
- Treatment
- Prevention

Synonyms: Botfly, berne, bot

Key features:

- Zoonosis caused by dipterous larvae
- Furunculoid, creeping lesions or wound infestations are the most common clinical features
- There is a history of travel or exposure

Introduction

Myiasis is a zoonosis derived from the Greek (mya, or fly) that covers a variety of associations between dipterous larvae and mammals. It is the infestation of live humans or vertebrate animals with dipterous larvae that, at least for a certain period, feed on the host's dead or living tissue, liquid body substance, or ingested food.[1] The distribution is worldwide with more species and greater abundance in tropical, subtropical, and warm temperate areas. Disease of domestic animals is a global agricultural problem. Nosocomial infestation has rarely been reported. The appropriate travel or exposure history in a compatible clinical setting should alert the clinician to the possibility of myiasis.[2]

Classification

The order Diptera (two-winged flies) is divided into three sub-orders. The first, Nematocera, contains most families of blood-feeding flies that serve as vectors for a variety of viral, protozoan, and helmintic disease. The suborder Brachycera causes facultative myiasis. The third, Cyclorrhapha, contains all groups that cause obligate myiasis as well as several groups that cause facultative myiasis.[3]

The various forms of myiasis may be classified from an entomologic or clinical point of view. Entomologically, flies may be classified into:[1]

- Specific (obligatory): produced by larvae that can only develop in human or animal living tissue and start pathologic processes.
- Semispecific (facultative): produced by larvae that breed normally in garbage, feces, or corpses but occasionally attack living tissue.
- Accidental: produced by larvae that are rarely found in the human body, usually occurring in the digestive system or another cavitary organ. This is not part of the fly's life cycle.

Cyclorrapha Dipterus: the flies

Cyclorrapha are important in producing and transmitting many diseases. The wings, which are important for classifying the flies, differ between families and classes. The female puts the egg on the exterior; and some species have a dilatation of the vaginal canal (i.e. the uterus) where the egg remains until the larval stage is reached.

Typically the larvae are worm-shaped. They have three segments. In the third segment posterior respiratory spiracles create different outlines for each species, and can be used to classify the larvae.

The vast majority of Cyclorrapha larvae eat organic detritus. Some grow on human corpses. These are of particular interest for forensic medicine; it is possible to estimate by computing the age of larvae how long the body has been exposed to flies and thereby calculate the minimum number of days since death. Other species need living tissue to feed. They are considered true parasites and are called protelian parasites because when they reach the end of the larval stage the host is left behind and they go to the ground to pupate.[4]

Cyclorrapha classification

The subclass Cyclorrapha is composed of three series of flies: Aschiza, Schizophora, and Pupipara:[4]

1. In the series Aschiza only one species has been claimed to cause human myiasis: *Eristalis tenax*, of the family Syrphidae.
2. Schizophora includes the true flies. These are subclassified in two sections: (a) the first section is called Acalyptratae and there are two families (Drosophilidae and Choropidae) but none is known to cause myiasis; (b) the second section is called Caliptratae. The most important families are:Muscidae, Cuterebridae, Calliphoridae, Sarcophagidae, Tachinidae, Oestridae, Gasterophilidae, and Glossinidae.
3. The Pupipara series is not important for human medicine.

Myiasis-inducing flies are members of the superfamily Oestrodiae. This superfamily consists of three major families: Oestridae, which includes four subfamilies (Oestrinae, Gasterophilinae, Hypodermatinae, and Cuterebrinae), Calliphoridae, and Sarcophagidae. All Oestridae, at least 151 species, are obligate parasites. The families Calliphoridae, greater than 1000 species, and Sarcophagidae, greater than 2000 species, contain both obligate and facultative organisms. Only a limited number of species actually cause disease.[2]

Muscidae family

The Muscidae family is of the Schizophora series. Eggs of *Fannia canicularis* (lesser house fly) and *Musca domestica* (house fly) may be deposited on ulcers and give rise to wound myiasis.

Oestridae family

Dermatobia hominis (Fig. 31.1), also known as human or tropical botfly or berne, is a fly about 12 mm long of the Cuterebrinae subfamily, which is endemic to tropical Mexico, South America, Central America, and Trinidad. Bot is the term sometimes used for the invading larvae.

When the female botfly is ready to lay eggs it captures blood-sucking arthropods and attaches the eggs to the abdomen of the carrier insect – a method of egg delivery called phoresis.[5] The usual intermediary is a mosquito (*Psonophora*). After 1 week, when the insect approaches a warm-blooded animal, the heat induces the larvae to hatch. Larvae try to grab the skin or hair of the animal with a lid. If it succeeds the larvae leaves the egg, otherwise it returns to the interior. The maggots have 20 days to grab a host. The first instar or stage I larva painlessly penetrates the skin and gains access to the dermis and subcutaneous tissue. Within 5–10 weeks, the organism goes to second instar or stage II, then third instar or stage III larvae (Fig. 31.2). After leaving the host, the larva pupates in the ground, to form flies in 2–3 weeks.[2]

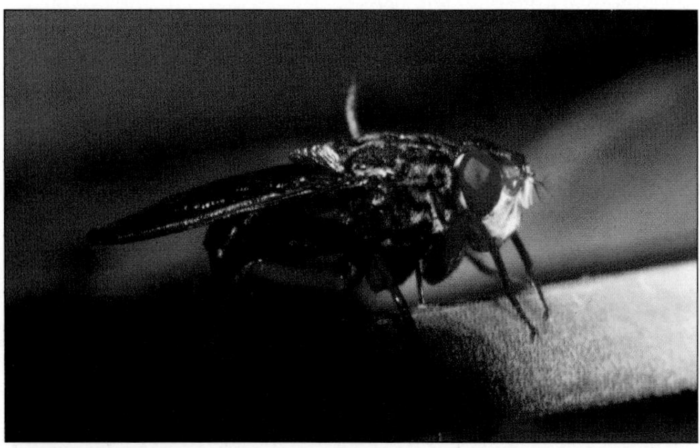
Figure 31.1 Adult fly of *Dermatobia hominis*.

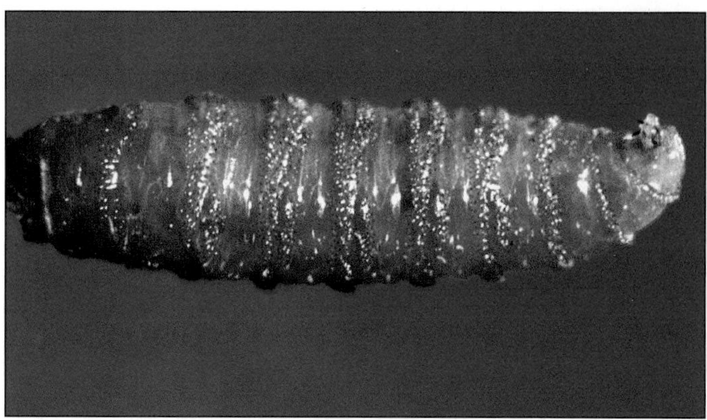
Figure 31.2 *Dermatobia hominis* larvae.

Dermatobia hominis and their vectors are silvestrian, inhabiting forests and woods. Cattle are the animals attacked the most, and humans and dogs are occasionally infested. While going through the skin a sensation of pruritus is felt. After some time, an inflammatory reaction occurs, with edema and erythema. Eventually a furuncle-like lesion develops with a central hole which drains a serosanguineous fluid. Sometimes it is possible to visualize the posterior end of the maggot. Some patients feel pain or a sensation of movement.

Gasterophilus spp.

A form of migratory cutaneous myiasis known as "creeping eruption" is caused by *Gasterophilus* spp. (the horse botfly) larvae. The Gasterophilidae are mainly parasites of the alimentary tract of horses. On occasion, however, especially in warmer climates, the eggs are laid on human skin, and the emerging larvae burrow into the skin, wandering aimlessly about and producing a curious pattern of allergies that somewhat simulates the clinical picture of classic creeping eruption due to the dog hookworm.[1]

Hypoderma bovis (cattle botfly) is found in temperate regions, including North America and Europe; it is a major cause of morbidity in cattle. Humans are occasionally infested. Humans are abnormal hosts and the larvae do not mature fully. After penetrating the skin the larvae produce migratory subcutaneous swellings. They may also invade the eye, producing severe damage.[2]

Cuterebra spp. is a large bee-like rabbit-parasitizing obligatory fly. It occurs in North America and rarely causes cutaneous myiasis and ophthalmomyiasis in humans; it occurs especially in children. Eggs are laid on leaves and stems of underbrush, during the spring and early summer, from where the first-stage larvae can enter its host. The larvae then migrate to a dermal site, where continuous growth occurs for 3–5 weeks. The larva pupates in the soil during the winter. The adult fly emerges from the pupa the next winter.[3]

Oestrus ovis, the sheep nasal botfly, is found in all major sheep-raising regions, and has been particularly implicated in ophthalmomyiasis. Female flies directly deposit first-instar larvae in the nostrils of sheep for obligate development in the upper respiratory tract. The condition is relatively common among shepherds of Middle-Eastern countries.[2]

Rhinoestrus purpureus, which parasitizes horses, is responsible for human myiasis, especially ophthalmomyiasis. The head botfly of horses causes similar conditions to *Oestrus ovis* in Europe, Africa, and Asia.[1]

Calliphoridae family

Cordylobia anthropophaga, the tumbu fly, is endemic to sub-Saharan Africa. The flies are 8–11 mm in length and dull-yellow with two broad dark longitudinal stripes. Female flies deposit eggs on shaded soil or drying clothes, preferably contaminated with urine or feces. The female lives for 2–3 weeks and, during this time, produces 300–500 eggs. Within 1–3 days, larvae hatch and remain near the soil surface until activated by heat. Larvae from eggs deposited on clothes have direct access to the host when the clothes are worn.

In many parts of Africa wild animals have been infested by the larvae of the tumbu fly: especially rats, mice, monkeys, mongooses, squirrels, leopards, boars, and antelopes. Of all domestic animals, it is the dog that is particularly affected by this disease, and that, next to the rat, is an important reservoir for the infection of humans. As rivers widen, in the rainy period, the rats (*Rattus novergicus*) approach human settlements. Transfer of the infection to house rats or dogs is then only a matter of time. It is especially when dogs suffer from disease that the infection is carried to the immediate environment of humans.[6]

The reason why children are more affected by tumbu-fly-myiasis than adults is principally the thin texture of their skin, through which the larvae can easily bore.

A relative, temporary immunity to this infection seems to develop, lasting for about a year in larger mammals, including humans.

The sylvan myiasis larvae of *Cordylobia rodhaini*, the Lund's fly, are adapted to various thin-skinned forest mammals in tropical Africa, and the few reported attacks on humans have occurred in tropical humid forest areas. The female lays about 500 eggs in sand or soil containing feces or urine, or on sun-exposed washing. The eggs hatch after 2–4 days and on contact with the skin of a suitable host the minute larvae penetrate to a depth of several millimeters. After 12–15 days development, the larvae reach a size of 1–1.5 cm or more causing furuncular lesions. Mature larvae then emerge spontaneously.[7]

The *Cochliomyia hominivorax* (New World screwworm) are obligatory parasites found in the tropics and warm temperate zones, and are endemic in the southern USA, Caribbean, and most of Latin America (Fig. 31.3). The infestation may be serious, and death may occur in a significant percentage of patients. Contact with infested domestic animals is the usual source of human disease. This proliferation is a particular problem in cattle breeding.

The adult flies are attracted by discharge from an open wound, particularly the nose, where a gravid female may lay as many as 300 eggs in a few minutes. In less than 24 h, the maggots hatch and start eating living tissue. They mature in approximately 1 week, but occasionally require 3 weeks. They finish their cycle on the ground. Some decompose in the tissue. The larvae are unable to penetrate intact human skin. They do not remain in necrotic foci, but burrow

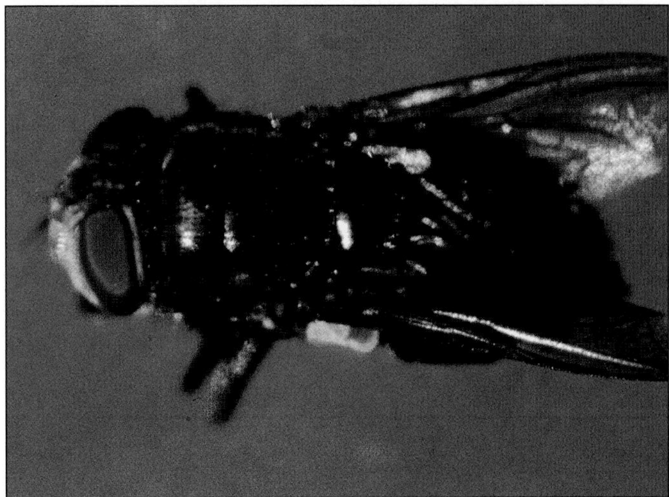

Figure 31.3 Adult fly of *Cochliomyia hominivorax*.

deeply into living tissue, even into cartilage and bone. When in the nose or ears the fatality rate is approximately 8%.[1]

Callitroga macellaria larvae often occur together with *C. hominivorax* in the same lesion. However, *C. macellaria* are essentially harmless, living on necrotic tissue and serving more to clean up the primary lesion than extend it.

Chrysomyia bezziana (Old-World screwworm) are obligatory parasites of the wound found in Africa, India, the Arabian Peninsula, Indonesia, Philippines, and New Guinea, where they are not only an important pest of sheep but also the cause of a disfiguring human myiasis. *C. bezziana* lay their eggs at the periphery of wounds or lacerations or in moist and exudative areas. After hatching, the larvae penetrate the wounds or even the intact epidermis, feeding on live or necrotic tissue. They are able to erode bone, similar to the New-World screwworm.[1]

Auchmeromyia senegalensis, the Congo floor maggot, is a unique obligate parasite of sub-Saharan Africa that is primarily a human parasite. Eggs are laid in the soil or sand floors of traditional huts. The larvae hatch in 1–3 days to emerge at night (they lie buried in the day). The Congo floor maggot feeds on sleeping individuals, doing so rapidly (in about 20 min) once every 24 h up to 16 times to complete its development. All three larval stages are blood-sucking. The bite may be slightly painful and some patients experience considerable local edema. The maggot is unable to climb and therefore cannot feed on persons on elevated structures. Prevention is by sleeping off the ground.[1]

Facultative wound myiasis may be due to several frequent Calliphoridae animal pests: *Luicilia* spp., the ubiquitous greenbottle flies; *Calliphora* spp., the ubiquitous bluebottle flies; and *Phormia regina*, the black blow fly of North America.

Sarcophagidae family

Wohlfartia magnifica is an obligate flesh fly of the Mediterranean basin, Near East, and Eastern, and Central Europe. The females give birth to active first-stage maggots which penetrate unbroken skin. These are deposited on wounds and mucous membranes (ear, eye, or nose) and may cause extensive destruction of healthy tissue. Infants are most often infected and fatal cases in humans have been reported.

W. vigil and *W. opaca* are North American species whose females deposit larvae on the skin in young animals. Human infestation only occurs in young babies, as the larvae are unable to penetrate adult skin.

Pathophysiology

Once the larvae have reached the tissues, they may remain at the site of penetration, causing a local reaction that betrays their presence. Certain species with an affinity for particular organs may migrate towards them and try to adapt to the unfavorable surroundings. Others, with great migratory potential, travel through the body, causing serious damage.

A study of microflora in the furuncular lesions of cattle caused by *D. hominis* demonstrated that only bacteria belonging to skin wounds were isolated on the external surface of larvae, increasing the number of isolations from second to third instars. The results from the internal parts of the body indicated that wound bacteria were not significantly isolated and internal bacteria were never significantly isolated from wounds. Similar results have been found in other species. Although capable of producing pyoderma, *Staphylococcus aureus* when found in furuncles of myiasis, does not cause secondary infection. Nevertheless, when the parasite attacks other host tissues, a secondary bacterial infection is seen. This suggests that the skin has an inhibitory effect on bacteria present in the wound. Another possibility is a larval substance with bactericidal properties in *D. hominis* (as suggested by the data of Picasso 1935) and in other warble flies,[8] as Baba et al. have shown with the antibacterial effect of sarcotoxins I, II, and III from flesh flies. Likewise, Coronado (1989) observed the bactericidal effect of the larval extracts from *D. hominis* against *S. aureus*, *S. epidermidis*, and *Streptococcus*. These findings may explain the lack of secondary infections in furuncular lesions of myiasis.[9]

Clinical manifestations

There are some predisposing ecological factors for acquiring myiasis, including an abundance of exposed preexisting suppurative lesions that attract and stimulate the deposit of eggs by the female insect; habits of the population, such as sitting or lying on the ground; some religious rites; poor personal hygiene; and climatic conditions. With the increase in international travel, cases are also encountered outside the endemic region, in both North America and Europe. In the native countries, this is a familiar condition that is easily recognized, but for travelers, the physician may need to be familiar with such conditions.[1]

Cutaneous myiasis is the most frequently encountered clinical form. The cutaneous form is further subclassified according to the nature of the manifestation, such as a furunculoid, subcutaneous infestation with tunnel formation, a wound infestation, and a subcutaneous infestation with subcutaneous swellings. Nasopharyngeal myiasis has been reported to include infestation of the nose, mouth, sinuses, ear, or eye (ophthalmomyiasis). Intestinal myiasis includes enteric disease caused by ingestion of organisms and anal disease. Urogenital myiasis encompasses urethral, vaginal, and bladder infestations.[2]

Furunculoid lesions

D. hominis and *Cordylobia anthropophaga* are the most common offending agents causing furunculoid myiasis. The lesions are characterized by cutaneous nodules, occurring singly or multiply, in general containing one larva (Figs 31.4 and 31.5). The term "warble" is synonymous with a furunculoid lesion. A central punctum usually develops that may exude serosanguineous or purulent fluid. Frequently, patients are aware of movements within the nodule; pruritus is common. The presence of the parasite may be evidenced by either bubbles in serous discharge or by visualization of the tail of the larvae with the two spiracles simulating tiny black eyes (Fig. 31.6). *D. hominis* infestations are associated with local pain, perhaps because of the larval hooklets. Sometimes history of a preceding insect bite can be elicited. *D. hominis* favors scalp, face, and extremities, whereas C. *anthropophaga* is more likely to affect the trunk, buttocks, and thighs; in children a palpebral lesion is

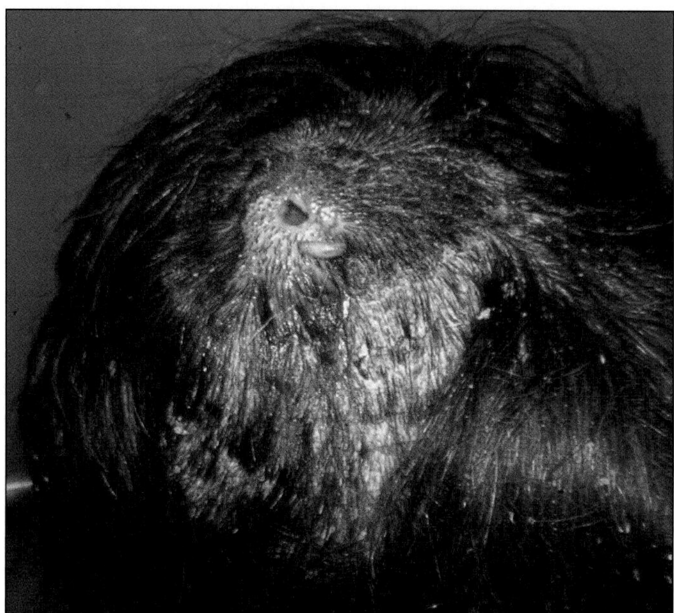

Figure 31.4 Furunculoid myiasis of the scalp caused by *Dermatobia hominis*.

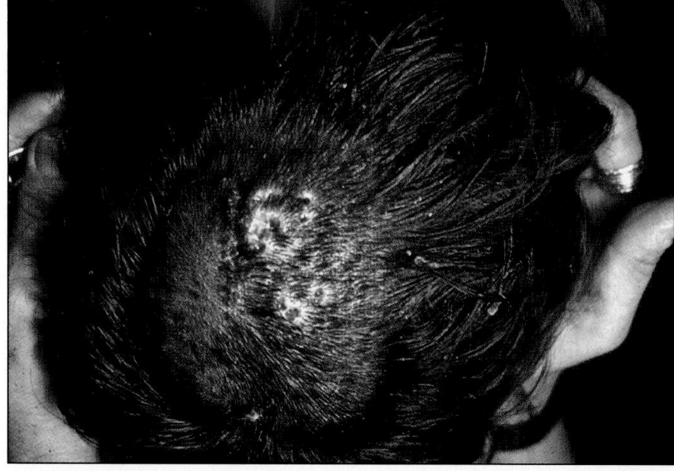

Figure 31.5 Furunculoid myiasis of the scalp.

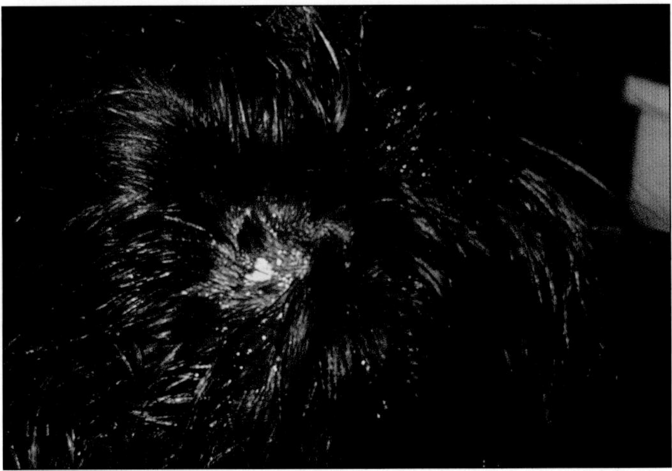

Figure 31.6 Furunculoid myiasis of the scalp.

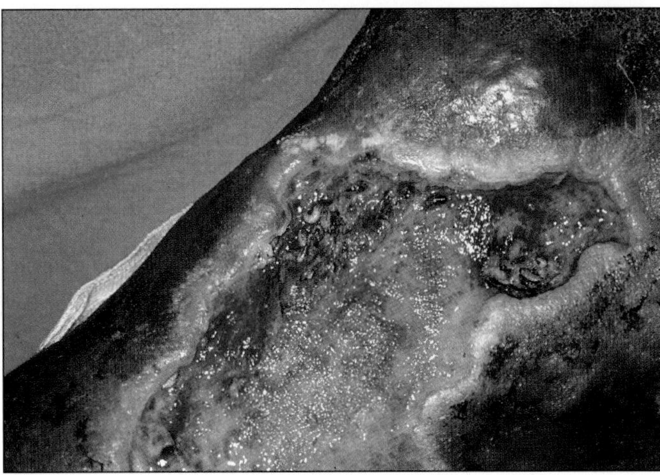

Figure 31.7 Wound myiasis caused by *Cochliomyia hominivorax*.

not uncommon. C. *rodhaini* is similar to C. *anthropophaga*, but the lesion is larger and more painful.

Associated findings include regional lymphadenopathy, malaise, and fever. Secondary bacterial infection may be present and a thick purulent discharge may suggest a typical staphylococcal furunculosis. Clinical variants can take the form of lesions that are vesicular, bullous, pustular, erosive, ecchymotic, and ulcerative, especially in malnourished children. Almost always the lesions heal completely without leaving any trace. Sometimes hyperpigmentation and scarring can occur. Severe cicatricial outcomes have only been observed in malnourished children.

Rarer causes may be rodent and rabbit botflies of the genus *Cuterebra*. *Wohlfartia magnifica* have also occasionally caused furunculoid disease.

Subcutaneous infestation with tunnel formation

Gasterophilus intestinalis and G. *haemorrhoidalis* are responsible for migratory myiasis, the so-called "creeping eruption," as larvae slowly migrate through the skin. The clinical correlation is the development of a pruritic, painful, erythematous lesion in a serpiginous configuration. Recurrent disease tends to form larger pustules or nodules. Botfly larvae may survive for months in human skin, creating a tortuous, telltale inflammatory ridge or line to mark the path of their migrations. Rarely the larvae may appear in the lungs and cause nodular parenchymal lesions.

Subcutaneous infestation with migratory swelling

The cattle botflies, or cattle grub, *H. bovis* and *H. lineatum*, affect humans occasionally causing disease similar to *Gasterophilus* infestations but more characteristically involving the formation of furunculoid lesions as larvae mature. On hatching the larvae penetrate the subcutaneous tissue more deeply than *Gasterophilus*, producing an inflamed and painful swelling resembling a boil. Mature larvae may thus emerge through puncta as with *D. hominis* infestation. When located superficially, they may travel very fast, 125–150 cm per 12 h. They sometimes migrate considerable distances and have been reported to invade the nervous system, eye, and ear, with reported cases of blindness, paralysis, and death. As with other parasites too large to be phagocytosed, peripheral eosinophilia may occur. A drop or two of mineral oil applied just in advance of the visible line of inflammation will generally reveal the parasite.

Migratory myiasis from botflies is usually distinguishable from migratory helmintiasis from hookworms because the migrations in the former are generally more restricted and extend more slowly. In addition, the fly larvae, being larger, can generally be visualized, whereas round worms cannot.

Wound myiasis

C. *hominivorax* and C. *bezziana*, New-World and Old-World screwworms, respectively, may cause an obligatory wound myiasis. More mature larvae are often more invasive, readily leaving necrotic tissue for viable tissue, leading to significant local destruction and secondary bacterial infection (Fig. 31.7). Similarly, *W. magnifica* may parasitize wounds in an obligatory manner. *Lucilia sericata* and *Musca domestica* may facultatively infest wounds when gravid females deposit eggs in and around wounds. Clinical manifestations include secondary infection and fistula formation.

Myiasis of body cavities

Myiasis of this type includes infestation of the eye, auditory canal, nasopharynx, and associated sinuses. Ophthalmomyiasis is usually caused by *Oestrus ovis*. It occurs in cooler latitudes of the northern and southern hemispheres in rural areas. Ophthalmomyiasis interna involves the eyeball, whereas ophthalmomyiasis externa is a relatively mild disease, characterized by conjunctivitis, lid edema, and superficial punctate keratopathy in response to movement of the larvae across the external surface of the eyeball. Patients commonly complain of acute foreign-body sensation with lacrimation, often with abrupt onset. Mild pain and inflammation follow for 10 days, but the infestation is self-limited and benign. Invasion of the eyeball and severe external inflammation occasionally occur. Non-O. *ovis* eye disease may be more severe. Larvae may appear within the cornea, lens, anterior chamber, or vitreous, but rarely undergo continued development when the eyeball has been entered. A rare devastating consequence is retinitis involving the macula, with fibrosis leading to blindness. Occasionally, enucleation or exenteration is required.

In nasal myiasis, the initial symptoms are swelling, tickling pain, and nasal obstruction, associated with a sensation of "crawling." Epistaxis is common, but the discharge soon becomes purulent and fetid. The most important species of flies in nasal myiasis are C. *hominivorax*, C. *bezziana*, and D. *hominis*. Extensive tissue destruction may follow. External auditory myiasis is usually seen in infants and debilitated individuals. Local irritation is the rule, with invasion of the tympanic membrane being rare. Infestation of the nose and ears is extremely dangerous because of the possibility of penetration into the brain: the fatality rate is approximately 8%. Nasal myiasis may complicate leprosy patients: first, the loss of the sneezing reflex and second, the inability to clean the nose properly on account of severe hand deformity.

Accidental myiasis

Ingestion of fly larvae in food can lead to fecal passage of live maggots. Some infestations result in local irritation, vomiting, or diarrhea. Sometimes these larvae will migrate up to the body orifices. True enteric myiasis does not occur in humans. Intestinal myiasis can be a public health problem when the source of contamination is the water supply of the region.[10] The genitourinary infestation is infrequent and accidental. Preexisting urinary tract infection is a predisposing factor for men.

Pathology

All the dipteran larvae are found in the dermis within a purulent cystic sinus tract. The surrounding inflammatory infiltrate is mainly composed of lymphocytes with an admixture of eosinophils, fibroblasts, histiocytes, basophils, mast cells, plasma cells, and Langerhans cells.[11]

A cuticle of variable thickness that is covered with spines characterizes botfly larvae. Striated muscle is found directly under the entire cuticle. The large central tubular cavity is most likely the primitive alimentary canal.[12]

Diagnosis

Usually clinical diagnosis is easily made, especially in endemic countries. In other countries the history is very important to identify one of the predisposing factors. Ultrasound is a method of confirming the diagnosis when the site is unusual or for control of the complete removal of the larvae.[13] Laboratory examination is usually normal, but in chronic cases the host may respond with eosinophilia in the tissues and blood. Immunoglobulin E may also be elevated.

After removing the larvae from the host, the larvae should be killed in hot water or ethanol to retain their overall shape. The posterior respiratory spiracles are an important means of identification. Larvae should be preserved in 80% alcohol. Identification of accidental or facultative parasites is often difficult, as many species may be involved. In contrast, identification of an obligate parasite is easier. Identification is greatly eased if larvae are reared to adults on small pieces of meat.[1]

Treatment

Therapy consists of three general techniques: (1) application of toxic substance to the larvae and eggs; (2) a method producing localized hypoxia to force the emergence of the larvae; and (3) mechanical or surgical debridement.

Furunculoid and migratory myiasis

The goal of treatment is complete removal of larvae from parasitized tissue. C. *anthropophaga* is reported to be easier to remove than D. *hominis*. Expression of C. *anthropophaga* may be adequate; use of wooden spatulas may be preferred because attempts to squeeze with the fingers may cause the larvae to rupture.[14] Numerous reports have noted successful eradication of D. *hominis* by occluding the punctum with a substance to prevent gas exchange. To avoid asphyxiation, the organism emerges far enough to be grasped by the forceps of a vigilant patient or physician. Occluding substances have included petrolatum, bacon, fingernail polish, pork fat, makeup cream, adhesive tape, and others. Polymyxin B is a sterile occlusive option.[15] Reportedly, occlusion may have to be maintained for 24 h or more to have the desired effect. The risk of attempted occlusion is that the organism may asphyxiate without emerging and the retained larvae may elicit an inflammatory response: a foreign-body granuloma eventually forms that may progress to calcification. Injection of 1% lidocaine (2 ml per nodule) is sometimes used to paralyze the larvae, making the extraction easier.[16]

Surgical excision is usually unnecessary for treatment; some advocate a cruciate incision which prevents damage to the larva and allows easier extraction without leaving remnants in the wound. Surgical excision is almost always required for migratory forms of the disease. When it is migrating deep, there is no known treatment. Antibiotic therapy may be necessary for secondary bacterial infection.

Wound myiasis

Treatment requires manual removal of all visible larvae, followed by debridement. Irrigation may be particularly useful. Fifteen percent chloroform in olive or other oil or ether may help to immobilize the larvae. Topical treatment with 1% ivermectin in a propylene glycol solution (a maximum of 400 µg/kg is reported to be safe) applied directly to the affected area for 2 h and washed with saline solution.[17] Most larvae die. Extensive wound exploration may be mandated by the degree of involvement. There is one report of oral ivermectin (200 µg/kg) in a case of *Hypoderma lineatum* with spontaneous emigration of the maggots.[18]

Ophthalmomyiasis

External manifestations are managed by mechanical removal of larvae from the surface of the anesthetized eyeball using fine, non-toothed forceps. Slit-lamp examination facilitates the process, but viable larvae have the tendency to avoid bright light. The use of lidocaine or cocaine as an anesthetic has the additional benefit of maggot immobilization, which facilitates removal. Occlusion with a thick ointment may assist removal by encouraging egress of organisms from the conjunctival sac, if it is involved.[2]

The management of internal infestation is more variable and highly dependent on the clinical situation. Dead larvae unassociated with significant inflammation can usually be left in place and eventually regress. Inflammation requires management with topical corticosteroids and mydriatics with close follow-up. The presence of persistently viable larvae may require surgical removal, particularly when critical structures are at risk. Living organisms in the appropriate location, such as the subretinal space, may be amenable to destruction by laser photocoagulation.

Prevention

Appropriate precautions will help avoid infestations. The use of screens and mosquito nets is essential to prevent flies from reaching the skin. *D. hominis* infestation may be thwarted by the application of insect repellents containing diethytoluamide (DEET). Drying clothes in bright sunlight and ironing them is an effective method of destroying occult eggs laid in clothing, especially by *C. anthropophaga*. Other general precautions include wearing long-sleeved clothing, covering wounds, and avoiding falling asleep out of doors.

A field control of flies is extremely important. All available methods should be used, including aerial sprays, destruction of animal carcasses, elementary sanitary and hygiene practices, and clearing debris and rubbish near houses. Inactivation of females by the release of large numbers of males previously sterilized by ionizing radiation has been highly successful. Reports on the control of *Cochliomyia* infestation in sheep with the use of ivermectin, which has been reported to be 100% effective in controlling existing infestations and as prophylaxis, suggest that this may be the route of the future.

References

1. Noutsis C, Milikan LE. Myiasis. Dermatol Clin 1994; 12:729–736.
2. Mandell GL, Bennett JE, Dolin R. Principles and practice of infectious diseases, 5th edn. New York: Churchill Livingstone; 2000:2976–2979.
3. Schiff TA. Furuncular cutaneous myiasis caused by *Cuterebra larva*. J Am Acad Dermatol 1993; 28:261–263.
4. Rey L. Bases da parasitologia médica. Rio de Janeiro: Guanabara Koogan; 1992:296–303.
5. Gordon PM, Hepburn NC, Willians AE et al. Cutaneous myiasis due to *Dermatobia hominis*: a report of six cases. Br J Dermatol 1995; 132:811–814.
6. Günther S. Clinical and epidemiological aspects of the dermal tumbu-fly-myiasis in Equatorial Africa. Br J Dermatol 1971; 85:226–231.
7. Pampiglione S, Schiavon S, Fioravanti ML. Extensive furuncular myiasis due to *Cordylobia rodhaini* larvae. Br J Dermatol 1992; 126:418–419.
8. Beesley WN. Symposium on the problems of the warble fly and its eradication in the UK. Veterinarian 1968; 5:177–179.
9. Sancho E, Caballero M, Ruiz-Martinez I. The associated microflora to the larvae of human bot fly *Dermatobia hominis* L.Jr. (Diptera: Cuterebridae) and its furuncular lesions in cattle. Mem Inst Osw Cruz 1996; 91:293–298.
10. Kun M, Kreiter A, Semenas L. Gastrointestinal human myiasis caused by *Eristalis tenax*. Rev Saude Publica 1998; 32:367–369.
11. Grogan TM, Payne CM, Payne TB et al. Cutaneous myiasis. Immunohistologic and ultrastructural morphometric features of a human botfly lesion. Am J Dermatopathol 1987; 9:232–239.
12. Baker DJ, Kantor GR, Stietorfer MB et al. Furuncular myiasis from *Dermatobia hominis* infestation. Diagnosis by light microscopy. Am J Dermatopathol 1995; 17:389–394.
13. Olumide YM. Cutaneous myiasis: a simple and effective technique for extraction of *Dermatobia hominis* larvae. Int J Dermatol 1994; 33:148–149.
14. Szczurko C, Dompmartin A, Moreau A. Ultrasonography of furuncular cutaneous myiasis: detection of *Dermatobia hominis* larvae and treatment. Int J Dermatol 1994; 33:282–283.
15. Richards KA. Brieva. Myiasis in a pregnant woman and an effective, sterile method of surgical extraction. Dermatol Surg 2000;26:955–957.
16. Lonng PTL, Lui H, Buck W. Cutaneous myiasis: a simple and effective technique for extraction of *Dermatobia hominis* larvae. Int J Dermatol 1992; 31:657–659.
17. Victori J, Trujillo R, Barreto M. Myiasis: a successful treatment with topical ivermectin. Int J Dermatol 1999; 38:142–144.
18. Jelinek T, Nothdurft HD, Rieder N et al. Cutaneous myiasis: review of 13 cases in travelers returning from tropical countries. Int J Dermatol 1995;34:624–626.

Part 3

Non-infectious conditions

Chapter 32

Nutritional diseases

Ana Maria Mosca de Cerqueira and Wânia Mara del Favero

Introduction

Appropriate qualitative and quantitative nutrition helps to prevent disease and to develop physical and mental potential. The limits of appropriate nutrition are variable due to genetic and metabolic differences between individuals.

Appetite and hunger have very distinct meanings. While appetite means a desire to eat that is not directly connected to basic organic needs, hunger is characterized by an organic sensation, with urgency for food, making the individual eat any kind of food. Appetite makes people continue to eat even if they do not feel hungry, which may often lead to obesity.

History

In Greece, doctors, followers of Hippocrates, practiced a kind of dietary medicine. Although they did not know the chemical nature of food, they believed that it contained just one unique nutritional principal – food. This theory persisted until the beginning of the nineteenth century, when researchers proclaimed the concept of nutritional essentiality.

Etiology and epidemiology

Brazil is a country with great problems in the field of health. It is evident that this area is fairly complex, certainly on account of the size of the country. One issue is the question of food fortification, as part of the solution for a lack in micronutrients.

The decision to add certain vitamins and minerals to food of mass consumption, with the aim of fighting off nutritional deficiencies, has been a strategy used for many decades in different countries. In 1931 the USA introduced niacin in wheat flour in a voluntary program of food fortification in view of the high incidence of pellagra in the population. In 1942 legislation was created to mandate fortification of all cereals, eradicating pellagra at that time.[1]

In the 1940s several European countries also adopted a program of food fortification. In Central and South America (Chile, El Salvador, Guatemala, Honduras, Panama) several movements appeared in favor of the compulsory fortification of wheat flour with iron, aiming to prevent iron-deficiency anemia.[1]

In Brazil this issue has been discussed, although effective measures have not yet been adopted. In the states of São Paulo and Rio de Janeiro, in government schools, some counties have adopted programs of food supplementation of the school meal, successfully reducing the prevalence of iron-deficiency anemia.[2] Compulsory fortification of iodine in salt was instituted in 1953, although legislation on enrichment of kitchen salt with iodine was not approved until 1974. Nowadays endemic goiter is practically eradicated in the country.[1]

Obesity

Synonyms: Excess weight

Key features:

- Overweight
- Bodymass index

Introduction

Obesity is an excess of body fat in comparison with the lean mass of the body as a consequence of a chronic instability between energy ingestion and expenditure.[2]

History

Like malnutrition, obesity is part of human history. However, in the same way that malnutrition has always been connected to poverty, obesity has always been associated with abundance, wealth, and health, and considered a model of beauty in some societies.

Etiology

Obesity is considered a multifactorial illness superimposed by genetic,[3] behavioral, and environmental factors. It is classified as endogenous (caused by endocrine illness in 5% of cases)[2] and exogenous (caused by nutritional errors).[4]

Obesity in childhood is not a disease, but a complex of symptoms which presents an association with adult obesity, with correlation of increased mortality, cardiovascular illness, hypertension, hyperlipidemia, hepatic illness, cholelithiasis, and diabetes which begins in adulthood.

A common denominator is the occurrence of a positive energy balance, stored as adipose tissue for long periods. Some known factors include an excessive ingestion of food rich in energy, inadequate exercise in relation to age, more sedentary activity, low metabolic rate in relation to the composition of body mass, elevation of the respiratory quotient in repose, and altered sensitivity to insulin. Obese children do not always eat in a different way or ingest more food including fast-food or nitrogen than non-obese children of the same age. No specific evidence shows that the greater prevalence of obesity is solely related to a direct increase in ingestion of calories.

Obese individuals may become insulin-resistant, leading to an increase of levels of circulating insulin. Insulin decreases lipolysis, increasing the synthesis and captivation of lipids. An obese individual responds to a meal of carbohydrates with an increase of insulin secretion and reduced use of free fatty acids.[2]

Epidemiology

Childhood obesity is associated with variables within a physical environment (climate, region, and population density). Obesity in children and adolescents is also more predominant in winter and spring than in summer and fall. Cultural factors such as differences in the amount of clothes worn and their effect on the perception of body appearance represent reasonable hypotheses. The incidence of childhood obesity strongly relates to family variables. Children of parents with more sport activity tend to be thinner than children of the same age who are sedentary. More time spent watching television, participating in video-games, or browsing on the internet may correlate with a high incidence of childhood obesity, which may originate, not only from the sedentary nature of the pastime, but also from the subtle effects of promotion of food consumption in advertisements of food products, especially those of low nutritional value, such as snacks rich in sugar, lipids, and salt. In highly urbanized areas, the reduced access to exercise facilities or excessive concern with security may lessen the opportunity for activities.[5]

Clinical manifestations

Obesity may appear in any age group, but we often note predominance in the first year of life, from 2 years of age, and in adolescence.[6] Adiposity in boys in the mammary region frequently suggests development of breasts. The abdomen tends to hang, with white or purple striae. Boys' external genital organs seem disproportionately small, but are in fact of medium size. The penis is surrounded by pubic adiposity. The obesity of the limbs is usually greater in the arms and thighs and is sometimes limited to these regions. The hands may be relatively small and the fingers slender. In the lower limbs the presence of genu varum is common.

The effects of obesity are not only connected to esthetic and psychological problems. It presents a greater tendency to metabolic alteration. In the skin, there is a predisposition to develop more illnesses related to metabolic alteration, such as acanthosis nigricans, insulin resistance, hyperandrogenia, and possible fungal infections.

Diagnosis

The body mass index (BMI) is recommended for the definition of populations with obesity and overweight, based on measuring the weight divided by the height^2 (BMI = w/h_2). Overweight is defined as BMI ≥ 85% and obesity as BMI ≥ 95% for age and gender.[7]

Another screening tool includes the following areas of risk to health:

1. Positive family background for cardiovascular disease.
2. Parents' high cholesterol level.
3. Type 2 diabetes or parenteral obesity.
4. Infantile arterial hypertension.
5. High level of total cholesterol, higher than 5.2 mmol/l or 200 mg/dl.
6. Large annual additional increase of BMI, above 2 units.
7. Concern with weight, that is, perception about excess weight.[8]

Differential diagnosis

Children with high BMI must undergo a careful medical assessment looking for illnesses which may have a primary association with obesity. Such illnesses, quoted below, represent less than 1% of all cases of childhood infantile obesity.

Treatment

The involvement of the family in the treatment of infantile and adolescent obesity is decisive because the patient is rarely responsible for the purchase, preparation, and presentation of food.

As obesity may perpetuate itself for psychological or physiological reasons, obese children and children of obese parents, or those who have obese siblings, must be encouraged to follow a systematic program of vigorous exercise and a well-balanced diet for their level of energy expenditure.

Early attempts to change behavior from the first months of life, such as feeding infants when needed soon after birth, only offering food in the first year when there are signs of hunger, the absence of suggestions showing tasty food or establishing rigid timetables for meals and encouraging the child to eat only when hungry may prevent excessive feeding and obesity. Once childhood obesity is established, it is very hard to implement an effective plan to reduce and maintain weight without the active participation of the child and the family.

Successful treatment requires attention to the following components:[2]

- Change in diet and calorie content
- Definition and use of programs of appropriate exercises
- Change in the child's behavior
- Involvement of the family in the treatment.

Regardless of the severity of the obesity, the first consideration in any obese individual is to maintain weight. For some children, for example, those who weigh 120% of their ideal weight, keeping the same weight for 1 year may be the only measure needed to reach the ideal weight for height. However, aggressive therapy must be considered above 200% of ideal weight. With such patients, more aggressive therapies, such as pharmacotherapy or gastric bypass surgery, may be justified. Unfortunately, the experience of these therapies in adolescents is limited.

Prognosis

The results of changes in diet or exercise have only been successful short-term. Exercise without controlling the diet or diet without intensifying exercise almost always results in failure. Although there are no programs of mass screening to control obesity, it is prudent, and to the benefit of all motivated patients, that the physician should establish a treatment based on food and a wise choice of exercise combined with change in behavior and family therapy. The purpose should be to facilitate substantial social and psychological support.

Excess of protein

When a patient ingests an excessive quantity of protein without water, dehydration fever may result. The signs of excess protein are rare, but may be seen in premature infants with a diet rich in protein. It may also occur in marasmic infants who receive a diet rich in protein during the recovery phase, developing hyperammonemia.

In patients with hepatic disease, protein toxicity may also be noted. Weight-reducing diets that include a high protein content may also be responsible.

Anorexia nervosa and bulimia

Synonyms: Nervous lack of appetite, spontaneous induction of vomiting and purging

Key features:

- Psychiatric disturbance
- Undernourishment
- Compulsive eating

Introduction

Anorexia nervosa and bulimia are psychiatric disturbances characterized by abnormal patterns of food consumption and by the search for thinness as the primary goal.

Weight-loss diets are endemic, especially among young people, and one of the reasons is mass propaganda in the media, with thinness as the model of beauty. Most adolescents, when interviewed, are not happy with their bodies. Patients usually have a distorted view of their own image. When they look in the mirror they do not see their real image, defining themselves as fatter than they are.

Etiology

Anorexia (lack of appetite) is the condition where the individual does not spontaneously ingest the quantity of food needed for normal growth and development. There is instability between the satisfaction of the patient's psychic need for food and the organic need, causing undernourishment, which may be serious in some cases.

In bulimia there is a serious disturbance, characterized by compulsive eating and frequent purging, associated with a loss of control over eating and excessive and persistent concern about shape and body weight. These patients turn to vomiting or purging through abuse of laxatives and diuretics to keep their body weight low.

Epidemiology

This illness occurs in women, usually at the beginning of puberty, and is rare in men. It usually occurs in young women, who often present with normal weight, but who are greatly concerned with how they look. This behavior is commonly noted in ballet dancers, who need to be slender and light, and individuals who work in fashion, such as models.

Several biological, psychological, and social determinants are implied in the pathogenesis of anorexia nervosa and bulimia. It is believed that there is a depressive personality in the dynamics of these diseases.

Clinical manifestations

Visible cutaneous signs are related to inappropriate nutrition. Some examples are gingival bleeding, gingivitis, and thin, easily broken hair. In the lower limbs there may be edema with Russell's sign. Apathy and excess sleep may be caused by nutritional deficiency.

Treatment

Antidepressive medication seems to be effective in the therapy of both conditions, as well as long-term psychiatric treatment.

Undernutrition

Synonyms: Protein–energy malnutrition

Key features:

- Marasmus
- Kwashiorkor
- Polydeficit syndrome

Introduction

Protein–energy malnutrition (PEM) is a clinical syndrome characterized by a multiple and progressive worsening of nutritional deficiencies. It includes a broad spectrum of clinical manifestations conditioned by the relative intensity of protein or energy deficiency, the gravity and duration of deficiencies, the age of the host, the cause of the deficiency, and the association with other nutritional or infectious diseases. When the deficiency is predominantly protein, clinical kwashiorkor syndrome occurs, and when the deficiency is predominantly of energy, marasmus occurs.

History

At the beginning of the nineteenth century the descriptions of PEM paid special attention to the dermatological signs and this led to the belief that the illness was caused by tropical parasites or a vitamin deficiency. In 1920 and 1930, several authors disputed this theory. Cicely Williams studied the real nature of the disease carefully, describing kwashiorkor.[9] This term was used by the Ga tribe on the Gold Coast (nowadays Ghana)[10] when describing the illness in infants during weaning associated with inappropriate diet. In 1940 researchers showed that most patients had low concentrations of blood proteins, which could also be related to the quality of protein in the diet. From 1950 on, several authors described this clinical syndrome as polydeficit syndrome of childhood, indicating that mainly young children were affected and that there was a deficiency of several nutrients. Today we use the more widely accepted comprehensive term PEM: serious forms are called marasmus (non-edematous PEM), kwashiorkor (edematous PEM), and marasmic kwashiorkor. The lay term undernourishment is generally used to refer to PEM.

Etiology

The causes of undernourishment may go back as far as the prenatal phase, with particular reference to the family's socioeconomic situation and poor distribution of food proteins, according to age, the cultural practice of inadequate diet, as well as emotional, cognitive, and physical factors.

Epidemiology

An epidemiological analysis of 53 developing countries showed that 56% of deaths of children aged 6 to 59 months were caused by undernourishment as a precipitating factor in infectious disease and that light or moderate undernourishment was involved in 83% of those deaths. About 99% of children showed a growth and development deficit and a greater propensity to infection, while only 0.1% developed the classical syndrome of malnutrition.[10]

There are about 800 million undernourished people in the world. Most live in developing countries, about 17% in the south and east of Asia, 33% in sub-Saharan Africa, and 8% in Latin America and the Caribbean.[9,10]

Consequently, 36% of children (193 million) under the age of 5 in the world are below their weight for age, 43% (230 million) are underdeveloped, and 9% (50 million) are physically weak.

In Brazil, in December 2000, Fagundes et al.[11] studied 164 Indian children in the Upper Xingu, selected at random, in four villages, by anthropometry and measurement of bioelectric impedance. The results showed low rates of undernourishment and obesity (1.8% and 3.0%, respectively). These findings prove that the nutritional conditions of the children in the Indian reservation of Xingu have maintained their qualities for the last three decades. The BMI of the population studied was significantly lower than the BMI found among North-American Indians.[12,13] In these studies, the children's good nutritional state reflects the good nutritional condition of the upper Xinguana population. This is related to that population's cultural identity, which makes it possible to sustain their nutritional habits and healthy life, at least until today, preserving the environment of the reservation area, and controlling infectious diseases in the region. These results contrast with other studies carried out with the native populations of the Americas: generally there are high incidences of nutritional damage, especially undernourishment, in Brazil and Latin America, and obesity in the USA and Canada. This is likely due to poor sanitation and poverty in the Latin–American Indian population, and the incorporation of western eating habits in North-Americans.[12–14]

Pathogenesis

Undernourishment favors the appearance of opportunistic infections and is related to the disease prognosis. Nutrition is an important determinant of the immune response. Poor nutrition reduces cellular immunity, phagocyte function, and the complement system. It also causes a decrease in antibody concentration (immunoglobulin A (IgA), IgM and IgG) and in cytokine production, as well as a deficiency of specific micronutrients, such as iron, zinc, selenium, copper, vitamins A, C, and B-complex, and folic acid, which play an important role in the modulation of the immune response. Although a considerable number of moderately or severely undernourished children are affected by acute diarrhea, there are other associated infections: pneumonia, tuberculosis, malaria, and human immunodeficiency virus (HIV). Between 50% to 90% of patients affected by HIV suffer during the development of their disease from some level of undernourishment.[9,10]

Diagnosis

The clinical, biochemical, and physiological characteristics of PEM vary with the severity of the disease, the patient's age, the presence of other nutritional deficits, infections, and the predominance of energy or protein deficiency.

The severity of malnutrition is mainly determined by anthropometry. The classification of the illness as acute and chronic is also accomplished through anthropometry, assessing the present nutritional state and the grade of delay in the children's development. The dietary denominations of the protein and energy deficit in light and moderate forms of PEM are mainly evaluated by a dietary history of the individual or the dietary habits and food availability of the population.

Kwashiorkor

Synonyms: Edematous PEM

Key features:

- PEM
- Subcutaneous edematous
- Flag sign

Introduction

This is a serious form of PEM. It occurs when the body's requirements for proteins, fuel for energy, or both cannot be satisfied through diet.

Etiology and pathogenesis

Kwashiorkor is not frequent in the first months of life, when the infant is exclusively fed with its mother's milk. When there is a serious lack of food, endocrine adjustments activate fatty acids in the adipose tissue and amino acids in the muscular tissue. The concentration of plasma proteins may remain normal, but glyconeogenesis is increased. The increased ingestion of carbohydrate and decreased protein induces the liberation of insulin. The reduced synthesis of plasma proteins in the liver, especially albumins, reduces the oncotic intravascular pressure. The plasma water diminishes and accumulates in the extravascular tissues, tissue pressure increases, and cardiac output decreases. This contributes to the physical appearance or increase of edema.

An excess of carbohydrates, with an increase in hepatic synthesis of fatty acids, leads to infiltration of the liver and consequent hepatomegaly.[10]

Epidemiology

Kwashiorkor occurs especially in children aged 1–3 years. It is common in poor regions, where the basic diet is carbohydrates and is deficient in proteins.

Clinical manifestations

The child looks weak; the weakness is especially noted in the muscles of the arms and legs. This fact may be hidden by the soft edema, and depressions in the skin when pressed, which is painless: this is the most important manifestation of the disease.

Invariably there are mental changes. The child seems apathetic and uninterested in what is happening and shows irritation, crying easily, especially when disturbed. The child has a tormented sad look. He/she may be pale, with cold cyanotic extremities.

In the majority of cases there are skin lesions, with lack of pigmentation; these are often mistaken for pellagra, especially in areas of friction, edema, and continuous pressure. The skin may be erythematous and shiny, mainly in edematous regions. Area's of dryness, hyperkeratosis, and hyperpigmentation has a tendency to confluence. The skin attracts attention with large scales, exposing underlying tissues which are easily infected (Fig. 32.1).

The hair changes texture and color, breaks easily, is opaque, and easily pulled out painlessly. Curly hair becomes straight and the pigmentation usually changes to opaque chestnut, red, or even yellowish-white. On the same hair can be seen alternate strips of unpigmented hair and normal hair: this is called the flag sign (signe de la bandera),[10,15] representing periods of bad ingestion of protein and periods of better ingestion. The subcutaneous fat is present, in contrast with marasmus, and serves as a parameter of the level of calorie deficiency. Some muscular atrophy may be present. Weight loss, after discounting edema weight, is not usually as serious as in marasmus. The height may be normal or slowed, depending on the chronicity of the present episode and on the past history.

In the feces undigested food can be found, sometimes appearing liquefied and with blood. Anorexia, postprandial vomiting, and diarrhea are common. The abdomen often protrudes on account of the stomach and intestines being distended. The liver usually appears augmented due to fatty infiltration.

Treatment

It is essential to treat immediately any acute problem, like intense diarrhea, renal insufficiency, and shock. Initial treatment consists of milk meals diluted in low volumes, containing nutrient supplements such as zinc, magnesium, manganese, selenium, iodine, copper and multivitamins, especially vitamin A, or mineral supplements of potassium, magnesium, and zinc. The recommendations vary from 4.0 to 8.0 mmol/kg per day at the start of therapy to 7.7 mmol/kg per day in the recovery phase, increasing progressively until milk rich in energy and supplements can be given. Intravenous liquids are necessary in the treatment of serious dehydration. Children with lactose intolerance should be given cow's milk or yogurt, with 50 g of sugar/l. Diets rich in calories and protein should not be given too soon because of abdomen distension and liver enlargement, as well as slow clinical improvement. Vegetable lipids are better absorbed than the lipids in cow's milk. Intolerance to glucose improves in some children with daily administration of 250 mg chromium chloride. Iron and folic acid generally cure anemia.[10]

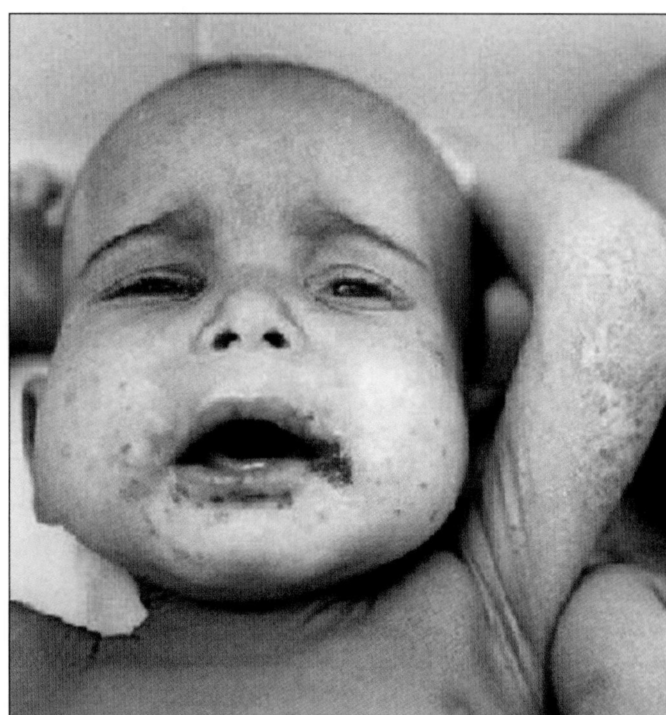

Figure 32.1 Kwashiorkor. Edema of the face, typical skin lesions, fissuring of lips, and hair changes.

After treatment has begun, the patient may lose weight for a few weeks, due to loss of edema, whether this is evident or not. The intestinal and blood enzymes normalize and the intestinal absorption of lipids and protein increases.

If growth and development are extensively damaged, mental and physical retardation may be permanent.

Marasmus

Synonyms: Non-edematous PEM

Key features:

- Inadequate caloric rate
- Emaciation

Introduction

These are patients who present with a generalized absence of subcutaneous fat, not edematous, and prominence of skin and bones. Marasmic patients often have 60% or less of expected weight for their height. Children have a marked retardation in longitudinal growth.

Etiology

The clinical picture of marasmus originates from an inadequate caloric rate due to insufficient diet with lack of food, incorrect nutritional habits, inadequate nutritional technique, and precarious hygiene. Another common cause is the relation between parents and children, which presents psychological problems, in which we note false anorexia or behavioral anorexia. Pseudoanoretic patients refuse food on account of problems such as difficulty chewing and/or deglutition, presence of aphthae, palatine fissure, stomatitis, or other conditions that make eating difficult, leading to acute impairment and causing malnutrition.

Epidemiology

Marasmus is more common in children under 1 year of age, although it is not restricted to this age group. It occurs in almost all developing countries, and the most common cause is early withdrawal of lactation, and replacement with formulas deficient in calories, often diluted in order to reduce financial expenditure but without meeting the energy needs of the child.

This, combined with ignorance about hygiene, frequently leads to the development of gastrointestinal infections, which start the vicious circle leading to marasmus.

Clinical manifestations

Initially there is an inability to gain weight, until emaciation develops, with loss of skin turgor. Growth deficiency, extreme muscular atrophy, little subcutaneous fat, and wrinkled skin, especially in the buttocks and thighs, can be seen. There is no edema. The cheeks are hollow on account of the disappearance of Bichat's adipose pads, which are among the last subcutaneous adipose deposits to disappear (Fig. 32.2). This thinness gives the face of the marasmic child the appearance of a monkey or an aged person. It presents marked weakness and often the child cannot get up without help.

The skin is dry, thin, wrinkled, and with little elasticity. The hair is sparse, thin, dry, without its normal brightness, and is easily pulled out painlessly.

Patients are apathetic but generally attentive and have an anxious look. Some patients are anorexic, while others are voraciously hungry, but they rarely tolerate great quantities of food and vomit easily. The infant is usually constipated, but so-called diarrhea by inanition may occur, with frequent evacuation of small quantities of feces containing mucus.

Cardiac frequency, arterial pressure, and body temperature may be low, but tachycardia may be present. Hypoglycemia may occur, often together with hypothermia of 35.5° C or less. The viscera are usually small. Abdominal distension may be present. The lymphatic ganglia are easily palpable.

Differential diagnosis

The differential diagnosis is all pathologies which present with PEM, secondary to diseases which weaken the body, such as acquired immunodeficiency syndrome (AIDS) and others.

Treatment

Treatment will vary if the patient is in hospital or a primary care center. In hospital, the most important aim is to keep the patient alive for long enough to treat the underlying cause and to allow sufficient time for nutritional recovery. Often the primary concern will be control of infection. Even when no apparent sign of systemic infection is detected, this possibility must not be discarded. Even if clinical and laboratory indicators of systemic infection are not apparent on the initial report.[9]

In addition to implementing the treatment of the infectious cause, the physician must pay attention to reestablishing and maintaining hydration and electrolyte balance. Early nutrition helps in the recovery of villous atrophy and normalization of disaccharidase activity. Oral nutrition must be carefully introduced because there is a grade of intolerance to carbohydrates, which may cause hyperosmolar diarrhea. As a general rule, energy may be initially provided as 50 kcal/kg per day and water 125–150 ml/kg per day, with protein comprising 10–12% of total energy. One single dose of 5000 IU vitamin A must be given right from the beginning; iron must be supplemented at a dose of 1–3 mg/day and zinc 1 mg/day must be administered until recovery.

The nutritional, emotional, and intellectual recovery of the child may take place inside or outside the hospital.[9]

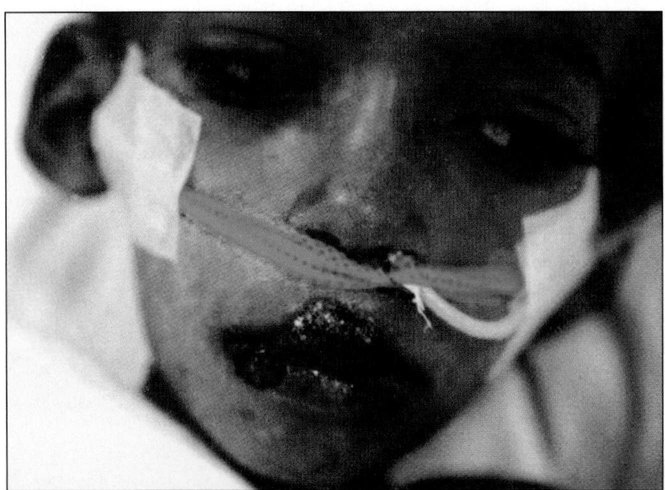

Figure 32.2 Marasmus. The disappearance of Bichat's adipose pads on the cheeks.

Deficiency of essential fatty acids

Synonyms: Polyunsaturated fatty acid (PUFA)

Key features:

- PUFA *n*-3
- PUFA *n*-6
- Gamma-linoleic

Introduction

The essential fatty acids (EFA) act throughout the organism, protecting the cellular membranes. In the external layer, they select absorption through the cells, allowing entry of nutrients and preventing access of harmful substances.

Etiology

EFA deficiency is noted in patients with chronic poor absorption, such as in the short intestine syndrome, and in those maintained on oral food formulas deficient in EFA and on long-term parenteral nutrition devoid of lipids.

Pathogenesis

The influence of fatty acids on the immune function of the cells and on the immune response has been researched for over 30 years. A deficiency in EFA impairs the immunity mediated by the cells, which diminishes while the content of fat in the diet grows.

The first studies of the effects of fatty acids on the immune system were connected with the family of polyunsaturated fatty acids (PUFA) *n*-6, also known as omega-6 fatty acid. They are found in wholesome fats, which are part of many vegetable oils.

Recently, there has been interest in the effects of the alpha-linolenic acid, known as an omega-3 fatty acid or PUFA *n*-3, found in fish oil and flaxseed. Gamma-linoleic acid is an essential fatty acid, which the body converts into compounds similar to hormones called prostaglandins, which regulate many of the body functions.

Clinical manifestations

Manifestations of EFA deficiency include a series of alterations in the organism. Notable features of omega-6 EFA deficiency include a delay in growth, sparse growth of body hair, thin desquamation of the trunk skin, and eczema, which generally begins in the nasolabial folds and eyebrows, and extends to the face and neck. Slow healing of wounds, increased susceptibility to infection, thrombocytopenia, anemia, and hepatosplenomegaly are part of the picture. On microscopy, the stratum corneum of the skin is fissured and impaired, showing an increase disturbance of the transepiderm barrier.

In the omega-3 EFA deficiency neurological alterations have been noted, including paresthesia, weakness and inability to walk, pain in the legs, and cloudy vision.

Treatment

An adequate diet containing lipids, such as fish oil and flaxseed. Vegetable oils, also found in flaxseed, such as linoleic acid, must also be offered.

Vitamin A deficiency

Synonyms: Retinoic acid

Key features:

- Phrynoderma (follicular hyperkeratosis)
- Keratomalacia
- Bitot's spots
- Xerophthalmia

Introduction

Vitamin A constitutes a nutritional term, which describes a family of essential fat-soluble food compounds whose structures relate to retinol lipoid alcohol and which share biological activities.

History

In the past, Egyptian and Greek physicians[16] may have understood the healing value of liver tissue, as a rich source of vitamin A for nocturnal blindness. This kind of blindness represents the ocular manifestation of vitamin A deficiency.

In the 1920s, several researchers made fundamental discoveries about the relation between vitamin A deficiency and the development of xerophthalmia, normal tissue differentiation, and resistance to infection. Between 1920 and 1930, Karrer et al., in Switzerland, elucidated the chemical structure of vitamin A as all-*trans*-retinol. At the end of 1940, Arens and Van Dorp described the synthesis of the vitamin A acid, known today as retinoic acid.[16]

Etiology

The term vitamin A is a generic label for all derivatives of the provitamin-A carotenoids.[16]

Vitamin A is initially processed in the intestine, through several cycles of hydrolysis and reesterification, which are characteristic of the metabolism of vitamin A.

At birth, the liver possesses a low content of vitamin A, which quickly increases because colostrums and the mother's milk provide great quantities. Full-fat cow's milk is also a satisfactory source of vitamin A. Other food, like vegetables, fruit, eggs, butter, and liver, also provide this vitamin. The risk of vitamin A deficiency is low in children who receive a well-balanced diet, but it may frequently occur in weaned infants and in chronic intestinal disturbances.

Pathogenesis

The retinoids are essential to cellular differentiation, to activation of the genes responsive to retinoic acid and to the stability of the membranes. Both an excess and a deficiency of vitamin A bring about the rupture of the lysosomal membranes, with liberation of hydrolyses. The typical alterations in the epithelium include proliferation of basal cells and hyperkeratosis.

In the retina, vitamin A maintains normal differentiation of the cells of the membrane of the conjunctiva, cornea, and other ocular structures, preventing xerophthalmia. There are two distinct systems of photoreceptors: the rods, which are sensitive to low-intensity light, and the cones, sensitive to colors and to high-intensity light.

Clinical manifestations

The ocular lesions appear insidiously. Initially, the back segment of the eye is affected with impairment of the adaptation to darkness, which results in nocturnal blindness. Later they present conjunctival and corneal xerosis, which develops into wrinkling and opacification of the cornea, known as keratomalacia. Dry silver-gray plaques may arise in the bulbar conjunctiva, also known as Bitot's spots, with follicular hyperkeratosis and photophobia.

The skin is dry and with exfoliation, and sometimes one finds follicular hyperkeratosis, especially in the extensor surfaces of the limbs, trunk, and buttocks (Fig. 32.3). The vaginal epithelium, may become like the skin, and the epithelial metaplasia of the urinary system may contribute to pyuria and hematuria.

A chronic deficiency of vitamin A may cause delays in physical and mental development, with signs of apathy.

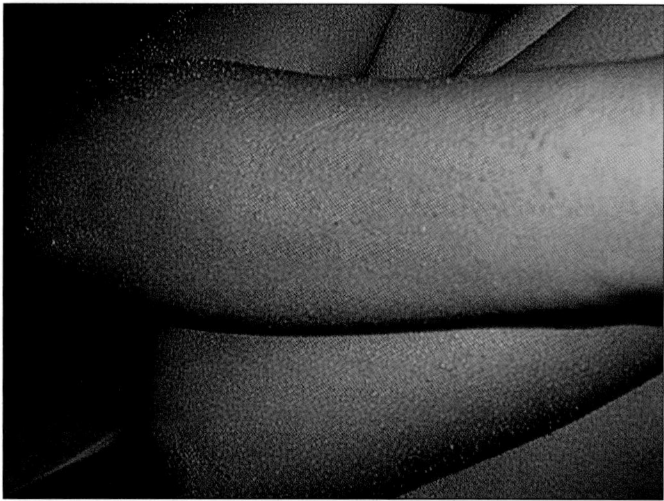

Figure 32.3 Vitamin A deficiency. Perifollicular hyperkeratosis on the arm.

Diagnosis

The clinical exam suggests the diagnosis. In the ophthalmic exam, the tests of adaptation to darkness may be conclusive. The conjunctival xerosis is detected on biomicroscopic examination of the conjunctiva. Examination of the eye lesions and the vagina are recommended to aid the diagnosis.

Treatment

For therapeutic reasons, diets poor in lipids may be supplemented with vitamin A. In cases of latent deficiency, a daily supplement of 1500 µg vitamin A is sufficient. It is estimated that infants aged 6–11 months must receive supplements with 30 000 µ (100 000 IU) of vitamin A; children aged 12 months to 6 years should receive 60 000 µ (200 000 IU), provided orally in a hydrosoluble base every 4 months.[16] In xerophthalmia, 1500 µ/day is given orally, and, later, daily intramuscular injections of 7500 µ of vitamin A are administered until recovery.

Hypervitaminosis A

Synonyms: Carotenemia

Key features:

- Bulging of the fontanel
- Pseudotumor cerebri
- Diplopia

Introduction

The acute form of hypervitaminosis A occurs in infants who ingest 100 000 µ or more of vitamin A. Symptoms are related to rising intracranial pressure: in serious cases diplopia, papillary edema, paralysis of the cranial nerves, and signs mimicking brain tumors may be seen. The skin demonstrates marked desquamation.

The chronic form occurs after excessive ingestion of vitamin A for several weeks or months. In the skin we note dryness, with itching and desquamation, perhaps presenting with fissures in the angles of the mouth, gingival discoloration, and alopecia with dry hair.

The cranial junctions are wider in small children. Craniotabes are common. Serious congenital malformations may occur in a newborn of a mother who has consumed more than 10 000 IU vitamin A before the seventh week of pregnancy.[16] The excessive ingestion of carotenoids may cause hypercarotenosis. Yellow or orange discoloration of the skin, called carotenoderma, and xanthosis of the cutis may be seen. It appears in the areas where the fatty secretions are more intense, especially in the nasolabial folds, forehead, armpits, areas between the legs and keratinized surfaces, like the palms of the hands and soles of the feet. What distinguishes the hypercarotenosis from jaundice is that the scleral and buccal membranes are not affected.

Thiamin deficiency

Synonyms: Vitamin B_1

Key features:

- Beriberi
- Polyneuropathy
- Wernicke–Korsakoff encephalopathy

Introduction

Thiamin is a B-group vitamin that helps to convert carbohydrates into energy and is also important in maintaining sensory nerve conduction.

History

The first reports of beriberi are from Neiching, a Chinese doctor in 2697 BC, but this disease was not attributed to thiamin deficiency. In 1890, Eijkman reported a polyneuropathy in birds fed only with rice; the condition was similar to those reported in humans with beriberi. Thiamin was not synthesized until 1936.[17]

Etiology and pathogenesis

Thiamin chlorhydrate is a white substance, soluble in water, alcohol, and acetone but not fat-soluble. Thiamin is not accumulated and is eliminated in its free form in urine and in less amounts in bile.

Thiamin plays an important role in neurotransmission and nerve conduction and can be found in many foods, whether animal or mineral. Main sources are vegetables, cereals, and yeast. Milk, seafood, green vegetables, and fruits are not a good source of this vitamin.

Epidemiology

Dietary deficiency and alcoholism are the most common risk factors for beriberi. In Asia a diet based only on carbohydrates and rice is most common. Alcoholism is the most frequent cause of thiamin deficiency in western countries.[17]

A mother with chronic thiamin deficiency raises her baby's risk for thiamin deficiency.

Clinical manifestations

There is an adult and infantile form of beriberi. The infantile form usually occurs between 2 and 3 months of age and cardiac involvement is acute and fatal. In severe forms death can occur within hours if thiamin is not administered.

The aphonic form of beriberi is characterized by the intensity of crying, varying from hoarse to aphonic.

The adult form of beriberi can be divided into three types: dry, wet, and cerebral.

1. The dry form is found in adults and rarely in children and is characterized by peripheral neuropathy.[17,18]
2. In the wet form cardiac involvement is found in addition to peripheral neuropathy. Edema, cardiomegaly, and cardiac failure are associated symptoms.
3. The cerebral form or Wernicke–Korsakoff encephalopathy has been associated with other conditions such as alcoholism.[17,18]

Treatment

A dietary supplement of 1.4 mg is sufficient to prevent thiamin deficiency. Therapeutic doses include 200 mg/day in cardiac insufficiency, 100 mg/day in peripheral neuropathy, and 150 mg/day in alcoholism.

Thiamin is better absorbed when administered with meals. The doses should be divided throughout the day or thiamin will be promptly eliminated.

Riboflavin deficiency

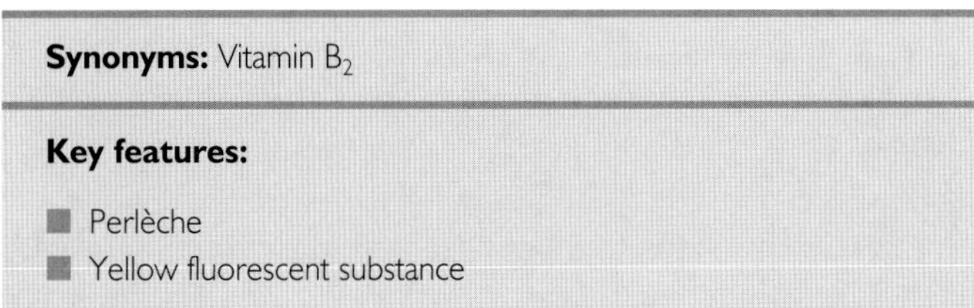

Synonyms: Vitamin B_2

Key features:

- Perlèche
- Yellow fluorescent substance

Introduction

Riboflavin plays an important role in many areas, such as repair and cicatrization, prevention of cataracts, aids in thyroid hormone synthesis, reduces acne rosacea, and reduces the frequency of migraine attacks.

History

In 1879 a fluorescent substance was discovered in milk. Emmett and Luros, in 1920, described a heat-stable substance and attributed it to a second factor, called vitamin B_2. It was not until 1933 that riboflavin was identified as a yellow fluorescent substance, water-soluble, and present in many natural materials such as milk, egg, and liver.[19]

Epidemiology

Despite the presence of riboflavin in many kinds of food, its isolated deficiency is rarely seen and it is commonly present in many nutritional deficiencies. Riboflavin deficiency is seen all over the world.

Etiology and pathogenesis

Riboflavin is absorbed in the proximal bowel by a transportation system. Bile plays a role in its absorption.

Milk, cheese, yogurt, liver, meat, fish, bread, eggs, and cereals are good sources of riboflavin.

A deficiency can occur due to a reduced intake, utilization, or both. Anorexia is a good example of reduced intake. Reduced utilization can be found in many conditions that increase peristaltic (infectious enteritis, irritable colon, lactose intolerance) or reduced absorption (celiac disease, bowel resections, tropical sprue, and glucose-6-phosphate dehydrogenase deficiency).

Clinical manifestations

Skin and mucous membranes are affected. On the skin, regions with many sebaceous glands are more affected, especially on the nasolabial area, ears, internal and external eyelid angles, the scrotal region on men, and vulvar regions on women. These parts became squamous, fatty, reddish, painful, and pruriginous. The desquamations are rough with sebaceous secretions accumulating on hair follicles. On mucous membranes, during the acute phase, painful clefts in the lip angles are described and these are termed angular stomatitis. In a chronic stage, those clefts are called cheilosis or perlèche.

Fungal infection by *Candida albicans* is frequently associated with the perlèche appearance. The tongue may be painful, swollen, and reddish.

These lesions are not pathognomonic of riboflavin deficiency. Other nutritional deficiencies can present similar lesions and elderly people may also have similar lesions due to chronic wetting of the lips and loss of teeth.

Other symptoms include photophobia, lacrimation, and conjunctivitis. The blood and central nervous system are occasionally affected.

Treatment

The riboflavin dietary supplement is 1.6 mg for adults. The therapeutic doses include 25 mg/day for cataract prevention, 200 mg/day in migraine, and 50 mg/day in patients with rosacea.

Mixed formulations of vitamin B usually contain 50 or 100 mg riboflavin. Other supplements can have greater doses. Riboflavin excess is not harmful. Any excess is eliminated by the urine which may change in color: this is an inoffensive adverse reaction.

Niacin deficiency

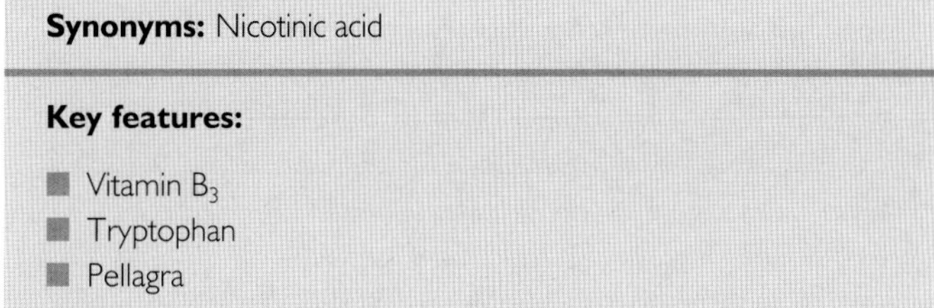

Synonyms: Nicotinic acid

Key features:

- Vitamin B_3
- Tryptophan
- Pellagra

Introduction

Niacin, also called nicotinic acid, is a well-known member of the group-B vitamins. It is considered the main factor in reducing cholesterol and its deficiency is called pellagra.

History

Pellagra motivated the study of this vitamin. The first description of this nutritional deficiency was made by Casal in 1735, who called it Rose's disease, due to the classic symptoms of diarrhea, dermatitis, and dementia.

In 1937, Elvehjem et al. reported a cure of pellagra in dogs with the administration of nicotinic acid. In the same year, Foust et al. reported the possibility of remission of human pellagra by niacin administration.[20]

Epidemiology

The disease occurs mainly in rural areas with poor population and in undeveloped countries where protein intake is low and dietary habits include large amounts of corn with poor use of vegetables and fruits. This disease is endemic in India and some parts of China and Africa.[20]

In countries like Mexico and others in Central America, pellagra has a very low prevalence. This is attributed to the alkalization of the corn to prepare tortillas: this process raises the availability of niacin.[20]

Chronic alcoholism, consumptive disorders, large-bowel resections, and anorexia due to reduced intake or malabsorption increase the risk for pellagra.

Pathogenesis

Niacin is absorbed through the intestinal mucus by simple diffusion.

Tryptophan is a precursor amino acid of niacin. Niacin and nicotinamide are metabolized in different ways and are excreted in the urine.

Niacin can be found in meats (especially red meat), liver, vegetables, milk, egg, cereals, yeast, fish, and corn.

In the transformation of tryptophan into nicotinic acid many nutrients are required, such as vitamins (B_6) and minerals (copper).

Clinical manifestations

In the later stages, pellagra is characterized by dermatitis, diarrhea, and dementia.

In earlier stages anorexia, weakness, abdominal pain, diarrhea, photosensitivity and sensory abnormalities are the main features.

The dermatitis is characterized by a pigmented eruption on sunlight-exposed areas. It evolves symmetrically on the face, neck, fists, and hands. The erythema may be associated with itching. The lesions worsen in summer and improve in winter. The pellagroid nose is characteristic, with erythema with soft desquamation and a seborrheic dermatitis appearance. On the neck extending to the sternal portions there is dermatitis in a necklace form, called the Casal's necklace.[21]

The mucous membranes are affected with painful clefts and ulcers. On the tongue, dermatitis is very characteristic, resembling fresh meat, with swelling and pain. In the terminal stages neurological symptoms are more evident than cutaneous.

Tuberculosis therapy with isoniazide can induce niacin deficiency by pyridoxine depletion. Other treatments, with similar effects, include mercaptopurine, 5-fluorouracil, sulfonamides, antiepileptic drugs, and antidepressives.[21]

Hartnup syndrome is an autosomal recessive disease characterized by deficiency of cellular transport. This deficiency leads to a decrease in absorption and/or increase in elimination of tryptophan. These patients have dermatitis similar to pellagra. The carcinoid syndrome may have similar lesions to pellagra.[21]

Diagnosis

The diagnosis is usually made in the later stages and is essentially clinical with a therapeutic test.

Histological features include hyperkeratosis with parakeratosis. There is vasodilatation in the upper dermis associated with collagen swelling and perivascular histiocytic infiltration.

Treatment

When associated with malnutrition, dietary correction including increases in animal protein uptake, eggs, milk, and vegetables are beneficial in association with supplements of nicotinamide 100 mg four times per day. The use of tryptophan is controversial because the correct ratio of tryptophan to niacin is not well established. It has been reported that 60 mg tryptophan is converted to 1 mg niacin.[20]

Biotin deficiency

Synonyms: Vitamin B_5

Key features:

- Group-B vitamin
- Egg intake
- Chronic alcoholism

Introduction

Biotin was recently recognized as part of the group-B vitamins and it plays a role in the synthesis of enzymes that act in many organic reactions to facilitate carbohydrate, lipid, and protein metabolism, and also participates in glucose utilization. Biotin is indicated to keep hair and nails healthy.

History

Biotin's structure was identified by Kogl and du Vigneaud in the early 1940s. Boas[22] was the first to show that mammals need a factor called biotin.

Etiology and pathogenesis

Biotin is a cofactor to four biotin-dependent carboxylases: each one of these enzymes plays an important role in many basic metabolic reactions.

Biotin is absorbed from the bowel and is transported to the liver and other tissues.

It is also transferred by the placenta, where it accumulates and is gradually released to the fetus. In human milk 95% of biotin is in its activated form.

Biotin deficiency is present in patients with fatty acid oxidation diseases, malabsorption syndromes, those receiving parenteral nutrition, in chronic alcoholism, or in individuals with a large intake of uncooked egg whites.[22]

Biotin can be found in liver, soy, nuts, oats, rice, barley, vegetables, and wheat.

Clinical manifestations

Individuals with biotin deficiency have dry, scaly, and shiny skin, and fragile nails; in adults, urticaria and alopecia are also described. The oral cavity and tongue can be painful and swollen. Also, hair loss, pale mucous membranes, irritability, torpor, and mild hypotonia are described.

Treatment

Most individuals can get enough biotin from multivitamins or

B-complex formulations. Food supplementation with polysaturated fatty acid *n*6 prevents cutaneous manifestations. Using 10–200 mg/day PO or 20 mg/day IV will treat biotin deficiency.

Pyridoxine deficiency

Synonyms: Vitamin B_6

Key features:

- Pyridoxal
- Pyridoxamine

Introduction

Pyridoxine is an important nutrient involved in more reactions than any other vitamin or mineral and it acts as a coenzyme.

History

Gyorgy and Lepkovsky were the first researchers to isolate the crystalline form of pyridoxine. Snell et al., 10 years later, contributed to the understanding of the many forms of pyridoxine and developed microbiological analytic techniques to determine these forms in biological systems.[23]

Etiology and pathogenesis

Vitamin B_6 includes pyridoxal, pyridoxine, and pyridoxamine and is present in 75% of foods such as greens, vegetables, beans, nuts, cereals, and some fruits (such as bananas and alligator-pear). The three primary forms of vitamin B_6 are absorbed by non-saturable passive diffusion, mainly in the jejunum. Vitamin B_6 is metabolized in the liver and transported in plasma and the erythrocytes.[23]

Its deficiency is related to a low immune function as a result of reduced synthesis of interleukins and low lymphocyte proliferation. Litwack et al.[23] have demonstrated the pyridoxol interaction with steroid receptors (androgenic, estrogenic, corticoid, and progesterone) and the B_6 status that can be involved in endocrine dysfunctions.

Pyridoxine also plays an important role in the central nervous system. Its function as a coenzyme is very important for neurotransmitters such as serotonin, dopamine, norepinephrine (noradrenaline), histamine, and γ-aminobutyric acid.

Clinical manifestations

Pyridoxine deficiency induces severe symptoms only in rare cases. The cutaneous lesions are similar to seborrheic dermatitis on the face, cheek, neck, and perineum. On the mucous membranes, glossitis and angular stomatitis are described. Peripheral neuropathy can also be seen.

Large doses of pyridoxine can cause sensory neuropathy with progressive ataxia and loss of vibration sensitivity.

Treatment

For treatment of pyridoxine deficiency, 50 mg/day is recommended. Higher doses can be used to treat premenstrual tension (100 mg/day), convulsions due to pyridoxine deficiency (100 mg intramuscularly), or carpal tunnel syndrome (50 mg/day).

Cyanocobalamin deficiency

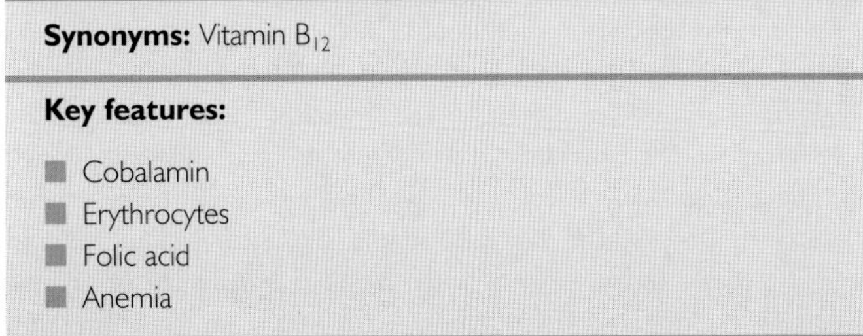

Synonyms: Vitamin B_{12}

Key features:

- Cobalamin
- Erythrocytes
- Folic acid
- Anemia

Introduction

Cobalamin is an essential vitamin for cell replication (especially erythrocytes), myelin synthesis, and it helps to convert food into energy and plays an important role in DNA and RNA synthesis.

History

James Coombe revealed its relevance to medicine in 1824. Paul Ehrlich, in 1880, described megaloblastic anemia. In 1926, George Minot and William Murphy showed anemia remission by dietary supplement of liver.

It was not until 1979 that cobalamin could be synthesized pharmacologically.

Etiology and pathogenesis

Bacteria are the only source of vitamin B_{12}. It can be found in many other animal tissues, but is not present in vegetables or greens. Animals obtain vitamin B_{12} indirectly from bacteria and store large amounts in tissues, mainly the liver.[24]

Cobalamin deficiency is found in gastrointestinal dysfunctions that reduce its absorption, such as achlorhydria, pancreatic disorders, celiac disease, chronic alcoholism, and in elderly people due to atrophic gastritis.

Clinical manifestations

Symmetric hyperpigmentation is found in exposed areas such as the face and hands. Dark nails may occur. The tongue may swell and appear shiny, with ulcerations and atrophy.

Treatment

Daily dietary intake should be 1 mg/day. As a special supplement, the recommended dose is 100–400 mg/day in adults. In patients with clinical deficiency 1000 mg/day should be given together with folic acid (400 mg/day). When absorption is impaired in individuals with gastrointestinal disorders, parenteral administration should be considered.[24,25]

Vitamin C deficiency

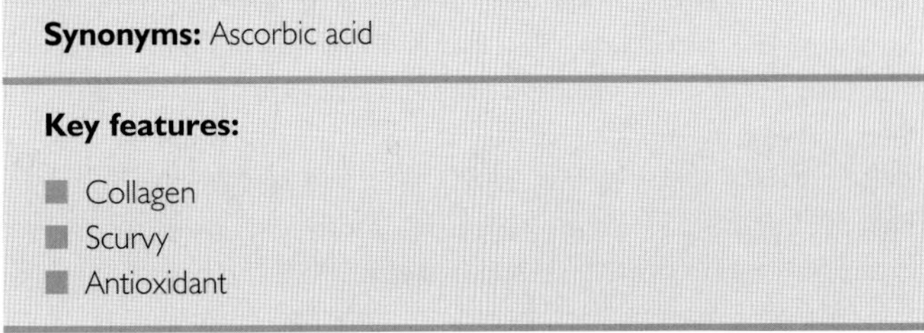

Synonyms: Ascorbic acid

Key features:

- Collagen
- Scurvy
- Antioxidant

Introduction

Ascorbic acid is essential to the formation of normal collagen, and is responsible for the protection of cells.

History

The symptoms of ascorbic acid deficiency are characteristic enough and have been described since the ancient civilizations of the Egyptians, Greeks, and Romans. In the sixteenth and eighteenth centuries, sailors presented with bloody and necrosed gums, inflamed edematous articulations, dark spots in the skin, and muscular weakness. In 1747, James Lind, the surgeon, through his experiments, discovered that dietary supplements contained in oranges and lemons prevented the appearance of scurvy. However, it was not until 1928 that Albert Szent-György, in Hungary, and Glen King, in the USA, published, independently, the wholesome component in the lemon juice, identified as vitamin C, or hexuronic acid, also called ascorbic acid.[26]

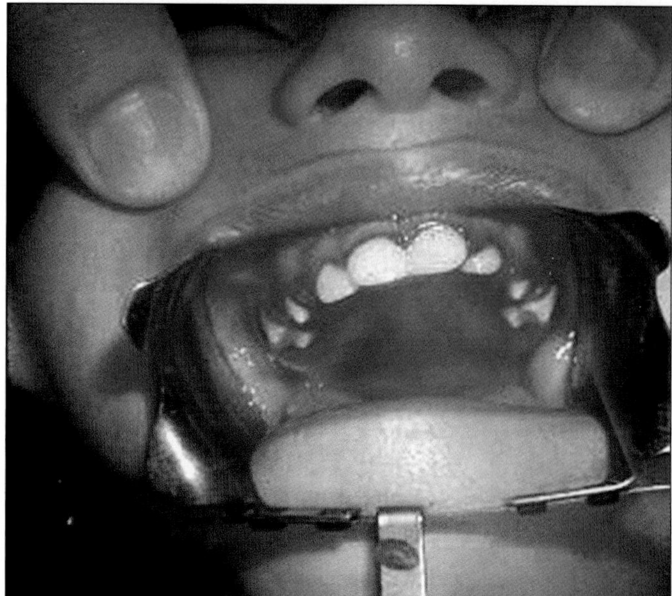

Figure 32.4 Vitamin C deficiency. Hemorrhages in mucous membranes. (Courtesy of Dr. Pedro Carlos Pinheiro.)

Etiology

Ascorbic acid constitutes the enolic form of an α-ketolactone. Other terms include hexuronic acid, cevitamic acid, xyloascorbic, and vitamin C. Currently, vitamin C is used as a generic denomination for all compounds, which qualitatively show the biological activity of ascorbic acid.[26,27]

Ascorbic acid is absorbed in the human intestine by means of an active dependent process of energy, that is saturable and dose-dependent. An infant is only born with adequate reserves of ascorbic acid if the mother's intake is satisfactory.[26,27]

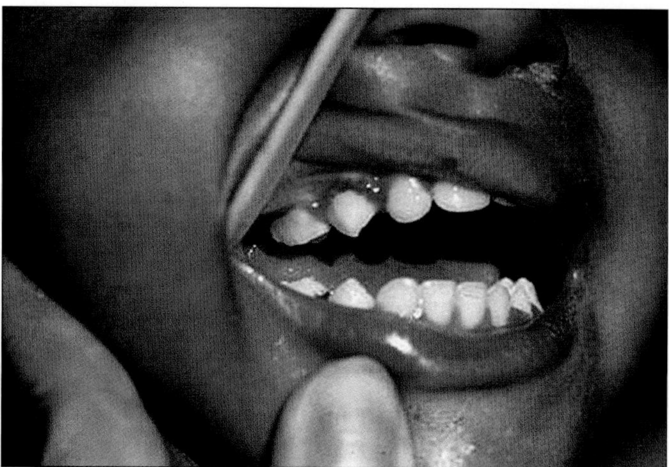

Figure 32.5 Vitamin C deficiency. Hemorrhages in mucous membranes. (Courtesy of Dr. Pedro Carlos Pinheiro.)

Pathogenesis

Ascorbic acid also influences the cellular secretion of procollagen and the biosynthesis of other components of the conjunctiva.

It is believed that ascorbic acid is the most versatile and effective of the dietary water-soluble antioxidants. High levels provide antioxidant protection in the eyes against free radicals generated photolytically in several fluids and ocular tissues, including the crystalline lens, cornea, vitreous humor, and the retina. Ascorbic acid was also noted in the neutrophils as an intracellular antioxidant. Ascorbic acid seems to be important in the protection of the DNA against oxidative damage associated with mutagenesis and the initiation of carcinogenesis.[26]

Clinical manifestations

When food ingestion of ascorbic acid is insufficient, humans show a set of reproducible conditions, called scurvy.

Scurvy may occur at any age, but it is rare in the newborn. The majority of cases affect children aged 6–24 months. The clinical manifestations are insidious, with vague symptoms of irritability, tachypnea, digestive alterations, and lack of appetite. The facial expression is of anxiety. The gums show purple-bluish spongy tumefactions of the mucosa, becoming bloody after trauma, in general above the upper incisors.

Hemorrhages may occur in the skin and mucous membranes (Figs 32.4 and 32.5). Hemorrhages by multiple fragmentation may form a half-moon near the distal extremities of the nails.

Hematuria, melena, and orbital or subdural hemorrhages may arise. Anemia may reflect the inability to use iron or impairment of folic acid metabolism. Bleeding in the viscera or the brain leads to convulsions and shock. Death may occur abruptly.

A distinctly apparent characteristic of the disease in the adult is the presence of perifollicular hemorrhages and follicular hyperkeratosis, as well as Sjögren's syndrome, which is usually associated with collagen disturbances and includes xerostomia, dry keratoconjunctivitis, and salivary gland changes.

The hair is broken and curly, with an appearance of what is called corkscrew hairs, resulting from the fact that they are transversely flat instead of round. The face has acne, of a different form from that which appears in adolescents' faces, and this precedes the defects that occur in the body hair.[26,27]

The localized signs are sensitivity and swelling, more markedly on the knees and ankles. The pain causes pseudoparalysis and the lower limbs take on a typical frog-like position, in which the hips and knees are half-bent and the feet are turned sideways (Fig. 32.6).

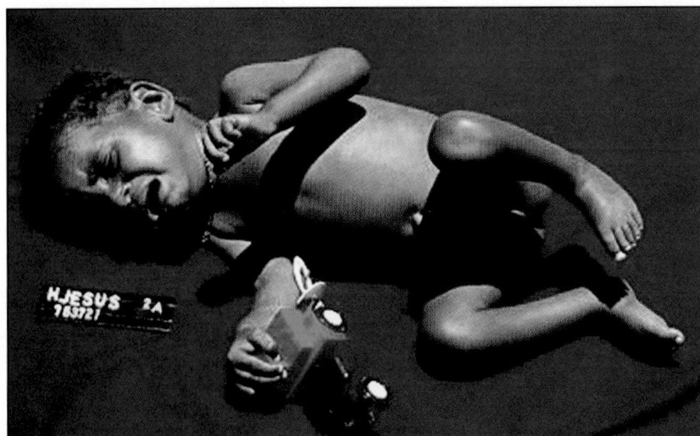

Figure 32.6 Vitamin C deficiency. Frog-like position. (Courtesy of Dr. Pedro Carlos Pinheiro.)

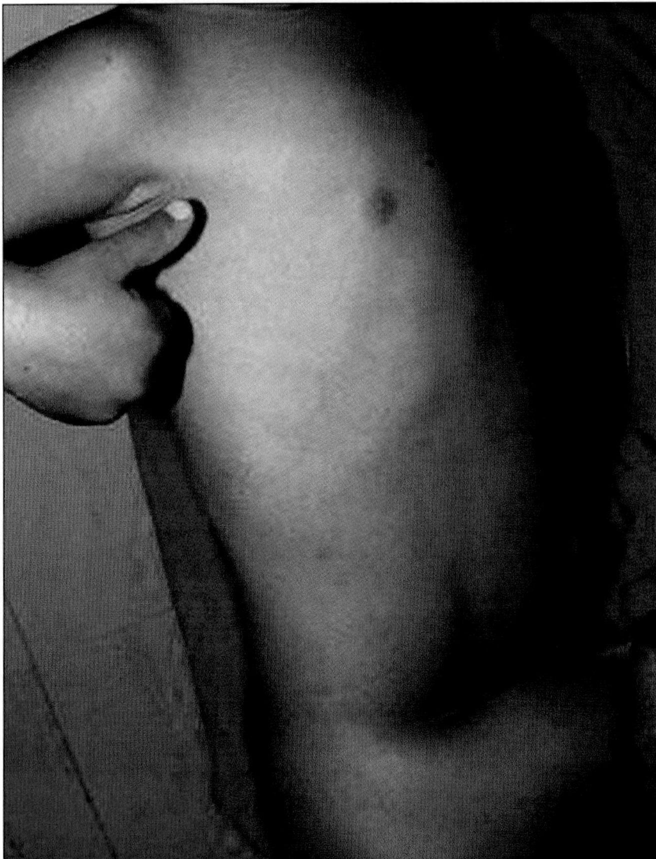

Figure 32.7 Vitamin C deficiency. Scurvy rosary. (Courtesy of Dr. Pedro Carlos Pinheiro.)

A temporary calcification zone causes a dense spot in the periphery of the centers of ossification. This appearance, similar to a ring, is better noticed on the knees, and is very characteristic of scurvy. While the deficiency develops, spontaneous fractures, in the rarefaction areas, may cause temporary calcification. The augmentation of the costochondral junctions produces a scurvy rosary (Fig. 32.7). The subperiosteal hemorrhage is not visible on X-ray, and is usually felt in the extremity of the femur. However, during resolution the high periosteum calcifies and the affected bone takes the form of a dumbbell or cudgel.[27]

Diagnosis

This is based on the clinical picture, the radiological appearance, and a history of deficient ingestion of vitamin C. Rare cases of scurvy in infants are caused by mothers offering boiled fruit juice.

Laboratory tests for scurvy are unsatisfactory. A fasting plasma level of vitamin C above 0.6 mg/dl helps to exclude scurvy, but a lower level does not prove its presence.

Differential diagnosis

The limb pain and the pain caused by frequent movements lead to a mistaken diagnosis of arthritis, suppurative acrodynia, and osteomyelitis.

The patient's age helps to differentiate scurvy from rheumatic fever, because it is rare in children younger than 2 years of age. The pseudoparalysis of syphilis usually occurs at an earlier age than that of scurvy and is usually accompanied by other specific signs. A radiological examination may help in the diagnosis. Other less common differential diagnoses include Henoch–Schönlein's purpura, thrombocytopenic purpura, leukemia, meningitis, and nephritis.[26,27]

Treatment

The daily administration of 90–120 ml citrus fruit produces a quick resolution, but ascorbic acid is preferable. The daily therapeutic dose is 100–120 mg or more, by the oral or parenteral route.

As prevention, infants fed formula milk must receive 35 mg ascorbic acid daily. Breast-feeding mothers must receive 100 mg; children and adults need 45–60 mg/day. High doses of vitamin C, more than 2000 mg/day, may cause undesirable gastrointestinal effects (flatulence, soft feces, and diarrhea).

Vitamin D deficiency

Synonyms: Calciferol, cholecalciferol

Key features:

- Rickets
- Calcium gluconate
- Undermineralized matrix

Introduction

The term rickets, derived from the Greek, means deformation of the spinal column. It describes the clinical syndrome originating from an excess of bone matrix undermineralized in the bone in development. In general, it results from a deficiency in vitamin D metabolism.[28,29]

Historical background

Although historians affirm that rickets has occurred in human beings since the second century AD, the illness was not considered a significant health problem until the industrialization of southern Europe. In 1949, Velluz et al. described a new photoproduct of esterol, which they called previtamin D_3. It was thermolabile and underwent rearrangements of its double bonds to form vitamin D_3 in a thermodependent process.[28]

Etiology

The main causes of acquired deficiency originate from an inadequate diet, undernourishment, and lack of sunlight.

Children with celiac disease, steatorrhea, cystic fibrosis, or who use anticonvulsives (phenytoins or phenobarbital) may experience problems in the metabolism of vitamin D.

In practice, we consider two forms of vitamin D to be significant: D_2 and D_3. Vitamin D_2 or calciferol, available as irradiated ergosterol, is present mainly in fish liver oils, such as cod liver oil. Vitamin D_3, synthetically available, is naturally present in the human skin in provitamin form. It is activated photochemically in cholecalciferol and transferred to the liver.

Pathogenesis

Osteocytes, covered by bone, reabsorb and redeposit calcium. The new bone formation is started by the osteoblast, which is responsible for the deposition of the matrix and its mineralization. The osteoblast discharges collagen and, in the presence of adequate calcium and phosphorus, there follows alterations of the polysaccharide, phospholipids, alkaline phosphatase, and pyrophosphatase until mineralization occurs.

The factors that affect growth are not fully understood, but phosphorus, calcium, fluoride, and growth hormone exert some influence. Parathormone and calcitonin also participate in the homeostasis of calcium and phosphorus in liquids and body tissues.

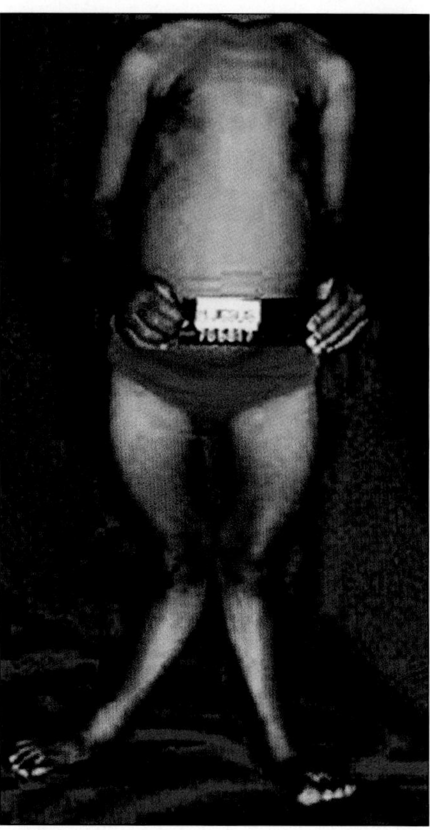

Figure 32.8 Vitamin D deficiency. Deformities of the limbs: knock-knees rickets. (Courtesy of Dr. Pedro Carlos Pinheiro.)

Clinical manifestations

The long bones present with softening and deformity. In the cranial region after finger pressure, we can see the presence of a curve called craniotabes, which is a result of the thinness of the outer table of the skull. With nutritional recovery there is a flattening and permanent asymmetry of the head. The front fontanel is larger than normal and closure may be delayed until after the second year of life. The central parts of the parietal and frontal bones are usually thick, forming protuberances and swellings, which give the head the appearance of a box, called caput quadratum.

In the region of the expansion of the costochondral junctions, a deformity is seen with the aspect of a "rachitic rosary." Retraction of the softened ribs along the insertion of the diaphragm produces a concavity called Harrison's groove.[29] Affected children frequently have a deformity in the pelvis, in which development is retarded. In girls, if these alterations persist to maturity, the risk may increase during childbirth.

The thickening of the wrists and ankles is initial evidence of bone alteration, while the rickets process develops genu varo or genu valgo. The spontaneous greenstick fracture of long bones may progress to genu varum or genu valgum. Deformities of the spinal column, pelvis, and lower limbs result in a smaller stature, called rachitic nanism (Figs 32.8–32.11). The laxity of the ligaments is also responsible for the bone deformities. The muscles are not very developed and hypotonic and, as a consequence, children have difficulty in standing and walking.[30,31]

Patients with a blood level of calcium lower than 7 mg/dl may develop clinical manifestations of tetany, which appear with muscular irritability, laryngospasm, and convulsions.[28,29,30]

Diagnosis

The diagnosis is based on a history of inadequate ingestion of vitamin D, the clinical picture, and the radiologic examination. The biochemical examination presents normal or low blood levels of calcium, phosphorus, levels lower than 4 mg/dl, and a high level of alkaline phosphatase. The urinary level of cyclic adenosine monophosphate is high and the serum 25-hydroxycholecalciferol is reduced.[28]

Treatment

Nutritional treatment makes use of oral supplements of vitamin D and correction of predisposing risk factors. Daily administration of vitamin D_3 50–150 mg or 0.5–2 mg 1.25-dihydroxycholecalciferol is recommended until the solution is confirmed by X-rays.[29]

Other forms of therapy for cases resistant to vitamin D include the administration of 15 000 μg calcium in one dose. When oral administration of the medicine is not feasible, calcium gluconate 5–10 ml in 10% solution is given intravenously.[29]

Prevention is through health education, with well-balanced diets, vitamin D supplementation and exposure to sunlight for 10 min/day, at adequate times (until 10:00 and after 16:00 h).

Ingestion of excessive quantities of vitamin D may result in signs and symptoms of hypercalcemia, characterized by hypersensitivity to vitamin D, which may arise 1–3 months after ingestion. Hypotonia, anorexia, irritability, constipation, polydipsia, polyuria, and paleness are seen.

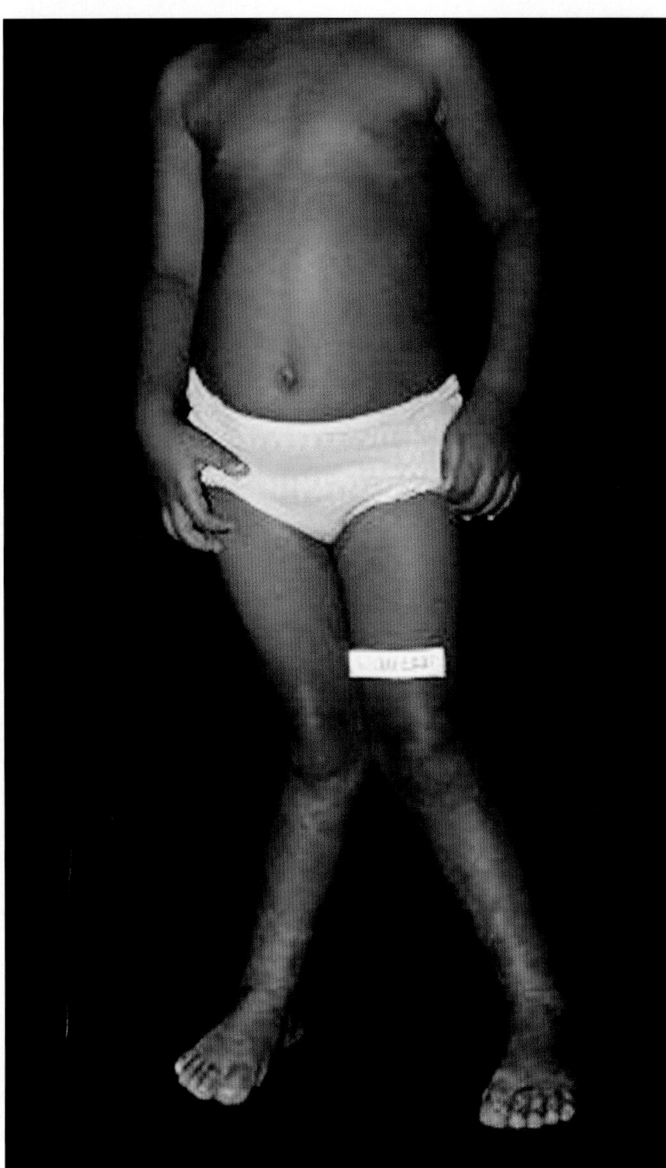

Figure 32.9 Vitamin D deficiency. Deformities of the spine (kyphosis) and legs (knock-knees). (Courtesy of Dr. Pedro Carlos Pinheiro.)

Vitamin E deficiency

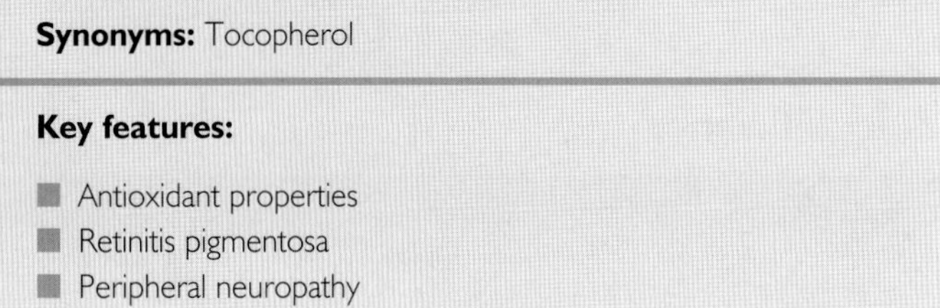

Synonyms: Tocopherol

Key features:

- Antioxidant properties
- Retinitis pigmentosa
- Peripheral neuropathy

Introduction

Vitamin E is a fat-soluble antioxidant. It protects against cardiomyopathy, some cancers, and cataracts. It also plays a role in cicatrization and in immunological reactions.

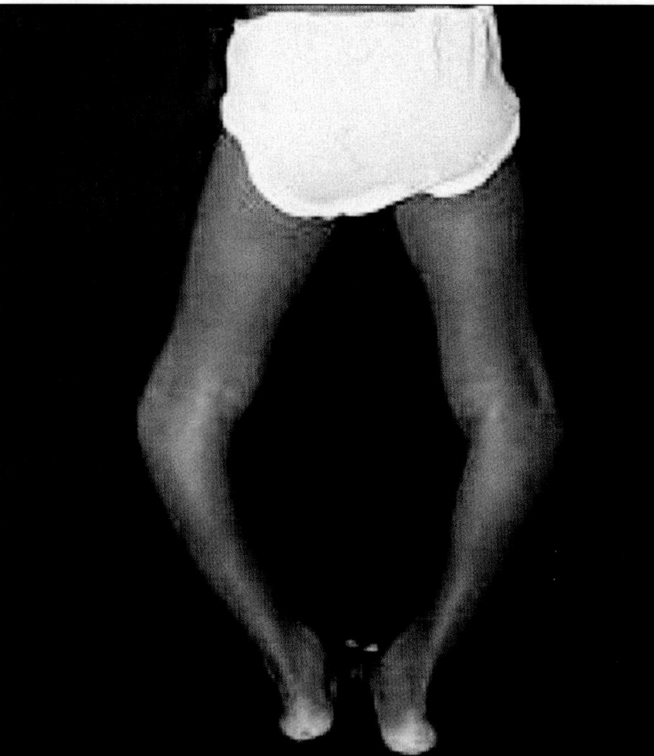

Figure 32.10 Vitamin D deficiency. Deformities of the legs: overextension of the knee joints. (Courtesy of Dr. Pedro Carlos Pinheiro.)

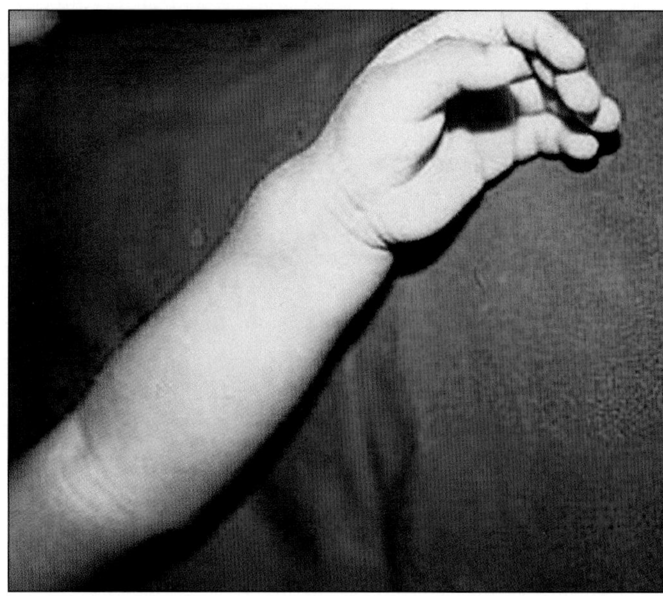

Figure 32.11 Vitamin D deficiency. Deformities of arms: enlargement of the wrist. (Courtesy of Dr. Pedro Carlos Pinheiro.)

History

In 1922 at the University of California, Evans and Bishop first described vitamin E deficiency but it was not until 1960 that Sokol first described vitamin E deficiency in children with fatty malabsorption disease due to a cholestatic disorder.[32]

Etiology and pathogenesis

Vitamin E is a group of substances called tocopherols which occur in four main forms: alpha, beta, gamma, and delta. The alpha one is the most common and most potent.

Vitamin E absorption is linked to fat digestion and absorption. It is transported on plasma bound to lipoproteins and is transferred to tissues.

Vitamin E can be stored in several tissues, especially the liver and fat, for long periods and is excreted by bile, urine, and stool.

Pancreatic enzymes and biliary acids are necessary for fat absorption. Vitamin E deficiency can occur in patients with pancreatic or hepatic disorder, genetic disorder, and in undernutrition.

Vitamin E may be important in cancer prevention due to its antioxidant properties. It may also help prevent cardiovascular and cerebrovascular disease by reducing the low-density lipoprotein concentrations, leading to reduced vascular risk.

Vitamin E may be found in wheat, vegetable oils, dry fruits, greens, and in seeds like hazelnut, almond, and sunflower seeds.

Clinical manifestations

Primary vitamin E deficiency includes symptoms like spinocerebellar ataxia, myopathy, retinitis pigmentosa, and ophthalmoplegia. The peripheral neuropathy is progressive with distal involvement. Axonal myelin from sensitive tracts is the main target of vitamin E deficiency.

Diagnosis

Vitamin E deficiency is best detected by a serum ratio of alpha-tocopherol to lipid of less than 0.8 mg/g and/or erythrocyte hemolysis in hydrogen peroxide of more than 10%. Three days should elapse before determination of blood levels because orally administered vitamin E may circulate for 1–2 days. Thus, blood levels within 3 days of vitamin E administration may not reliably reflect vitamin E status.[32]

Treatment

Intake should be 7 IU/day. In premature infants 15–25 IU/day can be used. Large oral or parenteral doses of vitamin E may prevent permanent neurological abnormalities in children with biliary atresia or abetalipoproteinemia.

As additional advice, vitamin E administration during meals reduces gastric irritation and increases its absorption.

Vitamin K deficiency

Synonyms: Naphthoquinone

Key features:

- Coagulation
- Hemorrhagic factor
- Hypoprothrombinemia

Introduction

Vitamin K plays an important role in the process of coagulation and is also helpful in cicatrization, to prevent neonatal hemorrhagic disease, and in bone development.

History

In 1930 Danish researchers reported that chicks that did not have a fat intake suffered a hemorrhagic disease. A lipid-soluble antihemorrhagic factor was described. In 1934 Dam et al. isolated vitamin K and related it to coagulation.

Nowadays scientists know that most vitamin K is obtained from bacteria in the intestine and only 20% comes from food.

Etiology and pathogenesis

Pancreatic enzymes and biliary salts are necessary in vitamin K effectiveness. Vitamins belonging to the K-group are naphthoquinones. It is absorbed in the small bowel and, linked to chylomicrons, is transferred to cells of liver, bone, and spleen.

Vitamin K can be found in milk, eggs, meat, fat, onion, cereals, and nuts.

Deficiency of vitamin K or hypoprothrombinemia should be considered in all patients with a hemorrhagic disturbance.

The organism produces most of the body's needs; in healthy individuals, vitamin K deficiency is rare. It is found in patients with hepatic disorders (that reduces prothrombin synthesis) and in intestinal disorders, malnutrition, and in the neonatal period. Neonatal hemorrhagic disease can be attributed to immaturity of the fetus, the placenta's reduced ability to transfer lipids, and low vitamin K concentration in human milk.

Clinical manifestation

Hemorrhagic diastasis is the most important symptom. Spontaneous ecchymoses, epistaxis, hemorrhagic striae under the nails and conjunctiva, melena, hematemesis, and hematuria are also described.

High doses of vitamin A and E can block vitamin K, leading to severe hemorrhagic symptoms.

Diagnosis

The diagnosis is made according to the clinical history, 50% reduced plasma prothrombin, and other coagulation factors that are vitamin K-dependent (VII, IX, and X).

Treatment

The total vitamin K amount is obtained both from bacteria in the intestine and from food. Genetic factors may lead to different gender needs. Males need more than females.

The mean daily intake is 0.5 mg/kg per day and the recommended daily intake is 80 mg/day.

Zinc deficiency

Key features:

- Acrodermatitis enteropathica
- Chronic diarrhea

Introduction

Animal products provide about 70% of zinc consumed by people. In vegetable products cereals are the main source.

History

Zinc was recognized as a distinct element in 1509. In 1934, Todd et al. demonstrated evidence of its essentiality. In 1943, Danbolt and Closs described the first hereditary zinc disorder.[33]

Pathogenesis

Excretion of zinc, especially intestinal, is increased in acute diarrhea, in poor absorption syndromes, and in situations where metabolism is increased. An increased need for the mineral also occurs in situations of fast growth, such as in nutritional recovery or during growth of a low weight newborn child.

Etiology

Acrodermatitis enteropathica is a rare recessive autosomal disturbance, caused by inability to absorb sufficient zinc from the diet. It may also be noted, in patients with total parenteral nutrition, after a long time without zinc, and in syndromes of chronic poor absorption.

An exanthema similar to that of acrodermatitis enteropathica was also described in infants fed with mother's milk poor in zinc and in those with a deficiency of EFA, in serious protein malnutrition, and cystic fibrosis.

Clinical manifestations

The symptoms of zinc deficiency depend on the severity of the deficiency and on other factors. The cutaneous lesions have a characteristic distribution, especially in the extremities and in parts adjacent to the orifices of the body, with the possibility of generalization. Erythematous, vesicular, blistering, eczematous, pustular, scaly, or psoriasiform eruptions have been described.

The body hair may become hypopigmented and acquire a reddish shade, with focal loss of hair.

There appears photophobia, conjunctivitis, blepharitis, dystrophy of the cornea and opacity. A moderately dry conjunctivitis, associated with bilateral xerosis and keratomalacia, may appear.

Chronic diarrhea is a frequent complication, in addition to anorexia and behavioral alterations. More developed lesions may leave sequelae, after zinc replacement therapy. Other intercurrent manifestations include stomatitis, glossitis, paronychia, ungual dystrophy, delay in the cicatrization of wounds, bacterial infections, and secondary infection with *Candida albicans*.

Treatment

The US Environmental Protection Agency established a reference oral dose for zinc of 0.3–0.5 mg/kg per day using zinc sulfate.

Acute zinc intoxication may occur as a result of consuming food and beverages contaminated with zinc liberated from galvanized recipients. The excess of zinc in the organism may cause epigastric pain, diarrhea, nausea, vomiting, lethargy, anemia, and depression of plasma high-density lipoprotein.

References

1. Queiroz SS. Fortificação de alimentos e suas implicações. Temas de nutrição em pediatria. Rio de Janeiro: Sociedade Brasileira de Pediatria-Departamento de Nutrição; 2001:22–44.
2. Oliveira NAL. Obesidade: como lidar com as doenças crônicas mais comuns, 59° curso. Nestlé de Atualização em Pediatria-Sociedade Brasileira de Pediatria 2002; 14:245–250.
3. Ukkola O, Bouchard C. Fatores genéticos e obesidade infantil. Anais Nestlé 2002; 62:12–21.
4. Oliveira FLC, Escrivão MAMS. Obesidade exógena na infância e na adolescência. Temas de nutrição em pediatria. Rio de Janeiro: Sociedade Brasileira de Pediatria-Departamento de Nutrição; 2001:45–49.
5. Donohoue PA. Obesity. In Behrman RE, Kliegman RM, Jenson HB, eds. Nelson textbook of pediatrics, 17th edn. Philadelphia: Saunders; 2003:173–177.
6. Abrantes MM, Lamounier JA, Colosimo EA. Overweight and obesity prevalence among children and adolescents from northeast and southeast regions of Brazil. J Pediatr 2002; 78:335–340.
7. Oliveira AMA, Cerqueira EMM, Oliveira AC. Prevalence of overweight and childhood obesity in Feira de Santana-BA: family detection × clinical diagnosis. J Pediatr 2003; 79:325–328.
8. James WPT. Tendências globais da obesidade infantil – consequências a longo prazo. Anais Nestlé 2002; 62:1–11.
9. Williams CD. The story of kwashiorkor. Courrier 1973; 13:361–363.
10. Heird WC. Food insecurity, hunger, and undernutrition. In: Behrman RE, Kliegman RM, Jenson HB, eds. Nelson textbook of pediatrics, 17th edn. Philadelphia: Saunders; 2003:167–177.
11. Fagundes U, Oliva CAG, Fagundes-Neto U. Evaluation of the nutrition status of Indian children from Alto Xingu Brazil. J Pediatr 2002; 78:383–388.
12. Lohman TG, Caballero B, Himes JH et al. Body composition assessment in American Indian children. Am J Clin Nutr 1999; 69 (suppl. 4):764–766.
13. Bustos MP, Amigo CH, Letlelier P et al. Déficit de crescimiento en escolares de procedência indígena. Rev Child Nutr 1995; 23:42–47.
14. Hauck FR, Gallaher M, Yang-Oshida M et al. Trends in anthropometric measurements among Mescalero Apache Indian preschool children. 1968 through 1988. Am J Dis Child 1992; 146:1194–1198.
15. Lissauer T, Clayden G, Vasconcelos MM. Nutrition. In: Lissauer T, Clayden G, eds. Illustrated textbook of paediatrics. Rio de Janeiro: Guanabara Koogan; 1998:113–122.
16. Ross AD. Vitamina A. In Shils ME, Olsom JÁ et al., eds. Tratado de nutrição moderna na saúde e na doença. Rio de Janeiro: Manole; 2003:325–350.
17. Tanphaichitr V. Tiamina. In Shils ME, Olsom JA et al., eds. Tratado de nutrição moderna na saúde e na doença. Rio de Janeiro: Manole; 2003:407.
18. Heird W. Vitamin deficiencies and excesses. In Behrman RE, Kliegman RM, Jenson HB, eds. Nelson textbook of pediatrics, 17th edn. Philadelphia: Saunders; 2003:181–182.
19. McCormick DB. Riboflavina. In Shils ME, Olsom JA et al., eds. Tratado de nutrição moderna na saúde e na doença. Rio de Janeiro: Manole; 2003:417–424.
20. Cervantes-Laurean D, McElvaney N, Moss J. Niacina. In Shils ME, Olsom JA et al., eds. Tratado de nutrição moderna na saúde e na doença. Rio de Janeiro: Manole; 2003:427–438.

21. Heird W. Vitamin deficiencies and excesses. In Behrman RE, Kliegman RM, Jenson HB, eds. Nelson textbook of pediatrics, 17th edn. Philadelphia: Saunders; 2003:182–183.
22. Mock DM. Biotina. In Shils ME, Olsom JA et al., eds. Tratado de nutrição moderna na saúde e na doença. Rio de Janeiro: Manole; 2003:489–497.
23. Leklem JE. Vitamina B_6. In Shils ME, Olsom JA et al., eds. Tratado de nutrição moderna na saúde e na doença. Rio de Janeiro: Manole; 2003:439–449.
24. Weir DG, Scott JM. Vitamina B_{12} "cobalamina." In Shils ME, Olsom JA, et al., eds. Tratado de nutrição moderna na saúde e na doença. Rio de Janeiro: Manole; 2003:477–486.
25. Glader B. Anemias of inadequate production. In Behrman RE, Kliegman RM, Jenson HB, eds. Nelson textbook of pediatrics, 17th edn. Philadelphia: Saunders; 2003:1612–1613.
26. Ross AD. Manifestações clínicas de distúrbios humanos de minerais e vitaminas. In Shils ME, Olsom JA et al., eds. Tratado de nutrição moderna na saúde e na doença. Rio de Janeiro: Manole; 2003:529–532.
27. Heird W. Vitamin deficiencies and excesses. In Behrman RE, Kliegman RM, Jenson HB, eds. Nelson textbook of pediatrics, 17th edn. Philadelphia: Saunders; 2003:184–186.
28. Holick MS. Vitamina D. In Shils ME, Olsom JA et al., eds. Tratado de nutrição moderna na saúde e na doença. Rio de Janeiro: Manole; 2003: 351–368.
29. Heird WC. Vitamin deficiencies and excesses. In Behrman RE, Kliegman RM, Jenson HB, eds. Nelson textbook of pediatrics, 17th edn. Philadelphia: Saunders; 2003:186–189.
30. Amoedo A, Pinheiro CM, Martire T. Aspectos clínicos e radiológicos do escorbuto – Hospital Municipal Jesus (RJ) 1973–1983 – análise de 13 casos. J Pediatr 1985; 58:157–162.
31. Bianco S, Pinheiro CM, Correa MG. Raquitismo: uma visão ortopédica 1994; 29:11–12.
32. Traber MG. Vitamina E. In Shils ME, Olsom JA et al., eds. Tratado de nutrição moderna na saúde e na doença. Rio de Janeiro: Manole; 2003:369–385.
33. Danbolt M, Closs K. Acrodermatitis enteropathica. Act Dermatol Venereol (Stockh) 1943;23:172.

Further reading

Calder PC. O efeito dos ácidos graxos da dieta sobre a resposta imune e a suscetibilidade à infecção. Nestlé Nutrition Workshop Series 2001; 45:20.

Farthing MJ. Anorexia e citocinas na resposta da fase aguda à infecção. Nestlé Nutrition Workshop Series 2001; 45:35–37.

Lissauer T, Clayden G, Vasconcelos MM. Emoções e comportamento (anorexia nervosa). In Lissauer T, Clayden G, eds. Illustrated textbook of paediatrics. Rio de Janeiro: Guanabara Koogan; 1998:245–258.

Maldonado LA, Castro IRR, Azevedo AMF et al. Evaluation of the "Com gosto de saúde" project: an initiative of health promotion through nutritional education of schools. Saúde Foco 2002; 23:105–117.

Marcos A, Monteiro A, Lopez-Varela S et al. Distúrbio de conduta na alimentação (obesidade, anorexia nervosa, bulimia nervosa). Imunidade e infecção. Nestlé Nutrition Workshop Series 2001; 45:26–28.

Meydani SN, Fawzi W, Han SN. O efeito da dficiência de vitaminas (E e A) e da suplementação sobre a infeção eresposta imune. Nestlé Nutrition Workshop Series 2001; 45:23–25.

Motta MEFA, Silva GAP. Obesity and malnutrition in children: profile of a low-income community. J Pediatr 2001; 77:288–293.

Chapter 33

Fogo selvagem (endemic pemphigus foliaceus)

Evandro Rivitti, Valeria Aoki, Gunter Hans Filho, Julio Hilario-Vargas and Luis A. Diaz

Introduction

The term pemphigus encompasses a group of human autoimmune diseases characterized by blisters and erosions on the skin and/or mucous membranes. These diseases include pemphigus vulgaris (PV), pemphigus foliaceus (PF), the endemic form of PF known as fogo selvagem (FS), drug-induced pemphigus, and two new variants recently described: paraneoplastic pemphigus (PNP) and immunoglobulin A (IgA) pemphigus.[1–3]

Autoantibodies against stratified-epithelial-specific desmosomal glycoproteins are found in all forms of pemphigus. Two of these transmembrane glycoproteins, known as desmoglein 1 (Dsg1) and desmoglein 3 (Dsg3), are recognized by PF and PV autoantibodies, respectively. These autoantibodies against the extracellular domain of Dsg1 and Dsg3 proved to be pathogenic when passively transferred into experimental mouse models, since these animals reproduce the clinical and histopathological features of these human diseases.[4,5]

The unique aspect of FS is based on its epidemiologic features, since the disease shares the same clinical, histopathological, and immunological characteristics of the classic form of PF, first described by Cazenave in 1844. Therefore, FS represents an interesting scientific challenge, since many possible etiologic factors may regulate or trigger the autoimmune response in an individual living in endemic sites.

Pathogenesis and etiology

Multiple factors involving autoimmunity, environmental and genetic influences may contribute to FS onset, and are described below.

Fogo selvagem: an environmentally triggered form of pemphigus foliaceus

Although FS was originally reported, and is still most frequently found in Brazil,[6–8] there are reports of other foci of endemic PF in Colombia and Tunisia.[9,10] The clinical, histological, and immunological features of FS are similar to those of the non-endemic form of PF seen in the USA and around the world. Similar to the non-endemic form of PF, FS is characterized by superficial, subcorneal blisters, and pathogenic autoantibodies that are specific for the ectodomain of Dsg1.[11] FS, however, shows several unique and remarkable features such as the geographic and temporal clustering of cases, the increased frequency of cases among young adults and children, the increased frequency of familial cases, and an association with certain distinct human leukocyte antigen (HLA)-DR alleles.[12]

We have described two settlements of Amerindian natives in Brazil that exhibit a high prevalence of FS: a Xavante reservation located in the eastern region of the state of Mato Grosso and the Terena reservation of Limao Verde.[13,14] The Limao Verde reservation has a population of 1200 individuals with a prevalence of FS of 3.2% and an incidence of 1–4 new cases per year. We evaluated the presence of specific anti-Dsg1 autoantibodies in the sera of FS patients from the Limao Verde reservation and from a large group of normal donors from the USA, Japan, and Brazil using a highly sensitive and specific Dsg1-enzyme-linked immunosorbent assay (ELISA).[15] Controls from Brazil included samples from cities located at different distances from the Limao Verde reservation. Anti-Dsg1 autoantibodies were absent in the control sera from outside the endemic sites. Intriguingly, anti-Dsg1 autoantibodies were detected not only in the sera of FS patients, but also in the sera of several normal controls from the reservation and from Brazilian cities. The percentage of ELISA-positive sera among the normal control population was inversely related to the distance from the endemic focus of Limao Verde. In five FS cases followed in Limao Verde for several years, anti-Dsg1 autoantibodies were present in blood samples obtained 1–5 years prior to the onset of the disease. However, the titers of anti-Dsg1 antibodies increased severalfold once the disease was clinically apparent. These results suggest that, in an area endemic for FS, such as the Limao Verde reservation, certain members of the population become sensitized to an environmental antigen or antigens producing anti-Dsg1 autoantibodies that, in the course of several years, can lead to FS. The molecular mechanisms of anti-Dsg1 formation and the putative environmental antigen or antigens in FS remain to be determined. It is feasible that epidermal Dsg1 and the environmental antigens may share certain cross-reactive epitopes that are relevant to the immunopathogenesis of this disease.

T- and B-cell autoimmune response in FS is directed against desmosomal antigens

Eyre and Stanley[16] demonstrated by immunoprecipitation techniques that the sera of patients with PF and FS recognize Dsg1, while those with PV recognize Dsg3. Sequence analysis of Dsg1 and Dsg3 revealed that both antigens belong to the cadherin family of calcium-dependent cell adhesion molecules (CAMs). These desmosomal cadherins share extensive homology with other members of this gene superfamily of CAMs, such as desmocollins, and E and P cadherins. Dsg1 and Dsg3 are glycoproteins with an ectodomain that contains six putative calcium-binding sites, a transmembrane region, and an intracellular domain that is linked to the keratinocyte cytoskeleton via desmosomal plaque proteins.[17]

Autoantibody response in FS

It has been known that the autoantibody response in FS is mediated by IgG antiepidermal autoantibodies, and is predominantly of the IgG4 subclass, even though an IgG1 response might be present as well. Total IgG4, and F(ab')2 and Fab' fragments of FS IgG were all pathogenic in the mouse model of FS. Additional studies have demonstrated that the autoantibody response in FS exhibits a limited heterogeneity, consisting of all oligoclonal IgG1 and IgG4 banding, when tested with epidermal antigens by affinity immunoblotting.[18,19]

We have extended the seroepidemiological studies of the Terena reservation of Limao Verde, Brazil, to include the IgG subclass of anti-Dsg1 autoantibodies present in FS patients and controls using an IgG-subclass-specific anti-Dsg1 ELISA. These studies revealed that normal controls from endemic areas show low levels of IgG1 and IgG4 anti-Dsg1 autoantibodies, whereas FS patients have the same levels of IgG1, but 19.3 fold higher IgG4 response. Moreover, in preclinical disease and remission, FS patients show a predominant IgG1 anti-Dsg1 response, in contrast with disease activity, where IgG4 anti-Dsg1antibodies are the main antibody isotype involved.[20]

Elegant studies performed by Li et al.[21] with the same population described above and utilizing domain-swapped Dsg1 and Dsg3 revealed that anti-Dsg1 antibodies from healthy controls and FS patients under remission show an exclusive response to the EC5 domain of the molecule, whereas FS patients with active disease reveal a major reactivity against the EC1–2 domains of Dsg1. When analyzing preclinical stages of FS, EC-5 remains the major domain involved in the autoimmune response; however, intramolecular spreading may occur at the disease onset, leading to a EC1–2-oriented IgG response. Hence, EC1 and 2 may be the drivers of the pathogenic process, rather than IgG heterogeneity.

The mechanisms involved in triggering epidermal cell detachment in FS still remain under intense investigation. Postulated mechanisms include impairment of Dsg1 or Dsg3 adhesive function, as suggested by studies demonstrating that the Fab fragments of PV and PF IgG are also pathogenic.[22] Recent observations suggest that binding of pemphigus autoantibodies to the epidermis may alter the normal distribution of Dsg1 and Dsg3 and trigger acantholysis. This compensation theory proposes that binding of Dsg1 on the upper layers of epidermis by anti-Dsg1 antibodies, unique to PF or FS, induces subcorneal vesicles because, in these regions, a lack of Dsg3 to compensate for the loss of function of Dsg1 may occur.[23] It has also been proposed that binding of PV or PF autoantibodies to Dsg3 or Dsg1 may trigger phosphorylation and activation of transmembrane signaling pathways, leading to release of effector molecules such as plasminogen activator. These findings have been challenged by other studies that demonstrate that acantholysis induced by PV autoantibodies in mice is seen in animals depleted of plasminogen activator.[24,25]

T cells from FS patients recognize Dsg1 extracellular epitopes

Recent studies show that T cells from patients with FS recognize epitopes located on the ectodomain of Dsg1.[26] T cells from 13 of 15 FS patients responded to recombinant Dsg1. The proliferation of FS T cells to Dsg1 was antigen-specific, since they did not respond when incubated with other epidermal antigens, such as BP180. Conversely, T cells from control groups, including patients with bullous pemphigoid (BP), lupus, psoriasis, as well as normal individuals, remained unresponsive to Dsg1. Dsg1-responsive T-cell clones were developed from five patients. These T-cell clones specifically responded to Dsg1, but not to other epidermal antigens such as Dsg3 and BP180. The proliferative response of these T-cell clones was blocked by anti-DR antibodies, but not by anti-DQ or -DP antibodies, suggesting that the Dsg1-specific response of FS T cells is restricted to HLA-DR. The FS T-cell clones expressed CD3, CD4, CD45RO, and TCRα/β, but not CD8, CD19, or CD45RA, suggesting that they are CD4 memory T cells. The T-cell clones derived from FS patients produce IL-4, IL-5, and IL-6, but not γ-interferon, suggesting that they secrete a Th2-like cytokine profile. These cytokines may promote the production of anti-Dsg1 autoantibodies of the IgG4 subclass.

Therefore, in FS, antigen-specific Th2 cell lines and clones produce type II cytokines on stimulation with Dsg1. These findings strongly suggest that the ectodomain of Dsg1 is the target for both pathogenic autoantibodies and regulatory T cells. The type II cytokines such as IL-4 might be relevant in modulating the IgG subclass response in these patients.

Environmental factors

A possible role of hematophagous insects, especially black flies (simuliid) has been hypothesized for many years. In our first hospital-based epidemiological case-control study, it was reported that black fly bites were 4.7 times more frequent in individuals developing FS than in control individuals. Interestingly, a predominant black fly species (*Simulium nigrimanum*) in the Terena reservation of Limao Verde was found, and this species is rarely seen in non-endemic areas of Brazil.[27] Recent data resulting from a case–control study performed in the same Terena village suggest that individuals living in this endemic area might be at risk of developing FS if they live in rustic houses with thatched roofs and adobe walls; moreover, FS chances might be increased if these individuals are exposed to hematophagous insect bites (kissing bugs or bed bugs).[28]

Genetics

Genetic influence in FS has been the focus of many studies that demonstrate that certain major histocompatibility complex type II (MHC II) genes are frequently linked to FS. There have been previous studies in FS documenting the familial nature of the disease. For example, in a series of 2686 patients reported from the Hospital for Pemphigus in Goiania (Brazil), 18% were familial cases.[8] Ninety-three percent of these familial cases were found in genetically related family members. Recent studies have reported that the expression of DRB1 0404, 1402, or 1406 alleles is significantly linked to FS (relative risk: 14). The hypervariable region of the DRB1 gene of these alleles at the level of residues 67–74 shares the same sequence, i.e., LLEQRRAA. This shared epitope may confer susceptibility to develop FS, as is hypothesized for rheumatoid arthritis.[12]

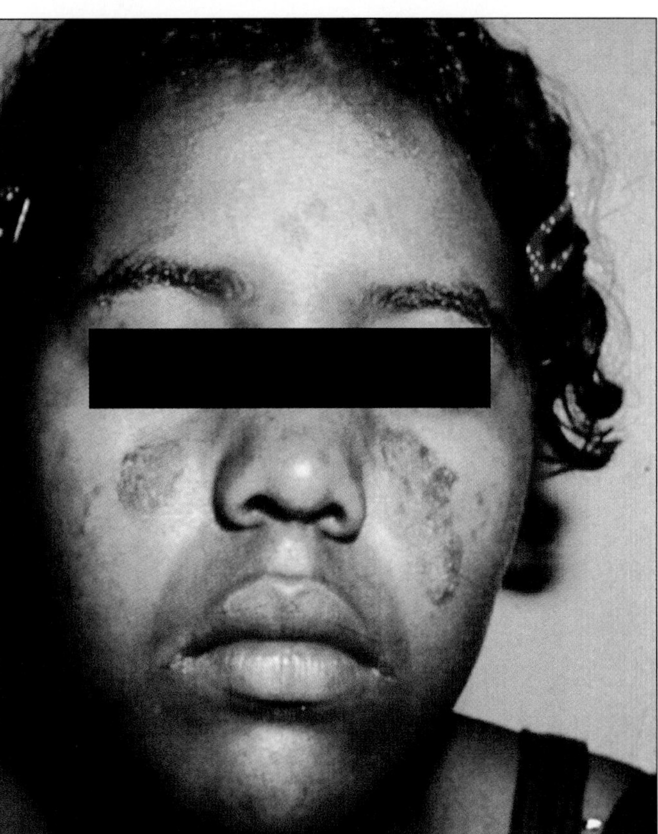

Figure 33.1 Localized form of fogo selvagem. Oval, keratotic plaques with crust resembling lupus erythematosus.

Clinical findings

The primary cutaneous lesion is a superficial blister, which may be filled with clear fluid or yellowish content, resembling impetigo. These lesions rupture easily, leaving superficially denuded areas. The initial lesions occur in seborrheic areas of the head (scalp and face), and on the anterior aspect of the neck and upper trunk. In all active clinical forms of FS, the Nikolsky sign is easily elicited. Mucosal blisters or erosions are not observed, even in cases with generalized disease. In most patients the disease begins gradually, with cutaneous lesions evolving over a period of several weeks or months. In rare cases FS can be acute and fulminant, with extensive bullae erupting over a period of 1–3 weeks.[1] The clinical presentations that are commonly observed in FS are described below.

Localized forms of FS (forme fruste)

The lesions are small vesicles that rupture easily, leaving secondary erosions and crusts that are distributed on seborrheic areas of the face and trunk. Individual lesions appear as round or oval keratotic plaques with a yellow-brown surface. In other patients, the lesions may be erythematous, violaceus, or hyperpigmented papules and plaques, distributed in the same seborrheic areas, and may resemble discoid lupus erythematosus (DLE); however, FS lesions lack the follicular prominence ("carpet tack" sign), the epidermal atrophic changes, and hypopigmentation usually seen in DLE lesions (Fig. 33.1).

Localized FS may remain unchanged for months or years; sometimes they may present in spontaneous remission, or evolve to an acral spreading, involving the trunk and extremities and leading patients to a severe, generalized form of the disease.

Generalized forms of FS

The generalized forms of FS fall into three distinct clinical syndromes:

1. Vesiculobullous forms: these include patients with acute, aggressive disease, in which there is a predominance of widespread bullous lesions (Fig. 33.2). The lesions usually become confluent on the trunk, and remain isolated on the arms and legs. Fever, arthralgias, and general malaise are associated with the onset of the vesicular eruption, but bacteremia or sepsis are not usually observed. Patients with the generalized form of FS may develop life-threatening Kaposi's varicelliform eruption, if exposed to the herpes simplex virus (Fig. 33.3). Vesicles are superficial, and pustular lesions can be seen in active, untreated disease. Occasionally the vesicles form circinate or annular patterns, and after rupturing, produce exfoliation resembling tinea imbricata.
2. Exfoliative erythrodermic forms: superficial blisters appear on the erythrodermic surface, and after their rupture, the skin surface becomes eroded and moist (Fig. 33.4). Due to the keratin maceration, a characteristic odor occurs. Other causes of exfoliative dermatitis must be eliminated before diagnosing FS. In these patients, confluent superficial erosions with crusting and serum exudate are the prominent features of the disease. Secondary infections such as dermatophytosis, scabies, warts, and others are also reported as a complication of generalized FS.

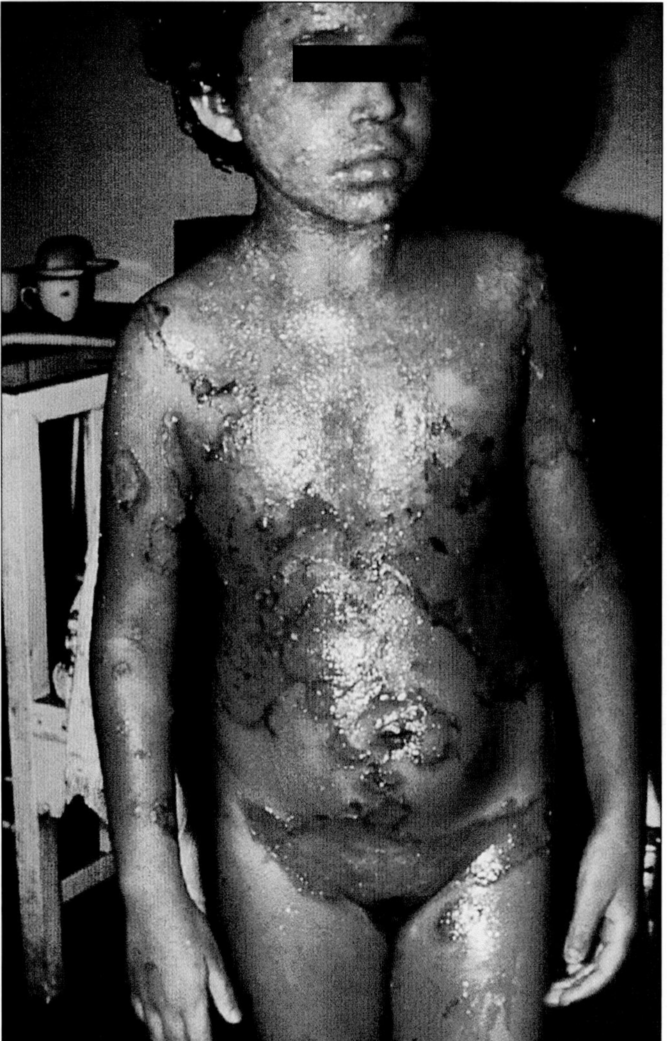

Figure 33.2 Generalized fogo selvagem, vesiculobullous form. Widespread erosions due to rupture of bullous lesions.

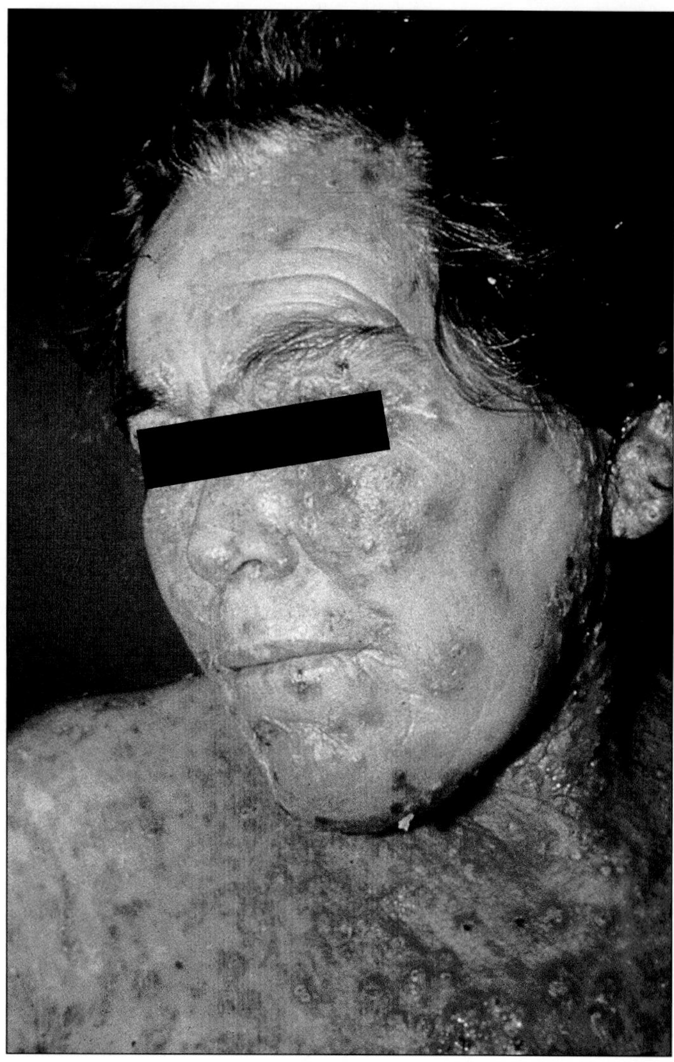

Figure 33.3 Generalized fogo selvagem and herpes simplex infection. Umbilicated pustules on the eyelids and face.

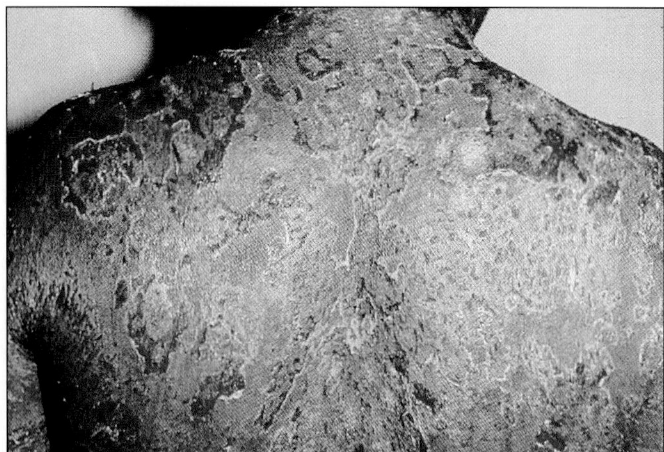

Figure 33.4 Generalized fogo selvagem, exfoliative erythrodermic form. Erythrodermic surface with erosions and crusts.

3. Keratotic forms: disseminated, keratotic plaques and nodular lesions, similar to those seen in chronic, localized forms of the disease, are observed in some rare patients (Fig. 33.5). These patients may comprise a small proportion of FS resistant to therapy.

Other rare clinical forms of FS include the hyperpigmented variant which is often seen in patients undergoing remission. It may be restricted to areas of previous lesions, or it may be diffuse, involving previously unaffected skin (Fig. 33.6). Before the introduction of systemic treatment with corticosteroids, diffuse hyperpigmentation was considered an early indicator of spontaneous remission or cure of FS. The authors observed several patients undergoing clinical remission who would experience dramatic changes in their skin color: white-skinned patients became as dark-skinned as mulattos (mixed Caucasian and black), mulattos became black, and black patients acquired a deep grayish-blue color.

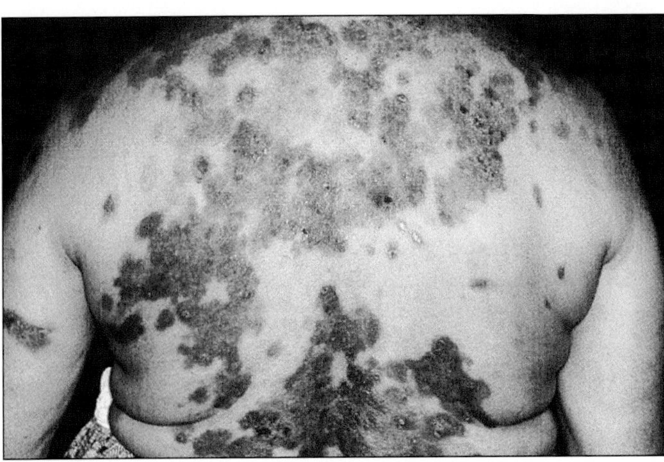

Figure 33.5 Generalized fogo selvagem, keratotic form. Disseminated keratotic and hyperpigmented plaques with erosions and crusts.

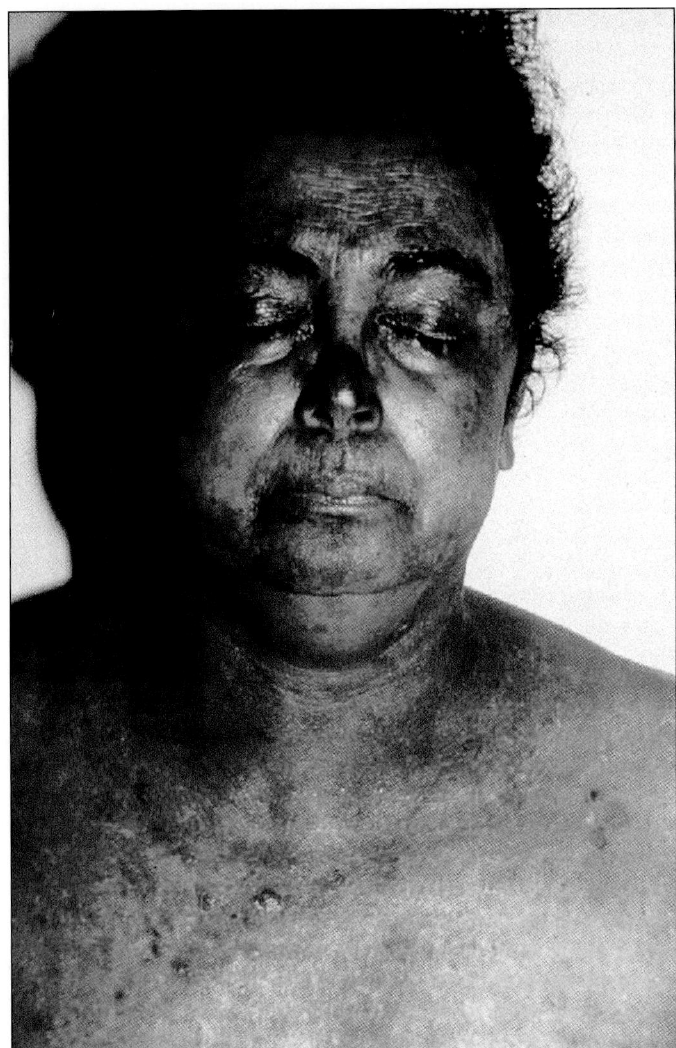

Figure 33.6 Fogo selvagem, hyperpigmented form. Diffuse hyperpigmentation with nodular keratotic lesions on the trunk.

Pemphigus herpetiformis has been described as a clinical variant of PF, FS, or PV.[29] It is characterized by vesicles or pustules in a herpetiform arrangement, eosinophilic spongiosis, and may either precede or follow typical FS lesions. Immunochemical analysis of pemphigus herpetiformis autoantigens demonstrated reactivity against either Dsg1 or Dsg3. Transition forms from PF into PV[30] have been described; however, this progression appears to be extremely rare.

There are also curious complications of FS that remain unexplained: some children, when affected by the disease, show growth retardation; if the disease remains untreated for long periods, they may suffer from dwarfism. On the other hand, if they are treated with oral corticosteroids, they may paradoxically achieve normal stature. A possible explanation for this dwarfism is the intense protein depletion due to chronic exudation and scaling, with low levels of albumin, since endocrine studies performed in these children did not reveal any alterations. Azoospermia in adults who had FS during childhood is reported as a late complication, but so far there are no explanations for this condition.

Laboratory evaluation

Blister formation in FS results from a progressive epidermal cell (keratinocyte) detachment also known as acantholysis, detected either by a Tzanck test or by histopathological analysis (hematoxylin and eosin: H&E). In FS, the cleavage occurs below the stratum corneum (subcorneal vesicles)[1] (Fig. 33.2). Electron microscopic examination of FS cases shows separation of desmosomes with widening of the epidermal intercellular spaces. The keratinocytes round up and exhibit retraction of intermediate filaments around the nucleus. By immunofluorescence (IF) techniques, patients with FS exhibit anti-Dsg autoantibodies, bound to perilesional epidermis and circulating in the patients' serum (Fig. 33.3). Circulating autoantibody titers roughly correlate with disease activity and extent of skin involvement. Laboratory evaluation at a molecular level, utilizing recombinant Dsg1 as the source of antigen, may be performed, when the diagnosis of FS cannot be established by the usual parameters (clinical features, epidemiology, H&E, and IF); most techniques include ELISA, which is a useful tool for screening and patient follow-up, immunoblotting (IB), and immunoprecipitation (IP).

Treatment

Systemic steroids are the first-choice treatment, especially prednisone. Initial doses vary from 0.5 to 1 mg/kg per day. In prednisone-resistant cases, triamcinolone may be administered in equivalent doses, with a good response.[1] When circulating autoantibody titers are high, plasmapheresis may be helpful, and antimalarials are useful in those cases with lesions that predominate in sun-exposed areas, but are always associated with systemic steroids. Dapsone and gold are also cited as adjuvant therapies; however, their value is limited.[1] More recently, mycophenolate mofetil, a 2-morpholinoethyl ester of mycophenolic acid with immunosuppressant properties, has been used to treat several autoimmune diseases, including pemphigus. Our experience shows that it may be helpful as a steroid-sparing drug in refractory FS cases.

Prognosis

Before the introduction of systemic corticosteroids, mortality rates in FS were around 40–60%; currently, death occurs in 5–10% of FS patients, and results from complications of prolonged systemic steroid therapy or secondary infections (bacterial or parasitic, particularly strongyloidiasis). Careful and constant monitoring of glucose and blood pressure levels and the early signs of any infections or osteoporosis should be performed.[1]

References

1. Sampaio SAP, Rivitti EA, Aoki V et al. Brazilian pemphigus foliaceus, endemic pemphigus foliaceus, or fogo selvagem (wild fire). Dermatol Clin 1994; 12:765–776.
2. Anhalt GJ, Nousari HC. Paraneoplastic autoimmune syndromes. In: Rose NR, Mackay IR, eds. The autoimmune diseases, 3rd edn. New York: Academic Press; 1998:795–804.
3. Oliveira JP, Gabbi TG, Hashimoto T et al. Two Brazilian cases of IgA pemphigus. J Dermatol 2003; 30:886–891.
4. Anhalt GJ, Labib RS, Voorhees JJ et al. Induction of pemphigus in neonatal mice by passive transfer of IgG from patients with the disease. N Engl J Med 1982; 306:1189–1196.
5. Roscoe JT, Diaz L, Sampaio SA et al. Brazilian pemphigus foliaceus autoantibodies are pathogenic to BALB/c mice by passive transfer. J Invest Dermatol 1985; 85:538–541.
6. Auad A. Penfigo foliaceo Sul-Americano no estado de Goias, Brazil. Rev Patol Trop 1972; 1:293–346.
7. Diaz LA, Sampaio SAP, Rivitti EA et al. Endemic pemphigus foliaceus (fogo selvagem). I. Clinical features and immunopathology. J Am Acad Dermatol 1989; 20:657–669.
8. Diaz LA, Sampaio SAP, Rivitti EA et al. Endemic pemphigus foliaceus (fogo selvagem): II. Current and historic epidemiologic studies. J Invest Dermatol 1989; 92:4–12.
9. Robledo MA, Prada SC, Jaramillo D et al. South-American pemphigus foliaceus: study of an epidemic in El Bagre and Nechi, Colombia 1982 to 1986. Br J Dermatol 1988; 118:737–744.
10. Morini JP, Jomaa B, Gorgi Y et al. Pemphigus foliaceus in young women. An endemic focus in the Sousse area of Tunisia. Arch Dermatol 1993; 129:69–73.
11. Emery DJ, Diaz LA, Fairley JA et al. Pemphigus foliaceus and pemphigus vulgaris autoantibodies react with the extracellular domain of desmoglein-1. J Invest Dermatol 1995; 104:323–328.
12. Moraes ME, Fernandez-Viña M, Lazaro A et al. An epitope in the third hypervariable region of the DRB1 gene is involved in the susceptibility to endemic pemphigus foliaceus (fogo selvagem) in three different Brazilian populations. Tissue Antigens 1997; 49:35–40.
13. Friedman H, Campbell I, Rocha-Alvarez R et al. Endemic pemphigus foliaceus (fogo selvagem) in native Americans from Brazil. J Am Acad Dermatol 1995; 32:949–956.
14. Hans-Filho G, dos Santos V, Katayama JH et al. An active focus of high prevalence of fogo selvagem on an Amerindian reservation in Brazil. J Invest Dermatol 1996; 107:68–75.
15. Warren SJP, Lin MS, Giudice GJ et al. The prevalence of antibodies against desmoglein 1 in endemic pemphigus foliaceus in Brazil. N Engl J Med 2000; 343:23–30.
16. Eyre RW, Stanley JR. Identification of pemphigus vulgaris antigen extracted from normal human epidermis and comparison with pemphigus foliaceus antigen. J Clin Invest 1988; 81:807–812.
17. Buxton RS, Cowin P, Franke WW et al. Nomenclature of the desmosomal cadherins. J Cell Biol 1993; 121:481–483.
18. Rock B, Labib RS, Diaz LA. Monovalent Fab' immunoglobulin fragments from endemic Pemphigus foliaceus autoantibodies reproduce the human disease in neonatal BALB/c mice. J Clin Invest 1990; 85:296–299.
19. Allen EM, Giudice GJ, Diaz LA. Subclass reactivity of pemphigus foliaceus autoantibodies with recombinant human desmoglein. J Invest Dermatol 1993; 100:685–691.
20. Warren S, Arteaga LA, Rivitti EA et al. The role of IgG subclass switch in the pathogenesis of fogo selvagem. J Invest Dermatol 2003; 120:104–108.
21. Li N, Aoki V, Hans-Filho G et al. The role of intramolecular epitope spreading in the pathogenesis of endemic pemphigus foliaceus (fogo selvagem). J Invest Dermatol Symp Proc 2004; 9:34–40.
22. España A, Diaz LA, Mascaro JM Jr et al. Mechanisms of acantholysis in pemphigus foliaceus. Clin Immunol Immunopathol 1997; 85:83–89.
23. Mahoney MG, Wang Z, Rothenberger K et al. Explanations for the clinical and microscopic localization of lesions in pemphigus foliaceus and vulgaris. J Clin Invest 1999; 193:461–468.
24. Anhalt GJ, Patel HP, Labib RS et al. Dexamethasone inhibits plasminogen activator activity in experimental pemphigus in vivo but does not block acantholysis. J Immunol 1986; 136:113–117.
25. Mahoney MG, Wang ZH, Stanley JR. Pemphigus vulgaris and pemphigus foliaceus antibodies are pathogenic in plasminogen activator knockout mice. J Invest Dermatol 1999; 113:22–25.
26. Lin M-S, Fu C-L, Aoki V et al. Development and characterization of desmoglein-1 specific T lymphocytes from patients with endemic pemphigus foliaceus (fogo selvagem). J Clin Invest 2000; 105:207–213.
27. Hans-Filho G, dos Santos V, Katayama JH et al. An active focus of high prevalence of fogo selvagem on an Amerindian reservation in Brazil. J Invest Dermatol 1996; 107:68–75.
28. Aoki V, Millikan RC, Rivitti EA et al. Environmental risk factors in endemic pemphigus foliaceus (fogo selvagem). J Invest Dermatol Symp Proc 2004; 9:34–40.
29. Santi CG, Maruta CW, Aoki V et al. Pemphigus herpetiformis is a rare clinical expression of nonendemic pemphigus foliaceus, fogo selvagem and pemphigus vulgaris. J Am Acad Dermatol 1996; 34:40–46.
30. Kawana S, Hashimoto T, Nishikawa T et al. Changes in clinical features, histologic findings, and antigen profiles with development of pemphigus foliaceus from pemphigus vulgaris. Arch Dermatol 1994; 130:1534–1538.

Acknowledgment

This work was supported in part by US Public Health Service grants AR32081 (LAD) and AR32599 (LAD).

Chapter 34

Pigmentary disorders

Antoine Mahé

Introduction[1]

The scope of this chapter refers first to diseases specific to tropical areas, but, actually, one should be aware that ubiquitous disorders, such as vitiligo or pityriasis alba (PA), are statistically more common in these tropical areas, and may present with certain particularities in this environment. In addition, certain diseases that do not present with pigmentary changes on so-called Caucasian types of skin might present some on dark skin, an especially important issue as the majority of people in the tropics do have more or less marked pigmentation of the epidermis.[2] Finally, from a pathophysiologic perspective, disorders can be classified as either primary or secondary to various processes. Tables 34.1 and 34.2 list the main pigmentary disorders that may be encountered in tropical areas. Certain diseases might be either hypo- or hyperchromic, or both conditions may coexist in the same patient. In this chapter, a pragmatic approach to pigmentary disorders may help health care workers diagnose and treat these problems.

Hypochromic disorders

Classically, the topic of hypochromia in the tropics was dominated by leprosy, but today most hypochromic lesions do not have any relationship with leprosy. Nevertheless, this disease remains a diagnostic challenge, especially in its early identification.

Epidemiology

A study conducted in rural Mali in children of less than 15 years of age found that the prevalence of hypochromic patches was 4% (personal data). The main causes were: tinea versicolor (about 1.5%), PA (1%), naevus achromicus (1%), and other rarer causes (vitiligo, scar). Thus, if the prevalence of leprosy is estimated at about 1/10 000, as it is now in many tropical countries, this disease should be considered as statistically 400 times less common than the other causes of hypochromia.

Morphological diagnosis[2]

Due to the multiplicity of causes of depigmentation, it is important to know about more subtle variants of this feature. Firstly, hypochromia should be differentiated from achromia (Table 34.1). Leprosy never produes achromia, and achromic disorders are much less numerous than hypochromic ones. Naevus achromicus is a misnomer since it is generally only hypochromic. Punctuated achromia, with persisting pigment at the collar of hair follicles, is an unusual variant that can be observed in a limited number of disorders, mainly systemic sclerosis, vitiligo (when repigmentation occurs from hair follicles), and chronic pruritus, such as in onchocerciasis. Postinflammatory hypochromia refers to circumstances in which an usually transient hypochromia follows the resolution of other features; it may be dramatic in disorders with an epidermal erosion such as many bullous disorders.

Main causes of hypochromia and/or achromia

Synonym:

- Tinea versicolor, pityriasis versicolor

Tinea versicolor is generally easily identified based on the presence of wide geographical hypochromic areas involving mostly the trunk and upper limbs, with a slight superficial desquamation that may be revealed by gentle scraping. Although considered classically as unusual, facial involvement is commonly isolated, especially in teenagers (Fig. 34.1). Other common variants are follicular, hyperchromic, or those without visible scales. A useful procedure in difficult cases is to perform a microscopic examination of an adhesive tape applied to the skin in order to see typical aggregated yeasts. Many topical applications are active against the responsible yeast, but recurrences are common under tropical humid climates.

Pityriasis alba

PA results from excessive drying of the skin, and may be associated with atopic dermatitis. There is often a history of aggressive use

Table 34.1 Main causes of hypochromia or achromia in the tropics (many of these disorders only appear hypochromic on dark skins)

Disorders with achromia[a]	Disorders commonly hypochromic	Disorders rarely hypochromic
Secondary		
Chronic lupus erythematosus	Pityriasis alba	Sarcoidosis
Systemic sclerosis[b]	Seborrheic dermatitis	Mycosis fungoides
Lichen sclerosus	Tinea versicolor	Pityriasis rosea
Lichen simplex chronicus[b]	Psoriasis	Darier's disease
Onchocerciasis[b,c]	Pityriasis lichenoides	Secondary syphilis
Endemic treponematoses[c]	Lichen striatus	
Chemical injuries	Leprosy[c]	
Scar	Bleaching compound application	
Postlesional achromia	Postlesional hypochromia	
Primary		
Vitiligo[b]	Tuberous sclerosis (ash-leaflet macules)	
Naevus achromicus	Creole dyschromia	
Idiopathic guttate hypomelanosis		
Albinism		
Piebaldism		

[a]Hypochromia possible in certain cases; [b]punctuated achromia possible; [c]tropical diseases.

Table 34.2 Main causes of hyperchromia in the tropics

Ubiquitous causes of hyperchromia (in all skin pigmentation types)	Other causes of hyperchromia (mainly on dark skins)	
Secondary	Common causes	Unusual causes
Photoreactions (fragrances, plants)	Contact dermatitis	Psoriasis[a]
Drug reactions Fixed drug eruption Other variants: antimalarials, silver (argyrism), minocycline, bleomycin	Prurigo Lichen simplex chronicus Irritant dermatitis	Pityriasis rosea Pityriasis alba[a] Seborrheic dermatitis[a]
Mastocytosis	Chronic friction	Treponematoses
Melanoderma	Acne	Leprosy[a] (during type I reactions)
Acanthosis nigricans	Dermatophytoses	Tinea nigra
Tumoral causes	Lichen planus	
	Erythema multiforme	
	Lupus erythematosus	
Primary	Vasculitis	
Melasma	Lichenoid melanodermatitis	
Café-au-lait spots	Ashy dermatitis	
Becker's nevus	Exogenous ochronosis	
	Postlesional hyperchromia	

[a]More often hypochromic.

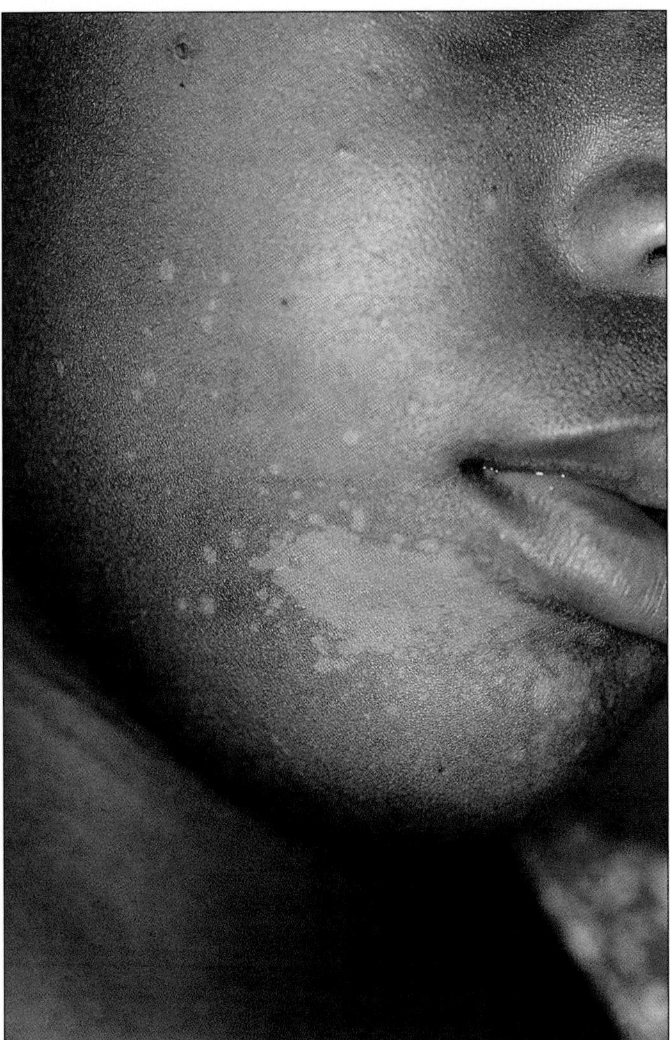

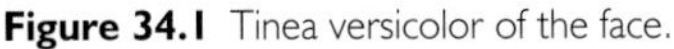

Figure 34.1 Tinea versicolor of the face.

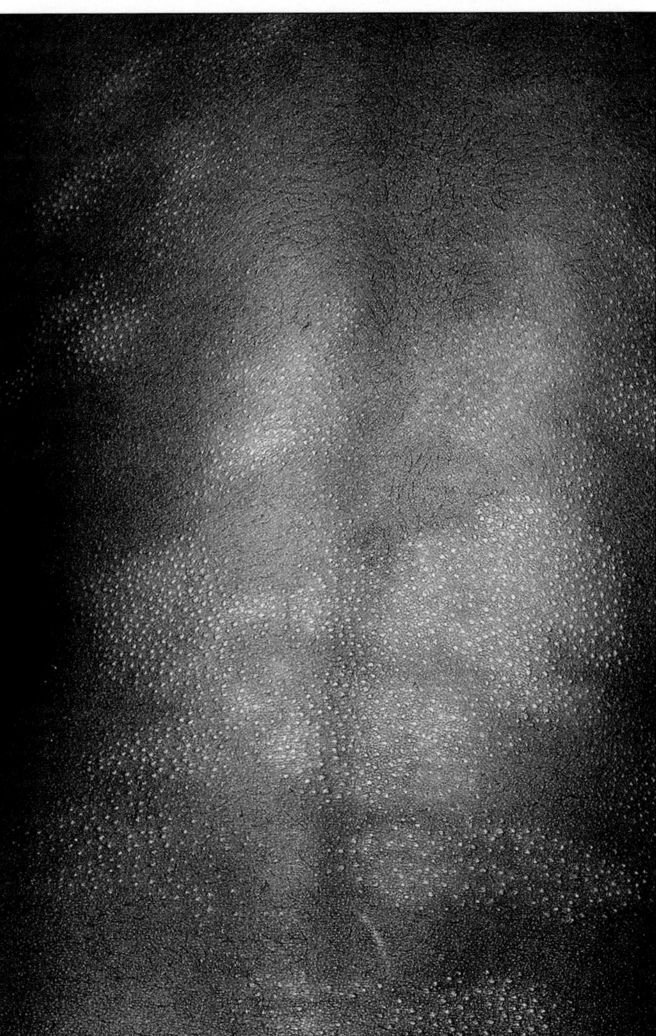

Figure 34.2 Widespread pityriasis alba with prominent follicular keratosis.

of soap or washing procedures. It is common on the face, trunk, or limbs. Lesions might be solitary or multiple. In addition to hypochromia, typical features are dryness of the skin and follicular involvement (Fig. 34.2). Treatment relies on reducing the use of harsh soaps, application of emollients, and transient use of low-potency topical steroids.

Seborrheic dermatitis

Seborrheic dermatitis can be seen in infants under 3 months of age, in whom it involves the scalp, diaper area, and possibly other sites (face and folds), with rarely an erythrodermic evolution; in adults, it may involve the scalp, eyebrows, perinasal area, retroauricular folds, and, rarely, other large body folds. It presents with scaling, hypochromia, and erythema; this last feature can become visible on dark skin because of depigmentation. In areas where human immunodeficiency virus (HIV) prevalence is high, severe seborrheic dermatitis in adults might be a revealing sign of this infection. Treatment relies on antimycotic topicals and emollients in children, to which low-potent topical steroids may be added in adults. Postinflammatory hypochromia may be dramatic, especially in children, but is reversible (Fig. 34.3).

Naevus achromicus

Naevus achromicus is a congenital lesion, common on the trunk, limbs, or face, that presents with hypochromia and well-delineated margins. It may be small, limited to a particular part of the body, or large, eventually with a disposition along Blaschko's lines.

Vitiligo

Vitiligo exhibits the same frequency on every type of skin, and probably in every geographical setting, but is much more visible on dark skin. In addition, several variants are more evident on those types of skin: trichrome vitiligo (Fig. 34.4), with the presence of intermediate skin tints between normal skin and complete achromia; and minor vitiligo, in which depigmentation is partial, and may be difficult to distinguish from other causes of hypochromia if isolated. A skin biopsy may be necessary in order to eliminate other potentially serious causes.

Leprosy

There is a strong need to make a diagnosis of leprosy at very early stages, before definite disability occurs. However, it is more difficult to make the diagnosis early on in the disease.

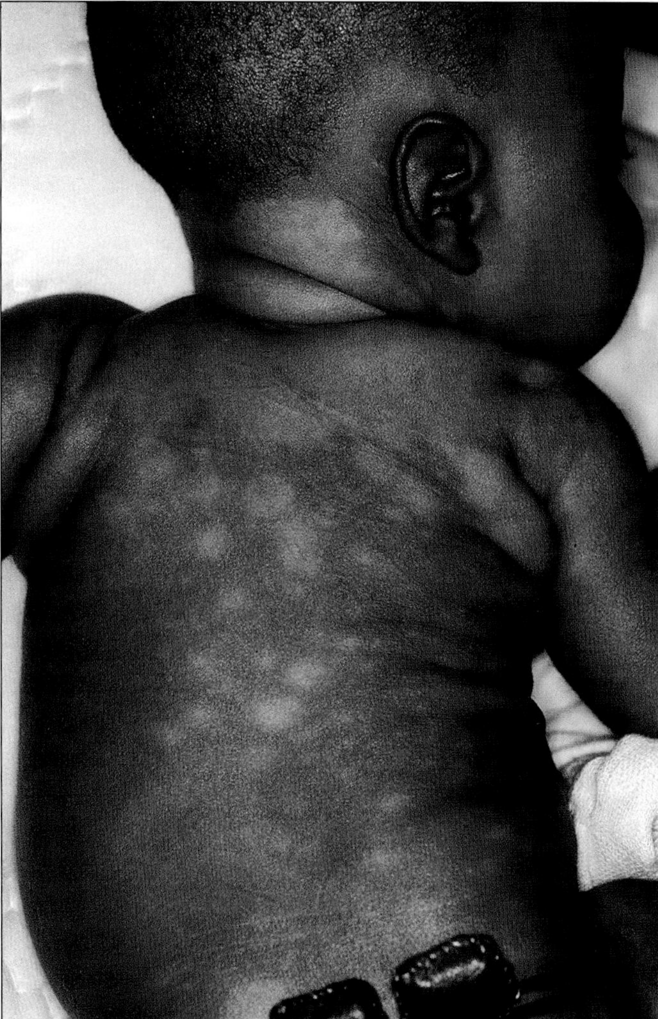

Figure 34.3 Transient postlesional hypochromia following resolution of seborrheic dermatitis in a young child.

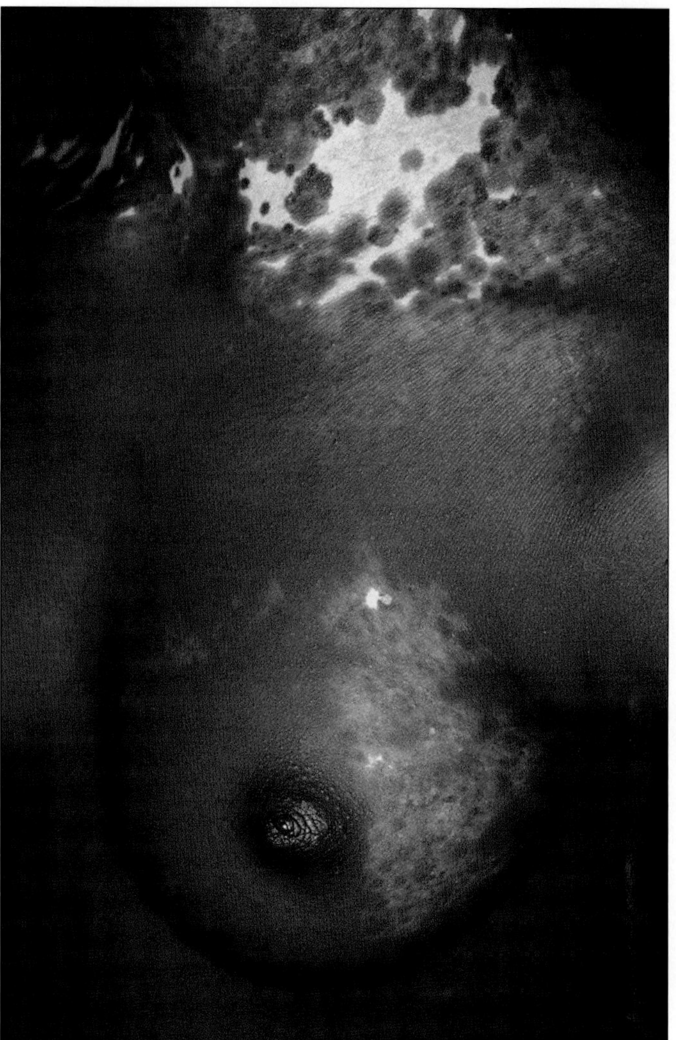

Figure 34.4 Trichrome vitiligo.

It is therefore important to think of leprosy when one, or several, hypochromic patches present in a patient living in, or originating from, a tropical area (Fig. 34.5). Hypochromia may be very discrete, and even hardly visible. There is typically a loss of sensation in skin lesions, but this pathognomonic sign may be lacking in early forms, especially on the face; it must be investigated with extreme care, since it may be mild. In addition, it is often absent in multibacillary forms. A general examination, including palpation and inspection of superficial nerves, is needed. Skin smears are only positive for acid-fast bacilli in multibacillary forms. A skin biopsy is diagnostic when it shows perineural and/or perisudoral infiltrates, especially if they are granulomatous; a Fite–Faraco stain is mandatory. It should be remembered that, on occasion, skin lesions of leprosy are not hypochromic; this is especially the case on lightly pigmented skin, in which lesions can appear erythematous, or during reversal reactions in which the skin lesions may be frankly hyperchromic.

Creole dyschromia

Synonym:

- Hypomélanose maculeuse confluente et progressive du métis mélanoderme

This variance of normality, rather than true disease, is common in populations with a mixed heritage, African and European.[3] It is characterized by the presence in young adults of multiple hypopigmented patches on the lower trunk, with indistinct margins, located mostly in the lumbar area but sometimes also on the anterior or lateral sides of the lower abdomen (Fig. 34.6). No other symptom is present. Many patients report multiple unsuccessful treatments for tinea versicolor, which is the main differential diagnosis. No treatment, except exposure to the sun in order to decrease contrast in skin color, is known for this benign disorder, that often fades spontaneously during the patient's fifth decade.

Idiopathic guttate hypomelanosis

This benign and common disorder is characterized by the presence of multiple achromic, circular and sharply demarcated, small patches, involving the inferior limbs or sometimes the trunk, in middle-aged to older persons. No treatment is necessary, but patients, who are often anxious about the possibility of vitiligo, should be reassured.

Oculocutaneous albinism

Tyrosinase-positive albinism is not rare in certain groups of populations from sub-Saharan Africa, a continent in which it can be

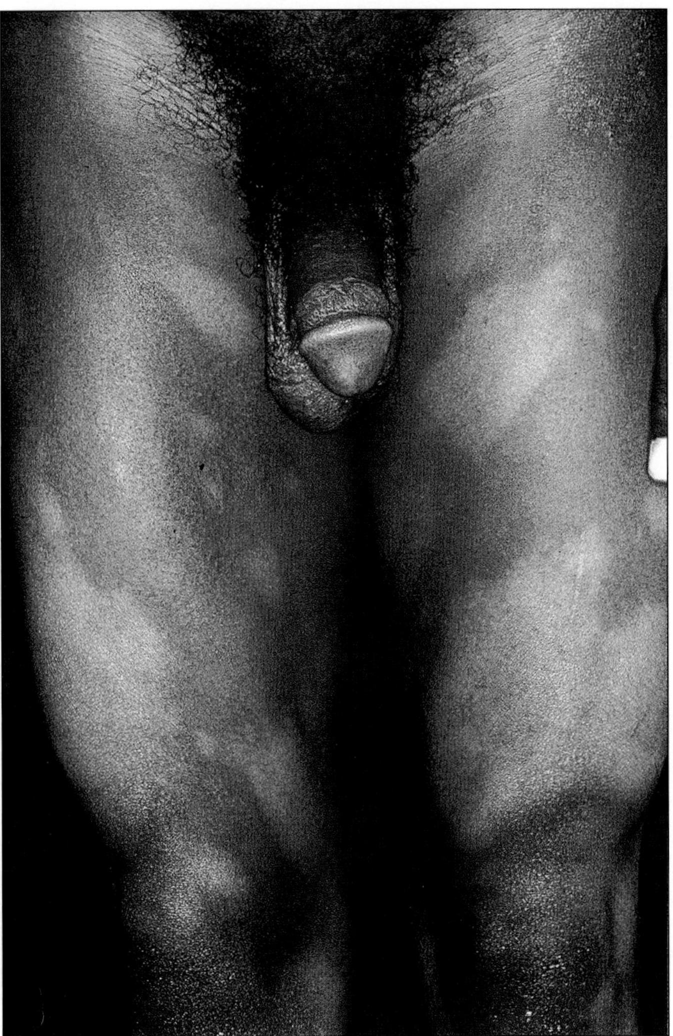

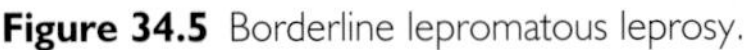

Figure 34.5 Borderline lepromatous leprosy.

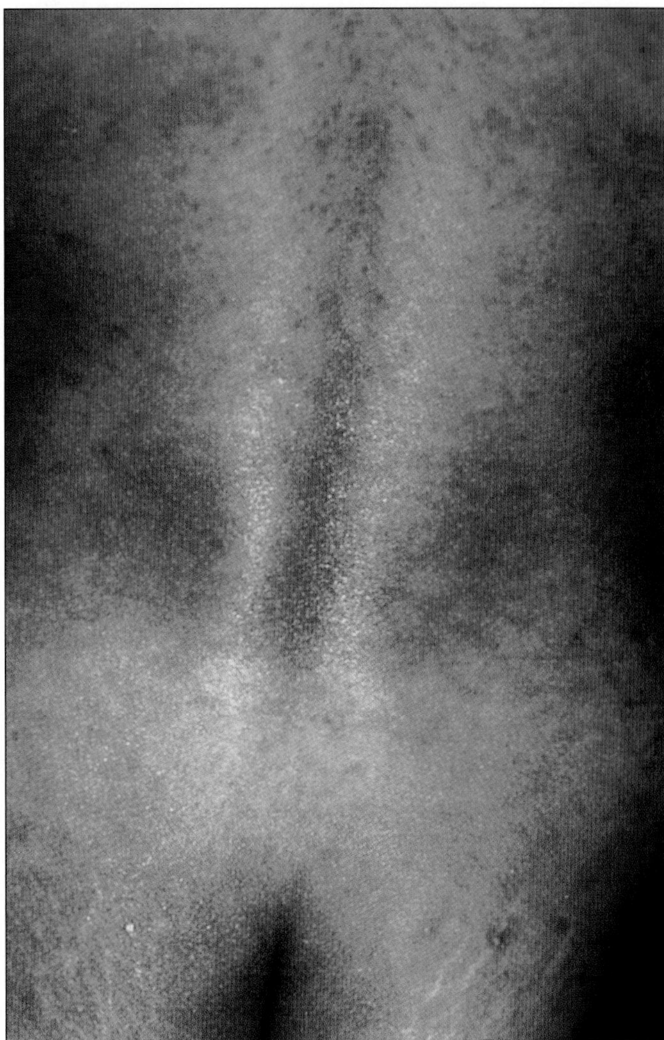

Figure 34.6 Creole dyschromia.

considered as the most common genodermatosis; prevalences as high as 1/2000 have been reported in several areas.[4] This disease is transmitted through a recessive autosomal pattern, and, in certain areas, the birth of a white child from parents with black skin can be interpreted negatively. The clinical picture is generally obvious since birth, with very clear skin and high sun susceptibility (however, often with a residual low capacity for light tanning), yellow hair, and clear irises associated with ocular nystagmus. Pigmented macules, that have been compared to "ink spots," are common on sun-exposed areas, and may attest that some areas of the skin have some tanning capacity. There is a high risk of epidermal skin cancer in affected people.[5] Limitation of sun exposure, with protective clothing and sunscreens from early childhood, appears essential to limit skin cancers, but may be difficult to implement for cultural or economic reasons. Tyrosinase-negative albinism seems more unsual. Other more rare variants, that seem specific to Africa, include erythematous and brown albinism.

Other less common causes of hypochromia

Hypochromia is a common accompanying sign of psoriasis on dark skin.

In discoid lupus erythematosus, there is often achromia associated with scaling, hyperchromia, erythema, and scarring. There is a vitiligo-like, macular variant, in which symptoms other than achromia are discrete. Although often dramatic, achromia may resolve slowly with specific treatment (such as antimalarials).

Despite the association of deformities of the hand with areas of skin depigmentation, systemic sclerosis should not be confused with leprosy. The diagnosis is easy, due to the usual presence of typical achromia with punctuated perifollicular pigmentation (Fig. 34.7), while deformities of the hands are related to sclerosis of skin and joints without frank neurologic signs.

Sarcoidosis may present with hypochromia, either associated with otherwise typical papules, or possibly purely macular (Fig. 34.8). It is more common among patients originating from the Caribbean. Confusion with leprosy is possible, but the search for acid-fast bacilli is negative – a fact that, in the presence of multiple lesions, excludes leprosy.

Onchocerciasis, that remains a significant health problem in only a minority of tropical areas, may present with punctuated achromia on the anterior legs ("leopard skin," a non-specific sign that may be observed in any chronic itching disorder) associated with other cutaneous and ocular symptoms of disease.

In endemic treponematosis, dyschromic features are classical, especially in pinta. A triangular achromia on the anterior side of the wrist is considered consistent with bejel.

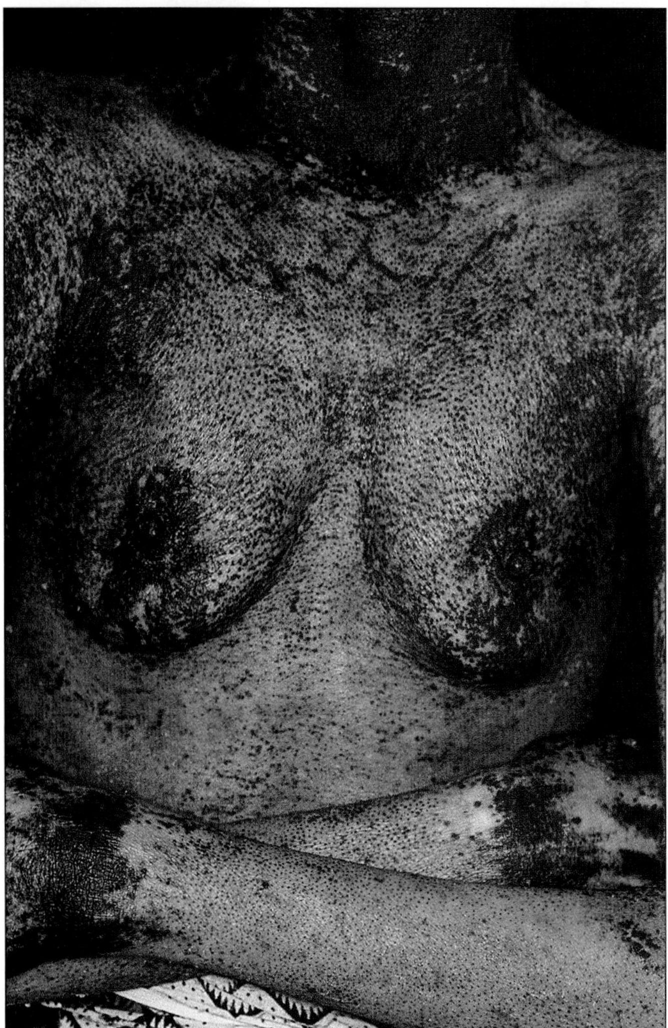

Figure 34.7 Systemic sclerosis with typical punctuated achromia.

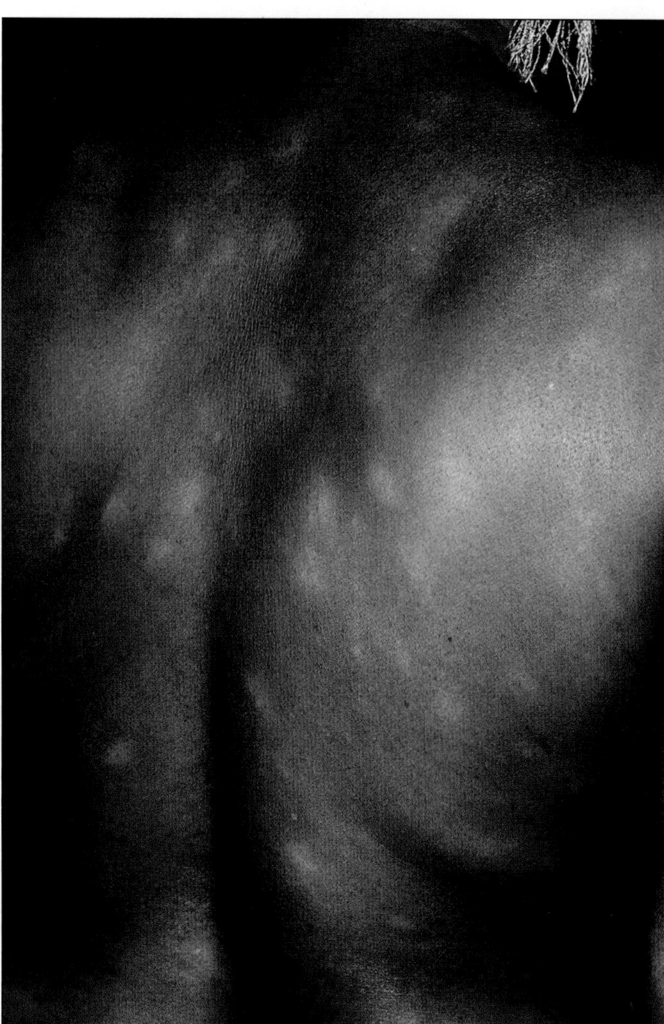

Figure 34.8 Hypopigmented variant of sarcoidosis.

Mycosis fungoides has a hypochromic, macular variant that appears to have a better prognosis than the non-depigmenting type.[6] Rarely, a similar aspect may be seen in adult T-cell leukemia/lymphoma associated with human T-lymphotropic virus-1 (HTLV-1) infection.

A contact leukomelanosis (hyperpigmentation associated with confetti-like hypopigmentation) on the face, induced by the application of leaves of the plant *Piper betle* followed by sun exposure, has been reported.[7] This presentation seems very similar to that observed after application of phenolic-related compounds.

Steroid use, either topically or by local infiltration, is often responsible for transient hypochromia on dark skins.

Management of patients presenting with localized hypochromia

The very common circumstance of seeing a patient for one or several "clear spots" should be addressed carefully. Tinea versicolor, PA, and naevus achromicus should be easily identified. In other situations, testing of superficial sensitivity, added to palpation of superficial nerves, should be performed. Skin biopsy is a key procedure in equivocal situations. A strategy for early identification of leprosy cases by primary healthcare workers, based on the assessment of several signs that are easy to evaluate (presence of a clear patch, superficial sensitivity testing, evaluation of the duration of the lesion), and referral of suspected cases, has been proposed.[8]

Hyperchromic disorders

Epidemiology

Compared with hypochromic disorders, many skin problems on dark skin are accompanied by, or resolve through, hyperchromia. This is especially true for acne, in which mottled hyperchromia is a main symptom on dark skins (and often constitutes the main complaint of patients), many cases of contact dermatitis, superficial mycoses, or even simple chronic irritation (Table 34.2).

Morphological diagnosis[2]

Hyperchromia may present a more distinctive picture related to lesions involving the basal layer of the epidermis (junctional hyperchromia). In these situations, hyperchromia that results from pigmentary incontinence appears particularly dark, with well-delineated margins. Diseases exhibiting this presentation include lichen planus, lupus erythematosus (noticeably in its subacute variant), erythema multiforme, and severe drug reactions.

Noteworthy causes of hyperchromia

Lichen planus

For unknown reasons, lichen planus is much more common in tropical areas than in temperate countries. Diagnosis is generally easy in the presence of firm papules, with a typical shiny surface, and associated hyperpigmentation of a more or less marked intensity (Fig. 34.9). Tints vary from purple on light skin, to grey, brown, or deep black; pigmentation might be more noticeable after resolution of lesions. There is a purely macular pigmenting variant, that seems more common in India.[9] Itching varies from mild to severe. Buccal or ungual locations are uncommon; however, there is a purely ungual variant of lichen planus. There are multiple other morphological variants of lichen planus, e.g., annular, hypertrophic, erythrodermic, or bullous. Diagnosis is generally easy, but secondary syphilis should be carefully ruled out. In difficult cases, skin biopsy is diagnostic. Treatment consists of topical potent or superpotent steroids; in the most severe cases, transient systemic steroid therapy may be indicated. Several medications may be the source of drug-induced lichen planus, such as antituberculous drugs (ethionamide or isoniazid), antimalarial agents, or cyclines. Although an association with hepatitis C has been reported in certain zones, such an underlying infection appears very unusual in our African experience. In every variant, postlesional hyperchromia is common and often marked, but usually fades with time.

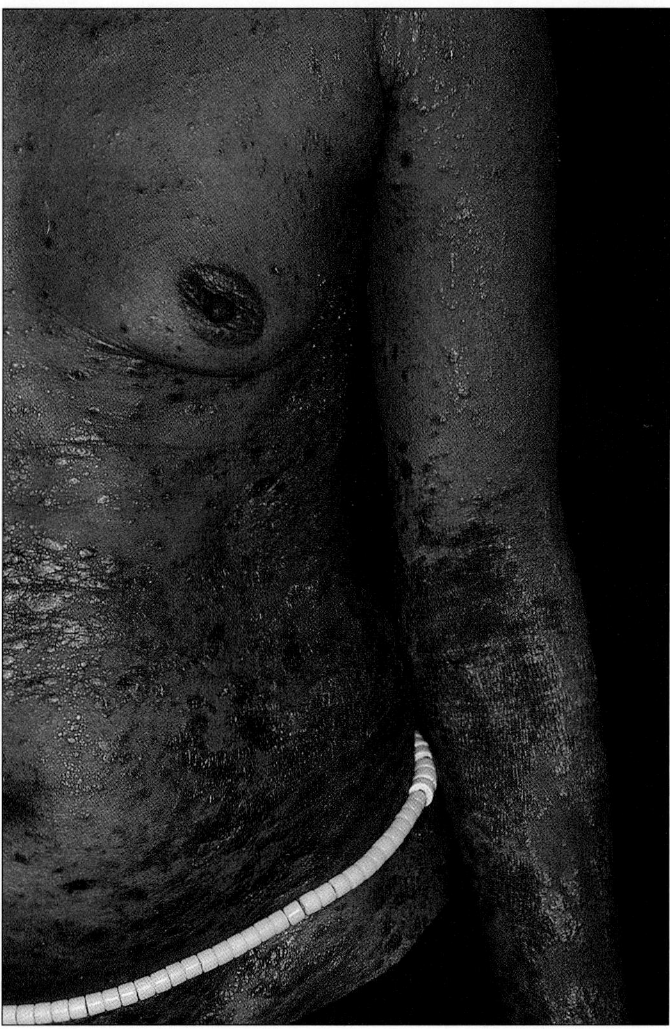

Figure 34.9 Lichen planus with prominent associated hyperchromia.

Melasma

Synonyms:

- Melasma, chloasma

Melasma is common on light- and intermediate-pigmented skins. It is mainly observed in women, but men may be affected, without any hormonal explanation.[10] It is easily identified by the presence of dark macules on malar areas and cheeks, or, more rarely, the upper lip, lateral sides of mandibular areas, or the forehead. Differential diagnosis mainly includes sunlight-related reactions to various topical compounds, such as perfumes or plants (berloque dermatitis), or, quite commonly today, hydroquinone-based cosmetics. Treatment is difficult, and relies on suppression of any predisposing factors such as estrogen intake, high-level sun protection, and careful use of topical lightening agents such as hydroquinone, tretinoin, or the association of both with topical steroids.

Fixed drug reaction

This is a common variant of drug reaction to various compounds after oral or parenteral intake, characterized by the occurrence of round to oval pigmenting macules, either isolated or multiple, that at each intake of a specific drug present inflammatory, eventually bullous, exacerbations (Fig. 34.10). In the tropics, the drugs most commonly responsible are antimicrobial agents (especially sulfonamides), antipyretics, or antiinflammatory agents. The only treatment is to withhold any intake of the responsible drug.

Exogenous ochronosis

This is a common complication of the chronic, long-lasting use of skin-lightening products containing hydroquinone. Occurrence has been reported to be high in certain areas such as South Africa, yet it seems less important in other geographical zones despite wide use of those type of compounds.[11] It is characterized by the occurrence on certain sun-exposed areas (mainly the neck, shoulder, and face) of very dark areas with progressive thickening of the skin, that becomes rough on palpation, with a typical "caviar-like" superficial aspect (Fig. 34.11).[12] "Punched-out" zones of normal-looking skin may be present among ochronotic areas. Histology, which in general is not necessary for diagnosis, typically shows the presence of dysmorphic ochronotic fibers in the dermis, with strange shapes; rarely, there may be a granulomatous infiltrate, that should raise suspicion of associated sarcoidosis. There is no treatment for this disfiguring disease, except stopping use of lightening procedures; in general this will allow the lesions to be less visible due to suppression of the contrast with adjacent skin.

Syphilis

Although the hypochromic variant of secondary syphilis is classic (collier de Vénus), it appears that, more often, lesions can be deeply pigmented on dark skin (Fig. 34.12). The presentation can be very close to that of lichen planus. Clinical suspicion relies

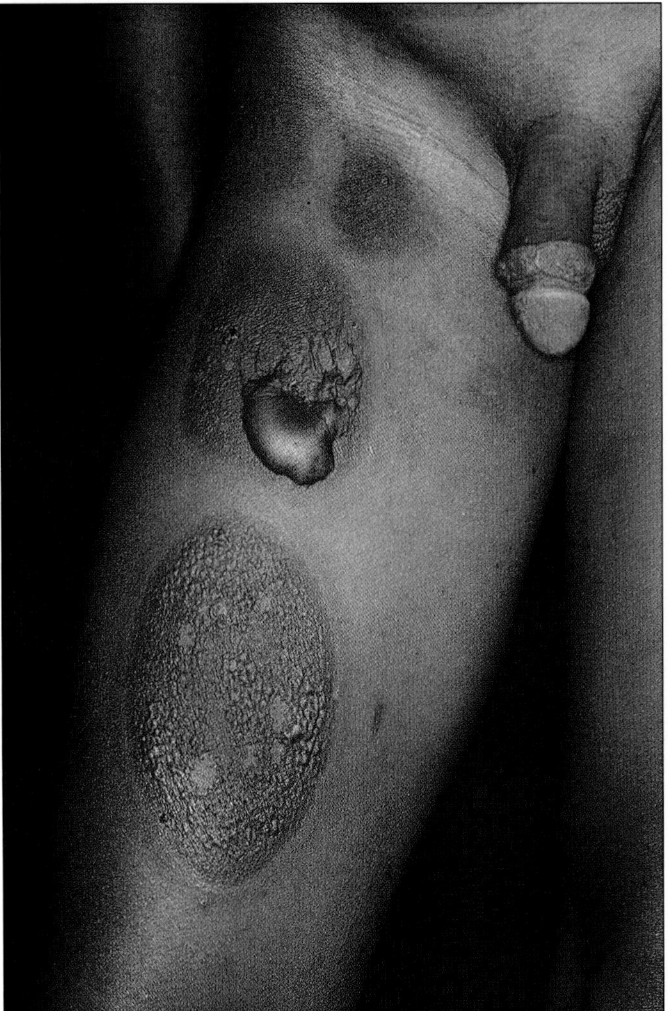

Figure 34.10 Fixed drug eruption at various stages.

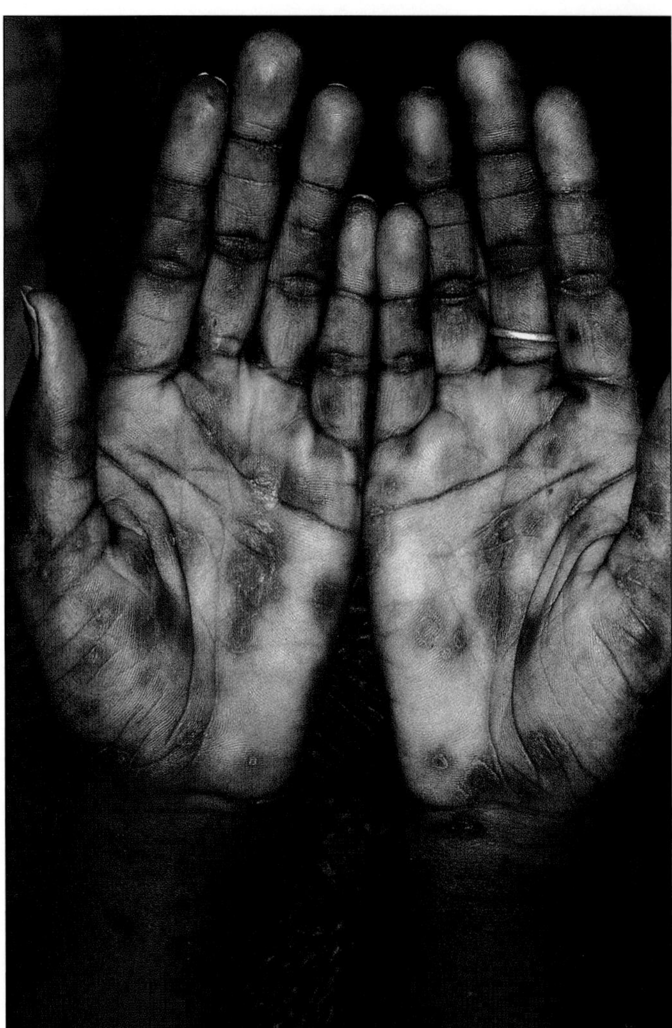

Figure 34.12 Typical palmar pigmenting papular lesions of secondary syphilis.

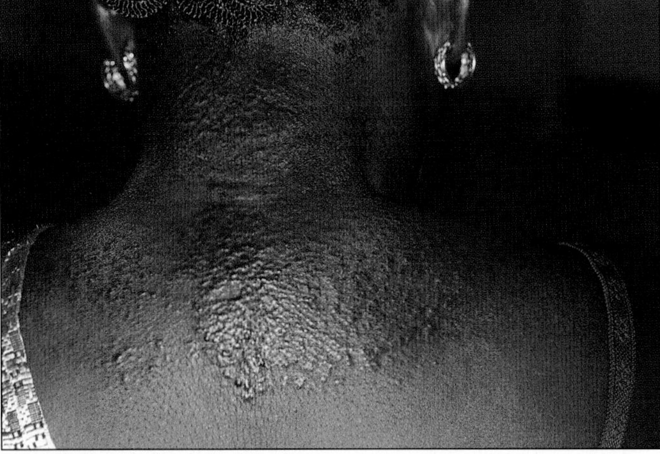

Figure 34.11 Exogenous ochronosis in a long-standing user of hydroquinone-based bleaching products.

on other characteristic signs of the disease, i.e., involvement of palms and soles or genitalia, presence of papules with a coppery aspect, annular shape of lesions, mucosal involvement, or general symptoms. It may be difficult to differentiate physiologic palmoplantar pigmented macules from syphilitic lesions, but one should remember that physiologic macules are much less numerous on palms, and are never papular. Serological tests for syphilis are indicated, if this diagnosis is suspected.

Melanoderma

In the tropics and/or on dark skin, several causes should be included on the list of internal disorders possibly associated with melanoderma, mainly pernicious anemia (with a typical dark pigmentation of palms and soles) and HIV infection. In HIV infection, pigmentation may be generalized, or restricted to nail folds. A distinctive picture of "blue nails" has been described in Uganda in HIV-infected people (Fig. 34.13).[13] Zidovudine can also be responsible for this presentation, as can several antimitotic drugs.

Pellagra

Pellagra is related to severe lack of niacin intake. Pseudopellagra refers to changes in niacin metabolism in people with chronic and severe alcohol intake. The clinical presentation is usually that of hyperchromic areas with superficial scaling and well-delineated margins, involving sun-exposed areas, mainly the neck (Casal's necklace), dorsum of the hands, and forearms, but with the usual notable exception of the face. Other symptoms (diarrhea, dementia), are possible. Malnutrition is often severe.

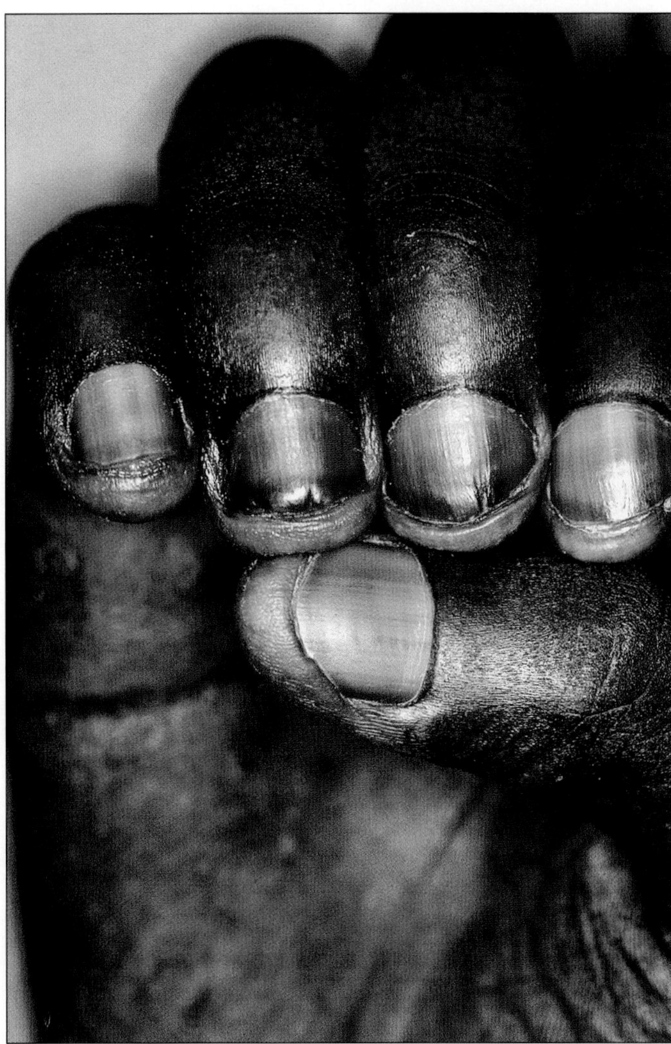

Figure 34.13 "Blue nails" associated with human immunodeficiency virus (HIV) infection.

Lichenoid melanodermatitis

Synonyms:
- Tropical lichen planus, actinic lichen planus

This rare disorder is characterized by the occurrence of rounded, pigmented maculopapular lesions typically encircled by a white halo, and occurring mainly on the face.[14] There is a pseudomelasma variant. It is observed in Northern Africa, the Middle East, and Kenya, but seems rare in other areas. The main differential diagnoses are classical lichen planus and lupus erythematosus.

Ashy dermatitis

Synonym:
- Erythema dyschromicum perstans

Cases of this disease have only been reported in South and Central America, where it seems to involve mainly people of mixed ethnic descent.[15] It is characterized by the occurrence over years of hyperpigmented areas, with a typically slightly raised border. The characteristic ashy tint, related to the migration of pigmentary incontinence deep into the dermis, however, is not always present and is not specific. Lupus erythematosus, especially in its subacute variant, should be excluded, as well as the macular variant of lichen planus.[9] Treatment is difficult, but the condition may improve with clofazimine.

Frictional dermal melanocytosis

Chronic friction of skin may be responsible on moderately pigmented skin for the occurrence of hyperpigmentation with an irregular pattern, mainly in front of bony prominences.[16]

Tumoral hyperchromias

Several tumoral disorders may be accompanied by intense pigmentation. Dermatosis papulosa nigra is an ethnic, topographical variant of seborrheic keratosis usually seen in middle-aged or older persons; it consists of small papules occurring on the face and upper trunk, often with a familial context. Basal cell carcinomas are rare on dark skin, on which they are generally hyperpigmented. The purple tint of Kaposi's sarcoma is often difficult to evaluate on dark skin, on which lesions present often with a dark, eventually black, tint. Bowen's disease and bowenoid papulosis should be differentiated from condyloma acuminatum, that are commonly pigmented.

The main concern with the occurrence of a dark macule on the soles or palms is malignant melanoma. The identification of this potentially lethal disease is difficult because of the common presence of physiologic pigmented macules on the same sites in people with dark skin. The recent occurrence of a pigmented lesion is an essential clue that the lesion should be biopsied, because classical features of malignancy often appear late in the course (Fig. 34.14). Tinea nigra is another possible differential diagnosis, that can be easily excluded by a simple mycologic examination. An early skin biopsy is the key for a diagnosis of malignant melanoma and for a chance of cure. The same is true for melanoma of the nail fold, that should be considered in the presence of any acquired isolated pigmented lesion under the nail in an adult.

The cosmetic use of skin-bleaching products

This has become a major dermatological issue in many sub-Saharan African countries, with growing importance.[17] The cosmetic use of products with the aim of lightening the skin has many dermatological consequences, including eventual occurrence of pigmenting disorders.

Epidemiology

Epidemiological studies in certain capitals of sub-Saharan African countries, such as Mali or Senegal, have found very high prevalence rates of the use of bleaching products among adult women (e.g., 25% of adult women in Bamako). In general, only dark-skinned women use these products, although certain men occasionally do also.

Current modalities of skin-bleaching in sub-Saharan Africa

The most frequently used bleaching products are hydroquinone preparations, often at high concentrations, topical superpotent steroids, caustic agents, and, more rarely today, mercury-based soaps. Products are generally applied on the whole body, once

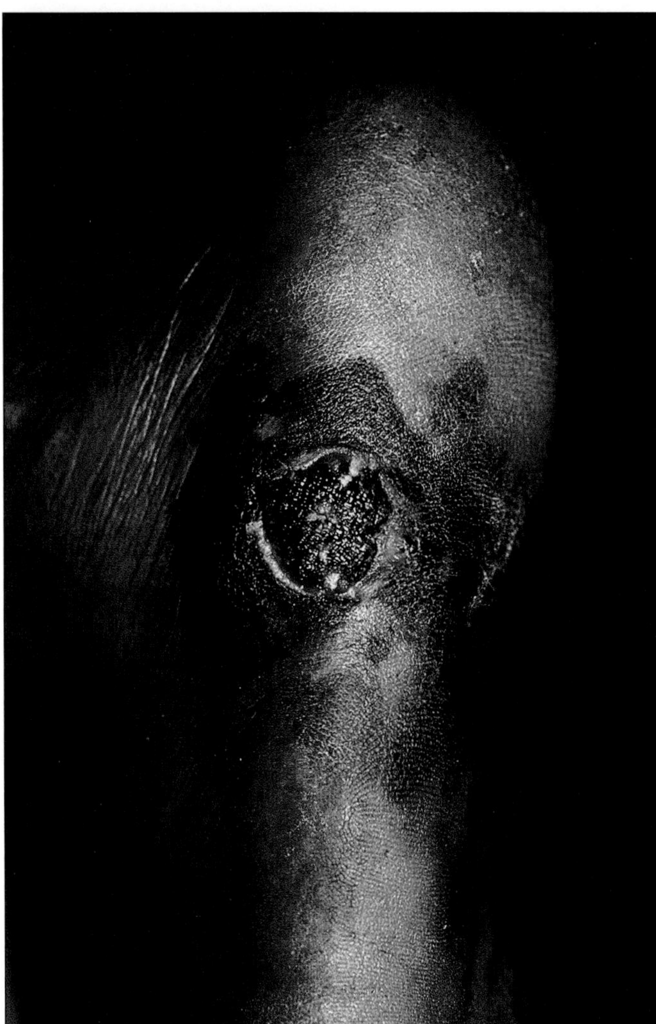

Figure 34.14 Late-stage malignant melanoma of the sole.

or twice a day, sometimes for years. The compounds are easily found in popular markets at low prices, with no need for a medical prescription.

Main complications

General complications

Nephrotoxicity and neurotoxicity of mercurial compounds are well-known. More recently, it has been suggested that cosmetic steroid use may be a risk factor for hypertension and diabetes mellitus.[18]

Dermatologic complications[17]

Pigmenting disorders are common: hyperchromic exogenous ochronosis, periocular berloque dermatitis-like hyperpigmentation, and achromic vitiligo-like lesions are the main variants; poikilodermic aspects at the base of the neck are also possible. Today, due to the wide use of superpotent steroids, common complications of this practice are widespread dissemination of superficial mycoses or scabies, or eventually serious bacterial sepsis, such as cellulitis. Another type of complication consists in the modifications of the presentation of coincidental skin diseases, resulting in the hiding of characteristic features, such as hypochromia in leprosy.[19]

References

1. Olumide YM. Depigmentation in black African patients. Int J Dermatol 1990; 29:166–174.
2. Mahé A, ed. Dermatologie sur peau noire. Paris, France: Doin; 2000.
3. Guillet G, Hélénon R, Gauthier Y et al. Progressive macular hypomelanosis of the trunk: primary acquired hypopigmentation. J Cutan Pathol 1988; 15:286–289.
4. Barnicot NA. Albinism in south western Nigeria. Ann Eugen 1952; 17:38–73.
5. Luande J, Henschke CL, Mohammed N. The Tanzanian human albino skin. Natural history. Cancer 1985; 55:1823–1828.
6. Lambroza E, Cohen SR, Phelps R et al. Hypopigmented variant of mycosis fungoides: demography, histopathology, and treatment of seven cases. J Am Acad Dermatol 1995; 32:987–993.
7. Liao YL, Chiang YC, Tsai TF et al. Contact leukomelanosis induced by the leaves of Piper betle L. (Piperaceae): a clinical and histopathologic survey. J Am Acad Dermatol 1999; 40:583–589.
8. Mahé A, Faye O, Thiam N'Diaye H et al. Definition of an algorithm for the management of common skin diseases at a primary health care level in sub-Saharan African. Trans R Soc Trop Med Hyg 2005; 99:39–47.
9. Bhutani LK, Bedi TR, Pandhi RK et al. Lichen planus pigmentosus. Dermatologica 1974; 149:43–50.
10. Vazquez M, Maldonado H, Benmaman C et al. Melasma in men. Int J Dermatol 1988; 27:25–27.
11. Hardwick N, Van Gelder LW, Van der Merwe CA et al. Exogenous ochronosis: an epidemiological study. Br J Dermatol 1989; 120:229–238.
12. Findlay GH, Morrison JGL, Simson IW. Exogenous ochronosis and pigmented colloid milium from hydroquinone bleaching creams. Br J Dermatol 1975; 93:613–622.
13. Sheppard B. Blue nails are a sign of HIV infection. Int J STD AIDS 1999; 10:479–482.
14. Verhagen ARHB, Koten JW. Lichenoid melanodermatitis. Br J Dermatol 1979; 101:651–658.
15. Knox JM, Dodge BG, Freeman RG. Erythema dyschromicum perstans. Arch Dermatol 1968; 97:262–272.
16. Sharquie KE, Al-Dorky MK. Frictional dermal melanosis (Lifa disease) over bony prominences. J Dermatol 2001; 28:12–15.
17. Mahé A, Ly F, Aymard G et al. Skin diseases associated with the cosmetic use of bleaching products in women from Dakar, Senegal. Br J Dermatol 2003; 148:493–500.
18. Raynaud E, Cellier C, Perret JL. Dépigmentation cutanée à visée cosmétique: enquête de prévalence et effets indésirables dans une population féminine sénégalaise. Ann Dermatol Venereol 2001; 128:720–724.
19. Mahé A, Ly F, Badiane C et al. Irrational use of skin-bleaching products can delay the diagnosis of leprosy. Int J Lepr 2002; 70:119–121.

Chapter 35

Environmental causes of dermatitis

- **Plant dermatitis** ▪ *Joao Paulo Niemeyer-Corbellini and Omar Lupi*
- **Tropical bites and stings** ▪ *Dirk M. Elston*
- **Marine/freshwater dermatology** ▪ *Mathijs Brentjens, Karan K. Sra, Vidal Haddad Junior, Patricia Lee and Stephen K. Tyring*

Plant dermatitis

Joao Paulo Niemeyer-Corbellini and Omar Lupi

Synonym: Plant dermatitis

Key features:

- Plant dermatitis may be produced by different plant species
- It is increasing in incidence worldwide
- It may be classified as mechanical injury, primary irritant (toxic) dermatitis, allergic phytodermatitis, and contact urticaria
- Acute cases present as linear urticarial, erythematous, and blistering lesions that may leave hyperpigmented macules
- Chronic cases present as lichenified, scaling dermatitis
- Diagnosis includes a history and physical examination, identification of plant species, and patch testing
- Treatment is symptomatic, including wet soaks, topical steroids, and antihistamines. More severe cases need systemic steroids

Introduction

Plant dermatitis or phytodermatitis is a skin eruption produced by different plant species.[1] It has been known to humans since it was first recorded by ancient farmers, such as the Assyrians, 4000 years ago.[2] Trees, flowers, grasses, vegetables, fruits, weeds, and air-borne pollens may produce it. However, those plants known to cause phytodermatitis belong to just a few families and plant sensitizers belong to closely related chemicals.[3] Plant dermatitis is more common in hot climates, not only because of greater exposure as less clothes are worn, but also because hot-climate plants seem to have a wider variety of chemicals.[3]

Almost everyone is subject to exposure to plants every day, whether at work or to those plants used as food or ornaments. Exposure at work represents an occupational dermatitis affecting mostly farmers, gardeners, carpenters, florists, and field workers. There has been an increasing number of cases of plant dermatitis as more and more plant-derived products are used in health care and beauty.[4] Although some plant families have worldwide distribution, many have only been reported in tropical and subtropical areas, and this should be considered when dealing with individuals who have been in these areas. The reaction may be classified, in accordance with its mechanism, as mechanical injury (including pharmacological injury), primary irritant (toxic) dermatitis, allergic phytodermatitis, or contact urticaria.[1–6]

Mechanical injury

Lesions are produced directly by thorns, spines, and hairs present on the surface of the plant; palms, cacti, grasses, and cereals, etc. are sources. In addition to the injuries caused by their spines, cacti may contain structures called glochids that may produce allergic or granulomatous reactions. *Opuntia ficus indica*, prickly pear or sabra of the USA, Mexico, and the Mediterranean region, causes dermatitis through its glochids. Some families and genera of plants that have been reported to cause mechanical injury in tropical areas are shown in Table 35.1.[7]

The wound may be complicated by secondary infection, either bacterial or fungus, such as sporotrichosis. Thorns and spines near to joints may cause septic arthritis and when near bone may mimic bone tumors.[2] Pharmacological injury is the term used for lesions produced by some plant species, especially from the Urticaceae family,[2] that contain glandular hairs which inoculate pharmacologically active substances such as histamine, acetylcholine and 5-hydroxytryptamine, producing mechanical effects enhanced by the substance reaction.[5]

Contact dermatitis

Substances produced by the plant cause primary irritant (toxic) and allergic contact dermatitis. Commonly, the substance responsible for the dermatitis is a secondary product, not participating directly in the plant metabolism. The distribution of the substance in the plant is important for the occurrence of the reaction. It may be present on the surface of the plant, and a simple or casual contact

Table 35.1 Major families of tropical plants known to cause plant dermatitis[13]

Family	Example	Type of reaction	Distribution
Acanthaceae	Acanthus	M	Tropics and Mediterranean
Actinidiaceae	Actinidia chinensis Planchon (Kiwi fruit)	A/I/U	Tropical regions of eastern Asia, northern Australia, and the USA
Agavaceae	*Agave americana* L. (American aloe)	A/I/M	Tropics and subtropics
Alangiaceae		A/M	Tropical Africa and Asia
Alliaceae	*Allium sativum* L. (garlic) and *A. cepa* L. (onion)	A/I	Worldwide
Alstroemeriaceae	*Alstroemeria* L. (Peruvian lily)	A	Central and South America
Amaranthaceae	Amaranth	A/M	Tropical and temperate regions
Amaryllidaceae	Amaryllis	I	Tropics and subtropics
Anacardiaceae	*Anacardium occidentale* L. (cashew-nut tree), *Lithraea brasiliensis* (aroeira), and *Mangifera indica* L. (mango)	A	Tropical and warm temperate regions
Annonaceae	*Annona* spp. (custard apple, graviola, sugar apple)	I	Tropical USA
Apocynaceae	*Aspidosperma* spp.	A/I/M	Tropics
Araceae	*Philodendron* spp. and *Dieffenbachia* spp.	I	Tropics
Araliaceae	*Panax ginseng* C. Meyer (ginseng)	A	Tropical regions, particularly in Indo-Malaysia and tropical USA
Araucariaceae	*Araucaria angustifolia* Kuntze (Brazilian pine)	A/M	Southern hemisphere
Asteraceae (formerly Compositae)	*Parthenium hysterophorus* L. (feverfew, carrot weed) and some species of *Ambrosia*	A	Worldwide
Balanitaceae	*Balanites aegyptica* Del. (desert date)	M/P	Tropical Africa to Myanmar
Bignoniaceae	*Jacaranda brasiliana* Pers. (jacaranda)	A/I	Tropics
Bombacaceae	*Adansonia digitata* L. (baobab, sour gourd)	M	Tropical areas, especially in Americas
Bromeliaceae	*Ananas comosus* Merrill (pineapple)	I/M	Tropical USA and the West Indies
Cactaceae	*Opuntia ficus-indica* Miller (Indian fig cactus, common sabra)	M	Arid regions of Americas
Cannabaceae	*Cannabis sativa* L. (marijuana)	A	Tropical and temperate regions
Caricaceae	*Carica papaya* L. (papaya)	I	Tropical regions of USA and Africa
Cecropiaceae	*Cecropia Loefl.* (trumpet tree)	I	Tropical USA
Cleomaceae	*Cleome* L. spp. (spider plant)	I	Tropics and subtropics
Crypteroniaceae	*Dactylocladus stenostachya* Oliver (jongkong, medang tabak)	I	Tropical Asia
Cucurbitaceae	Gourds, squashes, pumpkins and cucumbers	I	Tropics
Dilleniaceae	*Davilla rugosa* Poiret (fire vine)	I	Tropics and subtropics
Dioscoreaceae	*Dioscorea* spp.	I	Tropical and warm temperate regions
Ehretiaceae	*Cordia goeldiana* Huber (Brazilian walnut)	A	Tropics and subtropics
Erythroxylaceae	*Erythroxylum coca* Lam. (cocaine)	I	Tropics
Euphorbiaceae	*Hevea brasiliensis* Muell. Arg. (rubber)	A/I/M	Worldwide
Ginkgoaceae	*Ginkgo biloba*	A	Widely cultivated and perhaps found wild in eastern China
Graminae	Most food grains such as rice, oat, corn, and wheat	A/I/M/U	Worldwide
Iridaceae	*Iris* spp.	A/I	Southern Africa and tropical USA
Jubulaceae	*Frullania* sp. (liverworts)	A	Tropics and subtropics
Lecythidaceae	*Bertholletia excelsa* (Brazil-nut tree)	A	Tropical USA
Leguminosae	*Dalbergia nigra* (Brazilian rosewood) and *Mucuna pruriens* (buffalo bean)	I	Worldwide

Continued

Table 35.1 Major families of tropical plants known to cause plant dermatitis[13]—cont'd

Family	Example	Type of reaction	Distribution
Liliaceae	*Aloe* spp., *Asparagus* spp.	A	Worldwide
Lythraceae	*Lawsonia inermis* (henna tree)	I/U	Worldwide
Malvaceae	*Gossypium hirsutum* (cotton)	A/PP	Tropics and subtropics
Meliaceae	*Khaya* spp. (African mahogany)	A	Warm regions
Moraceae	*Ficus carica* (fig)	A/P	Tropics and subtropics
Palmae or Arecaceae	*Cocos nucifera* L. (coconut), *Copernicia cerifera* (wax palm, carnauba palm)	I	Tropics and subtropics
Rutaceae	Citrus limon (lemon)	P	Tropics and temperate regions
Solanaceae	*Capsicum annuum* (cayenne pepper, paprika, chilli, tabasco)	I	Central and South America
Urticaceae	Nettles	U	Tropical and temperate regions
Zingiberaceae	*Zingiber officinalis* (ginger)	I	Tropical regions, especially Indo-Malaysia

A, allergic phytodermatitis; I, primary irritant contact dermatitis; M, mechanical injury; P, phytophotodermatitis; PP, pseudophytophotodermatitis; U, contact urticaria.

may be sufficient to cause dermatitis, or it may be situated deeper in the plant structure or in its root, and in this case, the plant needs to be crushed in order to produce the disease.[1,2,6] Equally important is the relative quantity of these substances, and this depends on different factors such as stage of maturity, hydration level, soil type, and climatic conditions.[1]

Primary irritant contact dermatitis is produced by direct chemical irritation, without an allergic mechanism. Everyone who is exposed is expected to react, unless the degree of exposure, including concentration of the chemical and duration of contact, is not sufficient. Irritation is caused by chemicals present in the plant such as proteolytic enzymes (i.e., Bromeliaceae family), oxalic, formic and acetic acids, glycosides, isothiocyanates, and crystals of calcium oxalate.[8] *Mucuna pruriens*, also known as itch plant, produces a proteolytic enzyme named mucunine, which is used by practical jokers as the major ingredient of "itching powder."[3] Pineapple (*Ananas comosus*), which contains calcium oxalate and a proteolytic enzyme called bromelin, is a common cause of occupational phytodermatitis in less-developed tropical countries, where workers contract hand dermatitis as a result of fruit juice handling.[2] *Dieffenbachias* spp. and *Philodendrons* spp. are genera of tropical plants of Central and South America that produce irritant dermatitis by bundles of needle-like calcium oxalate known as raphides.[6,7] Some families and genera of plants that have been reported to cause primary irritant contact dermatitis in tropical areas are shown in Table 35.1.[7]

First described in 1942 by Klaber, phytophotodermatitis is a very common skin disease within the irritant contact dermatitis group. It consists of an acute phototoxic reaction, usually caused by contact with substances known as furocoumarins (5-methoxypsoralen, limettin, isopimpinellin, bergapten, and xanthotoxin) followed by sun exposure, specifically in the ultraviolet A (UVA) range, which is 320–400 nm.[8] Many cases are occupational in nature, but nowadays this disorder is becoming more widespread as more people apply to their skin products varying from home remedies to trademark preparations that contain photosensitizing agents.[9] In the tropics, these substances have mostly been found in plants of the Rutaceae and Moraceae families. Citrus fruits such as lime (*Citrus aurantifolia*), lemon (*C. limon*), and grapefruit (*C. paradisi*) of the Rutaceae family and fig (*Ficus carica*) of the Moraceae family are commonly occurring plants that contain these photosensitizing substances.[7,9] Furocoumarins in lime pulp are 13–182 times less concentrated than those in the peel.[9] Berloque dermatitis results from the application of perfumes or colognes containing oil of bergamot which comprises 5-methoxypsoralen.[2]

Fig, a member of the Moraceae family, has been described as an important causative agent of burns and bullous dermatitis during the summer months in countries of the Middle East and Mediterranean, as well as tropical and subtropical areas of the USA.[10] In Brazil, fig leaves have long been used as a tanning agent, resulting in several cases of phototoxic dermatitis being seen in dermatologic clinics (Fig. 35.1).[10]

Sometimes the furocoumarin substance is not produced by the plant itself, but, for example, by fungi infecting the plant. This is called pseudophytophotodermatitis.[2] Table 35.1 shows some families and genera reported to cause phytophotodermatitis in tropical areas.

Many cases fall in the group of allergic phytodermatitis, which is a type IV hypersensitivity reaction (delayed reaction). Previous contact with the plant or a phylogenetically correlated species must have occurred in order for the hypersensitivity to have taken place. The sensitization may occur in 7–10 days after the first contact with the plant, as well as several years after exposure. The sensitizing agent is usually present in the oleoresin fraction which may be distributed throughout the plant and in the pollen.[3] The oleoresin is a mixture of aldehydes, aromatic alcohols, terpenic compounds, aliphatic and aromatic esters, and phenols, including catechols, resorcinols, and hydroquinones.[6]

In the Americas, the great majority of cases occurs after contact with plants of the Anacardiaceae family, which contains potent hydroxylated benzenes (catechols).[1] The antigenic substance is the urushiol or 3-*n*-pentadecyl-catechol. Several genera may be

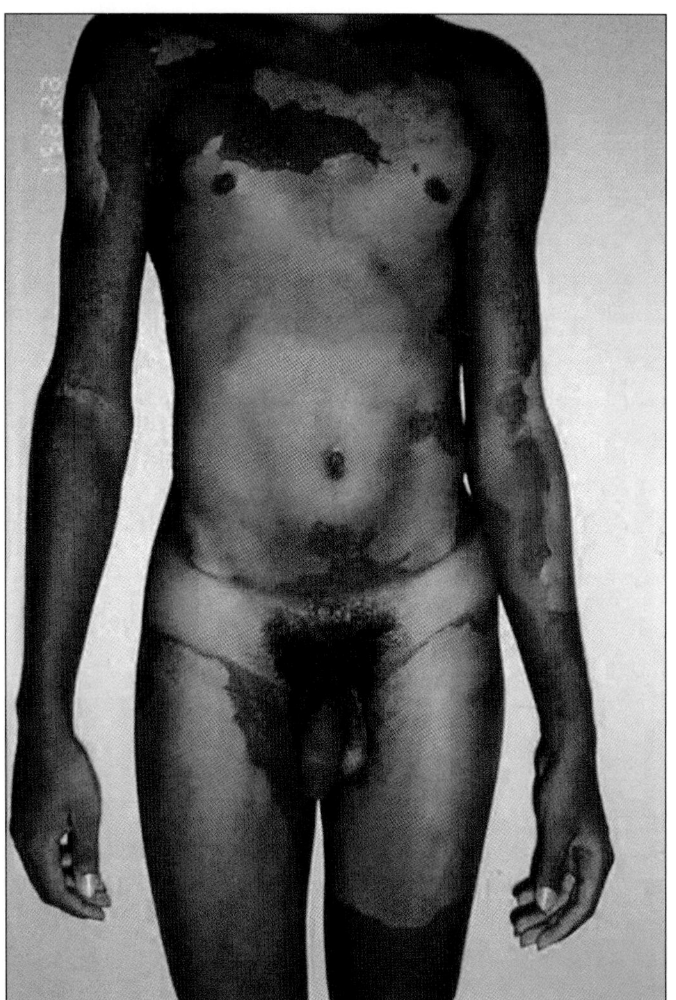

Figure 35.1 Severe case of phototoxic dermatitis due to fig leaves (*Ficus carica*).

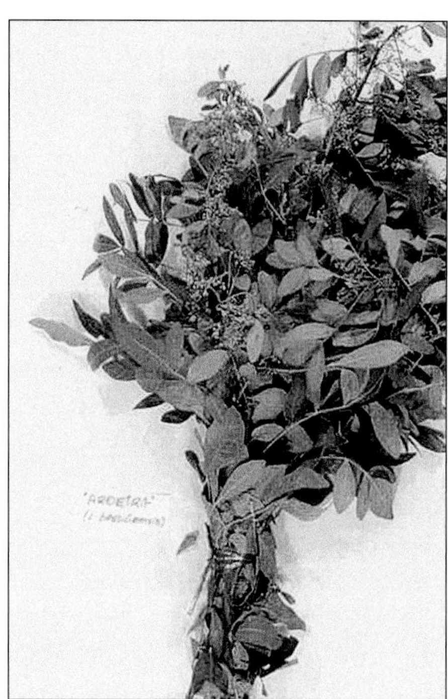

Figure 35.2 Aroeira (*Lithraeae brasiliensis*), used in popular medicine to relieve pruritus.[14]

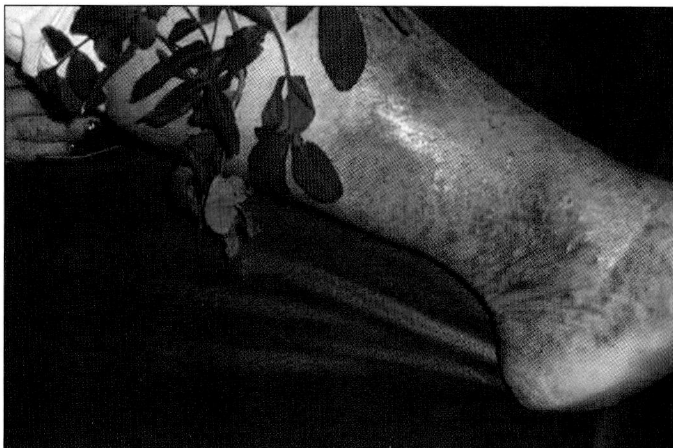

Figure 35.3 Contact dermatitis on lower limb due to aroeira.

found in tropical areas of South America, the most studied being Lithraeae (Fig. 35.2). Other members of the family include cashew nut tree (*Anacardium occidentale*), mango (*Mangifera indica*), Brazilian pepper tree (*Schinus terebinthifolius*), Indian marking nut tree (*Semecarpus anacardium*), Japanese lacquer tree (*Toxicodendron verniciflua*), *S. coriacea* in the Indian subcontinent, *Rhus verniciflua*, and *R. succedaneum* in Australia and New Zealand.[4,7,11]

The ginkgo tree (*Ginkgo biloba*) that belongs to the Ginkyoaceae family also contains urushiol and is considered together with members of the Anacardiaceae family.[7] In Brazil some reactions are due not only to working exposure but also to its use in popular medicine. In these particular cases, aroeira (*Lithraeae brasiliensis*) is use most frequently, for wound care as well as in the treatment of ulcerative lesions in lower limbs (Fig. 35.3), joint pain, diarrhea, and bronchitis. Cross-reactivity may occur with other members of the Anacardiaceae family, due to structural similarity, including the *Toxicodendron* (formerly *Rhus*) genus, which is quite common in the USA.[1]

The Asteraceae (formerly Compositae) family includes some genera that may be found in tropical regions and in which the sensitizers are sesquiterpene lactones.[2] *Parthenium hysterophorus* (carrot-weed) was accidentally introduced in India, where it is now an important source of cases of allergic phytodermatitis, affecting up to 4% of the exposed population.[2] The liverwort (*Frullania* spp.) is responsible for reactions mostly in forest workers of tropical and subtropical regions.[7] The antigen is also sesquiterpene lactones, which cross-react with members of the Asteraceae family. *Philodendron* spp., a member of the Araceae family, may cause allergic dermatitis: the sensitizer substance is resorcinols.[12]

Balsam of Peru may cause allergic dermatitis, and shows cross-reactivity with perfumes and cinnamon, orange, and other flavors. Exposure may occur as early as in baptismal procedures from chrism oil.[3]

Fig trees contain a milky sap which may produce allergic dermatitis.[3] In Africa, bee glue (propolis), which is used as wood and leather varnish, and as a base for ointments, cosmetics, and polishes may produce allergic dermatitis.[3]

An erythema multiforme-like eruption from Brazilian rosewood (*Dalbergia nigra*) was reported in a carpenter in whom a patch test with wood dust produced a positive reaction.[13]

Some families and genera of plants that have been reported to cause allergic phytodermatitis in tropical areas are shown in Table 35.1.[7]

Contact urticaria

This type of reaction may have two different mechanisms. Non-immune contact urticaria is an immunoglobulin E (IgE)-independent reaction, which may be induced by nettles, and plant extracts such as cinnamic aldehyde, cinnamic acid, and balsam of Peru.[7] On the other hand, allergic contact urticaria is an IgE-dependent reaction that may be produced by plant extracts such as natural rubber, which is derived from *Hevea brasiliensis*. Individuals sensitive to rubber may cross-react with banana and apple.[4] *Actinidia chinensis* Planchon (kiwi fruit) has been reported to cause type I hypersensitivity in tropical areas of eastern Asia, northern Australia, and the USA.[7]

Ingested plants may induce urticarial lesions and anaphylaxis, as occurs in individuals who are allergic to peanuts.[4] Atopic patients are more prone to this kind of reaction.[4,5]

Table 35.1 shows some families and genera reported to cause contact urticaria in tropical areas.[7]

Clinical features

A detailed history is necessary to determine the likely source of exposure. It usually involves the hands, forearms, and face, including the eyelids. The perioral region is most affected in reactions caused by fruits, such as in dermatitis caused by mango.[6,11] In mechanical lesions, the clinical manifestations depend on agent shape and injury mechanism. In lesions produced by the Indian fig (*Opuntia ficus indica*), glochids present at its surface, penetrate the skin, and a tinea corporis-like dermatitis is formed, sometimes with granuloma formation – a condition called sabra dermatitis.[8] In pharmacological dermatitis the lesion assumes the characteristic physiologic changes of the active substance in the contact area.

In other cases, individuals present with acute urticarial, erythematous, and/or vesicobullous dermatitis. They usually present as linear or bizarre lesions, reflecting the contact with the plant. Chronic cases present as lichenified lesions and chronic fissuring or scaling dermatitis (Fig. 35.4). Fissuring and hyperkeratosis of the fingertips and subungual hyperkeratosis may be the only manifestation. This is the case, for example, for lesions provoked by onion (*Allium cepa*) and garlic (*A. sativum*).[11] The dermatitis may be that of a volatile pattern, such as in air-borne pollen dermatitis, with lesions involving mostly the exposed areas and resembling a light-aggravated dermatitis.[3,5] Patients who evolved to an actinic chronic dermatitis following the acute phase of disease have been reported.[1] Contact dermatitis from some wood-dust can resemble seborrheic dermatitis or neurodermatitis.

In phytophotodermatitis the clinical picture is that of sunburn, ranging from mild erythema to severe blistering at the site of exposure. Residual hyperpigmented, linear streaks represent the final stage of the disease and may remain for a long time.[8,9] Stinging or burning sensations usually accompany it. Individuals of skin type IV–VI may present with just hyperpigmentation without any previous signs or symptoms of acute dermatitis.[9]

In photoallergic contact dermatitis the clinical features are those of an allergic contact dermatitis which is aggravated by sun exposure and that occurs especially in sun-exposed areas.

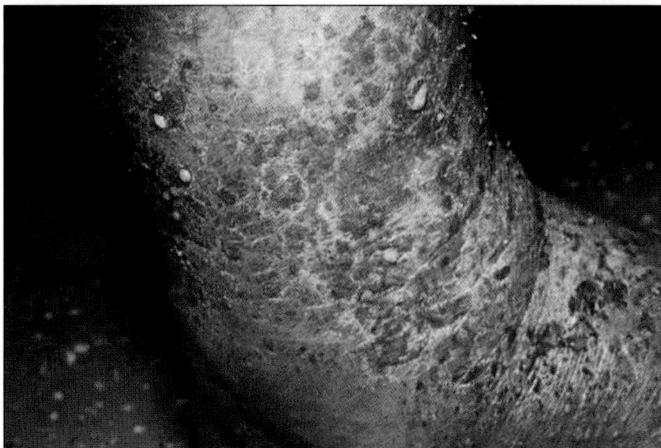

Figure 35.4 Chronic case of contact dermatitis due to aroeira, manifest as lichenified lesions and scaling dermatitis.

Diagnosis

The diagnosis may not be evident when the patient does not present with the typical manifestations. Therefore, a history of working and leisure exposure to tropical plants or plant derivatives such as herbal remedies, spices and foods, woods, and fragrances is important in the diagnosis of phytodermatitis. When suspected, samples of the contacting plant, if available, should be obtained and brought to the physician. This sample should be divided into three parts. One part is used to identify the plant: this may be carried out by an expert botanist. The other parts are used for patch testing and for additional chemical studies. The first patch test should be limited to the group of plant families usually reported to cause plant dermatitis, in order to prevent unnecessary patch testing with popular but innocuous plants. If this is negative, subsequent testing may be necessary for diagnosis. Testing with known irritant plants should be avoided. When testing an unknown plant, several control volunteers are necessary to consider the value of a positive patch testing. The leaves are usually used for patch testing; however, sometimes the antigen is located in a different organ of the plant, in which case this plant part should be used for testing.[5] In the setting of a photoallergic contact dermatitis, photopatch testing is an important tool to confirm the diagnosis.[1]

Histological examination shows an upper dermal perivascular infiltrate rich in both eosinophils and lymphocytes, lymphocytic exocytosis, and epidermal spongiosis (Fig. 35.5).

The occurrence of cross-sensitization is a real problem; however true cases are not common and most cases represent false cross-sensitivity. This may occur when the same sensitizing chemical is present in two or more plant species.[5]

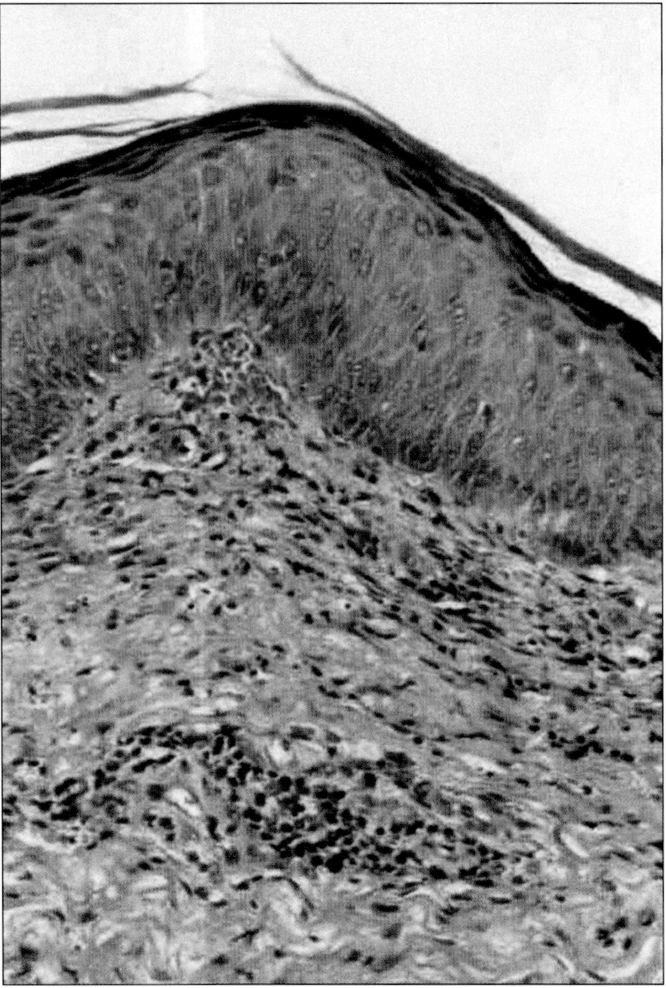

Figure 35.5 Contact dermatitis due to plants with a mild acanthosis and upper dermal perivascular infiltrate rich in both eosinophils and lymphocytes.

Differential diagnosis

In some cases the dermatitis may have not been produced by the plant itself, but herbicides, pesticides, fungicides, or fungi and arthropods infesting the plant may be the source of antigen.[5] This condition is called pseudophytodermatitis.[2,3] Appropriate history and physical examination and allergic testing should exclude other contact dermatitis and acute localized blistering diseases.

Prevention

Individuals should avoid contact with plants known to cause the dermatitis. Clothes and gloves do not always give complete protection. Workers with occupational dermatitis may stop working with one variety of plant or change to a job that does not involve contact with the allergen. A new topical product containing quaternium-18 bentonite, called Ivy Block, that interferes with cutaneous absorption of urushiol, is available in the USA for the prevention of poison-ivy dermatitis. It may be extrapolated that this product may be useful for dermatitis caused by other members of the Anacardiacae family. The dermatitis may persist or recur due to contact with cross-reacting chemicals present in other products or as a result of unwitting contact with the allergen.[5]

Management

Treatment involves avoidance and a symptomatic approach. Avoidance of further contact with the allergen remains the cornerstone of management. Acute dermatitis is treated with wet soaks and soothing creams. Topical steroids in a cream base may be tried to alleviate the burning and stinging sensation, but do not seem to alter the course of the disease. Oral antihistamines may help stop the pruritus. Severe cases require systemic steroids. Chronic and subacute cases should be treated with topical steroids in an ointment base and oral antihistamines. For hyperpigmentation following phytophotodermatitis, sunscreens may be of help and may be used as a prophylactic measure for individuals at high-risk. Resistant cases and patients who develop chronic actinic dermatitis may need to use azathioprine, cyclosporin, and psoralens and long-wave ultraviolet light (PUVA). Hyposensitization can be tried when reexposure cannot be avoided, but is difficult to achieve.[2,5]

References

1. Santos OR, Filgueira AL. Dermatites fitogenicas: a proposito de dois casos de fotossenbilizacao por aroeira. An Bras Dermatol 1994; 69:291–295.
2. Stoner JG, Rasmussen JE. Plant dermatitis. J Am Acad Dermatol 1983; 9:1–15.
3. Mitchell JC, Fisher AA. Dermatitis due to plants and spices. In: Fisher AA, ed. Contact dermatitis. Philadelphia, PA: Lea & Febiger; 1986:418–453.
4. Lovell CR. Phytodermatitis. Clin Dermatol 1997; 15:607–613.
5. Wilkinson JD, Shaw S. Contact dermatitis – allergic. In: Champion RH, ed. Textbook of dermatology. Oxford: Blackwell Science; 1998:733–819.
6. Sasseville D. Phytodermatitis. J Cutan Med Surg 1999; 3:263–279.
7. Botanical Dermatology Database website. Available online at: http://bodd.cardiff.ac.uk (accessed March 27, 2004).
8. Adams RM. Occupational skin disease. In: Freedberg IM, ed. Fitzpatrick's dermatology in general medicine. New York: McGraw-Hill; 1999:1609–1632.
9. Dominguez-Soto L, Hojyo-Tomoka MT, Vega-Memije E et al. Photodermatoses in tropical countries. Clin Dermatol 1999; 17:237–243.
10. Serpa SS, Lupi O, Oliveira WN et al. Queimaduras extensas provocadas pela folha da figueira (*Ficus carica*). An Bras Dermatol 1996; 71:443–446.
11. Sampaio SAP, Rivitti EA. Dermatoses ocupacionais. In: Sampaio SAP, Rivitti EA, eds. Dermatologia. Sao Paulo: Artes Medicas; 2000:991–998.
12. Knight TE. Philodendron-induced dermatitis: report of cases and review of the literature. Cutis 1991; 48:375–378.
13. Martin P, Bergoend H, Piette F. Erythema multiforme-like

eruption from Brazilian rosewood. 5th International Symposium on Contact Dermatitis. Barcelona; 1980.

14. Lupi O, Figueira A. Aroeira-induced photosensitization, Int J Dermatol 1994; 33(3): 222.

Tropical bites and stings

Dirk M. Elston

Tropical arthropods as vectors of disease

Key features:

- Tropical arthropods carry bacterial, protozoan, and helminthic pathogens
- Mosquitoes are the most important group of vectors
- Preventive strategies include repellents, insecticides, bed nets, and infrastructure improvement

Introduction

In tropical regions, arthropod vectors are responsible for huge numbers of deaths each year. Malaria remains a major cause of death in much of the world, and has been reintroduced into areas of the USA. In areas of Africa with high transmission rates, most severe cases occur in infants under 1 year of age and the clinical picture is dominated by severe anemia. In areas with lower transmission rates, cerebral malaria is more common.[1] Interventions such as insecticide-treated bed nets are critical to reduce the high death rate, especially in the first year of life.

Epidemiologic patterns of malaria are related to variations in the population of anopheline mosquitoes. The entomologic inoculation rate (EIR) is the product of the bite rate times the percentage of infected mosquitoes. This product serves as a predictor of malaria risk in a given area. In most areas, there is a linear relationship between the logarithm of the EIR and malaria prevalence. In areas with more than 15 infective bites per year, the prevalence of disease is >50%. The goal for vector-control programs is fewer than one infective bite per person per year.[2]

Yellow fever, transmitted by *Aedes aegypti* mosquitoes, caused epidemics in American cities during the seventeenth, eighteenth, and nineteenth centuries. In the twentieth and twenty-first centuries, it has mostly been found in tropical regions. The eradication of yellow fever from Cuba and Panama in the early part of the twentieth century was accomplished by means of vector control. One central principle in these eradication programs was the elimination of standing water where mosquitoes could breed.

Buruli ulcer is the third most common mycobacterial disease in humans, only surpassed in frequency by tuberculosis and leprosy. The bacterium is found in stagnant water, especially in rural areas where deforestation has led to flooding. Most patients are children who are infected either by direct inoculation through cuts and abrasions or via arthropod vectors. Implicated vectors include mosquitoes and aquatic bugs (Naucordiae) that harbor the bacterium in their salivary glands.

Scrub typhus, carried by chigger mites, affects an estimated one million people each year. The causative organism, *Orientia tsutsugamushi*, is no longer classified with the genus *Rickettsia*.[3] Severe systemic illness, including pneumonitis, can occur. Vector control is difficult, and control efforts center on personal protection.

Onchocerciasis (river blindness), is caused by *Onchocerca volvulus*, and transmitted by black flies, which breed in fast-flowing rivers. The disease has been endemic in tropical areas of Africa, Central America, and South America, but a global eradication campaign (the Onchocerciasis Control Program) has reduced the burden of disease. Adult worms reproduce for up to 14 years, creating microfilariae to be ingested by the vector. Vector control is the central strategy for disease reduction. Weekly helicopter spraying of larvacide as well as the contribution of free medication (i.e. ivermectin) for some 16 million people by Merck has almost eradicated the disease in the seven original target countries in Africa. An estimated 600 000 cases of blindness have been prevented.[4]

Pathogenesis

Not only does the vector spread the disease, but it may also influence the disease manifestations. When *Bartonella* organisms are transmitted by a flea, cat-scratch disease or bacillary angiomatosis occurs. In contrast, when *Bartonella* is transmitted by a louse, it is more likely to produce endocarditis.

Clinical features

Clinical features vary widely, depending on the disease that is transmitted. The bite itself may present as papular urticaria, but many are relatively asymptomatic. In tropical areas, individuals have high degrees of exposure to biting arthropods, and relative immune tolerance to the bites often occurs.

Pathology

The initial bite or sting is characterized by a wedge-shaped perivascular lymphoid infiltrate with eosinophils. These features are highly variable, and those who demonstrate immune tolerance to the bite demonstrate little histologic reaction.

Treatment

Prevention of disease transmission requires a knowledge of the vectors involved. Some vectors respond poorly to control efforts, and personal protection against bites is the mainstay of disease prevention. Other vectors can be controlled by area spraying and control of standing water. When traveling to malaria-endemic areas, mosquito netting, screening, protective clothing, repellents and chemoprophylaxis are important components of an effective disease prevention strategy. The vast majority of travelers who acquire malaria abroad have not complied with recommended steps for disease prevention, including the recommended chemoprophylactic drug regimen.[5] In endemic areas, mosquito-control programs have an excellent record of reducing the risk of mosquito-borne illness. Appropriate use of insecticides plays an important role in vector control, and has a favorable risk–benefit profile for those in the community.[6] The importance of window screens and avoidance of arthropods when they are feeding should be stressed. During a recent outbreak of Dengue virus in Mexico and South Texas, the incidence of disease was much higher in Mexico, although the mosquito vector was more abundant in Texas.[7] Anopheline mosquitoes that carry malaria tend to bite at night, while *Culex* mosquitoes tend to bite during the day. Prevention programs must consider the feeding habits of important disease vectors in the area.

Protective long-sleeved light-weight clothing can be treated with permethrin to provide a measure of protection against both crawling and flying arthropods. Permethrin is also used to treat screens and mosquito netting. Treated clothing can be combined with the use of a repellent to minimize the risk of disease. DEET (*N,N*-diethyl-3-methylbenzamide, previously called *N,N*-diethyl-*m*-toluamide) is effective against a wide range of arthropods. It can be applied to skin and clothing.

Consistent use of the repellent as well as other personal protective measures is essential while in a disease-endemic area. A study of 955 Australian Defense Force soldiers in East Timor showed that, although 84% of soldiers used repellents, only 19% used them daily. Bed net usage also differed significantly between groups of soldiers, and consistent use of bed nets was associated with a lower incidence of malaria.[8]

Although some evidence suggests that children are not any more sensitive than adults to toxic effects of DEET, the American Academy of Pediatrics recommends concentrations of 30% or less in products intended for use in children. As many such products are available, it seems prudent to adhere to these guidelines in most circumstances. Repeated applications of high concentrations of DEET have been associated with signs of toxic encephalopathy in some individuals. DEET can also occasionally produce erythematous or bullous irritant dermatitis.[9] Extended-duration formulations reduce the need for repeated applications.

Picaridin in concentrations of 9.3% picaridin or 19.2% picaridin compares favorably to 35% DEET gel, 20% controlled-release DEET, and 33% DEET in a polymer formulation (US Army Extended Duration Repellent). The higher concentration of picaridin performed better than the lower concentration.[10]

Neem oil has been used effectively in areas endemic for malaria.[11] Kerosene-burning lamps used to vaporize transfluthrin, a pyrethroid insecticide, can provide significant protection against *Culex* mosquitoes, and are useful during the pre-bedtime hours before mosquito nets are used.[12] Citronella candles have limited efficacy.[13]

Additional mosquito-control strategies include elimination of standing water, and stocking ponds and water barrels with selected fish or turtles to consume mosquito larvae. For limited areas, mosquito traps are helpful for area control. Mosquitoes are attracted to the trap by carbon dioxide, light, heat, and chemical attractants. Although octenol is commonly employed, some mosquitoes respond best to combinations of attractants, and some *Culex* mosquitoes are repelled by octenol. Propane-powered units are the most versatile and are effective for control of mosquitoes in limited areas.[14]

Arachnids

Mites (Arachnida: acarina)

Key features:

- Mesostegmatid mites infest mammals and birds
- Mites are ubiquitous in the environment and many can cause dermatologic disease
- In tropical countries, scabies infestation is a common cause of refractory impetigo

Introduction

Mites infest rodents (Fig. 35.6), wild birds, livestock, cheese, produce, and grains. They are widespread in the environment, and humans are commonly affected. Some mites act as disease vectors. Scabies infestation is a common cause of impetigo in tropical climates. The impetigo is typically refractory to treatment until the scabies infestation is treated.

Clinical features

Eschars at the site of a bite suggest a rickettsial disease. Honey-crusted lesions of impetigo commonly obscure the burrows of scabies infestation in tropical climates. Cutaneous reactions include papular, papulovesicular, bullous, urticarial, and morbilliform eruptions. Secondary infection is common. Bullous eruptions may

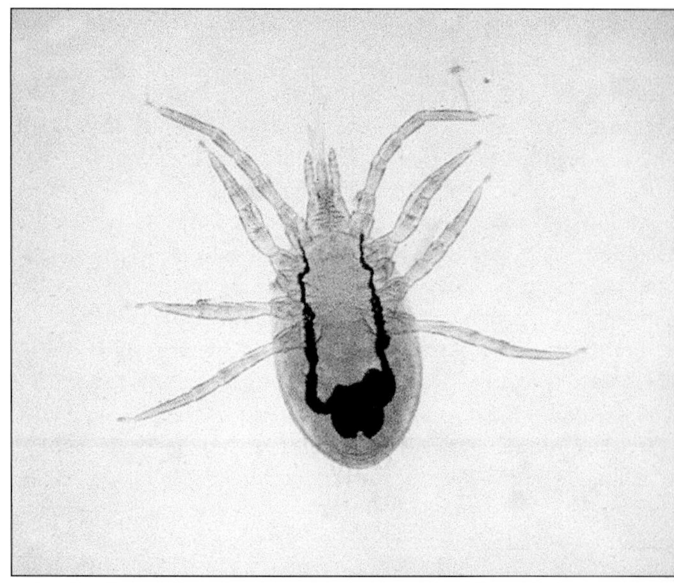

Figure 35.6 Tropical rat mite.

mimic bullous pemphigoid, even with positive immunofluorescent findings, and a high index of suspicion should be maintained.

Scrapings can identify scabies mites, and the burrows can become more apparent after the application of India ink or gentian violet and cleaning with alcohol. Zoonotic mites can be treated with lactic acid or lactophenol to improve visibility of identifying structures. Hoyer's medium is used for mounting. A qualified acarologist can be of immense help with identification. To prepare the mounting medium, 30 g of Arabic gum is mixed with 50 ml of distilled water. Chloral hydrate (200 g) is then added, followed by 20 g of glycerin. The mixture is filtered through cheese cloth.

Treatment

Some mites remain attached to the skin, and scabies mites burrow. Most mites simply "bite and run" on human skin, and the resulting hypersensitivity reaction is treated in a manner similar to other bites. Scabies mites are generally treated with topical agents such as permethrin, lindane, benzyl benzoate, and precipitated sulfur in petrolatum. Bird and bat roosts may have to be eliminated or treated with an insecticide. Some species are protected, which may complicate control efforts. Infested pets and livestock should be evaluated by a veterinarian. Personal protection with repellents and permethrin-treated clothing is important, especially in preventing infestation with a disease vector. Topical antipruritics containing camphor and menthol can be of immense value for symptomatic relief. Some topical anesthetics are potential contact allergens. Pramoxine has a low risk of contact allergy and is found in a wide variety of products. Class I topical corticosteroids are helpful for persistent cutaneous reactions. Intralesional triamcinolone may also be useful.

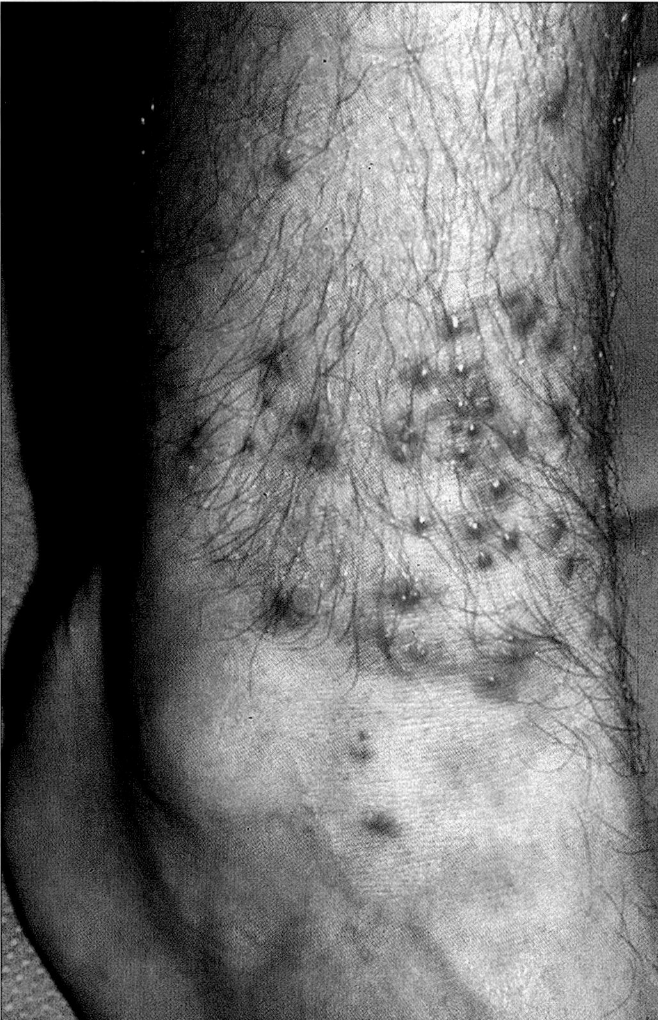

Figure 35.7 Chigger bites.

Chiggers

Introduction

Trombiculid chigger mites are a common cause of mite-induced dermatitis in brushy areas. The larval, six-legged mite is most commonly found attached to the host. The eight-legged nymph and adult stages are free-living, and found less commonly.

Clinical features

Chigger bites present as intensely pruritic grouped erythematous papules on the lower extremities (Fig. 35.7), waistline, and genitalia. Any area of constricted clothing impedes the progress of the mite and is a common site for bites. Genital lesions may be prominent, and may mimic scabies nodules. In children, dysuria may be a prominent symptom.

Treatment

Potent topical corticosteroids are commonly needed, and may have to be occluded. As the lesions tend to be widespread and multiple, intralesional injection may be difficult, but may be the only successful intervention. Topical antipruritics and anesthetics may be helpful. Clothing impregnated with permethrin is very effective in the prevention of chigger bites.

Ticks

Key features:

- Ticks are disease vectors in most climates
- They cause devastating economic losses from death of cattle
- Some cause tick paralysis

Ticks carry disease in tropical regions, just as they do in temperate zones. Rickettsial fevers are often associated with a black eschar at the site of the tick bite (Fig. 35.8). *Ornithodoros* ticks carry borrelial relapsing fever in tropical regions, as they do in other parts of the world. *Boophilus microplus* transmits *Anaplasma marginale* and babesiosis. It is an important cause of economic losses for those

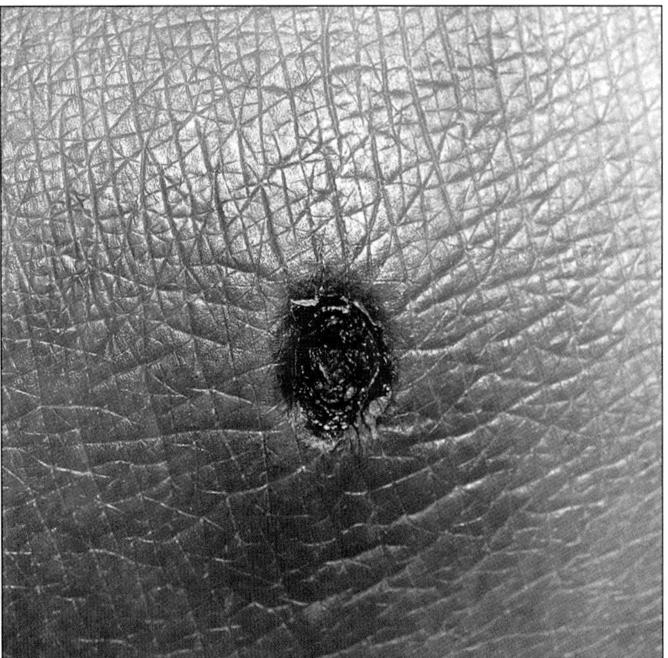

Figure 35.8 Rickettsial eschar.

dependent on cattle in the tropical areas of Central and South America. *Aponomma hydrosauri* is associated with Australian reptiles, and carries *Rickettsia honei*, the etiologic agent of Flinders Island spotted fever. In Australia, *Ixodes holocyclus* is an important cause of tick paralysis. *I. rubicundus* is the South African Karoo paralysis tick.

Prevention of tick infestation depends on a comprehensive program of environmental strategies and personal protection with permethrin-treated clothing and repellents. In many tropical areas, tick eradication programs have been successful and have reduced disease and economic losses.

Spiders (Arachnida: Araneae)

Key features:

- Spiders are widely distributed
- They may cause local necrosis or systemic symptoms

Introduction

Spider bites commonly produce necrotic skin reactions. Disseminated intravascular coagulation and neurotoxic effects may also be seen with some species. A wide variety of spiders produces local cutaneous reactions, and most are not well characterized. Brazilian *Phoneutria nigriventer* spiders (armed spiders) contain neurotoxins that produce cerebral changes and breakdown of the blood–brain barrier. Bites may be fatal in children.

Sparassidae

Key features:

- Sparassidae are widely distributed in tropical climates
- Their local effects tend to be self-limited
- Systemic symptoms are generally mild and transient

Sparassidae spiders occur in tropical regions worldwide. Sparassid spider bites tend to occur during the day in the warmer months of the year. These spiders are generally not aggressive and must be provoked in order to bite. Pain, swelling, bleeding, and itching are common at the site of the bite. Systemic effects are usually mild, and include headache and nausea. Genera of medical importance include *Isopeda, Isopedella, Neosparassus, Heteropoda, Delena,* and *Holconia*.[15]

Widow spiders (Theridiidae)

Key features:

- Black and brown widow spiders are a problem in many tropical climates
- The females are large with a bulbous shiny round abdomen
- Systemic symptoms are secondary to a neurotoxin, and mimic an acute abdomen
- Severe tetany may be associated with rhabdomyolysis
- In general, black widow toxins are more potent than brown widow toxins

Introduction

Black widows are web-building spiders commonly found under outhouse seats, in woodpiles and window wells. *Latrodectus mactans*, the common black widow, is distributed throughout North America and may be found in the Caribbean. *L. curacavienis* is native to South America, and *L. indistinctus* is found in Africa. The brown widow, *L. geometricus,* is native to southern Africa and Madagascar. Australia and New Zealand have related red-black spiders (*L. mactans hasselti*).

Pathogenesis

Latrotoxins are neurotoxins that produce uncontrolled nerve depolarization, increasing intracellular calcium and stimulating uncontrolled exocytosis of and release of neurotransmitters.

Clinical features

As symptoms commonly mimic an acute surgical abdomen, unnecessary exploratory laparotomy may be performed. Tetany may be severe and prolonged, lasting for days.

Treatment

Antivenin is highly effective, but presents some risk of serum sickness. Benzodiazepines and intravenous calcium gluconate are used to treat associated tetany.

Brown spiders (Loxoscelidae)

Key features:

- Brown spiders may cause extensive local necrosis and disseminated intravascular coagulation
- Brown spiders are found throughout the western hemisphere

Introduction

Loxosceles spiders are found throughout the Americas. In South America, *Loxosceles laeta* has a wide distribution. Brown spiders are hunting spiders, and are commonly found in woodpiles and where trash and debris accumulate.

Pathogenesis

Sphingomyelinase D, the major toxin in brown spider venom, causes local neutrophil activation and endothelial damage. Absorption of the toxin can produce widespread endothelial damage and disseminated intravascular coagulation.

Clinical features

Most bites are associated with mild symptoms that can be treated with rest, ice and elevation. Severe local necrotic reactions may require extensive debridement. Patients with minor appearing reactions may be at greater risk for disseminated manifestations and must be monitored.

Funnel web spiders

Key features:

- Funnel web spiders are large, hairy, and aggressive spiders, found in dark, moist areas
- They are common in Australia
- They make funnel-shaped webs
- These are aggressive spiders that produce severe dermonecrotic reactions

Introduction

Funnel web spiders in Australia include *Atrax robustus* and a small number of related *Hadronyche* species. The most toxic spiders are found in the vicinity of Sydney. Related spiders are found in northwestern USA, Canada, and Europe.

Clinical features

Extensive local necrosis and life-threatening systemic reactions have been reported. Sydney funnel web spider bites can be fatal. Hemolysis and thrombocytopenia may also occur.

Treatment

Antivenin can be effective for a variety of related species. Supportive medical and surgical management is dictated by clinical signs and symptoms.

Tarantulas (Lycosidae: theraphosidae)

Key features:

- These are typically large, hairy spiders; they can measure up to 15 cm in diameter
- Normally they are non-aggressive
- They have urticating hairs, that are thrown at skin and eyes
- They are an important cause of ophthalmia nodosa

Introduction

Spiders of the family Theraphosidae occur in most tropical regions. Most are large, hairy, hunting spiders.

Clinical features

Most tarantula bites do not produce severe systemic toxicity, but bites may be associated with severe local pain. Bleeding from the puncture wounds may occur. Although reports of severe human toxicity are rare, dogs bitten by *Phlogellius* and *Selenocosmia* spiders often die.[16]

Many species of tarantula possess urticating hairs on the dorsal abdomen. These hairs are used in a defensive fashion to drive predators from the spider's burrow. Urticating hairs form a characteristic dorsal patch on the abdomen. Vibrations of the hind legs are used to flick hairs at the perceived attacker. Itching at the site of hair penetration may persist for several weeks after exposure. Urticating hairs are absent on most African and Asian species.

Pathology

Urticating tarantula hairs penetrate the stratum corneum and epidermis and may extend as deep as the reticular dermis. Hairs that penetrate the cornea can result in ophthalmia nodosa, a chronic granulomatous reaction that may result in loss of vision.

Scorpions (Arachnida: scorpionida)

Key features:

- Scorpions have large anterior claws
- They have a long tail curved upward to sting when threatened

Introduction

Many toxic scorpions exist worldwide. The most venomous species include *Tityus serrulatus*, found in Brazil, *Buthotus (Buthus) tamulus*, found in India, *Leiurus quinquestriatus* and *Androctonus crassicauda*, found in North Africa and southwest Asia, and *Centruroides suffussus*, found in Mexico. Scorpions are frequently found under table tops, in woodpiles, and in shoes. In several studies, most stings have been found to occur in the home.

Clinical features

Common symptoms include paresthesia, pain, and edema. Systemic neurological complications depend on the species, and include autonomic storm, myoclonus, dysarthria, ataxia, tachycardia, vomiting, abdominal pain, diaphoresis, excessive salivation, seizures, coma, hypertension, and priapism.

Treatment

Cardiac monitoring and supportive treatment for cardiac events are critical. Antiarrhythmics, antiadrenergic agents, vasodilators, and calcium-channel blockers have been used. Antivenin represents the most definitive treatment. Most preparations are still made from horse serum. The safety profile of these agents has been good, although serum sickness is possible, and there is a theoretical risk of transmitting infectious viruses or prions. These risks are generally outweighed by the risk of mortality from untreated envenomation and the low cost and history of safe use of the antivenin.

Ants (Hymenopterids)

Key features:

- Red ant venom contains formic acid
- Imported fire ants have become widespread in Latin America and the southern USA

In tropical areas, ant stings are usually benign, and result in temporary symptoms of pain and pruritic hypersensitivity reactions. Severe allergic reactions can occasionally occur, including urticaria and anaphylactic shock.[17]

Fire ants swarm when their mound is disturbed. Multiple stings typically occur simultaneously (Fig. 35.9), as the ants grasp the skin with their mandibles, and pivot their rear stinging apparatus to sting repeatedly in a rosette. The burning sensation lasts for several minutes, and is frequently accompanied by a wheal-and-flare reaction. Later, sterile pustules appear in a rosette pattern. The pustules are extremely pruritic, but non-tender. The presence of tenderness suggests secondary infection.

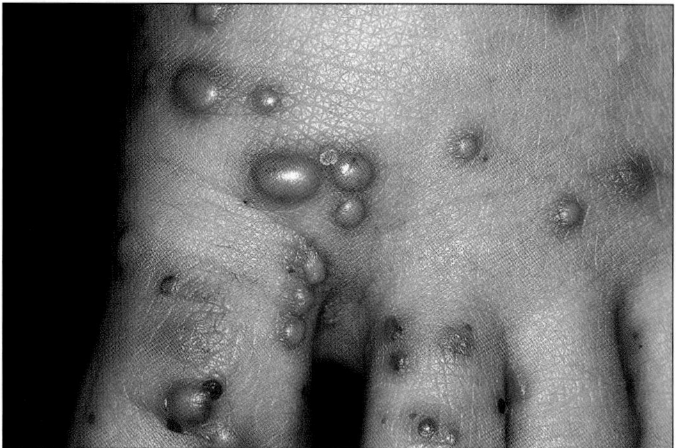

Figure 35.9 Fire ant stings.

Fire ant venom causes release of histamine from mast cells. It also causes aggregation of platelets and attracts neutrophils. Anaphylaxis may occur in those sensitized by previous stings or by yellow jacket venom.

Clinical features

The presence of the characteristic pruritic pustules is usually diagnostic in an endemic area. Widespread pustules may be seen when an inebriated individual falls asleep on a fire ant mound.

Treatment

Treatment is largely symptomatic, except in the case of anaphylaxis, when epinephrine (adrenaline) must be administered and platelets should be refused for desensitization. Cold compresses, rest, and elevation provide some relief. Potent fluorinated topical steroids and topical anesthetics can be helpful to relieve itching.

For control of fire ants in local areas, ant baits resembling breadcrumbs and containing hydramethylnon and sulfuramid are spread in the area to be protected. Other insecticides, parasitic microsporidia (*Thelohania solenopsae*), and decapitator flies can also be used.

Bedbugs (Cimicids)

Key features:

- Bedbugs have a red-brown, flat oval body
- They are about the size of a tick
- Their forewings are reduced to sclerotic shoulder pads; hind wings are absent

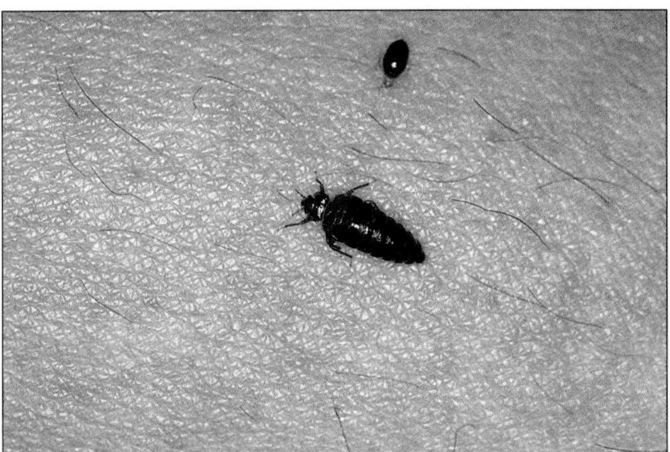

Figure 35.10 Tropical bedbug.

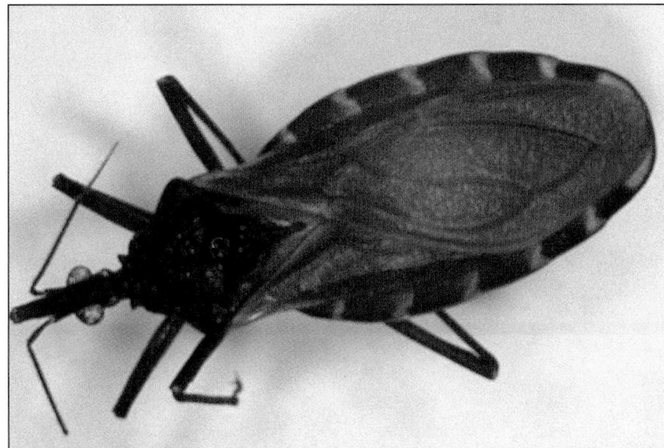

Figure 35.11 Triatome bug.

Introduction

Bedbugs are reddish-brown, with a flat body pointed in the rear. They are similar in size to a tick. The mouth parts are retroverted and only visible when the bug is feeding or if it is turned over. The eyes are widely separated. The sclerotic proximal portion of the wings is retained, but the hind wings are absent. This contrasts with other true bugs that have overlapping membranous hind wings. A small semicircular to triangular sclerotic dorsal scutellum is present. The abdominal segments expand during feeding to expose intersegmental membranes.

Bedbugs hide during the day in cracks and crevices of plaster or mud and daub walls. They also infest thatched rooves. Bedbugs feed at night, often inflicting several bites in a row ("breakfast, lunch, and dinner").

Cimex hemipterus (Fig. 35.10) is the most common species in tropical climates, and is longer than C. *lectularius*. Hybrid forms also occur.[18]

Bedbugs may act as vectors for hepatitis B and American trypanosomiasis (Chagas disease).[19,20] Control of bedbugs includes the repair of walls, and the use of insecticides. Pyrethroid-treated bed nets can be effective, but must be used in the entire village or camp to prevent the emergence of resistance.

The intermediate hosts include swallows and bats. As many species are protected, or serve valuable roles in mosquito control, disruption of their habitat must often be avoided. Cracks in walls should be sealed when possible, and insecticides such as dichlorvos can be used inside the house. Microencapsulation of some insecticides enhances persistence, especially on mud and straw walls.[21]

Triatome reduviids

Key features:

- These are true bugs with prominent stripes often noted on the abdomen
- The distal membranous halves of the wings overlap
- They are vectors for American trypanosomiasis

Introduction

Unlike bedbugs, triatome reduviids have retained the distal membranous portion of their wings. As the overlapping wings fail to cover the lateral portions of the abdomen, the abdominal markings are plainly visible (Fig. 35.11). A prominent triangular pronotum is present behind the head. The labium (sucking mouth piece) is straight and composed of three segments.

Clinical features

Triatome reduviids are the most important vector for American trypanosomiasis (Chagas disease). Although triatomes also occur in more temperate climates, tropical triatome bugs are more efficient vectors of the disease. Triatome bugs are shy, and prefer to feed under cover of darkness. The bites are typically painless, although some species are also capable of delivering a more painful defensive bite. Large urticarial plaques (Fig. 35.12) may develop, and central clearing may be noted as the lesions spread. Unilateral eyelid swelling may be noted after a nighttime triatome bite, and this is referred to as Romaña's sign. Chagas disease may result in cardiomegaly and megacolon.

Blister beetles (coleoptera)

Synonyms: Spanish fly, rove beetle

Key features:

- Long thin beetles with blunt ends
- Antennae are composed of multiple short segments
- Canthardin is discharged from leg joints in some species
- Crushed beetles may produce severe reactions

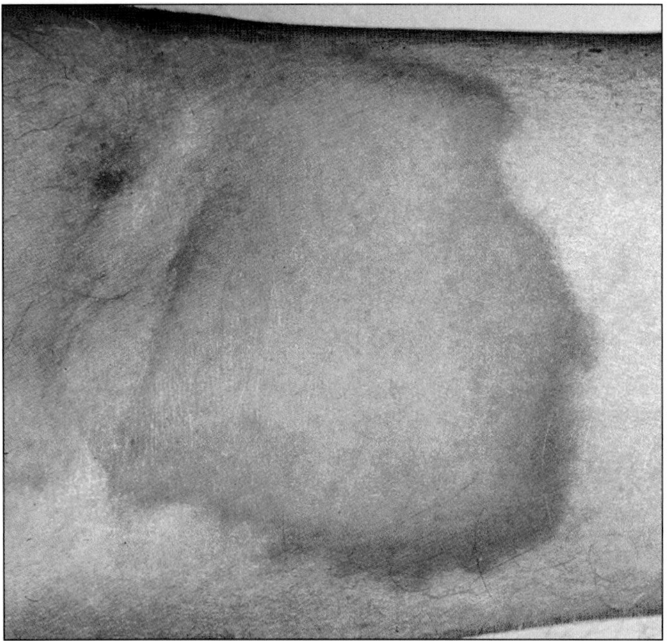

Figure 35.12 Reduviid bite. (Courtesy of Brooke Army Medical Center teaching file.)

Introduction

Blister beetle families (Fig. 35.13) include Meloidae and Staphylinidae beetles. Meloidae beetles are distributed worldwide and account for most cases of blister beetle dermatosis. Oedemeridae beetles, or "false" blister beetles, can also produce blistering. Cantharidin may protect the beetle from being eaten. Cantharidin is transferred from male to female during mating, and the strategy has been referred to as a "mate or die" strategy.

Clinical features

Vesicles, pustules, extensive erythema, and bullae may occur. Epidemics of bullous skin disease in hospital wards have been described in tropical climates, where windows are left open at night. "Nairobi eye," "night burn," or rove beetle blistering is related to *Paederus eximius*, a blister beetle found in Northern Kenya.

Pathology

Blisters form as a result of acantholysis of suprabasal keratinocytes. Eosinophilic necrosis occurs as the blister ages.

Treatment

Screens will prevent the light-seeking behavior of some species, and help to keep them outdoors. Crushed blister beetles used as a folk remedy for various skin disorders have resulted in severe blistering. These practices should be avoided.

Fleas

Key features:

- Fleas have laterally compressed bodies with large hind legs
- They are vectors for melioidosis, erysipeloid, endemic typhus, bubonic plague, and brucellosis

Introduction

The human flea (Fig. 35.14), *Pulex irritans*, is a combless flea commonly found in refugee populations, where it can serve as an important disease vector. During the great plague epidemics, the disease is thought to have spread from the enzootic focus by means of rat fleas, then spread from human to human by *Pulex* fleas, and ultimately by pneumonic transmission. *Ctenocephalides* dog and cat fleas (Fig. 35.15) are combed fleas that are common in households all over the world. The genal and pronotal combs resemble a mustache and mane of hair (Fig. 35.16). C. *canis*, the dog flea, has a more rounded head and eight hair-bearing notches on the dorsal hind tibia. C. *felis* has a flatter head and six notches.

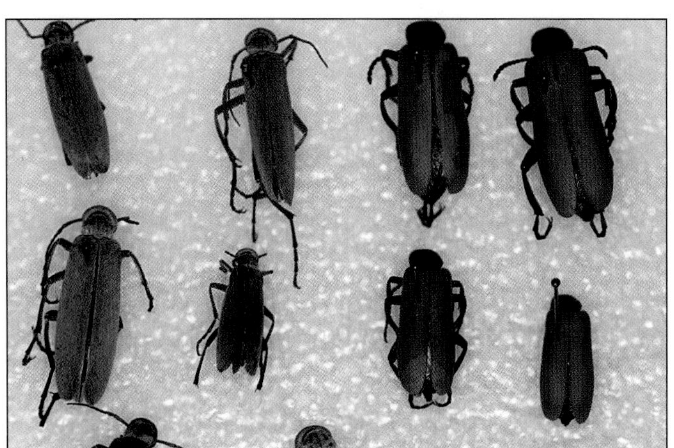

Figure 35.13 Blister beetles.

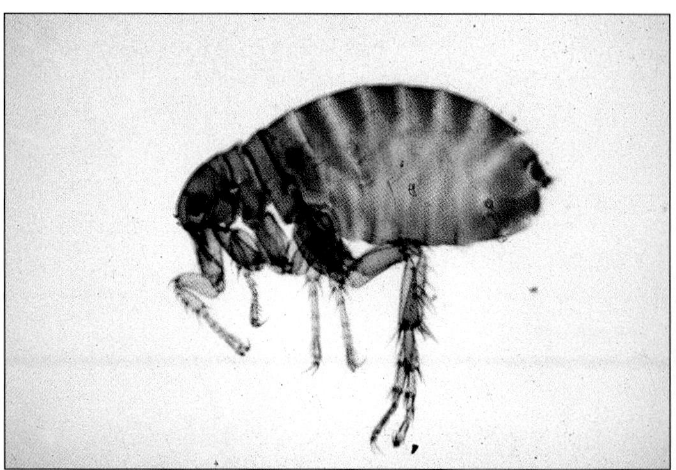

Figure 35.14 *Pulex irritans*.

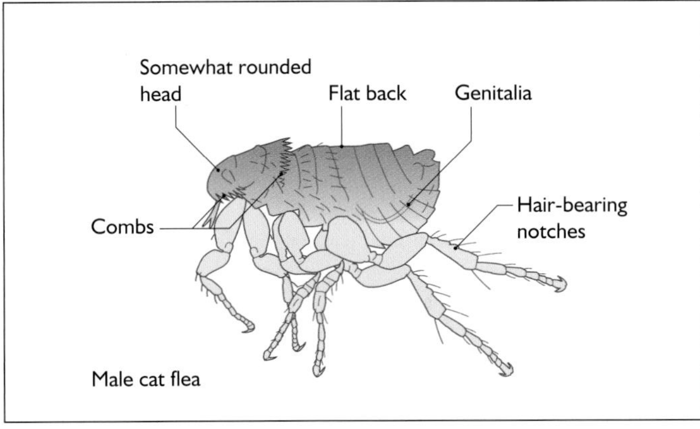

Figure 35.15 Cat flea. (Courtesy of *Cutis*.)

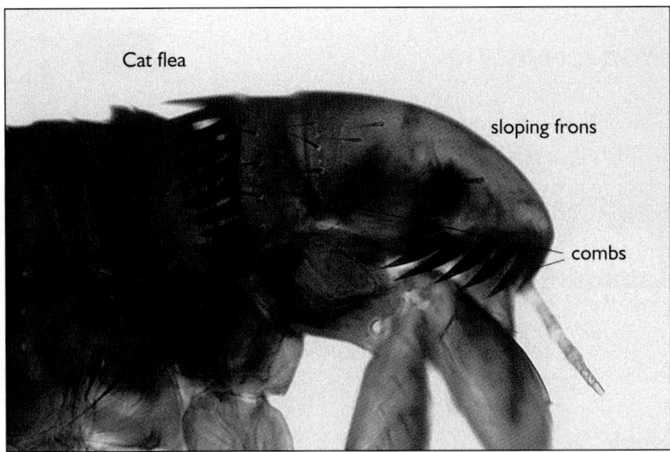

Figure 35.16 Cat flea combs. (Reprinted courtesy of *Cutis*.)

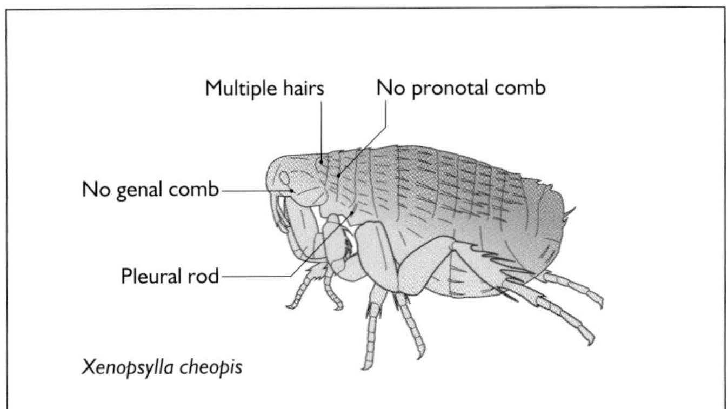

Figure 35.17 Oriental rat flea. (Courtesy of *Cutis*.)

The oriental rat flea is a combless flea with a pleural rod (Fig. 35.17). The stick-tight flea (Fig. 35.18) is recognizable by its flattened frons (forehead) and the broad serrated mouth part that allows it to "stick tight".

Clinical features

Fleas transmit a variety of diseases, including plague, brucellosis, melioidosis, erysipeloid and endemic typhus. The bites appear

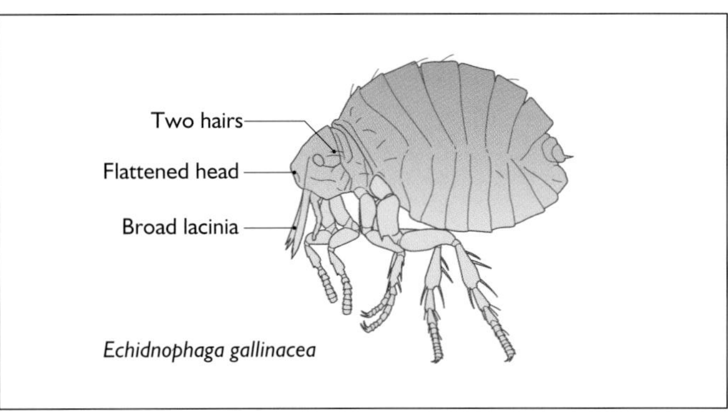

Figure 35.18 Stick-tight flea. (Courtesy of *Cutis*.)

as pruritic papulovesicles on the lower legs, or anywhere the flea has an opportunity to bite. They cannot fly, but can jump several centimeters.

Treatment

Topical fipronil is commonly used to prevent flea infestation in pets. Lufenuron, which makes the fleas sterile, can be used orally or by injection. Boric acid, growth regulators such as pyriproxyfen, and various insecticides have been used to rid the environment of fleas. Refugees often harbor fleas in their clothing, and these must be laundered or treated with insecticide. Fleas may also reside on the body, and other ectoparasites are also commonly present.

Centipedes and millipedes (Chilopoda, diplopoda)

Key features:

Centipedes

- Centipedes have long flat bodies, with one pair of legs on each segment
- The venom generally produces self-limited symptoms

Millipedes

- Millipedes have long cylindrical bodies, with two pairs of legs on each segment
- They can result in chemical burns

Clinical features

Centipedes can inject a neurotoxic venom through venom ducts in their jaws (Fig. 35.19). The bite often has a characteristic chevron shape. Pain, paresthesia, erythema, and edema (Fig. 35.20) are usually self-limited, but bleeding may be profuse. Millipedes have long cylindrical bodies (Fig. 35.21). They lack venomous jaws, but secrete caustic substances that may result in deep brown discoloration of the skin or local burns. Millipede burns often occur when the millipede is trapped in an article of clothing.

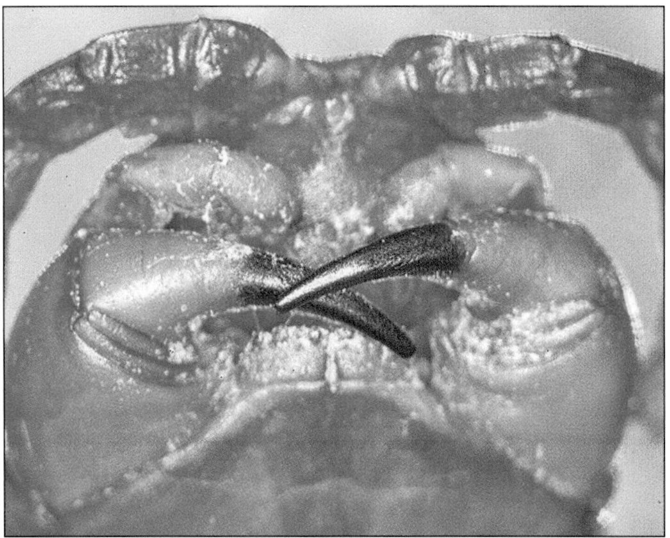

Figure 35.19 Centipede jaws inflict a chevron-shaped wound.

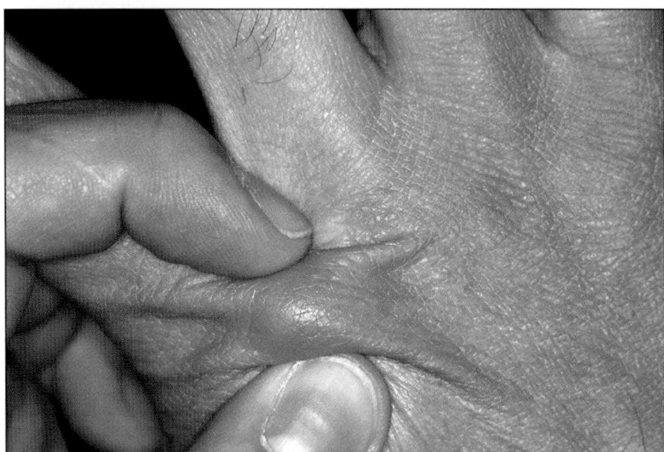

Figure 35.20 Centipede bite.

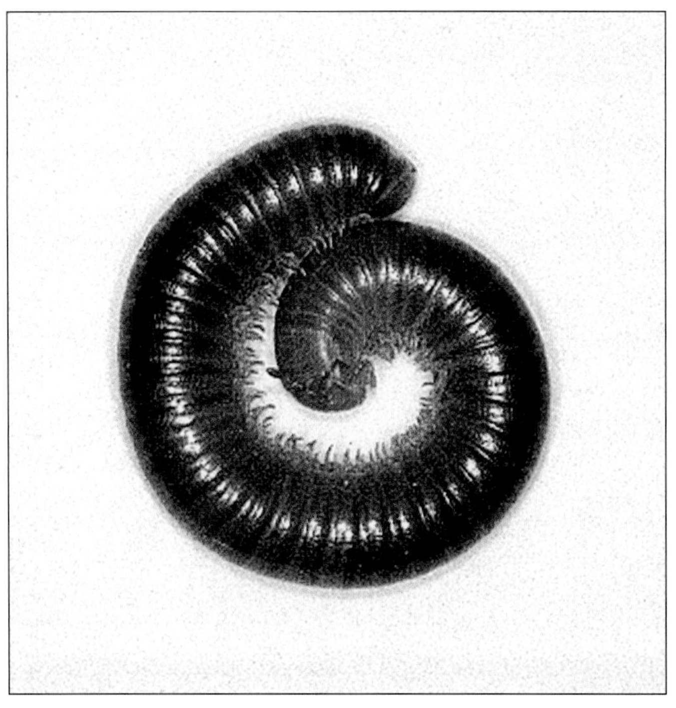

Figure 35.21 Millipede.

Caterpillars, butterflies, and moths

Key features:

- Moths and caterpillars can cause dermatitis or systemic reactions (lepidopterism)
- Ophthalmia nodosa (involvement of the cornea) may also occur
- There have been epidemics of lepidopterism aboard ships that have docked in the Venezuelan port of Caripito

Introduction

A wide variety of caterpillars, butterflies, and moths can cause lepidopterism. Hairs embedded in the cocoons can also cause disease.

Pathogenesis

The hairs embed themselves in the cornea and skin, where toxin-mediated reactions may be mediated by histamine, kinins, and plasminogen activators.

Clinical features

Clinical manifestations include intense itch, pain, erythema, hemorrhage, papules, or urticaria, depending on the species. In Latin America, the caterpillar *Lonomia achelous* can cause a fatal bleeding diathesis. Caripito itch has been described in sailors whose ship docked in the port city of Caripito. Adult female *Hylesia* moths are responsible for the eruption. The hairs circulate in the ventilation system of the ship, and the itch may be difficult to eradicate. Ocular manifestations include ophthalmia nodosa, keratoconjunctivitis, and vitreoretinal involvement.

Treatment

Topical anesthetics and camphor and menthol preparations can provide some symptomatic relief. Tape stripping can remove many of the caterpillar hairs.

References

1. Snow RW, Marsh K. The consequences of reducing transmission of *Plasmodium falciparum* in Africa. Adv Parasitol 2002; 52:235–264.
2. Beier JC, Killeen GF, Githure JI. Short report: entomologic inoculation rates and *Plasmodium falciparum* malaria prevalence in Africa. Am J Trop Med Hyg 1999; 61:109–113.
3. Watt G, Parola P. Scrub typhus and tropical rickettsioses. Curr Opin Infect Dis 2003; 16: 429–436.
4. Vieta F. River blindness. Protection for 54 cents a year. UN Chron 1998; 1:12–13.
5. Filler S, Causer LM, Newman RD et al. Malaria surveillance – United States, 2001. MMWR Surveill Summ 2003; 52:1–14.

6. Surveillance for acute insecticide-related illness associated with mosquito-control efforts – nine states, 1999–2002. MMWR Morb Mortal Wkly Rep 2003; 52:629–634.
7. Reiter P, Lathrop S, Bunning M et al. Texas lifestyle limits transmission of dengue virus. Emerg Infect Dis 2003; 9:86–89.
8. Frances SP, Auliff AM, Edstein MD et al. Survey of personal protection measures against mosquitoes among Australian defense force personnel deployed to East Timor. Mil Med 2003; 168:227–230.
9. McKinlay JR, Ross V, Barrett TL. Vesiculobullous reaction to diethyltoluamide revisited. Cutis 1998; 62:44.
10. Frances SP, Van Dung N, Beebe NW et al. Field evaluation of repellent formulations against daytime and nighttime biting mosquitoes in a tropical rainforest in northern Australia. J Med Entomol 2002; 39:541–544.
11. Caraballo AJ, Mosquito repellent action of Neemos. J Am Mosq Contr Assoc 2000; 16:45–46.
12. Pate HV, Line JD, Keto AJ et al. Personal protection against mosquitoes in Dar es Salaam, Tanzania, by using a kerosene oil lamp to vaporize transfluthrin. Med Vet Entomol 2002; 16:277–284.
13. Lindsay LR, Surgeoner GA, Heal JD et al. Evaluation of the efficacy of 3% citronella candles and 5% citronella incense for protection against field populations of *Aedes* mosquitoes. J Am Mosq Contr Assoc 1996; 12:293–294.
14. Kline DL. Evaluation of various models of propane powered mosquito traps. J Vector Ecol 2002; 27:1–7.
15. Isbister GK, Hirst D. A prospective study of definite bites by spiders of the family Sparassidae (huntsmen spiders) with identification to species level. Toxicon 2003; 42:163–171.
16. Isbister GK, Seymour JE, Gray MR et al. Bites by spiders of the family Theraphosidae in humans and canines. Toxicon 2003; 41:519–524.
17. Rodriguez-Acosta A, Reyes-Lugo M. Severe human urticaria produced by ant (*Odontomachus bauri*, Emery 1892) (Hymenoptera: Formicidae) venom. Int J Dermatol 2002; 41: 801–803.
18. Newberry K. Production of a hybrid between the bedbugs *Cimex hemipterus* and *Cimex lectularius*. Med Vet Entomol 1988; 2:297–300.
19. Jorg ME. *Cimex lectularius*, L (la chinche comun de cama) tranmisor de *Trypanosoma cruzi*. Rev Soc Bras Med Trop 1992; 25:277–278.
20. Jupp PG, McElligott SE. Transmission experiments with hepatitis B surface antigen and the common bedbug (*Cimex lectularius* L). S Afr Med J 1979; 56:54–57.
21. Gao YT, Shen PY, Wang BH et al. Controlled release effect of insecticide microcapsules and their results in common household insect pest control. J Microencapsulation 1984; 1:307–315.

Marine/freshwater dermatology

Mathijs Brentjens, Karan K. Sra, Vidal Haddad Junior, Patricia Lee and Stephen K. Tyring

Introduction

Human contact with an aquatic environment is very common. People are now able to vacation relatively cheaply in tropical destinations, and the increasing popularity of home marine and freshwater aquariums has also contributed to exposures not otherwise seen in non-tropical locations.

Injury after exposure to a marine environment may occur as a result of infection, contact or allergic dermatitis, physical trauma, or envenomation. Cutaneous manifestations result from contact with various marine organisms, including bacteria (*Erysipelothrix rhusiopathiae, Vibrio vulnificus, Aeromonas hydrophila, Mycobacterium marinum*), plants, sponges, coelenterates (hydroids, fire corals, Portuguese man-of-war, corals, sea anemones, box and true jellyfish), worms, echinoderms (starfish, sea cucumbers, and sea urchins), mollusks (shellfish and octopi), arthropods, and fish.

Although acute injuries resulting from marine exposure are most often seen by urgent care or emergency room personnel, both dermatologists and primary care physicians should be familiar with common manifestations of aquatic injuries. Usually, the late manifestations of injuries caused by cnidarians, sea urchins, and fishes are observed by dermatologists and the early signs and symptoms are treated by emergency professionals. Patients presenting with unusual histories or clinical presentations should be asked about recent contact with a marine environment (vacation or exposure to marine aquaria). Most injuries caused by aquatic animals present with characteristic cutaneous manifestations. The dermatologist should recognize these lesions and diagnose injuries from aquatic animals with no difficulty. This section addresses the dermatologic manifestations of marine and freshwater exposures.

Marine bacteria

Although the most frequent marine-acquired infections are due to common skin pathogens *Staphylococcus* and *Streptococcus*, inoculation by other bacteria such as *E. rhusiopathiae, V. vulnificus, A. hydrophila*, and *M. marinum* can cause cutaneous disease. There are diseases caused by fungi, such as sporotrichosis acquired by fishermen from *Tilapia* spp. In addition, we reported a patient who acquired sporotrichosis while cleaning his domestic aquarium.[1]

Erysipeloid, caused by the Gram-positive organism *E. rhusiopathiae*, is a self-limited, localized infection occurring most commonly on the hand 24–72 h after inoculation resulting from injury or trauma (Fig. 35.22). The infection can occur in fresh or salt water and is commonly seen in workers who handle seafood or fish. Similar to erysipelas, erysipeloid typically manifests as a pruritic and/or painful well-demarcated erythematous plaque.[2] However, unlike erysipelas, constitutional signs and symptoms such as fever, chills, and regional lymphadenopathy are not usually present. Although the infection is usually self-limited, hematologic dissemination can occur, resulting in sepsis, septic arthritis, and endocarditis. Localized infection can be treated with oral antibiotics such as penicillin, ampicillin, erythromycin, and first-generation

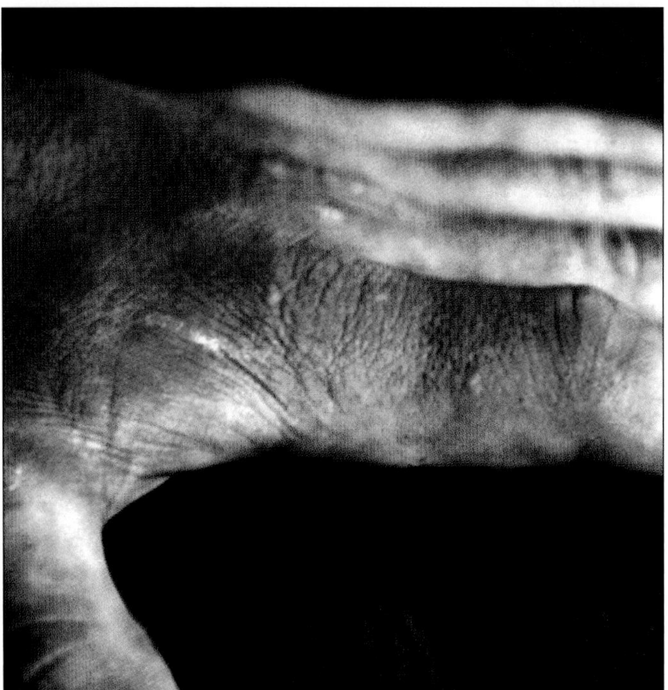

Figure 35.22 Erysipeloid (*Erysipelothrix rhusiopathiae*) in a fisherman. (Courtesy of Dr. Vidal Haddad Junior.)

cephalosporins. Disseminated disease often requires more aggressive treatment with intravenous antibiotics. However, vancomycin should not be used because *E. rhusiopathiae* is resistant to this antibiotic.

V. vulnificus, a Gram-negative rod, can be acquired by ingesting infected raw or undercooked seafood (i.e., oysters, shellfish) or via direct inoculation injury in salt water. Ingestion of the virulent organism results in vomiting, diarrhea, or abdominal pain. In immunocompromised individuals and those with liver disease, septic shock can occur, with an associated mortality rate of around 50%. Necrotic bullae, petechiae, and purpura can be seen in patients with sepsis. Primary cutaneous infection with *V. vulnificus* can manifest as cellulitis, ulceration, and/or necrosis (Fig. 35.23).

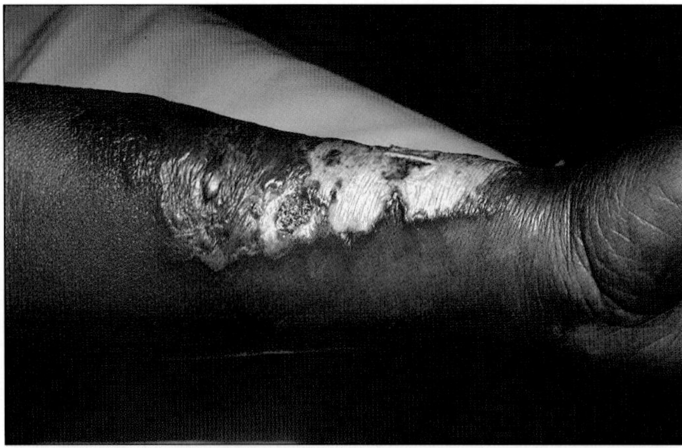

Figure 35.23 Hemorrhagic bullae and necrosis resulting from *Vibrio vulnificus* cellulitis of the left arm of a 62-year-old diabetic and alcoholic fisherman one week following minor trauma while cleaning shellfish. (Courtesy of Dr. Juan Pedro Lonza.)

In immunocompromised individuals, cutaneous inoculation may lead to more serious complications as a result of bacteremia. The diagnosis can be made via history or with wound or blood cultures, and doxycycline, tetracycline, and/or third-generation cephalosporins (i.e., ceftazidime) can be used to treat infected patients.

A. hydrophila, a Gram-negative anaerobic rod, is found in fresh and salt water and is a common pathogen of fish and amphibians. Most infections caused by *Aeromonas* spp., however, are observed in freshwater environments. Like *V. vulnificus*, *A. hydrophila* can be acquired by infection of open wounds, the ingestion of contaminated food (shellfish, fish, beef, and poultry), or by drinking water. Ingestion of the organism can cause gastroenteritis, and in some individuals (especially those who are immunocompromised) sepsis, pneumonia, and meningitis can occur. Cutaneous inoculation of the organism can result in cellulitis, abscesses, and even gangrene. Also, similar to *V. vulnificus*, immunocompromised patients and those with liver disease are at an increased risk for developing disseminated disease. Diagnosis of infection can be aided by history and wound or blood cultures. *A. hydrophila* can be treated with antibiotics such as trimethoprim–sulfamethoxazole, fluoroquinolones, tetracycline, doxycycline, chloramphenicol, or third-generation cephalosporins.

M. marinum, an acid-fast mycobacterium, is seen in individuals who swim in fresh or salt water, along with individuals who handle fish, seafood, or aquaria. The skin is the most common site of inoculation which often occurs at sites of trauma or injury. Cutaneous manifestations of the organism often appear several weeks to months after initial inoculation. Characteristically, a small papule or nodule presents at the site of inoculation. Enlargement of the lesion with necrosis and ulceration, along with lymphangitic spread in a sporotrichoid manner, is not uncommon. Joint and bone involvement can also occur, resulting in septic arthritis and osteomyelitis. Infection with *M. marinum* most commonly causes localized disease, although several rare cases of disseminated infection have been reported. Diagnosis can be made through history or biopsy and culture of cutaneous lesions. Treatment consists of antibiotics such as rifampin, ethambutol, minocycline, trimethoprim–sulfamethoxazole, clarithromycin, or ciprofloxacin. Because the organism does not tolerate temperatures above 33° C,[3] hot compresses can be used in conjunction with antibiotics. Surgical excision has also been used in the treatment of this infectious disease.

Plants

Red tide is caused by dinoflagellates such as *Gymnodinum brevis* that contain neurotoxins called brevetoxins. This toxin can be released into the water or air (via water droplets) where it is known to have adverse affects on fish and humans. In fish, the toxin is deadly in small concentrations, whereas in humans direct exposure can result in contact dermatitis, coughing, sneezing, and conjunctivitis. *Pfiesteria piscicida*, another toxic dinoflagellate, is commonly found in lakes, rivers, and estuaries. It also contains a toxin which is deadly to fish. In humans, exposure to *P. piscicida* can cause contact dermatitis, pain, burning, eye or respiratory irritation, confusion, problems with memory, and impaired cognitive function. Exposed individuals typically develop symptoms shortly after exposure (within 2 weeks), and signs and symptoms may persist for weeks, months, or indefinitely. Avoiding areas in which they are known to be endemic can prevent exposure to such dinoflagellates.

Cyanobacteria, or blue-green algae, are found in both marine and freshwater habitats. There are over 50 different genera of freshwater blue-green algae, and more than a third produce toxins (neurotoxins, hepatotoxins, and other non-specific toxins). When exposed to these toxins, gastroenteritis, nausea, vomiting, and respiratory irritation can occur. Dermatologic manifestations include contact or irritant dermatitis, which is most prominent around the site of the bathing suit due to retention of algae microfilaments. The eruption can begin within minutes of exposure and prompt removal of the bathing suit, along with showering and rinsing with rubbing alcohol, can prevent this seaweed dermatitis.[4] Treatment is typically targeted towards symptomatic care. However, topical corticosteroids may be used to minimize the inflammatory response.

Sponges

There are over 10 000 species of sponges that belong to the phylum Porifera. Sponges get their structure from hard rods known as spicules. The spicules are made from silica or calcium carbonate and function to protect the organism. In addition to spicules, many sponges produce toxins that are found on the surface of the organism or secreted into the water. These spicules and toxins can cause pain, edema, pruritus, erythema, vesicles, and paresthesia at the site of contact.[5] Although rare, systemic symptoms such as nausea, vomiting, and malaise can occur. Treatment options include soaking the affected area in vinegar, using the sticky side of adhesive tape to remove spicules, and low-potency topical corticosteroids. The cutaneous eruption usually resolves spontaneously in several days.

Cnidarians

Cnidarians are aquatic animals characterized by the presence of defense cells, known as cnidocytes, that contain nematocysts. Nematocysts, also known as stinging capsules, contain a coiled filament which discharges after contact with a foreign body or by osmotic mechanisms. After the filament punctures the skin, nematocysts release toxins causing both local and systemic reactions. Although the amount of toxin contained in a single nematocyst is not large, typical contact involves the discharge of thousands to millions of nematocysts, leading to clinical symptoms. Nematocysts may survive for an extended period of time after the death of the organism. Jellyfish and Portuguese man-of-war washed up on a beach should be handled with extreme caution in order to prevent envenomation.

Injuries by cnidarians are of two types: toxic (the initial effects) and allergic, with early and late reactions, like anaphylaxis, urticaria, persistent papular lesions, and granulomas. The toxins contained in nematocysts include a variety of enzymes and polypeptides capable of inducing anaphylactic or cytotoxic reactions. Envenomation by cnidarians most often results in local tissue reactions, including necrosis, erythema, edema, piloerection, and localized lymphadenopathy. Long-term sequelae include keloid formation, hyperpigmentation, fat atrophy, and gangrene. Systemic effects are less often seen and may include fever, malaise, nausea and vomiting, urticaria, hypersensitivity reactions, respiratory acidosis, muscle spasms, arthralgias, and convulsions. Rarely, death occurs secondary to cardiac or respiratory arrest, hepatotoxicity, delayed renal failure, or anaphylaxis.[6]

Cnidaria contain four classes which have species capable of causing toxic reactions in humans: (1) Hydrozoa (hydroids, fire corals, and *Physalia* spp.); (2) Anthozoa (corals and sea anemones); (3) Cubozoa (box jellyfish); and (4) Scyphozoa (true jellyfish).

Hydrozoa

Hydroids, fire corals, and *Physalia* belong in the class Hydrozoa. Hydroids or fire-weed (*Aglaophenia cupresina*) and a great number of hydroids are found on reefs, rocks, coral, seaweed, docks, and pilings.[7]

Direct cutaneous exposure can cause an erythematous patch, burning, pain, urticaria, and sometimes lymphadenopathy. The reaction can last from hours to several weeks. Treatment for hydroid infection is focused on symptomatic care.

Fire-coral dermatitis

While coral dermatitis is caused by corals, fire coral, a hydrozoan, is most frequently seen in scuba divers and is commonly caused by contact with Red Sea coral, also known as stinging or fire coral (*Millepora* spp.). Organelles located on the tentacles of corals release toxins such as catecholamines, proteins, and histamines. Direct physical contact with fire coral allows the tentacles and nematocysts to penetrate the skin and cause cutaneous symptoms. Cutaneous manifestations of the organism in the acute phase can vary, as lesions can be vesicular, bullous, hemorrhagic, necrotic, ulcerative, and/or urticarial. Subacute granulomatous dermatitis and chronic lichenoid dermatitis can also be present several weeks after initial infection with the nematocysts, and complete healing may take up to 15 weeks.[8] Because type IV hypersensitivity reaction is also associated with fire-coral dermatitis, some individuals may develop a delayed or recurrent reaction after exposure to the nematocysts. As a result of the variety of possible cutaneous manifestations of fire-coral dermatitis, an accurate diagnosis can be difficult. In addition to history, the presence of constitutional symptoms such as pain, fever, malaise, nausea, vomiting, and abdominal pain may aid in the diagnosis. Initial treatment begins with adequate cleansing and debridement of the area with soap and water, alcohol, or vinegar. Tetanus prophylaxis, antihistamines, topical antibiotic ointment, oral antibiotics, and topical corticosteroids are also commonly employed to treat the symptoms and possible superimposed infection.

P. physalis, commonly known as the Atlantic Portuguese man-of-war, is one of the most toxic cnidarians. It consists of a bladder with a cock-comb crest, which floats on the surface of the water. Underneath the bladder are numerous tentacles, which may grow as long as 50 m and contain nematocysts capable of penetrating even rubber wetsuits (Fig. 35.24). The toxin from the Portuguese man-of-war consists of a heat-labile protein complex which can act as a paralytic and cardiotoxic substance. Acute symptoms include severe local and muscle pain, intense burning, anxiety, nausea, weakness, and bradycardia. Anaphylaxis may also occur. Although

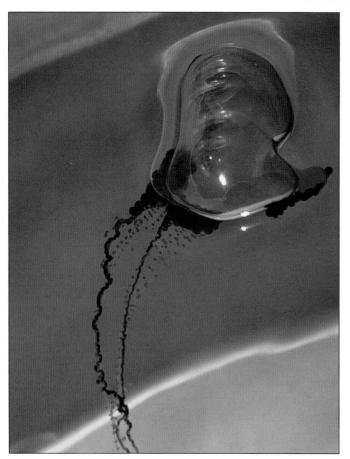

Figure 35.24 *Physalia physalis*, the Atlantic Portuguese man-of-war. (Courtesy of Ed Robinson, Hawaiian Water Colours.)

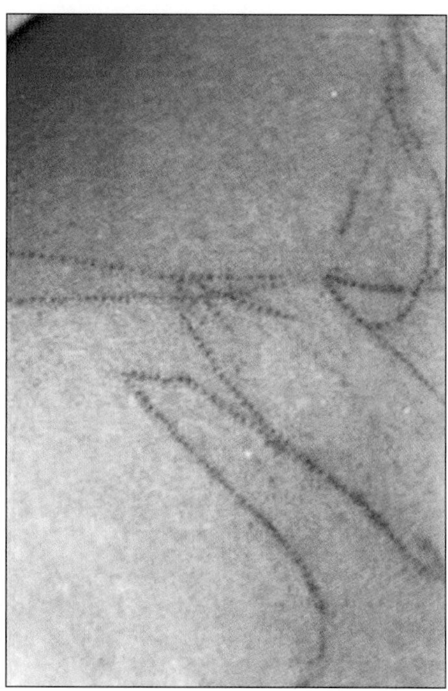

Figure 35.25 Linear plaques, erythema, and edema in a girl following contact with the tentacles of a Portuguese man-of-war. (Courtesy of Dr. Vidal Haddad Junior.)

rare, the reaction is sometimes fatal.[9] Dermatologic symptoms of minor *Physalia* envenomations appear similar to those of true jellyfish stings, with linear wavy erythematous papules and plaques (Fig. 35.25). The linear plaques caused by box jellyfish and Portuguese man-of-war are longer than those of true jellyfish. This is an important clinical sign distinguishing the more severe injuries caused by box jellyfish and Portuguese man-of-war from those caused by true jellyfish.[10–12]

Urticarial reactions are also common. Lesions may develop ulceration or hemorrhage. Treatment for acute stings includes cardiac and respiratory support if necessary, rinsing the affected areas with sea water (or vinegar), removal (with tweezers) of tentacles still stuck to the skin, and ice compresses to the skin for pain control. It is very important to note that cold freshwater compresses should not be applied. The cnidocytes also use osmotic mechanisms, and freshwater compresses can precipitate this effect. The use of vinegar or meat tenderizer may be beneficial in order to inactivate remaining nematocysts on tentacle remnants. Vinegar use is supported by some scientific evidence; it inactivates the firing of the nematocyst, not the venom. However, using fresh water, urine, or alcohol to rinse affected sites or rubbing affected areas in sand is not recommended as these actions may cause the activation of remaining nematocysts via pressure or osmotic mechanisms. Nematocysts remaining on the skin may be shaved off after they have been inactivated. Local wound care may include topical steroids, antibiotics for ulcerated lesions, and antihistamines for pruritus. Steroids, however, do not affect the initial phase of envenomation.

Anthozoa

True corals belong to the class Anthozoa, which contains two orders: Alcyonaria and Zoantharia. Soft corals and sea ferns belong to the class Alcyonaria, whereas sea anemones and hard corals are in the class Zoantharia. Serious injury can result from touching true corals, as they have a sharp calcium carbonate skeleton that can abrade or cut the skin. Corals also possess nematocysts, which can cause a stinging sensation together with an erythematous inflammatory cutaneous response. The wounds caused by corals are chronic and severe. Treatment begins with adequate cleansing of the wound, along with the removal of remaining nematocysts. Secondary infection can be treated with appropriate antibiotics and tetanus prophylaxis is recommended.

Sea anemones are flower-like coelenterates that contain numerous nematocysts on their tentacles (Figs 35.26–35.28). The majority of sea anemones are harmless. However, some sea anemones can cause a cutaneous reaction, especially if tentacles come into contact with sensitive areas such as the face, lips, and underarms. Pain, pruritus, erythema, and bullae can occur at the site of contact (Figs 35.29 and 35.30). More serious reactions, such as cutaneous ulceration lasting several months, have been reported with sea anemones such as *Actinodendron plumosum* and *Triactis producta*. Treatment after contact with sea anemones is symptomatic.

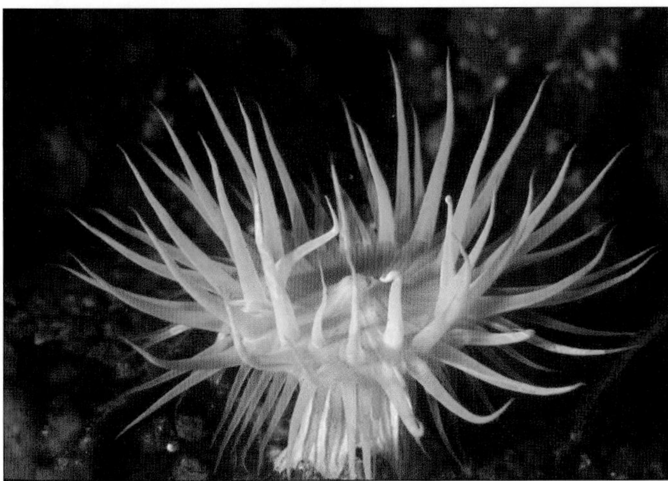

Figure 35.26 *Anthoethoe chilensis*, the sea anemone, in the resting state. (Courtesy of Dr. Juan Pedro Lonza.)

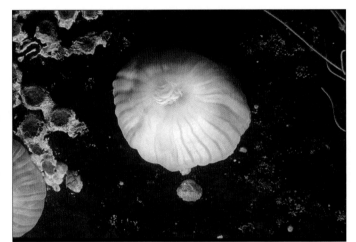

Figure 35.27 The sea anemone contracting after being disturbed. (Courtesy of Dr. Juan Pedro Lonza.)

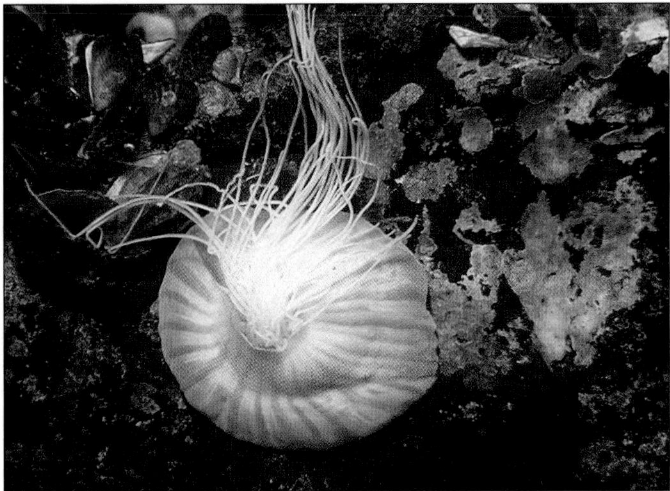

Figure 35.28 The sea anemone releasing acontios (threads) full of nematocytes as a defensive mechanism. (Courtesy of Dr. Juan Pedro Lonza.)

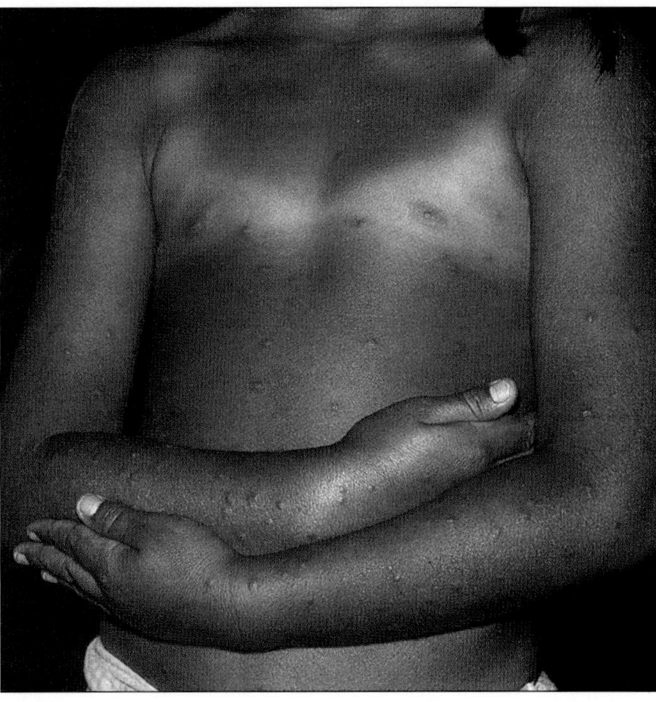

Figure 35.29 Erythematous, pruritic papules (and some vesicles) on the skin of a child exposed to the nematocytes of the sea anemone while playing in shallow water in a Chilean harbor. (Courtesy of Dr. Juan Pedro Lonza.)

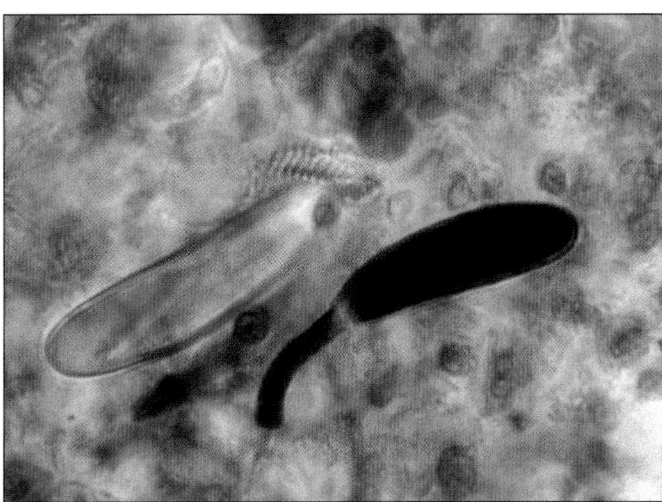

Figure 35.30 Discharged and undischarged nematocysts of the sea anemone. (Courtesy of Dr. Juan Pedro Lonza.)

Cubozoa

Box jellyfish (*Chironex fleckeri*, *Chiropsalmus quadrigatus*, and *C. quadrumanus*) are the most toxic marine animals and envenomation usually results in a medical emergency. They have a transparent cube-shaped body with underlying tentacles. The venom of box jellyfish contains hemolytic, neurotoxic, and cardiotoxic elements. Additional toxins may cause massive dermal necrosis. Acute symptoms consist of intense pain and the development of brown-purple lines across areas that come into contact with the tentacles. Cardiorespiratory arrest may result within minutes. If the patient survives, the acute envenomation, the dermatonecrotic component of the box jellyfish toxin, often results in skin necrosis and eventual scarring.

Treatment of box jellyfish stings involves acute supportive care and the use of *Chironex fleckeri* antivenom if indicated. Indications for antivenom use include cardiorespiratory arrest, arrhythmias, difficulty with breathing, severe pain, or extensive skin lesions. Additionally, affected areas should be immobilized to prevent spread of the toxins. As with other jellyfish stings, great care should be taken to remove tentacle components after nematocyst inactivation with vinegar or sea water. Analgesia and treatment with topical or systemic steroids may be warranted. Additionally, infection prophylaxis is indicated, especially with dermal necrosis.

The Irukandji syndrome results from contact with the jellyfish *Carukia barnesi*. It is characterized by the presence of severe pain at the sting site, headache, backache, joint pains, nausea, and vomiting. Pulmonary edema and heart failure may ensue. Less severe cases will resolve spontaneously within 1–2 days.[13]

On the Atlantic coast, from Brazil to the USA, dangerous species of jellyfish such as *Tamoya haplonema* and *Chiropsalmus quadrumanus* are found. The latter species has resulted in two deaths in Texas, the only ones reported for this species. Another species, *Chironex fleckeri*, has been responsible for about 200 deaths in the world, mostly in Australia.

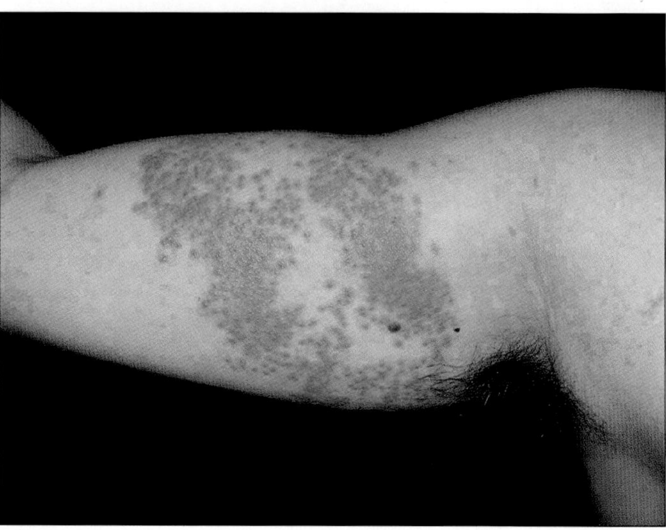

Figure 35.32 Papules and vesicles resulting from exposure to the tentacles of *Chrysaora plocamia*. (Courtesy of Dr. Juan Pedro Lonza.)

Scyphozoa

Scyphozoa, or true jellyfish (Fig. 35.31), have cutaneous manifestations similar to those of box jellyfish and *Physalia*. However, they generally have fewer systemic symptoms. Immediate reactions to true jellyfish include pain, itching, and burning. Linear wheals and vesicular eruptions appear within hours after exposure (Figs 35.32 and 35.33). Generalized urticaria and allergic cutaneous responses may also be seen after envenomation. Rarely, systemic manifestations occur, depending on the degree of contact and the size of the patient (children more frequently demonstrate systemic symptoms after exposure). These include fever, malaise, weakness, and muscle spasms. Acute local therapy for jellyfish stings should be instituted as above for box jellyfish. Jellyfish stings are usually self-limited

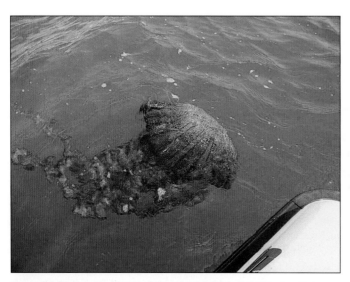

Figure 35.31 *Chrysaora plocamia*, a true jellyfish. (Courtesy of Dr. Juan Pedro Lonza.)

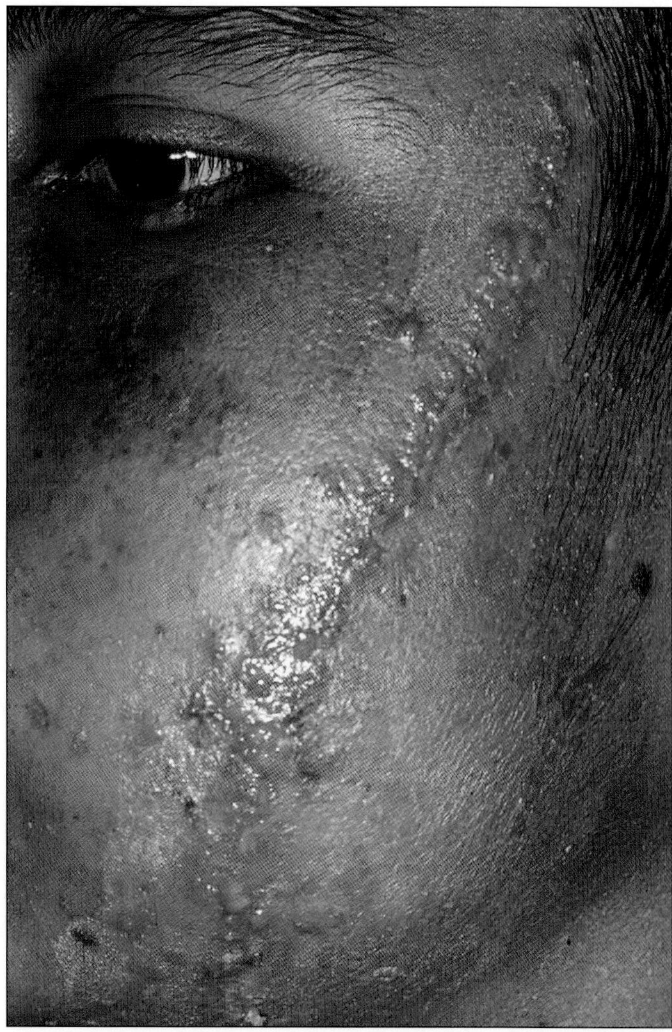

Figure 35.33 Linear vesicles of the face resulting from exposure to the tentacles of *Chrysaora plocamia*. (Courtesy of Dr. Juan Pedro Lonza.)

and resolve within a few weeks. Symptomatic treatment may be necessary until lesions resolve.

Seabather's eruption

Seabather's eruption is a relatively common dermatitis, which occurs after swimming in sea water. This eruption results after cnidarian larvae (*Linuche* spp.) become trapped in the bathing suits of swimmers. Pressure from the bathing suit or wetsuit results in toxin release. Clinically, multiple pruritic erythematous papules and macules develop within hours of sea bathing. New lesions may occur for days after the initial exposure. In general, these lesions are distributed over areas that were covered by clothing while the victim was swimming. Rapid removal of swimwear followed by bathing may limit the severity of the outbreak. Otherwise, treatment is symptomatic (topical steroids may be useful), and usually resolves in a week. The lesions are very difficult to prevent, because they do not begin immediately after contact and the nematocysts fire for several minutes before the victim notices the symptoms.[14]

Worms

Bristleworms are one of the more dangerous species of marine worms, and they can be found under corals and rocks and in aquaria. The aquatic worms can cause injuries by three mechanisms: (1) bites with the mandibles (traumatic lesions); (2) envenomation; and (3) traumatic lesions through the corporal bristles. The lesions or bites are common in persons who harvest mussels. Bristleworms have hair-like filaments along their body which can break off when touched. Although these bristles are generally not toxic, injury can be inflicted with these bristles or via the worm bite. Cutaneous signs and symptoms following injury include pain, erythema, edema, and numbness. Treatment includes the use of tweezers or tape to remove the bristles, applying topical vinegar or isopropyl alcohol (controversial), topical or oral antibiotics in cases of superimposed bacterial infection, and pain relievers. Other marine worms that are capable of biting include bloodworms, which are named for their deep-red color, and clamworms. Clamworms are frequently found in marine flats, and both worms can cause an irritant dermatitis with their bite. Treatment for the bite includes adequate cleansing of the area and symptomatic care.

Cercarial dermatitis (swimmer's itch)

Cercarial dermatitis, also known as swimmer's itch, is caused by cutaneous infestation by the larval stage of trematodes of the genera *Schistosoma* and *Trichobilharzia*. Aquatic bird species (i.e., ducks and geese) in freshwater lakes are typical definitive hosts for schistosomes, as the adult fluke uses the intestinal wall of these animals for laying eggs. These eggs are then excreted with feces in the water where they hatch into developed larvae (miracidiae) and infect snails. Five to six weeks later, hundreds of cercariae or free-swimming sporocysts are excreted by the infected snail. These cercariae can penetrate the human host skin, with infestation resulting in the termination of the organism's life cycle. Typically, symptoms such as pain, prickling, and pruritus develop several hours after initial infection. Erythematous macules and urticaria may be seen around sites of penetration. Signs and symptoms of the disease typically worsen 12–24 h after exposure, as vesicles and pustules can develop as a result of scratching from intense pruritus. The intensity of the response can vary from individual to individual, and those with previous exposure to the organism are more likely to develop severe signs and symptoms.

The differential diagnosis for these lesions includes seabather's eruption, which can be distinguished from swimmer's itch by its occurrence after exposure to cnidarians in salt water and because it involves the area limited to the bathing suit. Although most reported cases of cercarial dermatitis occur after exposure in freshwater lakes, it has been documented in individuals after contact with aquaria.[15]

Treatment of cercarial dermatitis is usually not necessary, as most signs and symptoms resolve without intervention within 5–14 days. However, cool compresses, topical corticosteroids, and antihistamines may be used for symptomatic relief. Prevention includes avoidance of known contaminated areas and towel-drying or showering after possible exposure.

Cutaneous larva migrans

Larvae of cat or dog hookworms such as *Ancylostoma caninum*, *A. braziliense*, and *Toxocara canis* can cause cutaneous larva migrans in humans. Eggs of these hookworms hatch after being passed through the host's feces. These larvae can then penetrate and migrate through human skin. The larvae can remain in the skin for weeks to months, and their movement can be tracked by the intense inflammatory pruritic response that results. Infection by this parasite typically occurs on sandy beaches where infected feces of dogs or cats may be present. Although the infection is usually self-limiting, topical or oral tiabendazole is frequently used for treatment. Alternatives to tiabendazole include albendazole, mebendazole, and ivermectin. Oral or topical antibiotics may also be used if secondary bacterial infection occurs.

Echinoderms

Echinoderms are composed of a group of slow-moving animals, including starfish, sea urchins, and sea cucumbers. Some of these have long, sharp spines which may cause puncture wounds. Additionally, most echinoderms produce toxins, and this can result in cutaneous manifestations. Rarely, systemic symptoms occur. Long-term sequelae of contact with these animals typically result from retained foreign materials embedded in the skin. Envenomation by starfish is unusual. However, injury by *Acanthaster planci* (the crown-of-thorns starfish) often results in cutaneous manifestations. This starfish has unusually long sharp dorsal spines (Fig. 35.34). Contact usually occurs by stepping on them or by careless handling. Immediately after skin penetration, victims notice a sharp burning pain. The pain may persist for several hours and is accompanied by edema, bleeding, and ecchymosis at the puncture site. Systemic symptoms, including nausea, vomiting, and paralysis, have been reported.

Sea urchins have numerous sharp, mobile spines, which can cause penetrating injuries when carelessly handled or stepped on (Fig. 35.35). Their spines also contain toxins, which are introduced

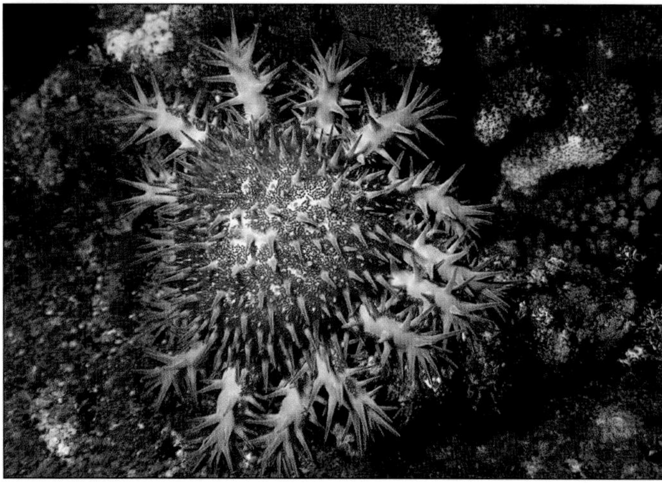

Figure 35.34 *Acanthaster planci*, the crown-of-thorns starfish. (Courtesy of Ed Robinson, Hawaiian Water Colours.)

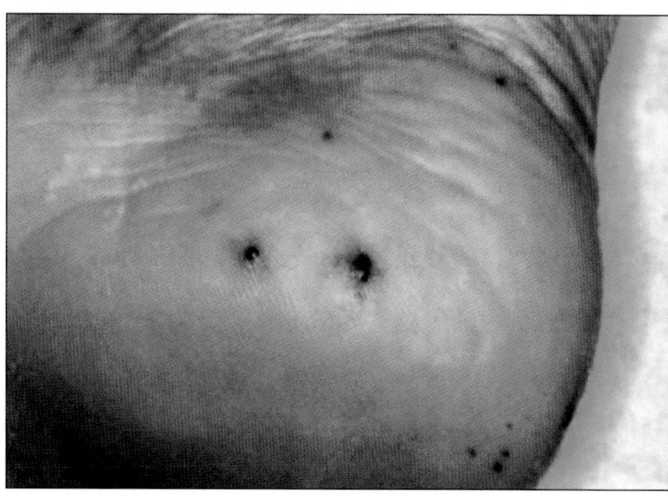

Figure 35.36 Puncture wounds from a sea urchin. (Courtesy of Dr. Vidal Haddad Junior.)

into the body after spines break off. Local reactions include an immediate sharp pain, which may last for hours, followed by edema and erythema (Fig. 35.36). Copious bleeding may also occur. Tenosynovitis, fasciitis, and bursitis have also been reported following sea urchin injuries.[16] Systemic symptoms are rare, but may include muscle pain, torpor, and breathlessness. Envenomation by echinoderms is rare, but the most common genus that causes envenomation is *Diadema*. Early extraction of the spines is very important to prevent sequelae.[17]

Acute treatment for starfish and sea urchin injuries includes soaking the affected area in hot water to inactivate possible thermolabile toxins (this measure is controversial, because there is no proof that the venom of those animals is thermolabile), symptomatic care, and the removal of all retained spine fragments. Radiographs and a surgical consultation may be necessary to ensure complete removal of foreign bodies from the wound. Depending on the level of wound contamination and the depth of spine penetration, prophylactic antibiotics may be warranted (see above). Infections and granuloma formation secondary to retained spinal fragments may result after either starfish or sea urchin injuries. The extraction of the spines of sea urchins is a very painful process and uses two large-caliber needles as tweezers. The extraction is difficult and small spines are easily broken and may stay in the epidermis. Another problem is that some spines do not penetrate, they just tattoo the skin.

Sea cucumbers do not contain spines, but may cause cutaneous reactions by secretion of a toxic visceral solution (Figs 35.37 and 35.38). This solution acts as a contact irritant to skin and eyes and can cause blindness (Fig. 35.39).

Mollusks

Mollusks include the following classes: bivalves, shells, and cephalopods (octopus, squid, and cuttlefish). Bivalves do not possess toxins harmful to humans but may cause traumatic injuries due

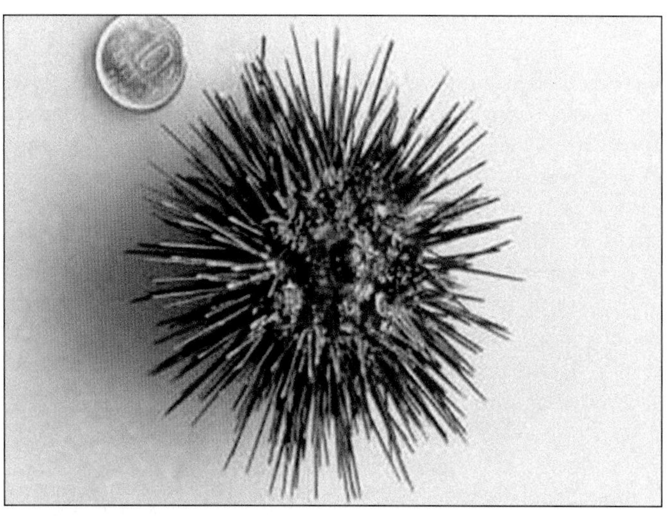

Figure 35.35 *Tetrapygus niger*, a sea urchin. (Courtesy of Dr. Vidal Haddad Junior.)

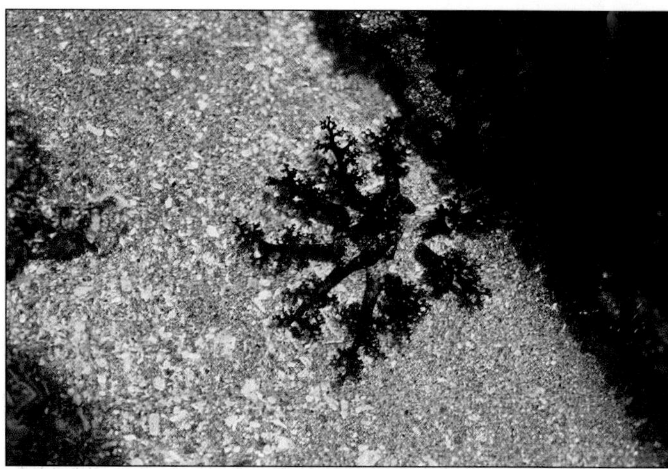

Figure 35.37 *Athyoniduim chilensis*, a sea cucumber extending its green tentacles above the surface of the sandy bottom, where it lies buried in close contact with banks of clams. (Courtesy of Dr. Juan Pedro Lonza.)

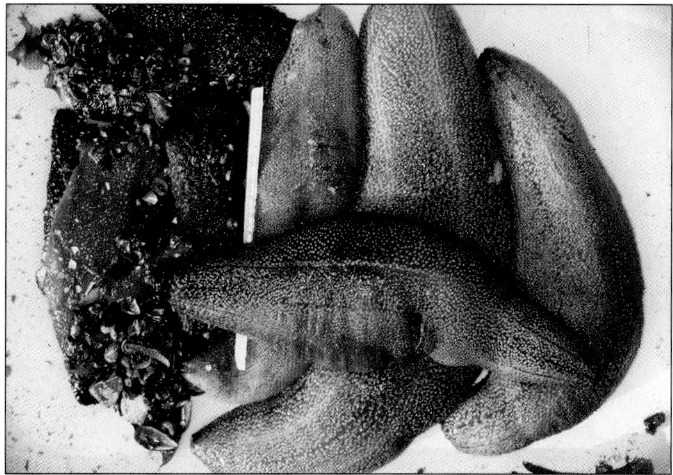

Figure 35.38 *Athyoniduim chilensis* and *Patallus molli*, two species of sea cucumbers. (Courtesy of Dr. Juan Pedro Lonza.)

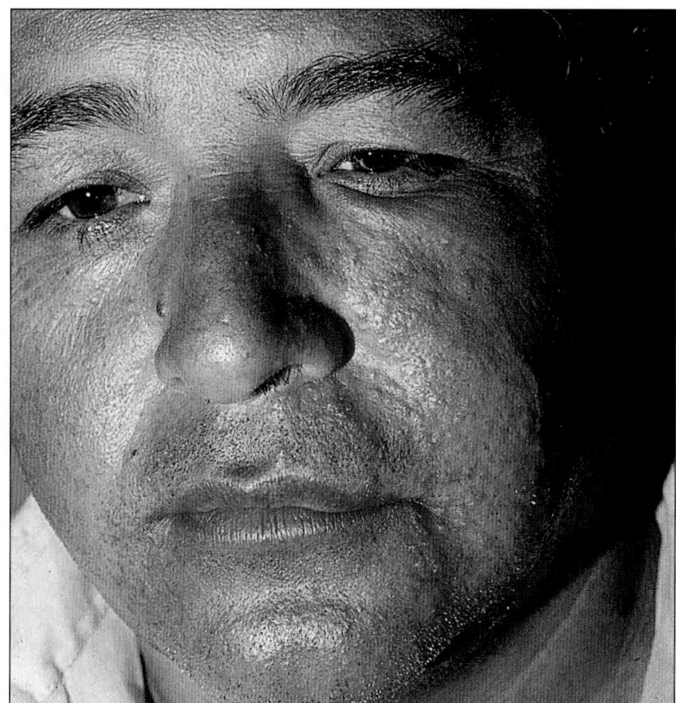

Figure 35.39 Acute vesicular dermatitis from a jet of digestive secretions of *Athyonidium chilensis* in a man who was digging clams and who disturbed the adjacent sea cucumber. (Courtesy of Dr. Juan Pedro Lonza.)

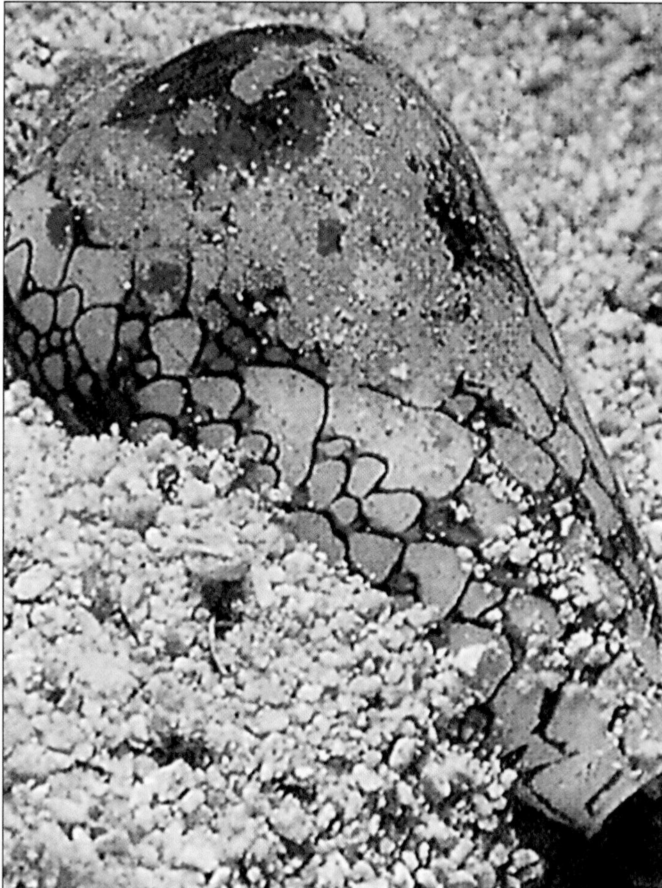

Figure 35.40 *Conus textile*, the poisonous cone shell, is widely distributed from the Red Sea to Polynesia. Several species have a potentially fatal venom apparatus that discharges through the barbed radular tooth that passes through the proboscis. (Reproduced from Peters W and Pasvol G (eds). Tropical Medicine and Parasitology, 5th edition, Mosby, London 2002. image 1044.)

to their sharp shells. Gasteropods (shells) include the Conidae family, which produces toxins that can be extremely harmful to humans. Injuries due to cone shells are common, since their shells are attractive and avidly collected (Fig. 35.40). Envenomation occurs by means of a hollow tooth which can be thrust into exposed tissue, releasing toxins. Toxin composition is variable among Conidae species but generally includes a potent neurotoxin, which paralyzes its victim. Immediately after toxin injection, victims feel an excruciating burning sensation, numbness, and tingling at the wound site. The affected area quickly becomes edematous and erythematous. This frequently spreads over the whole body with pronounced tingling of the oral area. Wound ischemia, muscle paralysis, and heart failure may all ensue within 6 h of the initial sting. If the patient survives, most systemic symptoms will subside within 1–2 days, although skin findings may persist. No specific treatments exist for Conidae stings, but local pressure and immobilization may limit the spread of the toxin. Therapy is otherwise supportive.

Although octopi are generally not considered toxic to humans, the blue-ringed octopus (*Hapalochlaena maculosa*) produces a toxin that may be fatal to humans (Fig. 35.41). This small octopus is found off the coast of Australia, and is characterized by distinctive blue rings on its body. Initially, a bite from the octopus may be painless, but severe pain, pruritus, and urticarial lesions develop within a few minutes (Fig. 35.42). Erythema and edema may affect the entire extremity. Respiratory paralysis may ensue, leading to death. Treatment is supportive, with pressure immobilization to reduce venom spread and intubation, if necessary. With appropriate therapy, paralysis will improve within the first few days after envenomation.

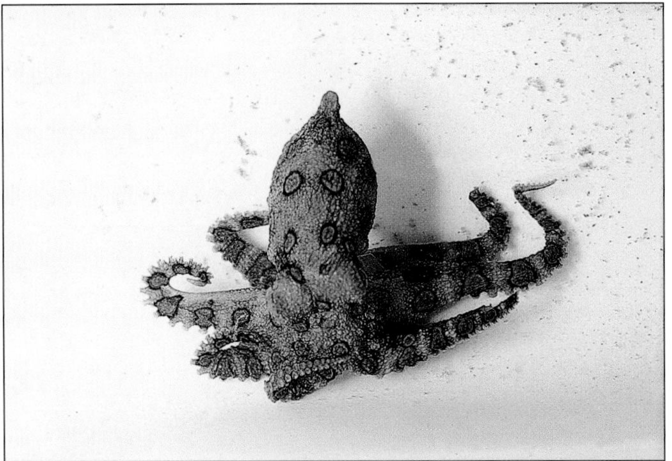

Figure 35.41 *Octopus lunulatus*, one of the two species of small octopi in the Indian and Pacific oceans which contains a potentially fatal tetrodoxin in its bite; the other species is *O. (Hapalochlaena) maculosus*. (Reproduced from Peters W and Pasvol G (eds). Tropical Medicine and Parasitology, 5th edition, Mosby, London 2002. image 1045.)

Fish

Fish may cause cutaneous manifestations due to trauma or envenomation. Traumatic injuries may be caused by catfish (Figs 35.43) (as well as injury due to venom), sharks, barracudas, groupers, piranha (Figs 35.44 and 35.45), and eels. They will not be considered further in this chapter.

Venomous fish

Envenomation by vertebrates is commonly seen in those with frequent exposure to the marine environment. Nearly 250 fish possess organs capable of causing toxic injury in humans.[18] Most injuries caused by marine vertebrates result from contact with stingrays (class Chondrichthyes) or class Osteichthyes (catfishes, weeverfish, and scorpionfish).

Stingrays

Stingray injuries occur through both traumatic and toxic mechanisms. These fish have flat bodies and a long tail containing up

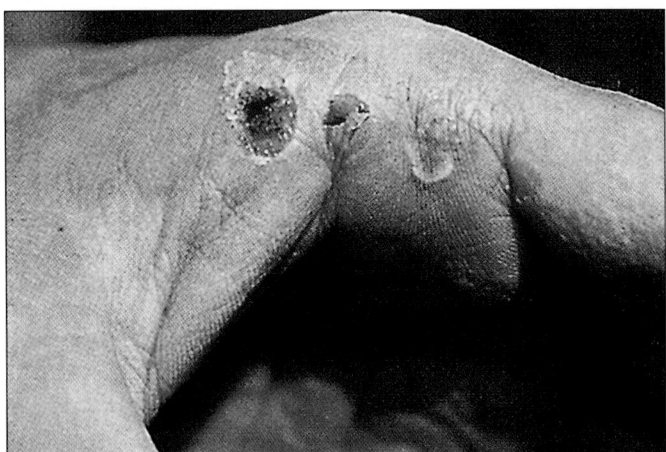

Figure 35.42 The beak of an octopus can produce severe wounds. (Reproduced from Peters W and Pasvol G (eds). Tropical Medicine and Parasitology, 5th edition, Mosby, London 2002. image 1046.)

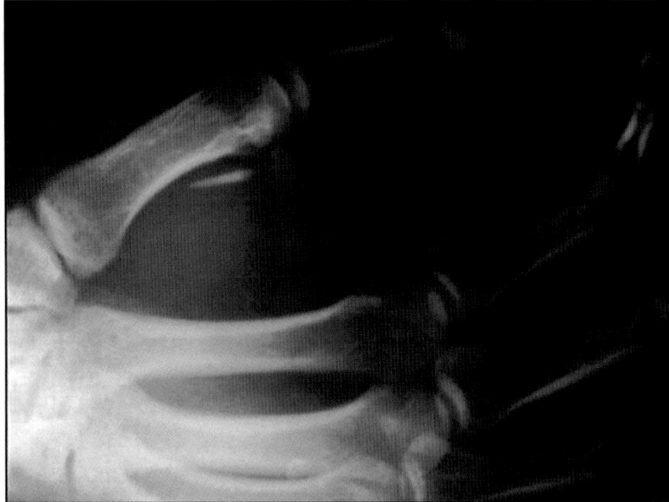

Figure 35.43 Radiograph of the hand of a patient who experienced a puncture wound from a catfish; notice the fragment of the spine in the first finger. (Courtesy of Dr. Vidal Haddad Junior.)

Crustaceans

Crustaceans (lobster, crabs, shrimp, and barnacles) belong to the Arthropod class. Unlike their land-based relatives (scorpions, spiders, and insects), crustaceans usually do not produce venom, and injuries resulting from contact with crustaceans are largely traumatic. If ingested, however, crustaceans which have tetrodotoxin, saxitoxin, and other neurotoxins can cause severe envenomation. Crab and lobster bites should be treated with regular wound care. Barnacles may cause cutting wounds because of their hard outer shells. With both bites and cutting wounds, secondary infection is a concern, and close monitoring of wound sites is essential. Prophylactic antibiotics may be warranted depending on the severity of the trauma and the general health of the victim. Contact dermatitis may also occur after contact with crustaceans.

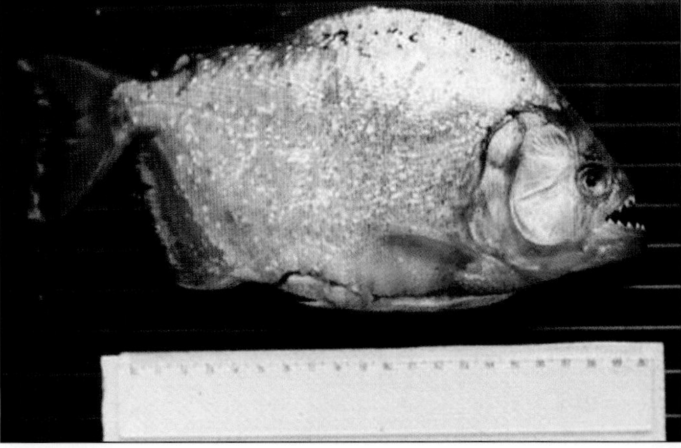

Figure 35.44 *Serrassalmus spilopleura*, the piranha. (Courtesy of Dr. Vidal Haddad Junior.)

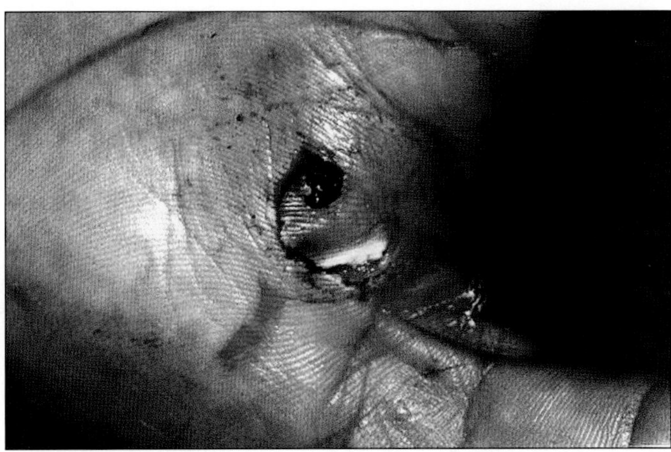

Figure 35.45 A piranha bite on the hand of a fisherman. (Courtesy of Dr. Vidal Haddad Junior.)

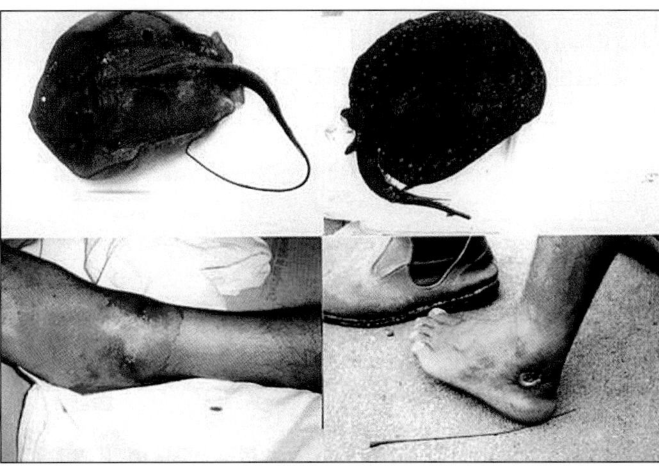

Figure 35.47 Freshwater stingrays and the resulting ulcers from their barbs. (Courtesy of Dr. Vidal Haddad Junior.)

to four venomous spines (Figs 35.46–35.48). Injury usually follows a bather inadvertently stepping on a stingray. Stingrays will rapidly whip their tails against an offending leg, thereby causing the tail spine to break the skin. The epithelium of the spine contains glandular structures, which subsequently secrete venom. This venom has dermatonecrotic, cardiotoxic, and neurotoxic properties and may cause respiratory distress. Stingray injuries are usually found on the feet and lower legs. More severe cutaneous necrosis is caused by South American freshwater stingrays, that have high levels of hyaluronidase in their venom.[19]

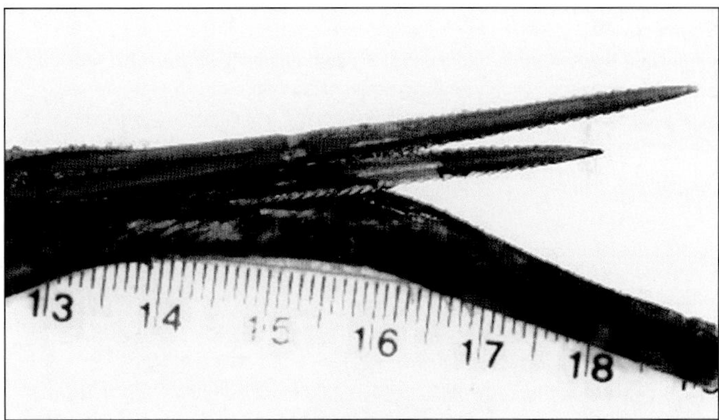

Figure 35.48 Serrated barbs of a marine stingray. (Courtesy of Dr. Vidal Haddad Junior.)

Osteichthyes

Freshwater and marine catfish are commonly encountered in the nets of fishermen and on the beaches and they cause about 80% of injuries provoked for venomous fishes in humans in marine and freshwater environments throughout the world. In a survey of 250 injuries from marine fish and 200 for freshwater fish, catfish caused the large majority of the injury, followed by stingrays and scorpionfish.

Weeverfish are only observed in the Mediterranean and on the African coast of the Atlantic. They cause severe injuries (Fig. 35.49), but they are less frequent than those from catfish, and the envenomation is less severe than that caused by stingrays or scorpionfish. Weeverfish are relatively small fish which have sharp spines on the body capable of injecting venom. As with stingrays, injury most often occurs after stepping on the fish. Not much is known about the weeverfish venom, but is does have potent cardiotoxic effects.

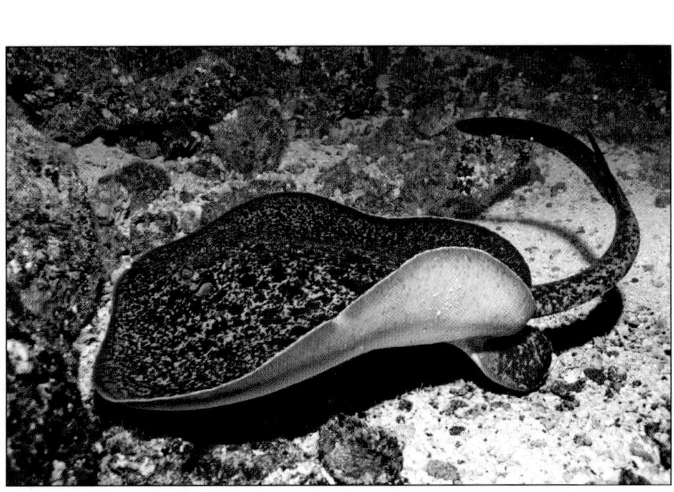

Figure 35.46 A stingray.

The Scorpaenidae family includes scorpionfish (Fig. 35.50), stonefish (Fig. 35.51), and lionfish. These animals have anal, pelvic, and dorsal spines, which contain potent toxins. Exposure is often accidental as both stonefish and scorpionfish have excellent camouflage. Envenomations also occur after careless handling of these fish. Lionfish are stunningly beautiful and are greatly sought after for marine aquariums. Therefore, lionfish stings are becoming increasingly more common with saltwater aquarium enthusiasts.[20] Of the three species, lionfish appear to have the mildest stings. This appears to be due to their long thin spines which deliver a correspondingly reduced venom load.

Clinical manifestations and treatment of fish envenomations are relatively uniform. Initially, patients present with severe pain, often out of proportion with the apparent extent of the injury. For stingray injuries, the affected area may be large and presents either

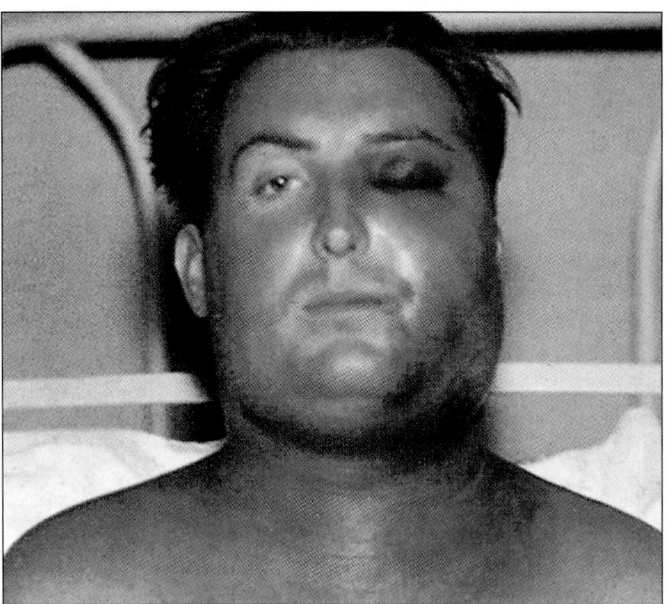

Figure 35.49 Hemorrhagic effects of a weeverfish sting. The venom is both neurotoxic and hemotoxic. Weeverfish are found in the Mediterranean sea and along the African coast of the Atlantic ocean. (Reproduced from Peters W and Pasvol G (eds). Tropical Medicine and Parasitology, 5th edition, Mosby, London 2002. image 1050.)

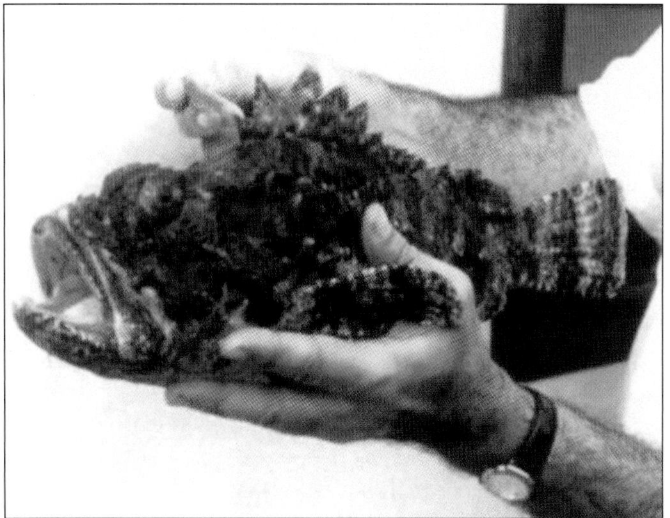

Figure 35.50 *Scorpaena plumieri*, the scorpionfish. (Courtesy of Dr. Vidal Junior Haddad.)

as a long laceration or a deep puncture wound. For weeverfish and members of the class Scorpaenidae, the affected area initially manifests as a small puncture wound which rapidly becomes edematous and erythematous. Initial local vasoconstriction is followed by intense erythema, edema, and local tissue necrosis. Patients may also develop purpura and local hemorrhagic bullae. Local numbness, tingling, and pruritus may ensue. Gastrointestinal symptoms frequently occur, and headaches and arthralgias are common. Severe envenomation may lead to hypotension, paralysis, and arrhythmias. Associated systemic symptoms may include nausea, vomiting, respiratory distress, abdominal pain, and seizures.[21,22]

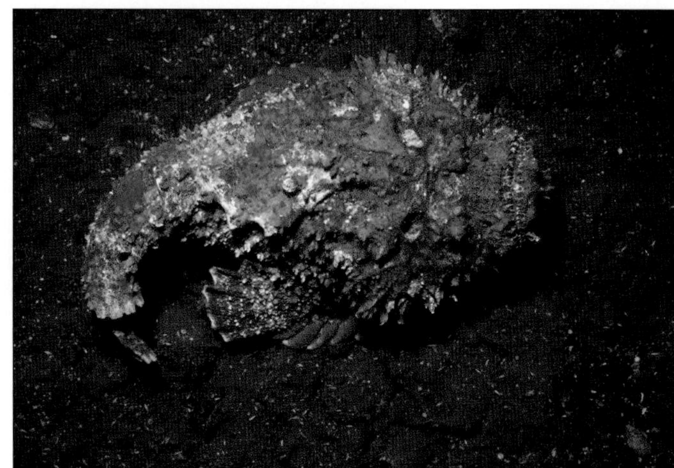

Figure 35.51 A stonefish. (Courtesy of Ed Robinson, Hawaiian Water Colours.)

Acute treatment for vertebrate envenomation includes immersing the affected area in hot water and supportive care with analgesia. Immersion of the affected area in hot water both inactivates heat-labile toxins and results in transient symptomatic pain relief. For severe systemic symptoms after stonefish injury, antivenom is available. Pain and systemic symptoms usually begin to subside within 24–48 h. Wound debridement with removal of spine remnants is necessary. Long-term sequelae include infection and the development of foreign-body granulomas at the puncture site if complete removal of spines is not achieved. Prophylactic antibiotic therapy may be indicated depending on the severity of the injury and the health status of the victim.

Other aquatic dermatoses

Contact dermatitis may result from various marine exposures. Among these are exposure to fish bait (such as sea worms), and diving equipment (masks, wetsuits, fins). Perioral contact dermatitis may result from the use of snorkels or scuba equipment. Contact dermatitis due to marine contact usually resolves with the use of mid- to high-potency topical steroids. Aquagenic urticaria may result from contact with water, and cold urticaria results from contact with cold water or other substances. Both forms of urticaria may be effectively treated with antihistamines.

Conclusion

Dermatoses caused by marine organisms are frequently seen in dermatology clinics. Cutaneous injuries after exposure to marine environments include bacterial infections, irritant or allergic contact dermatitis, physical trauma, and envenomations. These contacts may result in mild local reactions or more acute systemic reactions. An unusual history or atypical clinical presentation should alert the dermatologist to inquire about a patient's recent travel history, exposure to marine environments, or ownership of a marine aquarium.

References

1. Haddad VJ, Miot HA, Bartoli LD et al. Localized lymphatic sporotrichosis after fish-induced injury (*Tilapia* sp.). Med Mycol 2002; 40:425–427.
2. Barnett JH, Estes SA, Wirman JA et al. Erysipeloid. J Am Acad Dermatol 1983; 9:116–123.
3. Johnston JM, Izumi AK. Cutaneous *Mycobacterium marinum* infection ("swimming pool granuloma"). Clin Dermatol 1987; 5:68–75.
4. Burke WA. Cutaneous hazards of the coast. Dermatol Nurs 1997; 9:163–170; quiz 171–172.
5. Burke W. Cutaneous reactions to marine sponges and bryozoans. Dermatol Ther 2002; 15:26–29.
6. Burnett JW, Bloom DA, Imafuku S et al. Coelenterate venom research 1991–1995: clinical, chemical and immunological aspects. Toxicon 1996; 34:1377–1383.
7. Marques AC, Haddad V Jr, Migotto AE. Envenomation by a benthic Hydrozoa (Cnidaria): the case of *Nemalecium lighti* (Haleciidae). Toxicon 2002; 40:213–215.
8. Addy JH. Red sea coral contact dermatitis. Int J Dermatol 1991; 30:271–273.
9. Burnett JW, Gable WD. A fatal jellyfish envenomation by the Portuguese man-o'-war. Toxicon 1989; 27:823–824.
10. Haddad V Jr, Silveira FL, Cardoso JLC et al. A report of 49 cases of cnidarian envenoming from southeastern Brazilian coastal waters. Toxicon 2002; 40:1445–1450.
11. Haddad V Jr, Silva G, Rodrigues TC et al. Injuries with high percentage of systemic findings caused by the cubomedusa *Chiropsamus quadrumanus* (Cnidaria) in southeast region of Brazil: report of 10 cases. Rev Soc Bras Med Trop 2003; 36:84–85.
12. Haddad V Jr. Animais aquáticos de importância médica. Rev Soc Bras Med Trop 2003 ; 36:591–597.
13. Little M, Mulcahy RF. A year's experience of Irukandji envenomation in far north Queensland. Med J Aust 1998; 169:638–641.
14. Haddad V Jr, Cardoso JLC; Silveira FLS. Seabather's eruption: report of five cases in the southeast region of Brazil. Rev Inst Med Rrop S Paulo 2001; 43:171–172.
15. Folster-Holst R, Disko R, Rowert J et al. Cercarial dermatitis contracted via contact with an aquarium: case report and review. Br J Dermatol 2001; 145:638–640.
16. Guyot-Drouot MH, Rouneau D, Rolland JM et al. Arthritis, tenosynovitis, fasciitis, and bursitis due to sea urchin spines. A series of 12 cases in Reunion Island. Jt Bone Spine 2000; 67:94–100.
17. Haddad V Jr, Novaes SPMS, Miot HA et al. Accidents caused by sea urchins – the efficacy of precocious removal of the spines in the prevention of complications. An Bras Dermatol 2002; 77:123–128.
18. Angelini G, Bonamonte D. Aquatic dermatology. Milan: Springer; 2001.
19. Haddad V Jr, Garrone Neto D, Paula Neto JB et al. Freshwater stingrays: study of epidemiologic, clinic and therapeutic aspects based in 84 envenomings in humans and some enzymatic activities of the venom. Toxicon 2004; 43:287–294.
20. Aldred B, Erickson T, Lipscomb J. Lionfish envenomations in an urban wilderness. Wilderness Environ Med 1996; 7:291–296.
21. Haddad V Jr, Pardal PPO, Cardoso JLC et al. The venomous toadfish *Thalassophryne nattereri* (niquim or miquim): report of 43 injuries provoked in fishermen of Salinópolis (Pará state) and Aracaju (Sergipe state). Rev Inst Med Trop São Paulo 2003; 45:221–223.
22. Haddad V Jr, Martins IA, Makyama HM. Injuries caused by scorpionfishes (*Scorpaena plumieri* Bloch, 1789 and *Scorpaena brasiliensis* Cuvier, 1829) in the southwestern Atlantic ocean (Brazilian coast): epidemiologic, clinic and therapeutic aspects of 23 stings in humans. Toxicon 2003; 42:79–83.

Further reading

Numerous websites have indepth articles regarding marine dermatoses as well as photographs of both marine animals and cutaneous reactions. The list below is by no means exhaustive.

Haddad Jr V. Atlas of dangerous aquatic animals of Brazil: a guide of identifications and treatment. São Paulo: Editora Roca; 2000.

http://library.thinkquest.org/C007974

http://scuba-doc.com/

www.advancedaquarist.com/issues/april2003/feature1.htm

www.aloha.com/~lifeguards

www.dangerousaquaticanimals.com.br

www.emedicine.com

www.ucihs.uci.edu/biochem/steele/general_information.html

Index

Notes:
  Abbreviations
    AIDS = acquired immunodeficiency syndrome
    DEET = diethyltoluamide
    HAART = highly active anti-retroviral therapy
    HIV = human immunodeficiency virus
    HTLV-1 = human T-cell lymphotrophic virus type 1
  Page numbers followed by f refer to figures
  Page numbers followed by t refer to tables or boxes

B

D

F

G

I

J

M

U

V